ZOONOSES and Communicable Diseases Common to Man and Animals

SECOND EDITION

Pedro N. Acha
D.V.M., M.P.H., Dr.H.C.

Boris Szyfres
D.V.M.

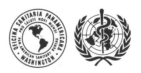

Scientific Publication No. 503

PAN AMERICAN HEALTH ORGANIZATION
Pan American Sanitary Bureau, Regional Office of the
WORLD HEALTH ORGANIZATION
525 Twenty-third Street, N.W.
Washington, D.C. 20037, U.S.A.

1987

First edition 1980

Published also in Spanish (1986) with the title:
Zoonosis y enfermedades transmisibles comunes
al hombre y a los animales, segunda edición
ISBN 92 75 31503 5

ISBN 92 75 11503 6

©Pan American Health Organization, 1987

CONTENTS

PART II: MYCOSES

PART III: CHLAMYDIOSES AND RICKETTSIOSES

PART IV: VIROSES

PART V: PARASITIC DISEASES

Section A: PROTOZOOSES

Section B: HELMINTHIASES

1. Trematodiases

2. Cestodiases

3. Acanthocephaliasis and Nematodiases

Section C: ARTHROPODS

APPENDIXES

LIST OF TABLES AND ILLUSTRATIONS

BACTERIOSES

Tables

Figures

MYCOSES

Map

CHLAMYDIOSES AND RICKETTSIOSES

Figures

VIROSES

Tables

Figures

Maps

PARASITIC ZOONOSES

PROTOZOOSES

Tables

Figures

Maps

HELMINTHIASES

1. Trematodiases

Figures

Maps

2. Cestodiases

Figures

3. Acanthocephaliasis and Nematodiases

Figures

Map

ARTHROPODS

Figures

PROLOGUE

Zoonoses and communicable diseases common to man and animals—at once the subject and title of this publication—represent an important threat to the health and well-being of the world's population. In spite of substantial recent progress in disease control and the extension of health care, these diseases continue to register high rates of incidence in urban, periurban, and rural areas of developing countries in all regions. They are also prevalent in many animal species on which man depends for food. Consequently, they have a potentially great impact on many national economies whose foreign trade and stability depend on the reliability of disease-free food exports. These diseases thus illustrate, perhaps better than any similar problem, the close relationship between public health, the environment, and socioeconomic well-being. It is for this reason that they constitute a priority concern of the Pan American Health Organization.

As an important element of its program of technical cooperation with the countries of the Americas, PAHO gives special emphasis to the management of knowledge. This function serves as a means for the timely dissemination of important information on advances in research and development in health, medicine, and related sciences, so that this information can be applied effectively to improve public health. It is in this spirit and context that PAHO has published this work.

This second English edition of *Zoonoses and Communicable Diseases Common to Man and Animals* appears seven years after the first. In that period, many advances have been achieved in the knowledge of these diseases, and new frontiers have been opened in technology, epidemiology, ecology, and the other biological and social sciences. The purpose of this volume is to summarize in a single source what is known at present about these diseases as a result of recent progress.

Consequently, the original version of this book, which was warmly received and was reprinted several times, has been considerably updated, amplified, and improved in the present edition. It is hoped that this work will provide scientists and health workers with a better understanding of these diseases, in order to aid the fight against them and permit their eradication wherever possible.

CARLYLE GUERRA DE MACEDO
DIRECTOR

PREFACE TO THE FIRST ENGLISH EDITION

This book considers two groups of communicable diseases: those transmitted from vertebrate animals to man, which are—strictly speaking—zoonoses; and those common to man and animals. In the first group, animals play an essential role in maintaining the infection in nature, and man is only an accidental host. In the second group, both animals and man generally contract the infection from the same sources, such as soil, water, invertebrate animals, and plants; as a rule, however, animals do not play an essential role in the life cycle of the etiologic agent, but may contribute in varying degrees to the distribution and actual transmission of infections.

No attempt has been made to include all infections and diseases comprised in these two groups. A selection has been made of some 150 that are of principal interest, for various reasons, in the field of public health. The number of listed zoonoses is increasing as new biomedical knowledge is acquired. Moreover, as human activity extends into unexplored territories containing natural foci of infection, new zoonotic diseases are continually being recognized. In addition, improved health services and better differential diagnostic methods have distinguished zoonoses previously confused with other, more common diseases. A number of diseases described in this book have only recently been recognized, examples of which include the Argentine and Bolivian hemorrhagic fevers, angiostrongyliasis, rotaviral enteritis, Lassa fever, Marburg disease, and babesiosis.

The principal objective in writing this book was to provide the medical professions a source of information on the zoonoses and communicable diseases common to man and animals. Toward that end, both medical and veterinary aspects, which have traditionally been dealt with separately in different texts, have been combined in a single, comprehensive volume. As a result, physicians, veterinarians, epidemiologists, and biologists can all gain an overview of these diseases from one source.

This book, like most scientific works, is the product of many books, texts, monographs, and journal articles. Many sources of literature in medicine, veterinary medicine, virology, bacteriology, mycology, and parasitology were consulted, as were a large number of reports from different biomedical disciplines, in order to provide up-to-date and concise information on each disease. It is expected that any errors or omissions that may have been committed can, with the collaboration of the readers, be corrected in a future edition.

Where possible, explanations were attempted with special emphasis on the Americas, particularly Latin America. An effort was made, one which was not always successful, to collect available information on diseases in this Region. Data on the incidence of many zoonoses are fragmentary and frequently not reliable. It is hoped that the establishment of control programs in various countries will lead to improved epidemiologic surveillance and disease reporting.

More space has been devoted to those zoonoses having greatest impact on public health and on the economy of the countries of the Americas, but information is also included on those regionally less important or exotic diseases.

xv

The movement of persons and animals over great distances adds to the risk of introducing exotic diseases that may become established on the American continent given the appropriate ecologic factors for existence of the etiologic agents. Today, public health and animal health administrators, physicians, and veterinarians must be familiar with the geographic distribution and pathologic manifestations of the various infectious agents so that they can recognize and prevent the introduction of exotic diseases.

We, the authors, would like to give special recognition to Dr. Joe R. Held, Assistant Surgeon-General of the United States Public Health Service and Director of the Division of Research Services of the U.S. National Institutes of Health, who gave impetus to the English translation and reviewed the bacterioses sections.

We would also like to express our utmost appreciation to the experts who reviewed various portions of this book and offered their suggestions for improving the text. These include: Dr. Jeffrey F. Williams, Professor in the Department of Microbiology and Public Health, Michigan State University, who reviewed the chapters dealing with parasitic zoonoses; Dr. James Bond, PAHO/WHO Regional Adviser in Viral Diseases, who read the viroses; Dr. Antonio Pío, formerly PAHO/WHO Regional Adviser in Tuberculosis and presently with WHO in Geneva, and Dr. James H. Rust, PAHO/WHO Regional Adviser in Enteric Diseases, both of whom reviewed the bacterioses; and Dr. F. J. López Antuñano, PAHO/WHO Regional Adviser in Parasitic Diseases, who read the metazooses.

We would like to thank Dr. James Cocozza, PAHO/WHO Veterinary Adviser, for his review of the translation and Dr. Judith Navarro, Editor in the Office of Publications of PAHO, for her valuable collaboration in the editorial revision and composition of the book.

PEDRO N. ACHA
BORIS SZYFRES

PREFACE TO THE SECOND ENGLISH EDITION

The fine reception accorded the Spanish, English, and French versions of this book has motivated us to revise it in order that it still may serve the purpose for which it was written: to provide an up-to-date source of information to the medical profession and allied fields. This book has undoubtedly filled a void, judging by its wide use in schools of public health, medicine, and veterinary medicine, as well as by bureaus of public and animal health.

The present edition has been considerably enlarged. In the seven years since the first edition was published, our knowledge of zoonoses has increased broadly and rapidly, and new zoonotic diseases have emerged. Consequently, most of the discussions have been largely rewritten, and 28 new diseases have been added to the original 148. Some of these new diseases are emerging zoonoses; others are pathologic entities that have been known for a long time, but for which the epidemiologic connection between man and animal has been unclear until recently.

The use this book has received outside the Western Hemisphere has caused us to abandon the previous emphasis on the Americas in favor of a wider scope and geomedical view. Moreover, wars and other conflicts have given rise to the migration of populations from one country or continent to another. A patient with a disease heretofore known only in Asia may now turn up in Amsterdam, London, or New York. The physician must be aware of these diseases in order to diagnose and treat them. "Exotic" animal diseases have been introduced from Africa to Europe, the Caribbean, and South America, causing great damage. The veterinary physician must learn to recognize them to be able to prevent and eradicate them before they become entrenched. It must be remembered that parasites, viruses, bacteria, and other agents of zoonotic infection can take up residence in any territory where they find the ecologic conditions suitable. Ignorance, economic or personal interests, and human customs and needs also favor the spread of these diseases.

Research in recent years has demonstrated that some diseases previously considered to be exclusively human have their counterparts in wild animals, which in certain circumstances serve as sources of human infection. On the other hand, these animals may also play a positive role by providing models for research, such as in the case of natural leprosy in nine-banded armadillos or in nonhuman primates in Africa. Of no less interest is the discovery of *Rickettsia prowazekii* in eastern flying squirrels and in their ectoparasites in the United States, and the transmission of the infection to man in a country where epidemic typhus has not been seen since 1922. A possible wild cycle of dengue fever is also discussed in the book. Is Creutzfeldt-Jakob disease a zoonosis? No one can say with certainty, but some researchers believe it may have originated as such. In any case, interest is aroused by the surprising similarity of this disease and of kuru to animal subacute spongiform encephalopathies, especially scrapie, the first known and best studied of this group. Discussion of human and animal slow viruses and encephalopathies is included in the spirit of openness to possibilities and the desire to bring the experience of one field of medicine to another. In view of worldwide concern over acquired immunodeficiency syndrome (AIDS), a brief section on retroviruses has also been added, in which the relationship between the human disease and feline and simian AIDS is noted. Another topic deeply interesting to researchers is the mystery of the radical antigenic changes of type A influenza virus, a cause of explosive pandemics that affect millions of persons around the world. Evidence is mounting that these changes result from recombination with a virus of animal origin (see Influenza).

That this should occur is not surprising, given the constant interaction between man and animals. As a rule, zoonoses are transmitted from animal to man, but the reverse may also occur, as is pointed out in the chapters on hepatitis, herpes simplex, and measles. The victims in these cases are nonhuman primates, which may in turn retransmit the infection to man under certain circumstances.

Among emerging zoonoses we cite Lyme disease, which was defined as a clinical entity in 1977; the etiologic agent was found to be a spirochete (isolated in 1982), for which the name *Borrelia burgdorferi* was recently proposed. Emerging viral zoonoses of note in Latin America are Rocio encephalitis and Oropouche fever; the latter has caused multiple epidemics with thousands of victims in northeast Brazil. Outstanding among new viral disease problems in Africa are the emergence of Ebola disease and the spread of Rift Valley fever virus, which has caused tens of thousands of human cases along with great havoc in the cattle industry of Egypt and has evoked alarm around the world. Similarly, the protozoan *Cryptosporidium* is emerging as one of the numerous agents of diarrheal diseases among man and animals, and probably has a worldwide distribution.

As the English edition was being prepared, reports came to light of two animal diseases not previously confirmed in humans. Three cases of human pseudorabies virus infection were recognized between 1983 and 1986 in two men and one woman who had all had close contact with cats and other domestic animals. In 1986, serologic testing confirmed infection by *Ehrlichia canis* in a 51-year-old man who had been suspected of having Rocky Mountain spotted fever. This is the first known occurrence of *E. canis* infection in a human. These two diseases bear watching as possible emerging zoonoses.

The space given to each zoonosis is in proportion to its importance. Some diseases that deserve their own monographs were given more detailed treatment, but no attempt was made to cover the topic exhaustively.

We, the authors, would like to give special recognition to **Dr. Donald C. Blenden**, Professor in the Department of Medicine and Infectious Diseases, School of Medicine, and Head of the Department of Veterinary Microbiology, College of Veterinary Medicine, University of Missouri; and to **Dr. Manuel J. Torres**, Professor of Epidemiology and Public Health, Department of Veterinary Microbiology, College of Veterinary Medicine, University of Missouri, for their thorough review of and valuable contributions to the English translation of this book.

We would also like to recognize the support received from the Pan American Health Organization (PAHO/WHO), the Pan American Health and Education Foundation (PAHEF), and the Pan American Zoonoses Center in Buenos Aires, Argentina, which enabled us to update this book.

We are most grateful to Dr. F. L. Bryan for his generous permission to adapt his monograph "Diseases Transmitted by Foods" as an Appendix to this book.

Mr. Carlos Larranaga, Chief of the Audiovisual Unit at the Pan American Zoonosis Center, deserves our special thanks for the book's artwork, as do Ms. Iris Elliot and Mr. William A. Stapp for providing the translation into English. We would like to express our most sincere gratitude and recognition to Ms. Donna J. Reynolds, editor in the PAHO Editorial Service, for her valuable collaboration in the scientific editorial revision of the book.

PEDRO N. ACHA
BORIS SZYFRES

INTRODUCTION

This book is divided into five parts on the basis of the etiologic agent's position in biological classification. For practical reasons, several types of pathogens—for example, chlamydiae and rickettsiae—have been placed in the same division.

To facilitate reference, the reader will find disease names arranged in alphabetical order within each division. Any difficulty in finding a subject may be overcome by referring to the alphabetical index, which also includes synonyms and names of the etiologic agents.

The present edition lists the number corresponding to the World Health Organization's International Classification of Diseases (*International Classification of Diseases*, Ninth Revision, 1975; Geneva, WHO, 1977) following the title of each disease. In this regard, it should be noted that some zoonoses, fortunately those of lesser importance, have not been included in the aforementioned classification, and therefore are difficult to classify within the present scheme.

Wherever possible, each discussion of a disease or infection includes information about synonyms, etiology, geographic distribution, occurrence in man, occurrence in animals, the disease in man, the disease in animals, the source of infection and mode of transmission, the role of animals in the epidemiology, diagnosis of the disease, and its control. Treatment of patients (man or other species) lies outside the scope of this book. Nevertheless, the medicine(s) of choice are indicated for many diseases, especially but not exclusively when they are applicable to prophylaxis. Particular attention is given to epidemiologic and ecologic aspects so that the reader will obtain an idea of the factors necessary for producing infection or disease. Many of the discussions include diagrammatic illustrations of the mode of transmission of the etiologic agent; they permit rapid visualization of the basic cycle, indicated by solid lines, and of accidental infections of man and other animals, indicated by dotted lines. The diagrams are simple, but it is hoped they will clarify for the reader the animals that maintain the cycle of infection in nature and the principal transmission mechanisms of the agent. Similarly, this edition includes maps, graphs, and tables that will provide an easy guide for the reader regarding the prevalence and geographic distribution of certain zoonoses.

Data on the occurrence of infection in man and animals, as well as information on its geographic distribution, can be useful in judging the relative impact of each of the diseases on public health and the livestock economy of different regions of the world. In this regard, it can be stated that a wide gamut of variation exists in the significance of different zoonoses. Foot-and-mouth disease, for example, is very important from the economic standpoint, but of small importance to public health, if animal protein losses are not considered. On the other hand, Argentine and Bolivian hemorrhagic fevers are important human diseases, but their impact on the economy is minimal, if treatment costs and loss of man-hours are not taken into account. Many other disease entities, such as brucellosis, leptospirosis, salmonellosis, and equine encephalitis, are important from both the public health and economic points of view.

The bibliography following each topic includes mainly books, monographs, and revisions, complemented by more recent studies from many different periodicals.

For this reason, many important scientific contributions are not expressly mentioned, but can be found in the bibliographies of the works cited.

We have included in this edition, at the ends of the respective divisions, summaries of the bacterial, rickettsial, viral, and parasitic zoonoses prepared by the WHO Expert Committee, with the participation of FAO (Geneva, WHO, Technical Report Series 637, 1979, and 682, 1982). At the end of the book is found Appendix I, "Zoonoses and Diseases Common to Man and Animals Transmitted by Foods," which is an adaptation of a monograph by the well-known specialist in diseases of food origin, Dr. Frank L. Bryan, and which constitutes an excellent guide for persons working in this field. Finally, Appendix II contains a list of definitions of terms currently used in epidemiology, as formulated by the American Public Health Association with the objective of precisely defining each word to create a unified terminology.

"But it should be borne in mind that while zoonoses study is an avowedly anthropocentric discipline, epidemiology certainly is not. It is just as important to the epidemiologist to be able to recognize the differences between each species as it is for him to see the similarities among them."

CALVIN W. SCHWABE

Part I

BACTERIOSES

ACTINOMYCOSIS

(039)

Synonyms: Actinophytosis, lumpy jaw, ray fungus disease.

Etiology: *Actinomyces israelii* is the principal etiologic agent in man, and *A. bovis* in animals. Other species—*A. naeslundii, A. viscosus,* and *Arachnia propionica (Actinomyces propionicus)*—are isolated less often; however, *A. viscosus* plays an important role in canine actinomycosis. Some reports indicate isolation of *A. israelii* from animals and *A. bovis* from man. Actinomyces are higher bacteria with many characteristics of fungi. They are gram-positive, non–acid-fast, range from anaerobic to microaerophilic, and are part of the normal flora of the mouth.

Geographic Distribution: Worldwide.

Occurrence in Man: Infrequent. The historical ratio of two cases in men to one in women is probably no longer valid because of the number of cases of genital actinomycosis in women using intrauterine contraceptive devices (IUDs).

Occurrence in Animals: The frequency of the disease varies widely between regions and is also influenced by different livestock management practices. The disease usually appears as sporadic cases. Small outbreaks have occurred in some marshy areas of the USA and the USSR.

The Disease in Man: *A. israelii,* the main causal agent in human beings, is a normal component of the buccal flora. As a result of wounds or surgery, it can enter the soft tissues and bones where it causes a suppurative granulomatous process that opens to the surface through fistulas. Several clinical forms have been identified according to their location: cervicofacial, thoracic, abdominal, and generalized. Cervicofacial, which is the most common, begins with a hard swelling under the mucous membrane of the mouth, beneath the periosteum of the mandible, or in the skin of the neck. At a later stage, softened areas, depressions, and openings to the exterior with a purulent discharge are evident. The secretions usually contain the characteristic "sulphur granules," which are actinomyces colonies. The thoracic form is generally caused by breathing the pathogen into the bronchial tubes where it establishes a chronic bronchopneumonia clinically similar to pulmonary tuberculosis. As the disease progresses, invasion of the thoracic wall and its perforation by fistulous tracks may occur. The abdominal form usually originates as an encapsulated lesion and often becomes localized in the cecum and the appendix, where it produces hard tumors that adhere to the abdominal wall. The generalized form is infrequent and results from the erosive invasion of blood vessels and lymph ducts.

In recent years, reports of actinomycosis in the genital tract of women using intrauterine contraceptive devices have multiplied, with the rate of infection increasing in proportion to the duration of IUD use. In one study (Valicenti *et al.,* 1982), the infection was found in 1.6% of women in the general population of IUD users and in 5.3% of those attending a particular clinic. Another study of 478 women using the IUD found a rate of infection of 12.6% based on Papanicolau smears (Koebler *et al.,* 1983). In the vast majority of cases, colonization by the actinomyces produces only a superficial infection.

The Disease in Animals: *A. bovis* is the principal agent of actinomycosis in bovines and occasionally in other animal species. In bovines it centers chiefly in the maxillae where it forms a granulomatous mass with necrotic areas that develop into abscesses. The latter open via fistulous passages and discharge an odorless, viscous, yellow pus. The pus contains small yellow granules called "sulphur granules," which are rosette-shaped when viewed under a microscope. In some cases chewing becomes very difficult; the animal stops eating and loses weight.

In swine, the etiologic agent locates principally in the udder of the female where it gives rise to abscesses and fistulas. Its pathway of penetration is the lesion caused by the teeth of suckling pigs.

In dogs the disease produces cervicofacial abscesses, empyema accompanied by pleurisy and osteomyelitis, and, more rarely, abdominal abscesses and cutaneous granulomas. The most common agent encountered in recent years has been *A. viscosus* (Hardie and Barsanti, 1982).

Source of Infection and Mode of Transmission: The infection is endogenous in origin. Actinomyces develop as saprophytes within and around carious teeth, in the mucin on dental enamel, and in the tonsillar crypts. In studies carried out in several countries, actinomyces have been found in 40% of excised tonsils; they have also been isolated from 30 to 48% of saliva samples or material from decayed teeth, as well as from the vaginal secretions of 10% of women using IUDs (American Public Health Association, 1985). Infections and pathologic developments are the product of tissue trauma, lesions, or prolonged irritation. It has not been possible to isolate the agent of actinomycosis from the environment. It is believed that the organism penetrates the tissues of the mouth through lesions caused by coarse foods or foreign objects, or by way of dental defects. From the oral cavity the bacteria can be swallowed or can be breathed into the bronchial tubes.

The Role of Animals in the Epidemiology of the Disease: The species of *Actinomyces* which attack man are different from those affecting animals, with rare exceptions. The infection in animals is not transmitted to man, nor is it transmitted from person to person or animal to animal.

Diagnosis: The clinical syndrome may be confused with other infections such as actinobacillosis, nocardiosis, and staphylococcosis as well as neoplasia and tuberculosis. The first step in confirming the diagnosis is to obtain pus, sputum, or tissue samples for microscopic examination and culture. Filament masses are visible by direct observation. In smears of crushed granules or pus stained by the Gram and Kinyoun methods, gram-positive and non–acid-fast filaments or pleomorphic forms, occasionally with bacillary-sized branching, may be seen (Cottral, 1978). It is possible to identify the species of actinomyces causing the disease only by culture and typing of the isolated microorganism. In testing women with IUDs, direct immunofluorescence has given good results (Valicenti *et al.*, 1982).

Control: Prevention in man consists of proper oral hygiene and care after dental extractions or other surgery in the oral cavity. No practical means have yet been established to prevent actinomycosis in animals.

Bibliography

Ajello, L., L. K. Georg, W. Kaplan, and L. Kaufman. *Laboratory Manual for Medical Mycology*. Washington, D.C., U.S. Government Printing Office, 1963. (Public Health Service Publication 994.)

American Public Health Association. *Control of Communicable Diseases in Man,* 14th ed. (Ed. by A. S. Benenson). Washington, D.C., APHA, 1985.

Brunner, D. W., and J. H. Gillespie. *Hagan's Infectious Diseases of Domestic Animals,* 6th ed. Ithaca, New York, Cornell University Press, 1973.

Cottral, G. E. (Ed.). *Manual of Standardized Methods for Veterinary Microbiology.* Ithaca, New York, Cornell University Press, 1978.

Dalling, T., and A. Robertson (Eds.). *International Encyclopaedia of Veterinary Medicine*. Edinburgh, Scotland, Green, 1966.

Hardie, E. M., and J. A. Barsanti. Treatment of canine actinomycosis. *J Am Vet Med Assoc* 180:537-541, 1982.

Koebler, C., A. Chatwani, and R. Schwartz. Actinomycosis infection associated with intrauterine contraceptive devices. *Am J Obstet Gynecol* 145:596-599, 1983.

Pier, A. C. *The Actinomycetes. In:* Hubbert, W. T., W. F. McCulloch, and P. R. Schnurrenberger (Eds.), *Diseases Transmitted from Animals to Man,* 6th ed. Springfield, Illinois, Thomas, 1975.

Valicenti, J. F., Jr., A. A. Pappas, C. D. Graber, H. O. Williamson, and N. F. Willis. Detection and prevalence of IUD-associated *Actinomyces* colonization and related morbidity. A prospective study of 69,925 cervical smears. *JAMA* 247:1149-1152, 1982.

ANIMAL ERYSIPELAS AND HUMAN ERYSIPELOID

(027.1)

Synonyms: Rosenbach's erysipeloid, erythema migrans, erysipelotrichosis, rose disease (in swine), fish-handler's disease (in man).

Etiology: *Erysipelothrix rhusiopathiae (E. insidiosa)*. Twenty-two different serotypes are recognized (1 to 22). Type 1 is further subdivided into two subtypes, 1a and 1b. Serotypes 1 and 2 are the principal and perhaps the only agents of acute swine erysipelas. No other serotypes have been isolated from this form of the disease up to this time. Serotyping is also important in the immunization of swine, since only a few strains of serotype 3 (Dedié's serotype B) produce effective bacterins against swine erysipelas (Wood and Harrington, 1978; Wood *et al.*, 1981).

Geographic Distribution: The etiologic agent is distributed on all continents among many species of mammals and birds, domestic as well as wild. It has also been isolated from aquatic animals such as dolphins, alligators, American crocodiles, and sea lions.

Occurrence in Man: Human erysipeloid is for the most part an occupational disease of workers in slaughterhouses and commercial fowl-processing plants, fishermen and fish-industry workers, and those who handle meat (especially pork) and seafood products. It is not a notifiable disease and little is known of its incidence. The best data derive from the USSR, where from 1956 to 1958 almost 3,000 cases were recorded in 13 slaughterhouses in the Ukraine, and in 1959, 154 cases in the Tula region. From 1961 to 1970, the Centers for Disease Control of the USA confirmed diagnosis of 15 cases in that country. A few isolated cases have occurred in Latin America. In the USSR, the USA, and on the southern Baltic coast, some epidemic outbreaks have occurred.

Occurrence in Animals: The disease in swine (rose disease, swine erysipelas) is important in Europe, Asia, Canada, the USA, and Mexico. It has also been observed in Jamaica, Guatemala, Guyana, Suriname, Brazil, Chile, and Peru, but the incidence is low in these countries. However, the disease seems to be increasing in importance in Chile (Skoknic *et al.*, 1981).

The Disease in Man: It is a cutaneous infection and is called erysipeloid to differentiate it from erysipelas caused by a hemolytic streptococcus. The incubation period varies from a few hours to 7 days. Erysipeloid localizes primarily on the hands and fingers. It consists of an erythematous, edematous skin lesion with violet coloration around a wound (inoculation point) that may be a simple abrasion. Arthritis in the finger joints occurs with some frequency. The patient experiences a burning sensation, a pulsating pain, and at times an intense pruritus. The course of the disease is usually benign and the patient recovers in 2 to 4 weeks. If the infection becomes generalized, septicemia, and endocarditis may cause death. Septicemia in man is rare.

The Disease in Animals: Many species of mammals and birds, domestic as well as wild, are hosts to the etiologic agent. In several animal species, *E. rhusiopathiae* produces pathologic processes. Swine are the most affected species.

SWINE: Swine erysipelas is an economically important disease in many countries. In several Central European countries, swine can only be raised profitably where systematic vaccination is practiced. Morbidity and mortality vary a great deal from one region to another, perhaps due to differences in the virulence of the etiologic agent. At the moment, acute forms are infrequent in western Europe and in North America.

The incubation period lasts from 1 to 7 days. There are two main clinical forms: acute and chronic. These forms may exist simultaneously in a herd or appear separately. The acute variety begins suddenly with a high fever. Some animals suffer from prostration, anorexia, and vomiting, while others continue to feed in spite of the high fever. In some animals, characteristic cutaneous lesions appear between 24 and 48 hours later in the form of red urticarial plaques, shaped like rhomboids and varying in size. In other animals, the edematous eruption is more diffuse and more difficult to observe. These lesions are found especially on the abdomen, the inside of the thighs, the neck, and the ears. The disease has a rapid course: the animals either recover or die. In the last phase of septicemic erysipelas, dyspnea and diarrhea are the most evident symptoms. Mortality varies, but at times the disease may decimate a herd. Necropsy reveals petechiae in many parts of the organism.

The spleen and lymph glands are very inflamed and often hemorrhagic. The septicemic acute form is almost always due to serotypes 1 and 2.

The chronic form is characterized by arthritis. At first, the joints swell and movement is painful; later, ankylosis may develop. Economic losses from arthritis are considerable because the animals' development and weight gain are affected and because they may be confiscated from abattoirs. The chronic form may also manifest itself in endocarditis, with progressive emaciation and sudden death.

SHEEP AND CATTLE: *E. rhusiopathiae* causes arthritis in lambs, usually after tail docking or sometimes as a result of an umbilical infection. The infection becomes established about 2 weeks after tail docking or birth, and the main symptoms are difficulty in movement and stunted growth. Recovery is slow.

In Chile, Argentina, Brazil, New Zealand, and Great Britain, a cutaneous infection caused by *E. rhusiopathiae* has been observed on the hooves of sheep a few days after they have undergone a benzene hexachloride dip. The lesions consist of laminitis and the animals experience difficulty in walking. The disease lasts nearly 2 weeks. Like human erysipeloid, the infection gains entry through small skin abrasions. It can be prevented by adding a disinfectant such as a 0.03% solution of cupric sulfate to the dip.

Arthritis has been observed in calves, and the agent has been isolated from the tonsils of adult cows.

BIRDS: A septicemic disease caused by *E. rhusiopathiae* occurs in many species of domestic and wild fowl; turkeys are the most frequently affected. The symptomatology includes general weakness, diarrhea, cyanosis, and a reddish purple, swollen comb. The disease characteristically attacks males in particular. Mortality varies between 2.5 and 25%. The lesions consist of large hemorrhages and petechiae of the pectoral and thigh muscles, serous membranes, intestine, and gizzard. The spleen and liver are enlarged. Symptoms and lesions are similar in chickens, turkeys, and pheasants.

Source of Infection and Mode of Transmission (Figure 1): Many animal species harbor *E. rhusiopathiae*. The principal reservoir seems to be swine; the etiologic agent has been isolated from the tonsils of up to 30% of apparently healthy pigs. In a study carried out recently in Chile, the agent was isolated from tonsil samples of 53.5% of 400 swine in a slaughterhouse (Skoknic *et al.*, 1981). *E. rhusiopathiae* was isolated from 25.6% of soil samples where pigs live and from their feces (Wood and Harrington, 1978). A great variety of serotypes may be isolated from swine, with serotypes 1, 2, 5, and 6 predominating in countries where these studies have been carried out. Fish, mollusks, and crustaceans constitute an important source of infection. The etiologic agent has been isolated from fish skin. In the USSR an epidemic of erysipeloid was caused by handling fish brought in by several different boats; on the Baltic coast there was an outbreak of 40 cases. In Argentina, where swine erysipela has not been confirmed but where cases of human erysipeloid have been discribed, the agent was isolated from two out of nine water samples from the Atlantic coast and from one out of 40 samples of fish integument (de Diego and Lavalle, 1977). Subsequently, these strains were identified as belonging to serotypes 21 and 22.

In meat and poultry processing plants, rodents can be important reservoirs and disseminators of the infection.

Figure 1. Animal erysipelas and human erysipeloid (*Erysipelothrix rhusiopathiae*). Mode of transmission.

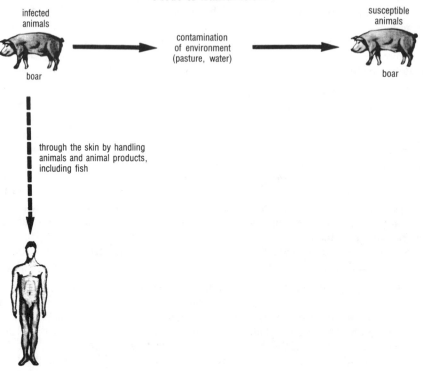

E. rhusiopathiae can survive a long time outside the animal organism, both in the environment and in products of animal origin, which contributes to its perpetuation.

Man is infected through wounds and skin abrasions, but is very resistant to other penetration routes. The infection is contracted by handling animals and products of animal origin, including fish. Cases among veterinarians have resulted from needle punctures when using the simultaneous method of vaccination (virulent culture and hyperimmune serum). In Chile, a case of human endocarditis was attributed to the ingestion of smoked fish sold in the street (Gilabert, 1968).

Carriers of swine erysipelas harbor the agent in the pharyngeal region and contaminate the environment by shedding it in the feces, thus constituting the reservoir and the source of infection. The routes of infection are believed to be digestive and cutaneous, through abrasions and wounds and perhaps through arthropod bites. The long survival of the agent in the environment ensures endemism in affected areas. Other animals and fowl also may contribute to maintaining the infection and to causing outbreaks.

Role of Animals in the Epidemiology of the Disease: Man is an accidental host who contracts the infection from sick animals, carriers, animal products, or objects contaminated by animals.

Diagnosis: Clinical diagnosis, based on the patient's occupation and on the characteristics of the cutaneous lesion, can be confirmed by isolation and identification of the etiologic agent. *E. rhusiopathiae* can be isolated from biopsies of liquid aspirated from the lesion.

In septicemic cases in animals, the etiologic agent can be isolated from the bloodstream or from internal organs. In cases of arthritis or skin infections, cultures are made from the localized lesions. Isolations from contaminated materials are accomplished through inoculation of mice, which are very susceptible.

Diagnosis of animal erysipelas makes use of several serologic tests, such as agglutination, growth inhibition, passive hemagglutination, and complement fixation. Bearing in mind the prevalence in animals of subclinical infections and vaccination, serologic tests are at times difficult to interpret. In a comparative study between the growth inhibition test and the complement fixation test, it was concluded that the latter is more useful in diagnosis, since it eliminates low titers caused by subclinical infection or vaccination (Bercovich *et al.*, 1981).

Control: In persons exposed as a result of their occupations, prevention of erysipeloid consists of hygiene, namely, frequent hand washing with disinfectant and appropriate treatment of wounds. Establishments where foods of animal origin are processed should control rodent populations.

The control of swine erysipelas depends mostly on vaccination. Two vaccines have given excellent results: a bacterin adsorbed on aluminum hydroxide and a live avirulent vaccine (EVA = "erysipelas vaccine avirulent"). Vaccination provides immunity for 5 to 6 months. The bacterin is first administered before weaning, followed by another dose 2 to 4 weeks later. The avirulent vaccine is also administered orally in the drinking water. The vaccines are not entirely satisfactory in preventing chronic erysipelas, and it is even suspected that vaccination may contribute to arthritic symptoms (Gillespie and Timoney, 1981). In the case of an outbreak of septicemic erysipelas, carcasses should be destroyed immediately and the premises disinfected. Sick animals should be treated with penicillin and the rest of the herd with anti-erysipelas serum. Rotation of the animals to different pastures and environmental hygiene measures are also of great help in control.

Bacterins are used on turkey-raising establishments, where the infection is endemic. At present, a live vaccine administered orally in the drinking water is being developed and has given good preliminary results (Bricker and Saif, 1983).

Bibliography

Bercovich, Z., C. D. Weenk van Loon, and C. W. Spek. Serological diagnosis of *Erysipelothrix rhusiopathiae:* a comparative study between the growth inhibition test and the complement fixation test. *Vet Q* 3:19-24, 1981.

Blood, D. C., and J. A. Henderson. *Veterinary Medicine*, 4th ed. Baltimore, Maryland, Williams and Wilkins, 1974.

Bricker, J. M., and Y. M. Saif. Drinking water vaccination of turkeys, using live *Erysipelothrix rhusiopathiae*. *J Am Vet Med Assoc* 183:361-362, 1983.

Castro, A. F. P. de, O. Campedelli Filho, and C. Troise. Isolamento de *Erysipelothrix rhusiopathiae* de peixes maritimos. *Rev Inst Med Trop S Paulo* 9:169-171, 1967.

de Diego, A. I., and S. Lavalle. *Erysipelothrix rhusiopathiae* en aguas y pescados de la costa atlántica de la provincia de Buenos Aires (Argentina). *Gac Vet (B Aires)* 39:672-677, 1977.

Gilabert, B. Endocarditis bacteriana producida por *Erysipelothrix*. Primer caso humano verificado en Chile, *Bol Hosp San Juan de Dios (Santiago)* 15:390-392, 1968. Cit. in Skoknic *et al.*, 1981.

Gillespie, J. H., and J. F. Timoney. *Hagan and Bruner's Infectious Diseases of Domestic Animals*, 7th ed. Ithaca, Cornell University Press, 1981.

Gledhill, A. W. Swine erysipelas. *In*: Stableforth, A. W., and I. A. Galloway (Eds.), *Infectious Diseases of Animals*, London, Butterworths, 1959.

Levine, N. D. Listeriosis, botulism, erysipelas, and goose influenza. *In*: Biester, H. E., and L. H. Schwarte (Eds.), *Diseases of Poultry*, 4th ed. Ames, Iowa State University Press, 1959.

Skoknic, A., I. Díaz, S. Urcelay, R. Duarte, and O. González. Estudio de la erisipela en Chile. *Arch Med Vet (Valdivia)* 13:13-16, 1981.

Shuman, R. D., and R. L. Wood. Swine erysipelas. *In*: Dunne, H. W. (Ed.), *Diseases of Swine*, 3rd ed. Ames, Iowa State University Press, 1970.

Wood, R. L. Erysipelothrix infection. *In*: Hubbert, W. T., W. F. McCulloch, and P. R. Schnurrenberger (Eds.), *Diseases Transmitted from Animals to Man*, 6th ed. Springfield, Illinois, Thomas, 1975.

Wood, R. L., and R. Harrington. Serotypes of *Erysipelothrix rhusiopathiae* isolated from swine and from soil and manure of swine pens in the United States. *Am J Vet Res* 39:1833-1840, 1978.

Wood, R. L., R. Harrington, and D. R. Hubrich. Serotypes of previously unclassified isolates of *Erysipelothrix rhusiopathiae* from swine in the United States and Puerto Rico. *Am J Vet Res* 42:1248-1250, 1981.

ANTHRAX

(022)

Synonyms: Malignant carbuncle, charbon, malignant pustule, malignant edema, woolsorters' disease.

Etiology: *Bacillus anthracis*. This organism is found in a vegetative state in man and animals. When exposed to oxygen in the air, it forms spores that are highly resistant to physical and chemical agents.

Geographic Distribution: Worldwide, with some areas of enzootic and sporadic occurrence.

Occurrence in Man: The infection in humans is correlated with the incidence of the disease in domestic animals. In countries with advanced economies, where animal anthrax has been controlled, it occurs only occasionally among humans. Some cases stem from the importation of contaminated animal products. Human anthrax is most common in enzootic areas in developing countries among those who work with livestock, eat insufficiently cooked meat from infected animals, or work in establishments where wool, goatskins, and pelts are stored and processed. The incidence of the human illness in developing countries is not well known because those sick with the disease do not always see a doctor, nor do doctors always report the cases; in addition, many times the diagnosis is based only on the clinical syndrome.

According to data from recent years, epidemic outbreaks continue to occur in spite of the availability of excellent preventive methods for animal anthrax and, therefore, for the disease in humans. There are some hyperendemic areas, as was shown in Haiti when an American woman contracted the infection after acquiring some goatskin drums. Careful compilation of data in that country revealed a high incidence of human anthrax in the southern peninsula, Les Cayes, with a population of approximately 500,000 people. From 1973 to 1977, 1,587 cases were recorded in the 31 clinics in that region (La Force, 1978).

In enzootic areas, the human disease is usually endemosporadic with epidemic outbreaks. The most recent outbreaks have been due to ingestion of meat, in some instances by many people, from animals dying of anthrax when slaughtered or from those already dead from it (Rey *et al.*, 1982; Fragoso and Villicaña, 1984; Sirisanthana *et al.*, 1984). In 1978 in a region of the Republic of Mali, there were 84 cases with 19 deaths. A high mortality was also seen in Senegal in 1957, with 237 deaths out of 254 cases. The high mortality was possibly due to intestinal anthrax (Simaga *et al.*, 1980).

In 1979 an epidemic outbreak occurred in Sverdlovsk, USSR, which gave rise to a controversy between that country and the United States. According to the USSR, fewer than 40 persons died from gastric anthrax in this epidemic, while US intelligence sources claimed that several hundred to a thousand people perished from pulmonary anthrax within a few weeks. The controversy centered on whether the epidemic was natural or man-induced, since the US intelligence source suspected that an accident had occurred at a plant presumably engaged in biological warfare projects. If so, this would have indicated an infringement of the 1975 treaty against biological weapons. In any case, the suspicion could not be confirmed (Wade, 1980). Sverdlovsk is located in an enzootic area, and the Soviet authorities, for their part, proposed that the farmers had sold infected animals on the black market.

Occurrence in Animals: Anthrax is common in enzootic areas where no control programs have been established.

The Disease in Man: The incubation period is from 2 to 5 days. Three clinical forms are recognized: cutaneous, pulmonary or respiratory, and gastrointestinal.

The cutaneous form is the most common and is contracted by contact with infected animals (usually carcasses) or contaminated wool, hides, and fur. The exposed part of the skin begins to itch and a papule appears at the inoculation site. This papule becomes a vesicle and then evolves into a depressed, black eschar. Generally, the cutaneous lesion is not painful or only slightly so; consequently, some patients do not consult a doctor in time. If left untreated, the infection can lead to septicemia and death. The case fatality rate for untreated cutaneous anthrax is from 5 to 20%.

The pulmonary form is contracted by inhalation of *B. anthracis* spores. At the onset of the illness, the symptomatology is mild and resembles that of a common upper respiratory tract infection. Some 3 to 5 days later the symptoms become acute, with fever, shock, and resultant death. The case fatality rate is high.

Gastrointestinal anthrax is contracted by ingestion of meat from infected animals and is manifested by violent gastroenteritis with vomiting and bloody stools. Mortality ranges from 25 to 75% (Brachman, 1984).

B. anthracis produces a powerful toxin composed of three parts (factor I, or the edema factor; factor II, protective antigen; and factor III, lethal factor). The toxin has been obtained both *in vitro* and *in vivo*. Death by anthrax is caused by the toxin, but its mechanism of action is still under discussion.

The Disease in Animals: It takes three forms: apoplectic or peracute; acute and subacute; and chronic. The apoplectic form is seen mostly in cattle, sheep, and goats, and it occurs most frequently at the beginning of an outbreak. The onset is sudden and death ensues rapidly. The animals show signs of cerebral apoplexy and die suddenly.

The acute and subacute forms are common in cattle, horses, and sheep. The symptomatology consists of fever, a halt to rumination, excitement followed by depression, difficulty in breathing, uncoordinated movements, convulsions, and death. Bloody discharges from the natural orifices as well as edemas in different parts of the body are sometimes observed.

Chronic anthrax occurs mainly in less susceptible species such as pigs, but is also seen in cattle, horses, and dogs. During an outbreak in a herd of swine, some animals fall victim to the acute form, but most suffer from chronic anthrax. The main symptom of this form is pharyngeal and lingual edema. Frequently, a foamy sanguinolent discharge from the mouth is observed. The animals die from asphyxiation. Another localized chronic form in pigs is intestinal anthrax.

Anthrax also affects free-roaming wild animals and those in zoos and national parks. In Etosha National Park in Namibia, South West Africa, anthrax killed 1,635 animals from among 10 species, causing 54% of all mortality between January of 1966 and June of 1974. The source of infection was artificial wells (Ebedes, 1976).

Autopsies of acute cases reveal bloody exudate in the natural orifices. Decomposition is rapid and the carcass is bloated with gases. Rigor mortis is incomplete. Hemorrhages are found in the internal organs; splenomegaly is almost always present, the pulp being dark red or blackish with a soft or semifluid consistency; the liver, kidneys, and lymph nodes are congested and enlarged; and the blood is blackish with little clotting tendency.

Source of Infection and Mode of Transmission (Figure 2): For man the source of infection is always infected animals, contaminated animal products, or environmental contamination by spores from these sources.

Cutaneous anthrax is contracted by inoculation during the process of skinning or butchering an animal or by contact with infected leather, pelts, wool, or fur. Broken skin makes transmission easier. Products made from contaminated hair (for example, shaving brushes), skins (e.g., drums), or bone meal (e.g., fertilizers) may continue to be sources of infection for many years. Transmission from animal to man is possible by means of insects acting as mechanical vectors, but documented cases are few.

Pulmonary anthrax comes from inhaling spores from contaminated wool or animal hair.

The source of infection for the gastrointestinal form is domestic and wild animals that died from anthrax. The pathway of transmission is through the digestive tract. Cases have been observed in Asia, Africa, and the Americas. Animals contract the infection mainly by ingestion of pasture or water contaminated with *B. anthracis* spores, especially in places near anthrax-infected carcasses. An animal dying from anthrax produces an enormous quantity of *B. anthracis* in its tissues, and if the

Figure 2. Anthrax. Transmission Cycle.

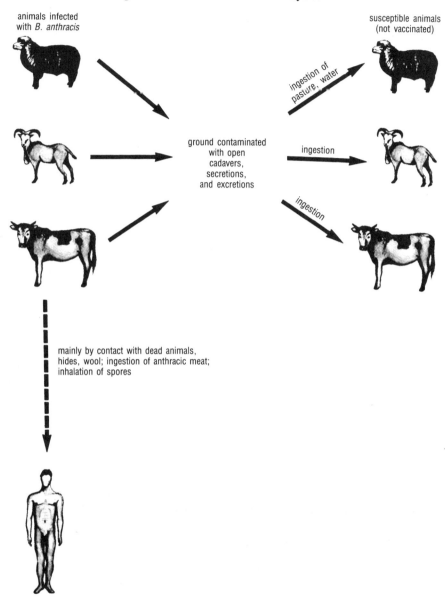

carcass is opened, the bacilli sporulate, contaminating the soil, grass, and water. Animals that graze the contaminated area become infected themselves and produce new foci of infection. Carrion-feeding animals and birds can transport the infection some distance. The most serious outbreaks occur during dry summers after heavy rains. The rain washes spores loose and concentrates them in low spots, forming so-called "cursed fields"—usually damp areas with glacial calcareous soils containing abundant organic material and having a pH above 6 (Van Ness, 1971). Nevertheless, outbreaks of anthrax may occur in acid soil, as happened in the 1974 epizootic in Texas in the United States, during which 218 cattle, six horses, and one mule died. Eighty-three per cent of the pasture where the outbreak took place had acid soil and 94% had subsoil with an alkaline pH (Whitford, 1979).

Contaminated animal by-products, especially bone meal and blood meal used as food supplements, can also give rise to distant foci of infection.

Another mode of transmission is cutaneous entry through insect bites, but this is considered of minor importance epidemiologically.

Role of Animals in the Epidemiology of the Disease: Animals are essential for its transmission. Anthrax is transmitted to humans by animals or animal products. Transmission between human beings is exceptional.

Diagnosis: The presence of the etiologic agent must be confirmed by microscopic examination of stained smears of vesicular fluid (in man), edemas (in swine), or blood (in other animals); by culturing the microorganism from the liquid aspirated from malignant pustules or from blood specimens of a dying or recently dead animal; or by inoculation of laboratory animals (guinea pigs and mice). If the material is contaminated, cutaneous inoculation (by scarification) should be employed. The use of antibiotics quickly reduces the possibility of isolating the pathogen.

The fluorescent antibody technique applied to fresh stains or blood smears can prove useful for presumptive diagnosis.

Ascoli's test may be useful for examining hides and pelts. Recently, specific serologic tests have been developed that use protective antigen (obtained from a concentrated culture filtrate free of bacterial cells). These tests, such as the indirect hemagglutination test, the agar-gel precipitation test, and the Farr test (using antigen marked with iodine 131), are promising for future use in diagnosis of the more slowly progressing forms of anthrax.

Control: In man, the prevention of anthrax is based mainly on: a) control of the infection in animals; b) prevention of contact with infected animals and contaminated animal products; c) environmental and personal hygiene in places where products of animal origin are handled (including adequate ventilation and work clothing); d) prompt medical care for cutaneous lesions; and e) disinfection of fur and wool with hot formaldehyde. Occupational groups at high risk may benefit from vaccination with the protective antigen.

In animals, anthrax control is based on systematic vaccination in enzootic areas. Sterne's avirulent spore vaccine is indicated because of its potency and safety; it can be used to vaccinate all species of animals. In general, one vaccination per year is sufficient; only in hyperenzootic areas is vaccination at shorter intervals recommended. Immunity is established in approximately 1 week in cattle, but takes longer in horses. In regions where anthrax occurs sporadically, mass vaccination is not justified and should be limited to affected herds. Rapid diagnosis, with isolation and treatment of sick animals with antibiotics (penicillin), is important.

Autopsies should not be performed on animals that have died from anthrax. An unopened carcass decomposes rapidly and the vegetative form of *B. anthracis* is destroyed in a short time. For confirmation of the diagnosis, blood should be taken from a peripheral vessel with a syringe and sent to the laboratory in a sterile container. Dead animals should be destroyed where they lie as quickly as possible, preferably by incineration. The alternative is to bury them 2 meters deep and cover them with a layer of lime.

Affected herds should be placed in quarantine for 2 weeks after the last case is found, with no animal or animal product allowed out.

If anthrax is suspected at a slaughterhouse, all operations should be halted until the diagnosis is confirmed. If positive, all exposed carcasses must be destroyed and the premises carefully disinfected (with a 5% caustic lye solution for 8 hours) before operations are resumed.

Bibliography

Bhat, P., D. Nagamani Mohan, and H. Srinivasa. Intestinal anthrax with bacteriological investigation. *J Infect Dis* 152:1357-1358, 1985.

Brachman, P. S. Anthrax. *In:* Warren, K. S., and A. A. F. Mahmoud (Eds.). *Tropical and Geographical Medicine.* New York, McGraw-Hill Book Co., 1984.

Ebedes, H. Anthrax epizootics in wildlife in the Etosha Park, South West Africa. *In:* Page, L. A. (Ed.), *Wildlife Diseases.* New York, Plenum Press, 1976.

Fragoso, R., and H. Villicaña Fuentes. Antrax en dos comunidades de Zacatecas, México. *Bol Of Sanit Panam* 97:526-533, 1984.

Gainer, R. S. Epizootiology of anthrax and nyasa wildebeest in the Selous Game Reserve, Tanzania. *J Wildl Dis* 23:175-178, 1987.

La Force, F. M. Report to the Pan American Sanitary Bureau. Haiti, 1978.

Okolo, M. I. Studies on anthrax in food animals and persons occupationally exposed to the zoonoses in Eastern Nigeria. *Int J Zoonoses* 12:276-282, 1985.

Rey, J. L., M. Meyran, and P. Saliou. Situation épidémiologique de charbon humain en Haute Volta. *Bull Soc Pathol Exot* 75:249-257, 1982.

Simaga, S. Y., E. Astorquiza, M. Thiero, and R. Baylet. Un foyer de charbon humain et animal dans le cercle de Kati (République du Mali). *Bull Soc Pathol Exot* 73:23-28, 1980.

Sirisanthana, T., M. Navachareon, P. Tharavichitkul, V. Sarisanthana, and A. E. Brown. Outbreak of oral-pharyngeal anthrax: an unusual manifestation of human infection with *Bacillus anthracis. Am J Trop Med Hyg* 33:144-150, 1984.

Sirol, J., Y. Gendron, and M. Condat. Le charbon humain en Afrique. *Bull WHO* 49:143-148, 1973.

Sterne, M. Anthrax. *In:* Stableforth, A. W., and I. A. Galloway (Eds.). *Infectious Diseases of Animals.* London, Butterworths, 1959.

Van Ness, G. B. Ecology of anthrax. *Science* 172:1303-1307, 1971.

Wade, N. Death at Sverdlovsk: a critical diagnosis. *Science* 209:1501-1502, 1980.

Whitford, H. W. Anthrax. *In:* Stoenner, H., W. Kaplan, and M. Torten (Section Eds.). *CRC Handbook Series in Zoonoses.* Section A, vol. 1. Boca Raton, Florida, CRC Press, 1979.

World Health Organization. *Joint FAO/WHO Expert Committee on Zoonoses. Third Report.* Geneva, 1967. (Technical Report Series 378.)

Wright, G. G. Anthrax. *In:* Hubbert, W. T., W. F. McCulloch, and P. R. Schnurrenberger (Eds.), *Diseases Transmitted from Animals to Man,* 6th ed. Springfield, Illinois, Thomas, 1975.

BOTULISM

(005.1) Botulinum poisoning
(008.4) Infant botulism
(041.8) Wound botulism

Synonyms: Allantiasis; "lamziekte" = bovine botulism in South Africa; "limber-neck" = botulism in fowl.

Etiology: Toxins produced by *Clostridium botulinum,* which are the most potent known. *C. botulinum* is an obligate, spore-forming anaerobe. It has been sub-classified (Smith, 1977) into four groups (I-IV), according to culture and serologic characteristics. Seven different types of botulinum antigens have been identified (A-G) according to their serologic specificity. Classic botulism results from preformed toxins ingested with food. In wound botulism, toxins form in contaminated injured tissue. In 1976 a new clinical type, infant botulism, was identified. It is caused by colonization of an infant's intestinal tract by *C. botulinum* and the resultant production and absorption of toxins.

Geographic Distribution: Occurs on all continents, with a marked regional distribution that probably reflects the presence in the soil of the microorganism and its different types of toxins.

Occurrence in Man: Botulism poisoning occurs both sporadically and among groups of people that ingest the same food containing the preformed toxin. From 1953 to 1973, an average of 15.1 outbreaks occurred annually in the United States of America, with 2.4 cases per outbreak. In that period there were only three outbreaks affecting more than 10 people, but in 1977 an outbreak of 59 cases involving type B botulinum toxin was described, caused by food eaten in a restaurant (Terranova *et al.,* 1978). Figure 3 illustrates the reported cases and deaths by year in the USA during the period 1960-1980 (Pan American Health Organization, 1982). More than half the cases reported since 1899 from 45 states occurred in five western states. Table 1 shows the foods and type of botulinum toxin that caused the illness. In Canada between 1979 and 1980, fifteen incidents were investigated (Pan American . Health Organization, 1982). In Argentina during the period 1967-1981, 139 cases were reported (Figure 4). In 1958 several suspected cases of botulism occurred in Brazil when six members of the same family died and others became ill after eating home-canned boiled fish. In 1981, two other suspected cases appeared in Rio de Janeiro, caused by ingestion of an industrially processed food.

In Eurasia the occurrence of the illness varies from one country to another. In Poland, which seems to be the country hardest hit by botulism on that continent, the majority of cases have occurred in rural areas, as they have in other countries. From 1959 to 1969, the incidence oscillated between 0.5 and 1.5 cases per 100,000 inhabitants. In 1933 in Dniepropetrovsk, the USSR, the largest outbreak known to date took place, with 230 cases and 94 deaths. More recently, about 14 outbreaks per year have occurred. In France, botulism is infrequent, with about four outbreaks annually. However, during World War II 500 outbreaks were recorded with more that a thousand people affected. Germany is second to Poland in the incidence of the illness. In the rest of Europe botulism is rare. During the period 1951-1968, 57

Figure 3. Botulism (transmitted by foods). Reported cases and deaths per year in the United States of America, 1960-1980.

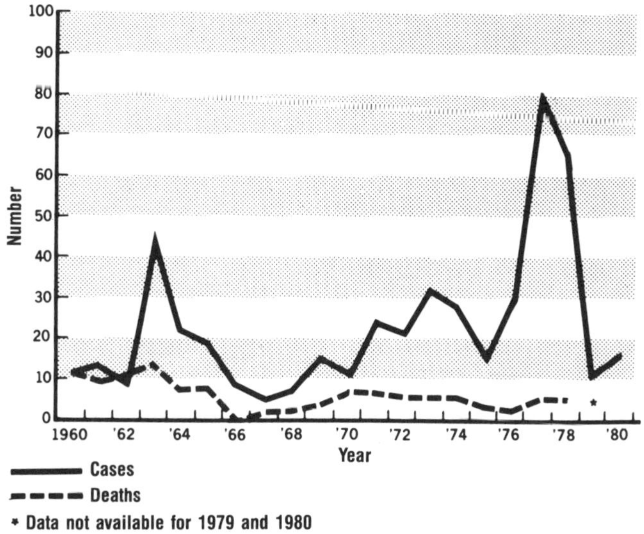

Cases
Deaths
* Data not available for 1979 and 1980

Source: PAHO Epidemiol Bull 3(4):2, 1982.

outbreaks with 321 cases and 85 deaths took place in Japan. In the rest of Asia, in Africa, and in Australia, few cases have been identified (Smith, 1977).

Infant botulism was recognized for the first time in the United States and then in Canada, several European countries, and Australia. From 1976 to 1980, 184 cases were recorded in the US, 88 of which occurred in California and 96 in 25 other states. Almost all the cases were seen in children younger than six months (Morris, 1983).

The first case of wound botulism was recognized in the same country in 1943. By 1982, 27 cases were recorded, 20 of them in states west of the Mississippi (Centers for Disease Control of the USA, 1982).

Occurrence in Animals: Botulism in bovines is type C beta or type D. It is economically important in some areas, affecting large numbers of animals. Such areas, generally poor in phosphorus, are found in the southwestern United States, Corrientes Province in Argentina, and Piauí and Matto Grosso in Brazil; however, bovine botulism occurs even more frequently in South Africa ("lamziekte") and Australia. It is also important in Senegal, where it is believed to cause more cattle loss than any other disease. In other countries sporadic outbreaks and cases occur, primarily caused by ingestion of fodder and silage containing the preformed toxins (Smith, 1977).

Botulism in sheep is due to type C and is known only in western Australia and South Africa.

In horses botulism cases are sporadic and for the most part are caused by *C. botulinum* type C, as described in Israel. The disease has been diagnosed in these animals in several European countries, the United States of America, Israel, Australia, and South Africa.

Table 1. Foods giving rise to botulism, and number of outbreaks in the United States of America, 1899-1977.[a, b]

Type of botulinum toxin	Vegetables	Fish and fish products	Fruits	Condiments[c]	Beef[d]	Milk and milk products	Pork	Fowl	Others[e]	Unknown[e]	Total
A	115	11	22	17	6	3	2	2	8	9	195
B	31	4	7	5	1	2	1	2	3	3	59
E	1	25							3	1	30
F					1						1
A and B	2										2
Unknown[e]	2	1		1						6	10
Total	151	41	29	23	8	5	3	4	14	19	297

[a] For the period 1899-1973, only outbreaks in which the type of toxin was confirmed are included; for 1974-1977, all outbreaks are included.

[b] Prepared by the Centers for Disease Control, Atlanta, Georgia, USA.

[c] Includes outbreaks caused by tomato condiments, hot sauces, and salad dressings.

[d] Includes one type F outbreak caused by venison, and one type A outbreak caused by mutton.

[e] Categories added for the period 1974-1977.

Source: PAHO Epidemiol Bull 3(4):2, 1982.

Figure 4. Reported cases of botulism in Argentina, 1967-1981.

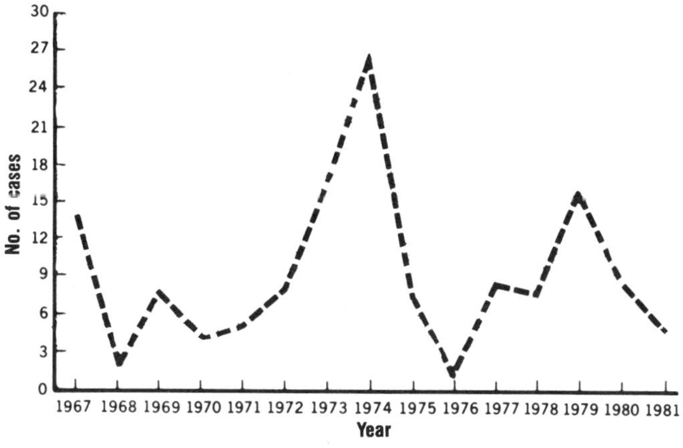

Source: PAHO Epidemiol Bull 3(4):2, 1982.

Botulism in swine is rare because of the natural high resistance of this species to botulinum toxin. Outbreaks diagnosed in Senegal and Australia were caused by type C beta, and one in the United States by type B.

Botulism in mink can be an important problem owing to their eating habits, if they are not vaccinated as recommended. Mink are highly susceptible to type C, which causes almost all outbreaks.

Botulism in fowl occurs practically worldwide and is caused principally by type C alpha. Outbreaks of types A and E have been recorded in waterfowl. In the western United States, type C is responsible for massive outbreaks in wild ducks during the summer and early fall. Many other species of wild fowl are susceptible to botulism, and outbreaks also occur in domestic chickens and farm-bred pheasants (Smith, 1977).

The Disease in Man: a) Botulinum poisoning by foods is produced primarily by types A, B, E, and F. Outbreaks in man described as type C have not been confirmed, as the toxin has not been found in the patients' blood or feces nor in foods they ate. An outbreak of type D was identified in Chad, Africa, among people who had eaten raw ham (Smith, 1977). A new toxicogenic type, *C. botulinum* type G, was isolated from the soil in Argentina in 1969 (Giménez and Ciccarelli, 1970). Recently, the first human cases were identified in Switzerland (Sonnabend *et al.*, 1981). The microorganism was isolated in autopsy specimens from four adults and an 18-week-old child, and the toxin was present in the blood serum of three of these persons who died suddenly at home. The symptoms were similar to those of classic botulism.

The incubation period is usually from 18 to 36 hours, but the illness can show up within a few hours or as long as 8 days after ingestion of the contaminated food, depending on the quantity of toxin ingested. The clinical signs of the different types vary little, although the mortality rate seems to be higher for type A. The disease is afebrile, and gastrointestinal symptoms such as nausea, vomiting, and abdominal pain precede neurologic symptoms. Neurologic manifestations are always symmetrical, with weakness or descending paralysis. Diplopia, dysarthria, and dysphagia are common. Consciousness and sensibility remain until death. The immediate cause of death is usually respiratory failure. The mortality rate in botulinum poisonings is high, the highest being registered in patients with short incubation periods, that is, those who have ingested a high dose of toxin. In the United States the fatality rate has been reduced from 60% in 1899-1949 to 15.7% in 1970-1977, by means of early and appropriate treatment. In patients who survive, complete recovery, especially of ocular movement, may take as long as 6 to 8 months.

b) Infant botulism is an intestinal infection caused by the ingestion of *C. botulinum* spores, which change in the intestine into the vegetative form, multiply, and produce toxins. Of 96 cases studied by Morris *et al.* (1983) that occurred in the United States outside California, 41 were caused by *C. botulinum* type A, 53 by type B, one by type F, and another by type B together with F. Type A appeared almost exclusively in western states, while type B predominated in the East. This distribution is similar to that of the spores in the environment (see Source of Poisoning or Infection and Mode of Transmission).

The disease in infants begins with constipation followed by lethargy and loss of appetite, ptosis, difficulty in swallowing, muscular weakness, and loss of control of the head. Neuromuscular paralysis may progress from the cranial nerves to the peripheral and respiratory muscles, resulting in death. The severity of the illness varies from moderate to life-threatening, causing sudden death of the child. It has been estimated that infant botulism is responsible for at least 5% of cases of sudden infant death syndrome (American Public Health Association, 1985).

c) Wound botulism is clinically similar to classic botulism in its neurologic syndrome. Of the 22 cases known, 15 were associated with type A, five with type B, one with both A and B, and one was undetermined.

The Disease in Animals: Botulism in domestic mammals is caused primarily by types C and D, and in fowl by type C. Outbreaks in bovines are usually associated with a phosphorus deficiency and resultant osteophagia and compulsive consumption of carrion ("pica") containing botulinum toxins. In locations where types C beta and D are found, such as South Africa, *C. botulinum* spores multiply rapidly in carrion and produce toxins to which bovines are very susceptible. The main symptom is the partial or complete paralysis of the locomotor, masticatory, and swallowing muscles. The animals have difficulty moving, stay motionless or recumbent for long periods of time, and, as the illness progresses, cannot hold their heads up and so bend their necks over their flanks. The mortality rate is high.

In sheep, botulism is also associated with pica and the symptomatology is similar to that seen in bovines.

In horses, as in other mammals, the incubation period varies widely according to the amount of toxin ingested. In very acute cases, death may ensue in 1 or 2 days. When the course is slower, the disease generally begins with paralysis of the hind quarters which progresses to other regions of the body until it produces death by respiratory failure.

Outbreaks with high death rates have been observed on mink farms. Food poisoning in these animals is due primarily to type C.

In ducks and other waterfowl, the first symptom of poisoning is paralysis of the wings which then extends to other muscles, finally those of the neck. The birds drown when they can no longer hold their heads above water.

The illness in chickens is produced mainly by type C alpha. The name "limber-neck" derives from the flaccid paralysis of the neck frequently observed in afflicted birds.

Source of Poisoning or Infection and Mode of Transmission. The reservoir of *C. botulinum* is the soil, river and sea sediments, vegetables, and the intestinal tracts of mammals and birds. The bacterial spores are very resistant to heat and desiccation. The etiologic agent is distributed on all continents, though irregularly. The distribution of the toxicogenic types also varies according to region. In a study (Smith, 1978) carried out across the United States, subdividing it into four transverse sections, *C. botulinum* was found in 23.5% of 260 soil samples. Type A was most prevalent in the western states with neutral or alkaline soil. Type B had a more uniform distribution, but predominated in the East, a pattern which seems to be associated with highly organic soils. Type C was found in acid soils on the Gulf Coast, type D in some alkaline soils of the West, and type E in the humid soils of several states. In the USSR, *C. botulinum* was isolated from 10.5% of 4,224 soil samples, with type E accounting for 61% of all positive cultures. The greatest concentration of spores was found in the European section of the country south of latitude 52° N (Kravchenko and Shishulina, 1967).

The wide distribution of *C. botulinum* in nature explains its presence in food. Vegetables are contaminated directly from the soil; foods of animal origin are probably contaminated via the animals' intestinal tracts or by spores in the environment. The main source of botulinum poisoning for man as well as for animals is food in which the microorganism has multiplied and produced its powerful toxin. After ingestion, the toxin is absorbed through the intestine, primarily the upper portion, and carried by the bloodstream to the nerves where it produces the symptomatology described above.

Any food, whether of vegetable or animal origin, can give rise to botulism if conditions favor the multiplication of *C. botulinum* and, consequently, the production of toxin. The main requirements for the multiplication of *C. botulinum* are anaerobiosis and a pH above 4.5, but once the toxin is formed an acid medium can be favorable. Home-canned foods are generally responsible for the disease, although incorrectly sterilized or preserved commercial products are sometimes the cause. Poisoning ensues after eating a raw or insufficiently cooked product that was preserved some time earlier.

The types of foods responsible for the poisoning vary according to regional eating habits. The most common sources of types A and B botulism in the United States and Canada are home-canned fruits and vegetables. In Europe, on the other hand, meat and meat products seem to play the most important role. In Japan and the USSR, seafood, especially fish, is the principal cause.

In contrast to classic botulism (ingestion of preformed toxins), infant botulism begins as an intestinal infection in which *C. botulinum* in the intestine multiplies and produces the toxin, which is then absorbed through the intestinal wall. Honey has been implicated as a source of the infection, since it is frequently a supplementary food for the nursing child. However, results of research on the presence of the spores in this food, as well as epidemiological investigations, have been inconclusive. In any case, there is no doubt that the microorganism enters the body through the ingestion of food.

The source of wound botulism is the environment.

Botulism in bovines results from grazing ("lamziekte") or the consumption of bailed fodder or silage. Poisoning contracted while grazing usually occurs in areas lacking in phosphorus. Many species of animals in a given area will have *C. botulinum* in their intestinal flora; when an animal dies, these bacteria invade the whole organism and produce great quantities of toxin. Bovines suffering from pica may ingest animal remains containing the preformed toxin and contract botulism. After dying, these bovines constitute a source of poisoning for the rest of the herd. Mortality in cattle has also been ascribed to drinking water which contained the decomposed bodies of small animals. Botulism contracted through the consumption of fodder or silage is produced by the accidental presence of a small animal's body, usually a cat, and the diffusion of the botulinum toxin around it into the food (Smith, 1977). The sources of poisoning for other mammalian species are similar.

For wild ducks the source of poisoning is insect larvae that feed on the bodies of dead ducks. If the duck had *C. botulinum* in its intestinal flora, the bacteria invade the whole organism after its death. The larvae then absorb the toxin produced, constituting a source of toxin for birds that may eat them. It is estimated that a duck need only ingest a few such larvae for death by botulism to ensue.

Research on outbreaks among pheasants has found that they ate maggots from the bodies of small animals.

Role of Animals in the Epidemiology of the Disease: No epidemiological relationship beween human and animal botulism has been demonstrated. *C. botulinum* type A spores have been isolated from animal feces, and types A and B botulism microorganisms have been found in the intestine and liver of bovines that died from other causes. The microorganism has also been isolated from the intestine and bone marrow of healthy dogs. Thus the possibility exists that these animals are carriers of the microorganism and serve to transport and disseminate *C. botulinum* from one place to another.

Diagnosis: Clinical diagnosis should be confirmed with laboratory tests. The most conclusive evidence is the presence of botulinum toxin in the serum of the patient. Stomach contents and fecal material of persons exposed to the suspected food should also be examined for the toxin. Cultures should be made of the food in question to isolate and identify the microorganism. When a wound is the suspected origin of the poisoning, aspirated fluid and biopsies should be examined bacteriologically.

Control: With regard to man, control measures include a) regulation and inspection of industrial bottling, canning, and food-preserving processes, and b) health education to point out the dangers of home canning and to make the public aware of important factors in the preservation of canned products, such as duration, pressure, and temperature of sterilization. Home-canned foods should be boiled before being served. Foods from swollen cans or food altered in taste, smell, or appearance should not be eaten even after cooking.

Immediate epidemiologic investigation and prompt diagnosis of an outbreak are essential to both the prevention of new cases and the recuperation of the patients.

In areas where botulism in animals is a problem, the diet of livestock should be supplemented with feed rich in phosphorus to avoid osteophagia or pica, and vaccination of animals with the appropriate toxoid can be used with good results.

Bibliography

American Public Health Association. *Control of Communicable Diseases in Man,* 14th ed. (Ed. by A. S. Benenson). Washington, D.C., APHA, 1985.

Arnon, S. S. Infant botulism: anticipating the second decade. *J Infect Dis* 154:201-206, 1986.

Centers for Disease Control of the USA. *Botulism in the United States, 1899-1973. Handbook for Epidemiologists, Clinicians, and Laboratory Workers.* Atlanta, Georgia, 1974.

Centers for Disease Control of the USA. Wound botulism associated with parenteral cocaine abuse. *Morb Mortal Wkly Rep* 31:87-88, 1982.

Centers for Disease Control of the USA. Update, international outbreak of restaurant-associated botulism. *Morb Mortal Wkly Rep* 34:643, 1985.

Divers, T. J., R. C. Bartholomew, J. B. Messick, R. H. Whitlock, and R. W. Sweeney. *Clostridium botulinum* type B toxicosis in a herd of cattle and a group of mules. *J Am Vet Med Assoc* 188:382-386, 1986.

Giménez, D. F., and A. S. Ciccarelli. Another type of *Clostridium botulinum. Zentralbl Bakteriol [Orig A]* 215:221-224, 1970.

Giménez, D. F., and A. S. Ciccarelli. *Clostridium botulinum* en Argentina: presente y futuro. *Rev Asoc Argent Microbiol* 8:82-91, 1976.

Ingram, M., and T. A. Roberts. *Botulism 1966.* London, Chapman and Hall, 1967.

Kravchenko, A. T., and L. M. Shishulina. Distribution of *C. botulinum* in soil and water in the USSR. *In:* Ingram, M., and T. A. Roberts (Eds.). *Botulism 1966.* London, Chapman and Hall, 1967.

Morris, J. G., J. D. Snyder, R. Wilson, and R. A. Feldman. Infant botulism in the United States: an epidemiological study of cases occurring outside of California. *Am J Public Health* 73:1385-1388, 1983.

Pan American Health Organization. *Bol Epidemiol* 3(4):1-3, 1982.

Prévot, A. R., A. Turpin, and P. Kaiser. *Les bactéries anaérobies.* Paris, Dunod, 1967.

Riemann, H. Botulism—Types A, B, and F. *In:* Riemann, H. (Ed.), *Food-borne Infections and Intoxications.* New York and London, Academic Press, 1969.

Smith, L. D. Clostridial diseases of animals. *Adv Vet Sci* 3:463-524, 1957.

Smith, L. D. *Botulism: The Organism, Its Toxins, the Disease.* Springfield, Illinois, Thomas, 1977.

Smith, L. D. The occurrence of *Clostridium botulinum* and *Clostridium tetani* in the soil of the United States. *Health Lab Sci* 15:74-80, 1978.

Sonnabend, O., W. Sonnabend, R. Heinzle, T. Sigrist, R. Dirnohofer, and U. Krech. Isolation of *Clostridium botulinum* type G and identification of type G botulinal toxin in humans: report of five sudden unexpected deaths. *J Infect Dis* 143:22-27, 1981.

Terranova, W., J. G. Breman, R. P. Locey, and S. Speck. Botulism type B: Epidemiologic aspects of an extensive outbreak. *Am J Epidemiol* 108:150-156, 1978.

BRUCELLOSIS

(023.0) Infection by *B. melitensis*
(023.1) Infection by *B. abortus*
(023.2) Infection by *B. suis*
(023.3) Infection by *B. canis*

Synonyms: Undulant fever, Malta fever, Gibraltar fever, Mediterranean fever (in man); contagious abortion, abortus fever, infectious abortion, epizootic abortion (animals), Bang's disease (cattle), ram epididymitis (sheep).

Etiology: Six species are presently known in the genus *Brucella: B. melitensis, B. abortus, B. suis, B. neotomae, B. ovis,* and *B. canis.*
The first three species (called "classic brucella") have been subdivided into biotypes which are distinguished by their different biochemical characteristics and/ or reactions to the monospecific A (*abortus*) and M (*melitensis*) sera. Thus *B. melitensis* is subdivided into three biotypes (1-3), *B. abortus* into eight (1-9, since biotype eight was discarded), and *B. suis* into four (1-4). In this last species, a new biotype has been proposed for strains isolated from rodents in the USSR; these differ from the four biotypes already recognized. From the epidemiologic point of view, the taxonomic system of the genus *Brucella* has eliminated confusion arising from the naming of new species or subspecies that did not agree with epidemiologic reality. Moreover, typing by biotypes constitutes a useful research tool in that field.

Geographic Distribution: Worldwide. The distribution of the different species of *Brucella* and their biotypes varies with geographic areas. *B. abortus* is the most widespread; *B. melitensis* and *B. suis* are irregularly distributed; *B. neotomae* was isolated from desert rats (*Neotoma lepida*) in Utah (USA) and its distribution is limited to natural foci, the infection never having been confirmed in man or domestic animals. In recent years, infection by *B. canis* has been confirmed in many countries on several continents, and its worldwide distribution can be asserted. *B. ovis* seems to be found in all countries where sheep raising is an important activity.

Occurrence in Man: Each year about a half million cases of brucellosis occur in humans (World Health Organization, 1975). The prevalence of the infection in animal reservoirs provides a key to its occurrence in humans. *B. abortus* and *B. suis* infections usually affect occupational groups, while infections from *B. melitensis* occur more frequently than the other types in the general population. The greatest prevalence in man is found in those countries with a high incidence of *B. melitensis* infection among goats, sheep, or in both species. The Latin American countries with the largest number of recorded cases are Argentina, Mexico, and Peru. The same pattern holds true for countries on the Mediterranean, Iran, the southwestern USSR, and Mongolia.
Programs for the control and eradication of bovine brucellosis markedly reduce the incidence of the disease in humans. For example, in the United States, 6,321 cases were recorded in 1947, while in the period 1972-1981 the annual average was 224 cases (Centers for Disease Control of the USA, 1982). In Denmark, where some 500 cases per year were notified between 1931 and 1939, human brucellosis had disappeared by 1962 as a result of the eradication of the infection in animals. In

Uruguay, where there is no animal reservoir of *B. melitensis* and where the few foci of *B. suis* have been eliminated, the disease in humans has almost disappeared since compulsory vaccination of calves was begun in 1964.

Occurrence in Animals: Bovine brucellosis is found worldwide, but it has been eradicated in, among other countries, Finland, Norway, Sweden, Denmark, the Netherlands, Belgium, Switzerland, the Federal Republic of Germany, Austria, Hungary, Czechoslovakia, Romania, and Bulgaria (Timm, 1982; Kasyanov and Aslanyan, 1982). Likewise, Great Britain, Ireland, Poland, Canada, the United States, Cuba, Panama, Australia, and New Zealand have freed the great majority of their herds and large tracts of their territory from brucellosis and are close to eradicating it. In the rest of the world, rates of infection vary greatly from one country to another and between regions within a country. The highest prevalence is seen in dairy cattle. In many countries, including most of those Latin American countries that have no control program, the data are unreliable. Nevertheless, available information indicates it is one of the most serious diseases in Latin America as well as in other developing areas. Official estimates put annual loses in Latin America from bovine brucellosis at approximately US$600 million, which explains the priority given by animal health services to control of this disease.

Swine brucellosis is infrequent and occurs sporadically in most of Europe, Asia, and Oceania. In many European countries it shows an epidemiologic relationship to brucellosis caused by *B. suis* biotype 2 in hares (*Lepus europaeus*). The disease has never been present in Finland, Norway, Great Britain, or Canada. Many predominantly Muslim countries are probably free of *B. suis* infection as a result of religious beliefs that have limited swine raising (Timm, 1982).

In most of Latin America, swine brucellosis is enzootic and, though the available data have little statistical value, this region is thought to have the highest prevalence in the world. Nevertheless, recent surveys of breeding operations for pure breds and hybrids in Argentina and Rio Grande do Sul in Brazil have shown the percentage of infected herds to be low. The problem is possibly rooted in commercial operations where animals of different origins are brought together. Canada has always been free of swine brucellosis, and Uruguay apparently was able to eradicate the few foci that stemmed from importation of infected pigs. Thus far, only biotype 1 of *B. suis,* which predominates worldwide, has been confirmed from Latin America. Biotype 2 is limited to pigs and hares in central and western Europe, while biotype 3 is restricted to the corn belt of the United States and to some areas of Africa and Asia. The United States and Cuba have successful national eradication programs.

Goat and sheep brucellosis constitute a significant problem in the Mediterranean basin of Europe and Africa, the southeastern Soviet Union, Mongolia, and the Middle East. In Latin America, the prevalence of *B. melitensis* infection in goats is high in Argentina, Mexico, and Peru. Sheep infection with *B. melitensis* has been identified only in flocks living together with infected goats. In the goat-raising region of Venezuela, the infection has not been reliably investigated. Goat brucellosis does not appear to exist in Brazil, which has a sizable number of goats. *B. melitensis* was recently isolated from goats in Chile, where the disease was thought to have been eradicated. Other American countries, including the United States, are apparently free of goat brucellosis at the present time.

Ram epididymitis caused by *B. ovis* is widespread. It has been confirmed in New Zealand, Australia, Africa, and Europe. It is present in Argentina, Brazil (Rio Grande do Sul), Chile, Peru, Uruguay, and the United States, that is, in all American countries where sheep are raised on a large scale. The prevalence is high.

Infection of dogs with *B. canis* has been found in almost every country in the world where it has been studied. Prevalence varies according to region and diagnostic method used. It constitutes a problem for some dog breeders since it causes abortions and infertility, but the infection is also found in family dogs and strays. In the latter, the incidence of infection is usually higher. In a study carried out in Mexico, for example, 12% of 59 stray dogs were positive in the isolation of the etiologic agent (Flores-Castro *et al.*, 1977).

The Disease in Man: Man is susceptible to infection caused by *B. melitensis*, *B. suis*, *B. abortus*, and *B. canis*. No human cases caused by *B. ovis* or *B. neotomae* have been confirmed. The most pathogenic and invasive species for man is *B. melitensis*, followed in order by *B. suis*, *B. abortus*, and *B. canis*.

In general, the incubation period is 1 to 3 weeks, but sometimes may be several months. The disease is septicemic with sudden or insidious onset and is accompanied by continued, intermittent, or irregular fever. The symptomatology of acute brucellosis, like that of many other febrile diseases, includes chills, profuse sweating, and elevation of temperature. An almost constant symptom is weakness, and any exercise produces pronounced fatigue. The temperature can vary from normal in the morning to 40°C in the afternoon. Sweating characterized by a peculiar odor occurs at night. Common symptoms are insomnia, sexual impotence, constipation, anorexia, headache, arthralgia, and general malaise. This disease has a marked effect on the nervous system, evidenced by irritation, nervousness, and depression. Many patients have enlarged peripheral lymph nodes or splenomegaly and often hepatomegaly, but rarely jaundice. *Brucella* organisms localize intracellularly in tissues of the reticuloendothelial system, such as lymph nodes, bone marrow, spleen, and liver. Tissue reaction is granulomatous. The duration of the disease can vary from a few weeks or months to several years. Modern therapy has considerably reduced the duration as well as the incidence of relapses. At times it produces serious complications such as encephalitis, meningitis, peripheral neuritis, spondylitis, suppurative arthritis, and vegetative endocarditis. A chronic form of the disease occurs in some patients and may last many years, with or without the presence of localized foci of infection. The symptoms are associated with hypersensitivity. Diagnosis of chronic brucellosis is difficult.

In enzootic brucellosis areas, especially in the case of bovine brucellosis, asymptomatic infections occur.

The Disease in Animals: The principal symptom in all animal species is abortion or premature expulsion of the fetus.

CATTLE: The main pathogen is *B. abortus*. Biotype 1 is universal and predominant among the eight occurring in the world. The distribution of the different biotypes varies geographically. In Latin America biotypes 1, 2, 3, and 4 have been confirmed, with biotype 1 accounting for more than 80% of the isolations. In the United States biotypes 1, 2, and 4 have been isolated. In eastern Africa biotype 3 predominates and affects native cattle as well as buffalo (Timm, 1982). Biotype 5, which occurs in cattle in Great Britain and Germany, has biochemical and serologic characteristics similar to those of *B. melitensis*. This similarity was a source of confusion for years until new methods of species identification (oxidative metabolism and phagocytolysis) established the biotype as *B. abortus*. The other biotypes also have a more or less marked geographic distribution. Cattle can also become infected by *B. suis* and *B. melitensis* when they share pasture or facilities with infected pigs, goats, or sheep. The infection in cattle caused by heterologous species of *Brucella* may be more transient than that caused by *B. abortus*. However, such cross-infections are a serious public health threat, since these brucellae, which are more highly pathogenic for man, can pass into cow's milk. Infection caused by *B. suis* is not very common. By contrast, infections by *B. melitensis*, with a disease course similar— according to some authors—to that caused by *B. abortus*, have been observed in several countries.

In natural infections it is difficult to measure the incubation period of the disease (from the time of infection to abortion or premature birth), since it is not possible to determine the moment of infection. Experiments have shown that the incubation period varies considerably and is inversely proportional to fetal development: the more advanced the pregnancy, the shorter the incubation period. If the female is infected orally during the breeding period, the incubation period can last some 200 days, while if she is exposed 6 months after being bred, incubation time is approximately 2 months. The period of "serologic incubation" (from the time of infection to the appearance of antibodies) may be from several weeks to several months. The incubation period varies according to such factors as the virulence and dose of bacteria, route of infection, and susceptibility of the animal.

The predominant symptom in pregnant females is abortion or premature or full-term birth of dead or weak calves. In general, abortion occurs during the second half of the pregnancy, often with retention of the placenta and resultant metritis, which may cause permanent infertility. It is estimated that the infection causes a loss of 20 to 25% in milk production as a result of interrupted lactation due to abortion and delayed conception. Cows artificially inseminated with infected semen come into estrus repeatedly, as in the case of vibriosis or trichomoniasis. Nonpregnant females show no clinical symptoms and, if infected prior to breeding, often do not abort.

In bulls brucellae may become localized in the testicles and other genital organs. When the clinical disease is evident, one or both testicles may become enlarged, with decreased libido and infertility. Sometimes a testicle may atrophy due to adhesions and fibrosis. Seminal vesiculitis and ampullitis are common. Occasionally, hygromas and arthritis are observed in cattle.

Upon infection, brucellae multiply first in the regional lymph nodes and are carried by the lymph and blood to different organs. Some 2 weeks after experimental infection, bacteremia can be detected and it is possible to isolate the agent from the bloodstream. Brucella organisms are most commonly found in lymph nodes, uterus, udder, spleen, liver, and, in bulls, the genital organs. Large quantities of erythritol, a carbohydrate that stimulates the multiplication of brucellae, have been found in cow placentas. This could explain the high susceptibility of bovine fetal tissues.

Individual animals within a herd manifest differing degrees of susceptibility to the infection depending on their age and sex. Male and female calves less than 6 months of age are not very susceptible and generally experience only transitory infections. A bull calf fed milk containing brucella organisms can harbor the agent in its lymph nodes, but after 6 to 8 weeks without ingesting the contaminated food, the animal usually rids itself of the infection.

Heifers kept separate from cows, as is routine in herd management, often have lower infection rates than adult cows. Heifers exposed to infection before breeding can become infected, but generally do not abort. In view of this, at the beginning of the century heifers were inoculated before breeding with virulent strains or with strains of unknown virulence to prevent future abortion. This practice had to be abandoned, however, when it was found that a large number of animals remained infected.

Cows, especially when pregnant, are the most susceptible; infection is common and abortion frequently results.

Bulls are also susceptible, though some researchers maintain that they are more resistant to infection than females. However, this conclusion may owe more to herd management procedures than to natural resistance in males, since bulls are usually kept separate from cows. On the other hand, neutered male and female animals do not play a role in the epizootiology of brucellosis, since they cannot transmit brucellae to the exterior environment.

In addition to age and sex, it is important to take individual susceptibility into account. Even in the most susceptible categories—cows and heifers—some animals never become infected, or if they do, their infection is transient. Some less susceptible cows have generalized infections and suffer losses in reproductive function and milk production for one or more years, but then gradually recover. In such animals the agglutination titers may become negative, shedding of brucella organisms may cease, and both reproductive function and milk production return to normal. In most infected cows, however, the agglutination titers remain positive for many years or for life and, although after one or two abortions they may give birth normally and resume normal production of milk, many continue to carry and shed brucellae. Other cows remain totally useless for reproduction and milk production.

In a previously uninfected herd, brucellosis spreads rapidly from animal to animal, and for one or two years there are extensive losses from abortions, infertility, decrease in milk production, and secondary genital infections. The acute or active phase of the disease is characterized by a large number of abortions and a high rate of reactors to the agglutination test. Because of individual differences in susceptibility, not all animals become infected and not all those that are serologically positive abort. After a year or two, the situation stabilizes and the number of abortions decreases. It is estimated that only between 10 and 25% of cows will abort a second time. In this stabilization phase, it is primarily the heifers—not previously exposed to the infection—that become infected and may later abort. A third stage, the decline phase, can be observed in small and self-contained herds. In this phase, the infection rate will gradually decrease, and most of the cows return to normal reproduction and milk production. Nevertheless, when a sufficient number of susceptible animals accumulates—either heifers from the same herd or newly introduced animals—a second outbreak can occur. In large herds there are always enough susceptible animals to maintain the infection, and abortions continue. The trading and movement of animals also help maintain active infections.

SWINE: The main etiologic agent of brucellosis in swine is *B. suis*. In Latin America, only biotype 1 infection has been confirmed, while in the United States both 1 and 3 have been involved. In Europe, biotype 2 plays an important role. Infection by biotypes 1 and 3 is spread directly and indirectly from pig to pig. In contrast, biotype 2 (or Danish biotype) is often transmitted to pigs by the European hare (*Lepus europaeus*). Pigs can also be infected by *B. abortus,* although it is less pathogenic for pigs and is apparently not transmitted from one animal to another; these infections are generally asymptomatic, with the organisms limited to the lymph nodes of the head and neck.

When brucellosis is introduced into a previously healthy herd, the symptoms are those of acute disease: abortions, infertility, birth of weak piglets, orchitis, epididymitis, and arthritis. In small herds the infection tends to die out or decrease in severity because of a lack of susceptible animals owing to the normal marketing of some pigs as well as spontaneous recovery from the infection by others. In large herds the infection is persistent, being transmitted from one generation to the next.

Early abortions, which occur when the female is infected during coitus, generally go unnoticed under open-range conditions. The aborted fetuses are eaten by pigs, and the only abnormality that may be noticed by the owner is the sows' repeated estrus. Abortions usually occur in the second half of gestation when the females are infected after one or more months of pregnancy. Affected sows seldom have a second abortion, and females infected before sexual maturity rarely abort.

The infection is usually temporary in suckling pigs; however, a few may retain the infection and become carriers. It rarely results in recognizable clinical symptoms. Occasionally, arthritis is observed, but transient bacteremia and low agglutination titers may be found.

In infected pigs abscesses of different sizes frequently occur in organs and tissues. Spondylitis is often found.

Infection of the genital organs lasts for a shorter period of time in the female than in the male. In the latter it may last for the life of the animal.

GOATS: The main etiologic agent in goats is *B. melitensis* with its three biotypes. Infection by *B. suis* and *B. abortus* has occasionally been found.

The symptomatology is similar to that observed in other species of animals and the main symptom is abortion, which occurs most frequently in the third or fourth month of pregnancy. Hygromas, arthritis, spondylitis, and orchitis are also observed. In contrast to brucellosis in females of other domestic species, mastitis is a common symptom in goats and may be the first noticeable sign in a flock. Clotting in milk and small nodules in the mammary glands may be observed. In chronically infected flocks the signs of the disease generally are not very apparent. Gross pathologic lesions are also not usually evident, though the pathogen can frequently be isolated from a number of tissues and organs.

Several researchers have observed that young goats can be born with the infection or become infected shortly after birth. Most of them recover spontaneously before reaching reproductive age, but in some the infection may persist longer.

The primitive conditions under which goats are raised constitute one of the most important factors in maintenance and spread of the infection in Latin America (Argentina, Mexico, Peru, and probably Chile) and in the rest of the world. In goat-raising areas it is common to find community-shared pastures, a lack of hygiene in makeshift corrals, nomadic flocks, and owners with little understanding of herd management.

SHEEP: Two disease entities are distinguishable in sheep: classic brucellosis and ram epididymitis. Classic brucellosis is caused by *B. melitensis* and constitutes a public health problem equally as or even more important than goat brucellosis in areas where the agent is found outside the American continent. In Latin America, the infection in sheep has been confirmed only in some mixed goat and sheep flocks remote from intensive sheep-raising areas.

While sheep brucellosis is similar in its symptomatology to the disease in goats, sheep appear to be more resistant to infection, and in mixed flocks fewer sheep than goats are found to be infected. Abortions are also less common. The infection tends to disappear spontaneously, and the high prevalence of the disease in some areas can best be attributed to poor herd management.

Occasionally, sheep have been found to be infected by *B. suis* (biotype 2 in Germany) and *B. abortus* (in various parts of the world). These agents are not very pathogenic for sheep, are acquired as a result of contact with infected animals of other species, and are not transmitted from sheep to sheep.

Ram epididymitis is caused by *B. ovis*. The clinical signs consist of genital lesions in rams, associated with varying degrees of sterility. Sometimes the infection in pregnant ewes can cause abortion or neonatal mortality. Ram epididymitis is generally unilateral but can be bilateral, and the tail of the organ is most commonly affected. Adhesions may occur in the tunica vaginalis testis, and the testicle may be atrophied with varying degrees of fibrosis. Lesions cannot be seen or palpated in many infected rams, even though *B. ovis* may be isolated from their semen. Some of these animals develop lesions when the course of the disease is more advanced. Early in the infection the semen contains many brucellae, but with time the number decreases, and eventually the semen may be free of the infectious agent. When localized in the kidneys, *B. ovis* is also shed through the urine.

HORSES: *B. abortus* and *B. suis* have been isolated from this species. The disease usually manifests itself in the form of fistulous bursitis, "poll evil" and "fistulous withers." Abortions are rare. *B. abortus* has been isolated from horse feces, but this is uncommon. Horses acquire the infection from cattle and swine, but transmission from horses to cattle has also been proven. Man can contract the infection from horses with open lesions. In general, horses are more resistant to the infection. Cases of horse-to-horse transmission are unknown. In areas where there is a high rate of infection, it is common to find horses with high agglutination titers.

DOGS AND CATS: Sporadic cases of brucellosis caused by *B. abortus*, *B. suis*, and *B. melitensis* occur in dogs. They acquire the infection by eating contaminated material, especially fetuses, afterbirth, and milk. The course of the infection is usually subclinical, but sometimes the symtomatology can be severe, with fever, emaciation, orchitis, anestrus, arthritis, and at times abortion. The disease is self-limiting and transmission from canine to canine is rare. Several human cases have been described in which the source of infection was dogs (especially fetuses).

A canine disease which occurs worldwide and can reach epizootic proportions is that caused by *B. canis*. This form of brucellosis is characterized by a prolonged, afebrile bacteremia, embryonic death, abortions, prostatitis, epididymitis, scrotal dermatitis, lymphadenitis, and splenitis. Abortion occurs about 50 days into gestation. The pups may be stillborn at full term or die a few days after birth. Survivors usually have enlarged lymph nodes and often have bacteremia.

Man is susceptible to *B. canis,* though less so than to classic brucellae. Several cases have been confirmed in the United States, Mexico, Brazil, and Argentina in laboratory and kennel personnel as well as in members of families with infected dogs.

Cats are resistant to *Brucella* and no cases of natural disease occurrence are known.

OTHER DOMESTIC MAMMALS: Brucellosis caused by *B. abortus* occurs in domestic buffaloes (*Bubalus bubalis*) and in yaks (*Bos grunniens*) with symptomatology similar to that in cattle. The disease has also been observed in Old World camels (*Camelus bactrianus*), in dromedaries (*Camelus dromedarius*), and in American Camelidae. An outbreak of brucellosis caused by *B. melitensis* biotype 1, accompanied by abortions and neonatal death, occurred on an alpaca (*Lama pacos*) ranch in the high plateau (altiplano) region of Peru; a serious outbreak also occurred in the human population of that ranch (Acosta *et al.,* 1972).

WILD ANIMALS: Natural infections caused by *Brucella* occur in a wide range of wild species. There are natural foci of infection, for example, among the desert rats of the United States (*Neotoma lepida*), which are the reservoir of *B. neotomae.* In Kenya, biotype 3 of *B. suis* has been isolated from two species of rodents (*Arvicanthis niloticus* and *Mastomys natalensis*). In Australia and the USSR, as yet unclassified biotypes of *Brucella* occur in various species of rodents. In Europe, the hare (*Lepus europaeus*) is the reservoir of *B. suis* biotype 2 and is responsible for transmission of the disease to domestic swine. The caribou (*Rangifer caribou*), a reservoir of *B. suis* biotype 4 in Alaska, can transmit the infection to man and to sled dogs. The infection can also be transmitted in the opposite direction, from domestic animals to wild animals. This is the case in Argentina, where infection of foxes (*Dusicyon gymnocercus, D. griseus*) and of grisons (*Galictis furax-huronax*) is caused by *B. abortus* biotype 1, of the European hare (*Lepus europaeus*) by *B. suis* biotype 1, and of the oppossum (*Didelphis azarae*) by both *B. abortus* biotype 1 and *B. suis* biotype 1. Carnivores acquire the infection by eating fetuses and afterbirth. There is no evidence that the infection is transmitted from one individual to another among carnivores, and it probably dies out when brucellosis is controlled in domestic animals. The situation is different when domestic animals transmit the infection to wild ruminants, such as the steppe antelope (*Saiga tatarica*) or the American bison (*Bison bison*), in which brucellosis persists.

Fur-bearing animals such as minks and silver foxes may contract brucellosis when fed viscera of infected animals, and they may in turn transmit this infection to man.

The etiologic agent has been isolated from many species of arthropods. Ticks can harbor the organism for lengthy periods and transmit the infection through biting. They also eliminate the bacteria in their coxal gland secretions. Nevertheless, the number of ticks harboring brucellae is insignificant (in one study done in the USSR, eight strains of *Brucella* spp. were isolated from 20,000 ticks) and there are few brucellae per tick. The species which have been isolated from arthropods are *B. melitensis* and *B. abortus.* Recently, *B. canis* was isolated in Brazil from *Rhipicephalus sanguineus* attached to a bitch suffering from brucellosis (Peres *et al.,* 1981). There is consensus that arthropods play a small role, if any, in the epidemiology of brucellosis.

FOWL: In a few cases, *Brucella* has been isolated from naturally infected domestic fowl. The symptomatology described is quite varied, and no certainty exists that it always involves brucellosis. While the infection may pass unnoticed, symptoms can include weight loss, reduction in egg production, and diarrhea; the course of the disease may even be acute. Fowl do not play a role in maintaining the infection in nature. *Brucella* has been isolated from some wild bird species, such as corvids (*Corvus cornix* and *Tripanscorax fragilecus*).

Source of Infection and Mode of Transmission: The natural reservoirs of *B. abortus, B. suis,* and *B. melitensis* are, respectively, cattle, swine, and goats and sheep. The natural host of *B. canis* is the dog and that of *B. ovis* is the sheep.

INFECTION IN HUMANS: Man is infected by animals through direct contact or indirectly by ingestion of animal products as well as by inhalation of airborne agents. The relative importance of mode of transmission and pathway of penetration of the etiologic agent varies with the epidemiologic area, the animal reservoirs, and the occupational groups exposed to the risk. Fresh cheese and raw milk from goats and sheep infected with *B. melitensis* are the most common vehicles of infection and can cause multiple cases of human brucellosis. Sometimes more widespread outbreaks occur when infected goat's milk is mixed with cow's milk. Cow's milk infected by *B. suis* has also been known to produce outbreaks of epidemic proportions. Cow's milk and milk products containing *B. abortus* may give rise to sporadic cases. The organisms rarely survive in sour milk, sour cream, butter, and fermented cheeses aged over 3 months.

In arctic and subarctic regions cases have occurred as a result of the habit of eating bone marrow or raw meat from reindeer or caribou infected with *B. suis* biotype 4. Brucellae are resistant to pickling and smoke curing, thus giving rise to the possibility that some meat products so prepared could cause human infection; however, this mode of transmission has never been verified.

It is also possible for raw vegetables and water contaminated with the excreta of infected animals to serve as sources of infection.

Transmission by contact predominates in areas where bovine and porcine brucellosis are enzootic. Human brucellosis is, for the most part, an occupational disease of stockyard and slaughterhouse workers, butchers, and veterinarians. The infection is usually contracted by handling fetuses and afterbirth, or by contact with vaginal secretions, excreta, and carcasses of infected animals. The microorganism enters through skin abrasions as well as through mucous membranes, including the conjunctiva, by way of the hands. In slaughterhouses prevalence of the disease is higher among recently employed staff. The practice in some companies of employing workers with negative serology is mistaken, since an individual who is asymptomatic but has a positive serology is less likely to become sick.

In areas where goat and sheep brucellois is enzootic, transmission by contact also occurs when shepherds handle newborn animals or fetuses. In some countries with hard winters, goats share the beds of goatherds and their families for protection against the cold, which results in infection of the whole family (Elberg, 1981).

Airborne transmission has been proved by experimentation and research. In laboratories, centrifugation of brucellosis suspensions poses a special risk when done in centrifuges that are not hermetically sealed. An epidemic outbreak of 45 cases occurred among students at Michigan State University in the United States in 1938-39. The 45 students were attending classes on the second and third floors of a building which housed a brucellosis research laboratory in the basement. In the ensuing investigation, it was shown that the only possible means of transmission was by aerosol particles. Recent epidemiologic studies have supplied proof that airborne transmission in lockers and slaughterhouses plays an important role, and perhaps is more frequent than transmission by direct contact with infected tissue. When air from the killing area is allowed to spread out, it gives rise to high rates of infection among workers in adjoining areas. The minimum infective dose for man by way of the respiratory passages seems to be small. When the killing area is completely separate, or maintained at a negative air pressure, the risk to surrounding areas is reduced (Kaufman *et al.*, 1980; Buchanan *et al.*, 1974).

INFECTION IN CATTLE (Figure 5): The main sources of the infection for cattle are fetuses, afterbirth, and vaginal discharges containing large numbers of brucellae. To a lesser extent, farm areas can be contaminated by fecal matter of calves fed on contaminated milk, since not all the organisms are destroyed in the digestive tract.

Figure 5. Bovine brucellosis (*Brucella abortus*). Mode of transmission.

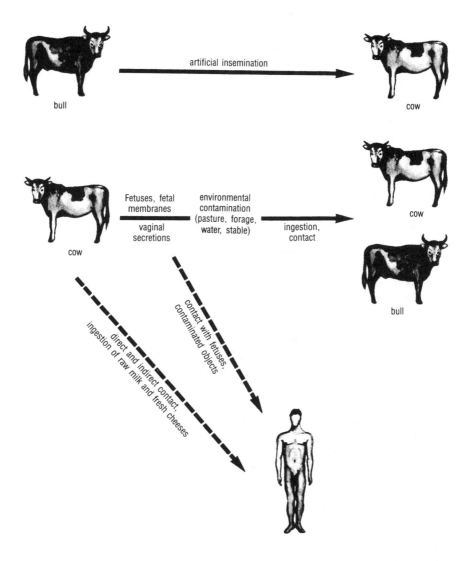

   The most common portal of entry is the gastrointestinal tract following the ingestion of contaminated pasture, feed, fodder, or water. Moreover, cows customarily lick afterbirth, fetuses, and newborn calves, all of which may contain a large number of the organisms and constitute a very important source of infection. Cows' habit of licking the genital organs of other cows also contributes to transmission of the infection.

   It has been shown experimentally that the organism may penetrate broken and even intact skin. The extent to which this mode of transmission is involved in natural infection is not known.

Bang and others experimentally reproduced infection and disease by way of the vaginal route. The results of those experiments indicate that a large number of brucellae are necessary to infect a cow by that means. However, there is no doubt that the intrauterine route used in artificial insemination is very important in transmitting the infection. The use of infected bulls for artificial insemination constitutes an important risk, since the infection can thus be spread to many herds.

In closed environments it is likely that infection is spread by aerosols; airborne infection has been demonstrated experimentally.

A new discovery, the magnitude of which is still being evaluated, is that of congenital infection and the so-called latency phenomenon. An experiment was carried out (Plommet *et al.*, 1973) in which calves born to cows artificially infected with a high dose of *B. abortus* were separated from their mothers and raised in isolation units. At 16 months of age, the heifers were artificially inseminated. In six experiments (Fensderbank, 1980) using 55 heifers born to infected cows, five were infected, brucellae being isolated during calving and/or after butchering 6 weeks later. At 9 and 12 months of age, two of these animals had serologic titers which were unstable until pregnancy. The other three heifers did not have serologic reactions until the middle or end of the pregnancy (latency). The authors of the experiment admit that under natural range conditions the frequency of the latency phenomenon could be much lower. In herds where vaccination of calves is systematically carried out, the phenomenon may go unnoticed. In a similar vein, other research projects (Lapraik *et al.*, 1975; Wilesmith, 1978) have been undertaken on the vertical transmission of brucellosis accompanied by a prolonged and serologically inapparent phase of the infection. In a retrospective study of highly infected herds, Wilesmith (1978) found that 8 of 317 heifers (2.5%), born to reactive cows tested serologically positive. The extent of the latency phenomenon is still not known, but it has not prevented the eradication of bovine brucellosis in vast areas and many countries. On the other hand, it undeniably has slowed its eradication in some herds.

INFECTION IN SWINE (Figure 6): In swine, the sources of infection are the same as in cattle. The principal routes of transmission are digestive and venereal. Contrary to the situation in cattle, natural sexual contact is a common and important mode of transmission. The infection has often been introduced into a herd following the acquisition of an infected boar. Pigs, because of their eating habits and the conditions in which they are raised, are very likely to become infected through the oral route. It is also probable that they become infected by aerosols entering via the conjunctiva or upper respiratory tract.

INFECTION IN GOATS AND SHEEP (Figure 7): Goats and sheep are infected with *B. melitensis* in a manner similar to cattle. The role of the buck and ram in transmission of the infection is not well established. Infection of goats *in utero* is not unusual, and the young can also become infected during the suckling period; such infection may persist in some animals.

In the case of the ram epididymitis caused by *B. ovis,* semen is the main and possibly the only source of infection. The infection is commonly transmitted from one ram to another by rectal or preputial contact. Transmission may also occur through the ewe when an infected ram deposits his semen and another ram breeds her. The infection is not very common in ewes, and when it occurs it is contracted by sexual contact. *B. ovis* does not persist very long in ewes and is generally eliminated before the next lambing period.

Figure 6. Swine brucellosis (*Brucella suis*). Mode of transmission.

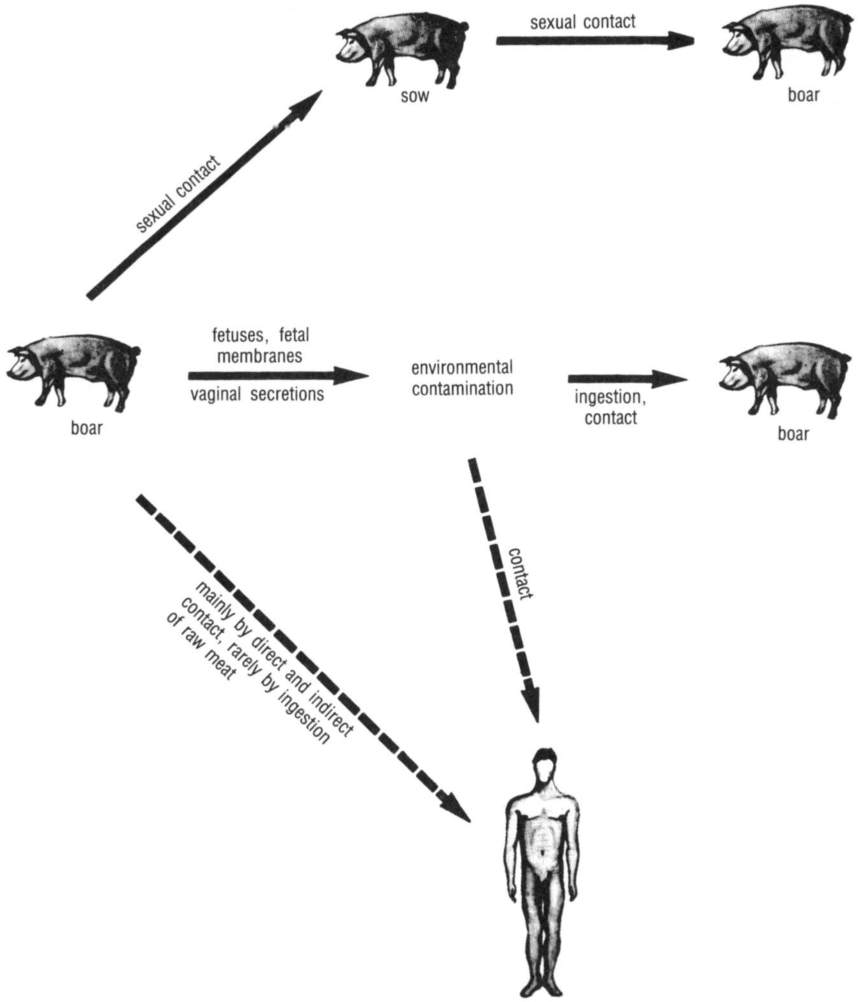

INFECTION IN DOGS: The transmission of *B. canis* occurs as a result of contact with vaginal secretions, fetuses, and fetal membranes. Infected males may transmit the infection to bitches during coitus. The milk of infected bitches is another possible source of infection. Human cases recorded in the literature amount to about 30. Many of these cases result from showing dogs that have recently aborted.

Role of Animals in the Epidemiology of the Disease: The role of animals is essential. Cases of human-to-human transmission are exceptional. Brucellosis is a zoonosis par excellence.

Diagnosis: In man, a clinical diagnosis of brucellosis based on symptoms and history should always be confirmed in the laboratory. Isolation and typing of the

Figure 7. Caprine and ovine brucellosis *(Brucella melitensis).* **Mode of transmission.**

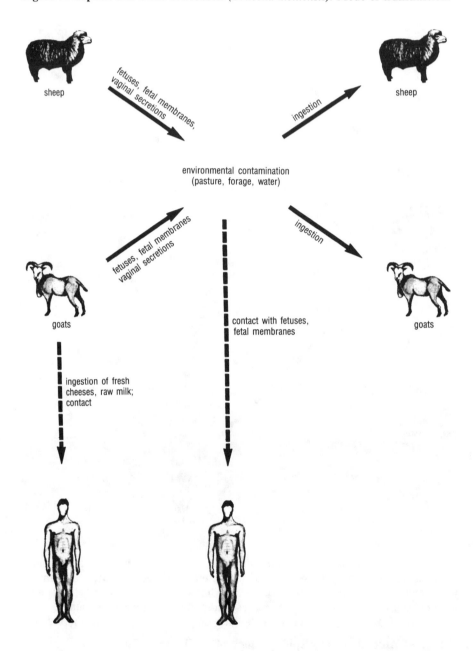

causal agent is definitive and, moreover, may indicate the source of the infection. Blood or sternal bone marrow taken while the patient is febrile is cultured in appropriate media. Culture material can also be taken from lymph nodes, cerebrospinal fluid, and abscesses. It is recommended that the cultures be repeated several times, especially in enzootic areas of *B. abortus*. Due to the widespread use of antibiotics before diagnosis in febrile patients, bacteriologic examinations often yield negative results, and serologic tests become increasingly necessary. The serum agglutination test is the simplest and most widely used procedure. A high titer (more than 100 international units, IU), with increasing titers in repeated serum samples, provides a good basis for diagnosis. Cross-reactions in serum agglutination have been observed in cases of cholera or tularemia (or as a result of vaccination against these diseases) and in infections caused by *Yersinia enterocolitica* type 9. The serum agglutination test reveals both M and G immunoglobulins. It is generally accepted that in an active stage of brucellosis IgG is always present. Thus, when low serum agglutination titers are found, tests that reveal the presence of IgG must be carried out. Such tests are the 2-mercaptoethanol test and the complement fixation test (in man, the IgG's fix complement, but often lack agglutinating power). These tests are of special interest in chronic brucellosis where, although agglutination titers return to low levels, active infection may continue. The intradermal test with noncellular allergens is useful for epidemiologic studies, but not for clinical diagnosis.

The 2-mercaptoethanol test (ME) is also useful in following the treatment and cure of the patient. In one study (Buchanan and Faber, 1980), the titers of 92 brucellosis patients were followed for 18 months with tube agglutination and ME tests. In spite of antibiotic treatments, the tube agglutination tests continued positive for 18 months in 44 (48%) of the patients, but at the end of 1 year the ME titers were positive in only eight (9%) of the patients and in four (4%) at 18 months. None of the 84 patients testing negative by ME at the end of a year had signs or symptoms, and none acquired chronic brucellosis. By contrast, four of the eight patients testing positive by ME after a year continued to have symptoms of brucellosis and had to continue treatment. Thus, a negative result by ME provides good evidence that a patient does not have chronic brucellosis and that the antibiotic treatment was successful. If effective treatment is begun early, it is possible that IgG antibodies (resistant to ME) never develop. Such was probably the case in three patients who contracted brucellosis in the laboratory and in whom infection was confirmed by blood culture. The diagnosis and treatment were so early in these patients that at no time during the 2-year follow-up did they show antibodies resistant to ME (García Carrillo and Coltorti, 1979).

Other useful methods for the diagnosis of human brucellosis are the rose bengal test and counterimmunoelectrophoresis. In a study of 222 cases (Díaz *et al.*, 1982), rose bengal was the most sensitive test, with 98.3% positive results. Counterimmunoelectrophoresis was positive in 84.9% of the acute cases and in 91.6% of the chronic.

In serologic diagnosis of humans or animals, it is necessary to bear in mind that at the outset of the infection only IgM antibodies are produced; consequently, the agglutination test provides a better standard for diagnosis, since ME will show negative. As the infection progresses IgG antibodies resistant to the ME test will appear, and will increase unless appropriate treatment is begun.

Diagnosis of infection caused by *B. melitensis, B. suis,* and *B. abortus* is carried out with a properly standardized antigen of *B. abortus* (Alton *et al.,* 1976). This antigen does not permit diagnosis of infection caused by *B. canis*, however, since this species of *Brucella* (like *B. ovis*) is found in a rugose phase (R), lacking the lipopolysaccharidic surface antigen that characterizes "classic brucellae" (for diagnosis of *B. canis* and *B. ovis* see below).

In cattle the diagnosis is primarily based on serology. A great many serologic tests are presently available, all of which are useful when applied with judgment. Both a serologic test reaction and the test's usefulness in each circumstance are a result of the sensitivity it shows to antibodies of different immunoglobulin types and of the seric concentration of each type of antibody (Chappel *et al.*, 1978). The most thoroughly studied immunoglobulins in bovine brucellosis are IgM and IgG_1 to IgG_2. Even though available tests are not qualitative enough to identify an individual immunoglobulin, they do give an indication of which predominates. In the diagnosis of bovine brucellosis the evolution of immunoglobulins during infection and vaccination is of special interest. In both cases, the IgM's appear first, followed by the IgG's. The difference is that in infected animals, the IgG's tend to persist and reach higher levels, while in calves that were vaccinated between 3 and 8 months of age, the IgG's tend to disappear about 6 months after vaccination. Based on this fact, complementary tests are used to distinguish infection from the agglutination titer, which may persist after vaccination with strain 19, and also from heterospecific reactions caused by bacteria which share surface antigens with the brucellae and which give rise to antibodies that, in general, are the IgM type.

According to their use in several countries, serologic tests may be classified as follows: 1) routine or operative, 2) complementary, 3) epidemiological surveillance, and 4) screening tests. A single test might serve as operative, as diagnostically definitive, as a screen, or as complementary, depending on the program employing it.

Serum agglutination tests (tube and plate) have been and continue to be widely used. They contributed greatly to the reduction of infection rates in Europe, Australia, and the Americas. Nevertheless, when the proportion of infected herds and worldwide prevalence is reduced, their limitations become apparent and it becomes necessary to use other tests to help eradicate the infection in so-called "problem" herds. The tests are internationally standardized, easy to carry out, and allow the examination of a great many samples. In agglutination tests, the IgM reaction predominates. Complementary tests are needed for clarification of suspect or marginally positive results. However, it is necessary to keep in mind that low agglutination titers could be due to recent infection and, consequently, it is advisable to repeat the test.

The rose bengal test (with buffered antigen) is fast, easy to do, and allows processing of many samples per day. It is qualitative and classifies animals as positive or negative. In regions where incidence of infection is low or where systematic vaccination of calves is practiced, the rose bengal test gives many "false positives," and so is unspecific if used as the only and definitive test. In many countries, such as Great Britain and Australia, it is used as a screening test. Animals showing a negative test result are so classified and those testing positive are subjected to other tests for confirmation. In regions of high incidence, results are satisfactory. Rose bengal may also be used as a complementary test for those animals classified as suspect by agglutination. Many suspect sera test negative to rose bengal, and since this test is very sensitive (there are few "false negatives") and detects the infection early, there is little risk of missing infected animals.

The principal complementary tests are complement fixation, 2-mercaptoethanol, and rivanol. Recently, new tests have been developed, such as indirect hemolysis, enzyme-linked immunosorbent assay (ELISA) for different types of immunoglobulins, and radial immunodiffusion with a polysaccharide antigen. These tests are used to distinguish antibodies caused by the infection from those left by vaccination or stimulated by heterospecific bacteria.

The complement fixation test is considered the most specific, but it is laborious, complicated, and involves many steps and variables. Moreover, it is not standardized internationally. Other, simpler tests can take its place, such as 2-mercaptoethanol and rivanol, which measure the IgG antibodies.

Epidemiological surveillance of brucellosis is carried out separately on dairy and meat-producing herds, since they require different diagnostic tests and strategic checkpoints. The objective in both cases is to identify infected herds and monitor healthy ones. For beef cattle, screening tests or other tests of presumed high sensitivity are used, such as rose bengal and its variants. Cattle markets and slaughterhouses are the strategic points for collecting samples. The sera that test positive are then subjected to standard tests and the animals are traced back to their points of origin. For dairy cattle, the milk-ring test is used. It is very simple and allows the examination of many herds in a short time. The composite samples are gathered from milk cans or tanks at collection points and dairy plants or on the dairy farm itself. If a positive sample is found, individual serologic examinations of the animals belonging to the source herd must then be carried out.

Bacteriologic examinations are of more limited use. The samples most often tested in this way are taken from fetuses, fetal membranes, vaginal secretions, milk, and semen. Infected cows may or may not abort, but a high percentage will eliminate brucellae from the genital tract beginning a few days before parturition and continuing some 30 days afterward. It is estimated that 85% of recently infected and more than 15% of chronically infected cows eliminate brucellae during calving. Since elimination through milk may be constant or intermittent, milk can be an excellent material for the isolation of *Brucella* if attempts are repeated. Serologic testing of bulls should be done using blood serum and seminal fluid. Bacteriologic examination of semen should be repeated if negative, since brucellae may be shed intermittently.

In swine, serologic tests are not indicated for individual diagnosis but rather to reveal the presence of herd infection. Agglutination (tube or plate), complement fixation, and buffered-acid antigen (rose bengal) tests can be used. The latter is preferable because it is negative in herds having animals with low and nonspecific tube and plate agglutination titers. For a herd to be classified as positive with the agglutination test (tube and plate), there must be one or more animals with titers of 100 IU or more.

In goats, serologic tests are also applied on a flock basis and not on individual animals. In infected flocks, one or more individuals are found with titers of 100 IU or more; in such cases titers of 50 IU should be adopted as indicative of infection. The complement fixation test is considered superior to the agglutination test, especially in herds vaccinated with *B. melitensis* Rev. 1, where agglutinating antibodies persist for long periods. The 2-mercaptoethanol test has also given very good results in vaccinated flocks. Results from the buffered-acid antigen (rose bengal) test are promising, but experience with it is limited and definite conclusions cannot be drawn at this time.

In diagnosing infections caused by *B. melitensis* in sheep, the Coombs' test (antiglobulin test), modified by Hajdu, can reveal 70% of infected animals. Agglutination and complement fixation tests give less satisfactory results and, in using them, adoption of significant titer levels lower than those for other species is recommended. Counterimmunoelectrophoresis would detect antibodies against intracellular antigens that appear late in the serum but remain a long time. Consequently, its use would be appropriate for sheep with chronic brucellosis that test negative by agglutination, rose bengal, or complement fixation tests (Trap and Gaumont, 1982). In the diagnosis of ram epididymitis, antigen prepared with *B. ovis* should be used, the preferred tests being gel diffusion and complement fixation. Bacteriologic examination of semen is an appropriate diagnostic method, but it should be kept in mind that brucellae may be shed intermittently.

For dogs infected with *B. canis,* the surest diagnostic method is the isolation of the etiologic agent from blood, vaginal discharges, milk, semen, fetal tissues, or placentas. Bacteremia can last 1 or 2 years, but after the initial phase it may become intermittent and thus a negative blood culture does not exclude the possibility of brucellosis.

The most common serologic tests for *B. canis* are tube or plate agglutination using *B. canis* antigens and immunodiffusion in agar gel with antigens extracted from the cell wall. To a greater or lesser degree, all these tests give nonspecific reactions. Zoha and Carmichael (1982) showed that the immunodiffusion test using sonicated antigens (internal cellular antigens) is satisfactory shortly after the onset of bacteremia and can detect infected animals for up to 6 months after it disappears, that is, when other tests give equivocal results.

Control: The most rational approach for preventing human brucellosis is the control and eradication of the infection in animal reservoirs, as has been demonstrated in various countries of Europe and America. Some human populations are protected by mandatory milk pasteurization. Prevention of infection in occupational groups (cattlemen, abattoir workers, veterinarians, and others who come into contact with animals or their carcasses) is more difficult and should be based on health education, the use of protective clothing whenever possible, and medical supervision.

Protection of refrigerator plant and slaughterhouse workers against brucellosis assumes particular interest because they constitute the occupational group at highest risk. Protection is achieved in part by separating the slaughter area from other sections and controlling air circulation. In countries having eradication programs, slaughter of reactive animals is limited to one or more designated slaughterhouses (cold storage plants) per region with official veterinary inspection. These animals are butchered at the close of the workday with special precautions and proper supervision to protect the workers. Employees should be instructed in personal hygiene and provided with disinfectants and protective clothing. For disinfecting installations after slaughter, a 5% solution of chloramine or an 8 to 10% solution of caustic soda should be used (Elberg, 1981). Instruments should be sterilized in an autoclave or boiled for 30 minutes in a 2% solution of caustic soda. Clothes may be disinfected with a 2% solution of chloramine or a 3% solution of carbolic acid soap followed by washing. Hands should be soaked for 5 minutes in a solution of 1% chloramine or of 0.5% caustic soda, then washed with soap and water.

The immunization of high-risk occupational groups is practiced in the USSR and China. In the Soviet Union, good results have apparently been obtained with the use of a vaccine prepared from strain 19-BA of *B. abortus* (derived from strain 19 used for bovine brucellosis vaccination), applied by skin scarification (World Health Organization, 1971). Annual revaccination is carried out for those individuals not reacting to serologic or allergenic tests. In China an attenuated live vaccine made from strain 104M of *B. abortus* is applied percutaneously. These vaccines are not used in other countries because of possible side effects. In the USSR and France promising trials have been made using antigenic fractions of *Brucella*.

Vaccination is recommended for control of bovine brucellosis in enzootic areas with high prevalence rates. The vaccine of choice is *B. abortus* strain 19, confirmed by its worldwide use, the protection it gives for the useful lifetime of the animal, and its low cost. To avoid interference with diagnosis, it is recommended that vaccination be limited (by legislation) to young animals (calves of 3 to 8 months), as these animals rapidly lose the antibodies produced in response to the vaccine. It is estimated that 65 to 80% of vaccinated animals derive long-term protection against infection. The antiabortive effect of the vaccine is pronounced, thus reducing one of the principal sources of infection, the fetuses. In a systematic vaccination program, the best results are obtained with 70 to 90% annual coverage in calves of the proper age for vaccination. Male calves and females over 8 months of age should not be vaccinated. Where possible, this upper limit should be 6 months. Revaccination is not recommended. The objective of a systematic and compulsory program of vaccination of calves in a given area or country is to reduce the infection rate and obtain herds resistant to brucellosis, so that eradication of the disease may then begin. It is estimated that 7 to 10 years of systematic vaccination are necessary to achieve this objective.

In regions or countries with a low prevalence of the disease, an eradication program can be carried out by repeated serologic diagnostic tests applied to the entire herd, and elimination of reactors until all foci of infection have disappeared. This procedure can be used alone (in countries with a low prevalence) or in combination with the vaccination of calves. Epidemiologic surveillance and control of animal transport are very important in such programs.

Until a few years ago, the vaccination of adult cows with strain 19 was inadvisable because of the prolonged persistence of antibodies that could interfere with diagnosis. In the 1950's several researchers proved that vaccination of adult animals with a smaller dose could impart an immunity comparable to that of a full dose, while at the same time agglutination titers stayed lower and disappeared faster. In 1975, Nicoletti (1976) initiated a series of studies in the United States, using a reduced dose in highly infected herds, and concluded that vaccination decreases the spread of the infection within the herd, that antibodies disappear in about 6 months, and that only 1% of the females remained infected by the vaccine strain from 3 to 6 months after vaccination. Complementary tests were very useful in distinguishing between reactions due to infection and those due to vaccination. Other studies, done under both controlled and natural conditions, confirm these findings (Nicoletti *et al.*, 1978; Alton *et al.*, 1980; Viana *et al.*, 1982; Alton *et al.*, 1983). Vaccination of adult females may be considered in herds suffering acute brucellosis characterized by abortions and rapidly spreading infections, as well as in large herds where chronic brucellosis has proven hard to eradicate. The recommended dose is one to three billion cells of strain 19 *Brucella* administered subcutaneously. Only animals testing negative should be vaccinated and they should be indelibly marked under government supervision. At the beginning of the operation, reactors should be eliminated immediately. Vaccinated animals should be examined serologically 6 months later using rivanol, mercaptoethanol, and complement fixation tests, and those that have become infected should be sent to slaughter. Using periodic serologic examination, it is estimated that a problem herd can be free from infection in 18 to 24 months (Barton and Lomme, 1980). Oral vaccination with strain 19 is a new possibility being explored (Nicoletti and Milward, 1983).

The control of swine brucellosis consists of identifying and certifying brucellosis-free herds. If infection is diagnosed in pigs raised for market, it is advisable to send the entire herd to the abattoir and reestablish it with animals from a brucellosis-free herd. If the infected pigs are valuable for breeding or research, suckling pigs should be weaned at 4 weeks and raised in facilities separate from the main herd. Periodic serologic tests (such as rose bengal) are recommended to eliminate any reactor. Finally, when no brucellosis is found in the new herd and it is well established, the original herd should be sent to slaughter. There are no vaccines available for swine.

Control of the infection caused by *B. melitensis* in goats and sheep is based mainly on vaccination. The preferred vaccine is *B. melitensis* Rev. 1, which is administered to 3-to-6-month-old females. Adult female animals can receive a smaller dose of the same vaccine (20,000 times fewer bacterial cells than in the dose for young females). As goats are generally raised in marginal areas where the socioeconomic conditions are very poor, it is difficult to carry out eradication programs. In these areas, reinfection occurs constantly, flocks are often nomadic, and animal-raising practices make sanitary control difficult. Experience with vaccine Rev. 1 for goats in Italy, Turkey, Iran, Mongolia, Peru, and the Caucasian Republics of the USSR has proven it to be an excellent means of control. However, the control procedure of diagnosing and sacrificing reactor animals has produced satisfactory results in areas of low prevalence.

Ram epididymitis can be successfully controlled by a combination of the following measures: elimination of rams with clinically recognizable lesions; elimination of clinically normal rams positive to the gel diffusion or the complement fixation test; and separation of young rams (those not yet used for breeding) from adult males. In some countries (New Zealand and the United States) a bacterin prepared from *B. ovis* and adjuvants is used. Animals are vaccinated when weaned, revaccinated 1 or 2 months later, and annually thereafter. This vaccine produces antibodies against *B. ovis* but not *B. abortus*. *B. melitensis* Rev. 1 vaccine protects against epididymitis, but also produces *B. abortus* antibodies.

Brucellosis caused by *B. canis* in dog kennels can be controlled by repeated serologic tests and blood cultures, followed by elimination of reactor animals. No vaccines are yet available. Veterinary clinics should advise the owners of the risk of keeping a dog with brucellosis and should recommend the dog's being put to sleep.

Bibliography

Acosta, M., H. Ludueña, D. Barreto, and M. Moro. Brucelosis en alpacas. *Rev Invest Pecu (Lima)* 1:37-49, 1972.

Alton, G. G., L. M. Jones, and D. E. Pietz. *Las técnicas de laboratorio en la brucelosis,* 2nd ed. Geneva, World Health Organization, 1976. (Monograph Series 55.)

Alton, G. G., L. A. Corner, and P. P. Plackett. Vaccination of pregnant cows with low doses of *Brucella abortus* strain 19 vaccine. *Aust Vet J* 56:369-372, 1980.

Alton, G. G., L. A. Corner, and P. P. Plackett. Vaccination of cattle against brucellosis. Reduced doses of strain 19 compared with one and two doses of 45/20 vaccine. *Aust Vet J* 60:175-177, 1983.

Anczykowski, F. Further studies on fowl brucellosis. II. Laboratory experiments. *Pol Arch Weter* 16:271-292, 1973.

American Public Health Association. *Control of Communicable Diseases in Man,* 14th ed. (Ed. by A. S. Benenson). Washington, D.C., APHA, 1985.

Barg, L. Isolamento de *Brucella canis* em Minas Gerais, Brasil. Pesquisa de aglutininas em soros caninos e humanos. Thesis. Universidad Federal de Minas Gerais, Belo Horizonte, Brazil, 1975.

Barton, C.E., and J. R. Lomme. Reduced-dose whole herd vaccination against brucellosis: A review of recent experience. *J Am Vet Med Assoc* 177:1218-1220, 1980.

Buchanan, T. M., S. L. Hendricks, C. M. Patton, and R. A. Feldman. Brucellosis in the United States. An abattoir-associated disease. III. Epidemiology and evidence for acquired immunity. *Medicine* 53:427-439, 1974.

Buchanan, T. M., and L. C. Faber. 2-mercaptoethanol brucella agglutination test: Usefulness for predicting recovery from brucellosis. *J Clin Microbiol* 11:691-693, 1980.

Cargill, C., K. Lee, and I. Clarke. Use of an enzyme-linked immunosorbent assay in a bovine brucellosis eradication program. *Aust Vet J* 62:49-52, 1985.

Centers for Disease Control of the USA. Annual summary 1981: Reported morbidity and mortality in the United States. *Morb Mort Wkly Rep* 30:14, 1982.

Chappel, R. J., D. J. McNaught, J. A. Bourke, and G. S. Allen. Comparison of the results of some serological tests for bovine brucellosis. *J Hyg (Camb)* 80:365-371, 1978.

Charmichael, L. E., and J. C. Joubert. A rapid slide agglutination test for the serodiagnosis of *Brucella canis* infection that employs a variant (M−) organism as antigen. *Cornell Vet* 77:3-12, 1987.

Corbel, M. J. The serological relationship between *Brucella* spp., *Yersinia enterocolitica* serotype IX and *Salmonella* serotypes of Kauffman-White group. *J Hyg (Camb)* 75:151-171, 1975.

Díaz, R., E. Maravi-Poma, J. L. Fernández, S. García-Merlo, and A. Rivero-Puente. Brucelosis: Estudio de 222 casos. Parte IV: Diagnóstico de la brucelosis humana. *Rev Clin Esp* 166:107-110, 1982.

Elberg, S. S. The Brucellae. *In:* Dubos, R. J., and J. G. Hirsch (Eds.), *Bacterial and Mycotic Infections of Man,* 4th ed. Philadelphia and Montreal, Lippincott, 1965.

Elberg, S. S. Immunity to *Brucella* infection. *Medicine* 52:339-356, 1973.

Elberg, S. S. A guide to the diagnosis, treatment and prevention of human brucellosis. World Health Organization, 1981. VPH/81.31 Rev. 1. (Unpublished document.)

Fensderbank, R. Congenital Brucellosis in Cattle. World Health Organization, 1980. WHO/BRUC/80.352. (Unpublished document.)

Flores-Castro, R., F. Suárez, C. Ramírez-Pfeiffer, and L. E. Carmichael. Canine brucellosis: bacteriological and serological investigation of naturally infected dogs in Mexico City. *J Clin Microbiol* 6:591-597, 1977.

Fredickson, L. E., and C. E. Barton. A serologic survey for canine brucellosis in a metropolitan area. *J Am Vet Med Assoc* 165:987-989, 1974.

García Carrillo, C. Métodos para el diagnóstico de la brucelosis. *Gac Vet (B Aires)* 32:661-667, 1970.

García Carrillo, C. *Programa de erradicación de la brucelosis en California.* Buenos Aires, Pan American Zoonoses Center, 1975. (Scientific and Technical Monographs 9.)

García Carrillo, C., B. Szyfres, and J. González Tomé. Tipificación de brucelas aisladas del hombre y los animales en América Latina. *Rev Latinoam Microbiol* 14:117-125, 1972.

García Carrillo, C., and E. A. Coltorti. Ausencia de anticuerpos resistentes al 2-mercaptoetanol en tres pacientes de brucelosis. *Medicina (B Aires)* 39:611-613, 1979.

Garin, B., D. Trap, and R. Gaumont. Assessment of the EDTA seroagglutination test for the diagnosis of bovine brucellosis. *Vet Rec* 117:444-445, 1985.

George, L. W., and L. E. Carmichael. A plate agglutination test for the rapid diagnosis of canine brucellosis. *Am J Vet Res* 35:905-909, 1974.

Gilman, H. L. Brucellosis. *In:* Gibbons, W. J. (Ed.), *Diseases of Cattle.* Santa Barbara, California, American Veterinary Publication, 1963.

Hendricks, S. L., and M. E. Meyer. Brucellosis. *In:* Hubbert, W. T., W. F. McCulloch, and P. R. Schnurrenberger (Eds.), *Diseases Transmitted from Animals to Man,* 6th ed. Springfield, Illinois, Thomas, 1975.

Kasyanov, A. N., and R. G. Aslanyan. Epizootiology and clinical appearance of animal brucellosis. *In:* A. Lisenko (Ed.), *Zoonoses Control.* VII Centre Int Projects. Moscow, 1982.

Kaufmann, A.F., M. D. Fox, J. M. Boyce, D. C. Anderson, M. E. Potter, W. J. Martone, and C. M. Patton. Airborne spread of brucellosis. *Ann NY Acad Sci* 353:105-114, 1980.

Lapraik, R. D., D. D. Brown, and H. Mann. Brucellosis. A study of five calves from reactor dams. *Vet Rec* 97:52-54, 1975.

Lee, K., C. Cargill, and H. Atkinson. Evaluation of an enzyme-linked immunosorbent assay for the diagnosis of *Brucella ovis* infection in rams. *Aust Vet J* 62:91-93, 1985.

Manthei, C. A. Brucellosis as a cause of abortion today. *In:* Faulkner, L. C. (Ed.), *Abortion Diseases of Livestock.* Springfield, Illinois, Thomas, 1968.

Manthei, C. A. Brucellosis. *In:* Dunne, H. W. (Ed.), *Diseases of Swine,* 3rd ed. Ames, Iowa State University Press, 1970.

McCaughey, W. J. Brucellosis in wildlife. *In:* Diarmid, A. (Ed.), *Diseases in Free-living Wild Animals.* New York. Academic Press, 1969.

McCullough, N. B. Microbial and host factors in the pathogenesis of brucellosis. *In:* Mudd, S. (Ed.), *Infectious Agents and Host Reactions.* Philadelphia, Saunders, 1970.

Myers, D. M., L. M. Jones, and V. M. Varela-Díaz. Studies of antigens for complement fixation and gel diffusion tests in the diagnosis of infections caused by *Brucella ovis* and other *Brucella. Appl Microbiol* 23:894-902, 1972.

Nicoletti, P. A preliminary report on the efficacy of adult cattle vaccination using strain 19 in selected dairy herds in Florida. *Proc Annu Meet US Livest Sanit Assoc* 80:91-106, 1976.

Nicoletti, P., L. M. Jones, and D. T. Berman. Adult vaccination with standard and reduced doses of *Brucella abortus* strain 19 in a dairy herd infected with brucellosis. *J Am Vet Med Assoc* 173:1445-1449, 1978.

Nicoletti, P., and F. W. Milward. Protection by oral administration of *Brucella abortus* strain 19 against an oral challenge exposure with a pathogenic strain of *Brucella. Am J Vet Res* 44:1641-1643, 1983.

Pacheco, G., and M. T. De Mello. *Brucelose.* Rio de Janeiro, Brazil, Graphics Service, Brazilian Geographic and Statistical Institute, 1956.

Pan American Health Organization. *Guía para la preparación y evaluación de proyectos de ucha contra la brucelosis bovina.* Buenos Aires, Pan American Zoonoses Center, 1972. echnical Note 14.)

Peres, J. N., A. M. Godoy, L. Barg, and J. O. Costa. Isolamento de *Brucella canis* de apatos (*Rhipicephalus sanguineus*). *Arq Esc Vet UFMG* (*B Horizonte*) 33:51-55, 1981.

ommet, M., R. Fensderbank, G. Renoux, J. Gestin, and A. Philippon. Brucellose e expérimentale. XII. Persistance à l'age adulte de l'infection congénitale de la génisse. *ch Vét* 4:419-435, 1973.

met, M., and R. Fensderbank. Vaccination against bovine brucellosis with a low dose 19 administered by the conjunctival route. *Ann Rech Vét* 7:9-23, 1976.

ciotti, F. *Brucelosis.* Córdoba, Argentina, Edición del Autor, 1971.

e, C. W. *Veterinary Medicine and Human Health,* 2nd ed. Baltimore, Maryland, nd Wilkins, 1969.

. W. *The Nature of Brucellosis.* Minneapolis, University of Minnesota Press,

. Brucellosis (Undulant fever, Malta fever). *In:* Wyngaarden, I. B., and L. H. .), *Cecil Textbook of Medicine,* 16th ed. Philadelphia, Saunders, 1982.

a situación de la brucelosis en América Latina. *Bol Hig Epidemiol* (*La* 09, 1967.

onomía del género *Brucella. Gac Vet* (*B Aires*) 33:28-40, 1971.

Brucellosis. *Distribution in Man, Domestic and Wild Animals.* Berlin,

Trap, D., and R. Gaumont. Comparaison entre electrosynerèse et epreuves serologiques classiques dans la diagnostic de la brucellose ovine. *Ann Rech Vét* 13:33-39, 1982.

Van der Hoeden, J. Brucellosis. *In:* Van der Hoeden, J. (Ed.), *Zoonoses*. Amsterdam, Netherlands, Elsevier, 1964.

Viana, F. C., J. A. Silva, E. C. Moreira, L. G. Villela, J. G. Mendes, and T. O. Dias. Vacinação contra brucelose bovina com dose reduzida (amostra B_{19}) por via conjuntival. *Arq Esc Vet UFMG (B Horizonte)* 34:279-287, 1982.

Wilesmith, J. W. The persistence of *Brucella abortus* infection in calves: A retrospective study of heavily infected herds. *Vet Rec* 103:149-153, 1978.

Witter, J. F., and D. C. O'Meara. Brucellosis. *In:* Davis, J. W., L. H. Karstady, and D. O. Trainer, *Infectious Diseases of Wild Mammals*. Ames, Iowa State University Press, 1970.

World Health Organization. *Joint FAO/WHO Expert Committee on Brucellosis. Fifth Report*. Geneva, WHO, 1971. (Technical Report Series 464.)

World Health Organization. *Fifth Report on the World Health Situation, 1969-1972*. Geneva, WHO, 1975. (Official Record 225.)

Zoha, S. J., and L. E. Carmichael. Serological responses of dogs to cell wall and internal antigens of *Brucella canis* (*B. canis*). *Vet Microbiol* 7:35-50, 1982.

CAMPYLOBACTERIOSIS

(027.8)

The genus Campylobacter *(heretofore* Vibrio*) contains several species of importance for both public and animal health. The principal pathogenic species are* C. jejuni *and* C. fetus *subsp.* fetus *(previously subsp.* intestinalis*) and* C. fetus *subsp.* venerealis. *Occasionally,* C. coli *is the cause of enteritis in man. Bacteria of this genus are gram-negative, microaerophilic, and have a curved or spiral form.*

The increased medical interest since 1977 in enteritis caused by C. jejuni *and the enormous bibliography on this new zoonosis make it advisable to discuss this disease separately from those caused by the two subspecies of* C. fetus. *Furthermore, the disease caused by* C. jejuni *and those originating from* C. fetus *are clinically different.*

1. Enteritis caused by *Campylobacter jejuni*

Synonym: Vibrionic enteritis.

Etiology: *Campylobacter jejuni* and occasionally *C. coli*. Several schemes for serologic typing have been proposed and are in development. One of these (McMyne *et al.*, 1982) includes 45 different serotypes. When a uniform scheme is perfected, serotyping will be a great help in epidemiologic tracking of sources of the infection.

Geographic Distribution: Worldwide.

Occurrence in Man: At present *C. jejuni* is considered to be one of the principal bacterial agents causing enteritis and diarrhea in man, especially in developed countries. In these countries, the prevalence is similar to enteritis caused by *Salmonella*. As methods for isolation and culture have been perfected, the number of recorded cases caused by *C. jejuni* has increased. In Great Britain, the 200 public health and hospital laboratories had been reporting isolations of salmonellas exceeding those of *Campylobacter,* but beginning in 1981, the proportions were reversed: 12,496 isolations of *Campylobacter* as opposed to 10,745 of *Salmonella* (Skirrow, 1982). In Australia, Canada, the United States, the Netherlands, the United Kingdom, and Sweden, between 5 and 14% of diarrhea cases are caused by *C. jejuni* (American Public Health Association, 1985). Based on records from private medical practice, it has been estimated that 20% of office consultations for enteritis in Great Britain were associated with campylobacteriosis, and that there are a projected 600,000 cases annually at the national level (Skirrow, 1982). It is harder to establish the incidence in developing countries; because of deficiencies in hygiene, *C. jejuni* is isolated from 5 to 17% of persons without diarrhea (Prescott and Munroe, 1982) and from 8 to 31% of persons who have diarrhea. Thus, *Campylobacter* is probably an important cause of infantile diarrhea in the Third World (Skirrow, 1982).

The illness affects all age groups and appears sporadically and in epidemic outbreaks. The largest known epidemics originated from common sources such as contaminated milk or, as in two European cities, from a contaminated municipal water supply. In countries with a temperate climate, the disease is most prevalent in the hot months.

Occurrence in Animals: Wild and domestic mammals and birds constitute the large reservoir of *C. jejuni,* but it is often difficult to identify this pathogen with diarrheic disease in animals since there is a high rate of infection in clinically healthy animals.

The Disease in Man: Enteritis caused by *C. jejuni* is an acute illness. In general, the incubation period is from 2 to 5 days. The principal symptoms are diarrhea, fever, abdominal pain, vomiting (in one-third of the patients), and visible or occult blood (50 to 90% of sufferers). Many times the fever is accompanied by a general malaise, headache, and muscle and joint pain. The feces are liquid and frequently contain mucous and blood. The course of the illness is usually benign, and the patient recovers spontaneously in a week to 10 days. Symptoms may be more severe in some people, similar to those of ulcerative colitis or salmonellosis, and may lead to suspicion of appendicitis and a resultant exploratory laparotomy. In some cases septicemia has occurred, either simultaneous to the diarrheic illness or afterward. Complications are rare and consist of meningitis and abortions.

The Disease in Animals: *C. jejuni* has been identified as an etiologic agent in several illnesses of domestic animals (Prescott and Munroe, 1982).

CATTLE: Enteritis caused by *C. jejuni* in calves is clinically similar to that in man. Heifers suffer a moderate fever, and diarrhea may last up to 14 days. It is also possible that this agent causes mastitis in cows. This conclusion is demonstrated indirectly by the fact that man can get the disease from drinking unpasteurized milk. Moreover, experimental inoculation of the udder with a very few bacteria causes acute mastitis.

SHEEP: *C. jejuni* is a major cause of abortions in sheep, similar in importance to *C. fetus* subsp. *fetus (intestinalis)*. Sheep abort toward the end of their pregnancy or give birth at term to either dead young or weak lambs that die within a few days.

DOGS AND CATS: Puppies with diarrhea constitute a source of infection for their owners. Diarrhea is the predominant symptom and is also common. In cats, enteritis caused by *C. jejuni* is rare.

OTHER MAMMALS: Enteritis caused by *C. jejuni* probably occurs in many other animal species. It has been described in monkeys and in one outbreak in young horses.

FOWL: Fowl are an important reservoir of *C. jejuni*. Even though it is possible to cause diarrhea in 3-day-old chicks with *C. jejuni* administered orally, it is not known if the illness occurs naturally since a high proportion of healthy birds harbor the bacteria in their intestines. Vibrionic hepatitis has been described in fowl in northern Europe, and North and South America. The unspecified microaerophilic vibrio to which the disease has been attributed is probably *C. jejuni*. The disease is characterized by hemorrhagic and necrotic lesions of the liver. In adult birds, egg production decreases notably.

Source of Infection and Mode of Transmission (Figure 8): Mammals and birds, both domestic and wild, are the principal reservoir of *C. jejuni*. In studies by various authors (Skirrow, 1982; Prescott and Munroe, 1982), *C. jejuni* was found in the ceca of 100% of 600 turkeys and in the droppings of 38 out of 46 chickens and 83 out of 94 ducks that had large numbers of bacteria in their intestines prior to slaughter. The organism has been found in several species of wild birds, for example in 35% of migratory birds, 50% of town-dwelling pigeons, and in 20 to 70% of gulls. The agent has been isolated from the feces of 2.5 to 100% of healthy cows, from the gallbladder of 20 out of 186 sheep, from the feces of 0 to 30% of healthy dogs, and also from a wide variety of wild mammal species.

C. jejuni is found commonly in natural water sources, where it can survive for several weeks at low temperatures. It is interesting to note that it has always been found in the presence of fecal coliforms, and therefore the contamination presumably stems from animals (mammals and fowl) and, in some circumstances, from man. The immediate source of the human infection cannot always be determined. Even though in some cases the infection is contracted directly from animals or indirectly from animal products (raw milk, birds handled in the kitchen and eaten without proper cooking), or from contaminated water, in many outbreaks in humans the source of infection is unknown. Transmission from person to person may take place, but it is unusual. Among the few cases described was an intrahospital infection of children in Mexico (Flores-Salorio *et al.*, 1983). Untreated patients may eliminate *C. jejuni* for 6 weeks and a few for a year or more. As in the case of other enteric infections, entry is through the digestive tract.

Diagnosis: In the initial stage of the disease, the agent can be isolated from the blood and later from the feces. Diagnosis is through culture on selective media incubated in an atmosphere of 5% oxygen, 10% carbon dioxide, and 85% nitrogen, preferably at 43°C. Serologic diagnosis may be done using indirect immunofluorescence or other tests on paired sera.

In animals, because of the high rate of healthy carriers, isolation of the agent is inadequate proof that it is responsible for illness. It is important to confirm an increase in the titer with serologic testing.

Figure 8. Campylobacteriosis *(Campylobacter jejuni)*. **Mode of transmission.**

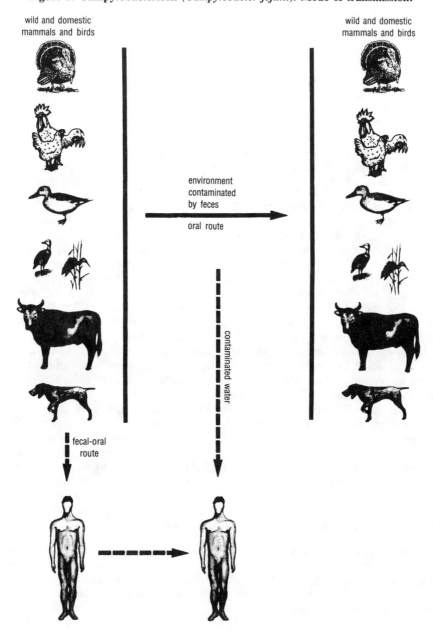

Control: According to present knowledge of the epidemiology of the illness, preventive measures can be only partial in scope. In a study of the risk factors in the state of Colorado (USA), where sporadic cases caused by *C. jejuni* occurred, it was estimated that about one-third of the cases could have been prevented by measures such as avoiding the consumption of untreated water, of unpasteurized milk, and of undercooked chicken (Hopkins *et al.*, 1984). People in contact with dogs and cats that have diarrhea should observe the rules of personal hygiene, such as thorough washing of the hands. Sick animals should not be in contact with children. Persons preparing food should take care to separate raw animal products, especially chicken, from other foods, and also to practice personal hygiene. Control of the infection in animals is clearly desirable, but is not presently feasible, owing to the wide diffusion of the agent and its presence in wild animal reservoirs.

Bibliography

American Public Health Association. *Control of Communicable Diseases in Man,* 14th ed. (Ed. by A. S. Benenson). Washington, D.C., APHA, 1985.

Blaser, M. J., G. Pérez Pérez, D. F. Smith, C. Patton, F. C. Tenover, A. J. Lastovica, and W. I. Wang. Extraintestinal *Campylobacter jejuni* and *Campylobacter coli* infections: host factors and strain characteristics. *J Infect Dis* 153:552-559, 1986.

Finch, M. J., and P. A. Blake. Food-borne outbreaks of campylobacteriosis: the United States experience, 1980-1982. *Am J Epidemiol* 122:262-268, 1985.

Flores-Salorio, S. G., V. Vázquez-Alvarado, and L. Moreno-Altamirano. *Campylobacter* como agente etiológico de diarrea en niños. *Bol Med Hosp Infant Mex* 40:315-319, 1983.

Hopkins, R. S., R. Olmsted, and G. R. Istre. Endemic *Campylobacter jejuni* infection in Colorado: Identified risk factors. *Am J Public Health* 74:249-250, 1984.

Hutchinson, D. N., F. J. Bolton, D. M. Hinchliffe, H. C. Dawkins. Evidence of udder excretion of *Campylobacter jejuni* as the cause of milk-borne campylobacter outbreak. *J Hyg (Camb)* 94:205-215, 1985.

Kaneuchi, C., K. Shishido, M. Shibuya, Y. Yamaguchi, and M. Ogata. Prevalences of *Campylobacter, Yersinia*, and *Salmonella* in cats housed in an animal protection center. *Jpn J Vet Sci* 49:499-506, 1987.

McMyne, P. M. S., J. L. Penner, R. G. Mathias, W. A. Black, and J. H. Hennessy. Serotyping of *Campylobacter jejuni* isolated from sporadic cases and outbreaks in British Columbia. *J Clin Microbiol* 16:281-285, 1982.

Prescott, J. M., and D. L. Munroe. *Campylobacter jejuni.* Enteritis in man and domestic animals. *J Am Vet Med Assoc* 181:1524-1530, 1982.

Rosenfield, J. A., G. J. Arnold, G. R. Davey, R. S. Archer, and W. H. Woods. Serotyping of *Campylobacter jejuni* from an outbreak of enteritis implicating chicken. *J Infect* 11:159-165, 1985.

Skirrow, M. B. Campylobacter enteritis—The first five years. *J Hyg (Camb)* 89:175-184, 1982.

2. Diseases caused by *Campylobacter fetus*

Synonyms: Vibriosis, vibrionic abortion, epizootic infertility, bovine genital vibriosis, epizootic ovine abortion.

Etiology: *Campylobacter* (*Vibrio*) *fetus* subsp. *fetus* (*intestinalis*) and *C. fetus* subsp. *venerealis.*

Geographic Distribution: Worldwide.

Occurrence in Man: Uncommon. The literature records at least 134 confirmed cases (Bokkenheuser and Sutter, 1981), most of them occurring in the United States and the rest in various parts of the world. The incidence is believed to be much higher than that recorded.

Occurrence in Animals: The disease is common in cattle and sheep and occurs worldwide.

The Disease in Man: The strains isolated from man have characteristics similar to those of *C. fetus* subsp. *fetus* (*intestinalis*), which causes outbreaks of abortion among sheep and sporadic cases in cattle. Generally, human campylobacteriosis accompanies a predisposing debilitative factor such as pregnancy, premature birth, chronic alcoholism, neoplasia, and cardiovascular disease. The majority of isolations are from pregnant women, premature babies, and men and women over 45 years of age. The proportion of cases is higher in men than in women.

Infection by *C. fetus* causes septicemia in man. The majority of cultures have been obtained from the bloodstream during fever, but the etiologic agent has also been isolated from the synovial and spinal fluids, as well as from the feces of patients with acute enteritis.

In pregnant women, the illness has been observed from the fifth month of pregnancy, accompanied by a sustained fever and often by diarrhea. The pregnancy may terminate in miscarriage, or premature or full-term birth. Premature infants and some full-term infants die from the infection, which presents symptoms of meningitis or meningoencephalitis. The syndrome may begin the day of birth with a slight fever, cough, and diarrhea; after 2 to 7 days the signs of meningitis appear. The case fatality rate is approximately 50%. Malnourished children, and at times apparently healthy ones, can develop bacteremia along with vomiting, anorexia, diarrhea, and fever. The patient usually recovers spontaneously or after antibiotic treatment. In adults, commonly those already weakened by other illness, the disease appears as a generalized infection with extremely variable symptomatology (Bokkenheuser and Sutter, 1981). *C. fetus* subsp. *fetus* is above all an opportunistic pathogen which gives rise to a systemic infection but rarely causes enteritis, in contrast to *C. jejuni*. Lately, some cases of gastroenteritis caused by *C. fetus* subsp. *fetus* have been noted in men with immune system dysfunction (Devlin and McIntyre, 1983; Harvey and Greenwood, 1983).

The Disease in Animals: In cattle and sheep, campylobacteriosis is an important disease that causes considerable losses due to infertility and abortions.

CATTLE: In this species, the principal etiologic agent is *C. fetus* subsp. *venerealis*, but subsp. *fetus* is involved to a lesser degree. Genital vibriosis is a major cause of infertility, giving rise to early embryonic death. The principal symptom is the repetition of estrus after service. During an outbreak, a high proportion of cows come into heat repeatedly for 3 to 5 months, but only 25 to 40% become pregnant after having been bred twice. Of the cows or heifers that finally become pregnant, 5 to 10% abort 5 months into gestation. An undetermined proportion of females harbor *C. fetus* subsp. *venerealis* during the entire gestation period and become a source of infection for bulls in the next breeding season. After the initial infection, cows acquire resistance to the disease and recover their normal fertility, that is, the embryo develops normally. Nevertheless, immunity to the infection is only partial, and the animals may become reinfected even though the embryos continue to develop normally. Resistance decreases substantially after 3 or 4 years.

The infection is transmitted by natural breeding or by artificial insemination. Bulls are the normal, though in most cases temporary, carriers of the infection. They play an important role in its transmission to the females. The etiologic agent is carried in the preputial cavity. Bulls may become infected while servicing infected cows, as well as by contaminated instruments and equipment in artificial insemination stations. The etiologic agent is sensitive to antibiotics that are added to semen used in artificial insemination.

C. *fetus* subsp. *fetus* is responsible for sporadic abortions in cattle. Some females are carriers of the infection, harboring the agent in the gallbladder and shedding it in their feces.

SHEEP: The principal agents of epizootic abortion in sheep are C. *fetus* subsp. *fetus* and C. *jejuni* and, to a lesser degree, C. *fetus* subsp. *venerealis*. The disease is characterized by fetal death and abortions in the final months of gestation, or by full-term birth of dead lambs or lambs that die shortly thereafter. The infection also gives rise to metritis and placentitis, both of which may result in septicemia and death of the ewe. Losses of 10 to 25% of lambs and 5% of ewes that abort are common. The rate of abortions varies and depends on the proportion of susceptible ewes. Infected animals acquire immunity. Ewes do not abort again for about 3 years. If the infection is recent in the flock, the abortion rate can be quite high, at times up to 70% of the pregnant ewes. The infection is transmitted orally; venereal transmission apparently plays no role.

Source of Infection and Method of Transmission (Figure 9): The reservoir of C. *fetus* is animals, but it is not clear how man contracts the infection. It is presumed that he can become infected by direct contact with infected animals, by ingestion of contaminated food or water, by transplacental transmission, by exposure during birth, and by sexual contact. It should be noted, however, that some patients have denied any contact with animals or even with products of animal origin.

The sources of infection for cattle are carrier bulls and also cows that remain infected from one parturition to the next. The mode of transmission is sexual contact.

The source of infection for sheep is environmental contamination. The placentas of infected ewes that abort or even of those that give birth normally, as well as aborted fetuses and vaginal discharges, all contain a high number of *Campylobacter*. A small portion of ewes become carriers by harboring the infection in the gallbladder and shedding the agent in fecal matter. Contaminated grass, tools, and clothing are vehicles of infection. Transmission is oral. Sexual transmission has not been demonstrated, but this subject requires further study.

Role of Animals in the Epidemiology of the Disease: Animals are the natural reservoir of C. *fetus*. The agent has been observed to lodge in the human gallbladder, but it is not known how often man may become a carrier and give rise to human foci of infection. It is probably an exceptional occurrence. The mechanism of transmission from animals to man is unclear.

Diagnosis: So far, diagnosis of campylobacteriosis in man has been largely fortuitous, upon discovery of C. *fetus* in hemocultures of patients in whom the disease was not suspected. During the febrile period, repeated blood samples should be taken for culture. In cases of meningitis, cultures of cerebrospinal fluid should also be made. For the isolation from vaginal fluid, repeated cultures on antibiotic media are recommended.

Figure 9. Campylobacteriosis (*Campylobacter fetus*). Probable mode of transmission.

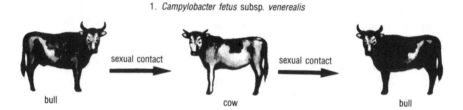

1. *Campylobacter fetus* subsp. *venerealis*

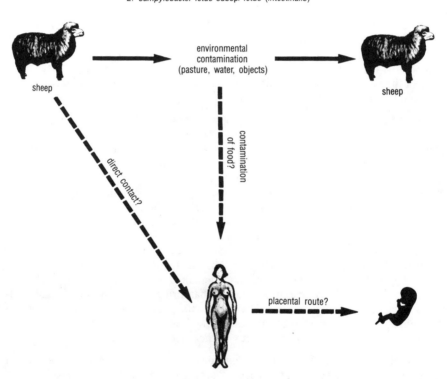

2. *Campylobacter fetus* subsp. *fetus* (*intestinalis*)

NOTE: It is not known how the disease is transmitted to humans; transmission is assumed to occur through direct contact, contamination of foods, or transplacental passage.

In cattle, diagnosis of epizootic infertility is based on the history of the herd, on the culture of the preputial secretion and semen from bulls and of vaginal mucus from nonpregnant cows and heifers, and also on the culture of tissue from aborted fetuses. All samples should be cultured within 6 hours of collection. The highest rate of isolation of *C. fetus* from the cervicovaginal mucus is obtained 2 days immediately before or after estrus.

When the existence of the infection is suspected in a herd of beef cattle, bacteriologic examination of the cervicovaginal mucus of about 20 heifers that were bred several times but remained barren is recommended. Samples should be taken 6 months after the start of the breeding season.

A good diagnostic technique for herd infection, though not for individual infection, is the agglutination test using cervicovaginal mucus. Another test in use is indirect hemagglutination, also employing vaginal mucus. Immunofluorescence is nonspecific in cows, since *C. fetus* subsp. *venerealis* gives cross-reactions with *C. fetus* subsp. *fetus*.

Individual diagnosis is difficult in bulls. An isolation obtained from the preputial secretion is conclusive if the culture is positive but not if it is negative. It is accepted that before a bull is introduced into an artificial insemination center, he must pass four consecutive bacteriologic tests at 1-week intervals or four immunofluorescence tests. An excellent test is to have him service virgin heifers and subsequently culture their cervicovaginal mucus.

In sheep, diagnosis is carried out primarily by culture of fetal tissue, afterbirths, and vaginal fluid.

Control: The few facts available at present on the epidemiology of the human infection are insufficient to allow control measures to be formulated. The best method of preventing epizootic infertility in cattle is artificial insemination using semen from bulls known to be free of the infection. In herds where this procedure is not practical, cows and heifers may be vaccinated annually some 2 or 3 months before breeding, using commercial bacterins with an adjuvant. Several trials offer evidence that vaccination with bacterins can also eliminate the carrier state in bulls and in cows. The curative properties of these vaccines thus provide a new perspective in control. Nevertheless, it must be borne in mind that while this method can reduce the infection in bulls under range conditions, vaccination of infected animals will not eliminate the infection from the herd. In one experiment (Vasquez *et al.*, 1983), *C. fetus* subsp. *venerealis* was isolated from two out of 10 artificially infected bulls 5 weeks after the administration of the recommended two doses a month apart.

In sheep, good control can be obtained based on the vaccination of the females with both monovalent (subsp. *fetus*) and bivalent (*fetus* and *venerealis*) bacterins with adjuvants, the combined product being preferable. In flocks where adult females have acquired natural immunity, good results have been attained by vaccinating only the yearly replacement ewes. Proper sanitary management is important, especially such measures as immediate removal of fetuses and afterbirths, isolation of aborting ewes, and protection of water from contamination.

Bibliography

Andrews, P. J., and F. W. Frank. Comparison of four diagnostic tests for detection of bovine genital vibriosis. *J Am Vet Med Assoc* 165:695-697, 1974.

Bokkenheuser, V. *Vibrio fetus* infection in man. I. Ten new cases and some epidemiologic observations. *Am J Epidemiol* 91:400-409, 1970.

Bokkenheuser, V. D., and V. L. Sutter. Campylobacter Infections. *In:* Balows, A., and W. J. Hausler, Jr. (Eds.), *Diagnostic Procedures for Bacterial, Mycotic and Parasitic Infections,* 6th ed. Washington, D.C., American Public Health Association, 1981.

Bouters, R., J. De Keyser, M. Fandeplassche, A. Van Aert, E. Brone, and P. Bonte. *Vibrio fetus* infection in bulls. Curative and preventive vaccination. *Br Vet J* 129:52-57, 1973.

Bryner, J. H. Vibriosis due to *Vibrio fetus*. *In:* Hubbert, W. T., W. F. McCulloch, and P. R. Schnurrenberger (Eds.), *Diseases Transmitted from Animals to Man,* 6th ed. Springfield, Illinois, Thomas, 1975.

Bryner, J. H., P. A. O'Berry, and A. H. Frank. Vibrio infection of the digestive organs of cattle. *Am J Vet Res* 25:1048-1050, 1964.

Bryner, J. H., P. C. Estes, J. W. Foley, and P. A. O'Berry. Infectivity of three *Vibrio fetus* biotypes for gall bladder and intestines of cattle, sheep, rabbits, guinea pigs, and mice. *Am J Vet Res* 32:465-470, 1971.

Carroll, E. J., and A. B. Hoerlein. Diagnosis and control of bovine genital vibriosis. *J Am Vet Med Assoc* 161:1359-1364, 1972.

Clark, B. L. Review of bovine vibriosis. *Aust Vet J* 47:103-107, 1971.

Clark, B. L., J. H. Duffy, M. J. Monsbourgh, and I. M. Parsonson. Studies on venereal transmission of *Campylobacter fetus* by immunized bulls. *Aust Vet J* 51:531-532, 1975.

Devlin, H. R., and L. McIntyre. *Campylobacter fetus* subsp. *fetus* in homosexual males. *J Clin Microbiol* 18:999-1000, 1983.

Firehammer, B. D., and W. W. Hawkings. The pathogenicity of *Vibrio fetus* isolated from ovine bile. *Cornell Vet* 54:308-314, 1964.

Harvey, S. M., and J. R. Greenwood. Probable *Campylobacter fetus* subsp. *fetus* gastroenteritis. *J Clin Microbiol* 18:1278-1279, 1983.

Hoerlein, A. B. Bovine genital vibriosis. *In:* Faulkner, L. C. (Ed.), *Abortion Diseases of Livestock.* Springfield, Illinois, Thomas, 1968.

Hoerlein, A. B., and E. J. Carroll. Duration of immunity to bovine genital vibriosis. *J Am Vet Med Assoc* 156:775-778, 1970.

Laing, J. A. Vibrio fetus *Infection of Cattle.* Rome, FAO, 1960. (Agricultural Studies 51.)

Miller, V. A. Ovine genital vibriosis. *In:* Faulkner, L. C. (Ed.), *Abortion Diseases of Livestock.* Springfield, Illinois, Thomas, 1968.

Manser, P. A., and R. W. Dalziel. A survey of *Campylobacter* in animals. *J Hyg (Camb)* 95:15-21, 1985.

Miner, M. L., and J. L. Thorne. Studies on the indirect transmission of *Vibrio fetus* infection in sheep. *Am J Vet Res* 25:474-477, 1964.

Osburn, B. I., and R. K. Hopkins. Experimentally induced *Vibrio fetus* var. *intestinalis* infection in pregnant cows. *Amer J Vet Res* 31:1733-1741, 1970.

Riley, L. W., and J. M. Finch. Results of the first year of national surveillance of *Campylobacter* infections in the United States. *J Infect Dis* 151:956-959, 1985.

Schurig, G. G. D., C. E. Hall, K. Burda, L. B. Corbeil, J. R. Duncan, and A. J. Winter. Infection patterns in heifers following cervicovaginal or intrauterine instillation of *Campylobacter (Vibrio) fetus venerealis. Cornell Vet* 64:533-548, 1974.

Schurig, G. G. D., C. E. Hall, L. B. Corbeil, J. R. Duncan, and A. J. Winter. Bovine venereal vibriosis. Cure genital infection in females by systemic immunization. *Infect Immun* 11:245-251, 1975.

Storz, J., M. L. Miner, A. E. Olson, M. E. Marriott, and Y. Y. Elsner. Prevention of ovine vibriosis by vaccination: effect of yearly vaccination of replacement ewes. *Am J Vet Res* 27:115-120, 1966.

White, F. H., and A. F. Walsh. Biochemical and serologic relationships of isolants of *Vibrio fetus* from man. *J Infect Dis* 121:471-474, 1970.

Vásquez, L. A., L. Ball, B. W. Bennet, G. P. Rupp, R. Ellis, J. D. Olson, and M. H. Huffman. Bovine genital campylobacteriosis (vibriosis): vaccination of experimentally infected bulls. *Am J Vet Res* 44:1553-1557, 1983.

CAT-SCRATCH DISEASE

(027.9)

Synonyms: Cat-scratch fever, benign inoculation lymphoreticulosis, cat-scratch syndrome.

Etiology: The causal agent of the disease is not known. Viral and chlamydial agents have been isolated from some patients, but it has not been possible to establish their relationship with the disease. Most investigators have been inclined to consider a viral etiology, involving a single or several viruses. Presently, there are strong indications that it is a bacterial disease. Histopathologic examination of lymph nodes from 39 patients with this illness revealed very small gram-negative bacilli in 34 of them, located in capillary walls or near areas of follicular hyperplasia and inside microabscesses. The observed bacilli were intracellular in the affected areas; they increased in number as lesions developed and diminished as they disappeared. The sera of three convalescent patients and human anti-immuno-globulin conjugated with peroxidase resulted in a precipitate with bacilli from the histologic sections of different patients, which demonstrates that they were serologically related (Wear *et al.*, 1983). However, until the causal agent is isolated, its true nature will remain uncertain.

Geographic Distribution: The disease appears sporadically. There have been 750 reported cases over the last 37 years (Wear *et al.*, 1983). About 75% of the cases were in children. Small epidemic outbreaks and familial clustering have been reported in several countries. When an outbreak occurs within a family, there are usually several familial contacts in whom intracutaneous tests will be positive to the Hanger-Rose antigen. It is possible that several endemic areas exist around Toronto (Canada), New York (USA), and Alfortville (France). Positive intracutaneous tests have been obtained in 10% of the population living in the vicinity of this last city.

The Disease in Man: From 7 to 20 or more days elapse between the cat scratch or bite (or other lesion caused by some inanimate object) and the appearance of symptoms. The disease is characterized by a regional lymphadenopathy without lymphangitis. In about 50% of the cases primary lesions are seen at the point of inoculation. These consist of partially healed ulcers surrounded by an erythematous area, or of erythematous papules, pustules, or vesicles. Lymphadenitis is generally unilateral and commonly appears in the epitrochlear, axillary, or cervical lymph nodes, or in the femoral and inguinal lymph glands. Swelling in the lymph glands, which is generally painful and suppurates in about 25% of patients, persists for periods ranging from a few weeks to a few months. A high proportion of patients shows signs of systemic infection, which consist of a low, short-lived fever and, less frequently, chills, anorexia, malaise, generalized pain, vomiting, and stomach cramps. Morbilliform cutaneous eruptions sometimes occur.

In general, the disease is benign and heals spontaneously without sequelae. Complications have been observed in a small proportion of the patients. The most common of these is Parinaud's oculoglandular syndrome; encephalitis, osteolytic lesions, and thrombocytopenic purpura are less frequent. The lymph gland lesions are not pathognomonic, but they follow a certain pattern, which helps in diagnosis.

Histopathologic studies have shown that alterations begin with hyperplasia of the reticular cells followed by an inflammatory granulomatous lesion. The center of the granuloma degenerates and becomes a homogeneous eosinophilic mass, in which abscesses and microabscesses later appear.

Most cases have occurred in children, who have more contact with cats.

In temperate climates the disease tends to be seasonal, with the majority of cases in fall and winter. In hot climates there are no seasonal differences.

Source of Infection and Mode of Transmission: The most salient fact in the epidemiology of this disease is its causal relation with a cat scratch. It is estimated that about 65% of patients were scratched or bitten by cats and that 90% of the cases had some contact with these animals. Nevertheless, cases have been observed in which the skin lesion was inflicted by such inanimate objects as splinters, thorns, or pins.

Without doubt, cats play an important role in the epidemiology, but there is doubt about whether it is as host for the etiologic agent or simply as a mechanical vector. Several observations—among them the fact that some cases were caused by inanimate agents—suggest that cats could be mechanical transmitters. Cats implicated in human cases were healthy animals, almost always young, that did not react to the Hanger-Rose intradermal test. It is also interesting to point out that cats inoculated with material from the lymph nodes of human patients did not develop illness. In summary, up to the present it has not been possible to show that cats are infected with the disease or are carriers of its causal agent, in spite of the many trials carried out. As long as the etiologic agent remains unisolated, the epidemiology of the disease cannot be clarified nor can a rational basis for its control be established.

Diagnosis: Cat-scratch disease (CSD) can be clinically confused with other diseases which cause regional lymphadenopathies, such as tularemia, brucellosis, tuberculosis, pasteurellosis, infectious mononucleosis, Hodgkin's disease, venereal lymphogranuloma, lymphosarcoma, and lymphoma. All these diseases must be excluded before considering a diagnosis of CSD. The above-described symptomatology, an initial lesion caused by a cat scratch or bite, the histopathology of biopsy material taken from the affected lymph node, and the Hanger-Rose intradermal test constitute the bases for diagnosis. The Hanger-Rose antigen is prepared by suspending pus taken from an abscessed lymph node in a 1:5 saline solution and heating it for 10 hours at 60°C. The antigen is very crude and difficult to standardize. The test is carried out by intradermal inoculation with 0.1 ml of the antigen. The reaction may be read in 48 hours. Edema measuring 0.5 cm and erythema of 1 cm in diameter are considered a positive reaction. The test is very useful, since 90% of 485 clinically diagnosed cases gave positive results to it, while only 4.1% out of 591 controls tested positive. The danger exists of transmitting viral hepatitis with this antigen; therefore, the preparation should be heat-treated for a lengthy period, as indicated above.

Control: Prevention is limited to avoiding cat scratches or bites.

Bibliography

Andrewes, C., and H. G. Pereira. *Viruses of Vertebrates,* 3rd ed. Baltimore, Maryland, Williams and Wilkins, 1972.

American Public Health Association. *Control of Communicable Diseases in Man,* 14th ed. (Ed. by A. S. Benenson). Washington, D.C., APHA, 1985.

Emmons, R. W., J. L. Riggs, and J. Schachter. Continuing search for the etiology of cat-scratch disease. *J Clin Microbiol* 4:112-114, 1976.

Gerber, M. A., A. Sedgwick, T. J. MacAlister, K. Gustafson, M. Ballow, and R. C. Tilton. The aetiological agent of cat-scratch disease. *Lancet* 1(8440), 1985.

Griesemer, R. A., and L. G. Wolfe. Cat-scratch disease. *J Am Vet Med Assoc* 158:1008-1012, 1971.

Macrae, A. D. Cat scratch Fever *In:* Graham-Jones, O. (Ed.), *Some Diseases of Animals Communicable to Man in Britain.* Oxford, Pergamon Press, 1968.

Rose, H. M. Cat-scratch Disease. *In:* Wyngaarden, J. B., and L. H. Smith, Jr. (Eds.), *Cecil Textbook of Medicine,* 16th ed. Philadelphia, Saunders, 1982.

Warwick, W. J. The cat-scratch syndrome, many diseases or one disease. *Prog Med Virol* 9:256-301, 1967.

Wear, D. J., A. M. Margileth, T. L. Hadfield, G. W. Fischer, C. J. Schlagel, and F. M. King. Cat-scratch disease: A bacterial infection. *Science* 221:1403-1404, 1983.

CLOSTRIDIAL FOOD POISONING

(005.2)

Synonyms: Clostridial gastroenteritis.

Etiology: *Clostridium perfringens* (*C. welchii*), an anaerobic, sporogenic, gram-positive bacillus. Five different toxigenic types are known, designated with the letters A through E.

Geographic Distribution: *C. perfringens* type A is ubiquitous in the soil and the intestinal tracts of man and animals throughout the world. Types B and E have a marked regional distribution.

Occurrence in Man: Outbreaks of food poisoning due to *C. perfringens* type A probably occur the world over, but the greatest amount of information comes from developed countries.

In Great Britain, where food poisoning is a notifiable disease, clostridial poisoning is estimated to cause 30% of all cases as well as a large portion of general and familial outbreaks, with an average of 37 people affected per outbreak.

In the United States during the period 1976-1980, 62 outbreaks affecting 6,093 persons were reported, representing 7.4% of all outbreaks of food toxicoses of known etiology and 14.8% of the total number of known cases in the country. The median of cases per outbreak was 23.5, but six outbreaks affected more than 200 persons (Shandera *et al.*, 1983).

Even in developed countries, cases are greatly underreported because the disease is mild and usually lasts no more than 24 hours. Moreover, laboratory diagnosis is difficult and not always possible, since it depends on obtaining food and stool samples.

Outbreaks affecting large numbers of people are the ones usually reported. These originate from meals prepared in restaurants and institutions.

In Germany and New Guinea, necrotic enteritis in man caused by *C. perfringens* type C has been confirmed.

Occurrence in Animals: In domesticated ruminants several types of enterotoxemia due to *C. perfringens* types B, C, D, and E are known. Enterotoxemia results from the absorption into the bloodstream of toxins produced in the intestine by the several types of *C. perfringens* that form part of the normal intestinal flora.

The Disease in Man: The disease is contracted upon ingestion of foods (especially red meat and fowl) in which *C. perfringens* type A has multiplied. It is now known that illness is caused by thermoresistant strains, which can survive at 100°C for more than an hour, as well as by thermolabile and hemolytic strains, which are inactivated in about 10 minutes at 100°C.

The incubation period is usually from 7 to 15 hours after ingesting the food, but in some persons it may last from 24 to 30 hours. The disease begins suddenly with abdominal cramps and diarrhea, but usually does not include vomiting and fever. It is of short duration, a day or less, and its course is benign except in debilitated persons, in whom it may prove fatal.

Necrotic enteritis, produced by ingestion of food contaminated by *C. perfringens* type C, is characterized by a regional gangrene in the small intestine, especially the jejunum.

On rare occasions, gastroenteritis due to *C. perfringens* type D has been confirmed in man. This type causes enterotoxemia in sheep.

The Disease in Animals: *C. perfringens* type A is a normal inhabitant of the intestine, where it does not usually produce its characteristic alpha toxin. A few cases of illness caused by type A have been confirmed in cattle. In California and Oregon (USA), a disease produced by type A in nursing lambs ("yellow lamb disease") has been described. The disease occurs in spring when there is a large population of nursing animals. The lambs show depression, anemia, jaundice, and hemoglobinuria. They die 6 to 12 hours after the onset of clinical symptoms (Gillespie and Timoney, 1981).

Type B is the etiologic agent of "lamb dysentery," which occurs in Great Britain, the Middle East, and South Africa. It usually attacks lambs less than 2 weeks old. It is characterized by hemorrhagic enteritis, frequently accompanied by ulceration of the mucosa. It also affects calves and colts.

Type C causes hemorrhagic enterotoxemia ("struck") in adult sheep in Great Britain, as well as hemorrhagic enteritis in calves, lambs, and suckling pigs.

Type D is the causal agent of enterotoxemia (pulpy kidney disease) in sheep. It is distributed worldwide and attacks animals of all ages. The disease is associated with abundant consumption of food, whether milk, pasture, or grains. Outbreaks have also been described in goats and, more rarely, in cattle.

Type E causes dysentery or enterotoxemia in calves and lambs.

Source of Infection and Mode of Transmission: The natural reservoir of *C. perfringens* type A is the soil and the intestinal tracts of man and animals. Some studies (Torres-Anjel *et al.*, 1977) have shown that man harbors higher numbers of *C. perfringens* than fowl or cattle and that some persons pass great quantities of bacteria, making man the most important reservoir of clostridial food poisoning.

The source of infection and poisoning for man is usually food contaminated with spores that have survived cooking. However, contamination with spores or the vegetative form of the bacteria may also take place after cooking. The food vehicle is almost always red meat or fowl, since they provide *C. perfringens* with the amino acids and vitamins it needs. Other foods such as pigeon peas, beans, mashed potatoes, cheeses, seafood, potato salad, noodles, and olives have occasionally given rise to the disease (Craven, 1980). Immersing meat in broth or cooking it in large pieces creates anaerobic conditions favorable for multiplication of the bacteria during cooling or storage. Food poisoning usually originates from foods prepared in great quantities by restaurants or dining halls and served later or the next day. Cooking and heating cause the spores to germinate. Spores of some strains of *C. perfringens* are destroyed by adequate cooking, but other spores are heat-resistant. Bacteria in the vegetative state multiply in food when it is allowed to cool at room temperature; high bacterial concentrations may be reached when cooling is prolonged at high ambient temperatures. Reheating food before serving may stimulate bacterial multiplication if the heating temperature is not high enough. It is now known that high concentrations of the vegetative form of *C. perfringens* in food cannot be destroyed by stomach acid. Consequently, they pass into the intestine where during sporulation they produce the enterotoxin that causes the disease. This enterotoxin, which is resistant to intestinal enzymes, is cytotoxic for the intestinal epithelium, affects the electrolyte transport system, and consequently causes diarrhea (Narayan, 1982).

It should be borne in mind that not all strains of *C. perfringens* are toxigenic. In one study of strains implicated in food poisonings, 86% were toxigenic, while in another study two strains out of 174 isolated from other sources produced the enterotoxin (cited in Narayan, 1982).

Other types of *C. perfringens* (B, C, D, E) that cause enterotoxemias in animals multiply rapidly in the intestine and produce toxins when animals are allowed sudden access to rich pastures or are given too much fodder.

Role of Animals in the Epidemiology of the Disease: Human food poisoning is brought about by foods contaminated by *C. perfringens,* usually foods consisting of mainly red meat or fowl. The animals themselves do not play a direct role in the epidemiology, since the etiologic agent is ubiquitous and may be found in the soil or in dust. Food of animal origin is important as a substrate for the multiplication of the bacteria and as a vehicle for the disease. Soil and the intestines of humans and animals constitute the reservoir of the etiologic agent.

Heat-resistant strains of *C. perfringens* may be found in the mesenteric lymph nodes of animals after slaughter. The rate of isolation is lower from animals that were allowed to rest 24 to 48 hours before butchering.

Diagnosis: The incubation period and clinical picture make it possible to distinguish between clostridial food poisoning, which is afebrile, and salmonellosis, shigellosis, and colibacillosis, which produce fever. Staphylococcal intoxication usually results in vomiting, while this symptom is rare with clostridial poisoning. Laboratory confirmation is based on the *C. perfringens* count in the implicated food and the patient's stool (within 48 hours of onset of illness). The existence of 10^5 cells per gram of food and 10^6 cells per gram of fecal material is considered significant. Serotyping of strains from food and feces with a battery of 70 sera has provided good results in epidemiologic research in Great Britain, but not in the United States, where only 40% of the strains received by the Centers for Disease Control could be typed. There is no proof that only certain serotypes are related to the disease (Shandera, 1983). Methods to detect the enterotoxin in the stool of patients by means of coagglutination, counterimmunoelectrophoresis, and enzyme-linked immunosorbent assay (ELISA) are being developed and should be evaluated in field investigations of outbreaks to determine their value (Dobosch and Dowell, 1983).

Laboratory diagnosis of animal enterotoxemias is done by mouse inoculation to demonstrate the presence of specific toxins. Some mice are inoculated with only intestinal contents and others with both intestinal contents and antitoxin.

Control: In man the control measures are as follows: Meat dishes should be served hot as soon as possible after cooking. If food must be kept for a while before eating, it should be rapidly refrigerated. If possible, meat should be cut into small pieces to cook. Broth should be separated from the meat. The use of pressure cookers is a good preventive measure. If necessary, food should be reheated at a temperature sufficiently high to destroy the agent's vegetative cells.

In animals, enterotoxemia control consists of good herd management, avoidance of a sudden change from poor to rich pasture, and active immunization by specific toxoids. Two doses of toxoid a month apart are recommended, followed by a booster at 6 months (type D) or a year (type C).

To protect lambs, ewes should be vaccinated with two doses, the second administered 2 weeks before lambing. To prevent lamb dysentery (caused by type B), ewes can be vaccinated with the specific toxoid or lambs can be passively immunized with antiserum at birth. In *C. perfringens* types B and C, the beta toxin predominates, and therefore a toxoid or antiserum made from one type will give cross-immunity.

Bibliography

Craven, S. E. Growth and sporulation of *Clostridium perfringens* in foods. *Food Technol* 34:80-87, 1980.

Dobosch, D., and R. Dowell. Detección de enterotoxina de *Clostridium perfringens* en casos de intoxicación alimentaria. *Medicina (B Aires)* 43:188-192, 1983.

Faich, G. A., and E. J. Gangarosa. Food poisoning, bacterial. *In*: Top, F. M., and P. F. Wehrle (Eds.), *Communicable and Infectious Diseases,* 7th ed. St. Louis, Missouri, Mosby, 1972.

Gillespie, J. H., and J. F. Timoney. *Hagan and Bruner's Infectious Diseases of Domestic Animals.* Ithaca, Cornell University Press, 1981.

Hobbs, B. C. *Clostridium perfringens* and *Bacillus cereus* infections. *In:* Riemann, H. (Ed.), *Food-borne Infections and Intoxications.* New York and London, Academic Press, 1969.

Narayan, K. G. Food-borne infection with *Clostridium perfringens* Type A. *Int J Zoonoses* 9:12-32, 1982.

Roberts, R. S. Clostridial diseases. *In:* Stableforth, A. W., and I. A. Galloway (Eds.), *Infectious Diseases of Animals.* London, Butterworths, 1959.

Rose, H. M. Diseases caused by *Clostridia*. *In:* Wyngaarden, J. B., and L. H. Smith, Jr. (Eds.), *Cecil Textbook of Medicine,* 16th ed. Philadelphia, Saunders, 1982.

Shandera, W. X., C. O. Tacket, and P. A. Blake. Food poisoning due to *Clostridium perfringens* in the United States. *J Infect Dis* 147:167-170, 1983.

Smith, L. D. S. Clostridial diseases of animals. *Adv Vet Sci* 3:463-524, 1957.

Torres-Anjel, M. J., M. P. Riemann, and C. C. Tsai. *Enterotoxigenic* Clostridium perfringens *Type A in Selected Humans: A Prevalence Study.* Pan American Health Organization, 1977. (Scientific Publication 350.)

Van Kessel, L. J. P., H. A. Verbruch, M. F. Stringer, and J. B. L. Hoekstra. Necrotizing enteritis associated with toxigenic type A *Clostridium perfringens. J Infect Dis* 151:974-975, 1985.

CLOSTRIDIAL WOUND INFECTIONS

(040.0; E999)

Synonyms: Gas gangrene, histotoxic infections, anaerobic cellulitis; malignant edema (in animals).

Etiology: Wound infection is characterized by mixed bacterial flora. The most important species are *Clostridium perfringens* (*welchii*), *C. novyi*, *C. septicum*, *C. bifermentans* (*sordellii*), *C. histolyticum,* and *C. fallax.* These bacteria produce potent exotoxins that destroy tissue. In human gas gangrene, the most important etiologic agent is *C. perfringens*, toxigenic type A. Infection by *C. septicum* predominates in animals.

Geographic Distribution: Worldwide.

Occurrence in Man: Formerly, gas gangrene was more prevalent in wartime than in peacetime. It has been estimated that during World War I 100,000 German soldiers died from this infection. Nevertheless, its incidence has diminished enormously during more recent wars. During the 8 years of the Vietnam War there were only 22 cases out of 139,000 wounds, while in Miami (USA) there were 27 cases in civilian trauma patients over a 10-year period (Finegold, 1977). The disease is relatively rare and occurs mainly in traffic and industrial accident victims; however, in natural catastrophes or other emergencies, it constitutes a grave problem. Gas gangrene also occurs after surgery, especially in elderly patients who have had a leg amputated. It may also develop in patients receiving intramuscular injections, especially of medicines suspended in an oil base.

Occurrence in Animals: The frequency of occurrence in animals is not known.

The Disease in Man: Pathogenic species of *Clostridium* may be found as mere contaminants in any type of traumatic lesion. When infection occurs, the microorganisms multiply and produce gas in the tissues. Gas gangrene is an acute and serious condition that produces myositis as its principal lesion. The incubation period lasts from 6 hours to 3 days after injury. The first symptoms are increasing pain around the injured area, tachycardia, and lowered blood pressure, followed by fever, edematization, and a reddish serous exudate from the wound. The skin becomes taut and discolored and is covered with vesicles. Crepitation is felt upon palpation. Stupor, delirium, and coma develop in the final stages of the disease. The infection may also begin in the uterus following an abortion or a difficult labor; these cases show septicemia, massive hemolysis, and acute nephrosis, with shock and anuria.

C. *perfringens* type A, alone or in combination with other pathogens, was the cause of 60 to 80% of gas gangrene cases in soldiers during the two world wars.

The Disease in Animals: C. *septicum* is the principal agent in clostridial wound infection, known as "malignant edema." This disease is characterized by an extensive hemorrhagic edema of the subcutaneous tissue and intermuscular connective tissue. The muscle tissue becomes dark red; little or no gas is present. The infected animal exhibits fever, intoxication, and lameness. The swellings are soft and palpation leaves depressions. The disease course is rapid and death can occur a few days after symptoms appear. Cattle are the most affected species, but sheep, horses, and swine are also susceptible. The infection is rare in fowl.

C. *perfringens* type A is sometimes responsible for infection of traumatic wounds in calves, lambs, and goats. As in man, the infection gives rise to gas gangrene. Edema with large quantities of gas develops around the injury site, spreads rapidly, and causes death in a short time.

In animals, as in man, other clostridia (such as C. *novyi*, C. *bifermentans*, and C. *histolyticum*) can cause wound infection, and the bacterial flora of the wound may be mixed.

Source of Infection and Mode of Transmission: Clostridia are widely distributed in nature—in the soil and in the intestinal tracts of most animals, including man. The sources of infection for man and animals are soil and fecal material. Transmission is effected through traumatic wounds or surgical incisions. Gas gangrene can also occur without any wound or trauma (spontaneous or endogenous gas gangrene) in patients weakened by malignant disease or those with ulcerative lesions either in the gastrointestinal or urogenital tract or in the bile ducts (Finegold, 1977). In animals the infection may originate in minor wounds such as those produced by castration, tail docking, or shearing.

Role of Animals in the Epidemiology of the Disease: Wound clostridiosis is a disease common to man and animals, not a zoonosis.

Diagnosis: Diagnosis is based mainly on clinical manifestations, such as the color around the lesion, swelling, toxemia, and muscle tissue destruction. The presence of gas is not always indicative of clostridial infection. A smear of exudate from the wound or a muscle tissue sample stained by Gram's method may be helpful in diagnosis if a high number of large gram-positive bacilli are found. The culture of anaerobic bacilli from human cases is generally of little value because of the time required and the urgency of diagnosis. Moreover, isolation of a potentially pathogenic anaerobe from a wound may only indicate contamination and not necessarily active infection (penetration and multiplication in the human or animal organism). In animals, culture and isolation of the responsible agent can be important in distinguishing the infection caused by C. *chauvoei* (symptomatic anthrax, blackleg, or emphysematous gangrene) from infections caused by C. *septicum*. The latter bacterium invades the animal's body rapidly after death, and for this reason the material used for examination should be taken before or very shortly after death.

The fluorescent antibody technique permits identification of the pathogenic clostridia in a few hours and can be very useful in diagnosis.

Control: Prevention of the infection consists of the prompt treatment and debridement of wounds. Special care must be taken to ensure that tourniquets, bandages, and casts do not interfere with circulation and thus create conditions favorable to the multiplication of anaerobic bacteria by diminishing the amount of oxygen reaching the area.

Combined vaccines of *C. chauvoei* and *C. septicum* are used for active immunization of calves and lambs.

Bibliography

Bruner, D. W., and J. H. Gillespie. *Hagan's Infectious Diseases of Domestic Animals,* 6th ed. Ithaca, New York, Cornell University Press, 1973.

Finegold, S. M. *Anaerobic Bacteria in Human Disease.* New York, Academic Press, 1977.

Joklik, W. K., H. P. Willett, and D. B. Amos (Eds.). *Zinsser Microbiology,* 18th ed. Norwalk, Connecticut, Appleton-Century-Crofts, 1984.

MacLennan, J. D. The histotoxic clostridial infections of man. *Bacteriol Rev* 26:177-274, 1962.

Prévot, A. R., A. Turpin, and P. Kaiser. *Les bactéries anaerobies.* Paris, Dunod, 1967.

Rose, H. M. Disease caused by clostridia. *In:* Wyngaarden, J. B., and L. H. Smith, Jr. (Eds.), *Cecil Textbook of Medicine,* 16th ed. Philadelphia, Saunders, 1982.

Rosen, M. M. Clostridial infections and intoxications. *In:* Hubbert, W. T., W. F. McCulloch, and P. R. Schnurrenberger (Eds.), *Diseases Transmitted from Animals to Man,* 6th ed. Springfield, Illinois, Thomas, 1975.

Smith, D. L. S. Clostridial diseases of animals. *Adv Vet Sci* 3:465-524, 1957.

Smith, L. D., and L. V. Holderman. *The Pathogenic Anaerobic Bacteria.* Springfield, Illinois, Thomas, 1968.

COLIBACILLOSIS

(008.0)

Synonyms: Colibacteriosis, colitoxemia, white scours, gut edema of swine.

Etiology and Physiopathogenesis: *Escherichia coli* belongs to the family Enterobacteriaceae. *E. coli* is a normal component of the intestinal flora of warm-blooded animals, including man. Pathogenic strains causing enteric disease are grouped in three categories: a) enterotoxigenic, b) enteroinvasive, and c) "enteropathogenic." At present the validity of this last category is in question, as is the usefulness of serotyping.

The enterotoxigenic *E. coli* (ETEC) have been the most intensely studied in the last few years. Research has not only added knowledge about the physiopathogenic action mechanisms of these bacteria, but has also provided means to prevent diarrheal disease in several animal species. Enterotoxigenic strains synthesize two types of toxin: thermolabile (LT) and thermostable (ST). There are some strains which produce both types of toxin and others which produce only one. Toxins are coded for in the plasmids, which may be transferred from one ETEC strain to others that lack them.

The ETEC strains are distributed heterogeneously among the different serotypes. ETEC strains make use of fimbriae or pili (nonflagellar, proteinic, filamentous appendages) to adhere to the mucous lining of the small intestine, multiply, and produce one or more toxins, which interact with the epithelial cells. These pili are called colonization factors and their synthesis is also plasmid-dependent. The antigenic characteristics of the pili differ in different animal species. In calves and lambs, the implicated pili are predominantly K99. Even though K88 and 987P have also been isolated, it is believed that they do not play a role in ETEC virulence in these species. In suckling pigs, the pili associated with enterotoxic colibacillosis are K88, K89, and 987P. In man the colonization factors are CFA I and CFA II, which were only recently identified.

Enteroinvasive *E. coli* invade the colon's mucous membrane and produce a dysenteric symptomatology similar to that of *Shigella*. These *E. coli* strains multiply within the colonic mucosa and cause colitis and inflammation. This category contains a limited number of serotypes.

The third category, the pathogenic role of which is questioned, is made up of specific enteropathogenic serotypes, identified on the basis of the Kaufmann-White serotypification scheme. The mechanism by which these strains cause diarrhea is not known. Several enteropathogenic serotypes produced diarrhea experimentally in volunteers (Lévine and Lanata, 1983; Binsztein, 1982; WHO Scientific Working Group, 1980).

Geographic Distribution: Worldwide; some endemic areas exist in developing countries.

Occurrence in Man: In developing countries, the enterotoxigenic *E. coli* group (ETEC) is made up of etiologic agents of diarrhea that are common in children under 2 years of age. After 4 years of age, these agents become less prevalent. ETEC is also the most common cause of "traveler's diarrhea," which occurs in adults from the industrialized world when visiting endemic countries. This epidemiologic characteristic suggests that the population in endemic countries acquires immunity, while in developed countries the population is little exposed to these agents and does not acquire immunity.

Enteroinvasive strains of *E. coli* are the cause of sporadic cases and of outbreaks of diarrhea in adults and school-age children. Several outbreaks have been reported in hospitals, schools, and in the population at large as a result of contamination of the water supply or consumption of contaminated cheese.

Several epidemics of infant enteritis have been attributed to enteropathogenic *E. coli* strains (EPEC), principally in poor socioeconomic groups in industrial cities. In developing countries, the disease possibly occurs in children over 6 months of age in the form of community outbreaks. Isolation of these strains from sporadic cases is difficult to interpret. In 1983 a special working group (Workshop on Enteropathogenic *E. coli*, 1983) changed the scope of the problem by providing data that showed that epidemic outbreaks caused by EPEC have occurred in many countries.

Occurrence in Animals: Common, especially in calves and suckling pigs.

The Disease in Man: The incubation period is from 12 to 72 hours. ETEC strains produce a syndrome closely resembling that caused by *Vibrio cholerae,* with profuse and watery diarrhea, abdominal colic, vomiting, acidosis, and dehydration. The feces do not contain mucus or blood and fever may or may not be present. The duration of the illness is short and in general the symptoms disappear in 2 days or less.

Enteroinvasive strains cause a dysenteric syndrome with mucoid diarrhea, at times tinged with blood.

Infant "enteropathogenic" strains have been characterized in the past by high mortality. However, in the last few years, the disease has tended to be benign in outbreaks occurring in nurseries. In one of the strains classified as "entero-pathogenic," O:128, the production of thermostable toxin was confirmed (Ryder *et al.*, 1979); however, other investigators (Robins-Browne *et al.*, 1982) could not detect enterotoxins in three strains of proven pathogenicity belonging to that group.

E. coli is also an important agent of urogenital infections.

The Disease in Animals: In addition to sporadic cases of mastitis, urogenital infections, abortions, and other pathological processes, *E. coli* is responsible for several important diseases.

Calf diarrhea (white scours) is an acute disease causing high mortality in calves less than 10 days old. It manifests itself as serious diarrhea, with whitish feces and rapid dehydration. Its course may last from a few hours to a few days. Calves not receiving colostrum are almost always victims of this disease. Colostrum, because of its high content of IgM antibodies, is essential in preventing diarrhea in calves. In the first 24 to 36 hours of the calf's life, the intestinal mucous membrane is permeable to immunoglobulins, which pass quickly into the bloodstream and protect the animal against environmental microorganisms.

Enterotoxigenic strains causing diarrhea in newborn calves generally produce a thermostable toxin, and the pili antigen is almost always type K99.

The septicemic form of colibacillosis in calves that did not receive colostrum includes diarrhea as well as signs of generalized infection. Surviving animals usually suffer from arthritis and meningitis (Gillespie and Timoney, 1981).

Mastitis caused by *E. coli* appears especially in older cows with dilated milk ducts. In milk free of leukocytes, coliforms multiply rapidly, causing an inflammatory reaction that destroys the bacteria and liberates a great quantity of endotoxins. This produces an acute mastitis with fever, anorexia, cessation of milk production, and weight loss. In the next lactation period, the mammary gland returns to normal functioning.

A disease with white diarrhea was reported in lambs in England and Australia. In South Africa, colipathogens were indicated as the cause of a septicemic illness in lambs, with neurologic symptomatology, ascites, and hydropericarditis, but without major gastrointestinal disorder.

A long-term study of horse fetuses and newborn colts found that close to 1% of abortions and 5% of deaths of newborns were due to *E. coli*.

Neonatal enteritis caused by *E. coli* in suckling pigs begins 12 hours after birth with a profuse watery diarrhea, and may end with fatal dehydration. The mortality rate is especially high among offspring of sows bearing for the first time. About 50% of isolated strains are toxicogenic and some produce both thermostable (ST) and thermolabile (LT) toxins (Gillespie and Timoney, 1981). Enteritis in weaned piglets is caused by hemolytic *E. coli* strains. The animals suffer from anorexia, depression, and diarrhea. Mortality is lower than in newborn suckling pigs and the pathogenesis may be similar.

Edema in suckling pigs (gut edema) is an acute disease that generally attacks between 6 and 14 weeks of age. It is becoming increasingly important in swine-producing areas. It is characterized by sudden onset, incoordination, and edema of the eyelids, the cardiac region of the stomach, and sometimes other parts of the body. Body temperature is usually normal. Morbidity varies from 10 to 35%, and the case fatality rate between 20 and 100%. The triggering factor in the disease seems to be stress caused by weaning, changes in diet, and vaccination against hog cholera. The disease mechanism could be an intestinal toxemia caused by specific types of *E. coli*.

During septicemic diseases of fowl, such as cases of salpingitis and pericarditis, pathogenic serotypes of *E. coli* have been isolated. A colibacillary etiology has also been attributed to Hjarre's disease (coligranuloma), which is a condition in adult fowl characterized by granulomatous lesions in the liver, cecum, spleen, bone marrow, and lungs. The lesions resemble those of tuberculosis, and mucoid strains of *E. coli* have been isolated from them. The disease can be reproduced in laboratory animals and chickens by parenteral inoculation but not by oral administration.

Source of Infection and Mode of Transmission: The main reservoir of human colibacillosis is man. The source of infection is the feces of infected persons (principally sick persons, secondarily carriers) and objects contaminated by them. The most common mode of transmission is the fecal-oral route. In the case of epidemic diarrhea in newborn infants in nurseries, airborne transmission by contaminated dust is possible.

Some serotypes are species-specific, others are not. Animals may be carriers of enteropathogenic *E. coli* serotypes similar to those that infect man. Milk, milk products, and meat products can contain pathogenic serotypes. Although pathogenic *E. coli* have been isolated from food, animals, and animal products, more studies are needed to determine the role played by food of animal origin in human infection. Nevertheless, awareness of this possibility is in order, since outbreaks of human colibacillosis that could have originated from a common food, such as cheese, have been described. In addition, several experiments carried out with volunteers suggested that food may be a source of infection.

In animals, the source of infection and mode of transmission follow the same patterns as in human infection. Animals with diarrhea constitute a very important source of infection.

Role of Animals in the Epidemiology of the Disease: The importance of animals has not yet been clearly defined. The discovery of the same entero-pathogenic serotypes of *E. coli* in children and in animals indicates that animals could serve as reservoirs and disseminators of the infective agent. Foods of animal origin (especially milk) and contact with dogs and cats have been indicated as sources of infection for children.

Diagnosis: Diagnosis is based on isolation of the etiologic agent and on tests that can identify it as enterotoxigenic, invasive, or as belonging to an enteropathogenic serotype. In sporadic cases, isolation of an enteropathogenic serotype has only relative importance and is difficult to interpret. The ELISA test may be used to examine the feces for K99 protein in bovines, K88 in hogs, or enterotoxigenic (LT) toxin in humans (Merson *et al.*, 1980; Mills *et al.*, 1983; Ellens *et al.*, 1979). The fluorescent antibody technique is a valuable eliminatory test once the etiologic agent has been established by conventional means.

Control: With respect to man, control measures include: a) personal cleanliness and hygienic practices, sanitary waste removal, and environmental sanitation; b) provision of maternal and child health and hygiene services; c) protection of food products, milk pasteurization, and compulsory veterinary inspection of meat; and d) special preventive measures in hospital nursery wards. These measures should include placing healthy newborn infants in a different room from sick nursing infants or older children. Nurses who tend the nurseries should not have contact with other wards, and those in charge of feeding bottles should not be involved with diaper changing. Special precautions should be taken in the laundry.

With regard to the prevention of colibacillosis in animals, the commonly accepted rules of herd management should be followed. In calves, colostrum is important for the prevention of white scours, and in pigs all unnecessary stress should be avoided during weaning.

Investigations over the last few years on factors permitting enterotoxigenic *E. coli* strains to colonize the small intestine have opened up new horizons in the prevention of colibacillosis in animals. Vaccines for bovines and hogs have been developed based on fimbria (pili) antigens. These vaccines act to inhibit *E. coli* from adhering to the mucous membrane of the small intestine. To this end, gestating cows and hogs are vaccinated with vaccines based on K99 and K88 antigens, respectively. Newborns acquire passive immunity via colostrum and milk, which contain antibodies against these factors. In the same way, good results have been obtained in protecting newborn lambs by vaccinating the ewe with K99. In addition, studies (Rutter *et al.,* 1976; Myers, 1978; Nagy, 1980) are being carried out with oral vaccines for humans using toxicogenic *E. coli* toxoids of both thermolabile and thermostable toxins as well as antiadherence factors made from purified fimbria. Genetic engineering is another approach being used to obtain vaccines with attenuated *E. coli* virulence (Lévine and Lanata, 1983).

Bibliography

American Public Health Association. *Control of Communicable Diseases in Man,* 14th ed. (Ed. by A. S. Benenson). Washington, D.C., APHA, 1985.

Biester, H. E., and L. H. Schwarte (Eds.). *Diseases of Poultry,* 4th ed. Ames, Iowa State University Press, 1959.

Binsztein, N. Estudio de la diarrea. Factores de virulencia y mecanismos fisiopatogénicos. *Bacteriol Clin Argent* 1:138-142, 1982.

Cooke, E. M. *Escherichia coli*—an overview. *J Hyg (Camb)* 95:523-530, 1985.

Edwards, P. R., and W. H. Ewing. *Identification of Enterobacteriaceae,* 3rd ed. Minneapolis, Minnesota, Burgess, 1972.

Ellens, D. J., P. W. de Leeuw, and H. Rosemond. Detection of the K99 antigen of *Escherichia coli* in calf feces by enzyme-linked immunosorbent assay (ELISA). *Vet Q* 1:169-175, 1979.

Gay, C. C. *Escherichia coli* and neonatal disease of calves. *Bacteriol Rev* 29:75-101, 1965.

Gillespie, J. H., and J. F. Timoney. *Hagan and Bruner's Infectious Diseases of Domestic Animals,* 7th ed. Ithaca, New York, Cornell University Press, 1981.

Hinton, M. The sub-specific differentiation of *Escherichia coli* with particular reference to ecological studies in young animals including man. *J Hyg (Camb)* 95:595-609, 1985.

Lévine, M. N., and C. Lanata. Progresos en vacunas contra diarrea bacteriana. *Adel Microbiol Enferm Infecc* 2:67-118, 1983.

Lovell, R. Coliform diseases. *In:* Stableforth, A. W., and I. A. Galloway (Eds.), *Infectious Diseases of Animals,* London, Butterworths, 1959.

Merson, M. H., R. M. Yolken, R. B. Sack, J. L. Forehlich, H. B. Greenborg, I. Hug, and R. W. Black. Detection of *Escherichia coli* enterotoxins in stools. *Infect Immun* 29:108-113, 1980.

Mills, K. W., K. L. Toetze, and R. M. Phillips. Use of enzyme-linked immunosorbent assay for detection of K88 pili in fecal specimens from swine. *Am J Vet Res* 44:2188-2189, 1983.

Myers, L. L. Enteric colibacillosis in calves: immunogenicity and antigenicity of *Escherichia coli* isolated from calves with diarrhea. *Infect Immun* 13:1117-1119, 1978.

Nagy, B. Vaccination of cows with a K99 extract to protect newborn calves against experimental enterotoxic colibacillosis. *Infect Immun* 27:21-24, 1980.

Robins-Browne, R. M., M. N. Lévine, B. Rowe, and E. M. Gabriel. Failure to detect conventional enterotoxins in classical enteropathogenic (serotyped) *Escherichia coli* strains of proven pathogenicity. *Infect Immun* 38:798-801, 1982.

Rowe, B., J. Taylor, and K. A. Betterheim. An investigation of traveller's diarrhoea. *Lancet* 1:1-5, 1970.

Rutter, J. M., G. W. Jones, G. T. H. Brown, M. R. Burrows, and P. D. Luther. Antibacterial activity in colostrum and milk associated with protection of piglets against enteric disease caused by K88-positive *Escherichia coli*. *Infect Immun* 13:667-676, 1976.

Ryder, R. W., R. A. Kaslow, and J. G. Wells. Evidence for enterotoxin production by a classic enteropathogenic serotype of *Escherichia coli*. *J Infect Dis* 140:626-628, 1979.

Saltys, M. A. *Bacteria and Fungi Pathogenic to Man and Animals.* London, Baillière, Tindall and Cox, 1963.

Siegmund, O. H., and L. G. Eaton (Eds.). *The Merck Veterinary Manual,* 3rd ed. Rahway, New Jersey, Merck, 1967.

Williams, L. P., and B. C. Hobbs. Enterobacteriaceae infections. *In:* Hubbert, W. T., W. F. McCulloch, and P. R. Schnurrenberger (Eds.), *Diseases Transmitted from Animals to Man,* 6th ed. Springfield, Illinois, Thomas, 1975.

Workshop on enteropathogenic *Escherichia coli*. *J Infect Dis* 147:1108-1120, 1983.

World Health Organization Scientific Working Group. *Escherichia coli* diarrhoea. *Bull WHO* 58:23-26, 1980.

Wray, C., and J. A. Morris. Aspects of colibacillosis in farm animals. *J Hyg (Camb)* 95:577-593, 1985.

CORYNEBACTERIOSIS

(040)

Etiology: The genus *Corynebacterium* includes species such as *C. diphtheriae* (type species), the agent of human diphtheria, and animal pathogens such as *C. pseudotuberculosis* (*C. ovis*), *C. equi,* and *C. pyogenes*. It also contains species that are pathogenic for plants and others that are saprophytes. In recent years, cases of human disease caused by these agents and also by *C. ulcerans* have been recognized. Corynebacteria, with the exception of *C. diphtheriae,* are called diphtheroids.

Geographic Distribution: Worldwide.

Occurrence in Man: Few cases have been recognized.

Occurrence in Animals: *C. pseudotuberculosis* (*C. ovis*) occurs in many parts of the world among sheep and goats. It is less frequent in horses and camels. Suppurative pneumonia caused by *C. equi* has been recognized in colts in Australia, the United States, and India, and probably occurs in other parts of the world. *C. bovis* is a commensal bacteria in the udder and urogenital tract of bovines. It may occasionally cause mastitis (Gillespie and Timoney, 1981). *C. ulcerans* is found in the nose and throat of man and horses (Wiggins *et al.*, 1981).

The Disease in Man: Only 12 cases of infection in humans caused by *C. equi* are known and 11 of these were in persons being treated with immunosuppressive drugs. The patients ranged in age from 9 months to 64 years. A pulmonary illness developed in 11 patients, and in seven of them X rays revealed cavitation. The symptoms developed insidiously over days or weeks, with fever, fatigue, and, in several, a dry cough. One patient manifested multiple cerebral abscesses. Mortality was high (Van Etta *et al.*, 1983).

The few cases recorded as caused by *C. bovis* revealed a highly varied pathology including acute nephritis, endocarditis, impaired functioning of the nervous system, chronic otitis, and a persistent ulcer on one leg (Vale and Scott, 1977).

Sporadic cases of the human disease are caused by *C. pseudotuberculosis* or *C. ulcerans* (which is intermediate between *C. pseudotuberculosis* and *C. diphtheriae* and produces toxins of both) and a mutant of *C. pyogenes*. These agents caused conditions such as ulcers, lymphadenitis, and tonsillitis (Rountree and Carne, 1967). In some cases, there was no clear identification of the *Corynebacterium* species.

The Disease in Animals: The corynebacterioses are much more important in veterinary medicine. Some of the diseases are described briefly below (Gillespie and Timoney, 1981).

C. pseudotuberculosis is the usual etiologic agent in caseous lymphadenitis in sheep and goats. It occurs in many parts of the world where these animal species are raised. The agent gains entry through wounds and concentrates in the regional lymph nodes, where a caseous greenish pus forms. Abscesses may also be found in the lungs, as well as in the mediastinal and mesenteric lymph nodes.

Two different pathological conditions have been found in horses. One is ulcerative lymphangitis, with metacarpal and metatarsophalangeal abscesses which contain a thick greenish pus and at times leave an ulceration that heals very slowly. The other consists of large and painful abscesses on the chest and in the inguinal and abdominal regions.

C. pseudotuberculosis produces an exotoxin as does *C. diphtheriae,* but the toxins are antigenically different. Nevertheless, *C. pseudotuberculosis* can synthesize a diphtheric toxin if lysogenized with a gentox$^+$ phage. With the exception of these two species of *Corynebacterium*, no other produces exotoxins (Willet, 1983).

C. equi produces a highly lethal bronchopneumonia in colts. Necropsy reveals bilateral suppurative bronchopneumonia with necrosis. Lymphadenitis is common. *C. equi* can cause uterine infections in mares.

In bovines *C. pyogenes* produces abscesses as well as suppurative infections in different organs and tissues, endometritis and pyometritis, and arthritis in calves. In addition, it is the agent of the udder infection known in Europe as summer mastitis. This disease also occurs in the USA in other seasons of the year. In sheep and goats the agent produces suppurative pneumonia and arthritis. In hogs it plays a role, together with other microorganisms, in pyogenic conditions.

Source of Infection and Mode of Transmission: *C. equi* has been isolated from the feces of a high proportion of healthy horses and the natural reservoir is probably the soil. The pulmonary localization in man as well as in colts would indicate that the infection is contracted by inhalation. Even though eight of the 12 human patients affected with *C. equi* were exposed to animals, the role of animals in the transmission of infection is doubtful.

C. pseudotuberculosis is transmitted from one animal with purulent lesions to another, especially during shearing. The agent can also survive in the environment and transmission can occur indirectly to animals with skin lesions.

C. pyogenes is an opportunistic commensal commonly found in the nasal cavities and udders of healthy animals; it invades tissue through open wounds, lesions, and the umbilicus.

C. bovis is a commensal organism in the reproductive tract of bovines and is frequently found in milk, though it only occasionally produces mastitis. In a survey carried out in 74 milk-producing establishments in Ontario, Canada, *C. bovis* was found in the milk of 36% of the cows (Brooks *et al.*, 1983).

C. ulcerans can be found in the nasal cavities and the throats of both humans and horses in good health.

Diagnosis: A confirmed diagnosis of human corynebacteriosis can only be done by isolation and identification of the species.

The same applies to animal corynebacteriosis, though in the case of caseous lymphadenitis in the surface lymph nodes of sheep and goats, the lesions, along with a smear stained by Gram's method, are sufficiently characteristic for diagnosis. Several serologic tests have been used to detect healthy carriers of *C. pseudotuberculosis*.

Control: The few human cases identified to date do not justify the establishment of special preventive measures. Nevertheless, correct diagnosis is important for effective treatment.

The several vaccines against *C. pyogenes* infection are of little use. To prevent caseous lymphadenitis caused by *C. pseudotuberculosis* it is important to avoid cuts during shearing and, if one does occur, to treat it promptly and correctly. Vaccinations against this disease are of questionable value. Control methods for infection caused by *C. equi* consist of general hygienic measures. Pregnant mares should be removed from infected areas.

Bibliography

Brooks, B. S., D. A. Barnum, and A. H. Meek. An observational study of *Corynebacterium bovis* in selected Ontario dairy herds. *Can J Comp Med* 47:73-78, 1983.

Gillespie, J. H., and J. F. Timoney. *Hagan and Bruner's Infectious Diseases of Domestic Animals,* 7th ed., Ithaca, Cornell University Press, 1981.

Rountree, P. M., and H. R. Carne. Human infection with an unusual *Corynebacterium. J Pathol Bacteriol* 94:19-27, 1967.

Vale, J. A., and G. W. Scott. *Corynebacterium bovis* as a cause of human disease. *Lancet* 2:682-684, 1977.

Van Etta, L. L., G. A. Filice, R. M. Ferguson, and D. N. Gerding. *Corynebacterium equi:* a review of 12 cases of human infection. *Rev Infect Dis* 5:1012-1018, 1983.

Wiggins, G. L., F. O. Sottnek, and G. Y. Hermann. Diphtheria and other corynebacterial infections. *In*: Balows, A., and W. J. Hausler, Jr. (Eds.), *Diagnostic Procedures for Bacterial, Mycotic and Parasitic Infections*, 6th ed. Washington, D.C., American Public Health Association, 1981.

Willet, H. P. *Corynebacterium. In*: Yoklik, W. K., H. P. Willet, and D. B. Amos (Eds.), *Zinsser Microbiology*, 18th ed. Norwalk, Connecticut, Appleton-Century-Crofts, 1984.

DERMATOPHILOSIS

(027.8)

Synonyms: Streptotrichosis, mycotic dermatitis (in sheep).

Etiology: *Dermatophilus congolensis* (*D. dermatonomus*, *D. pedis*) is a bacterium belonging to the order Actinomycetales and characterized by branched filaments with transverse and longitudinal septation. When the filaments mature, they fragment and liberate motile, flagellate spores, called zoospores, which constitute the infective agent. In turn, the zoospores germinate and form filaments that produce new zoospores, thus repeating the cycle.

Geographic Distribution: Dermatophilosis has been verified in many areas of Africa, Australia, New Zealand, in North and South America, and in the Caribbean region. Consequently, its worldwide distribution may be asserted.

Occurrence in Man: The first cases known were identified in 1961 in New York, USA, where four persons became ill after handling a deer with dermatophilosis lesions. Subsequently, several other cases were described: one in a student at the University of Kansas (USA), three cases in Australia, and two in Brazil (Kaplan, 1980; Portugal and Baldassi, 1980).

Occurrence in Animals: The disease has been observed in several species of domestic and wild animals. Those affected with the greatest frequency are cattle, sheep, and horses. This disease is most prevalent in tropical and subtropical climates. The importance of dermatophilosis lies in the economic losses it causes due to damage to leather, wool, and pelts. In some African countries, from 16% of cow hides (Kenya) up to 90% (Tanzania) have been damaged. In Great Britain it has been estimated that affected fine wool loses 20% of its commercial value. Moreover, shearing is difficult in chronically sick woolbearing animals.

The Disease in Man: In the few cases identified, the disease has been characterized by pimples and multiple pustules (from 2 to 25) on the hands and forearms, containing a serous or yellowish white exudate. Upon rupturing they left a reddish crateriform cavity. The lesions healed in 3 to 14 days, leaving a purplish red scab.

The Disease in Animals: In dermatophilosis or streptotrichosis in bovines, horses, or goats, a serous exudate at the base of hair tufts dries and forms a scab. When the scab comes off it leaves a moist alopecic area. The lesions vary in size; some may be very small and go unnoticed, but at times they are confluent and cover a large area. In general, they are found on the back, head, neck, and places where ticks attach. In sheep, the disease known as mycotic dermatitis (lumpy wool) begins with hyperemia and swelling of the affected area of skin, and an exudation that becomes hard and scablike. In chronic cases, conical hard crusts with a horny consistency form around tufts of wool. In mild cases, the disease is seen only during shearing, since it makes the operation difficult. Animals do not experience a burning sensation and are not seen to scratch themselves against posts or other objects. Secondary infections may cause death in lambs. Dermatophilosis is also a factor favoring semispecific myiases (see Myiases), caused in Australia by *Lucilia cuprina* (the principal agent of "body strike"). The fly not only prefers the moist areas affected by dermatophilosis above other moist areas in the fur for egg laying, but larval development is aided by the skin lesion caused by *D. congolensis* (Gherardi *et al.*, 1981).

A form of the disease confirmed in Great Britain is localized in the distal regions of the extremities of sheep and called proliferative hoof dermatitis. This form is characterized by extensive inflammation of the skin and formation of thick scabs. The scabs come loose, revealing small hemorrhagic dots that cause the lesion to resemble a strawberry, from which the disease's common name, "strawberry rot foot," is derived.

In dermatophilosis cases described in domestic cats, the lesions differ from those of other domestic species by affecting deeper tissues. In cats, granulomatous lesions due to *D. congolensis* have been found on the tongue, bladder, and popliteal lymph nodes (Kaplan, 1980).

Source of Infection and Mode of Transmission: The etiologic agent, *D. congolensis*, is an obligate parasite that has been isolated only from lesions in animals.

Human cases have arisen from direct contact with animal lesions. Man is probably quite resistant to the infection, as the number of human cases is small in spite of the frequency of the disease among animals.

The most common means of transmission between animals seems to be mechanical transport by arthropod vectors, including ticks, flies, and mosquitoes. The infective element is the zoospore. Most infections occur at the end of spring and in the summer, when insects are most abundant. An important factor in transmission is moisture, which permits detachment of the zoospore from the mycelium.

The most serious outbreaks occur during prolonged humid seasons. Sheep with long wool that retains moisture are most susceptible to the infection. During dry seasons, the agent can survive in moist spots on the body, such as the axilla or in folds of skin.

The infection may also be transmitted by means of objects, such as plant thorns or shears, that cause lesions on the extremities or on the lips.

Role of Animals in the Epidemiology of the Disease: The infection is transmitted from one animal to another and only occasionally from animal to man. The only known reservoirs of the agent are domestic and wild animals.

Diagnosis: Clinical diagnosis is confirmed by microscopic examination of stained smears (Giemsa, methylene blue, or Wright's stain) made from exudates or scabs. This is the simplest and most practical method. Immunofluorescence may be used on smears or tissue samples.

The isolation of the agent should be done in rich media, such as blood agar. This culture method may prove difficult because of contamination. To avoid this difficulty, passage through rabbits has been used.

Several serologic methods have been used to detect antibodies against *D. congolensis*. In a comparative study between passive hemagglutination, immunodiffusion in agar gel, and counterimmunoelectrophoresis, the last test gave the best results with respect to both sensitivity and specificity. This test could be useful for seroepidemiologic surveys once the results are confirmed with a larger number of samples (Makinde and Majiyagbe, 1982).

Control: Given the few cases of dermatophilosis in man, special control measures to protect against infection are not justified. Nevertheless, it would be prudent not to handle animals with lesions with bare hands (especially, if one has abrasions or skin wounds).

In Africa tick control has been demonstrated effective in preventing bovine dermatophilosis.

Sheep with mycotic dermatitis should be shorn last or, preferably, in a separate place. Affected wool should be burned. Satisfactory results have been obtained using 1% alum dips. In chronic cases, an intramuscular injection of 70 mg of streptomycin and 70,000 units of penicillin may be administered 2 months before shearing. This chemotherapy seems to be very effective and prevents difficulties in shearing.

The use of antibiotics (streptomycin, penicillin, and others) produced clinical improvement in affected animals, but did not always eliminate the causal agent.

The study of vaccination against dermatophilosis in animals is presently in an experimental stage.

Bibliography

Ainsworth, G. C., and P. K. C. Austwick. *Fungal Diseases of Animals*, 2nd ed. Farnham Royal, Slough, England, Commonwealth Agriculture Bureau, 1973.

Carter, G. R. *Diagnostic Procedures in Veterinary Microbiology*, 2nd ed. Springfield, Illinois, Thomas, 1973.

Dean, D. J., M. A. Gordon, C. W. Sveringhaus, E. T. Kroll, and J. R. Reilly. Strep-
tothricosis: a new zoonotic disease. *NY State J Med* 61:1283-1287, 1961.

Gherardi, S. G., M. Monzu, S. S. Sutherland, K. G. Johnson, and G. M. Robertson. The
association between body strike and dermatophilosis of sheep under controlled conditions.
Aust Vet J 57:268-271, 1981.

Gordon, M. A. The genus *Dermatophilus*. *J Bacteriol* 88:508-522, 1964.

Kaplan, W. Dermatophilosis in man and lower animals: a review. *In: Proceedings, Fifth
International Conference on the Mycoses.* Washington, D.C., Pan American Health Organization, 1980. (Scientific Publication 396.)

Makinde, A. A., and K. A. Majiyagbe. Serodiagnosis of *Dermatophilus congolensis*
infection by counterimmunoelectrophoresis. *Res Vet Sci* 33:265-269, 1982.

Mendoza, L., and E. Acosta. Dermatofilosis en Costa Rica. *Rev Costarricense Cienc Méd*
6:81-85, 1985.

Pier, A. C. Géneros *Actinomyces, Nocardia y Dermatophilus*. *In:* Merchant, I. A., and R.
A. Packer, *Bacteriología veterinaria*, 3rd ed. Zaragoza, Spain, Acribia, 1970.

Portugal, M. A. C. S., and L. Baldassi. A dermatofilose no Brasil. Revisão bibliográfica.
Arq Inst Biol (São Paulo) 47:53-58, 1980.

Roberts, D. S. *Dermatophilus* infection. *Vet Bull* 37:513-521, 1967.

DISEASES CAUSED BY NONTUBERCULOUS
MYCOBACTERIA

(031)

Synonyms: Mycobacteriosis, atypical tuberculosis, nontuberculous mycobacterial infection.

Etiology: The etiologic agents of nontuberculous mycobacteriosis form a group
separate from those that cause tuberculosis in mammals (*Mycobacterium tuberculosis, M. bovis*, and *M. africanum*). Heretofore termed anonymous, atypical, or
unclassified mycobacteria, they recently have been characterized and given specific
names.

The mycobacteria potentially pathogenic for man, many of which also affect
animals, are divided into two classes: a) slow growers and b) rapid growers. The
principal slow-growing species are the complex consisting of *M. avium-intracellulare-
scrofulaceum* (MAIS complex), *M. kansasii, M. ulcerans, M. marinum, M. xenopi,
M. szulgai,* and *M. simiae*. Among the fast-growing species are *M. fortuitum* and
M. chelonei (or the *M. fortuitum* complex).

The *M. avium-intracellulare-scrofulaceum* (MAIS) complex is composed of 31
serotypes, which are numbered from 1 to 28 (*M. avium* and *M. intracellulare*) and
from 41 to 43 (*M. scrofulaceum*). In turn, *M. fortuitum* includes two serotypes (1
and 2). Serologic identification of nontuberculous mycobacteria is valuable for
epidemiologic studies and sometimes can indicate the human or animal source of
infection.

Geographic Distribution: Their presence, distribution, and relative importance as a cause of disease have been studied primarily in the more developed countries, where the prevalence of tuberculosis is lower. Some species are distributed worldwide, while others predominate in certain areas. For example, the pulmonary disease in man caused by *M. kansasii* is prevalent in England and Wales in the United Kingdom, and in Kansas City, Chicago, and the state of Texas in the United States. On the other hand, the disease caused by *M. avium-intracellulare* is more frequent in the southeastern United States, western Australia, and Japan (Wolinsky, 1979). Distribution is similar in animals, since the infection comes from the environment. These agents are believed to be a greater problem in hot and humid areas than in temperate and cold climates.

Occurrence in Man: A distinction must be made between colonization and temporary sensitivity, infection, and cases of disease. Since diagnosis depends on the isolation and typing of the etiologic agent, most confirmations come from countries with a good system of laboratories. In Australia, the annual rate of pulmonary infection has been estimated at 1.7 to 4 cases per 100,000 people in Queensland, and 0.5 to 1.2 in the entire country. In the Canadian province of British Columbia, the annual rate for all nontuberculous mycobacterial infections grew from 0.17 to 0.53 per 100,000 people between 1960 and 1972 (Wolinsky, 1979).

In Argentina, 8,006 cultures from 4,894 patients were studied. Of these cultures, nontuberculous mycobacteria were identified in 113 (1.4%), representing 18 cases (0.37% of the total number of patients). The agents isolated were *M. kansasii* in eight cases, MAIS in eight others, *M. marinum* in one case, and a double infection by *M. tuberculosis* and *M. kansasii* in another. The localization was pulmonary in 16 cases and cutaneous in the other two (Di Lonardo *et al.*, 1983).

In Mexico, of 547 cultures from patients diagnosed as tubercular by bacilloscopy, 89.6% were identified as *M. tuberculosis* and 8.9% corresponded to potentially pathogenic nontuberculous mycobacteria, such as *M. fortuitum, M. chelonei, M. scrofulaceum,* and *M. kansasii.*

Occurrence in Animals: The same considerations that apply to man are also valid for animals. The disease has been confirmed in many species of animals, mammals as well as poikilotherms and birds. Among domestic animals, the disease in swine is economically important. Serotypes 1 and 2 of the MAIS complex are the most commonly isolated from swine. These two serotypes are also the ones responsible for avian tuberculosis. Serotype 8 is an important pathogen for animals as well as for man (Thoen, 1981).

The surveillance and identification of mycobacteriosis in animals is mainly carried out in countries where the problem of bovine tuberculosis has been controlled, for example, the United States. This does not mean that mycobacterioses do not exist in other areas, but rather that little information is yet available on the subject.

The Diseases in Man: The most common are a) pulmonary disease, b) lymphadenitis, and c) soft tissue lesions. Other organs and tissues may be affected and in some cases hematogeneous dissemination occurs (Wolinsky, 1979).

a) Chronic pulmonary disease resembling tuberculosis is the most important clinical problem caused by nontuberculous mycobacteria. The most common etiologic agents of this disease are *M. kansasii* and *M. avium-intracellulare; M. xenopi, M. scrofulaceum, M. szulgai, M. simiae,* and *M. fortuitum-chelonei* are found less frequently. As in the case of tuberculosis, the clinical picture varies greatly, ranging from minor lesions to an advanced disease with cavitation. Most of the cases appear in middle-aged people who have preexisting pulmonary lesions (pneumoconiosis, chronic bronchitis, and others). Persons taking immunosuppressant drugs or with acquired immune deficiency are also predisposed. Nevertheless, an appreciable proportion of patients contract the disease without having previous damage to the respiratory or immune systems (Wolinsky, 1979).

b) Mycobacterial lymphadenitis occurs in children from 18 months to 5 years of age. The affected lymph nodes are primarily those of the neck close to the jaw bone, generally on one side only. They soften rapidly and develop openings to the outside. The child's general health is not affected. Calcification and fibrosis occur during the healing process.

In British Columbia, Canada, the morbidity rate was 0.37 per 100,000 people, while that for tubercular lymphadenitis caused by *M. tuberculosis* was only 0.04 per 100,000 per year (Wolinsky, 1979).

The most common etiologic agents are various serotypes of *M. avium-intracellulare*, *M. scrofulaceum*, and *M. kansasii*. The prevalence of each of these mycobacteria varies according to region. Other mycobacteria are isolated from the lesions less often (Wolinsky, 1979).

c) Diseases of the skin and subcutaneous tissue are caused by *M. fortuitum-chelonei*, *M. marinum*, and *M. ulcerans*. They appear clinically as abscesses, cutaneous granulomas, and ulcers.

Localized abscesses ensue especially after injections, surgical interventions, war wounds, thorn penetration, and various traumas.

Granulomas (swimming pool granuloma, fish tank granuloma) develop on the extremities as a group of papules that ulcerate and scab over. Lesions may persist for months. Healing is usually spontaneous. The etiologic agent is *M. marinum (M. balnei)*, which inhabits and multiplies in fresh and salt water. In Glenwood Spring, Colorado (USA), 290 cases of granulomatous lesions were found among children who swam in a pool of tepid mineral water.

Infections caused by *M. ulcerans* occur in many tropical areas of the world, and particularly in central Africa. They start as erythematous nodules on the extremities and gradually become large indolent ulcers with a necrotic base. In Africa this lesion is known as "Buruli ulcer" and in Australia as "Bairnsdale ulcer."

Infections caused by nontuberculous mycobacteria have also been described in the joints, spinal column, urogenital tract, and as osteomyelitis of the sternum after heart operations. A generalized, highly lethal infection occurs mainly in leukemia patients or those undergoing treatment with immunosuppressants, or in patients with acquired immunodeficiency. Generalized infection has been demonstrated in patients with acquired immunodeficiency syndrome (AIDS).

The Diseases in Animals: Many species of mammals and birds are susceptible to nontuberculous mycobacteria. The most important etiologic agents are the different serotypes of the *M. avium-intracellulare* complex. The most frequent clinical form in mammals is lymphadenitis, but other tissues and organs may be affected (Thoen *et al.*, 1981).

CATTLE: In bovines, the most common nontuberculous mycobacterial infection affects the lymph glands. In the United States during the period 1973-1977, nontuberculous mycobacteria were isolated from more than 14% of specimens remitted to the laboratory because tuberculosis was suspected (Thoen *et al.*, 1979).

More than 50% of the isolations corresponded to serotypes 1 and 2 of the *M. avium* complex; the rest primarily consisted of serotypes from the same complex, and only 2.7% were other species, such as *M. fortuitum*, *M. paratuberculosis*, *M. kansasii*, *M. scrofulaceum*, and *M. xenopi*.

In São Paulo, Brazil, attempts at isolations from 28 lesions in cattle and 62 caseous lesions in slaughterhouse carcasses yielded 18 isolations of *M. bovis*, one of *M. tuberculosis*, one of *M. fortuitum,* and one of *M. kansasii* (Correa and Correa, 1973).

Even though nontuberculous mycobacteria usually cause lesions only in lymph nodes, they sometimes give rise to granulomas in other tissues.

The principal problem presented by nontuberculous mycobacteria in bovines lies in paraspecific sensitization for mammalian tuberculin, which causes confusion in diagnosis, as well as unnecessary sacrifice of animals.

SWINE: In swine, infection by *M. avium-intracellulare* causes serious economic losses in many parts of the world, especially through confiscation of animals from slaughterhouses and locker plants. In countries that have carried out successful programs to eradicate bovine tuberculosis, swine confiscated for "tuberculosis" are primarily infected by the *M. avium-intracellulare* complex. Serotypes 1, 2, 4, 5, and 8 of this complex are the principal causes of mycobacterial infection of hogs in the United States (Songer *et al.*, 1980). Serotype 8, especially, has caused outbreaks with great losses in several countries, including the United States, Japan, and South Africa. Lesions in these animals are usually restricted to cervical and mediastinal lymph glands, that is, near the digestive tract. Generalized lesions are usually caused by *M. bovis*, but nontuberculous mycobacteria may sometimes be responsible. In addition to the different *M. avium-intracellulare* complex serotypes, other nontuberculous mycobacteria, among them *M. kansasii* and *M. fortuitum,* have been isolated from swine. Recently, strains similar to *M. fortuitum* but differing in several biochemical characteristics were isolated from swine with lymphadenitis (Tsukamura *et al.*, 1983); the name *M. porcinum* has been proposed for these strains.

Bacteria belonging to the *M. avium-intracellulare* complex can at times be isolated from the lymph nodes of a large proportion of apparently healthy animals inspected at slaughterhouses (Brown and Neuman, 1979).

CATS AND DOGS: In cats, nodular lesions, with or without fistulation, are seen in the cutaneous and subcutaneous tissues, primarily on the venter. Among the mycobacteria identified is *M. fortuitum;* on one occasion, *M. xenopi* was also found. This disease should be distinguished from "cat leprosy," the etiologic agent of which is *M. lepraemurium* and which is possibly transmitted by rat bite. The cutaneous and subcutaneous nodules of "leprosy" can localize in any part of the body (White *et al.*, 1983). Skin infections caused by nontuberculous mycobacteria also occur in dogs.

OTHER SPECIES: In addition to infections caused by tuberculosis mycobacteria (*M. tuberculosis* and *M. bovis*), which are prevalent, nontuberculous mycobacterial infections by different serotypes of the *M. avium-intracellulare* complex also occur in nonhuman primates kept in colonies or in zoos. The infection is predominantly intestinal and manifests itself clinically as diarrhea and emaciation. Lesions in these animals differ from those caused by *M. tuberculosis* and M. *bovis* in that tubercles do not form and necrosis and giant cells are absent. The lamina propria of the intestine is infiltrated by epithelioid cells (Thoen *et al.*, 1981).

Nontuberculous mycobacterial infection also occurs in other species of animals kept in captivity. In cold-blooded animals, the disease may be caused by several species of mycobacteria, such as *M. chelonei*, *M. marinum*, *M. fortuitum*, and *M. avium*.

Recently, an infection caused by *M. ulcerans* in koalas (*Phascolarctos cinereus*) on Raymond Island, Australia, was described (Mitchell and Johnson, 1981). The animals manifested ulcers on the flexor muscles of the extremities. This is the first confirmation of *M. ulcerans* infection in animals other than man.

Disease among aquarium or aquiculture fish may be caused by several mycobacteria, especially *M. marinum* and *M. fortuitum*. Clinical signs vary and resemble those of other diseases, with emaciation, ascites, dermal ulcerations, hemorrhages, exophthalmos, and skeletal deformities. Necropsy discloses grayish white necrotic foci in the viscera. Exposure to *M. marinum* from aquarium fish can cause skin infections in man (Leibovitz, 1980; Martin, 1981).

Unculturable mycobacteria that can be confused with *M. leprae* have been found in several species of animals, such as frogs from Bolivia (*Pleurodema cinerea* and *P. marmoratus*) and water buffaloes in Indonesia (*Bubalus bubalis*). Owing to recently confirmed natural infection by *M. leprae* in the nine-banded armadillo (*Dasypus novemcinctus*) and in two nonhuman primate species (see Leprosy, Natural Infection in Animals), interest has been aroused by an agent that cannot be distinguished from *M. leprae* of human origin.

In the province of Buenos Aires, the lymph nodes of 67 apparently normal armadillos were cultured. Potentially pathogenic mycobacterial strains were isolated from 22 (53.7%) of 41 hairy armadillos (*Chaetophractus villosus*) examined. These strains included *M. intracellulare*, *M. fortuitum*, and *M. chelonei*. Mycobacterial cultures were not obtained from 26 *Dasypus hybridus* armadillos ("mulitas") (Kantor, 1978).

To avoid errors, leprologists doing experimental work with armadillos must take into account both identified mycobacteria from these animals as well as those insufficiently characterized to be identified (Resoagli *et al.*, 1982).

FOWL: Avian tuberculosis is due to *M. avium* serotypes 1, 2, and 3. Serotype 2 is the most common in chickens, and serotype 1 in wild or captive birds in the United States (Thoen *et al.*, 1981). The lesions are found mainly in the liver, spleen, intestine, and bone marrow, and infrequently in the lungs and kidneys. Avian tuberculosis is common; it has a high incidence on farms where chickens have been kept many years and the enclosures and grounds are contaminated. *M. avium* can survive in the soil for several years. In industrial establishments the infection is rare because of the rapid replacement of fowl, maintenance conditions, and hygienic measures.

Turkeys can contract tuberculosis by living in association with infected chickens. Ducks and geese are not very susceptible to *M. avium*.

The disease has been observed in several species of wild birds. It may affect any species kept in zoos. Among birds kept as family pets, tuberculosis infections have been found in parrots, with *M. tuberculosis* as the etiologic agent causing infection localized on the skin and in the natural orifices. This situation is exceptional among fowl.

Source of Infection and Mode of Transmission: Man and animals contract the infection from environmental sources, such as water, soil, and dust. Intrahuman transmission has never been reliably proved. *M. fortuitum* abounds in nature and the ability of this mycobacterium as well as *M. chelonei* to multiply in the soil has been confirmed experimentally. The natural hosts of the serotypes 1, 2, and 3 of *M. avium* are fowl. Other serotypes of the MAIS complex have been isolated repeatedly from water. In a recent study (Gruft *et al.*, 1981), MAIS complex bacteria were isolated from 25% of 250 water samples collected along the eastern coast of the US, predominantly from the warm waters of the southern part of the coast. Similarly, isolations were more abundant from estuarine water samples than from river or sea water. During this study *M. intracellulare* was isolated from aerosols, which would explain the method of transmission to man. Various serotypes of *M. avium-intracellulare-scrofulaceum* were isolated from soil and house dust in research carried out in Australia and Japan. *M. kansasii* and *M. xenopi* were isolated from drinking water supplies. The habitat of *M. marinum* is water, and it has been isolated from snails, sand, and infected aquarium fish.

The human pulmonary infections are probably contracted through the respiratory tract by means of aerosols. On the other hand, the location of affected lymph nodes suggests that lymphadenitis in man, bovines, and swine is contracted through the intestinal tract. Mycobacteria causing abscesses, cutaneous granulomas, and ulcers penetrate through skin lesions.

Avian tuberculosis is transmitted via the intestinal tract by contaminated food, soil, and water.

Role of Animals in the Epidemiology of the Diseases: Mycobacteriosis is not a zoonosis but a disease common to man and animals. Both acquire the infection from environmental sources.

M. avium-intracellulare often can be isolated from the macroscopically normal lymph nodes of swine, and a study was carried out to determine if the human disease was related to eating pork from these animals. When students who had consumed the pork and those who had not were given the tuberculin test with *M. intracellulare* PPD, there was no significant difference in the sensitivity of these two groups (Brown and Tollison, 1979).

Diagnosis: Although radiologic examination may suggest that the human pulmonary disease was caused by nontuberculous mycobacteria, diagnosis can only be made by culturing and identifying the causal agent. The possibility of environmental contamination of the culture medium should be taken into account. Also, the sputum, gastric juice, or saliva from healthy individuals may contain saprophytic mycobacteria as well as *M. intracellulare* and *M. fortuitum*. Repeated cultures with abundant growth of a potentially pathogenic species of *Mycobacterium* that was isolated from a patient with symptoms compatible with the disease should be considered significant. Diagnosis is certain when nontuberculous mycobacteria are isolated from biopsy specimens. Differential diagnosis between nontuberculous mycobacterial and pulmonary tuberculosis infections (*M. tuberculosis*, *M. bovis*, and *M. africanum*) is important, since *M. avium-intracellulare* is naturally resistant to antituberculosis medications, while *M. kansasii* is sensitive to rifampin and mildly resistant to other medications (Wolinsky, 1979). The other common forms of nontuberculous mycobacterial infections are less difficult to diagnose.

Infection in bovines and swine is usually diagnosed by culturing lymph nodes obtained from a slaughterhouse or locker.

Clinical diagnosis of avian tuberculosis can be confirmed by necropsy and laboratory procedures. The avian tuberculin test on the wattle is also useful for diagnosing the disease on the farm.

The enzyme-linked immunoassay test (ELISA) has good sensitivity for detecting mycobacterial antibodies in swine, fowl, bovines, and other animals (Thoen *et al.*, 1981).

Control: Prevention of the pulmonary disease in man would consist of the removal of environmental sources of infection, which are difficult to recognize. Consequently, the recommended alternative is prevention and treatment of predisposing causes. Specific measures for preventing lymphadenitis in children are not available either. On the other hand, proper skin care, adequate treatment of wounds, and avoidance of contaminated swimming pools can prevent dermal and subcutaneous tissue infections.

The source of infection in swine affected by lymphadenitis was determined on several occasions, such as in cases described in Australia, the United States, and Germany (Songer *et al.*, 1980). When other materials were substituted for sawdust and shavings used as bedding, the problem disappeared.

The control of avian tuberculosis should be centered above all on the farms. Given the long-term survival of *M. avium* in the environment contaminated with the droppings of tubercular fowl, the only remedy is to eliminate all existing birds on a farm and repopulate with new stock in an area not previously inhabited by fowl.

Similar measures are needed to control mycobacteriosis in fish. Infected fish should be destroyed and the aquarium disinfected. In addition, the introduction of contaminated fish or products should be avoided.

Bibliography

Acland, H. M., and R. H. Whitlock. *Mycobacterium avium* serotype 4 infection of swine: the attempted transmission by contact and the sequence of morphological changes in inoculated pigs. *J Comp Pathol* 96:247-266, 1986.

Blancarte, M., B. Campos, and S. Serna Villanueva. Micobacterias atípicas en la República Mexicana. *Salud Pública Méx* 24:329-340, 1982.

Brown, J., and M. A. Neuman. Lesions of swine lymph nodes as a diagnostic test to determine mycobacterial infection. *Appl Environ Microbiol* 37:740-743, 1979.

Brown, J., and J. W. Tollison. Influence of pork consumption on human infection with *Mycobacterium avium-intracellulare*. *Appl Environ Microbiol* 38:1144-1146, 1979.

Correa, C. N., and W. M. Correa. Micobacterias isoladas de bovinos e suinos em São Paulo, Brasil. *Arq Inst Biol (São Paulo)* 40:205-208, 1973.

Di Lonardo, M., N. C. Isola, M. Ambroggi, G. Fulladosa, and I. N. de Kantor. Enfermedad producida por micobacterias no tuberculosas en Buenos Aires, Argentina. *Bol Of Sanit Panam* 95:134-141, 1983.

Fry, K. L., D. S. Meissuer, and J. O. Falkinham III. Epidemiology of infection of nontuberculous mycobacteria. IV. Identification and use of epidemiologic markers for studies of *Mycobacterium avium*, *M. intracellulare* and *M. scrofulaceum*. *Am Rev Resp Dis* 134:39-43, 1986.

Gruft, H., J. O. Falkinham III, and B. C. Parker. Recent experience in the epidemiology of disease caused by atypical mycobacteria. *Rev Infect Dis* 3:990-996, 1981.

Kantor, I. N. de. Isolation of mycobacteria from two species of armadillos, *Dasypus hybridus* ("mulita") and *Chaetophractus villosus* ("peludo"). *In*: *The Armadillo as an Experimental Model in Biomedical Research*. Washington, D.C., Pan American Health Organization, 1978. (Scientific Publication 366.)

Leibovitz, L. Fish tuberculosis (mycobacteriosis). *J Am Vet Med Assoc* 176:415, 1980.

Martin, A. A. Mycobacteriosis: a brief review of a fish-transmitted zoonosis. *In*: Fowler, M. F. (Ed.), *Wildlife Diseases of the Pacific Basin and Other Countries*. 4th International Conference of the Wildlife Diseases Association, Sydney, Australia, 1981.

Mitchell, P., and D. Johnson. The recovery of *Mycobacterium ulcerans* from koalas in east Gippsland. *In*: Fowler, M. F. (Ed.), *Wildlife Diseases of the Pacific Basin and Other Countries*. 4th International Conference of the Wildlife Diseases Association, Sydney, Australia, 1981.

Resoagli, E., A. Martínez, J. P. Resoagli, S. G. de Millán, M. I. O. de Rott, and M. Ramírez. Micobacteriosis natural en armadillos, similar a la lepra humana. *Gac Vet (B Aires)* 44:671 676, 1982

Songer, J. G., E. J. Bicknell, and C. O. Thoen. Epidemiological Investigation of swine tuberculosis in Arizona. *Can J Comp Med* 44:115-120, 1980.

Thoen, C. O., E. M. Himes, W. D. Richards, and J. L. Harrington, Jr. Bovine tuberculosis in the United States and Puerto Rico. *Am J Vet Res* 40:118-120, 1979.

Thoen, C. O., A. G. Karlson, and E. M. Himes. Mycobacterial infections in animals. *Rev Infect Dis* 3:960-972, 1981.

Tsukamura, M., H. Nemoto, and H. Yugi. *Mycobacterium porcinum* sp. nov. a porcine pathogen. *Int J Syst Bacteriol* 33:162-165, 1983.

White, S. D., P. J. Ihrke, A. A. Stannard, C. Cadmus, C. Griffin, S. A. Kruth, E. J. Rosser, S. I. Reinke, and S. Jang. Cutaneous atypical mycobacteriosis in cats. *J Am Vet Med Assoc* 182:1218-1222, 1983.

Wolinsky, E. Nontuberculous mycobacteria and associated diseases. *Am Rev Resp Dis* 119:107-159, 1979.

ENTEROCOLITIC YERSINIOSIS

(027.8)

Etiology: *Yersinia enterocolitica* (*Bacterium enterocoliticum*), a gram-negative coccobacillus that is motile at 25°C and belongs to the family Enterobacteriaceae. This species includes a heterogeneous group of bacteria that differ a great deal in their biochemical properties.

For epidemiologic purposes the species has been subdivided into five biotypes and 34 serotypes. Serotyping is based on the somatic antigens (O). Most of the isolations from man have been serotypes O:3 and O:9, but the predominant serotype varies geographically. Type 3 predominates in Europe with type 9 in second place, while in the United States the predominant serotype is 8 with 5 in second place.

Geographic Distribution: Worldwide. The agent has been isolated from animals, man, foodstuffs, and water. The human disease has been confirmed on five continents and in more than 30 countries (Swaminathan *et al.*, 1982).

Occurrence in Man: There are marked differences in disease incidence between different regions and even between neighboring countries. The highest incidence rates are observed in Scandinavia, Belgium, several eastern European countries, Japan, South Africa, and Canada. On the other hand, the disease is less common in the United States, Great Britain, and France. In Belgium the agent was isolated from 3,167 patients between 1963 and 1978, with isolations increasing in the last three of those years. Of the strains isolated, 84% belonged to serotype 3, but serotype 9 rose in prevalence in more recent years (de Groote *et al.*, 1982). In Canada from 1966 to 1977, 1,000 isolations (serotype 3) were made from human patients, while in the United States from 1973 to 1976, 68 cases occurred and serotype 8 was predominant. Approximately 1 to 3% of acute enteritis cases in Sweden, the Federal Republic of Germany, Belgium, and Canada are caused by *Y. enterocolitica* (World Health Organization Scientific Working Group, 1980). Lack of laboratory facilities hinders knowledge of the disease incidence in developing countries. In tropical areas, *Y. enterocolitica* seems to be a minor cause of diarrhea (Mata and Simhon, 1982).

Most cases are sporadic or show up as small, familial outbreaks, but several epidemics have also been described. Three of these outbreaks occurred in Japan in 1972 and affected children and adolescents, with 189 cases in one, 198 in another, and 544 in the third. The source of infection could not be determined. In 1976, an outbreak in the state of New York affected 218 schoolchildren. The source of the infection was thought to be chocolate milk (possibly owing to contaminated chocolate syrup). An outbreak in 1982 in the United States affected three states (Tennessee, Arkansas, and Mississippi) and caused 172 patients to be hospitalized. From these patients were isolated serotypes 13 and 18 of *Y. enterocolitica*, serotypes that are very uncommon in the US. Statistical association indicated milk from a single processing plant as the source (Tacket *et al.*, 1984).

In Europe most cases occur in fall and winter, and in South Africa, from December to May.

Occurrence in Animals: *Y. enterocolitica* has been isolated from a great many domestic and wild mammals, as well as from some birds and cold-blooded animals. The serotypes isolated from most species of animals differ from those in man. Important exceptions are swine, dogs, and cats, from which serotypes 3 and 9, the most prevalent causes of the human infection in many countries, have been isolated. In addition, serotype 5 was found in swine and is common in people in Japan (Hurvell, 1981).

In some countries the rate of isolations from animals is very high. In Belgium, serotypes that affect man were isolated from 62.5% of pork tongues collected from butchers (de Groote *et al.*, 1982), and studies done in Belgium and Denmark revealed that 3 to 5% of swine carry the agent in their intestines.

The Disease in Man: *Y. enterocolitica* is mainly a human pathogen that usually affects children. The predominant symptom in small children is an acute enteritis with watery diarrhea lasting 3 to 14 days; blood is present in the stool in 5% of the cases. In older children and adolescents, the pseudoappendicitis syndrome predominates, with pain in the right iliac fossa, fever, moderate leukocytosis and a high rate of erythrosedimentation. The great similarity to acute appendicitis has sometimes led to surgery. In adults, especially in those over 40 years of age, an erythema nodosum may develop 1 to 2 weeks after enteritis. It goes away completely in almost all those affected, 80% of whom are women. Reactive arthritis of one or more joints is a more serious complication. About 100 cases of septicemia have been described, mainly in Europe. Other complications may be present, but are much rarer.

Of 1,700 patients with *Y. enterocolitica* infection in Belgium, 86% had gastroenteritis, nearly 10% had the pseudoappendicitis syndrome, and less than 1% had septicemia and hepatic abscesses (Swaminathan *et al.*, 1982).

An epidemic with 172 cases occurred in the United States in 1982 and was attributed to pasteurized milk. Of these patients, 86% had enteritis, and 14% had extraintestinal infections localized in the throat, blood, urinary tract, peritoneum, central nervous system, and wounds. Extraintestinal infections were more common in adults. In patients with enteritis, mostly children, the disease caused fever (92.7%), abdominal pains (86.3%), diarrhea (82.7%), vomiting (41.4%), sore throat (22.2%), cutaneous eruptions (22.2%), bloody stool (19.7%), and joint pain (15.1%). The last symptom was seen only in patients 3 years of age or older (Tacket *et al.*, 1984).

The Disease in Animals: In the 1960s several epizootics in chinchillas occurred in Europe, the United States, and Mexico, with many cases of septicemia and high mortality; these outbreaks were originally attributed to *Pasteurella pseudotuberculosis*, but the agent was later determined to be *Y. enterocolitica*, serotype 1 (biotype 3), which has never been isolated from man. The principal clinical symptoms consisted of sialorrhea, diarrhea, and loss of weight. In the same period, cases of septicemia were described in hares, from which serotype 2 (biotype 5) was isolated; this serotype also does not affect man. *Y. enterocolitica* has been isolated from several species of wild animals, in some of which intestinal lesions or hepatic abscesses were found. In Czechoslovakia and the Scandinavian countries, *Y. enterocolitica* has been isolated from 3 to 26% of wild rodents, but necropsy of these animals revealed no lesions. Similar results were obtained in the south of Chile, where the agent was isolated from 4% of 305 rodents of different species and from different habitats (Zamora *et al.*, 1979). Serotypes isolated from rodents are generally not those pathogenic for man.

Studies carried out on swine, dogs, and cats are of particular interest, since these animals harbor serotypes that infect man. The agent has been isolated from clinically healthy swine and from animals destined for human consumption. In one study, a much higher rate of isolations was obtained from swine with diarrhea than from apparently healthy animals. In another study, however, the agent was isolated from 17% of healthy swine and from 5.4% of swine tested because of various symptoms (Hurvell, 1981). Swine carrying serotypes of *Y. enterocolitica* that infect man have been observed principally in countries where incidence of the human disease is high, such as Scandinavia, Belgium, Canada, and Japan. The isolation rate from swine varies from one herd to another and depends on the degree of contamination of each establishment. On one farm the agent may be isolated only sporadically and at a low rate, while on another, isolations may be continuous and reach 100% of the groups examined (Fukushima *et al.*, 1981).

Serotypes of *Y. enterocolitica* were isolated from 5.5% of 451 dogs in Japan (Kaneko *et al.*, 1977), and from 1.7% of 115 dogs in Denmark (Pedersen, 1979). In contrast, the incidence of canine carriers in the United States and Canada is low. The disease seems to occur rarely in dogs, but it should be borne in mind that many clinical cases are not diagnosed because isolation is not attempted. In two cases of enteritis recently described in Canada, the dogs manifested neither fever nor abdominal pains, but they experienced frequent defecations covered with mucous and blood. The agent was isolated in both cases (Papageorges and Gosselin, 1983). *Y. enterocolitica* has also been isolated from apparently healthy cats.

Source of Infection and Mode of Transmission (Figure 10): The epidemiology of enterocolitic yersiniosis is not yet well understood. The agent is widespread in water, foods, many animal species, and man. Of greater interest is the fact that the serotypes isolated from water and food often do not correspond to the types that produce disease in man. This is also true of the serotypes found in the majority of

**Figure 10. Enterocolitic yersiniosis (*Yersinia enterocolitica*).
Supposed mode of transmission.**

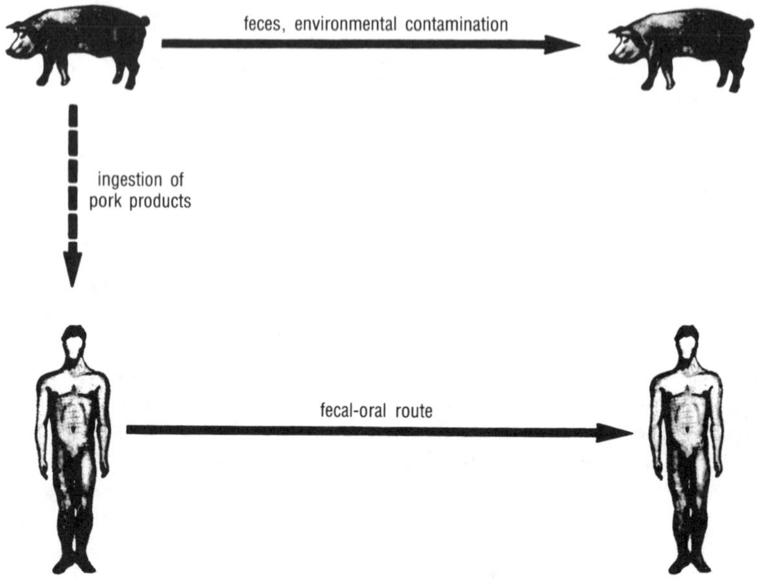

animal species, with the exceptions of pigs and, to some extent, dogs and cats. In countries with the highest incidence of human disease, pigs are frequently carriers of serotypes pathogenic for man. By contrast, in those countries where the incidence of human disease is low, such as the United States and Great Britain, serotypes pathogenic for man are rarely isolated (Wooley *et al.*, 1980; Brewer and Corbel, 1983).

Research carried out in Scandinavia, Canada, and South Africa strongly suggests that the probable reservoir of the agent is swine. In other countries, however, the reservoir is still unknown. Serotype 8, which predominates in the United States, was isolated from two of 95 asymptomatic individuals after an outbreak in New York State due to chocolate milk and caused by the same serotype. Serotype 8 was isolated from water and foods in Czechoslovakia, but no human cases were seen (Aldova *et al.*, 1981). Small nosocomial outbreaks indicate that human-to-human transmission is also possible. Some familial outbreaks were attributed to exposure to dogs. Nevertheless, dogs and cats are not considered to be important reservoirs.

The mode of transmission is not well known either, but it is widely accepted that the infection is contracted by ingestion of contaminated foodstuffs, as in the case of other enterobacterial diseases, as well as by contact with carrier animals and by human-to-human transmission. Even though pasteurization usually kills the agent, pasteurized milk can be a source of infection because some of the bacteria may survive if they were originally present in large numbers. In addition, *Y. enterocolitica* can multiply at refrigeration temperature. These factors are believed to have led to the 1982 epidemic in the United States (see Occurrence in Man) produced by pasteurized milk. This epidemic also reveals that serotypes other than 3, 5, 8, and 9 can give rise to the disease, though less commonly.

The Role of Animals in the Epidemiology of the Disease: Although not providing definitive proof, the accumulated data in countries with a high incidence of the human disease indicate that swine are probably an important reservoir of *Y. enterocolitica*.

Diagnosis: The agent can be isolated from the feces of patients; both biotype and serotype should be identified. The cold enrichment technique is useful, especially in the case of carriers, who may excrete few cells of *Y. enterocolitica*. To this end, samples are suspended in peptone culture broth or a buffered phosphate solution for 3 to 7 days at 4°C to encourage the growth of *Y. enterocolitica* and inhibit that of other bacteria. In cases of erythema nodosum, reactive arthritis, or suspected appendicitis, the possibility of *Y. enterocolitica* infection should be considered.

The serum agglutination test and, more recently, enzyme-linked immunosorbent assay (ELISA) can be employed with good results as additional diagnosis techniques. Active infections produce high titers, which decline with time. In countries where *Y. enterocolitica* serotype 9 is a common pathogen for man and is also harbored by swine, cross-reaction between *Brucella* and that serotype may cause difficulties.

Antibodies in swine against serotype 9 of *Y. enterocolitica* can be differentiated from those against *Brucella* by using flagellar antigens, which *Y. enterocolitica* has and brucellae do not. *Y. enterocolitica* also possesses the common enterobacterial antigen, which *Brucella* does not have and which therefore may also be used (Mittal *et al.*, 1984). Other animals that have been exposed to serotype 9 can also show cross-reactions with *Brucella*.

Control: For the present, observance of food hygiene rules constitutes the only measure that can be recommended.

Bibliography

Aldova, E., J. Sobotková, A. Brezinova, J. Cerna, M. Janeckova, J. Pegrimkova, and V. Pokorna. *Yersinia enterocolitica* in water and food. *Zentralbl Bakteriol Mikrobiol Hyg* [*B*] 173:464-470, 1981.

Brewer, R. A., and M. J. Corbel. Characterization of *Yersinia enterocolitica* strains isolated from cattle, sheep and pigs in the United Kingdom. *J Hyg (Camb)* 90:425-433, 1983.

Das, A. M., V. L. Paranjape, and S. Winblad. *Yersinia enterocolitica* associated with third trimester abortion in buffaloes. *Trop Anim Health Prod* 18:109-112, 1986.

De Groote G., J. Vandepitte, and G. Wauters. Surveillance of human *Yersinia enterocolitica* infection in Belgium: 1963-1978. *J Infect* 4:189-197, 1982.

Delmas, C. L., and D. J. Vidon. Isolation of *Yersinia enterocolitica* and related species from foods in France. *Appl Environ Microbiol* 50:767-771, 1985.

Fukushima, H., R. Nakamura, Y. Ito, and K. Saito. Ecological studies of *Yersinia enterocolitica* I. Dissemination of *Y. enterocolitica* in pigs. *Vet Microbiol* 8:469-483, 1983.

Hurvell, B. Zoonotic *Yersinia enterocolitica* infection: host range, clinical manifestations, and transmission between animals and man. *In*: E. J. Bottone (Ed.), *Yersinia enterocolitica*. Boca Raton, Florida, CRC Press, 1981.

Kaneko, K., S. Hamada, and E. Kato. Occurrence of *Yersinia enterocolitica* in dogs. *Jpn J Vet Sci* 39:407-414, 1977.

Kaneuchi, C., K. Shishido, M. Shibuya, Y. Yamaguchi, and M. Ogata. Prevalences of *Campylobacter, Yersinia*, and *Salmonella* in cats housed in an animal protection center. *Jpn J Vet Sci* 49:499-506, 1987.

Kawaoka, Y., K. Otsuk, T. Mitani, T. Kubota, and M. Tsubokura. Migratory waterfowl as flying reservoirs of Yersinia species. *Res Vet Sci* 37, 1984.

Mata, L., and A. Simhon. Enteritis y colitis infecciosas del hombre. *Adel Microbiol Enferm Infecc (B Aires)* 1:1-50, 1982.

Mittal, K. R., I. R. Tizard, and D. A. Barnum. Serological cross-reactions between *Brucella abortus* and *Yersinia enterocolitica* O9. *International Symposium on Human and Animal Brucellosis.* Taipei, Taiwan, 1984.

Papageorges, M., and Y. Gosselin. *Yersinia enterocolitica* enteritis in two dogs. *J Am Vet Med Assoc* 182:618-619, 1983.

Pedersen, K. B., and S. Winblad. Studies of *Yersinia enterocolitica* isolated from swine and dogs. *Acta Pathol Microbiol Scand B*87:137-140, 1979.

Swaminathan, B., M. C. Harmon, and I. J. Mehlman. *Yersinia enterocolitica. J Appl Bacteriol* 52:151-183, 1982.

Tacket, C. O., J. P. Narain, R. Sattin, J. P. Lofgren, C. Konigsberg, R. C. Rendorff, A. Rausa, B. R. Davis, and M. L. Cohen. A multistate outbreak of infections caused by *Yersinia enterocolitica* transmitted by pasteurized milk. *JAMA* 251:483-486, 1984.

Wooley, R. E., E. B. Shotts, and J. W. Connell. Isolation of *Yersinia enterocolitica* from selected animal species. *Am J Vet Res* 41:1667-1668, 1980.

World Health Organization Scientific Working Group. Enteric infections due to *Campylobacter, Yersinia, Salmonella*, and *Shigella. Bull WHO* 58:519-537, 1980.

Zamora, J., O. Alonso, and E. Chahuán. Isolement et caracterisation de *Yersinia enterocolitica* chez les rongeurs sauvages du Chili. *Zentralbl Veterinarmed B*26:392-396, 1979.

GLANDERS

(024)

Synonyms: Farcy (cutaneous glanders), equine nasal phthisis, maliasmus.

Etiology: *Pseudomonas (Malleomyces, Actinobacillus) mallei*, a nonmotile, gram-positive bacillus; it is not very resistant to environmental conditions and can survive only about 1 or 2 months outside the animal host.

Geographic Distribution: At one time the disease was distributed worldwide. It was eradicated in Europe and the Americas, but foci reappeared in 1965 in Greece, Romania, and Brazil (Food and Agriculture Organization of the United Nations *et al.*, 1972). The present distribution is not well known, but there are indications that it persists in some African and Asian countries; Mongolia is or was the area of greatest incidence.

Occurrence in Man: At present the disease in man is exceptional. Attenuated strains of *P. mallei* are found in Asia, where the infection persists.

Occurrence in Animals: According to various sources, incidence in solipeds is now low in Burma, China, India, Indonesia, Vietnam, and Thailand, and the disease is seen only occasionally. Sporadic cases used to occur in Pakistan and, rarely, in Iran. In June 1982, 826 foci with 1,808 cases were reported in solipeds in Turkey, and in 1984, 274 foci were reported (International Office of Epizootics, 1982,

1984). The incidence in Mongolia is believed to be high. The present situation in Ethiopia and the Central African Republic is not known, but cases have occurred in these countries in the past few years. The most recent information available is from the *Animal Health Yearbook* (Food and Agriculture Organization of the United Nations *et al.*, 1985) and *World Animal Health, Animal Health Status and Disease Control Methods, 1986* (International Office of Epizootics, 1987). In the period 1984-86, the following countries reported the continued, though rare, occurrence of this disease: Turkey, Afghanistan, India, Burma, Swaziland, Senegal, Lebanon, Iraq, Nepal, Mauritania, Indonesia, Pakistan, and Sudan.

The Disease in Man: The period of incubation is usually from 1 to 14 days. Cases of latent infection that became clinically evident after many years have been described. The disease course may be either chronic or acute. Similarly, subclinical infections have been discovered during autopsy.

In man as well as in animals, *P. mallei* tends to localize in the lungs and mucosa of the nose, larynx, and trachea. The disease is manifested clinically as pneumonia, bronchopneumonia, or lobar pneumonia, with or without bacteremia. Pulmonary abscesses may occur, as well as pleural effusion and empyema. In the acute disease, there is mucopurulent discharge from the nose, and in chronic processes, granulomatous nodular lesions are found in the lungs.

Ulcers appear in the nostrils and may also be found in the pharynx. Cellulitis with vesiculation, ulceration, lymphangitis, and lymphadenopathy is seen on the skin at the etiologic agent's point of entry. Mortality in clinical cases is high.

The Disease in Animals: Glanders is primarily a disease of solipeds. The disease course is predominantly chronic in horses and almost always acute in asses and mules. The acute form results in high fever, depression, dyspnea, diarrhea, and rapid loss of weight. The animal dies in a few weeks. The chronic form may last years; some animals recover, others die.

Chronic glanders is characterized by three clinical forms, occurring alone or simultaneously: pulmonary glanders, upper respiratory tract disease, and cutaneous glanders.

Pulmonary glanders can remain inapparent for lengthy periods. When clinical symptoms do appear, they consist of intermittent fever, cough, depression, and weight loss. In more advanced stages there is dyspnea with rales. Pulmonary lesions consist of nodules or pneumonic foci. The nodules are grayish white with red borders; in time, the center becomes caseous and soft, or undergoes calcification and becomes surrounded by grayish granulated or whitish fibrous tissue.

The upper respiratory disease is characterized by ulcerations of the mucous membrane (necrosis of the nodules is the initial lesion) of one or both nostrils and frequently of the larynx and trachea. The ulcers have a grayish center with thick, jagged borders. There is a mucous or mucopurulent discharge from one or both nostrils that forms dark scabs around them.

The cutaneous form (farcy) begins with superficial or deep nodules; these later become ulcers that have a gray center and excrete a thick, oily liquid that incrusts the hair. The lymph vessels form visible cords, and the lymph nodes are swollen.

Most authors consider upper respiratory glanders and cutaneous glanders as secondary forms of pulmonary glanders.

In zoos and circuses, carnivores have contracted glanders as a consequence of eating meat from infected solipeds.

Source of Infection and Mode of Transmission (Figure 11): Man contracts the infection by contact with sick solipeds, especially those kept in crowded conditions such as army stables. The portals of entry are the skin and the nasal and ocular mucosas. Nasal discharges, skin ulcer secretions, and contaminated objects constitute the source of infection.

Solipeds acquire the infection from conspecifics, mainly via the digestive route, but probably also through inhalation and wound infection.

Role of Animals in the Epidemiology of the Disease: The reservoir of *P. mallei* is solipeds. The great epizootics of glanders have occurred in metropolitan stables, especially during wartime. Horses with chronic or latent infection are responsible for maintaining the disease in an establishment or region, and their movement from one place to another contributes to its spread. Man and carnivores are accidental hosts.

Diagnosis: Diagnosis of glanders is based on a) bacteriologic examinations by means of culture or inoculation into hamsters of nasal or skin secretions or tissue from internal organs, especially the lungs; b) allergenic test with mallein (the intrapalpebral test is preferred); and c) serologic tests, especially complement fixation. Although this last test is considered specific, false positives have occurred.

Control: Prevention in humans consists primarily of eradication of the infection in solipeds. Greatly improved diagnostic methods have made successful eradication campaigns possible, as have the disappearance of stables from cities and the almost complete substitution of automobiles for horses. Eradication procedures consist of

Figure 11. Glanders. Mode of transmission.

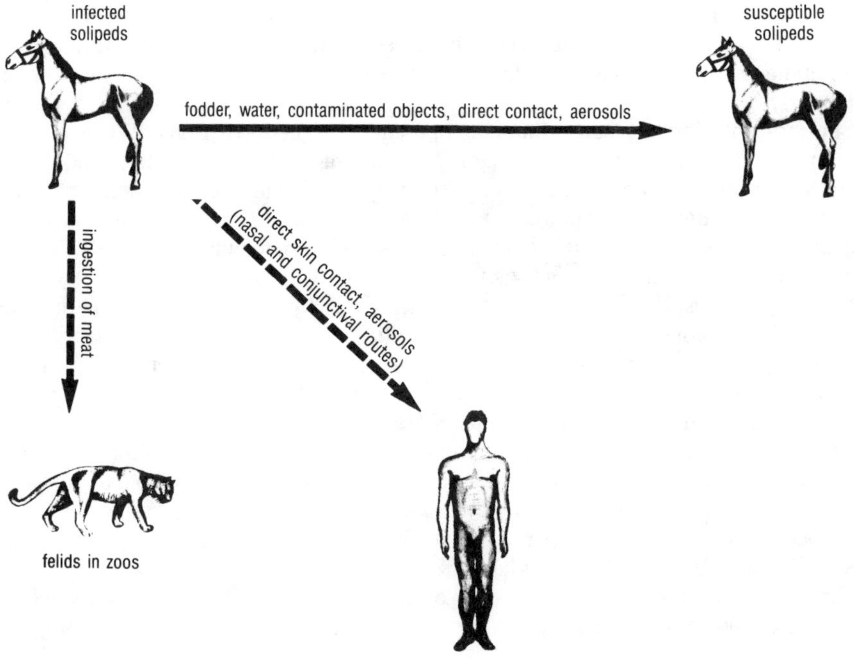

identification of infected animals with allergenic or serologic tests, and sacrifice of reactors. Installations and equipment must then be disinfected.

Bibliography

Blood, D. C., and J. A. Henderson. *Veterinary Medicine*, 4th ed. Baltimore, Maryland, Williams and Wilkins, 1974.

Bruner, D. W., and J. H. Gillespie. *Hagan's Infectious Diseases of Domestic Animals*, 6th ed. Ithaca, New York, Cornell University Press, 1973.

Cluff, L. E. Diseases caused by *Malleomyces*. *In*: Beeson, P., B. W. McDermott, and J. B. Wyngaarden (Eds.), *Cecil Textbook of Medicine*, 15th ed. Philadelphia and London, Saunders, 1979.

Food and Agriculture Organization of the United Nations/World Health Organization/International Office of Epizootics. *Animal Health Yearbook*. Rome, FAO, 1972.

Food and Agriculture Organization of the United Nations/World Health Organization/International Office of Epizootics. *Animal Health Yearbook, 1984*. Rome, FAO, 1985.

Hipólito, O., M. L. G. Freitas, and J. B. Figuereido. *Doenças Infeto-Contagiosas dos Animais Domésticos*, 4th ed. São Paulo, Melhoramentos, 1965.

International Office of Epizootics. *Enfermedades animales señaladas a la OIE, Estadísticas 1982*. Paris, OIE, 1982.

International Office of Epizootics. *World Animal Health, Animal Health Status and Disease Control Methods, 1986*. Paris, OIE, 1987.

Langeneger, J., J. Dobereiner, and A. C. Lima. Foco de mormo (Malleus) na região de Campos. Estado do Rio de Janeiro. *Arq Inst Biol Anim* 3:91-108, 1960.

Oudar, J., L. Dhennu, L. Joubert, A. Richard, J. C. Coutard, J. C. Proy, and F. Caillere. A propos d'un recent foyer de morve du cheval en France. *Bull Soc Sci Vet Med Comp (Lyon)* 67:309-317, 1965.

Van der Schaaf, and A. Malleus. *In*: Van der Hoeden, J. (Ed.), *Zoonoses*. Amsterdam, Elsevier, 1964.

Van Goidsenhoven, C., and F. Schoenaers. *Maladies Infectieuses des Animaux Domestiques*. Liège, Belgium, Desoer, 1960.

LEPROSY

NATURAL INFECTION OF ANIMALS BY *MYCOBACTERIUM LEPRAE*

(030)

Synonym: Hansen's disease.

Etiology: *Mycobacterium leprae*, a polymorphic acid-alcohol-fast bacillus that up to now has been impossible to culture on artificial laboratory media. *M. leprae* is hard to distinguish from other unculturable mycobacteria naturally infecting animals.

The failure of attempts to culture *M. leprae in vitro* constitutes a great barrier to better determining its biochemical characteristics for identification purposes as well

as for therapeutic and immunologic studies. In part, this difficulty has been overcome, first, by *in vivo* culture on mouse foot pads and, lately, by the discovery that
the leprosy organism can infect the nine-banded armadillo (*Dasypus novemcinctus*).
At present, the latter serves as a model for lepromatous leprosy and provides a large
number of bacilli for research.

In recent laboratory trials in the USA, researchers managed to isolate and culture
all the genes belonging to the leprosy bacillus (nearly 5,000) using recombinant
DNA (gene splicing) techniques. The genes control production of diverse substances, such as proteins that had never before been isolated. Five of these were
found to be the most potent substances known for stimulating the formation of
antibodies in animals vaccinated against leprosy.

The availability of antigens produced by recombinant DNA technology permits
tackling problems in leprosy that could not be approached by other means. Use of
these protein antigens should allow perfection of simple and specific seroepidemiologic techniques that can identify members of the population who produce antibodies
for antigenic determinants of *M. leprae*. This could make practicable rapid diagnosis
of leprosy, permitting early treatment to reduce transmission and prevent nerve
damage and deformities. Finally, identification of antigens related to cellular immunity could lead to perfection of a new generation of vaccines (Young *et al.*, 1985).

In identification of *M. leprae*, the dopa (3,4-dihydroxyphenylalanine) oxidation
test and extraction with pyridine are of value. Homogenate of human leproma
(granulomatous nodule rich in *M. leprae* and characteristic of lepromatous leprosy)
oxidizes dopa to indole. Extraction with pyridine eliminates the acid-fast quality of
M. leprae, but not of other mycobacteria. For criteria governing identification of *M.
leprae*, see section on nontuberculous mycobacterial diseases, where the identity of
mycobacteria isolated from animals is discussed.

In recent years, more precise identification of *M. leprae* has been achieved by
structural analysis of its mycolic acids, analysis by immunodiffusion of its antigens,
and interaction of leprosy bacilli with bacteriophages specific for mycobacteria
(Rastogi *et al.*, 1982).

Occurrence in Man: An estimated 12 million people are affected by leprosy. The
highest prevalence is in tropical and subtropical regions of Asia, Africa, Latin
America, and Oceania. Leprosy is very prevalent in India, Southeast Asia, the
Philippines, Korea, southern China, Papua New Guinea, and some Pacific islands.
Ninety percent of the cases reported in the Americas come from five countries:
Argentina, Brazil, Colombia, Mexico, and Venezuela (Brubaker, 1983). Chile is the
only South American country free of the infection. In the United States 2,500 cases
are known, most of them in immigrants. Autochthonous cases arise in Hawaii,
Puerto Rico, Texas, and Louisiana. The infection's prevalence is related to the
socioeconomic level of the population. The fact that the disease has practically
disappeared in Europe is attributed to the improved standard of living there.

The proportion of total leprosy cases represented by lepromatous leprosy (see The
Disease in Man) varies with the region. In Asia and the Americas this form makes
up between 25 and 65% of all cases, while in Africa it accounts for only 6 to 20%
(Bullock, 1982).

Occurrence in Animals: Natural infection has been found in nine-banded armadillos (*Dasypus novemcinctus*) in Louisiana and Texas (USA). By 1983, the infection had been observed in some 100 armadillos captured in Louisiana (Meyers *et al.*,

1983). Depending on their place of origin, between 4 and 29.6% of 1,033 armadillos examined were infected. On the Gulf Coast of Texas, leprosy lesions were found in 4.66% of 451 armadillos captured (Smith *et al.*, 1983). The disease form found in these animals was a lepromatous leprosy identical to the type produced by experimental inoculation with material from humans. On the other hand, the search for naturally infected armadillos carried out by other researchers in Louisiana, Texas, and Florida, as well as in Colombia and Paraguay, produced negative results (Kirchheimer, 1979).

In recent studies carried out in Louisiana by researchers at the state university, *M. leprae* infection was detected using serologic techniques (ELISA) in 17% of 84 captured wild armadillos and in 11% of 184 serum samples from armadillos captured a few years earlier (Trueman, 1984).

A spontaneous case of leprosy, similar to the borderline or dimorphous form, was described in a chimpanzee imported from Sierra Leone to the United States. Clinical and histopathologic characteristics (with invasion of dermal nerves by the etiologic agent) were identical to those of the human disease. Attempts to culture the bacteria were negative, and the chimpanzee did not react to tuberculin or lepromin, just as humans infected with lepromatous or borderline leprosy give a negative reaction. As with *M. leprae* of human origin, experimental inoculation of rats with the isolated bacillus produced neither disease nor lesions. The only difference between the agent of this case and *M. leprae* of human origin was negative results to the dopa oxidation and pyridine tests. On the other hand, the dopa oxidation test sometimes fails in animals inoculated experimentally with human *M. leprae* (Donham and Leininger, 1977). Results obtained by inoculating mouse foot pads were similar to those derived with *M. leprae* of human origin, that is, multiplication of the bacterium in 6 months up to a quantity similar to that of human *M. leprae* without dissemination from the inoculation point (Leininger *et al.*, 1978).

Another case of naturally acquired leprosy was discovered in a primate, *Cercocebus atys* or sooty mangabey monkey (identified in one publication as *Cercocebus torquatus atys*), captured in West Africa and imported in 1975 to the United States (Meyers *et al.*, 1980, 1981). The clinical picture and histopathology were similar to man's and the etiologic agent was identified as *M. leprae* based on the following criteria: invasion of the host's nerves, staining properties, electron microscopy findings, inability to grow in mycobacteriologic media, positive dopa oxidation reaction, reactivity to lepromin, patterns of infection in mice and armadillos, sensitivity to sulfones, and DNA homology (Meyers *et al.*, 1985). Simultaneous intravenous and intracutaneous inoculation succeeded in reproducing the infection and disease in other *Cercocebus* monkeys. The early appearance of signs (5 to 14 months), varying clinical disease forms, neuropathic deformities, bacillemia, and dissemination to various cool parts of the body make the mangabey monkey potentially the most complete model for the study of leprosy. It is the third animal species known to be able to acquire leprosy by natural infection (Walsh *et al.*, 1981; Meyers *et al.*, 1983, 1985).

The Disease in Man: The incubation period is usually 3 to 5 years, but it can vary from 6 months to 10 years or more (Bullock, 1982). Clinical forms of leprosy cover a wide spectrum, ranging from mild self-healing lesions to a progressive and destructive chronic disease. The polar form at one end of the spectrum is tuberculoid leprosy, and at the other, lepromatous leprosy. Intermediate forms are also found.

Tuberculoid leprosy is characterized by localized lesions of the skin and nerves, often asymptomatic. Basically, the lesions consist of a granulomatous, paucibacillary, inflammatory process. The bacilli are difficult to detect, and can be observed most frequently in the nerve endings of the skin. This form results from active destruction of the bacilli by the cellular immunity of the patient. On the other hand, serum antibody titers are generally low. Nerve destruction causes lowered conduction; heat sensibility is the most affected, tactile sensibility less so. Trophic and autonomic changes are common, especially ulcers on the sole and mutilation of body members (Toro-González et al., 1983).

Lepromatous leprosy is characterized by numerous symmetrical skin lesions consisting of macules and diffuse infiltrations, plaques, and nodules of varying sizes (lepromas). There is involvement of the mucosa of the upper respiratory tract, of lymph nodes, liver, spleen, and testicles. Infiltrates are basically histiocytes with a few lymphocytes. Cellular immunity is absent (negative reaction to lepromin) and antibody titers are high. In this form of the disease, as in the borderline, erythema nodosum leprosum (ENL) often appears.

The indeterminate form of leprosy has still not been adequately characterized from the clinical point of view; it is considered to be the initial stage of the disease. The first cutaneous lesions are flat, hypopigmented, and have ill-defined borders. If this form is not treated, it may develop into tuberculoid, borderline, or lepromatous leprosy. Bacilli are few, and it is difficult to confirm their presence.

Finally, the borderline form occupies a position intermediate between the two polar forms (tuberculoid and lepromatous), and shares properties of both; it is unstable and may progress in either direction. Destruction of nerve trunks may be extensive. Bacilli are observed in scrapings taken from skin lesions.

Two types of the disease were defined by a WHO study group, with the goal of improving treatment:

"1. *Paucibacillary*. This includes indeterminate (I) and tuberculoid (T) leprosy of the Madrid classification, and indeterminate (I), polar tuberculoid (TT), and borderline tuberculoid (BT) leprosy in the Ridley and Jopling classification, whether diagnosed clinically or histopathologically, but with a bacterial index of less than 2 according to the Ridley scale at all sites.

"2. *Multibacillary active*. This includes both lepromatous (L) and borderline (B) leprosy in the Madrid classification, and polar lepromatous (LL), borderline lepromatous (BL), and borderline (BB) leprosy in the Ridley and Jopling classification, and anyone with a bacterial index of 2 or greater at any site." (World Health Organization, 1985.)

An estimated one-third of clinical cases become incapacitated, half of them completely. Nevertheless, these proportions are now changing, due to both prevention/control programs and early implementation of effective treatments.

There is evidence that inapparent infection may occur with a certain frequency among persons, especially family members, in contact with patients.

The Disease in Animals: The disease in armadillos (*Dasypus novemcinctus*) is similar to the lepromatous form in man. Infection in these animals is characterized by macrophage infiltrates containing a large number of bacilli. Skin lesions vary from mild to severe. The small dermal nerves are invaded by the etiologic agent. Many bacilli are seen in the macrophages of the lymph tissue, in the pulp of the spleen, and in Kupffer's cells in the liver.

M. leprae is known to prefer the coolest parts of the human or mouse body. For this reason, armadillos were used as experimental animals even before natural infection was confirmed in them, since their body temperature is from 30 to 35°C. Experimental inoculation of armadillos with human leproma material reproduces the disease, characterized by broad dissemination of the agent, and involvement of lymph glands, liver, spleen, lungs, bone marrow, meninges, and other tissues, in a more intense form than is usually observed in man (Kirchheimer *et al.*, 1972).

The disease in the chimpanzee appeared as a progressive chronic dermatitis with nodular thickening of the skin of the ears, eyebrows, nose, and lips. Lesions of the nose, skin, and dermal nerves contained copious quantities of acid-fast bacteria (Donham and Leininger, 1977). The case was histologically classified as borderline 12 months after the clinical symptoms were first observed, and as lepromatous after a later biopsy (Leininger *et al.*, 1978).

In the case of the *Cercocebus* monkey, the initial lesion consisted of nodules on the face. Four months later, a massive infiltration and ulceration were seen on the face, and nodules appeared on the ear and the forearms. Sixteen months after cutaneous lesions were first observed, the animal began to suffer deformities and paralysis of the extremities. Histopathologic findings indicated the subpolar or intermediate lepromatous form, according to the Ridley and Jopling classification scheme. The disease was progressive, with neuropathic deformation of feet and hands. It seemed to regress when specific treatment was administered. The animal apparently contracted the disease from a patient with active leprosy. Experimental infections carried out to date have indicated that these animals may experience a spectrum of different forms similar to those in man (Walsh *et al.*, 1981; Meyers *et al.*, 1985).

Source of Infection and Mode of Transmission: Man is the principal reservoir of *M. leprae*. The method of transmission is still not well known due to the extended incubation period. Nevertheless, the principal source of infection is believed to be lepromatous patients, in whom the infection is multibacillary, skin lesions are often ulcerous, and a great number of bacilli are shed through the nose; similarly, bacilli are found in the mouth and pharynx. Consequently, transmission might be effected by contact with infected skin, especially through wounds or abrasions, and by aerosols, as is the case in tuberculosis. Lately, more importance has been attributed to aerosol transmission. Oral transmission and transmission by hematophagous arthropods are not discounted, but they are assigned less epidemiologic importance.

Until recently, leprosy was believed to be an exclusively human disease. But research in recent years has demonstrated that the infection and the disease also occur naturally in wild animals. Even though some researchers (Kirchheimer, 1979) have expressed doubt that the animal infection is identical to the human, at present an accumulation of evidence indicates that the etiologic agent is the same. Criteria (Binford *et al.*, 1982) used to identify the bacillus in animals as *M. leprae* are as follow: 1) selective invasion of the peripheral nerves by bacilli, since the only *Mycobacterium* known to date to invade the nerves is *M. leprae*; 2) failure to grow on laboratory media usual for mycobacteria; 3) positive pyridine test to eliminate acid-fastness; 4) positive dopa test; 5) characteristic multiplication in mouse foot pads and in armadillos; and 6) reactivity of lepromin prepared with animal bacilli compared to that of standard lepromin.

The origin of infection in animals is unknown. It is believed that armadillos contracted the infection from a human source, perhaps from multibacillary patients before the era of sulfones. In this regard, it should be pointed out that leprosy bacilli may remain viable for a week in dried nasal secretions and that armadillos are in close contact with the soil. The high disease prevalence in some localities would indicate armadillos can transmit the infection to one another, either by inhalation or direct contact. Another possible transmission vehicle is maternal milk, in which the agent has been detected (Walsh *et al.*, 1981).

It is difficult to demonstrate that armadillos are a source infection for man because of the long incubation period in humans and the impossibility of excluding a human source in an endemic area. In Texas, a case of human leprosy was attributed to a patient's practice of capturing armadillos and eating their meat (Freiberger and Fundenberg, 1981). Subsequently, another five cases with hand lesions were detected in natives of the same state who habitually hunted and cleaned armadillos but had no known contact with human cases (Lumpkin III *et al.*, 1983). To determine if there was a significant association between contact with armadillos and human leprosy in Louisiana, a group of 19 patients was compared with another group of 19 healthy individuals from the same area. Of those with leprosy, four had had contact with armadillos, as opposed to five in the control group; consequently, it was concluded that such an association did not exist (Filice *et al.*, 1977). However, this conclusion was questioned since the only valid comparison would be between persons who have handled armadillos and those who have had no contact with them (Lumpkin III *et al.*, 1983).

The prevalence of leprosy in armadillos in Louisiana and Texas suggests that these animals could serve as a reservoir of *M. leprae*; however, nothing is known about the frequency of infection in nonhuman primates and the role they may play in transmission of the disease. The sources of the cases of leprosy in these animals were probably people with lepromatous leprosy.

Diagnosis: Clinically, an anesthetic or hypoesthetic cutaneous lesion raises suspicion of leprosy, even more so if the nerves are enlarged. Diagnosis is confirmed by biopsy of the skin lesion, which in addition permits classification of the form of leprosy. For patients with lepromatous or borderline leprosy, diagnosis can be made by using the Ziehl-Neelson staining technique on a film of nasal mucosa scrapings or the interphase between erythrocytes and leukocytes from a centrifuged blood sample. Histopathologic preparations do not stain well using Ziehl-Neelson and consequently a Fite-Faraco stain is recommended. Also used is the simplified staining method consisting of eliminating acid-fastness by pyridine in order to differentiate *M. leprae* (Convit and Pinardi, 1972). In tuberculoid and other paucibacillary forms of leprosy, it is difficult and at times impossible to confirm the presence of the etiologic agent; nevertheless, examination of many histologic sections is recommended in order to detect any bacteria present, especially in the nerve endings.

Skin tests have no diagnostic value, but they serve as an aid to prognosis. Patients with tuberculoid or other paucibacillary forms of leprosy react positively to the intradermal lepromin or Mitsuda test (with dead *M. leprae* bacilli and a reading after 28 days), since their cellular immunity is generally not affected. In contrast, lepromatous and other multibacillary forms give negative results to the Mitsuda test. Researchers at Louisiana State University have developed an excellent and very sensitive ELISA serologic test for diagnosing leprosy in humans and armadillos, which may be of great value in epidemiologic studies (Hugh-Jones, 1985).

Control: Control is based on early detection and chemotherapy. In the face of multiple confirmed cases of resistance to dapsone, combination of this medication with rifampicin is presently recommended for paucibacillary leprosy, and the same two medications in combination with clofazimine for multibacillary leprosy. Rifampicin has a rapid bactericidal effect and eliminates contagion in patients in 1 to 2 weeks. The isolation of patients in leprosariums is no longer necessary, since the chemotherapy effectively eliminates infectiousness and thereby interrupts transmission of the disease.

Bibliography

Binford, C. H., W. M. Meyers, G. P. Walsh, E. E. Storrs, and H. L. Brown. Naturally acquired leprosy-like disease in the nine-banded armadillo (*Dasypus novemcinctus*). Histopathologic and microbiologic studies of tissues. *J Reticuloendothel Soc* 22:377-388, 1977.

Binford, C. H., W. M. Meyers, and G. P. Walsh. Leprosy—state of the art. *JAMA* 247:2283-2292, 1982.

Brubaker, M. El control de la lepra en las Américas. *In: Seminario Bolivariano sobre el Control de la Lepra*. Caracas, Pan American Health Organization, 1983. (PNSP/84-05.)

Bullock, W. E. Leprosy (Hansen's disease). *In*: Wyngaarden, J. B., and L. H. Smith, Jr. (Eds.), *Cecil Textbook of Medicine*, 16th ed. Philadelphia, Saunders, 1982.

Clark, K. A., S. H. Kim, L. F. Boening, M. J. Taylor, T. G. Betz, and F. V. McCasland. Leprosy in armadillos (*Dasypus novemcinctus*) from Texas. *J Wildl Dis* 23:220-224, 1987.

Convit, J., and M. E. Pinardi. A simple method for the differentiation of *Mycobacterium leprae* from other mycobacteria through routine staining technics. *Int J Lepr* 40:130-132, 1972.

Donham, K. J., and J. R. Leininger. Spontaneous leprosy-like disease in a chimpanzee. *J Infect Dis* 136:132-136, 1977.

Filice, G., R. N. Greenberg, and D. W. Fraser. Lack of observed association between armadillo contact and leprosy in humans. *Am J Trop Med Hyg* 26:137-142, 1977.

Fine, P. E. Leprosy: the epidemiology of a slow bacterium. *Epidemiol Rev* 4:161-188, 1982.

Freiberger, H. F., and H. H. Fundenberg. An appetite for armadillo. *Hosp Prac* 15:137-144, 1981.

Hugh-Jones, M. Department of Epidemiology and Community Health, School of Veterinary Medicine, Louisiana State University. Personal communication, July 1985.

Job, C. K., R. M. Sanchez, and R. C. Hastings. Manifestations of experimental leprosy in the armadillo. *Am J Trop Med Hyg* 34:151-161, 1985.

Job, C. K., E. B. Harris, J. L. Allen, and R. C. Hastings. Thorns in armadillo ears and noses and their role in the transmission of leprosy. *Arch Pathol Lab Med* 110:1025-1028, 1986.

Kirchheimer, W. F., E. E. Storrs, and C. H. Binford. Attempts to establish the armadillo (*Dasypus novemcinctus* Linn) as model for the study of leprosy. II. Histopathologic and bacteriologic postmortem findings in lepromatoid leprosy in the armadillo. *Int J Lepr* 40:229 242, 1972.

Kirchheimer, W. F. Leprosy (Hansen's Disease). *In*: Stoenner, H., W. Kaplan, and M. Torten (Section Eds.), *CRC Handbook Series in Zoonoses*. Section A, vol. 1. Boca Raton, Florida, CRC Press, 1979.

Leininger, J. R., K. J. Donham, and M. J. Rubino. Leprosy in a chimpanzee: morphology of the skin lesions and characterization of the organism. *Vet Pathol* 15:339-346, 1978.

Leininger, J. R., K. J. Donham, and W. M. Meyers. Leprosy in a chimpanzee. Postmortem lesions. *Int J Lepr* 48:414-421, 1980.

Lumpkin III, L. R., G. F. Cox, and J. E. Wolf, Jr. Leprosy in five armadillo handlers. *J Am Acad Dermatol* 9:899-903, 1983.

Martin, L. N., B. J. Gormus, R. H. Wolf, G. P. Walsh, W. M. Meyers, C. H. Binford, and M. Harboe. Experimental leprosy in nonhuman primates. *Adv Vet Sci Comp Med* 28:201-236, 1984.

Meyers, W. M., G. P. Walsh, H. L. Brown, Y. Fukunishi, C. H. Binford, P. J. Gerone, and R. H. Wolf. Naturally acquired leprosy in a mangabey monkey (*Cercocebus* sp.). *Int J Lepr* 48:495-496, 1980.

Meyers, W. M., G. P. Walsh, H. L. Brown, C. H. Binford, P. J. Gerone, R. H. Wolf, B. J. Gormus, and L. N. Martin. Leprosy in a mangabey monkey (*Cercocebus torquatus atys*, "sooty" mangabey). Summarized in *Int J Lepr* 49:500-502, 1981.

Meyers, W. M., G. P. Walsh, C. H. Binford, H. L. Brown, R. H. Wolf, B. J. Gormus, L. N. Martin, and P. J. Gerone. Multibacilar leprosy in unaltered hosts, with emphasis on armadillos and monkeys. Summarized in *Int J Lepr* 50:584-585, 1982.

Meyers, W. M., G. P. Walsh, C. H. Binford, R. H. Wolf, B. J. Gormus, L. N. Martin, G. B. Baskin, and P. J. Gerone. Modelos de lepra multibacilar en huéspedes no alterados: estado actual. *In: Seminario Bolivariano sobre Control de la Lepra*. Caracas, Pan American Health Organization, 1983. (PNSP/84-05.)

Meyers, W. M., G. P. Walsh, H. L. Brown, C. H. Binford, G. D. Imes, Jr., T. L. Hadfield, C. H. Schlagel, Y. Fukunishi, P. J. Gerone, R. H. Wolf, B. J. Gormus, L. N. Martin, M. Harboe, and T. Imaeda. Leprosy in a mangabey monkey—naturally acquired infection. *Int J Lepr* 53:1-14, 1985.

Portaels, F., K. DeRidder, and S. R. Pattyn. Cultivable mycobacteria isolated from organs of armadillos uninoculated and inoculated with *Mycobacterium leprae*. *Ann Inst Pasteur Microbiol* 136A:181-190, 1985.

Rastogi, M., C. Frehel, A. Ryter, and H. L. David. Comparative ultrastructure of *Mycobacterium leprae* and *M. avium* grown in experimental hosts. *Ann Microbiol (Paris)* 133B:109-128, 1982.

Smith, J. H., D. S. Folse, E. G. Long, J. D. Christie, D. R. Crouse, M. E. Tewes, A. M. Gaston, R. L. Erhardt, S. K. File, and M. T. Kelley. Leprosy in wild armadillos (*Dasypus novemcinctus*) of the Texas Gulf Coast: epidemiology and mycobacteriology. *J Reticuloendothel Soc* 34:75-88, 1983.

Stallknecht, D. E., R. W. Truman, M. E. Hugh-Jones, and C. K. Job. Surveillance for naturally acquired leprosy in a nine-banded armadillo population. *J Wildl Dis* 23:308-310, 1987.

Toro-González, G., G. Román-Campos, and L. Navarro de Román. *Lepra. Neurología Tropical*. Bogotá, Printer Colombiana, 1983.

Trueman, R. Hansen's Institute, Carville, Louisiana. Doctoral thesis. In press, 1985.

Truman, R. W., E. J. Shannon, H. V. Hagstad, M. E. Hugh-Jones, A. Wolfe, and R. C. Hastings. Evaluation of the origin of *Mycobacterium leprae* infections in the wild armadillo, *Dasypus novemcinctus*. *Am J Trop Med Hyg* 35:588-593, 1986.

Walsh, G. P., E. E. Storrs, W. M. Meyers, and C. H. Binford. Naturally acquired leprosy-like disease in the nine-banded armadillo (*Dasypus novemcinctus*). Recent epizootiologic findings. *J Reticuloendothel Soc* 22:363-368, 1977.

Walsh, G. P., W. M. Meyers, C. H. Binford, P. J. Gerone, R. H. Wolf, and J. R. Leininger. Leprosy—a zoonosis. *Lepr Rev* 52 (Suppl. 1):77-83, 1981.

World Health Organization. *Epidemiology of leprosy in relation to control*. Report of a WHO Study Group. Geneva, WHO, 1985. (Technical Report Series 716.)

Young, R. A., V. Mehra, D. Sweetser, T. Buchanan, J. Clark-Curtiss, R. W. Davis, and B. R. Bloom. Genes for the major protein antigens of the leprosy parasite *M. leprae*. *Nature* 316:450-452, 1985.

LEPTOSPIROSIS

(100)

Synonyms: Weil's disease, swineherd's disease, rice-field fever, cane-cutter's fever, swamp fever, mud fever, and other local names; Stuttgart disease, canicola fever (dogs).

Etiology: Two species of *Leptospira* are recognized: *Leptospira interrogans* and *L. biflexa*. The former is pathogenic for man and animal, while *L. biflexa* is a free-living saprophyte found in shallow water, and is seldom associated with infections in mammals. *L. illini*, a possible third species, is provisional and awaiting further study.

The species of interest as a zoonotic agent is *L. interrogans*. It has about 180 serologic variants, or serovars, the basic taxon. Serovars are grouped for convenience into 18 serogroups (which is not a recognized taxon) on the basis of the predominant agglutinogenic components they share (Faine, 1982).

Geographic Distribution: Worldwide. There are universal serovars such as *L. interrogans* serovar *icterohaemorrhagiae* and serovar *canicola*, and serovars that occur only in certain regions. Each region has characteristic serotypes, determined by its ecology. Leptospirosis has a high prevalence in tropical countries with heavy rainfall and neutral or alkaline soils.

Occurrence in Man: The incidence varies in different parts of the world. The disease may occur in sporadic form or in epidemic outbreaks. In general, outbreaks are caused by exposure to water contaminated with urine of infected animals. Several occupational groups are particularly at risk, such as workers in rice fields, sugarcane plantations, mines, sewer systems, and slaughterhouses, and animal caretakers and veterinarians.

Occurrence in Animals: The infection is common in rodents and other wild and domestic animals. Each serovar has its preferred animal host or hosts, but each animal species may be host to one or more serovars. Thus, for example, the serovar *pomona* has as its principal hosts pigs and cattle, but it may transitorily infect other animals. Dogs are the principal reservoir of *canicola*, but on occasion it may be found in foxes, swine, and cattle.

The Disease in Man: Man is susceptible to a large number of serovars. The incubation period lasts from 1 to 2 weeks, though cases with only a 2-day incubation period are known. The disease is characterized by two phases: the bacteremic phase, lasting 7 to 10 days, and the leptospiruric phase, lasting from a week to several months. Clinical manifestations are variable and have differing degrees of severity. Moreover, numerous cases transpire inapparently or subclinically. In general, two clinical types are distinguished: icteric and anicteric. The serious icteric or hepatonephritic type (Weil's disease) is much less frequent than the anicteric. It is often caused by *icterohaemorrhagiae*, but other serovars are also capable of producing this form. On the other hand, numerous infections caused by *icterohaemorrhagiae* occur in anicteric form. In the classical form of Weil's disease, the onset of symptoms is sudden, with fever, headache, myalgias, conjunctivitis, nausea, vomiting, diarrhea, and constipation. Prostration may be severe. Petechiae on the skin, hemorrhages in the gastrointestinal tract, and proteinuria are common. Hepatomegaly and jaundice, renal insufficiency with marked oliguria or anuria, azotemia, and electrolyte imbalance develop with the disappearance of leptospiremia and fever. If the patient improves, diuresis is reestablished and jaundice decreases. Convalescence lasts 1 or 2 months, during which time fever, cephalalgia, myalgias, and general malaise may reappear.

In anicteric cases the symptomatology is milder. The symptoms during leptospiremia (the first week of the disease) are fever, myalgias, conjunctivitis, stiffness in the neck, nausea, and sometimes vomiting. Often the disease resembles influenza. The anicteric form has a benign course and patients recover in about a month. Leptospiruria may continue for a week or several months after disappearance of the clinical symptoms.

The Disease in Animals

CATTLE: In the Americas the predominant serovars in cattle are *pomona, hardjo*, and *grippotyphosa*; at times infections caused by *canicola* and *icterohaemorrhagiae* as well as by other serovars, are found. At present, *pomona* and *hardjo* serovars seem to be universal. As laboratory methods have improved, outbreaks caused by the latter have been confirmed with increasing frequency. In recent years, serovars belonging to the *hebdomadis* group have been isolated more frequently.

The infection may provoke an acute or subacute disease or may remain clinically inapparent. The disease is manifested by a fever lasting 4 to 5 days, anorexia, conjunctivitis, and diarrhea. Infertility may be a sequela of the infection. Cows experience a sudden decrease in milk production and often an atypical mastitis, with flaccid udders and yellowish, viscous milk, at times tinged with blood. Serious cases include jaundice. Nevertheless, the most notable symptoms in a certain proportion of the animals are abortion and hemoglobinuria. Abortions usually occur between 1 and 3 weeks after the onset of the disease. Up to 20% of aborting animals retain the placenta.

Cattle of all ages are susceptible. The disease course is more severe in calves, which experience stunted growth and variable mortality rates.

Rapidly spreading epizootics are characterized by a high morbidity rate. It is possible that rapid passage of the leptospires from one animal to another intensifies their virulence. In slow-moving epizootics, the rate of inapparent infection varies from one herd to another.

SWINE: The serovars most often isolated from swine in the Americas and in the rest of the world are *pomona, tarassovi, grippotyphosa, canicola*, and *icterohaemorrhagiae*.

Swine are a very important reservoir of *pomona*, with abundant and prolonged leptospiruria. The clinical infection varies from one herd to another. In some cases infection occurs subclinically, though the animals may exhibit a fever lasting a few days; in others, the infection produces symptoms such as abortion and birth of weak piglets. Stunted growth of piglets, jaundice, hemoglobinuria, convulsions, and gastrointestinal upsets have also been seen. At times meningitis and nervous symptomatology are present. Abortion usually happens between 15 and 30 days after infection. The principal serovars causing abortions or stillborn piglets are *pomona, tarassovi,* and *canicola*. Infection that occurs during the last third of pregnancy is the most critical in interrupting gestation.

HORSES: Horses react serologically to many serotypes prevalent in the environment. *Pomona* has been isolated from these animals in the United States, and *hardjo* in Argentina. In Europe, *icterohaemorrhagiae, sejroe*, and *canicola* have been isolated in addition to *pomona*. Most infections are inapparent. Often the disease's sequela (periodic ophthalmia) is recognized instead of the acute febrile phase. The onset of periodic ophthalmia occurs when the febrile phase has disappeared, after a latent period that sometimes lasts several months. Leptospires have been detected in eye lesions of affected animals, and a high concentration of antibodies can be found in the aqueous humor. It should be borne in mind, however, that leptospirosis is not the only cause of periodic ophthalmia. Serious cases of leptospirosis with hepatonephritic and cardiovascular syndromes have been described in Europe.

SHEEP AND GOATS: Epizootics in these species are not very frequent. Various serovars, which appear to have come from other animal species in the same environment, have been isolated from sheep and goats in different countries (Faine, 1982), for example, *hardjo* in Australia and New Zealand, *pomona* in the United States and New Zealand, *grippotyphosa* in Israel, and *ballum* in Argentina.

As in other species of ruminants, the disease is characterized by fever, anorexia, and in some animals by jaundice, hemoglobinuria, anemia, abortion, birth of weak or stillborn animals, and infertility. The virulence of the infecting serovar and the condition of the animal determine the severity of the clinical picture.

DOGS AND CATS: The predominant canine serovars are *canicola* and *icterohaemorrhagiae*. In addition to these serovars, *pyogenes, paidjan*, and *tarassovi* have been isolated in Latin America and the Caribbean. The infection may vary from asymptomatic to severe. The most serious form is the hemorrhagic, which begins suddenly with a fever lasting 3 to 4 days, followed by stiffness and myalgia in the posterior limbs and hemorrhages in the oral cavity with a tendency toward necrosis and pharyngitis. In subsequent stages there may be hemorrhagic gastroenteritis and acute nephritis. Jaundice may occur with infection by *canicola* or by *icterohaemorrhagiae*, but especially in the case of the latter serovar. Case fatality is estimated at 10%.

The disease rarely occurs in cats.

WILD ANIMALS: Many wild animals, including rodents, are perfectly adapted to leptospires and show no symptoms or lesions.

Source of Infection and Mode of Transmission (Figure 12): After a week of leptospiremia, animals shed leptospires in their urine, contaminating the environment. The best reservoirs of the infection are animals, since they have prolonged leptospiruria and generally do not suffer from the disease themselves. Such is the case with rats, which harbor *icterohaemorrhagiae* but rarely have lesions. The infection in man and animals is contracted directly or indirectly, through the skin and the nasal, oral, and conjunctival mucosas. Indirect exposure through water, soil, or foods contaminated by urine from infected animals is the most common route.

People who work with livestock are often exposed to animal urine, directly or as an aerosol, which can contaminate the conjunctiva or nasal mucosa or abrasions on exposed skin. They may also become infected indirectly by walking barefoot where animals have urinated. In many countries, domesticated animals, especially swine and cattle, constitute important leptospire reservoirs and a source of infection for man.

Figure 12. Leptospirosis. Synanthropic transmission cycle.

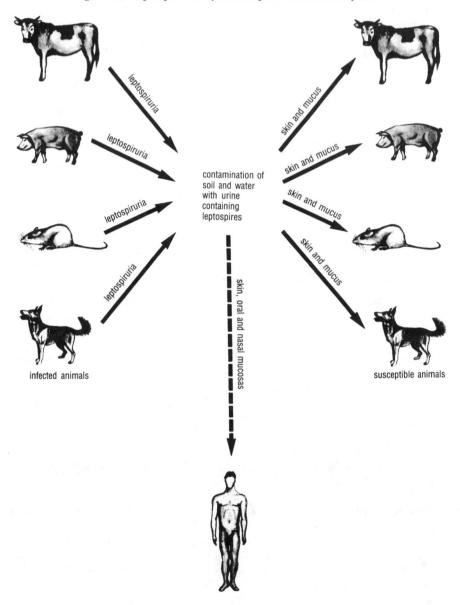

Rice-paddy workers are exposed to water contaminated by urine of rodents infesting the countryside. Sugarcane harvesters make up another high-risk group. Field mice nesting among vegetable crops are a source of infection for harvesters, whose hands may come in contact with dew mixed with rodent urine in early morning.

Among pets, the dog is a common source of infection for man by serovars *canicola* and *icterohaemorrhagiae*.

Tropical regions are endemic areas of leptospirosis and the highest case rates correspond to heavy rain zones. The greatest number of cases occur during the rainy season. Epidemic outbreaks erupt because of environmental changes, such as flooding, that cause rodents to move into cities. The epidemics in the city of Recife, Pernambuco Province, Brazil, are an illustrative example, in which 181 and 102 cases occurred in 1966 and 1970, respectively. The predominant serovar was *icterohaemorrhagiae*. Humidity, high temperatures, and an abundance of rats were the principal factors setting off these outbreaks as well as others in tropical regions. Small epidemic outbreaks are also caused by recreational activities such as swimming or diving in streams or ponds contaminated with the urine of infected animals, either domestic or wild species. Epidemic outbreaks caused by several different serovars have been produced in soldiers wading streams or camping by river banks during jungle maneuvers. Such epidemics occurred in Panama and Malaysia; in these cases, the source of infection was the urine of infected wild animals.

Animals, either secondary or primary hosts, contract the infection in a similar way. The density of the host population and environmental conditions in which it lives play important roles. On cattle ranches, the infection is usually introduced by animal carriers with leptospiruria and, at times, by flooding with water contaminated at a neighboring establishment.

Pathogenic leptospires (*L. interrogans*) do not multiply outside the animal organism. Consequently, in addition to carrier animals, existence of a leptospirosis focus requires environmental conditions favorable to the survival of the agent in the exterior environment. Leptospires need high humidity, a neutral or slightly alkaline pH, and suitable temperatures. Low, water-covered ground and artificial or natural freshwater receptacles (ponds, streams, reservoirs, etc.) are favorable to their survival, whereas salt water is deleterious. Soil composition, both its physiochemical and biological characteristics (microbe population), also act to prolong or shorten life for leptospires in the environment. Temperatures in the tropics constitute a very favorable factor for survival of leptospires, but cases of leptospirosis may also occur in cold climates, though they are less frequent.

Role of Animals in the Epidemiology of the Disease: Wild and domesticated animals are essential for the maintenance of pathogenic leptospires in nature. Transmission of the infection from animals to man is effected directly or indirectly.

Human-to-human transmission is rare. Man is an accidental host and only in very special conditions can he contribute to the maintenance of an epidemic outbreak. Such was the case in an epidemic described in the forest to the northeast of Hanoi, Vietnam. The outbreak occurred among soldiers occupied in logging and transport of logs by buffalo through a swampy area. Leptospiruria was observed in 12% of 66 convalescent soldiers. In contrast, among buffalo and rodents in the region the rate of infection was insignificant. The pH of the surface water was neutral, the soldiers worked barefoot, and their urine had a pH that fluctuated around 7 (their diet was vegetarian). Leptospiruria persisted in some of the soldiers for more than 6 months (Spinu *et al.*, 1963).

Diagnosis: In man, the etiologic agent can be isolated from the blood during the first week of the disease; afterwards, it can be isolated from the urine, either by direct culture or by inoculation into young hamsters. Repeated blood samples are necessary for serologic examination. The patient has no antibodies during the first week; they appear in 6 to 7 days and reach maximum levels in the third or fourth week. If the first sample is negative or low-titer and the second shows an appreciable increase in antibody titer (fourfold or more), leptospirosis is indicated.

The same diagnostic procedures are employed for animals as for man. Blood or urine may be used for the bacteriologic examination, in accordance with the stage of the illness. If a necropsy is performed on a sacrificed or dead animal, kidney cultures should be made. Examination of several tissue samples from the same individual is not always feasible in veterinary practice, but individual diagnosis of domestic animals is not as important as herd diagnosis. Discovery of high antibody titers in several members of a herd and a clinical picture compatible with leptospirosis indicate a recent infection.

Low titers may mean residual antibodies from a past infection or recently formed antibodies that have not yet reached a high level.

The serologic reference test that is used most for man as well as for animals is microscopic agglutination. This test should be carried out using representative serovars from different serogroups, especially those occurring in the region. It is necessary to bear in mind that cross-reactions are produced not only between different serovars of the same serogroup but, at the beginning of the infection (2 to 3 weeks), also between serovars of different serogroups, and a heterologous serovar titer may predominate. Reaction to the homologous serovar becomes more pronounced with time. Cross-reactions are more frequent in man than in animals.

The macroscopic plate test with inactivated antigens can be used as a preliminary or screening test for man and animals. It is fast and easy, and particularly useful for diagnosing disease in a herd.

Plate agglutination is a genus-specific test, which uses as an antigen the *patoc* strain of saprophytic leptospira (*L. biflexa*) to determine if the patient is suffering from leptospirosis (Mazzonelli *et al.*, 1974). Reaction to this test is marked during the acute phase of leptospirosis and then quickly becomes negative (Faine, 1982). Among more recent tests, those of interest are indirect immunofluorescence and ELISA. With both, the types of immunoglobulins (IgM or IgG) can be determined by using corresponding antigens. IgM appears after the first week of the disease and IgG after several weeks. In some human cases, IgG anibodies cannot be detected for reasons as yet unknown.

Control: In man, control measures include the following: a) personal hygiene; b) the use of protective clothing during farm work; c) drainage of lowlands when possible; d) rodent-proof structures; e) food protection and correct garbage disposal; f) control of infection in domestic animals; g) avoidance of swimming in streams and other fresh watercourses that may be contaminated; and h) vaccination of high-risk occupational groups.

Human immunization has not been widely applied. It has been used with promising results in Italy, Poland, and the USSR, but because of secondary effects, mainly allergic, its use has not spread. On the other hand, tests are under way of a vaccine made in a medium chemically defined as free of proteins (Shenberg and Torten, 1973). In China a similar vaccine is being used on a wide scale.

Even though the use of antibiotics in prophylaxis and treatment has given contradictory results, a recent investigation (Takafuji *et al.*, 1984) showed that doxycycline is effective in chemoprophylaxis; the same drug is probably also effective in treatment. It has been suggested (Sanford, 1984) that chemoprophylaxis can be justified in areas where incidence is 5% or greater. Mechanization of farm work has resulted in a decrease of outbreaks, for example, among rice-paddy workers.

Among domesticated animals, vaccination of pigs, cattle, and dogs is effective in preventing the disease, but it does not protect completely against infection. Vaccinated animals may become infected without showing clinical symptoms; they may even develop leptospiruria, though to a lesser degree and for a shorter time than unvaccinated animals. A few known human cases of leptospirosis were contracted from vaccinated dogs. There are bacterins to protect against the *pomona, hardjo*, and *grippotyphosa* serovars in cattle, against *pomona* in swine, and against *canicola* and *icterohaemorrhagiae* in dogs. Immunity is predominantly serovar-specific and therefore the serovar or serovars active in a focus must be known in order to correctly immunize the animals. Females should be vaccinated before the reproductive period to protect them during pregnancy. Young animals can be immunized after 3 or 4 months of age. Bacterins now in use require annual revaccination.

It has been demonstrated that vaccination with bacterins initially stimulates the production of IgM antibodies, which disappear after a few months to be replaced by IgG antibodies. Vaccination does not greatly interfere with diagnosis because of the quick disappearance of IgM antibodies, which are active in agglutination. IgG are the protective antibodies and can be detected by serum protection assays in hamsters or by the growth inhibition test in culture media.

Recently, a vaccine produced from the outer leptospiral envelope has given promising results in laboratory trials by providing resistance not only against the disease but also against the establishment of leptospiruria.

Chemotherapy is promising. Experiments have shown that a single injection of dihydrostreptomycin at a dose of 25 mg per kg of body weight is effective against leptospiruria in bovines and swine. The infection has been eradicated in several herds with antibiotic treatment and proper environmental hygiene. The combination of vaccination and chemotherapy for the control of swine leptospirosis has been proposed.

Proper herd management is important for control. It has been demonstrated many times that swine can transmit the *pomona* serovar to cows. Therefore, separation of these two species is important for prophylaxis.

Bibliography

Alexander, A. D., W. E. Gochenour, Jr., K. R. Reinhard, M. K. Ward, and R. H. Yagen. Leptospirosis. *In*: Bodily, H. L. (Ed.), *Diagnostic Procedures for Bacterial, Mycotic and Parasitic Infections*, 5th ed. New York, American Public Health Association, 1970.

Alston, J. M., and J. C. Broom. *Leptospirosis in Man and Animals*. Edinburgh and London, Livingstone, 1958.

Banlee, J., C. O. R. Everard, and J. D. Everard. Leptospires in vervet monkeys (*Cercopithecus aethiops safacus*) on Barbados. *J Wildl Dis* 23:60-66, 1987.

Cacchione, R. A. Enfoques de los estudios de la leptospirosis humana y animal en América Latina. *Rev Assoc Argent Microbiol* 5:36-53, 100-111, 143-154, 1973.

Diesch, S. L., and H. C. Ellinghausen. Leptospiroses. *In*: Hubbert, W. T., W. F. McCulloch, and P. R. Schnurrenberger (Eds.), *Diseases Transmitted from Animals to Man*, 6th ed. Springfield, Illinois, Thomas, 1975.

Ellis, W. A., P. J. McParland, D. G. Bryson, A. B. Thiermann, and J. Montgomery.

Isolation of leptospires from the genital tract and kidneys of aborted sows. *Vet Rec* 118:294-295, 1986.

Ellis, W. A., and A. B. Thiermann. Isolation of leptospires from the genital tracts of Iowa cows. *Am J Vet Res* 47:1694-1696, 1986.

Everard, C. O. R., A. E. Green, and J. W. Glosser. Leptospirosis in Trindad and Grenada, with special reference to the mongoose. *Trans R Soc Trop Med Hyg* 70:57-61, 1976.

Faine, S. (Ed.). *Guidelines for the Control of Leptospirosis.* Geneva, World Health Organization, 1982. (Offset Publication 67.)

Hanson, L. E., D. N. Tripathy, and A. H. Killinger. Current status of leptospirosis immunization in swine and cattle. *J Am Vet Med Assoc* 161:1235-1243, 1972.

Hart, R. J. C., J. Gallagher, and S. Waitkins. An outbreak of leptospirosis in cattle and man. *Br Med J* 288, 1984.

Mazzonelli, J. Advances in bovine leptospirosis. *Bull Off Int Epizoot* 3:775-808, 1984.

Mazzonelli, J., G. T. Dora de Mazzonelli, and M. Mailloux. Possibilité de diagnostique sérologique des leptospires á l'aide d'un antigène unique. *Med Mal Infect* 4:253, 1974.

Motie, A., and D. M. Myers. Leptospirosis in sheep and goats in Guyana. *Trop Anim Health Prod* 18:113-115, 1986.

Motie, A., D. M. Myers, and E. E. Storrs. A serologic survey for leptospires in nine-banded armadillos (*Dasypus novemcinctus* L.) in Florida. *J Wildl Dis* 22:423-424, 1986.

Myers, D. M. Equine leptospirosis: serological studies and isolations of serotype *hardjo* and *Leptospira biflexa* strains from horses of Argentina. *J Clin Microbiol* 3:548-555, 1976.

Public Health Laboratory Service, Leptospira Reference Unit, Communicable Disease Surveillance Centre. Leptospirosis in man, British Isles, 1983. *Br Med J* 288, 1984.

Sanford, J. P. Leptospirosis—time for a booster. *N Engl J Med* 310:524-525, 1984.

Shenberg, E., and M. Torten. A new leptospiral vaccine. I. Development of vaccine leptospires grown in a chemically defined medium. *J Infect Dis* 128:642-646, 1973.

Spinu, I., V. Topcin, Trinh Thi Hang Quy, Vo Van Hung, Mguyen Sy Quoe, Chu Xnan Long, Li Van Thuyen, and Nguyen Van An. L'homme comme reservoir de virus dans une épidémie de leptospirose survenue dans la jungle. *Arch Roum Pathol Exp* 22:1081-1100, 1963.

Stalheim, O. H. V. Chemotherapy of renal leptospirosis in swine. *Am J Vet Res* 28:161-166, 1967.

Stalheim, O. H. V. Chemotherapy of renal leptospirosis in cattle. *Am J Vet Res* 30:1317-1323, 1969.

Stalheim, O. H. V. Duration of immunity in cattle to viable avirulent *Leptospira pomona* vaccine. *Am J Vet Res* 32:851-854, 1971.

Sulzer, C. R., and W. L. Jones. *Leptospirosis Methods in Laboratory Diagnosis.* Atlanta, Georgia, Centers for Disease Control of the USA, 1974.

Szyfres, B. Leptospirosis as an animal and public health problem in Latin America and the Caribbean area. *In: VIII Inter-American Meeting on Foot-and-Mouth Disease and Zoonoses Control.* Washington, D.C., Pan American Health Organization, 1976. (Scientific Publication 316.)

Takafuji, E. T., J. W. Kirkpatrick, and R. N. Miller. An efficacy trial of doxycycline chemoprophylaxis against leptospirosis. *N Engl J Med* 310:524-525, 1984.

Tripathy, D. N., A. R. Smith, and L. E. Hanson. Immunoglobulins in cattle vaccinated with leptospiral bacterins. *Am J Vet Res* 36:1735-1736, 1975.

Van der Hoeden, J. Leptospirosis. *In:* Van der Hoeden, J. (Ed.), *Zoonoses.* Amsterdam, Netherlands, Elsevier, 1964.

Waitkins, S. A. From the PHLS: Update on leptospirosis. *Br Med J* 290, 1985.

World Health Organization. Research needs in leptospirosis. Memorandum. *Bull WHO* 47:113-122, 1972.

LISTERIOSIS

(027.0)

Synonyms: Leukocytosis, mononucleosis, listerial infection, listerellosis, listeriasis, circling disease (in animals).

Etiology: *Listeria* (*Listerella*) *monocytogenes*, a motile, gram positive aerobe that is a facultative intracellular parasite of the reticuloendothelial system. Among classified strains within this species there is great heterogeneity in antigens and pathogenicity. The current serotyping classification scheme is based on the different somatic and flagellar antigens; seven serotypes are recognized, and are in turn divided into subtypes.

It is of epidemiologic interest that 98% of infections in man and animals are caused by types 1 (subdivided in three subtypes: 1/2a, 1/2b, and 1/2c) and 4b.

Revision of the taxonomy of the genus *Listeria* is presently under way based on cross-hybridization studies. These studies allow subdivision of *L. monocytogenes* into five genomic groups. The virulent strains belong to two groups (*L. monocytogenes sensu stricto* and strains of serotype 5, also called *L. bulgarica*). Specific names proposed for the remaining groups are *L. innocua*, *L. welshimeri*, and *L. seeligeri* (Recourt *et al.*, 1983; Recourt and Grimont, 1983).

Geographic Distribution: Worldwide. *L. monocytogenes* is widely distributed in vegetation, soil, and human and animal intestines.

Occurrence in Man: Incidence is low. Greater concentrations of cases are reported from Europe and the United States, perhaps because medical personnel in these countries are on the alert and because better laboratory support is available. For the same reasons, the number of recorded cases has risen considerably in recent years, as shown by statistics from East and West Germany and the United States. From 1950 to 1959, a total of 500 cases were recorded in the two German republics, while almost 1,500 were registered from 1960 to 1966. In the USA between 1933 and 1958, only 184 cases were recorded, while from 1959 to 1966, 547 were reported. In developing countries few cases are reported. Sporadic cases have been seen in several Latin American countries. In a Mexican hospital, hemocultures were carried out during a 3-month period on all children whose mothers showed signs of amniotic infection; *L. monocytogenes* was isolated from four out of 33 newborns examined (Pérez-Mirabete and Giono, 1963). In Peru (Guevara *et al.*, 1979), serovars 4d and 4b of *L. monocytogenes* were isolated from three fatal cases of neonatal listeriosis and from five aborted fetuses.

A considerable rise in the number of listeriosis cases in renal transplant patients has been noted in recent years. From 1969 to 1980, 102 cases were recorded from among these patients (Stamm *et al.*, 1982). In addition to newborns, elderly people are also at risk of contracting listeriosis, especially those suffering from malignancies or other debilitating diseases or conditions. A review of English-language literature on the subject between 1968 and 1978 indicated that the average age of patients was 52 (Nieman and Lorber, 1980). A major epidemic in the United States, associated with consumption of pasteurized milk, occurred between June 30 and August 30, 1983, with 49 patients hospitalized and 14 deaths.

Occurrence in Animals: Listeriosis has a wide variety of host animals, both domestic and wild. The infection has been confirmed in a large number of domestic and wild mammals, in birds, and even in poikilotherms. The most susceptible domestic species is sheep, followed by goats and cattle. The frequency of occurrence in these animals is not known.

Outbreaks in sheep have been described in several Latin American countries. The disease has been confirmed in alpacas in Peru, in chickens in Argentina, and in canaries in Uruguay.

The Disease in Man: The most affected group is newborn children (they make up 50% of cases in France and 39% in the United States), followed by persons over 50 years of age. The disease is rare among those between 1 month and 18 years of age. According to data from two German obstetric clinics, listerial infection was the cause of 0.15 to 2% of perinatal mortality. Listerial abortion in women usually occurs in the second half of pregnancy. Symptoms that precede miscarriage or birth by a few days or weeks are chills, raised body temperature, cephalalgia, and mild dizziness. These symptoms may or may not recur in repeated episodes before birth of a stillborn fetus or a seriously ill full-term baby. After delivery the mother shows no disease symptoms, but *L. monocytogenes* can be isolated from the vagina, cervix, or urine for periods varying from a few days to several weeks. If the child is born alive, it dies shortly afterward from listerial septicemia. The main lesion is a focal hepatic necrosis in the form of small, grayish white nodules. Some children born apparently healthy fall ill with meningitis a few days to 3 weeks later; in these cases the infection was probably acquired *in utero* or during birth. In the United States neonatal meningitis is the most common clinical form, while in Europe perinatal septicemia prevails. Hydrocephalus is a common sequela of neonatal meningitis.

Meningitis or meningoencephalitis is the most common clinical form in adults, especially in those over 50. Listerial meningitis will often occur as a complication in debilitated persons, alcoholics, diabetics, or cancer patients. Before the existence of antibiotics, case fatality was 70%. Listerial septicemia also occurs among weakened adults, especially patients undergoing long-term treatment with corticosteroids or antimetabolites. In addition, listeriosis may result in endocarditis, external or internal abscesses, and endophthalmitis. A cutaneous eruption has been described among veterinarians who handled infected fetuses.

The Disease in Animals:

SHEEP, GOATS, AND CATTLE: Listeriosis manifests itself clinically in ruminants as encephalitis, neonatal mortality, and septicemia. The most common clinical form is encephalitis. In sheep and goats, the disease has a hyperacute course, and mortality may vary from 3% to more than 30%. In cattle, listerial encephalitis has a longer course, with the animals surviving for 4 to 14 days. In general, only 8 to 10% of a herd is affected.

A ruminant with encephalitis isolates itself from the herd and shows symptoms of depression, fever, incoordination, torticollis, spasmodic contractions and paralysis of facial muscles and throat, profuse salivation, strabismus, and conjunctivitis. The animal tries to lean against some support while standing and, if able to walk, moves in circles. In the final phase of the disease, the animal lies down and makes characteristic chewing movements when attempting to eat.

Listerial encephalitis can affect animals of any age, but it is more common in the first 3 years of life. Nevertheless, it does not appear before the rumen becomes functional. Septicemia is much more common among young animals than adults. Abortion occurs mainly during the last months of gestation and is generally the only symptom of genital infection, the dam showing no other signs of disease. If uterine infection occurs in the cow before the seventh month of pregnancy, the dead fetus is usually retained in the uterus for several days and has a macerated appearance, with marked focal necrotic hepatitis. In addition, the placenta may be retained and metritis may develop. If infection occurs in the last months of pregnancy, the fetus is almost intact and shows a minimum of lesions.

L. monocytogenes can also cause mastitis in cows. There are few described cases, either because the presence of this agent in cows has not been studied or because its occurrence really is rare. Mastitis caused by *Listeria* varies in severity from subclinical to acute and chronic. Elimination of the agent in the milk occurs over a long period of time and may have public health repercussions, especially since pasteurization does not offer a guarantee of complete safety if the viable bacteria count is high before heat treatment (Gitter, 1980).

A study carried out in 1970-71 in Victoria, Australia (Dennis, 1975), showed that listeriosis is an important cause of perinatal mortality in sheep. In 94 flocks, fetuses and lambs that died during the neonatal period were examined, and *L. monocytogenes* was found in 25%. The disease caused by this agent occurs mostly in winter. It has been estimated that the rate of abortion in flocks affected by listeriosis in Victoria varies from 2 to 20%.

OTHER MAMMALS: Listeriosis is rare in swine; when it does occur in the first few weeks of life, it usually takes the septicemic form. Few cases are known in dogs, in which the disease may be confused with rabies. In other domestic and wild species the disease generally appears as isolated cases and in the septicemic form. Outbreaks in rabbit and guinea pig breeding colonies have been described.

FOWL: Young birds are the most affected. Outbreaks are infrequent and mortality may vary on different farms from loss of a few birds to a high rate. The septicemic form is the most common, with degenerative lesions of the myocardium, pericarditis, and also focal hepatic necrosis. On rare occasion the meningoencephalitic form is found, with marked torticollis. Since the generalized use of antibiotics in poultry feed began, few cases of listeriosis in this species have been reported.

Source of Infection and Mode of Transmission: The causal agent is widely distributed, in animals and man as well as in the environment. *L. monocytogenes* has been isolated from different mammalian and avian species and from the soil, plants, mud, pasture, waste water, and streams. The presence of virulent and avirulent (for mice) strains in animals and in the environment complicates clarification of the epidemiology, but serotyping can be of considerable help. Cattle, sheep, and many other animal species eliminate the agent in feces. *L. monocytogenes* can also be isolated from the stool of a large proportion of healthy people. It has been isolated from the stools of 20 to 30% of pregnant women, and has also been found in the female genital tract. In addition to untypable strains, potentially pathogenic serotype 1 and serovar 4b have been recovered (Kampelmacher and Van Noorle Jansen, 1980). Consequently, the natural reservoir is wide and the number of hosts is large. In spite of this, few people contract the disease. Many women from whose stools the agent has been isolated give birth to healthy children. Concurrent conditions, such as stress and other predisposing causes, come into play in initiating the disease.

The reservoir and source of infection for the fetus and newborn is apparently the infected mother herself. It is believed that the almost inapparent disease course manifested by the mother is caused by a mild bacteremia. Airborne infection might play a role, as suggested by the influenzalike symptoms exhibited by the mother. The mother's genital tract is probably infected via the fecal route, while the fetus is infected via the bloodstream and placenta. The discovery of the causal agent in the semen of a man whose wife's genital organs were infected would indicate that in some cases the infection may be transmitted by sexual contact.

In other cases the infection is produced through oral transmission, such as in the recent epidemic in the United States (see Occurrence in Man) in which milk was the vehicle. It is interesting to note that the milk associated with the outbreak came from establishments where listeriosis had been diagnosed in the animals. The epidemic affected two very susceptible groups: newborn children and debilitated persons. Of 49 patients hospitalized with listerial septicemia and meningitis, seven were newborns and 42 were adults. All adults were suffering from other diseases or undergoing treatment with immunosuppressants.

An outbreak in the Maritime Provinces of Canada included 34 perinatal cases and seven cases in adults without antecedent illness or immunosuppressant use; the source of infection was coleslaw. The investigation showed that the cabbage came from a farm on which there was listeriosis in sheep whose dung had been used as fertilizer. *L. monocytogenes* serovar type 4b was isolated from the cabbage as well as from the patients. It is also worth noting that the farmer kept the cabbage refrigerated at 4°C, which allowed the etiologic agent to multiply at the expense of other contaminant microorganisms (Schlech *et al.*, 1983).

L. monocytogenes is an opportunistic bacteria, as is demonstrated by cases of the disease in patients whose immune response is suppressed because of illness or therapy, such as cancer victims, kidney transplant patients, and others (see Occurrence in Man).

Transmission between newborn children in nurseries has been described on several occasions. In Chile one such outbreak occurred recently in a neonatal ward (Garcia *et al.*, 1983). Nosocomial transmission among adults is also suspected to occur. Following admission of a patient with listerial septicemia and meningitis to a hospital, three septicemia cases appeared in other patients with suppressed immune systems; however, the mode of transmission could not be determined (Green and Macaulay, 1978).

A rise in listeriosis cases when animals feed on silage would indicate the digestive system as the portal of entry. The causal agent has been isolated from spoiled fodder that had a pH higher than 5. *L. monocytogenes* is distributed within populations of healthy animals and the disease can be produced when stress lowers the host's resistance.

Role of Animals in the Epidemiology of the Disease: The epidemiology of listeriosis is still not well known. Most researchers are inclined to consider it as a disease common to man and animals and not as a zoonosis *per se*. It is probable that animals contribute to maintenance of the agent in nature and especially to its distribution.

Studies carried out over the last few years suggest that man and animals can contract the infection in many ways and from many sources. In the United States, most human cases occur in urban areas where there is little contact with animals. Nevertheless, the latter may serve as a source of infection. In one case the infection was confirmed in a woman who drank raw milk; the same serotype of *Listeria* was isolated from the raw milk and from the woman's premature twins. The etiologic agent was isolated from the milk of 16% of cows that had listerial abortions. The above-described outbreaks originated by milk or vegetables contaminated with manure from listeria-infected animals demonstrate that animals may be an important source of infection.

In summary, the source of infection for man can be humans and animals as well as the environment (soil, plants, dust).

Diagnosis: Diagnosis can be made only through isolation of the causal agent. In septicemic cases, the agent may be isolated from the blood. In women it may be cultured from vaginal secretions and the stool. Isolations can be done from any organ of septicemic fetuses and from the cerebrospinal fluid of meningitis or meningoencephalitis cases. In sheep, goats, or cattle with encephalitis, samples of the medulla oblongata may be cultured, and in septicemic fowl, rodents, or neonatal ruminants, the blood or internal organs. Part of the material should be cultured immediately and part should be kept at 4°C to be cultured again every 2 weeks if the first test turns out negative. The "cold enrichment" method is used especially in epidemiologic investigations and is important for culture of highly contaminated specimens. Nevertheless, this method has no value for diagnosis of clinical cases because of the time it takes, since treatment with antibiotics (preferably ampicillin) should begin as soon as possible to be effective. Isolation by inoculation into mice or embryonated eggs is very useful.

A test has been developed to distinguish between pathogenic and nonpathogenic strains of *L. monocytogenes*. It is based on the potentiating and synergistic effect that the extrosubstance of *Rhodococcus equi* has for producing hemolysis in cultures of pathogenic *L. monocytogenes* (Skalka *et al.*, 1982).

In general, serologic tests are confusing and not useful because of cross-reactions with enterococci and *Staphylococcus aureus*, especially by serogroups 1 and 3 of *Listeria*.

Control: In regions where human neonatal listeriosis is common, a Gram stain can be made from the meconium of a newborn, and treatment with antibiotics rapidly initiated if bacteria suspected of being *Listeria* are encountered. Women who develop influenzalike symptoms in the final months of pregnancy should be carefully examined, and treated, if necessary, with antibiotics. The limited arsenal of defense against the infection includes such measures as the pasteurization of milk, rodent control, and common practices of environmental and personal hygiene.

Animals with encephalitis or those that have aborted should be isolated and their placentas and fetuses destroyed. Recently acquired animals should only be added to a herd after undergoing a reasonable period of quarantine.

Bibliography

Bojsen-Moller, J. Human listeriosis; diagnostic, epidemiological and clinical studies. *Acta Pathol Microbiol Scand (B), Suppl* 229, 1972.

Broadbent, D. W. Infections associated with ovine perinatal mortality in Victoria. *Aust Vet J* 51:71-74, 1975.

Centers for Disease Control of the USA. Listeriosis outbreak associated with Mexican-style cheese. California. *Morb Mortal Wkly Rep* 34:357-359, 1985.

Dennis, S. M. Perinatal lamb mortality in Western Australia. Listeric infections. *Aust Vet J* 51:75-79, 1975.

Fleming, D. W., S. L. Cochi, K. L. MacDonald, J. Brondum, P. S. Hayes, B. D. Plikaytis, M. B. Holmes, A. Audurier, C. V. Broome, and A. L. Reingold. Pasteurized milk as a vehicle of infection in an outbreak of listeriosis. *N Engl J Med* 312:404-407, 1985.

Franck, M. Contribution a l'Etude de l'Epidémiologie des Listerioses Humaines et Animales. Thesis. National Veterinary School, Lyon, France, 1974.

García, H., M. E. Pinto, L. Ross, and G. Saavedra. Brote epidémico de listeriosis neonatal. *Rev Chile Pediatr* 54:330-335, 1983.

Gitter, M., R. Bradley, and P. H. Blampied. *Listeria monocytogenes* infection in bovine mastitis. *Vec Rec* 107:390-392, 1980.

Gray, M. L., and A. H. Killinger. *Listeria monocytogenes* and listeric infections. *Bacteriol Rev* 30:309-382, 1966.

Green, H. T., and M. B. Macaulay. Hospital outbreak of *Listeria monocytogenes* septicemia: a problem of cross infection. *Lancet* 2:1039-1040, 1978.

Guevara, J. M., J. Pereda, and S. Roel. Human listeriosis in Peru. *Tropenmed Parasitol* 30:59-61, 1979.

Kampelmacher, E. H., and L. M. Van Noorle Jansen. Listeriosis in humans and animals in the Netherlands (1958-1977). *Zentralbl Bakteriol* [A] 246:211-227, 1980.

Killinger, A. H., and M. E. Mansfield. Epizootiology of listeric infection in sheep. *J Am Vet Med Assoc* 157:1318-1324, 1970.

Killinger, A. H. Listeriosis. *In:* Hubbert, W. T., W. F. McCulloch, and P. R. Schnurrenberger (Eds.), *Diseases Transmitted from Animals to Man*, 6th ed. Springfield, Illinois, Thomas, 1975.

Lamont, R. J., and R. Postlethwaite. Carriage of *Listeria monocytogenes* and related species in pregnant and non-pregnant women in Aberdeen, Scotland. *J Infect* 13:187-193, 1986.

Larsen, H. E. Epidemiology of listeriosis. The ubiquitous occurrence of *Listeria monocytogenes*. *In: Proceedings, Third International Symposium on Listeriosis.* Bilthoven, Netherlands, 1966.

Mair, N. S. Human listeriosis. *In:* Graham-Jones, O. (Ed.), *Some Diseases of Animals Communicable to Man in Britain.* Oxford, Pergamon, 1968.

Malinverni, R., J. Bille, C. Perret, F. Regli, F. Tanner, and M. P. Glauser. Epidemic listeriosis. *Schweiz Med Wochenschr* 115, 1985.

Moro, M. Enfermedades infecciosas de las alpacas. 2. Listeriosis. *Rev Fac Med Vet (Lima)* 16-17:154-159, 1961-62.

Nieman, R. E., and B. Lorber. Listeriosis in adults: a changing pattern. Report of eight cases and review of the literature, 1968-1978. *Rev Infect Dis* 2:207-227, 1980.

Pérez-Miravete, A., and S. Giono. La infección perinatal listérica en México. II. Aislamiento de *Listeria monocytogenes* en septicemia del recién nacido. *Rev Inst Salubr Enferm Trop* 23:103-113, 1963.

Recourt, J., J. M. Alonso, and H. P. R. Seeliger. Virulence comparée des cinq groupes génomiques de *Listeria monocytogenes (sensu lato)*. *Ann Microbiol (Inst Pasteur)* 134A:359-364, 1983.

Recourt, J., and P. A. D. Grimont. *Listeria welshimeri* sp. nov. and *Listeria seeligeri* sp. nov. *Int J Syst Bacteriol* 33:866-869, 1983.

Recourt, J., and H. P. R. Seeliger. Distribution des espèces du genre *Listeria*. (Classification of different *Listeria* species). *Zentralbl Bakteriol Mikrobiol Hyg* [A] 259:317-330, 1985.

Schlech, W. F., P. M. Lavigne, R. A. Bertolussi, A. C. Allen, E. V. Haldane, A. J. Worth, A. W. Hightower, S. E. Johnson, S. H. King, E. S. Nichols, and C. V. Broome. Epidemic listeriosis—evidence for transmission by food. *N Engl J Med* 308:203-206, 1983.

Seeliger, H. P. R. *Listeriosis.* New York, Hafner, 1961.

Skalka, B., J. Smola, and K. Elischerova. Routine test for *in vitro* differentiation of pathogenic and apathogenic *Listeria monocytogenes* strains. *J Clin Microbiol* 15:503-507, 1982.

Stamm, A. M., W. E. Dismukes, B. P. Simmons, C. Glenn Cobbs, A. Elliot, P. Budrich, and J. Harmon. Listeriosis in renal transplant recipients: report of an outbreak and review of 102 cases. *Rev Infect Dis* 4:665-682, 1982.

Weis, J., and H. P. R. Seeliger. Incidence of *Listeria monocytogenes* in nature. *Appl Microbiol* 30:29-32, 1975.

Young, S. Listeriosis in cattle and sheep. *In:* Faulkner, L. C. (Ed.), *Abortion Diseases of Livestock.* Springfield, Illinois, Thomas, 1968.

LYME DISEASE

(104.8)
(695.9)

Synonyms: Lyme arthritis, erythema chronicum migrans (ECM) with polyarthritis.

Etiology: The etiologic agent is a spirochete, recently isolated (Steere *et al.*, 1983), which to date does not have a specific name and for which the name of *Borrelia burgdorferi* has been proposed. The spirochete shares common characteristics with the treponemas and the borrelias (Johnson *et al.*, 1984).

Geographic Distribution: The disease was identified as a clinical entity in 1977 in the area of Lyme, Connecticut, USA. It is presently known to occur in 14 states of that country (Steere *et al.*, 1984). Its distribution is closely tied to the presence of the vector, which is a tick of the *Ixodes ricinus* complex (*I. dammini, I. pacificus*). Three different regions in the US are affected: the Northeast, the North Central (Wisconsin and Minnesota), and the Pacific Coast (northern California and Oregon) (Steere and Malawista, 1979). Cases have also been described in Europe (Scandinavia, Germany, Switzerland, France) and in Australia (Gester *et al.*, 1981; Charmot *et al.*, 1982; Schmid, 1985). Soviet literature cites cases of the disease in the Caucasus region.

Occurrence in Man: In 4 years, from November 1975 to August 1979, 512 cases were recorded (Steere and Malawista, 1979). Of the total during these 4 years, 242 cases (47%) appeared in the area of Lyme, where a system of epidemiological surveillance is in force; more recently, the total number of cases in this region amounted to 444, which represents 4% of the 12,000 residents (Steere *et al.*, 1983). Cases appear in summer when the tick *Ixodes dammini* and similar species are active and abundant.

Occurrence in Animals: In the natural foci of the infection, high rates of reactors to the indirect immunofluorescence test, using antigens from the etiologic agent, have been found in several wild animal species and in dogs. The prevalence of reactors in animals infested with *I. dammini* in the eastern part of Connecticut from 1978 to 1982 was as follows (Magnarelli *et al.*, 1984): white-tailed deer (*Odocoileus virginianus*), 27%; white-footed mice (*Peromyscus leucopus*), 10%; eastern chipmunks (*Tamias striatus*), 17%; gray squirrels (*Sciurus carolinensis*), 50%; opossums (*Didelphis virginiana*), 17%; raccoons (*Procyon lotor*), 23%; and dogs, 24%. The spirochete was isolated from the bloodstream of one out of 20 white-footed mice examined (Anderson and Magnarelli, 1983; Bosler *et al.*, 1984).

The Disease in Man: The characteristic cutaneous lesion, erythema chronicum migrans (ECM), appears from 3 to 20 days after the tick bite. This lesion begins with a red macula or papule that widens. The borders are clearly delineated, and as the center of the lesion pales, an annular erythema forms. The erythema may be recurrent, with secondary lesions appearing on other parts of the body. The cutaneous lesions may be accompanied for several weeks by malaise, fever, cephalagia, stiff neck, myalgias, arthralgia, or lymphadenopathy. After several weeks or months, some patients develop meningoencephalitis, neuropathology, myocarditis, and atrioventricular tachycardia. Some suffer arthritic attacks in the large joints which may recur for several years, at times taking a chronic course (Steere *et al.*, 1983). Treatment of these processes with penicillin has given very good results (Steere *et al.*, 1985).

It should be borne in mind that the connection between ECM and arthritis is not apparent, since several weeks or months transpire between the two episodes.

Of 405 patients showing ECM, 249 had later neurologic, cardiac, and articular symptoms (Steere and Malawista, 1979).

The Disease in Animals: The effect of the spirochete infection on wild animals and dogs is not known.

Source of Infection and Mode of Transmission: The etiologic agent is transmitted by a vector, which in the United States is the tick *Ixodes dammini* on the Northeast Coast and in the North Central states, and *I. pacificus* on the Pacific Coast (American Public Health Association, 1985). Recently, the tick *Amblyomma americanum* was recognized as a possible vector in the state of New Jersey (Schultze *et al.*, 1984). In Europe the vector is *I. ricinus*, and in Australia, possibly *I. holocyclus* (Stewart *et al.*, 1982).

The isolation of the etiologic agent from ticks verified their role as vectors. In fact, in the endemic area of Connecticut, a spirochete with the same morphological and antigenic characteristics as the one in Lyme disease patients was isolated from 21 (19%) of 110 nymphs and adult ticks (*I. dammini*). The high rate of infection of the vector was shown by direct immunofluorescence; in one locality, 30 (21%) of 143 *I. dammini* contained spirochetes, and in another, 17 (26%) of 66. Positive results were obtained only for nymphs and adults that had fed, while 148 larvae that had not fed were negative (Steere *et al.*, 1983).

Since the larvae are not infected, the tick must derive the infection from an animal reservoir. The serologic survey carried out on dogs and wild animals (see Occurrence in Animals) demonstrated that the infection is prevalent among these animals, which, together with ticks, could maintain the etiologic agent in natural foci.

Even though the ecology of the disease is not thoroughly understood, transmission seems to occur from an infected wild animal to another susceptible one through a tick's bite. Man is probably an accidental host in this cycle.

The survival of the infection in natural foci is assured by the high degree of infestation of wild animals by ticks (*I. dammini*). According to a recent study (Magnarelli *et al.*, 1984), this infestation varies from 21.4% among eastern chipmunks to 84.2% among opossums.

Man becomes infected by the bite of an infected tick, especíally in summer when ticks abound, when visiting a natural focus of infection. In addition, dogs may transport ticks to inhabited areas.

Role of Animals in the Epidemiology of the Disease: On the basis of present information, wild animals are presumed to be principally responsible for maintaining the infection in natural foci (Bosler *et al.*, 1984).

Diagnosis: Until recently, the diagnosis was based exclusively on the symptom complex, especially a history of ECM, and on epidemiologic information.

Although now possible, isolation of the infective agent by culture is still not very practical. In 1983, Steere *et al.* isolated the agent in only three patients, using a total of 142 clinical samples from 56 patients. On the other hand, the indirect immunofluorescence test with conjugated IgM and IgG sera gave good results. Patients with ECM had high titers of IgM antibodies only between the ECM phase and convalescence 2 or 3 weeks later. Patients with late manifestations of the disease (arthritis, cardiac, or neurologic anomalies) had elevated titers for IgG antibodies (Steere *et al.* 1983). Recently, the indirect immunofluorescence test has been perfected and an ELISA test has been developed, both of which have a high degree of sensitivity and specificity for diagnosis of the disease (Hazel and Wilkinson, 1984). Early treatment with antibiotics (penicillin or tetracycline), which shorten the duration of ECM and can prevent or at least attenuate late manifestations of the disease, may also reduce the number of antibodies.

Control: The only methods of prevention consist of avoiding endemic areas and tick bites. Persons entering natural foci should use protective footware and clothes, but this is not always possible. Repellents may give some protection. Moreover, it would be prudent to treat dogs with tickicides.

Bibliography

Anderson, J. F., R. C. Johnson, L. A. Magnarelli, F. W. Hyde. Involvement of birds in the epidemiology of the Lyme disease agent *Borrelia burgdorferi*. *Infect Immun* 51:394-396, 1986.

Anderson, J. F., and L. A. Magnarelli. Spirochetes in *Ixodes dammini* and *Babesia microti* on Prudence Island, Rhode Island. *J Infect Dis* 148:1124, 1983.

Anderson, J. F., and L. A. Magnarelli. Avian and mammalian hosts for spirochete-infected ticks and insects in a Lyme disease focus in Connecticut. *Yale J Biol Med* 57:627-641, 1984.

American Public Health Association. *Control of Communicable Diseases in Man*, 14th ed. (Ed. by A. S. Benenson). Washington, D.C., APHA, 1985.

Baranton, G., C. Edlinger, J. Mazzonelli, and Y. Dufresne. La borréliose dite de Lyme, maladie "nouvelle" identifiée depuis prés de 80 ans. *Med Mal Infect* 12:747-755, 1986.

Barbour, A. G. Isolation and cultivation of Lyme disease spirochetes. *Yale J Biol Med* 57:521-528, 1984.

Bosler, E. M., B. G. Ormiston, J. L. Coleman, J. G. Hanrahan, and J. L. Benach. Prevalence of the Lyme disease spirochete in populations of white-tailed deer and white-footed mice. *Yale J Biol Med* 57:651-659, 1984.

Bruhn, F. W. Lyme disease. *Am J Dis Child* 138:467-470, 1984.

Burgdorfer, W., A. G. Barbour, S. F. Hayes, J. L. Benach, E. Grunwaldt, and J. P. Davis. Lyme disease—a tickborne spirochetosis? *Science* 216:1317-1319, 1982.

Centers for Disease Control of the USA. Update: Lyme disease and cases occurring during pregnancy—United States. *Morb Mortal Wkly Rep* 34:376-378, 383, 1985.

Charmot, G., F. Rodhain, and C. Perez. Un cas d'arthrite de Lyme observé en France. *Nouv Presse Med* 11:207-208, 1982.

Fumarola, D., C. Marcuccio, F. Crovato, G. Nazzari, G. Rovetta, M. A. Cimmino, and G. Bianchi. Lyme disease in Italy: first reported case. *Bol Inst Sieroter Milan* 64:483-485, 1985.

Gester, J. C., S. Guggi, H. Perroud, and R. Bovet. Lyme arthritis appearing outside the United States: A case report from Switzerland. *Br Med J* 283:951-952, 1981.

Habicht, G. S., G. Beck, and J. L. Benach. Lyme disease. *Sci Am* 257:78-83, 1987.

Hanrahan, J. P., J. L. Benach, J. L. Coleman, E. M. Bosler, D. L. Morse, D. J. Cameron, R. Edelman, and R. A. Kaslow. Incidence and cumulative frequency of endemic Lyme disease in a community. *J Infect Dis* 150:489-496, 1984.

Hayes, S. F., W. Burgdorfer, and H. G. Barbour. A bacteriophage in *Ixodes* spirochete the etiologic agent of Lyme disease. *J Bacteriol* 154:1436-1439, 1983.

Hazel, W., and P. D. Wilkinson. Immunodiagnostic tests for Lyme disease. *Yale J Biol Med* 57:567-572, 1984.

Johnson, R. C., F. W. Hyde, A. G. Steigerwalt, and D. J. Brenner. *Borrelia burgdorferi* sp. nov.: Etiologic agent of Lyme disease. *Int J Syst Bacteriol* 34:496-497, 1984.

Johnson, R. C., F. W. Hyde, and C. M. Rumpel. Taxonomy of the Lyme disease spirochetes. *Yale J Biol Med* 57:529-537, 1984.

Levine, J. F., M. L. Wilson, and A. Spielman. Mice as reservoirs of the Lyme disease spirochete. *Am J Trop Med Hyg* 34:355-360, 1985.

Magnarelli, L. A., J. F. Anderson, W. Burgdorfer, and W. A. Chappel. Parasitism by *Ixodes dammini* (Acari: Ixodidae) and antibodies to spirochetes in mammals at Lyme disease foci in Connecticut, USA. *J Med Entomol* 21:52-57, 1984.

Magnarelli, L. A., J. F. Anderson, C. S. Apperson, D. Fish, R. C. Johnson, and W. A. Chappell. Spirochetes in ticks and antibodies to *Borrelia burgdorferi* in white-tailed deer from Connecticut, New York State and North Carolina. *J Wildl Dis* 22:178-188, 1986.

Magnarelli, L. A., J. F. Anderson, and A. G. Barbour. The etiologic agent of Lyme disease in deer flies, horse flies and mosquitoes. *J Infect Dis* 154:355-358, 1986.

Mazzonelli, J., and Y. Dufresne. Sérodiagnostic en immunofluorescence de la borréliose de Lyme avec la souche francaise 1P. *Med Mal Infect* 4:212-214, 1986.

Russell, H., J. S. Sampson, G. P. Schmid, H. W. Wilkinson, and B. Plikaytis. Enzyme-linked immunosorbent assay and indirect immunofluorescence assay for Lyme disease. *J Infect Dis* 149:465-470, 1984.

Schmid, G. P. The global distribution of Lyme disease. *Rev Infect Dis* 7:41-50, 1985.

Schmid, G. P., R. Horsley, A. C. Steere, J. P. Hanrahan, J. P. Davis, G. S. Bowen, M. T. Osterholm, J. S. Weisfeld, A. W. Hightower, and C. V. Broome. Surveillance of Lyme disease in the United States, 1982. *J Infect Dis* 151:1144-1149, 1985.

Schultze, T., G. S. Bowen, E. M. Bosler, M. F. Lakat, W. E. Parkin, R. Altman, B. G. Ormiston, and J. K. Shirler. *Amblyomma americanum*: A potential vector of Lyme disease in New Jersey. *Science* 224:601-603, 1984.

Stanek, G., G. Wewalka, V. Groh, R. Neuman, and W. Kristoferitsch. Differences between Lyme disease and European arthropod-borne Borrelia infections. *Lancet* 1(8425):401, 1985.

Steere, A. C., and S. E. Malawista. Cases of Lyme disease in the United States: Locations correlated with distribution of *Ixodes dammini*. *Ann Intern Med* 91:730-733, 1979.

Steere, A. C., R. L. Grodzicki, A. N. Kornblatt, J. E. Craft, A. G. Barbour, W. Burgdorfer, G. P. Schmid, E. Johnson, and S. E. Malawista. The spirochetal etiology of Lyme disease. *N Engl J Med* 308:733-744, 1983.

Steere, A. C., J. Green, R. T. Schoen, E. Taylor, G. J. Hutchinson, D. W. Rahn, and S. E.

Malawista. Successful parenteral penicillin therapy of established Lyme arthritis. *N Engl J Med* 312:869-874, 1985.

Steere, A. C., E. Taylor, M. L. Wilson, J. F. Levine, and A. Spielman. Longitudinal assessment of the clinical and epidemiological features of Lyme disease in a defined population. *J Infect Dis* 154:295-300, 1986.

Stevens, R., K. Hechemy, A. Rogers, and J. Benach. Fluoroimmunoassay (FIAX) for Lyme disease antibody. *Abstracts, Annual Meeting of the American Society for Microbiology*, March 3-7, 1985.

Stewart, A., J. Glass, A. Patel, G. Watt, A. Cripps, and R. Clancy. Lyme arthritis in the Hunter Valley. *Med J Aust* 1:139, 1982.

World Health Organization. Lyme disease: clinical, serological and epidemiological aspects. *Wkly Epidemiol Rec* 61(19):145-147, 1986.

MELIOIDOSIS

(025)

Synonyms: Whitmore's disease, rodent glanders.

Etiology: *Pseudomonas (Malleomyces) pseudomallei*, a small, aerobic, motile, pleomorphic bacillus closely related to *P. mallei*, the agent of glanders. In the laboratory, *P. pseudomallei* can survive in humid, clayey soil at room temperature and in the shade for 30 months (Thomas and Forbes-Faulkner, 1981).

Geographic Distribution: Most human and animal cases have been recorded in Southeast Asia (Burma, Thailand, Malaysia, and Indonesia), which is considered to be the principal endemic area. The disease has also been diagnosed in Korea, the Philippines, Turkey, Iran, Sri Lanka, Madagascar, northeastern Australia, Papua New Guinea, and Guam. In the Americas, the infection has been confirmed in Aruba (Netherlands Antilles), the Bahamas, Mexico, Panama, and Ecuador. More recent investigations have revealed the agent's presence in other areas (Peru, Brazil, Haiti, the Ivory Coast, Upper Volta, and France) by isolating it from people, animals, or soil or water samples. The agent's distribution is predominantly tropical. The epizootic that occurred in the "Jardin des Plantes" in Paris is the first reported outbreak in a temperate climate (American Public Health Association, 1985; Galimard and Dodin, 1982).

Occurrence in Man: Clinically apparent infection caused by *P. pseudomallei* is not very common. During the war in Indochina several hundred French, American, and Vietnamese soldiers became ill with melioidosis. In the period from 1965 to 1969, three cases per month occurred among US Army soldiers in Vietnam (Piggott, 1976). According to a serologic survey, 9% of the three million US personnel participating in the Vietnam conflict were exposed to the agent. Cases confirmed in the United States during the 1970s were almost all military personnel or travelers returning from Southeast Asia (Centers for Disease Control, 1977).

Occurrence in Animals: In endemic zones, sporadic cases have been reported in different animal species. Occasional outbreaks have occurred among sheep (Australia and Aruba), swine (Vietnam), and zoo animals.

The Disease in Man: The incubation period can be a few days, but in some patients the agent lies dormant for months or even years before clinical signs are seen. The infection may occur subclinically, as was shown by a serologic survey of war veterans, or the disease may take an acute fulminant, subacute, or chronic form. In the fulminant form, the patient dies in a few days, after suffering fever, pneumonia, and gastroenteritis. The disease generally appears as a respiratory illness that varies from mild bronchitis to severe and fatal pneumonia.

In septicemic cases of short duration, the principal lesion consists of small abscesses distributed throughout the body. When the septicemia is prolonged, large, confluent abscesses are found, often localized in one organ.

Lasting from a few months to many years, chronic melioidosis is characterized by localization in some organ, such as the lungs, lymph glands, skin, or bones. The lesion consists of a combination of necrosis and granulomatous inflammation. The central zone of necrosis contains a purulent or caseous exudate.

In northern Australian aborigines, a form of the disease has been observed in which primary localization is in the lower urogenital system. This localization was observed in six of 16 aborigines with melioidosis (Webling, 1980).

The infection may remain dormant several years and manifest itself if the host becomes debilitated.

The Disease in Animals: Many animal species are susceptible. Sporadic cases have been observed in sheep, goats, horses, swine, cattle, dogs, cats, nonhuman primates, wild and peridomestic rats, other wild animals, and laboratory guinea pigs and rabbits. The most susceptible species are sheep, swine, and goats, in which epidemic outbreaks have occurred.

In Aruba, the disease in sheep consisted primarily of abscesses of the viscera, joints, and lymph nodes. In a few weeks, 25 of 90 sheep died from the disease and many survivors suffered weight loss and polyarthritis (Sutmöller *et al.*, 1957). In cases in Australian sheep, cough and nervous symptoms were observed (Laws and Hall, 1964).

In swine, the symtomatology consists of fever, prostration, dyspnea, cough, and arthritis. In suckling pigs the disease is often fatal.

The symptomatology is not very characteristic, and the disease is difficult to diagnose in animal species where it appears sporadically. The lesions, which are similar to those in man, may suggest melioidosis and lead to its diagnosis.

Source of Infection and Mode of Transmission (Figure 13): Investigations carried out in recent years give increasing evidence that the reservoirs of *P. pseudomallei* are surface waters and soil, as corroborated by sampling done in Southeast Asia. The highest isolation rates were obtained in rice fields and newly planted oil palm plantations (14.5 to 33.3% of the isolations were from water samples). Seroepidemiologic studies also show that the highest reactor rates to the hemagglutination test came from workers or inhabitants of those areas. Human and animal infection occurs mainly during the rainy season. The etiologic agent can survive for many months in surface water and, with its low nutritional requirements, it can multiply in the hot, humid environment characteristic of endemic regions.

Figure 13. Melioidosis (*Pseudomonas pseudomallei*). Mode of transmission.

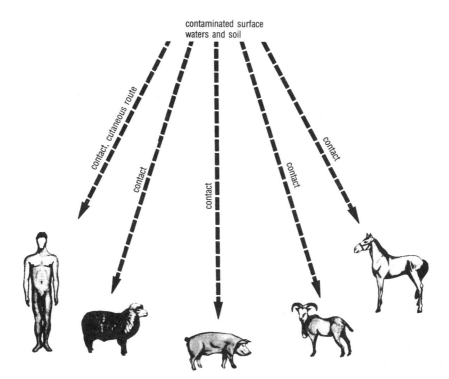

Transmission from animal to animal or from animal to man has not been proven, but it is thought that in some cases the infection may be passed from person to person. In addition to a case in which an American soldier in Vietnam with prostatitis seems to have transmitted the disease venereally to a woman, venereal transmission of the disease was also suspected among Australian aborigines with urogenital melioidosis. In accordance with tribal rituals, these aborigines smear their genitals with clay, and coitus normally takes place in contact with the soil (Webling, 1980).

Man and animals are believed to acquire the infection by contact with contaminated soil or water, primarily through skin abrasions, but also by inhalation of dust or ingestion of contaminated water. During the war in Indochina, the number of recorded human cases climbed considerably due to contamination of war wounds with mud, traversal of flooded countryside, or prolonged stay in trenches.

The rat flea *Xenopsylla cheopis* and the mosquito *Aedes aegypti* are capable of transmitting the infection experimentally to laboratory animals. The etiologic agent multiplies in the digestive tract of these insects. The role of these possible vectors in natural transmission has not yet been evaluated, but it is thought to be of little importance.

Role of Animals in the Epidemiology of the Disease: Recent findings indicate that melioidosis is a disease common to man and animals, with water and soil as reservoirs and sources of infection for both. Nevertheless, animals are believed to play a role as hosts in transporting the etiologic agent to new geographic areas.

Diagnosis: The only incontrovertible diagnostic method is isolation and identification of the etiologic agent, either by direct culture or inoculation of guinea pigs. *P. pseudomallei* can be isolated from abscesses, sputum, urine, and various tissues.

The allergenic test using melioidin may be useful for diagnosis in animals, but it gives many false negative results in swine and false positives in goats.

Of the serologic tests, the hemagglutination test with melioidin-sensitized erythrocytes has proved to be sufficiently sensitive and specific.

Control: Since it is an infrequent disease, specific preventive measures are not justified. The use of boots during outdoor work can give a certain amount of protection.

In animals, control of the infection is difficult, unless the environment is changed through such measures as drainage of low-lying, water-covered fields.

Bibliography

American Public Health Association. *Control of Communicable Diseases in Man*, 14th ed. (Ed. by A. S. Benenson). Washington, D.C., APHA, 1985.

Barnes, P. F., M. D. Appleman, and M. M. Cosgrove. A case of melioidosis originating in North America. *Am Rev Respir Dis* 134:170-171, 1986.

Biegeleisen, J. Z., Jr., M. R. Mosquera, and W. B. Cherry. A case of human melioidosis. Clinical, epidemiological and laboratory findings. *Am J Trop Med Hyg* 13:89-99, 1966.

Centers for Disease Control of the USA. Melioidosis—Pennsylvania. *Morb Mortal Wkly Rep* 25:419-420, 1977.

Galimard, M., and A. Dodin. Le point sur la melioidose dans le monde. *Bull Soc Pathol Exot* 75:375-383, 1982.

Hubbert, W. T. Melioidosis sources and potential. *Bull Wildl Dis Assoc* 5:208-212, 1969.

Kaufman, A. E., A. D. Alexander, A. M. Allen, R. J. Cronkin, L. A. Dillingham, J. D. Douglas, and T. D. Moore. Melioidosis in imported nonhuman primates. *J Wildl Dis* 6:211-219, 1970.

Ketterer, P. J., B. Donald, and R. J. Rogers. Bovine melioidosis in Southeastern Queensland. *Aust Vet J* 51:395-398, 1975.

Ketterer, P. J., W. R. Webster, J. Shield, R. J. Arthur, P. J. Blackall, and A. D. Thomas. Melioidosis in intensive piggeries in Southeastern Queensland. *Aust Vet J* 63:146-149, 1986.

Laws, L., and W. T. K. Hall. Melioidosis in animals in North Queensland. IV. Epidemiology. *Aust Vet J* 40:309-314, 1964.

Piggot, J. A. Melioidosis. *In*: Binford, C. H., and D. H. Connor (Eds.), *Pathology of Tropical and Extraordinary Diseases*. Washington, D.C., Armed Forces Institute of Pathology, 1976.

Piggot, J. A., and L. Hochoholzen. Human melioidosis. A histopathologic study of acute and chronic melioidosis. *Arch Pathol* 90:101-111, 1970.

Redfearn, M. S., and N. J. Palleroni. Glanders and melioidosis. *In*: Hubbert, W. T., W. F. McCulloch, and P. R. Schnurrenberger (Eds.), *Diseases Transmitted from Animals to Man*, 6th ed. Springfield, Illinois, Thomas, 1975.

Strauss, J. M., M. G. Groves, M. Mariappan, and D. W. Ellison. Melioidosis in Malaya. II. Distribution of *Pseudomonas pseudomallei* in soil and surface water. *Am J Trop Med Hyg* 18:698-702, 1969.

Sutmöller, P., F. C. Kraneveld, and A. van der Schaaf. Melioidosis (*Pseudomalleus*) in sheep, goats, and pigs in Aruba (Netherlands Antilles). *J Am Vet Med Assoc* 130:415-417, 1957.

Thomas, A. D., and J. C. Forbes-Faulkner. Persistence of *Pseudomonas pseudomallei* in soil. *Aust Vet J* 57:535-536, 1981.

Wehling, D. D'A. Genito-urinary infections with *Pseudomonas pseudomallei* in Australian aboriginals. *Trans R Soc Trop Med Hyg* 74:138-139, 1980.

NECROBACILLOSIS

(040.3)

Synonyms: Schmorl's disease, calf diphtheria, foot rot.

Etiology: *Fusobacterium necrophorum*, a nonsporulating, obligate anaerobe that is a pleomorphic, gram-negative bacillus of the family Bacteroidaceae. *F. necrophorum* is a component of the normal flora of the mouth and the urogenital and intestinal tracts of man and animals. Alone or acting together with other nonsporogenic anaerobic bacteria, it causes various diseases and pathologic conditions in man and animals. Different species of the genus *Bacteroides*, which belong to the same family as *F. necrophorum*, cause disease either by themselves (in man) or in combination and at times in synergistic action with *F. necrophorum* (in man and animals).

Geographic Distribution: Worldwide.

Occurrence in Man: Advances in laboratory technology for the isolation of anaerobes have led to greater recognition of their role in human pathology and, consequently, to an increase in the number of recorded cases in medical facilities.

Occurrence in Animals: Some diseases, such as foot rot in sheep, occur frequently in all countries where sheep are raised. Others, such as calf diphtheria (necrobacillary stomatitis), are less common. Bovine hepatic necrobacillosis causes appreciable economic losses in many countries due to confiscation of animals in slaughterhouses; it is more frequent in areas where cattle are fed grain (Gillespie and Timoney, 1981).

The Disease in Man: *F. necrophorum* causes a great variety of necrotic lesions, empyema, pulmonary abscesses, arthritis, and ovariosalpingitic sepsis. *Bacteroides fragilis* and *F. necrophorum* are important agents of cerebral abscesses and occasionally of meningitis, almost always as a consequence of an otitis media (Islam and Shneerson, 1980). The formerly high incidence of septicemia caused by *F. necrophorum* in children and adolescents who had suffered from tonsillitis (Lemierre's post-tonsillitic septicemia) has now diminished notably and constitutes only 1 to 2% of all bacteremias caused by anaerobes. Patients with septicemias usually exhibit exudative pharyngitis or a peritonsillar abscess, but these symptoms may disappear by the time some patients obtain medical attention (Seidenfeld *et al.*, 1982).

The Disease in Animals: *F. necrophorum* is more important in animal than in human pathology and is the cause of several common diseases.

SHEEP: Foot rot is the most common cause of lameness in sheep. The disease begins with interdigital dermatitis and progresses to the epidermal matrix of the hooves, next causing destruction of the interdigital skin along with detachment of the hoof. Environmental factors, such as wet soil and grass that soften the feet, are involved in producing the disease, along with two bacterial agents, *F. necrophorum* and *Bacteroides nodosus*. *F. necrophorum* establishes itself first and causes inflammation and destruction of the epidermis before penetrating to deeper layers. Hoof degeneration is due to the proteolytic properties of *B. nodosus*. The disease may appear in several forms: benign, usually caused by less virulent strains of *B. nodosus*; virulent, with deformation and detachment of the hoof; and chronic, which may last years, with or without producing lameness.

Other hoof diseases affecting sheep are interdigital dermatitis and infectious bulbar necrosis. The former, caused by *F. necrophorum*, is characterized by an edematous and erythematous inflammation of the interdigital skin, which may be covered by a layer of moist, gray, necrotic material. Infectious bulbar necrosis is caused by *F. necrophorum* and *Corynebacterium pyogenes*, and is characterized by abscesses and suppuration of the bulbar area of the hoof, particularly on the hind feet. The disease results from the interaction of both bacteria. *C. pyogenes* produces a factor that stimulates proliferation of *F. necrophorum*, and the latter protects *C. pyogenes* from phagocytosis by producing a leukocidin (Cottral, 1978).

CATTLE: Calf diphtheria (necrobacillary stomatitis) is caused by *F. necrophorum* and is characterized by sialorrhea, anorexia, and necrotic areas in the oral cavity. Infection can spread to the larynx and, by inhalation, to the lungs, where it causes abscesses and pneumonia. The disease only occurs in animals under 2 years of age; mature animals seem immune. It occurs in dairy operations with deficient hygiene. The same disease also affects young goats.

Hepatic necrobacillosis is discovered by veterinary inspection in slaughterhouses and results in confiscation of carcasses. Lesions on the liver are characterized by well delineated yellow areas with a firm consistency.

Foot rot in bovines is an acute or chronic necrotic infection of the interdigital skin and the coronary region. The chronic form frequently produces arthritis in the distal joint of the limb. *F. necrophorum* and *Bacteroides melaninogenicus* have been isolated from biopsy samples of foot rot lesions. A mixture of both bacteria administered by interdigital scarification or intradermal inoculation reproduced the typical lesions (Berg and Loan, 1975). Nevertheless, the etiology still has not been completely clarified, and it is possible that concurrent infection by *F. necrophorum* and other bacteria (*B. nodosus*, staphylococci) causes the disease (Gillespie and Timoney, 1981).

SWINE: Pathologies such as ulcerous stomatitis, necrotic enteritis, and necrotic rhinitis, have been described in this species.

Source of Infection and Mode of Transmission: *F. necrophorum* forms part of the normal flora of several mucous membranes in humans and animals. The infection is endogenous in origin, especially for man. The relative infrequency of the disease in man indicates that predisposing causes are necessary for it to occur. These causes are usually traumas and debilitating illnesses. A lowered oxidation-reduction potential (E_h) resulting from insufficient blood supply, together with tissue necrosis and the presence of facultative bacteria, creates a favorable environment for this and other anaerobic bacteria. Vascular disease, edema, surgery, and cold are some of the common factors favoring implantation and multiplication of anaerobes (Finegold, 1982).

An important predisposing factor in sheep and bovine foot rot is softening of the interdigital epidermis caused by moist ground, enabling *F. necrophorum* to implant itself and multiply. In addition, this bacteria abounds in humid environments (soil and grass contaminated by animal feces) and has been proved able to survive outside a host's body for several months. In contrast, *B. nodosus* is a parasite that can live for only a short time in the environment and is introduced to establishments by sick or carrier animals. *F. necrophorum* creates conditions necessary for the multiplication of *B. nodosus*. Thus, both bacteria are required to cause the disease.

As mentioned above, under different conditions other bacteria, such as *Corynebacterium pyogenes* (which causes infectious bulbar necrosis), interact synergistically with *F. necrophorum*.

Bovine hepatic necrobacillosis has an endogenous origin. The agent possibly penetrates by way of the hepatic portal circulation from epithelial lesions in the rumen, which in turn may be caused by excessive acidity due to provision of concentrated foods.

Calf diphtheria, or necrobacillary stomatitis, is prevalent in environments where hygienic practices are markedly poor.

Role of Animals in the Epidemiology of the Disease: None. Necrobacillosis is a disease common to man and animals.

Diagnosis: When a nonsporulating, anaerobic bacterium is suspected as the cause of infection in a human patient, specimens collected from the lesions for bacteriologic diagnosis must be free of contaminants from the normal flora, of which these anaerobes are natural components. Thus, for example, when anaerobic origin is suspected for human pulmonary infection, transtracheal aspiration with a needle or direct penetration of the lung must be used. By contrast, the patient's sputum would not be a suitable material for the examination. In the case of empyema or abscesses, obtaining pus under aseptic conditions is not a problem (Finegold, 1982).

In veterinary practice, diagnosis of hoof diseases in sheep and cattle is based on clinical characteristics. Samples for laboratory diagnosis of hepatic necrobacillosis can be collected without difficulty. In calf diphtheria, ulcerous, necrotizing lesions with a putrid odor point to the disease; if a bacteriologic examination is attempted, epithelial samples from the edges of the ulcer should be used (Guarino *et al.*, 1982).

Control: Prevention in man consists primarily of avoiding and properly treating predisposing conditions. It is not known if specific control measures are justified.

Control of sheep foot rot is the subject of continuing research. An important preventive measure is avoiding introduction of animals from places where the disease exists, since *B. nodosus* is an obligate parasite. As with other contagious diseases, a period of isolation is recommended for recently acquired animals before putting them with the flock. Once the disease is introduced, transmission may be reduced by chemoprophylaxis using a foot bath of 5% formalin. Studies are still under way to perfect a vaccine made with *B. nodosus*, but the existence of serogroups and serotypes within this bacterium complicates this task (Ribeiro, 1980). A recent work (Claxton *et al.*, 1983) pointed out that, in addition to eight serogroups (A-H), there are 16 or more serotypes. More than one serogroup of *B. nodosus* may exist in a single flock, and several serogroups are sometimes isolated from the hoof of a single sheep. Vaccines made from purified pili (which contain the principal protecting immunogen) of *B. nodosus* immunize satisfactorily against a homologous strain of the bacterium (Stewart *et al.*, 1983a). In addition to the pili, which only protect against homologous strains, there are two other immunogens that could give heterologous immunity. Vaccines made of whole cells tested against vaccines of purified pili (all having an equal pilus content) provided comparable protection. Although vaccines using whole cells are cheaper to produce and confer protection against heterologous strains, they are irritants and cause weight loss (Stewart, 1983b).

Prevention of calf diphtheria is achieved principally by maintaining hygienic standards.

Aureomycin has been effective in preventing hepatic necrobacillosis. A cytoplasmic fraction of *F. necrophorum* has also been effective in immunizing cattle (Gillespie and Timoney, 1981). An important preventive measure is avoidance of sudden changes from regular to concentrated food.

Bibliography

Berg, J. N., and R. W. Loan. *Fusobacterium necrophorum* and *Bacteroides melaninogenicus* as etiologic agents of foot rot in cattle. *Am J Vet Res* 36:1115-1122, 1975.

Claxton, P. D., L. A. Ribeiro, and J. R. Egerton. Classification of *Bacteroides nodosus* by agglutination tests. *Aust Vet J* 60:331-334, 1983.

Cottral, G. E. (Ed.). *Manual of Standardized Methods for Veterinary Microbiology*. Ithaca, Cornell University Press, 1978.

Finegold, S. M. Anaerobic bacteria. *In*: Wyngaarden, J. B., and L. H. Smith, Jr. (Eds.), *Cecil Textbook of Medicine*, 16th ed., Philadelphia, Saunders, 1982.

Gillespie, J. H., and J. F. Timoney. *Hagan and Bruner's Infectious Diseases of Domestic Animals*, 7th ed. Ithaca, Cornell University Press, 1981.

Guarino, H., G. Uriarte, J. J. Berreta, and J. Maissonave. Estomatitis necrobacilar en terneros. Primera comunicación en Uruguay. *In*: *Primer Congreso Nacional de Veterinaria*. Montevideo, Sociedad de Medicina Veterinaria del Uruguay, 1982.

Islam, A. K. M. S., and J. M. Shneerson. Primary meningitis caused by *Bacteroides fragilis* and *Fusobacterium necrophorum*. *Postgrad Med J* 56:351-353, 1980.

Ribeiro, L. A. O. Foot-rot dos ovinos: etiologia, patogenia e controle. *Bol Inst Pesqui Vet Finamor* 7:41-45, 1980.

Seidenfeld, S. M., W. L. Sutker, and J. P. Luby. *Fusobacterium necrophorum* septicemia following oropharyngeal infection. *JAMA* 248:1343-1350, 1982.

Stewart, D. J., B. L. Clark, J. E. Peterson, D. A. Griffiths, E. F. Smith, and I. J. O'Donell. Effect of pilus dose and type of Freund's adjuvant on the antibody and protective responses of vaccinated sheep to *Bacteroides nodosus*. *Res Vet Sci* 35:130-137, 1983a.

Stewart, D. J., B. L. Clark, D. L. Emery, J. E. Peterson, and K. J. Fahey. A *Bacteroides nodosus* immunogen, distinct from the pilus, which induces cross-protective immunity in sheep vaccinated against foot-rot. *Aust Vet J* 60:83-85, 1983b.

NOCARDIOSIS

(039.9)

Etiology: Three pathogenic species: *Nocardia asteroides, N. brasiliensis*, and *N. caviae*. The first has been proposed as the type species.

Nocardia are higher bacteria that resemble fungi in many characteristics. They are aerobic, gram-positive, weakly acid-fast, and they form long, branched filaments that fragment into coccoid and bacillary forms.

Geographic Distribution: Worldwide. *Nocardia* are common members of the soil flora and act to decompose organic matter. The species seems to have different distributions. *N. asteroides* has been identified all over the world, while *N. brasiliensis* is present mainly in tropical climates, especially in Central America (Pier, 1979). The geographic distribution of *N. caviae* has not been determined.

Occurrence in Man: Nocardiosis is not a notifiable disease, and there is no reliable information on its frequency. Cases are sporadic. In the United States (Beaman *et al.*, 1976), an estimated 500 to 1,000 cases occur each year. Between 1972 and 1974, 81.2% of the cases were due to *N. asteroides*, 5.6% to *N. brasiliensis*, 3% to *N. caviae*, and 10.2% to unspecified *Nocardia*. The majority of cases occurred in people from 21 to 50 years of age, and the male to female ratio was 3 to 1.

Occurrence in Animals: The frequency of animal nocardiosis is not well known. Different diseases due to *Nocardia* spp. have been described in cattle, sheep, dogs, cats, wild animals, marine mammals, and fish. In New Zealand, where little attention had been paid to this disease previously, 34 cases were reported between 1976 and 1978; 26 of these were manifested as bovine mastitis (Orchard, 1979).

The Disease in Man: The principal agent is *N. asteroides*. Nocardiosis is a chronic disease that usually begins with a primary pyogenic lesion, frequently in the lungs. Through hematogenous dissemination, the agent localizes in different organs and tissues. Cerebral abscesses are frequent. Between 20 and 38% of persons with nocardiosis show nervous symptomatology. The case fatality rate in patients with cerebral abscesses is around 50%. A few cases of cerebral abscesses caused by *N. caviae* have been reported (Bradsher *et al.*, 1982). Other localizations include subcutaneous tissue, bones, and various organs.

The incubation period is unknown. It most likely varies depending on the virulence and phase of multiplication of the *Nocardia* strain, as well as the host's resistance. Most (85%) of nocardiosis cases have occurred in immunologically compromised persons (Beaman *et al.*, 1976).

N. brasiliensis seldom causes pulmonary disease, but more frequently produces mycetomas.

The Disease in Animals: Cattle are the most affected species. *N. asteroides* and more rarely *N. caviae* are agents of bovine mastitis. The udder usually becomes infected 1 to 2 days after calving (Beaman and Sugar, 1983), but the disease may appear throughout lactation, frequently caused by unhygienic therapeutic infusions into the milk duct. The disease course varies from acute to chronic. The mammary gland becomes edematous and fibrotic. Fever is common. Pus forms, as do fistulas to the surface. There may also be lymphatic and hematogenous dissemination to other organs. Among animals with acute infection, mortality is high.

Bovine nocardiosis may also manifest itself as pulmonary disease (especially in calves under 6 months of age), abortions, lymphadenitis of various lymph nodes, and lesions in different organs.

Canines are the second most affected species. The principal agent is *N. asteroides*, but infections caused by *N. brasiliensis* and *N. caviae* have also been described. The clinical picture is similar to that in man, and the most common clinical form is pulmonary. Dogs exhibit fever, anorexia, emaciation, and dyspnea. Dissemination from the lungs to other organs occurs frequently and may affect the central nervous system, bones, and kidneys.

The cutaneous form is also common in dogs, with purulent lesions usually located on the head or extremities. Nocardiosis is most frequent in male dogs under 1 year old. The fatality rate is high (Beaman and Sugar, 1983).

Nocardiosis in cats is more unusual and is seen mostly in castrated males. Most cases are due to *N. asteroides*, but about 30% have been attributed to *N. brasiliensis* or to other similar nocardias.

Source of Infection and Mode of Transmission: Nocardias are components of the normal soil flora. These potential pathogens are much more virulent during the logarithmic growth phase than during the stationary phase, and it is believed that actively growing soil populations are more virulent for man and animals (Orchard, 1979).

Man probably acquires the infection by inhaling contaminated dust. Predisposing causes are important in the pathogenesis of the disease, since most cases occur either in persons with deficient immune systems or those taking immunosuppressant drugs. Mycetomas caused by *N. brasiliensis* may arise from a skin injury.

Animals probably contract pulmonary infections in the same way that man does. Mastitis occurring later in the lactation period is produced by contaminated catheters, but mastitis at the beginning of lactation is more difficult to explain. It is possible that the focus of infection already exists in the nonlactating cow and that when the udder fills with milk, the infection spreads massively through the milk ducts and causes clinical symptoms (Beaman and Sugar, 1983). The origin of the initial focus remains an enigma, but it could also be due to insertion of contaminated instruments. The multiple cases of nocardia-induced mastitis that are at times observed in a dairy herd are attributable to transmission of the infection from one cow to another by means of contaminated instruments or therapeutic infusions.

Role of Animals in the Epidemiology of the Disease: Nocardiosis is a disease common to man and animals; soil is the reservoir and source of infection. There are no known cases of transmission from animals to man or between humans.

Diagnosis: Microscopic examination of exudates can indicate nocardiosis, but only culture and identification of the agent provide a definitive diagnosis. Serologic (complement fixation, precipitation) and allergenic tests are not in common use.

Control: No specific control measures are available. Prevention consists of avoiding predisposing factors and exposure to dust (Pier, 1979). Environmental hygiene and sterilization of instruments are important.

Bibliography

Beaman, B. L., J. Burnside, B. Edwards, and W. Causey. Nocardial infections in the United States, 1972-1974. *J Infect Dis* 134:286-289, 1976.

Beaman, B. L., and A. M. Sugar. *Nocardia* in naturally acquired and experimental infections in animals. *J Hyg (Camb)* 91:393-419, 1983.

Bradsher, R. W., T. P. Monson, and R. W. Steele. Brain abscess due to *Nocardia caviae*. *Am J Clin Pathol* 78:124-127, 1982.

Orchard, V. A. Nocardial infections of animals in New Zealand, 1976-1978. *NZ Vet J* 27:159-165, 1979.

Pier, A. C. Actinomycetes. *In*: Stoenner, H., W. Kaplan, and M. Tortem (Section Eds.), *CRC Handbook Series in Zoonoses*. Section A, vol. 1. Boca Raton, Florida, CRC Press, 1979.

PASTEURELLOSIS

(027.2)

Synonyms: Shipping fever (cattle), hemorrhagic septicemia (cattle, lambs), pasteurella pneumonia (lambs), fowl cholera, snuffles (rabbits).

Etiology: *Pasteurella multocida* (syn. *P. septica*), *P. haemolytica*, *P. pneumotropica*, *P. ureae*. Pasteurellae are small, nonmotile, polymorphic, gram-positive bacilli with little resistance to physical and chemical agents.

Subdivision of *P. multocida* and *P. haemolytica* into serotypes is important in the areas of epidemiology and control (vaccines). Subclassification of *P. multocida* into serotypes is based on its capsular (A, B, D, and E) and somatic (1 to 16) antigens; the latter can occur in different combinations. *P. haemolytica* is subdivided into two biotypes (A and T) and 12 serotypes.

Geographic Distribution: *P. multocida* and *P. haemolytica* are distributed worldwide. The distribution of *P. pneumotropica* and *P. ureae* is not as well known.

Occurrence in Man: Uncommon. It is not a notifiable disease and its incidence is little known. According to laboratory records, 822 cases occurred in Great Britain from 1956 to 1965. A special survey in the United States revealed 316 cases caused by *P. multocida* from 1965 to 1968. Data on the occurrence of human pasteurellosis in other countries are scarce. The disease caused by *P. haemolytica*, *P. pneumotropica*, and *P. ureae* is uncommon.

Occurrence in Animals: Common in domestic and wild species.

The Disease in Man: The principal agent of human pasteurellosis is *P. multocida*. The main clinical symptoms consist of infected bites or scratches inflicted by cats or dogs (or occasionally by other animals), disease of the respiratory system, and localized infections in different organs and tissues. Cases of septicemia are exceptional.

The greatest number of clinical cases arise from infected wounds. Most cats and dogs are healthy carriers of *Pasteurella* and harbor the etiologic agent in the oral cavity. The microorganism is transmitted to the bite wound, and a few hours later produces swelling, reddening, and intense pain in the region. The inflammatory process may penetrate into the deep tissue layers, reaching the periosteum and producing necrosis. Septic arthritis and osteomyelitis are complications that occur with some frequency. Septic arthritis often develops in patients suffering from rheumatoid arthritis. Cases have been described in which articular complications appeared several months and even years after the bite (Bjorkholm and Eilard, 1983). Of 20 cases of osteomyelitis with or without septic arthritis, 10 developed as a consequence of cat bites, five from dog bites, one from bites of a dog and a cat, and four from wounds of unknown origin (Ewing *et al.*, 1980).

P. multocida may also aggravate certain respiratory tract diseases such as bronchiectasis, bronchitis, and pneumonia. In terms of case numbers, chronic respiratory conditions from which the agent is isolated are second in importance to infection transmitted by animal bite or scratch. Septicemia, meningitis, and endocarditis are extremely rare.

The age group most affected is persons over 40 years old, in spite of the fact that bites are more frequent in children and younger people.

The Disease in Animals: Pasteurellae have an extremely broad spectrum of animal hosts. Many apparently healthy mammals and birds can harbor pasteurellae in the upper respiratory tract. According to the most accepted hypothesis, pasteurellosis is a disease of weakened animals that are subjected to stress and poor hygienic conditions. In an animal with lowered resistance, pasteurellae harbored in the fauces or trachea may become pathogenic for their host. There is a marked difference in the level of virulence between different strains of *P. multocida*. In some diseases, *P. multocida* is the only and primary etiologic agent, and in others, it is a secondary invader that aggravates the clinical picture.

A relationship exists between the serotype of *Pasteurella*, its animal host, and the disease it causes. Therefore, serologic typing is important for epizootiologic studies as well as for control (by means of vaccination).

Bovine hemorrhagic septicemia is caused by *P. multocida* serotype 6:B in Asia, and by 6:E and 6:B in Africa. In fibrinous pneumonia ("shipping fever") in cattle, serotypes 2:A of *P. multocida* and 1 of *P. haemolytica* predominate.

CATTLE: Shipping fever, also called bovine respiratory disease complex, is a syndrome that causes large economic losses in the cattle industry of the Western Hemisphere. In the United States it causes annual losses estimated at more than US$25 million. Shipping fever is an acute respiratory disease that particularly affects beef calves and adult cows when they are subjected to the stress of prolonged transport. The symptomatology varies from a mild respiratory illness to a rapidly fatal pneumonia. Symptoms generally appear from 5 to 14 days after the cattle reach their destination, but some may be sick on arrival. The principal symptoms are fever, dyspnea, cough, nasal discharge, depression, and appreciable weight loss. The fatality rate is low.

The etiology of the disease has not been completely clarified, and it is noteworthy that the disease does not occur in Australia even when animals are transported long distances (Irwin *et al.*, 1979). Several concurrent factors are believed to cause the syndrome. Most prominent among these are stress factors such as fatigue, irregular feeding, exposure to heat and cold, and weaning. Viral infections, which occur constantly throughout a herd and are often inapparent, are exacerbated by factors such as overcrowding during transport. Moreover, susceptible animals suddenly added to a herd lead to increased virulence. The virus most often identified as the primary etiologic agent is parainfluenza virus 3 (PI3) of the genus *Paramyxovirus*. Infection by this virus alone usually causes a mild respiratory disease; however, damage it causes to the respiratory tract mucosa aids secondary invaders such as *P. multocida* and *P. haemolytica*, which aggravate the clinical picture. On the other hand, virulent strains of *Pasteurella* can originate the disease by themselves. Among pasteurellae frequently isolated in cases of shipping fever are *P. haemolytica* biotype A, serotype 1, and several serotypes belonging to group A of *P. multocida*. The fact that treatment with sulfonamides and antibiotics gives good results also indicates that a large part of the symptomatology is due to pasteurellae. Another important viral agent that acts synergistically with pasteurellae is the herpesvirus of infectious bovine rhinotracheitis. Similarly, the agent of viral bovine diarrhea as well as chlamydiae and mycoplasmas can take part in the etiology of this respiratory disease.

An important disease among cattle and water buffalo in southern and southeastern Asia is hemorrhagic septicemia. In many countries, it is the disease responsible for the most losses once rinderpest has been eradicated. Hemorrhagic septicemia also occurs in several African countries, including Egypt and South Africa, and less frequently, in southern Europe. The disease seems to be enzootic in the American bison, and several outbreaks have taken place (the last one in 1967) without the disease spreading to domestic cattle (Carter, 1982). In tropical countries, hemorrhagic septicemia occurs during the rainy season. The main symptoms are fever, edema, sialorrhea, copious nasal secretion, and difficulty in breathing. Mortality is high. Surviving animals become carriers and perpetuate the disease. It must be borne in mind that hemorrhagic septicemia is due to the specific *P. multocida* serotypes 6:B and 6:E. There is no evidence that the disease occurs in domestic cattle in the Americas.

P. multocida is also responsible for cases of mastitis.

SHEEP: *P. haemolytica* is the etiologic agent of two different clinical forms: pneumonia and septicemia. Biotype A, serotype 2 is the most prevalent agent of pasteurella pneumonia among lambs in Great Britain (Fraser *et al.*, 1982). As in cattle, pulmonary disease in sheep follows a viral infection (PI3), and even though *Pasteurella* is a secondary invader, it is the predominant pathogen. Occurrence of the disease is sporadic or enzootic. The main symptoms are a purulent nasal discharge, cough, diarrhea, and general malaise. Lesions consist of hemorrhagic areas in the lungs and petechiae in the pericardium. Pasteurella septicemia is caused by biotype T of *P. haemolytica* and appears in temperate climates in the fall, when the sheep's diet is changed (Gillespie and Timoney, 1981). *P. haemolytica* is the only etiologic agent of sporadic sheep mastitis in the western United States, Australia, and Europe (Blood *et al.*, 1979).

SWINE: Pasteurellosis appears in the form of pneumonia and, more unusually, as septicemia. *Pasteurella* may be a primary or secondary agent of pneumonia, particularly as a complication of the mild form of classic swine plague (hog cholera). The anterior pulmonary lobes are the most affected, with hepatization and a serofibrinous exudate on the surface. Serotype 3:A of *P. multocida* is the most prevalent in chronic swine pneumonia (Pijoan *et al.*, 1983). Recent studies have revealed evidence of the etiologic role of toxigenic strains of *P. multocida* serotype D in atrophic rhinitis. *Bordetella bronchiseptica* acting synergistically with toxigenic strains of *P. multocida* probably causes this disease, the etiology of which has been much debated (Rutter, 1983).

RABBITS: Pasteurellosis is common in rabbit hutches. The most frequent clinical manifestation is coryza. As in other animal species, the disease appears under stressful conditions. The principal symptoms are a serous or purulent exudate from the nose and sometimes from the eyes, sneezing, and coughing. The pathologic process may reach the lungs. Septicemia and death can occur. Males that are kept together may show pasteurella-infected abscesses produced by bites.

WILD ANIMALS: Pasteurellosis occurs in many wild animal species, among which occasional epizootic outbreaks take place. The etiologic agent is *P. multocida*; *P. haemolytica* has not been isolated so far. Two disease forms are found: hemorrhagic septicemia, in which the whole animal body is invaded by pasteurellae, and the respiratory syndrome or pulmonary pasteurellosis.

FOWL: Fowl cholera is an acute septicemic disease with high morbidity and mortality in all species of domestic fowl. In recent decades its incidence has diminished worldwide because of improved commercial poultry management practices. The disease usually appears on poultry farms where hygiene is deficient. Explosive outbreaks may occur 2 days after infected birds are introduced into a flock. Mortality is variable, at times reaching 60% of the poultry on a farm. Many of the survivors become carriers and give rise to new outbreaks. At the beginning of a hyperacute outbreak, fowl die without premonitory symptoms; mortality increases, but the only symptoms seen are cyanosis of the wattles and comb. Later, the spread of the disease slows down and respiratory symptoms appear. Cases of chronic or localized pasteurellosis may occur following an acute outbreak, or the disease may take this course from the outset of infection. The chronic disease is caused by attenuated strains of *P. multocida* and manifests itself mostly as "wattle disease" (edematization and later caseation of these appendages). Another localization can be the wing or foot joints. Fowl cholera is produced by *P. multocida* of serogroup A, predominantly serotypes 1 and 3 (Mushin, 1979); some strains of group D have also been isolated, but they seem to be less pathogenic. *P. multocida* causes outbreaks with high mortality among wild birds, especially waterfowl.

Source of Infection and Mode of Transmission: The reservoir is made up of animals and perhaps also man. The etiologic agent is harbored in the upper respiratory passages.

For human infections transmitted by animal bite or scratch, the source of the infection and the mode of transmission are obvious. Except in the case of bites, animal-to-man transmission is accomplished through the respiratory or digestive tract. An analysis of 100 cases of human pasteurella infections of the respiratory tract and other sites found that 69% of the patients had had contact with dogs or cats, or with cattle, fowl, or their products. Nevertheless, the remaining 31% of the patients denied all contact with animals; consequently, interhuman transmission is suspected to occur.

Among fowl, where *P. multocida* is without doubt the primary agent of infection, the source of the outbreaks is carrier fowl, and transmission occurs predominantly by means of aerosols. Dogs and cats rarely suffer from pasteurellosis (with the exception of wounds infected with pasteurellae in fights), and are healthy carriers. Other mammals acquire the disease from members of their species either through the respiratory or digestive tract, or by falling victim to the pasteurellae in their own respiratory tracts when stress lowers their defenses. There is much evidence that stress factors play an important enabling role in unleashing the respiratory syndrome of shipping fever, and that these factors permit multiplication of serotype 2 of *P. haemolytica* (Frank and Smith, 1983). Serotypes 6:B and 6:E, which cause hemorrhagic septicemia of cattle and water buffalo, are perpetuated by means of carriers and chronically ill animals that serve as a source of infection for their kind.

Role of Animals in the Epidemiology of the Disease: Pasteurellae survive only a very short time in the environment. It is certain that animals constitute the most important reservoir of *P. multocida*, *P. haemolytica,* and *P. pneumotropica.*

Diagnosis: In the case of human infection, diagnosis is made by isolating the etiologic agent from wounds or other sites.

In hemorrhagic septicemia or in fowl cholera, the etiologic agent can be cultivated from the blood or viscera. In pneumonia of domestic animals, a pure culture of pasteurellae may indicate their role in the pathology, but does not reveal whether these bacteria are primary or secondary agents of the disease.

Control: Measures to reduce the chance of bites, such as elimination of stray dogs, can prevent some cases of human infection.

Control in animals lies mainly in adequate management of herds or poultry farms. Bacterins as well as live attenuated vaccines are in use, or are being tested, against *P. multocida* and *P. haemolytica*. Protection against homologous serotypes is satisfactory, but protection is only partial or irregular against heterologous serotypes. In general, attenuated live vaccines give better immunity than bacterins. In Asia, extensive experimentation proved that a bacterin with an oil adjuvant can offer solid immunity against hemorrhagic septicemia. A single dose of live vaccine with a streptomycin-dependent, mutant strain conferred immunity against hemorrhagic septicemia on 66.6 to 83.3% of calves and on 100% of young buffalo (De Alvis and Carter, 1980).

The use of PI3 vaccine and *Pasteurella* (*P. multocida* and *P. haemolytica*) bacterin has been recommended for the control of shipping fever in beef calves, with vaccination at 4 months of age and revaccination a month later. Attenuated live vaccines of *P. haemolytica* are being tested. A bacterin containing multiple antigens of the prevalent serotypes, incorporated into a polyvalent anticlostridial biological with aluminum hydroxide adjuvant, has been tested against *P. haemolytica* pneumonia in lambs and has given satisfactory results (Wells *et al.,* 1984). Several live vaccines are available against avian cholera, some of which can be administered in the drinking water. Selection of *Pasteurella* strains within the serotypes that cause the disease is important in immunization.

Bovine hemorrhagic septicemia should be considered an exotic disease and appropriate measures should be taken to prevent its spread to disease-free areas.

Bibliography

Backstrand, J. M., and R. G. Botzler. Survival of *Pasteurella multocida* in soil and water in an area where avian cholera is enzootic. *J Wildl Dis* 22:257-259, 1986.

Bjorkholm, B., and T. Eilard. *Pasteurella multocida* osteomyelitis caused by cat bite. *J Infect* 6:175-177, 1983.

Blood, D. C., J. A. Henderson, and O. M. Radostitis. *Veterinary Medicine,* 5th ed., Philadelphia, Lea and Febiger, 1979.

Bruner, D. W., and J. H. Gillespie. *Hagan's Infectious Diseases of Domestic Animals,* 6th ed. Ithaca, New York, Cornell University Press, 1973.

Burdge, D. R., D. Scheifele, and D. P. Speert. Serious *Pasteurella multocida* infections from lion and tiger bites. *JAMA* 253:3296-3297, 1985.

Carter, G. R. Pasteurellosis: *Pasteurella multocida* and *Pasteurella haemolytica. Adv Vet Sci* 11:321-379, 1967.

Carter, G. R. Pasteurella infections as sequelae to respiratory viral infections. *J Am Vet Med Assoc* 163:863-864, 1973.

Carter, G. R. Whatever happened to hemorrhagic septicemia? *J Am Vet Med Assoc* 180:1176-1177, 1982.

De Alvis, M. C. L., and G. R. Carter. Preliminary field trials with a streptomycin-dependent vaccine against hemorrhagic fever septicemia. *Vet Rev* 106:435-437, 1980.

de Jong, M. F., and J. P. Akkermans. Investigation into the pathogenesis of atrophic rhinitis in pigs. I. Atrophic rhinitis caused by *Bordetella bronchiseptica* and *Pasteurella multocida* and the meaning of a thermolabile toxin of *P. multocida. Vet Q* 8:204-214, 1986.

Ewing, R., V. Fainstein, D. M. Musher, M. Lidsky, and J. Clarridge. Articular and skeletal infections caused by *Pasteurella multocida. S Med J* 73:1349-1352, 1980.

Frank, G. H., and R. G. Marshall. Parainfluenza-3 virus infection of cattle. *J Am Vet Med Assoc* 163:858-859, 1973.

Frank, G. H., and P. C. Smith. Prevalence of *Pasteurella haemolytica* in transported calves. *Am J Vet Res* 44:981-985, 1983.

Fraser, J., N. J. L. Gilmour, S. Laird, and W. Donachie. Prevalence of *Pasteurella haemolytica* serotypes isolated from ovine pasteurellosis in Britain. *Vet Rec* 110:560-561, 1982.

Gillespie, J. H., and J. F. Timoney. *Hagan and Bruner's Infectious Diseases of Domestic Animals,* 7th ed., Ithaca, New York, Cornell University Press, 1981.

Harshfield, G. S. Fowl cholera. *In*: Biester, H. E., and L. H. Schwarte (Eds.), *Diseases of Poultry,* 4th ed. Ames, Iowa State University Press, 1959.

Hoerlein, A. B. Shipping fever. *In*: Gibbons, W. J. (Ed.), *Diseases of Cattle,* 2nd ed. Santa Barbara, California, American Veterinary Publications, 1963.

Hubbert, W. T., and M. N. Rosen. *Pasteurella multocida* infection due to animal bite. *Am J Public Health* 60:1103-1108, 1970.

Hubbert, W. T., and M. N. Rosen. *Pasteurella multocida* infection in man unrelated to animal bite. *Am J Public Health* 60:1109-1117, 1970.

Irwin, M. R., S. McConnell, J. D. Coleman, and G. E. Wilcox. Bovine respiratory disease complex: a comparison of potential predisposing and etiologic factors in Australia and the United States. *J Am Vet Med Assoc* 175:1095-1099, 1979.

Mair, N. S. Some *Pasteurella* infections in man. *In*: Graham-Jones, O. (Ed.), *Some Diseases of Animals Communicable to Man in Britain.* Oxford, Pergamon Press, 1968.

Meyer, K. F. *Pasteurella* and *Francisella. In*: Dubos, R. J., and J. G. Hirsch (Eds.), *Bacterial and Mycotic Infections of Man,* 4th ed. Philadelphia, Lippincott, 1965.

Mushin, R. Serotyping of *Pasteurella multocida* isolants from poultry. *Avian Dis* 23:668-675, 1979.

Namioka, S., M. Murata, and R. V. S. Bain. Serological studies on *Pasteurella multocida*. V. Some epizootiological findings resulting from O antigenic analysis. *Cornell Vet* 54:520-534, 1964.

Pijoan, C., R. B. Morrison, and H. D. Hilley. Serotyping of *Pasteurella multocida* isolated from swine lungs collected at slaughter. *J Clin Microbiol* 17:1074-1076, 1983.

Quan, T. J., K. R. Tsuchiya, and L. G. Carter. Recovery and identification of *Pasteurella multocida* from mammals and fleas collected during plague investigations. *J Wildl Dis* 22:7-12, 1986.

Rimler, R. B., and M. Phillips. Fowl cholera: protection against *Pasteurella multocida* by ribosome-lipopolysaccharide vaccine. *Avian Dis* 30:409-415, 1986.

Rosen, M. N. Pasteurellosis. *In*: Davis, J. W., L. H. Karstad, and D. O. Trainer (Eds.), *Infectious Diseases of Wild Mammals*. Ames, Iowa State University Press, 1970.

Rutter, J. M. Virulence of *Pasteurella multocida* in atrophic rhinitis of gnotobiotic pigs infected with *Bordetella bronchiseptica*. *Res Vet Sci* 34:287-295, 1983.

Wells, P. W., J. T. Robinson, N. J. L. Gilmour, W. Donachie, and J. M. Sharp. Development of a combined clostridial and *Pasteurella haemolytica* vaccine for sheep. *Vet Rec* 114:266-269, 1984.

PLAGUE

(020)

Synonyms: Pest, black death, pestilential fever.

Etiology: The etiologic agent, heretofore named *Yersinia pestis*, is now called *Yersinia pseudotuberculosis* ssp. *pestis* on the basis of DNA hybridization studies that demonstrated its close relationship to *Y. pseudotuberculosis* (Bercovier *et al.*, 1980; International Committee on Systematic Bacteriology, List 7, 1981). *Y. pseudotuberculosis* ssp. *pestis* is a gram-negative, nonmotile bacterium, coccobacillary to bacillary in form, and not very resistant to physical and chemical agents. Three biological varieties are distinguished: orientalis (oceanic), antiqua (continental), and mediaevalis. This distinction has a certain epidemiologic significance, principally for nosography, but there is no difference in the biotypes' pathogenicities. For practical purposes and to avoid possible confusion, this text will continue to use the former, more familiar name, *Yersinia pestis*.

Geographic Distribution: Natural foci of infection persist on all continents except Australasia. In the Americas, sylvatic plague is maintained in rodents in the western third of the United States, the border region between Ecuador and Peru, southeastern Bolivia, and northeastern Brazil. Similarly, there are foci in north-central and southern Africa, including Madagascar; the Near East; the border area between Yemen and Saudi Arabia; Kurdistan Province, Iran; and in Central and

Southeast Asia, Burma, and Indonesia. There are several focal areas in the USSR (American Public Health Association, 1985).

Occurrence in Man: Since the dawn of the Christian era, there have been three great pandemics: the first began in the year 542 (Justinian plague) and is estimated to have caused 100 million deaths; the second began in 1346, lasted three centuries, and claimed 25 million victims; and the last began in 1894 and continued until the 1930s. As a result of the last pandemic, natural foci of infection were established in South America, West Africa, South Africa, Madagascar, and Indochina.

Urban plague has been brought under control in almost the entire world, and rural plague of murine origin is also on the decline. Nevertheless, epidemics have occurred in Indonesia, Nepal, and South Vietnam. In this last country, there were 5,274 cases in 1967 due to contact with domestic rats and their fleas.

From 1958 to 1979, 46,937 cases of human plague were recorded in 30 countries; if Vietnam is excluded, the total number is reduced to 15,785. The large number of cases in Vietnam is attributed to military operations there and consequent ecologic changes. Sixteen of the 30 countries reporting plague cases were in Africa. However, incidence of the disease on that continent was very low, less than 6% of the world total (Akeiv, 1982). Figure 14 shows the numbers of cases and deaths caused by human plague worldwide from 1971 to 1980.

In the Americas, 7,382 cases (15.7% of the world total) occurred in seven countries: Brazil, Bolivia, Peru, Ecuador, the United States, and occasional cases in Colombia and Venezuela (Akeiv, 1982). From 1971 through 1980, there were 2,312 cases in the Americas (Table 2), of which 1,551 occurred in Brazil, 316 in Peru, 247 in Bolivia, 123 in the United States, and 75 in Ecuador (Pan American Health Organization, 1981). In all the countries, the number of cases fluctuated greatly from year to year; at times, epidemic outbreaks have occurred. Plague continues to be a public health problem in the Americas because of the persistence of sylvatic plague and the link between domestic and wild rodents. In Ecuador an outbreak of seven cases occurred in May 1976 in Nizac, Chimborazo Province, a settlement of 850 inhabitants. The outbreak was preceded by a large epizootic in rats and mortality among guinea pigs raised in dwellings for food. The worst outbreak since 1966 occurred in 1984 in northern Peru, with 289 cases reported in 40 localities. An association was presumed between this outbreak and a great abundance of rodents, possibly the result of ecologic changes due to flooding (Rust, 1985).

In the USA, 35 cases were recorded from April to August of 1983, the greatest number of cases since 1925.

Occurrence in Animals: Natural infection by *Y. pestis* has been found in 230 species and subspecies of wild rodents. In natural foci sylvatic plague perpetuates itself by continuous cycling of the etiologic agent, transmitted by fleas from one rodent to another. It is generally believed that the survival of the etiologic agent in a natural focus depends on the existence of rodent species, or individuals within a species, with differing levels of susceptibility. The most resistant individuals are host to and infect the fleas, which in turn infect susceptible animals in the area and can spread to domestic rodents. Susceptible animals generally die, but they increase the population of infected fleas by means of their bacteremia. When the number of susceptible individuals is large and climatic conditions favorable, an epizootic may develop in which many rodents die. As the epizootic diminishes, the infection continues in enzootic form in the surviving population until a new outbreak occurs.

Figure 14. Number of cases and deaths from human plague worldwide, 1971-1980.

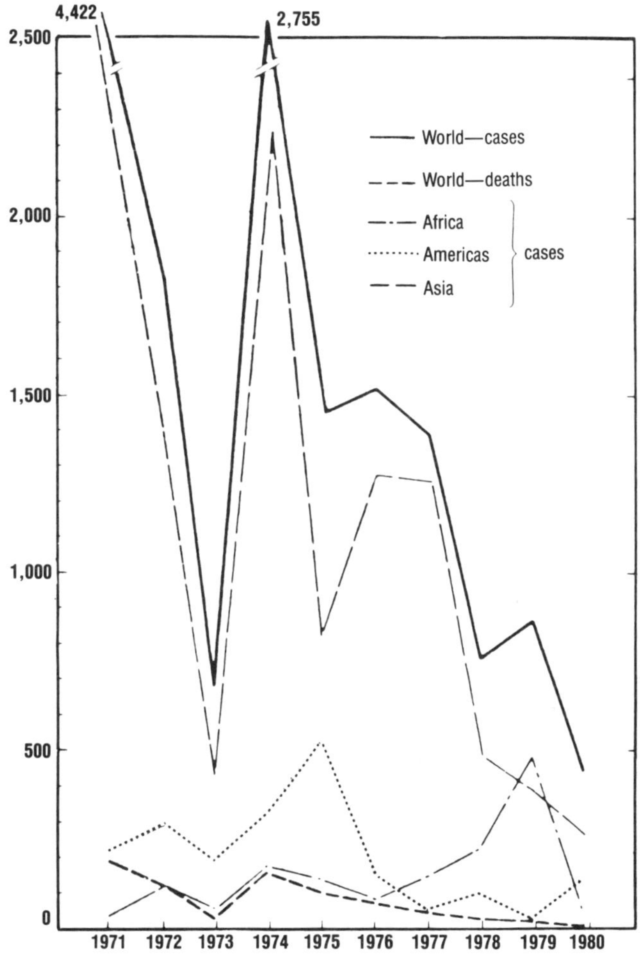

Source: *PAHO Epidemiol Bull* 2(6):4-5, 1981.

Infection may remain latent in enzootic foci for a long time, and the absence of human cases should not be interpreted as a sign that the natural focus is eliminated.

House cats that come into contact with rodents and/or their fleas can become infected and fall ill, and can transmit the infection to man. In the United States and South Africa several cases of the disease in cats have been described (Kaufmann *et al.*, 1981; Rollag *et al.*, 1981). There is also evidence that camels and sheep in enzootic plague areas can contract the infection and that, in turn, man can become infected when sacrificing these animals. Such cases occurred in recent years in Libya (Christie *et al.*, 1980).

Table 2. Number of cases and deaths from human plague in the Americas, 1971-1980.

Country	1971		1972		1973		1974		1975		1976		1977		1978		1979		1980	
	C	D	C	D	C	D	C	D	C	D	C	D	C	D	C	D	C	D	C	D
Bolivia	19	3	0	0	0	0	14	5	2	0	24	5	29	9	68	2	10	0	26	2
Brazil	146	2	169	13	152	...	291	...	496	5	97	...	1	...	11	...	0	0	98	0
Ecuador	27	0	9	0	1	1	0	0	0	0	8	1	0	0	0	0	0	0	0	0
Peru	22	5	118	15	30	2	8	2	3	0	1	0	0	0	6	1	0	0	0	0
United States of America[a]	2	0	1	0	2	0	8	1	20	4	16	3	18	2	12	2	13	2	18	5
Total	216	10	297	28	185	3	321	8	521	9	146	9	48	11	97	5	23	2	142	7

C = Cases.
D = Deaths.
... Data not available.
[a]Plague found in rodents.
Source: PAHO Epidemiol Bull 2(6):4-5, 1981.

The Disease in Man: The incubation period lasts from 2 to 6 days, though it may be shorter. Three clinical forms of plague are recognized: bubonic, septicemic, and pneumonic. The symptoms shared by all three are fever, chills, cephalalgia, nausea, generalized pain, diarrhea or constipation, and frequently toxemia, shock, arterial hypotension, rapid pulse, anxiety, staggering gait, slurred speech, mental confusion, and prostration.

Bubonic plague—the most common form in interpandemic periods—is characterized by acute inflammation and swelling of peripheral lymph nodes (buboes), which can become suppurative. There may be a small vesicle at the site of the flea bite. The buboes are painful and the surrounding area is usually edematous. Bacteremia is present at the beginning of the disease. The fatality rate in untreated cases is from 25 to 60%. At times the disease may take the form of a mild, localized, and short-lived infection (pestis minor).

In the septicemic form, nervous and cerebral symptoms develop very rapidly. Epistaxis, cutaneous petechiae, hematuria, and involuntary evacuations are present. The disease course lasts only 1 to 3 days, and mortality can reach nearly 100%.

Pneumonic plague may be a secondary form derived from the bubonic or septicemic forms by hematogenous dissemination, or it may be primary, produced directly by inhalation during contact with a pneumonic plague patient. In addition to the symptoms common to all forms, dyspnea, cough, and expectoration are present. The sputum may vary from watery and foamy to patently hemorrhagic. This is the most serious form.

Primary pneumonic plague, which has caused outbreaks and at times devastating epidemics, is exceptional. The pneumonic form seen in present times is secondary, resulting from septicemic dissemination. Since 1925, the United States has recorded only one case of primary pneumonic plague, which occurred in California in 1980 as a result of the patient's exposure to a kitten with pneumonia (Centers for Disease Control of the USA, 1982). Secondary pneumonic plague arises from invasion of the lungs of untreated patients, about 95% of whom die without becoming transmitters of the agent by aerosol. If left untreated, the small number of patients that do not die may give rise to other cases of pneumonic plague by airborne transmission (Poland and Barnes, 1979). In countries that maintain epidemiologic surveillance and where physicians and the general population are alert to the disease, the high fatality rates caused by all forms of plague have been largely arrested by early diagnosis and prompt treatment with antibiotics such as streptomycin, tetracyclines, and chloramphenicol.

The Disease in Animals: *Y. pestis* primarily infects animals of the order Rodentia; it affects wild as well as domestic rodents and, to a lesser degree, rabbits and hares (lagomorphs). The infection may be acute, chronic, or inapparent. Different species of rodents and different populations of the same species show varying degrees of susceptibility. In this regard, it has been observed that a population in an enzootic area is more resistant than another in a plague-free area, a phenomenon attributed to natural selection. Domestic (commensal) rats are very susceptible; *Rattus rattus* die in large numbers during epizootics. By contrast, susceptibility varies greatly between different species in natural foci and must be determined for each different situation. In the western United States, prairie dogs (*Cynomys* spp.) and the ground squirrel *Citellus beecheyi* are very susceptible, while certain species of *Microtus* and *Peromyscus* are resistant.

Lesions found in susceptible animals dead from plague vary with the course of the disease. In acute cases hemorrhagic buboes and splenomegaly are present without other internal lesions; in subacute cases the buboes are caseous, and punctiform necrotic foci are found in the spleen, liver, and lungs.

Recently, the natural infection in cats has come under close scrutiny, as they have been a source of infection for man in several instances. Feline plague is characterized by formation of abscesses, lymphadenitis, lethargy, and fever (Rollag *et al.*, 1981). Secondary pneumonia may also be present, as in the case at Lake Tahoe, California, where a kitten transmitted the infection to a man by aerosol. Fatality is over 50% among experimentally infected cats. In contrast, dogs inoculated with the plague agent react only with fever. Other carnivores are not very susceptible, with the exception of individuals with greater than normal susceptibility, as might be expected in any animal population.

Natural infection has been recorded in camels and sheep from the USSR and Libya (Christie *et al.*, 1980) and, more recently, in camels from Saudi Arabia (A. Barnes, personal communication).

Source of Infection of Mode of Transmission (Figure 15): Wild rodents constitute the natural reservoir. The maintenance hosts vary in each natural focus, but they are almost always rodent species with low susceptibility, that is, the animals become infected but do not die from the disease. Very susceptible species, in which many individuals die during an epizootic, are important in amplification and diffusion of the infection as well as in its transmission to man, but they cannot be permanent hosts. *R. rattus* is very susceptible, but the infection usually dies out rapidly in this species. In some circumstances it can serve as a temporary host, as it has in India, but not for many years. Consequently, the persistence of a focus depends on rodent species that have a wide spectrum of partial resistance.

In a natural focus the infection is transmitted from one individual to another by fleas. Different species of fleas vary greatly in their efficiency as vectors. Biological vectors of plague are characterized by the blocking phenomenon. When *Y. pestis* is ingested along with the septicemic host's blood, the agent multiplies in the flea's stomach and the proventriculum becomes blocked by the mass of bacteria. When a blocked flea tries to feed again, it regurgitates the bacteria into the bloodstream of the new host (this is the case with *Xenopsylla cheopis*, the domestic rat flea). Wild rodent fleas are generally less efficient and their capacity as biological vectors varies; it is believed that they may play an important role as mechanical vectors in natural foci. Also, these vectors are not very species-specific and can transmit the infection between different rodent species living in an enzootic area. The etiologic agent survives a long time in fleas; some have remained infected for a period of 396 days. For this reason fleas may be considered part of the natural reservoir, which would be an arthropod-vertebrate complex. More than 200 species of fleas have been implicated in the transmission of plague.

Infection from a natural focus may be passed to commensal rodents (domestic rats and mice) by members of ubiquitous rodent species that approach human dwellings and can thus initiate an outbreak of plague within households. In the same way, peridomestic rodents may come into contact with wild rodents. Transmission is effected by means of fleas. Other mammals (dogs, marsupials) may also serve as the link between the wild and domestic cycles by transporting fleas from one place to another. In northeastern Brazil, a marsupial (*Monodelphis domestica*) naturally infected with the plague agent via *Polygenis bohlsi jordani* (a principal vector of sylvatic plague in this region) has been found to live near and enter houses.

Figure 15. Plague. Domestic and peridomestic transmission cycle.

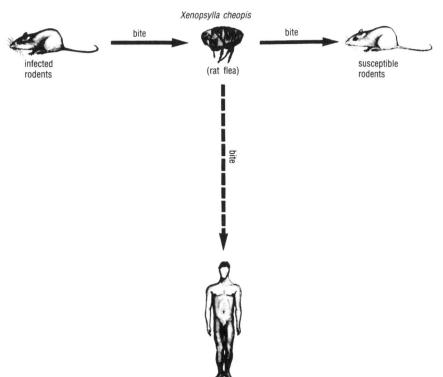

The natural foci can experience long periods of reduced activity, during which the proportion of infected rodents is small and no human cases occur. When these foci become active, epizootics among rodents and, at times, epidemic outbreaks can occur. Such could have been the case in the central Java, Indonesia, focus, where no human plague had occurred since 1959, but where 100 cases were reported in 1968 and 40 in 1971.

When man enters a natural focus, he may contract the infection through bites of fleas of wild rodents or lagomorphs, or through skin abrasions or bites when handling these animals. Human cases are sporadic under these circumstances. When plague penetrates the domestic and peridomestic environment, man is infected via fleas of commensal rodents, and epidemic outbreaks may result. The domestic rat flea (*Xenopsylla cheopis*) is the biological vector *par excellence* of plague. The name zootic plague has been given to plague transmitted by insects. Indirect interhuman transmission via human ectoparasites (*Pulex irritans* and *Pediculus humanis*) is rare and has only been observed in heavily infested environments. In some areas of the Andes, this mode of transmission occurs with some frequency, epecially during wakes for those who have died of plague. These outbreaks are almost always within families.

Cats have transmitted the infection in a small proportion of cases (in the USA, 2.2% from 1930 to 1979). Because buboes in cats are located in the head and neck region, it is thought that cats contract the infection by consuming infected rodents.

Transmission from cat to man has resulted from direct contact, bites, or scratches.

Secondary pneumonia as a complication of bubonic or septicemic plague may give rise to a series of primary pneumonic plague cases through interhuman transmission via the respiratory route. This is so-called demic plague. At present, bubonic plague is eminently zoonotic and occurs primarily in semi-arid areas.

Role of Animals in the Epidemiology of the Disease: Perpetuation of plague depends on the *Y. pestis*-rodents-fleas complex in natural foci. Plague in commensal rodents is usually a collateral phenomenon to sylvatic plague, and so, by extension, is demic plague.

Diagnosis: Early diagnosis is essential to protect the patient and the community. Diagnosis is confirmed in the laboratory by examining Gram- or Giemsa-stained gelatinous fluid collected from a punctured bubo or by culturing the fluid in appropriate media. The culture can be identified rapidly using specific phago-cytolysis or the immunofluorescence and agglutination tests.

An index case (the first case in a community), which may give rise to an outbreak, can be provisionally diagnosed with the rapid immunofluorescence test, using material from a bubo, and confirmed later by culture or inoculation in laboratory animals (guinea pigs and mice).

Hemoculture can be used in the initial, septicemic period of bubonic plague.

Inoculation of laboratory animals has proven superior to culture on culture media for plague research in rodents and fleas. Passive hemagglutination is of great value for epizootiologic studies of the infection, both in native rodent populations and in sentinel animals in natural foci. A resistant species, such as the dog, can fulfill the latter surveillance function. During a plague episode in which one man in south-eastern Utah, USA, died, the only evidence of the infection's activity was the discovery of positive titers in two of the family dogs. In the same country, the coyote is another animal that has proved useful as a sentinel. This animal rarely dies of plague, but produces antibodies against the disease agent; in addition, since it feeds on sick and dead rodents, examining a coyote is equivalent to examining several hundred rodents. A rapid serologic test (an enzymatic immunoassay) has been perfected for testing these animals (Willeberg *et al.*, 1979). The passive hemag-glutination test, employing specific Fraction-1 antigen (pesticin), is also useful in retrospective studies of plague in human communities in enzootic areas.

Control: Prevention of human plague is based on control of rodents and vectors. Eradication of the natural foci is a long-term, costly, and difficult task that can be achieved by a change in the ecology of the foci, such as dedicating an enzootic area to agriculture. In general, the objectives of prevention campaigns are more limited and consist mainly of emergency programs in situations that possess a high potential for human infection. In all areas where natural plague foci exist, continuous surveillance must be maintained (dogs have been used very successfully as sentinel animals) and emergency measures set in motion should cases of the disease develop. Essentially, these measures consist of the use of insecticides and rodenticides. Insecticides should be employed prior to or simultaneous with rodent poisons, but never after, since fleas abandon dead animal hosts and seek out new hosts, including man. During outbreaks, the main effort should be directed toward the control of fleas, which is very effective and economical. If human plague cases occur, patients must be isolated (stringent isolation is required for pneumonic patients) and treated. All contacts should be disinfested and kept under surveillance; if deemed necessary, chemoprophylaxis (tetracycline and sulfonamides) should be given for 6 days; control of fleas and rodents should be continued. In places where flea infestations on humans are prevalent, such as the Andes, prophylactic measures are recommended for persons attending funerals of plague victims, along with strict control of these cases to prevent human-to-human transmission.

Inactivated vaccine confers protection for less than 6 months, and vaccination is justified only for inhabitants of high-incidence areas, laboratory personnel who work with plague, and persons who must enter plague foci. It should be borne in mind that several doses are needed to achieve a satisfactory level of protection. Inactivated vaccine was used for US troops in Vietnam and is believed to have been effective in protecting them.

Plague is subject to control measures established under the International Sanitary Code (World Health Organization).

Bibliography

Akiev, A. K. Epidemiology and incidence of plague in the world, 1958-79. *Bull WHO* 60:165-169, 1982.

American Public Health Association. *Control of Communicable Diseases in Man*, 14th ed. (Ed. by A. S. Benenson). Washington, D.C., APHA, 1985.

Bercovier, H., H. H. Mollaret, J. M. Alonso, J. Brault, G. R. Fanning, A. G. Steigerwalt, and D. J. Brenner. Intra- and interspecies relatedness of *Yersinia pestis* by DNA hybridization and its relationship to *Yersinia pseudotuberculosis*. *Curr Microbiol* 4:225-229, 1980.

Butler, T. Plague. *In*: Warren K. S., and A. A. F. Mahmoud (Eds.), *Tropical and Geographical Medicine*, New York, McGraw-Hill Book Company, 1984.

Centers for Disease Control of the USA. Human Plague—United States, 1981. *Morb Mortal Wkly Rep* 31:74-76, 1982.

Christie, A. B., T. H. Chen, and S. S. Elberg. Plague in camels and goats: their role in human epidemics. *J Infect Dis* 141:724-726, 1980.

Davis, D. H. S., A. F. Hallett, and M. Isaacson. Plague. *In*: Hubbert, W. T., W. F. McCulloch, and P. R. Schnurrenberger (Eds.), *Diseases Transmitted from Animals to Man*, 6th ed. Springfield, Illinois, Thomas, 1975.

Dinger, J. E. Plague. *In*: Van der Hoeden, J. (Ed.), *Zoonoses*. Amsterdam, Netherlands, Elsevier, 1964.

Hudson, B. W., M. I. Goldenberg, J. D. McCluskie, H. E. Larson, C. D. McGuire, A. M. Barnes, and J. D. Poland. Serological and bacteriological investigations of an outbreak of plague in an urban tree squirrel population. *Am J Trop Med Hyg* 20:255-263, 1971.

International Committee on Systemic Bacteriology, List 7. Validation of the publication of new names and new combinations previously effectively published outside IJSB. *Int J Syst Bacteriol* 31:382-383, 1981.

Kartman, L., M. I. Goldenberg, and W. T. Hubbert. Recent observations on the epidemiology of plague in the United States. *Am J Public Health* 56:1554-1569, 1966.

Kaufmann, A. F., J. M. Mann, T. M. Gardiner, F. Heaton, J. D. Poland, A. M. Barnes, and G. C. Maupin. Public health implications of plague in domestic cats. *J Am Vet Med Assoc* 179:875-878, 1981.

Olsen, P. F. Sylvatic (wild rodent) plague. *In*: Davis, J. W., L. H. Karstad, and D. O. Trainer (Eds.), *Infectious Diseases of Wild Mammals*. Ames, Iowa State University Press, 1970.

Pan American Health Organization. *Plague in the Americas*. Washington, D.C., 1965. (Scientific Publication 115.)

Pan American Health Organization. *Health Conditions in the Americas, 1969-1972*. Washington, D.C., 1974. (Scientific Publication 287.)

Pan American Health Organization. *Inf Epidemiol Sem* 48:158, 1976.

Pan American Health Organization. Status of plague in the Americas, 1970-1980. *Epidemiol Bull* 2:5-8, 1981.

Pavlovsky, E. N. *Natural Nidality of Transmissible Diseases.* Urbana, University of Illinois Press, 1966.

Poland, J. D., and A. M. Barnes. Plague. *In*: Stoenner H., W. Kaplan, and M. Torten (Section Eds.), *CRC Handbook Series in Zoonoses.* Section A, vol. 1, Boca Raton, Florida, CRC Press, 1979.

Pollitzer, R. A review of recent literature on plague. *Bull WHO* 23:313-400, 1960.

Pollitzer, R., and K. F. Meyer. The ecology of plague. *In*: May, J. M. (Ed.), *Studies in Disease Ecology.* New York, Hafner, 1961.

Rollag, O. J., M. R. Skeets, L. J. Nims, J. P. Thilsted, and J. M. Mann. Feline plague in New Mexico: report of 5 cases. *J Am Vet Med Assoc* 179:1381-1383, 1981.

Rosser, W. W. Bubonic plague—zoonosis update. *J Am Vet Med Assoc* 191:406-409, 1987.

Rust, J. H. Plague research in northern Peru. PAHO/WHO Report, June 1985.

Stark, H. E., B. W. Hudson, and B. Pittman. *Plague Epidemiology.* Atlanta, Georgia, Centers for Disease Control of the USA, 1966.

Tirador, D. F., B. E. Miller, J. W. Stacy, A. R. Martin, L. Kartman, R. N. Collins, and R. L. Brutché. Plague epidemic in New Mexico, 1965. An emergency program to control plague. *Public Health Rep* 82:1094-1099, 1967.

Willeberg, P. W., R. Ruppaner, D. E. Behymer, H. H. Higa, C. E. Franti, R. A. Thomson, and B. Bohannan. Epidemiologic survey of sylvatic plague by serotesting coyote sentinels with enzyme immunoassay. *Am J Epidemiol* 110:328-334, 1979.

Williams, J. E., L. Arntzen, G. L. Tyndal, and M. Isaacson. Application of enzyme immunoassays for the confirmation of clinically suspect plague in Namibia, 1982. *Bull WHO* 64:745-752, 1986.

World Health Organization. *WHO Expert Committee on Plague.* Fourth Report. Geneva, 1970. (Technical Report Series 447.)

World Health Organization. Human plague in 1985. *Wkly Epidemiol Rec* 61(36):273-274, 1986.

PSEUDOTUBERCULOUS YERSINIOSIS

(027.8)

Etiology: *Yersinia pseudotuberculosis* ssp. *pseudotuberculosis.* In DNA hybridization studies the close relationship between the agent of plague and that of pseudotuberculosis was confirmed, for which reason they have been classified as different subspecies within the same species (Bercovier *et al.*, 1980).

Y. pseudotuberculosis ssp. *pseudotuberculosis* (or for the sake of simplicity *Y. pseudotuberculosis*) is subdivided on the basis of its somatic antigens (O) into six serotypes (I-VI), which in turn are divided, with the exception of serotypes III and VI, into subtypes A and B.

The bacterium has a coccobacillary form, is gram-negative, is motile at 25°C and nonmotile at 37°C, and can live a long time in soil and water. It belongs to the Enterobacteriaceae family.

Geographic Distribution: The distribution of the etiologic agent is probably worldwide. The greatest concentration of human and animal cases is found in Europe and the Soviet Far East.

Occurrence in Man: The disease occurs sporadically in Europe and in the Americas. A recent epidemic outbreak of 19 cases occurred in Finland (Tertii *et al.*, 1984). In the Soviet Far East, several thousand cases of a scarlatiniform illness have been described (Stovell, 1980). Serotype I predominates in human infections. Serotypes I, II, and III have been isolated in Asia, Europe, Canada, and the United States, and serotypes IV and V in Europe and Japan, while serotype VI has only been isolated from a few cases in Japan (Quan *et al.*, 1981).

Occurrence in Animals: A great many species of domestic and wild mammals, domestic and wild birds, and reptiles are naturally susceptible to the infection. The disease occurs sporadically in domestic animals. In Europe, devastating epizootics have been described in hares. Epizootic outbreaks have occurred in guinea pigs, wild birds, turkeys, ducks, pigeons, and canaries. Serotype I also predominates in animal disease.

The Disease in Man: The disease mainly affects children, adolescents, and young adults. The most common clinical form is mesenteric adenitis, or pseudoappendicitis, with acute abdominal pain in the right iliac fossa, fever, and vomiting. Only 20% of the patients experience diarrhea, whereas in the infection caused by *Y. enterocolitica* it is always a symptom. The disease lasted a week to 6 months in 19 patients studied in Finland (Tertii *et al.*, 1984). Twelve of these patients developed complications: six had erythema nodosum, four suffered from arthritis, one had iritis, and one developed nephritis.

The disease is more common in males. The length of the incubation period is still not precisely known, but it is thought to be from 1 to 3 weeks.

Septicemia caused by *Y. pseudotuberculosis* usually develops in weakened patients, especially the elderly.

In the Soviet Far East a scarlatiniform disease form has been described. The syndrome is characterized by fever, scarlatiniform eruption, and acute polyarthritis. The disease can be reproduced in volunteers given cultures of the agent isolated from patients (Stovell, 1980).

The Disease in Animals: Outbreaks of yersiniosis in guinea-pig colonies have occurred in several parts of the world with some frequency. The course of the disease in these animals is usually subacute. The mesenteric lymph nodes become swollen and caseous, and at times there are nodular abscesses in the intestinal wall, spleen, liver, and other organs. The animal rapidly loses weight and often has diarrhea. The disease lasts about a month. The septicemic form is rarer; the animal dies in a few days without showing significant symptoms. Fatality varies from 5 to 75%. Animals infected with *Y. pseudotuberculosis* that are apparently healthy and remain in the colony can perpetuate the infection and cause new outbreaks.

In cats, anorexia, gastroenteritis, jaundice, palpable mesenteric lymph nodes, and hypertrophy of the spleen and liver are frequently observed. Death can ensue 2 or 3 weeks after onset of the disease.

Outbreaks resulting in abortions, suppurative epididymo-orchitis, and high mortality have been recorded in sheep in Australia and Europe. Isolated cases with abortions and abscesses have been confirmed in sheep in several countries. The disease caused abortions and pneumonia in cattle in Canada. Cases of gastroenteritis have been observed in swine. *Y. pseudotuberculosis* has been isolated from the feces and especially from the tonsils of apparently healthy animals of this species.

Outbreaks in turkeys have been described in England and in the United States (Oregon and California). A recent outbreak occurred on four farms in California (Wallner-Pendleton and Cooper, 1983). The main symptoms were anorexia; watery, yellowish green diarrhea; depression; and acute locomotor impairment. The disease affected males 9 to 12 weeks of age, had a morbidity rate of 2 to 15%, and produced high mortality, principally owing to cannibalism. Administration of high doses of tetracyclines in food seemed to arrest the disease, but the animals were condemned in the postmortem inspection because of septicemic lesions. The principal lesions were necrotic foci in the liver and spleen, catarrhal enteritis, and osteomyelitis.

The pseudotuberculosis agent is the most common cause of death among hares (*Lepus europaeus*) in France and Germany. Rabbits (*Oryctolagus cuniculus*) and the ringdove (*Columba palumbus*) are also frequent victims of the disease. Epizootics have been described among rats (*Rattus norvegicus*) in Japan.

Source of Infection and Mode of Transmission (Figure 16): Many facets of the epidemiology of pseudotuberculous yersiniosis still need to be clarified. The broad range of animal and bird species naturally susceptible to the infection suggests that animals constitute the reservoir of the etiologic agent. In Germany and Holland, the agent was isolated from the tonsils of 5.8% and 4.3% of 480 and 163 clinically sound swine, respectively, indicating that this animal species can be a healthy carrier (Weber and Knapp, 1981a). The agent was also isolated from 0.58% of 1,206 swine feces samples examined over a period of 14 months. These isolations as well as the ones from tonsils were done in the cold months, corresponding to the season in which human cases occur (Weber and Knapp, 1981b). Several authors believe the soil is the agent's reservoir, but isolations from the soil in Europe have primarily yielded serotype II, which is rarely found in the human disease (Aldova *et al.*, 1979). However, in the focus of scarlatiniform pseudotuberculosis in the Soviet Far East, serotype I has been isolated from soil and water (possibly contaminated by animal feces), which would explain the large number of cases. In any event, animals and wild fowl undeniably contribute to environmental contamination. An epizootic or epornitic in one animal species has many repercussions in other species because the agent is excreted in the feces and contaminates the environment.

The mode of transmission is fecal-oral. The localization of the infection in the mesenteric lymph nodes indicates that the digestive tract is the bacteria's principal route of entry.

In repeated outbreaks of yersiniosis in guinea-pig colonies in Great Britain, the infection was transmitted by vegetables contaminated with the feces of the ringdove (*Columba palumbus*). In an outbreak of pseudotuberculosis in turkeys in California (Wallner-Pendleton and Cooper, 1983), two dead squirrels were found near the feeders. The etiologic agent was isolated from necrotic lesions in the liver and spleen of one of the squirrels. The immediate source of infection for man is often difficult to ascertain. A common source of infection was not found for an epidemic outbreak in 19 patients in Finland (Tertii, 1984). The more frequent occurrence of the disease in winter is attributed to stress factors.

Role of Animals in the Epidemiology of the Disease: The reservoir and source of the infection for man consists of wild animals (mainly rodents), domestic animals

Figure 16. Pseudotuberculous yersiniosis (*Yersinia pseudotuberculosis*). Probable mode of transmission.

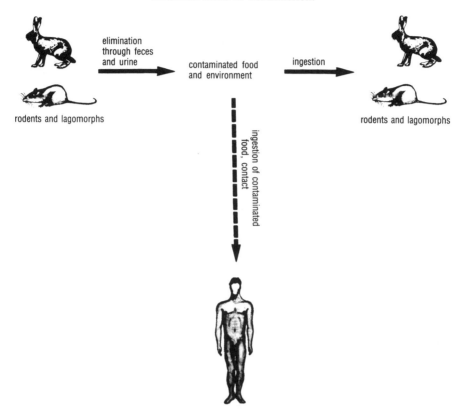

(swine), and wild birds. Indirect transmission is perhaps the most common means of transmission to man, occurring through contamination of the environment by feces. The agent can survive for a relatively long time on vegetables and inanimate objects. A case of transmission by dog bite is also known.

Diagnosis: Diagnosis can be confirmed only by isolating and identificating the causal agent. The most appropriate material for this examination is the mesenteric lymph nodes. Serotyping of the isolated strains is important from the epidemiologic standpoint. The serologic tests now in use to verify infection by *Y. pseudotuberculosis* are agglutination, hemagglutination, and, more recently, ELISA with the corresponding serotype; the last test is considered the most sensitive and specific. Results should be carefully evaluated, since several of the serotypes have antigens in common with other enterobacteria.

Control: The principal preventive measure consists of protecting food and water against fecal contamination by rodents and fowl. Also recommended is control of peridomestic rodent populations and limitation of the number of birds in public places.

Bibliography

Aldova, E., A. Brecinova, and J. Sobotkova. A finding of *Yersinia pseudotuberculosis* in well water. *Zentralbl Bakteriol [B]* 169:265-270, 1979.

Bercovier, H., H. H. Mollaret, J. M. Alonso, J. Brault, G. R. Fanning, A. G. Steigerwalt, and D. J. Brenner. Intra- and interspecies relatedness of *Yersinia pestis* by DNA hybridization and its relationship to *Yersinia pseudotuberculosis*. *Curr Microbiol* 4:225-229, 1980.

Joubert, L. La pseudo-tuberculose, zoonose d'avenir. *Rev Med Vet Lyon* 119:311-322, 1968.

Mair, N. S. Yersiniosis in wildlife and its public health implications. *J Wildl Dis* 9:64-71, 1973.

Mair, N. S. Yersiniosis (Infections due to *Yersinia pseudotuberculosis* and *Yersinia enterocolitica*). *In*: Hubbert, W. T., W. F. McCulloch, and P. R. Schnurrenberger (Eds.), *Diseases Transmitted from Animals to Man*, 6th ed. Springfield, Illinois, 1975.

Quan, T. J., A. M. Barnes, and J. D. Poland. Yersinioses. *In*: A. Balows, and W. J. Hausler, Jr. (Eds.), *Diagnostic Procedures for Bacterial, Mycotic and Parasitic Infections*, 6th ed. Washington, D.C., American Public Health Association, 1981.

Stovell, P. L. Pseudotubercular yersiniosis. *In*: Stoenner, H., W. Kaplan, and M. Torten (Section Eds.), *CRC Handbook Series in Zoonoses*. Section A, vol. 2. Boca Raton, Florida, CRC Press, 1980.

Tertii, R., K. Granfors, O. P. Lehtonen, J. Merisola, A. L. Makela, I. Valimaki, P. Haninem, and A. Toivanen. An outbreak of *Yersinia pseudotuberculosis* infection. *J Infect Dis* 149:245-250, 1984.

Wallner-Pendleton, E., and G. Cooper. Several outbreaks of *Yersinia pseudotuberculosis* in California turkey flocks. *Avain Dis* 27:524-526, 1983.

Weber, A., and W. Knapp. Uber die Jahreszeitliche Abhangigkeit des Nachweises von *Yersinia pseudotuberculosis* in Tonsillen gesunder Schlachtschweine. *Zentralbl Bakteriol Mikrobiol Hyg [A]* 250:78-83, 1981a.

Weber, A., and W. Knapp. Nachweis von *Yersinia enterocolitica* und *Yersinia pseudotuberculosis* in Kotproben gesunder Schlachtschweine in Abhangigkeit von der Jahreszeit. *Zentralbl Veterinarmed [B]* 28:407-413, 1981b.

Wetzler, T. F. Pseudotuberculosis. *In*: Davis, J. W., L. H. Karstad, and D. O. Trainer (Eds.) *Infectious Diseases of Wild Mammals*. Ames, Iowa State University Press, 1970.

RAT-BITE FEVER

(026.0)
(026.1)

Etiology: *Streptobacillus moniliformis* and *Spirillum minus*.

1. Infection due to *Streptobacillus moniliformis*

Synonym: Haverhill fever.

Geographic Distribution: Worldwide.

Occurrence in Man: Occasional. Of 13 cases of rat-bite fever on record in the United States since 1958, six were originated by the bite of laboratory rats. Twelve of the 13 cases in that country were caused by *S. moniliformis* (Anderson *et al.*, 1983).

Occurrence in Animals: The agent is isolated from the nasopharynx of a high percentage of healthy rats. Epizootics have been described in wild and laboratory mice. Some outbreaks have also occurred in turkeys, and isolated cases in other animals.

The Disease in Man: The incubation period lasts from 2 to 14 days. The disease begins with a symptomatology similar to that of influenza. The wound from the bite heals spontaneously without complications. Exanthema, regional lymphadenitis, migratory astralgias, and myalgias are common. In the most severe cases polyarthritis is observed. After a short time, body temperature returns to normal, but fever may recur. Endocarditis is a possible complication. In untreated cases, mortality reaches 10%.

The disease almost always appears in sporadic cases. An epidemic outbreak was described in Haverhill, USA, caused by consumption of raw milk, probably contaminated by rat fecal material.

The Disease in Animals: Rats are healthy carriers and harbor the etiologic agent in their nasopharynx. Purulent lesions have sometimes been observed in these animals. *S. moniliformis* is pathogenic for mice and has produced epizootics among these rodents both in laboratories and in their natural habitat. In one epizootic among laboratory mice, high morbidity and mortality rates were recorded, with symptoms such as polyarthritis, gangrene, and spontaneous amputation of members. In guinea pigs the agent can produce cervical lymphadenitis with large abscesses in the regional lymph nodes. Some outbreaks have been described among turkeys in which the most salient symptom was arthritis.

Source of Infection and Mode of Transmission: Rats constitute the reservoir of the infection. They harbor the etiologic agent in the nasopharynx and transmit it to humans by biting. In the Haverhill epidemic, the source of infection was milk. Infection among turkeys has been attributed to rat bites. It is suspected that infection in laboratory mice is produced by aerosols when mice are kept in the same environment with rats.

Role of Animals in the Epidemiology of the Disease: Rats constitute the reservoir of the infection and play an essential epidemiologic role.

Diagnosis: Diagnosis is accomplished by isolating *S. moniliformis* from the bloodstream or articular lesions on blood- or serum-enriched media.

Control: The principal means of prevention is control of the rat population. Other important measures are pasteurization of milk and protection of food against rodents. Laboratory mice, rats, and guinea pigs should be kept in separate environments, and personnel charged with their care should be instructed in proper handling techniques.

2. Infection due to *Spirillum minus*

Synonyms: Sodoku, spirillum fever.

Geographic Distribution: Worldwide.

Occurrence in Man: Occasional.

Occurrence in Animals: The incidence of the infection in rats varies in different parts of the world.

The Disease in Man: It is similar to the disease caused by S. *moniliformis.* Its incubation period is longer, from 1 week to 2 months. Fever begins suddenly and lasts a few days, but it recurs several times over a period of 1 to 3 months. A generalized exanthematous eruption may reappear with each attack of fever. Although the bite wound heals during the incubation period, it eventually exhibits an edematous infiltration and often ulcerates. Similarly, the lymph nodes become hypertrophic.

The Disease in Animals: The infection is inapparent in rats. The etiologic agent can be isolated from their blood.

Source of Infection and Mode of Transmission: The reservoir consists of rats and other rodents, whose saliva is the source of infection for man. Transmission is accomplished by bite.

Role of Animals in the Epidemiology of the Disease: Rats play the main role. Human infections originating from bites of weasels, dogs, cats, and other carnivores have been described. It is presumed that these animals were contaminated while catching rodents and therefore act as mechanical transmitters.

Diagnosis: Diagnosis is accomplished by dark-field microscopic examination of fluid aspirated from the wound. The most reliable diagnosis is obtained by intraperitoneal inoculation of mice with blood or infiltrate from the wound, followed by microscopic examination of their blood and peritoneal fluid some 2 weeks after inoculation. The bacteria do not grow on laboratory culture media.

Control: Control is based on reduction of the rat population and on construction of rat-proof dwellings.

Bibliography

Anderson, L. C., S. L. Leary, and P. J. Manning. Rat-bite fever in animal research laboratory personnel. *Lab Anim Sci* 33:292-294, 1983.

Bisseru, B. *Diseases of Man Acquired from His Pets.* London, Heinemann, 1967.

Boyer, C. I., D. W. Bruner, and J. A. Brown. A *Streptobacillus* the cause of tendo-sheat infection in turkeys. *Avian Dis* 2:418-427, 1958.

Ruys, A. C. Rat bite fevers. *In:* Van der Hoeden, J. (Ed.), *Zoonoses.* Amsterdam, Netherlands, Elsevier, 1964.

Yamamoto, R., and G. T. Clark. *Streptobacillus moniliformis* infection in turkeys. *Vet Rec* 79:95-100, 1966.

SALMONELLOSIS

(003)

Synonyms: Enteric epizootic typhoid, enteric infection, paratyphoid.

Etiology: The literature on the taxonomy of the genus *Salmonella* is confusing. The International Committee on Systematic Bacteriology accepts as valid the following species names: *S. typhi*, *S. cholerae-suis*, *S. enteritidis*, *S. typhimurium*, and *S. arizonae* (*Arizona hinshawii*) (Skerman *et al.*, 1980). In turn, *S. enteritidis* is subdivided into almost 2,000 serotypes and serovars according to different somatic and flagellar antigens. This subdivision is of interest in epidemiologic research. Specific names previously assigned to serotypes are no longer valid. Only a few serotypes are isolated wth any frequency from man and animals in a given region or country, and the predominant serotype may vary with time. Serotypes mentioned in this chapter belong to *S. enteritidis*.

S. typhi and *S. enteritidis* paratyphoid serotypes, *paratyphi A* and *paratyphi C*, are salmonellae specific to man. Serotype *paratyphi B* is less closely adapted to man and can be found in cattle, swine, dogs, and fowl.

S. cholerae-suis and several serotypes of *S. enteritidis* (such as *gallinarum, pullorum, abortus equi, dublin*) are adapted to animals, but are transmissible to man to varying degrees. The remaining numerous serotypes of *S. enteritidis* are parasites of a broad spectrum of animals, vertebrate and invertebrate, and are not species-specific.

S. arizonae comprises 300 serotypes.

Geographic Distribution: Worldwide. *S. typhimurium* is one of the most prevalent species in the world. *S. enteritidis* serotypes vary in different areas. In short periods of time (sometimes within 1 or 2 years), changes can be observed in the relative frequency of serotypes.

Occurrence in Man: It is very common. The true incidence is difficult to evaluate, since many countries do not have an epidemiologic surveillance system in place, and even where a system does exist, mild and sporadic cases are not usually notified. In countries with a reporting system, the number of outbreaks has increased considerably in recent years; this increase is in part real and in part due to better reporting.

In 1980 *Salmonella* was isolated from about 30,000 people in the United States (Centers for Disease Control of the USA, 1982). During the period 1973-1978, salmonellosis caused 40% of cases of food-borne disease and 23% of the outbreaks. In Canada the proportions were similar (Bryan, 1981). According to several authors' estimates, the number of human cases occurring each year in the United States probably varies between 740,000 and 5,300,000. Rates for reported cases are about 10 per 100,000 inhabitants in Denmark, 44 per 100,000 in Finland, and 43 per 100,000 in Sweden, one-third to two-thirds of which were probably contracted by international travelers (Silliker, 1982). In the Federal Republic of Germany, 33,215 cases were notified in 1978, 40,717 in 1979, and 48,607 in 1980 (Poehn, 1982).

It is difficult to evaluate the situation of this disease in developing countries because of a lack of epidemiologic surveillance data, but epidemic outbreaks are known to occur. In 1977 an extensive outbreak took place in Trujillo, Peru, among university students who lunched in the university dining hall. Of 640 students dining regularly in the hall, 598 (93%) became ill and 545 were hospitalized, which resulted in temporary overcrowding of community medical services. Serotype *thompson* was isolated from the patients' stools, and epidemiologic evidence pointed to eggs used in the food as the source of infection (Gunn and Bullón, 1980). In the period 1969-1974, 3,429 cases of acute diarrhea in Argentine children from Buenos Aires and environs were studied. Isolations of 932 *Salmonella* strains were obtained from 3,429 stool cultures. Between 1969 and 1972, isolations of *S. typhimurium* predominated, revealing the existence of an epidemic. The clinical picture was serious and the mortality rate was 14% of the 246 children studied. After 1972, isolations of the *oranienburg* serotype increased, and those of *S. typhimurium* decreased. In 73% of the children, the infection was acquired at home; 27% first showed symptoms in the hospital after being admitted for causes other than gastrointestinal disturbance (Binsztein *et al.*, 1982).

Occurrence in Animals: It is common. The rate of infection in domestic animals has been estimated at from 1 to 3%. In 1980, 16,274 strains of 183 serotypes of animal *Salmonella* were isolated in the Federal Republic of Germany (for diagnostic purposes during the veterinary inspection of slaughterhouses, from animal feed, and from water and other sources) (Pietzsh, 1982). The same year, 2,515 strains of nonhuman origin were isolated in the United States (Centers for Disease Control of the USA, 1982). Several surveys have found the incidence of avian salmonellosis to be lower than 1% in Sweden, around 5% in Denmark, and around 7% in Finland. Its incidence in other countries is higher. In Great Britain, there were 3,626 isolations in 1980 and 2,992 in 1981. Epidemiologic surveillance of animals is obviously of utmost importance, since the source of the large majority of nontyphic salmonellosis cases is food of animal origin. There are no data from developing countries in this regard.

The Disease in Man: With the exception of *S. typhi* and the paratyphoid serotypes (particularly A and C), which are species-specific for man, all other *Salmonella* infections may be considered zoonoses. Salmonellosis is perhaps the most widespread zoonosis in the world. *S. typhimurium* and all serotypes of *S. enteritidis* are potentially pathogenic for man.

Salmonellae of animal origin cause an intestinal infection in man characterized by a 6- to 72-hour incubation period after ingestion of the implicated food, and sudden onset of fever, myalgias, cephalalgia, and malaise. The main symptoms consist of abdominal pain, nausea, vomiting, and diarrhea. Salmonellosis normally has a benign course and clinical recuperation ensues in 2 to 4 days. The convalescent carrier may shed salmonellae for several weeks and, more rarely, for a few months. Conversely, the carrier state is persistent in infections due to *S. typhi* or paratyphoid salmonellae. Though salmonellosis may occur in persons of all ages, incidence is much higher among children and the elderly. Dehydration can be serious.

Serotypes adapted to a particular animal species are usually less pathogenic for man (*pullorum, gallinarum, abortus equi, abortus ovis*). An exception is *S. cholerae-suis*, which produces a serious disease with a septicemic syndrome, splenomegaly, and high fever a few days to a few weeks after the onset of gastroenteritis. Bacteremia is present in over 50% of patients with *S. cholerae-suis* infections, and the fatality rate may reach 20%. Serotypes *sendai* and *dublin* can also cause septicemia ("enteric fever") and often metastatic abscesses.

Antibiotics are not recommended for use against *Salmonella*-induced gastroenteritis without complications, except in cases of prolonged fever or septicemia, especially in small children and the elderly. The drugs are contraindicated because they may prolong the carrier period and cause antibiotic-resistant strains to emerge. In the last two decades, a high proportion of *Salmonella* with multiple antibiotic-resistance has been seen in many countries. The main cause of this phenomenon in industrialized countries has been the excessive use of antibiotics in animal feed as a growth enhancer, and also the indiscriminate prescription-drug treatment of people and animals. In Great Britain, the prophylactic use of antibiotics against bovine salmonellosis has resulted in the emergence of multiresistant strains of *S. typhimurium*, which have caused epizootics with high mortality. Outbreaks and epidemics of multiresistant strains of several serotypes have occurred in nurseries and pediatric clinics, with complications of septicemia or meningitis and high mortality. An epidemc caused by multiresistant strains of serotype *wien* originated in Algeria in 1969 and spread to several European and Asian countries; the source in the food chain was not discovered. Other epidemics extending to several countries were caused by *S. typhimurium* phage type 208 (WHO Scientific Group, 1980). In developing countries, the principal cause of the emergence of multiresistant *Salmonella* strains may be self-medication made possible by easy public access to non-prescription antibiotics.

An infrequent syndrome in human salmonellosis is localized infection in any part of the body, which may be either a sequela of bacteremia or the initial condition.

The Disease in Animals: Salmonellae have a large variety of animal hosts, domestic as well as wild. The infection may or may not be clinically apparent. In the subclinical form, the animal may have a latent infection and harbor the pathogen in its lymph nodes, or it may be a carrier and eliminate the agent with fecal material for a short while, intermittently or persistently. In domestic animals, there are several well-known clinical entities due to species-adapted serotypes, such as *pullorum* or *abortus equi*. Other clinically apparent or inapparent infections are caused by serotypes with multiple hosts.

CATTLE: The principal causes of clinical salmonellosis in cattle are serotype *dublin* (species *S. enteritidis*) and *S. typhimurium*. At times other serotypes can be isolated from sick animals.

Salmonellosis or paratyphoid in adult cattle occurs sporadically, but in calves it usually acquires epizootic proportions. Serotype *dublin*, adapted to cattle, has a focal geographic distribution. In the Americas, outbreaks have been confirmed in the western United States, Venezuela, and Brazil.

In adult cattle the disease begins with high fever, appearance of blood clots in the feces followed by profuse diarrhea, and then a drop in body temperature to normal or subnormal. Signs of abdominal pain are very pronounced. Abortion is common in pregnant cows. The disease may be fatal in a few days or the animal may recover, in which case it often becomes a carrier and new cases appear. Calves are more susceptible than adults, and in them the infection gives rise to true epidemic outbreaks, often with high mortality. The carrier state is less frequent among young animals than among adults. The infection is almost always spread by the feces of a cow that is shedding the agent, but it also may originate from milk.

SWINE: Swine are host to numerous serotypes of *Salmonella* and constitute the principal reservoir of *S. cholerae-suis*. Serotypes of *S. enteritidis* that attack swine are customarily isolated from the intestine and from the mesenteric lymph nodes, while *S. cholerae-suis* is very invasive, gives rise to septicemia, and may be isolated from blood or any organ. Swine are particularly susceptible and experience epidemic outbreaks between 2 and 4 months of age, but the infection also appears in mature animals, almost always as isolated cases.

Most of the time, swine paratyphoid, or necrotic enteritis, occurs in herds living under poor hygienic conditions and poor management. It is frequently associated with classic swine plague (cholera) and stress factors such as weaning and vaccination. The most frequent symptoms are fever and diarrhea. The infection usually originates from a carrier pig or contaminated food.

Infection by serotypes of *S. enteritidis* may sometimes give rise to serious outbreaks of salmonellosis with high mortality.

Because of the frequency with which swine are infected with different types of salmonellae, pork products have often been a source of human infection.

SHEEP AND GOATS: Cases of clinical salmonellosis in these species are not very frequent. The most common serotype found in gastroenteritis cases is *S. typhimurium*, but many other serotypes have also been isolated. Serotype *abortus ovis*, which causes abortions and gastroenteritis in sheep and goats, seems to be restricted to Europe.

HORSES: The most important pathogen among horses is *abortus equi*, which causes abortions in mares and arthritis in colts. Its distribution is worldwide. As in other types of salmonellosis, predisposing factors influence whether the infection manifests itself clinically. Pregnant mares are especially susceptible, particularly if other debilitating conditions are present. Abortion occurs in the last months of pregnancy, and the fetus and placenta contain large numbers of bacteria. The serotype *abortus equi* is adapted to horses and rarely found in other animal species.

Horses are also susceptible to other types of salmonellae, particularly *S. typhimurium*. *Salmonella* enteritis occurs in these animals, sometimes causing high mortality.

DOGS AND CATS: In recent years, a high prevalence of the infection, caused by numerous serotypes, has been confirmed among cats and dogs. These animals may be asymptomatic carriers or may suffer from gastroenteric salmonellosis of varying degrees of severity.

Dogs can contract the infection by eating the feces of other dogs, of other domestic or peridomestic animals, or of man. Dogs and cats can also be infected by contaminated food. Dogs can transmit the disease to man.

FOWL: Two serotypes, *pullorum* and *gallinarum*, are adapted to domestic fowl. They are not very pathogenic for man, although cases of salmonellosis caused by these serotypes have been described in children. Many other serotypes are frequently isolated from domestic poultry and for that reason these animals are considered one of the principal reservoirs of salmonellae.

Pullorum disease, caused by the serotype *pullorum*, and fowl typhoid, caused by *gallinarum*, produce serious economic losses on poultry farms if not adequately controlled. Both diseases have worldwide distribution and give rise to outbreaks with high morbidity and mortality. Pullorum disease appears during the first 2 weeks of life and causes high mortality. The agent is transmitted vertically as well as horizontally. Carrier birds lay infected eggs that contaminate incubators and hatcheries. Fowl typhoid occurs mainly in adult birds, and is transmitted by the fecal matter of carrier fowl. On an affected poultry farm, recuperating birds and apparently healthy birds are reservoirs of infection.

Salmonellae unadapted to fowl also infect them frequently. The infection in adult birds is asymptomatic, but during the first few weeks of life, its clinical picture is similar to pullorum disease (loss of appetite, nervous symptoms, and blockage of the cloaca with diarrheal fecal matter).

The most common agent in ducks and geese is *S. typhimurium*. The infection may be transmitted from the infected ovary to the yolk, as in pullorum disease, or by contamination of the shell when it passes through the cloaca.

Salmonellosis is frequent in wild birds. When 227 specimens of the herring gull (*Larus argentatus*) were examined, 8.4% were found to be salmonellae carriers, and the serotypes were similar to those in man. Wild birds were also considered vectors of disease caused by the *montevideo* serotype in outbreaks in sheep and cattle in Scotland (Butterfield *et al.*, 1982; Coulson et al., 1983).

OTHER ANIMALS: Rodents become infected with the serotypes peculiar to the environment in which they live. The rate of wild animal carriers is not very high. Rodents found in and around food processing plants can be an important source of human infection.

Of 974 free-living wild animals examined in Panama, 3.4% were found to be infected, principally by serotypes of *S. enteritidis* and less frequently by *S. arizonae* and *edwardsiella*. The highest rate of infection (11.8%) was found among the 195 marsupials examined. *Salmonella* was isolated from only eight of 704 spiny rats (*Proechimys semispinosus*).

Outbreaks of salmonellosis among wild animals in zoos or on pelt farms are not unusual.

Salmonella infection in cold-blooded animals has merited special attention lately. Because of the high rate of infection among little turtles kept as house pets in the United States, their importation was prohibited and a certificate stating them to be infection-free was required for interstate commerce.

An infection rate of 37% was found in 317 reptiles examined live or necropsied at the National Zoo in Washington, D.C. The highest rate of infection was observed in snakes (55%) and the lowest (3%) in turtles. The salmonellae isolated were 24 different serotypes of *S. enteritidis*, one strain of *S. cholerae-suis*, and 39 of *S. arizonae*. No disease was attributed to these bacteria, but they may act together with other agents to cause opportunistic infections (Cambre *et al.*, 1980).

Source of Infection and Mode of Transmission (Figure 17): *S. typhi* and the paratyphoid serotypes are predominantly human parasites. Animals form the reservoir of the other salmonellae. Practically any food of animal origin can be a source of infection for man. The most common vehicles are contaminated poultry, pork, beef, eggs, milk, and their products. Foods of vegetable origin contaminated by animal products, human excreta, or dirty utensils, in both commercial processing plants and household kitchens, have occasionally been implicated as vehicles of human salmonellosis. Contaminated public or private water supplies are important sources of infection in typhoid fever (*S. typhi*) and, less frequently, in other salmonella infections.

Man normally acquires the infection by consuming contaminated food. Important contributing factors are inadequate cooking, slow cooling of the food, lack of

Figure 17. Salmonellosis. Mode of transmission
(except *Salmonella typhi* and the paratyphoid serotypes).

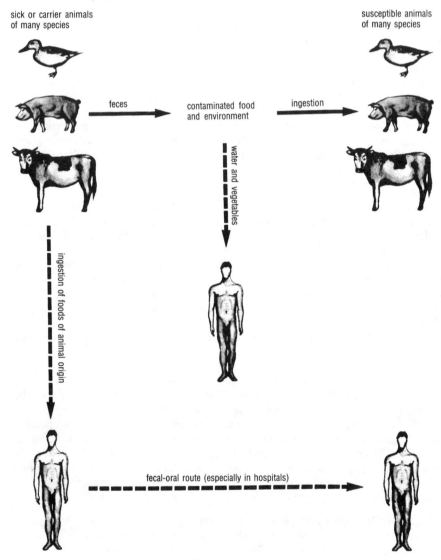

refrigeration for many hours, and inadequate reheating before serving. Large outbreaks are invariably due to inappropriate handling of food in restaurants and
institutional dining facilities. Man can also contract the infection directly, from
domestic animals or house pets such as dogs, turtles, monkeys, hamsters, and
others. Interhuman transmission is especially important in hospitals, and childen are
the principal victims. Insects, particularly flies, can serve as mechanical vectors in
highly contaminated environments.

Animal carriers perpetuate the animal-to-animal cycle by means of their excreta or, in the case of fowl, infected eggs. Feed contaminated mainly by such ingredients as meal made from bone, meat, or fish plays an important role as a vehicle of infection. Intensive cattle-raising in developed countries is a very important contributing factor in the epidemiology of salmonellosis. Close contact between animals and the use of concentrated feed or ingredients that may be contaminated create conditions favorable to outbreaks. In developing countries, the source of infection is mainly the contaminated environment and water sources where animals crowd together.

Animal-to-animal transmission occurs not only at the home establishment, but also during shipping, at auctions, and even at slaughterhouses prior to sacrifice. Meat can become contaminated in abattoirs by means of equipment and utensils during skinning and butchering. Contaminated water can be a source of infection for man and animals.

Non–species-specific serotypes spread easily from one animal species to another and also to humans.

Role of Animals in the Epidemiology of the Disease: Since animals constitute the reservoir of salmonellae (except *S. typhi* and the paratyphoid serotypes), they play an essential role in the epidemiology.

Diagnosis: In humans, clinical diagnosis of gastroenteritis due to *Salmonella* is confirmed by isolation of the etiologic agent from the patient's stool, serologic typing, and, when necessary, phage typing. In typhoid fever cases (caused by *S. typhi* and occasionally other salmonellae), the agent can be isolated from blood during the first week of illness and from feces in the second and third weeks.

Diagnosis of animal salmonellosis is also made by culturing fecal material. For infections caused by *pullorum* and *gallinarum* in fowl, serologic diagnosis is important to locate and eliminate individual carriers. Culture of mesenteric lymph nodes is the principal procedure used in postmortem examination of animals.

Surveillance of processed foods requires that cultures be made from product samples at different stages of preparation, and from utensils and surfaces that come into contact with the food. Special sampling methods have been developed for different kinds of foods.

Control: Given current conditions under which cattle and poultry are raised, transported, marketed, and slaughtered, as well as existing food processing practices, it is impossible to obtain salmonellae-free foods of animal origin. For the present, control is based on protecting man from infection and reducing its prevalence in animals. Veterinary meat and poultry inspection and supervision of milk pasteurization and egg production are important for consumer protection.

Another important control measure is the education of food handlers, both in commercial establishments and in the home, about correct cooking and refrigeration practices for foods of animal origin, and about personal and environmental hygiene.

Epidemiologic surveillance by health authorities is necessary to evaluate the magnitude of the problem in each country, locate the origins of outbreaks, and adopt methods designed to reduce risks.

In animals, salmonellosis control depends on a) elimination of carriers, which is possible at present for pullorum disease and fowl typhoid by means of serologic tests; b) bacteriologic control of foods, mainly of additives such as fish, meat, and bone meal; c) immunization; and d) proper management of herds and poultry farms.

Live attenuated vaccines against fowl typhoid and against *dublin* infection in cattle have been tested with promising results.

In general, studies of bacterins by several researchers have given contradictory results. A recent test evaluated a vaccine of *S. typhimurium* in which biosynthesis of aromatic compounds is genetically altered. Calves that were vaccinated intramuscularly or orally at 5 weeks of age and exposed orally to the agent were protected against serious or lethal disease (Smith *et al.*, 1984). The results of the many trials carried out to date indicate that vaccines and some bacterins can prevent the disease (particularly the severe form), but not infection or the carrier state.

A control measure known as Nurmi's method is being used on fowl in Finland. Salmonella-free cultures of fecal organisms from adult birds are administered orally to newly hatched chickens and turkey chicks. Treated chicks resist high doses of salmonellae. It is believed to work by competitive exclusion. The method is effective in preventing the disease, but it does not prevent the carrier state.

Bibliography

Ager, E. A., and F. H. Top, Sr. Salmonellosis. *In*: Top, F. H., Sr., and P. F. Wehrle (Eds.), *Communicable and Infectious Diseases*, 7th ed. St. Louis, Missouri, Mosby, 1972.

Anderson, J. M., and P. A. Hartman. Direct immunoassay for detection of salmonellae in foods and feeds. *Appl Environ Microbiol* 49:1124-1127, 1985.

Barker, R. M. Tracing *Salmonella typhimurium* infections. *J Hyg (Camb)* 96:1-3, 1986.

Binsztein, N., T. Eigher, and M. D'Empaire. Epidemia de salmonelosis en Buenos Aires y sus alrededores. *Medicina (B Aires)* 42:161-167, 1982.

Bryan, F. L. Current trends in food-borne salmonellosis in the United States and Canada. *J Food Protect* 44:394-402, 1981.

Butterfield, J., J. C. Coulson, S. V. Kearsey, and P. Monaghan. The herring gull *Larus argentatus* as a carrier of *Salmonella*. *J Hyg (Camb)* 91:429-436, 1983.

Buxton, A., and H. I. Field. Salmonellosis. *In*: Stableforth, A. W., and I. A. Galloway (Eds.), *Infectious Diseases of Animals*. London, Butterworths, 1959.

Cambre, R. C., E. Green, E. E. Smith, R. J. Montali, and M. Bush. Salmonellosis and arizonosis in the reptile collection at the National Zoological Park. *J Am Vet Med Assoc* 177:800-803, 1980.

Centers for Disease Control of the USA. *Salmonella* surveillance. *Annual Summary 1980*. Atlanta, Georgia. CDC, 1982.

Coulson, J. C., J. Butterfield, and C. Thomas. The herring gull *Larus argentatus* as a likely transmitting agent of *Salmonella montevideo* to sheep and cattle. *J Hyg (Camb)* 91:437-443, 1983.

Clarenburg, A. Salmonellosis. *In*: Van der Hoeden, J. (Ed.), *Zoonoses*. Amsterdam, Netherlands, Elsevier, 1964.

Edwards, P. R., and M. M. Galton. Salmonellosis. *Adv Vet Sci* 11:1-63, 1967.

Edwards, P. R., and W. H. Ewing. *Identification of Enterobacteriaceae*, 3rd ed. Minneapolis, Minnesota, Burgess, 1972.

Gunn, R. A., and F. Bullón. *Salmonella* enterocolitis: report of a large foodborne outbreak in Trujillo, Peru. *Bull Pan Am Health Organ* 13:162-168, 1979.

Kourany, M., L. Bowdre, and A. Herrer. Panamanian forest mammals as carriers of *Salmonella*. *Am J Trop Med Hyg* 25:449-455, 1976.

National Research Council of the USA. *An Evaluation of the Salmonella Problem*. Washington, D.C., National Academy of Sciences, 1969.

Peluffo, C. A. Salmonellosis in South America. *In*: Van Ove, E. (Ed.), *The World Problem of Salmonellosis*. The Hague, Netherlands, Junk, 1964.

Pietzsch, O. Salmonellose-Uberwachtung in der Bundesrepublik Deutchland einschl. Berlin (West). *Bundesgesundhbl* 25:325-327, 1982.

Poehn, H. P. Salmonellose-Uberwachtung beim Menschen in der Bundesrepublik Deutschland einschl. Berlin (West). *Bundesgesundhbl* 25:320-324, 1982.

Silliker, J. H. The *Salmonella* problem: current status and future direction. *J Food Protec* 45:661-666, 1982.

Skerman, V. B. D., V. McGowan, and P. H. A. Sneath. Approved list of bacterial names. *Int J Syst Bacteriol* 30:225-420, 1980.

Smith, B. P., M. Reina-Guerra, S. K. Hoiseth, B. D. Stocker, F. Habasche, E. Johnson, and F. Merrit. Aromatic-dependent *Salmonella typhimurium* as modified live vaccines for calves. *Am J Vet Res* 45:59-66, 1984.

Taylor, J., and J. H. McCoy. Salmonella and Arizona infections. *In*: Riemann, H. (Ed.), *Food-Borne Infections and Intoxications*. New York and London, Academic Press, 1969.

Thatcher, F. S., and D. S. Clark. *Análisis microbiológico de los alimentos*. Zaragoza, Spain, Acribia, 1973.

Weiss, S. H., M. J. Blaser, R. E. Black, M. A. Asbury, G. P. Carter, R. A. Feldman, and D. J. Brenner. Occurrence and distribution of serotypes of the Arizona subgroup of *Salmonella* strains in the United States from 1967 to 1976. *J Clin Microbiol* 23:1056-1064, 1986.

William, L. P., and B. C. Hobbs. Enterobacteriaceae infections. *In*: Hubbert, W. T., W. F. McCulloch, and P. R. Schnurrenberger (Eds.), *Diseases Transmitted from Animals to Man*, 6th ed., Springfield, Illinois, Thomas, 1975.

World Health Organization. *Microbiological Aspects of Food Hygiene*. Geneva, WHO, 1968. (Technical Report Series 399.)

World Health Organization Scientific Working Group. Enteric infections due to *Campylobacter*, *Yersina*, *Salmonella*, and *Shigella*. *Bull WHO* 58:519-537, 1980.

SHIGELLOSIS

(004)

Synonym: Bacillary dysentery.

Etiology: The type species is *Shigella dysenteriae*; other agents are *S. flexneri*, *S. boydii*, and *S. sonnei*. The first three species are subdivided into serotypes.

Geographic Distribution: Worldwide.

Occurrence in Man: It is frequent in tropical and subtropical developing countries. In 1969-1970, an extensive epidemic due to *S. dysenteriae* type 1 began in Central America and Mexico, producing high morbidity and mortality, especially in children, and resulting in the death of more than 13,000 patients. The infection reached the United States and caused 140 cases from 1970 to 1972. A similar epidemic occurred in Bangladesh in 1972 and in Sri Lanka in 1976 (World Health Organization Scientific Working Group, 1980). Shigellosis is endemic in many prisons in the United States.

Children are the principal victims in endemic areas. Resistance in adults is due to acquired immunity to the prevalent serotype. Adult travelers visiting endemic areas contract the disease because they have had no previous exposure. Similarly, when a new serotype is introduced into a susceptible population, the disease affects all age groups (Levine and Lanata, 1983).

Occurrence in Animals: It is common in captive nonhuman primates and rare in other animal species. All species of *Shigella*, including *S. dysenteriae* type 1, which is considered the most pathogenic for man, have been isolated from nonhuman primates (L'Hote, 1980).

The Disease in Man: It is seen most often in preschool-age children. A new serotype introduced into tropical areas where the population is undernourished provokes disease in all age groups, particularly children, the elderly, and debilitated individuals. Generally, the incubation period is less than 4 days. The disease begins with fever and abdominal pains, followed by diarrhea and dehydration for 1 to 3 days. A second phase of the symptomatology can last for several weeks. The main symptom is tenesmus; in serious cases, stools contain blood, mucus, and pus. The symptomatology is usually variable.

In many countries, strains of *Shigella* resistant to sulfonamides and to several antibiotics have been observed.

The Disease in Animals: A clinical picture similar to that in man occurs in monkeys.

Source of Infection and Mode of Transmission: The principal reservoir of the infection for man is other humans that are sick or carriers. The sources of the infection are feces and contaminated objects. The most common mode of transmission is the fecal-oral route. Outbreaks comprising numerous cases have had their origin in a common source of infection, such as foods contaminated by hands or feces of carrier individuals. Insects, particularly flies, can also play a role as mechanical vectors.

Bacillary dysentery is a serious disease with high mortality in nonhuman primates in captivity, but there is doubt that monkeys can harbor the etiologic agent in their natural habitat. Monkeys probably contract the infection by contact with infected humans. The infection spreads rapidly in nonhuman primate colonies because the monkeys defecate on the cage floor and also often throw their food there.

Role of Animals in the Epidemiology of the Disease: Of little significance. Cases of human bacillary dysentery contracted from nonhuman primates are known. The victims are mainly children. In highly endemic areas, dogs may shed *Shigella* temporarily.

The etiologic agent has also been isolated from horses, bats, and rattlesnakes. Nevertheless, animals other than nonhuman primates play an insignificant role.

Diagnosis: Definitive diagnosis depends on isolation of the etiologic agent by culture of fecal material on selective media. Serologic identification and typing are important from the epidemiologic viewpoint.

Control: In man, control methods include a) environmental hygiene, especially disposal of human waste and provision for potable water; b) personal hygiene; c) education of the public and of food handlers about the sources of infection and methods of transmission; d) sanitary supervision of the production, preparation, and preservation of foods; e) control of flies; f) reporting and isolation of cases and sanitary disposal of feces; and g) search for contacts and the source of infection.

A live, streptomycin-dependent vaccine, administered orally in three or four doses, has given good protection against the clinical disease for 6 to 12 months. Its use is indicated in institutions where shigellosis is endemic.

Indiscriminate use of antibiotics must be avoided in order to prevent the emergence of multiresistant strains and to ensure that these medications remain available for use in severe cases.

In animals, control consists of a) isolation and treatment of sick or carrier monkeys; b) careful cleaning and sterilization of cages; c) prevention of crowding in cages; and d) prompt disposal of wastes and control of insects.

Bibliography

American Public Health Association. *Control of Communicable Diseases in Man*, 14th ed. (Ed. by A. S. Benenson). Washington, D.C., APHA, 1985.

Edwards, P. R., and W. H. Ewing. *Identification of Enterobacteriaceae*, 3rd ed. Minneapolis, Minnesota, Burgess, 1972.

Fiennes, R. *Zoonoses of Primates*. Ithaca, New York, Cornell University Press, 1967.

Keusch, G. T., and S. B. Formal. Shigellosis. *In*: Warren, K. S., and A. A. F. Mahmoud (Eds.), *Tropical and Geographical Medicine*. New York, Mc-Graw-Hill Book Company, 1984.

L'Hote, J. L. *Contribution à l'étude des salmonelloses et des shigelloses des primates. Zoonoses*. Thesis, National Veterinary School of Lyon, 1980.

Levine, M. M., and C. Lanata. Progresos en vacunas contra diarrea bacteriana. *Adel Microbiol Enferm Infecc (B Aires)* 2:67-118, 1983.

Lewis, J. N., and E. J. Gangarosa. Shigellosis. *In*: Top, F. H., Sr., and P. F. Wehrle (Eds.), *Communicable and Infectious Diseases*, 7th ed. St. Louis, Missouri, Mosby, 1972.

Olson, L. C., D. Y. Bergquist, and D. L. Fitzgerald. Control of *Shigella flexneri* in Celebes black macaques (*Macaca nigra*). *Lab Anim Sci* 36:240-242, 1986.

Ruch, T. C. *Diseases of Laboratory Primates*. Philadelphia and London, Saunders, 1959.

Williams, L. P., and B. C. Hobbs. Enterobacteriaceae infections. *In*: Hubbert, W. T., W. F. McCulloch, and P. R. Schnurrenberger (Eds.), *Diseases Transmitted from Animals to Man*, 6th ed. Springfield, Illinois, Thomas, 1975.

World Health Organization Scientific Working Group. Enteric infections due to *Campylobacter*, *Yersinia*, *Salmonella*, and *Shigella*. *Bull WHO* 58:519-537, 1980.

STAPHYLOCOCCAL FOOD POISONING

(005.0)

Synonyms: Staphylococcal alimentary toxicosis, staphylococcal gastroenteritis.

Etiology: Coagulase-positive strains of *Staphylococcus aureus* that produce enterotoxins. Very few coagulase-negative strains are enterotoxigenic. The toxin is preformed in the food involved. To date, six types of enterotoxins are known: A, B, C, D, E, and F; of these A is the most prevalent in outbreaks. Enterotoxin F is implicated in toxic shock syndrome (TSS) (Bergdoll *et al.*, 1981). Some strains can produce two or even three different enterotoxins. The toxins are heat-resistant and can withstand a temperature of 100°C for 30 minutes.

Geographic Distribution: Worldwide.

Occurrence in Man: In some countries the disease constitutes an important cause of food poisoning. As it is benign and self-limiting, most sporadic cases are not recorded.

In the USA during the period 1977-1981, 131 outbreaks were reported, affecting 7,126 people. In the last 3 years of that 5-year period, only enterotoxin A was incriminated. At present, milk (the most common source of toxins C and D) and commercially packaged foods are the least common causes of the disease in the United States (Holmberg and Blake, 1984).

It has been suggested that a portion of the intestinal disorders frequently observed in developing countries are caused by staphylococcal food poisoning. Evidence is provided by the fact that titers of antibodies to enterotoxins are higher in residents of these countries than in travelers (Bergdoll, 1979).

Occurrence in Animals: Spontaneous cases of staphylococcal food poisoning in domestic animals are not known. The *Macaca mulatta* monkey is susceptible to enterotoxin introduced through the digestive tract and is used as an experimental animal to show the presence of the toxin in implicated foods. Cats and kittens have also been used for the same purpose by intravenous or peritoneal inoculation with the enterotoxin. Dogs possibly suffer from gastroenteritis similar to that in man.

Mastitis in cattle caused by staphylococci is of interest from the public health viewpoint. In modern milking systems, *S. aureus* is a common pathogen in cows' udders. The agent is transmitted by means of milking machines or the milker's hands, and enters through the milk duct or superficial lesions on the teat. Mastitis caused by *S. aureus* in cattle may vary from the prevalent subclinical form of the infection to a severe gangrenous form. Both forms are economically important because of the losses they cause in milk production (Gillespie and Timoney, 1981). Studies carried out over the last few years in five northern European countries and in Japan have isolated a large proportion of toxigenic staphylococci from cases of bovine mastitis. In Europe, 41.4% of 174 strains isolated were enterotoxin-producing, and of these, 48.6% produced A, 5.6% B, 29.2% C, and 33.3% D, either singly or in combination. In Japan, 34.4% of 1,056 strains isolated from cows with subclinical mastitis were toxigenic, and of these 31.1% were producers of enterotoxin A, 54.3% of C, 27% of D, and 10.7% of B, singly or in combination. Enterotoxins A, C, or D are the predominant types in staphylococcal poisoning in many countries (Kato and Kume, 1980). Nevertheless, types of enterotoxin produced by strains isolated from milk seem to vary in prevalence in different countries, perhaps because the strains studied have not been representative.

S. aureus is the most common agent in canine skin infections and causes pyoderma, impetigo, folliculitis, and furunculosis. It frequently is a complicating agent of demodectic mange, producing cellulitis in the deep layers of skin. Enterotoxigenic staphylococci were isolated from 13% of 115 domestic dogs in Japan. The strains isolated were enterotoxin producers (A, C, and D) that can cause food poisoning in man (Kaji and Kato, 1980).

In fowl, staphylococcal infection can cause diseases ranging from pyoderma to septicemia with different localizations (salpingitis, arthritis, and other disorders). Purulent staphylococcal synovitis is a disease causing appreciable losses in chickens and turkeys. In Czechoslovakia, one of the principal sources of staphylococcal food poisoning is thought to be infected poultry (Raska *et al.*, 1980). Staphylococcal strains isolated from poultry farms in that country and others produce enterotoxin D.

The Disease in Man: The incubation period is short, generally 3 hours after ingestion of the food involved. The interval between consumption of the enterotoxin and the first symptoms can vary from 30 minutes to 8 hours, depending on the quantity of toxin ingested and the susceptibility of the individual.

The major symptoms are nausea, vomiting, abdominal pains, and diarrhea. Some patients may show low pyrexia (up to 38°C). More serious cases manifest prostration, cephalalgia, abnormal temperature, and lowered blood pressure, as well as blood and mucus in the stool and vomit. The course of the disease is usually benign and the patient recovers without medication in 24 to 72 hours.

Recently, a toxic shock syndrome has been described. Symptoms consist of vomiting, diarrhea, high fever, erythroderma, edema, renal insufficiency, and toxic shock. Most patients are women who become ill during their menstrual period.

The above-described symptoms also are observed in association with abscesses and osteomyelitis caused by *S. aureus*. A staphylococcal enterotoxin designated F was isolated from 94% of these patients (Bergdoll *et al.*, 1981). In the Netherlands (De Nooij *et al.*, 1982), strains of *S. aureus* from nine patients with toxic shock were examined, and production of enterotoxin F was confirmed in eight of them; only 42% of 50 strains isolated from other hospitalized patients produced this toxin. Toxin F production was not found in 48 strains originating from animal clinical specimens. Of 24 strains from healthy human carriers, 25% produced the toxin.

Source of Infection and Mode of Transmission: The principal reservoir of *S. aureus* is the human carrier. A high proportion (from 30 to 35%) of healthy humans have staphylococci in the nasopharynx and on the skin. A carrier with a respiratory disease can contaminate foods by sneezing, coughing, or expectorating. Similarly, he may contaminate foods he handles if he has a staphylococcal skin lesion. However, even if not sick himself, the carrier may spread the agent by handling food ingredients, utensils, and equipment, or the finished food product. According to different authors, the proportion of enterotoxin-producing *S. aureus* strains of human origin varies between 18 and 75% (Pulverer, 1983). The proportion of toxigenic strains isolated from various sources (human, animal, and food) is very high.

Strains of human origin predominate in epidemics, but animals are also reservoirs of the infection. Milk from cow udders infected with staphylococci can contaminate numerous milk products. Many outbreaks have been produced by consumption of inadequately refrigerated raw milk or cheeses from cows whose udders harbored staphylococci. The largest outbreak affected at least 500 students in California between 1977 and 1981 and was traced to chocolate milk (Holmberg and Blake, 1984). In developing countries, where refrigeration after milking is often inadequate, milk and milk products may be an important source of staphylococcal intoxication.

According to recent investigations, a high proportion of strains isolated from staphylococcal mastitis produce enterotoxin A, which causes many outbreaks in humans.

In several investigations it was possible to isolate from skin lesions and cow's milk the *S. aureus* phage type 80/81, which is related to epidemic infections in man. One of the studies proved that phage type 80/81 produced interstitial mastitis in cows. The same phage type was found among animal caretakers, which indicates that the bacterium is intertransmissible between man and animals and that the latter may reinfect man.

Infected fowl and dogs (see Occurrence in Animals) may also give rise to and be a source of staphylococcal poisoning in man.

One subject that deserves special attention is the appearance of antibiotic-resistant strains in animals whose food includes antibiotics. Concern exists over the possible transmission of these strains to man. On several occasions, resistant strains have been found both in animals (cows, swine, and fowl) and in their caretakers, with the same antibiotic resistance. Moreover, "human" strains (phage typed) have on occasion been isolated from the nostrils and lesions of other species of domestic animals.

A variety of foods and dishes may be vehicles of the toxin. If environmental conditions are favorable, *S. aureus* multiplies in the food and produces enterotoxins. Once made, the toxin is not destroyed even if the food is subjected to boiling while being cooked. Consequently, the toxin may be found in the food whereas staphylococci are not.

An important causal factor in food-borne intoxications is holding food at room temperature, which permits multiplication of staphylococci. Lack of hygiene in food handling is another notable factor. Frequently, outbreaks of food poisoning may be traced to a single dish.

The Role of Animals in the Epidemiology of the Disease: Most outbreaks are caused by human strains, and to a lesser degree by strains from cattle and other domestic animals.

Animal products—such as meat, ham, milk, cheese, cream, and ice cream— usually constitute a good substrate for staphylococcal multiplication. Milk pasteurization offers no guarantee of safety if toxins were produced before heat treatment, as the toxins are heat-resistant. Outbreaks have been caused by reconstituted powdered milk, even when the dried product contained few or no staphylococci.

Diagnosis: The short incubation period between ingestion of contaminated food and appearance of symptoms is the most important clinical criterion. Laboratory confirmation, when possible, is based above all on demonstration of the presence of enterotoxin in the food. Biological methods (inoculation of cats with cultures of the suspect food, or of rhesus monkeys with the foodstuffs or cultures) are expensive and not always reliable. As substitutes, serologic methods such as immunodiffusion, immunofluorescence, hemagglutination inhibition, and, recently, ELISA are increasingly used.

Isolation of enterotoxigenic staphylococcal strains from foods and typing by phage or, more recently, by immunofluorescence have epidemiologic value. Quantitative examination of staphylococci in processed or cooked foods serves as an indicator of hygienic conditions in the processing plant and of personnel supervision.

Control: It includes the following measures: a) education of persons who prepare food at home or commercially in proper personal hygiene; b) exclusion from handling food of individuals with abscesses or other skin lesions; and c) refrigeration of all foods to prevent bacterial multiplication and formation of toxins. Foods should be kept at room temperature as little time as possible.

The veterinary milk inspection service should supervise dairy installations, ensuring that refrigeration units function correctly and are used immediately after milking, and that milk is refrigerated during transport to pasteurization plants.

The veterinary meat inspection service should be responsible for enforcing hygienic regulations before and after slaughter as well as during handling and production of meat products. Control of hygienic conditions in meat retail establishments is also important.

Bibliography

Bergdoll, M. S. The enterotoxins. *In*: Cohen, J. P. (Ed.), *The Staphylococci*. New York, Wiley, 1972.

Bergdoll, M. S. Staphylococcal intoxications. *In*: Riemann, H., and F. L. Bryan (Eds.), *Food-Borne Infections and Intoxications*, 2nd ed. New York, Academic Press, 1979.

Bergdoll, M. S., C. R. Borja, R. N. Robbins, and K. F. Weiss. Identification of enterotoxin E. *Infect Immun* 4:593-595, 1971.

Bergdoll, M. S., R. Reiser, and J. Spitz. Staphylococcal enterotoxin detection in food. *Food Technol* 30:80-83, 1976.

Bergdoll, M. S., B. A. Crass, R. F. Reiser, R. N. Robbins, and J. P. Davis. A new staphylococcal enterotoxin, enterotoxin F, associated with toxic-shock-syndrome *Staphylococcus aureus* isolates. *Lancet* 1:1017-1021, 1981.

Casman, E. P., and R. W. Bennett. Detection of staphylococcal enterotoxin in food. *Appl Microbiol* 13:181-189, 1965.

Cohen, J. O., and P. Oeding. Serological typing of Staphylococci by means of fluorescent antibodies. *J Bacteriol* 84:735-741, 1962.

De Nooij, M. P., W. J. Van Leeuwen, and S. Notermans. Enterotoxin production by strains of *Staphylococcus aureus* isolated from clinical and non-clinical specimens with special reference to enterotoxin F and toxic shock syndrome. *J Hyg (Camb)* 89:499-505, 1982.

Fluharty, D. N. Staphylococcosis. *In*: Hubbert, W. T., W. F. McCulloch, and P. R. Schnurrenberger (Eds.), *Diseases Transmitted from Animals to Man*, 6th ed. Springfield, Illinois, Thomas, 1975.

Gillespie, J. H., and J. F. Timoney. *Hagan and Bruner's Infectious Diseases of Domestic Animals*, 7th ed. Ithaca, Cornell University Press, 1981.

Holmberg, S. D., and P. A. Blake. Staphylococcal food poisoning in the United States. New facts and old misconceptions. *JAMA* 251:487-489, 1984.

Kaji, Y., and E. Kato. Occurrence of enterotoxigenic staphylococci in household and laboratory dogs. *Jpn J Vet Res* 28:86-94, 1980.

Kato, E., and T. Kume. Enterotoxigenicity of bovine staphylococci isolated from California mastitis test-positive milk in Japan. *Jpn J Vet Res* 28:75-85, 1980.

Live, I. Staphylococci in animals: differentiation and relationship to human staphylococcosis. *In*: Cohen, J. O. (Ed.), *The Staphylococci*. New York, Wiley, 1972.

Merchant, I. A., and R. A. Packer. *Bacteriología y virología veterinarias*, 3rd ed. Zaragoza, Spain, Acribia, 1970.

Mossell, D. A. A., and F. Quevedo. *Control microbiológico de los alimentos*. Lima, Peru, Universidad Nacional Mayor de San Marcos, 1967.

Pulverer, G. Libensmittelvergiftugen durch Staphylokokken. *Bundesgesundhbl* 26:377-381, 1983.

Răska, K., V. Matejovska, and L. Polak. To the origin of contamination of foodstuff by enterotoxigenic staphylococci. *Proceedings of the World Congress of Foodborne Infections and Intoxications*. Berlin, 1980.

Thatcher, F. S., and D. S. Clark. *Análisis microbiológico de los alimentos*. Zaragoza, Spain, Acribia, 1973.

STREPTOCOCCOSIS

(034)

(038)

(465)

(670)

(760)

Synonym: Streptococcocia.

Etiology: The genus *Streptococcus* comprises 21 species that display notable differences in their biological properties and especially in their pathogenicity for man and animals.

Lancefield's serologic classification is of great importance for the identification of these bacteria. Within this scheme, 20 serogroups are presently distinguished and identified with the letters A through V, excluding I and J. Specific names have not been given to many components of the serogroups.

Several serogroups produce additional antigens that serve to identify serotypes. Serotyping is useful in the epidemiology.

Within the same serogroup there may be strains that differ physiologically and biochemically; as a consequence, classification cannot be based exclusively on serology (Gillespie and Timoney, 1981). Moreover, there are strains that cannot be typed serologically in a serogroup and can only be identified on the basis of biochemical and physiological properties or by a combination of these characteristics plus serology (Kunz and Moellering, 1981).

A common initial technique for preliminary identification consists of dividing the streptococci by their hemolytic reactivity into alpha (incomplete hemolysis and greenish discoloration on blood-agar), beta (complete lysis of erythrocytes), and gamma (nonhemolytic). β-hemolytic streptococci are usually the cause of acute diseases and suppurative lesions, while α-hemolytic and Γ-streptococci cause sub-acute disease, with some exceptions.

S. pyogenes (serogroup A) is the type species of β-hemolytic streptococci.

Geographic Distribution: Streptococci have a worldwide distribution.

Occurrence in Man: Infections caused by group A (*S. pyogenes*) are common, with an apparently higher prevalence in temperate climates. For a long time, streptococci belonging to serogroup B (*S. agalactiae*) have been considered mainly pathogenic for animals. However, today these streptococci are recognized as being one of the principal causes of septicemia, pneumonia, and meningitis among human newborns. Similarly, serogroup D streptococci (*S. bovis*) are a frequent cause of endocarditis and bacteremia in man. Sporadic cases of disease are caused by members of the C, G, F, and H groups.

Occurrence in Animals: Some disease entities are very common and economically important, such as mastitis in cattle, caused by *S. agalactiae* (group B), and strangles in horses, caused by *S. equi* (group C).

The Disease in Man: *S. pyogenes* is the main pathogen among hemolytic streptococci. This agent frequently causes streptococcal sore throat and scarlet fever (streptococcal tonsillitis and pharyngitis), diverse suppurative processes, septicemia, puerperal fever, erysipelas, ulcerative endocarditis, and other localized infections. Streptococcal sore throat and scarlet fever are epidemiologically similar. The latter is differentiated clinically by the exanthema caused by strains producing an erythrogenic toxin. The disease is mild or inapparent in a large proportion of those infected. Rheumatic fever is a sequela of streptococcal sore throat or scarlet fever, and it may be caused by any strain of group A. Glomerulonephritis is another complication, produced only by certain nephritogenic strains of the same group.

The last two decades have witnessed the emergence of group B streptococci as important causal agents of neonatal disease. Group A streptococci and *Staphylococcus aureus* were displaced as principal causes of neonatal infection by *Escherichia coli* and group B streptococci. In infections caused by group B streptococci (*S. agalactiae*), two syndromes are distinguished depending on the age of the infant at onset of disease. The acute or early-onset syndrome appears between the first and fifth day of life and is characterized by sepsis and respiratory difficulty. The delayed-onset syndrome generally appears after the tenth day and is characterized by meningitis, with or without sepsis. Affected children show lethargy, convulsions, and anorexia. Mortality is high in both forms, but it is more so in the early-onset syndrome.

In older children and adults, group B streptococci cause a variety of clinical syndromes: urinary tract infections, bacteremia, gangrene, postpartum infection, pneumonia, endocarditis, empyema, meningitis, and other pathologies (Patterson and Hafeez, 1976).

Disease caused by group C streptococci (*S. equi*) is usually sporadic and rare in man. Nevertheless, in 1983 an epidemic outbreak occurred in New Mexico, USA, with 16 cases originating from consumption of cheese made at home with unpasteurized milk. The agent was identified as *S. zooepidemicus*, one of the four species that make up group C. The disease in these patients consisted of fever, chills, and vague constitutional symptoms, but five of them had localized infection which manifested itself in such varied symptoms as pneumonia, endocarditis, meningitis, pericarditis, and abdominal pains (Centers for Disease Control of the USA, 1983).

In sporadic cases, the most common clinical manifestation is exudative pharyngitis or tonsillitis. With some exceptions, the group C streptococci isolated from these cases belong to *S. equisimilis*, which causes septicemia in suckling pigs. An outbreak of group C streptococcal pharyngitis caused by consumption of raw milk was followed by a high incidence of glomerulonephritis (Duca *et al.*, 1969).

Group D streptococci, both enterococcal and nonenterococcal, cause serious diseases in man. *S. bovis* causes bacteremias and endocarditis, and enterococci cause urinary tract infections, abdominal abscesses, and an appreciable proportion of cases of bacterial endocarditis.

Streptococci belonging to other serogroups, as well as those not serologically grouped, cause a great variety of clinical manifestations, including dental caries and abscesses, meningitis, puerperal fever, wound infections, endocarditis, and other conditions (Kunz and Moellering, 1981).

Nonhemolytic streptococci and "viridans" type (α-hemolytic) can cause subacute endocarditis.

The Disease in Animals: *S. agalactiae* (*S. mastitidis*), in Lancefield's group B, is the principal agent of chronic catarrhal mastitis in milch cows. *S. dysgalactiae* (group C) and *S. uberis* (group E) cause sporadic cases of acute mastitis in bovines. *S. pyogenes*, a human pathogen, may infect the cow's udder, producing mastitis and leading to epidemic outbreaks in man.

Horse strangles, caused by *S. equi* (group C), is an acute disease of horses characterized by inflammation of the pharyngeal and nasal mucosa, with a mucopurulent secretion and abscesses of the regional lymph nodes.

S. equisimilis (group C) infects different tissues in several animal species. Group C streptococci that are adapted to animals and classified as *S. zooepidemicus* produce cervicitis and metritis in mares and often cause abortions. They also cause septicemia in colts. Similarly, they are pathogenic agents for bovines, swine, and other animals, in which they produce various septicemic processes.

Streptococci belonging to other groups cause abscesses and different disease processes in several animal species.

The many diseases caused by streptococci are clinically differentiated by the agent's portal of entry and the tissue it affects.

Source of Infection and Mode of Transmission: The reservoir of *S. pyogenes* is man. Transmission of this respiratory disease agent (septic sore throat, scarlet fever) results from direct contact between an infected person, whether suffering from the disease or a carrier, and another susceptible person. The disease is most frequent among children from 5 to 15 years old, but it also occurs at other ages.

In Iceland, Denmark, Germany, Great Britain, and the USA, important epidemic outbreaks have had their origin in the consumption of raw milk or ice cream made with milk from cows whose udders were infected with *S. pyogenes*. These epidemics were due to infection in the cows' udders contracted from infected milkers. Between 1920 and 1944, 103 such epidemics of septic sore throat and 105 of scarlet fever were recorded in the United States. In other instances, the milk was contaminated directly by persons with septic sore throat or with localized infections. In several epidemic outbreaks, the milk became contaminated after pasteurization.

According to the WHO Expert Committee on Streptococcal and Staphylococcal Infections, contamination of milk products has caused small outbreaks of streptococcal respiratory disease, but these are progressively less frequent.

Pasteurization has been the most important factor in the reduction of streptococcal outbreaks resulting from milk. In Third World countries, much milk is still consumed raw, and even in developed countries, outbreaks are produced by milk products made at home using raw milk.

In recent years, special attention has been given to neonatal sepsis caused by group B streptococci (S. agalactiae). Research has shown that S. agalactiae colonizes a high proportion of women (7 to 30% or more) in different locations, such as the intestinal tract, the cervicovaginal region, and the upper respiratory tract. The agent is possibly transferred from the rectal region to the vaginal canal, since most of the bacteria are intestinal. Infants can become infected in utero or during birth. Only a small proportion of the newborn (around 1%) become infected and ill, while in most, the agent colonizes the skin and mucous membranes without causing disease. The principal victims of the infection, especially in the case of the early-onset syndrome, are premature infants, those with low birthweight, and those born after a difficult labor. The principal reservoir of group B streptococci causing neonatal disease is clearly the mother. The S. agalactiae serotypes isolated from mothers and newborn are always the same. Although S. agalactiae is an agent of bovine mastitis and has also been isolated from other animal species, there is no proof that the infection is transmitted from animal to man. In general, human and animal strains differ in some biochemical, metabolic, and serologic properties. Human strains of S. agalactiae can produce mastitis experimentally in bovines (Patterson and Hafeez, 1976). In addition, some publications have suggested that a proportion of human infections could derive from a bovine source (Van Den Heever and Erasmus, 1980; Berglez, 1981) or that reciprocal intertransmission between humans and bovines takes place. However, the data from research so far indicate that if such transmission occurs, its importance is small.

The outbreak of disease caused by S. zooepidemicus (group C) in New Mexico (see The Disease in Man) clearly indicates that raw milk and unpasteurized milk products can be the source of infection for man. In the epidemiologic investigation of this outbreak, milk samples from cows on the establishment where the cheese was made and samples of the cheese itself were examined; S. zooepidemicus was isolated from many of the samples. In Europe there have also been cases of S. zooepidemicus infection caused by ingestion of raw milk. A case of pneumonia caused by S. zooepidemicus in a person caring for a sick horse has been described (Rose et al., 1980).

Animals can also transmit groups G, L, and M streptococci to man, but the epidemiology of these cross-infections has not been elucidated.

Role of Animals in the Epidemiology of the Disease: Animals are not maintenance hosts for S. pyogenes, but at times they can start important epidemic outbreaks by contracting the infection from man and retransmitting it by means of contaminated milk. There is no firm evidence that animals play a role of any importance in the transmission of group B streptococci causing neonatal sepsis.

Raw cows' milk can be a source of group C streptococcal infection for humans.

Diagnosis: If milk is suspected as the source of an epidemic outbreak in man, an attempt should be made to isolate the etiologic agent from it. Obviously, a correct identification of the agent is required.

From either a human or an animal source, it is advisable to identify the serogroup of streptococci involved, and to establish the species whenever possible. However, relatively few laboratories possess the human and material resources necessary for this task.

A method was recently described to identify pregnant women with heavy colonization of the genital tract by group B streptococci (Jones *et al.*, 1983). The goal of this procedure is implementation of chemotherapy in the newborn immediately after birth to reduce morbidity and mortality caused by group B streptococcal neonatal sepsis.

Control: Prevention of human infection transmitted through milk is achieved mainly by pasteurization. Infected persons should be prevented from taking part in milking or handling milk or other foods.

The prevention of neonatal sepsis has been attempted by active immunization of pregnant women with capsular polysaccharides of group B streptococci, as well as by passive immunization with immunoglobulin preparations given intravenously. Both methods are still in the experimental stage. Promising results have been obtained with prophylactic intravenous administration of ampicillin to women in labor. In this way, a significant level of antibiotic is obtained in the amniotic fluid and in samples of the umbilical cord. Among the newborn of obstetric patients receiving this treatment, only 2.8% were colonized by group B streptococci and none became ill, while in the control group, 35.9% of the infants were colonized and four developed the early-onset syndrome (National Institute of Allergy and Infectious Diseases, 1983).

To reduce the prevalence of mastitis caused by *S. agalactiae* in dairy herds, cows testing positive to the CMT (California mastitis test) are treated with penicillin by either intramammary infusion and/or parenteral administration. However, this procedure does not eradicate the infection, probably due to reinfection. Application of antiseptic creams to teat lesions can help prevent mastitis caused by S. *dysgalactiae* and S. *zooepidemicus*.

Several bacterins have been tried for prevention of equine strangles caused by *S. equi*. Although they confer satisfactory immunity, they produce a local and systemic reaction (Gillespie and Timoney, 1981).

Bibliography

Berglez, I. Comparative studies of some biochemical properties of human and bovine *Streptococcus agalactiae* strains. *Zentralbl Bakteriol Mikrobiol Hyg [B]* 173:457-463, 1981.

Centers for Disease Control of the USA. Group C streptococcal infections associated with eating homemade cheese, New Mexico. *Morb Mortal Wkly Rep*, Oct. 7, 1983.

Davies, A. M. Disease of man transmissible through animals. *In*: Van der Hoeden, J. (Ed.), *Zoonoses*. Amsterdam, Netherlands, Elsevier, 1964.

Duca, E., G. Teodoroviei, C. Radu, A. Vita, P. Talasman-Niculescu, E. Bernescu, C. Feldi, and V. Rosca. A nephritogenic streptococcus. *J Hyg (Camb)* 67:691-698, 1969.

Eickhoff, T. C. Group B streptococci in human infection. *In*: Wanmaker, L. W., and M. Matsen (Eds.), *Streptococci and Streptococcal Diseases: Recognition, Understanding and Management*. New York, Academic Press, 1972.

Fluharty, D. M. Streptococcosis. *In*: Hubbert, W. T., W. F. McCulloch, and P. R. Schnurrenberger (Eds.), *Diseases Transmitted from Animals to Man*, 6th ed. Springfield, Illinois, Thomas, 1975.

Gillespie, J. M., and J. F. Timoney. *Hagan and Bruner's Infections Diseases of Domestic Animals*, 7th ed. Ithaca, Cornell University Press, 1981.

Jones, D. E., E. M. Friedl, K. S. Kanorek, J. K. Williams, and D. V. Lim. Rapid identification of pregnant women heavily colonized with group B streptococci. *J Clin Microbiol* 18:558-560, 1983.

Kunz, L. J., and R. C. Moellering. Streptococcal infections. *In*: A. Balows, and W. J. Hausler, Jr. *Diagnostic Procedures for Bacterial, Mycotic and Parasitic Infections*, 6th ed. Washington, D.C., American Public Health Association, 1981.

MacKnight, J. F., P. J. Ellis, K. A. Jensen, and B. Franz. Group B streptococci in neonatal deaths. *Appl Microbiol* 17:926, 1969.

Merchant, I. A., and R. A. Packer. *Bacteriología y virología veterinaria*, 3rd ed. Zaragoza, Spain, Acribia, 1970.

National Institute of Allergy and Infectious Diseases. Workshop on group B streptococcal infection. *J Infect Dis* 148:163-166, 1983.

Onile, B. A. Is group B *Streptococcus* a zoonosis? *Trans R Soc Trop Med Hyg* 80:673, 1986.

Patterson, M. J., and A. E. B. Hafeez. Group B streptococci in human disease. *Bacteriol Rev* 40:774-792, 1976.

Rose, H. D., J. R. Allen, and G. Witte. *Streptococcus zooepidemicus* (group C) pneumonia in a human. *J Clin Microbiol* 11:76-78, 1980.

Stollerman, G. H. Streptococcal diseases. *In*: Beeson, P. B., and W. McDermott (Eds.), *Cecil-Loeb Textbook of Medicine*, 12th ed. Philadelphia and London, Saunders, 1967.

Van Den Heever, L. W., and M. Erasmus. Group B *Streptococcus*—Comparison of *Streptococcus agalactiae* isolated from humans and cows in the Republic of South Africa. *J S Afr Vet Assoc* 51:93-100, 1980.

World Health Organization. *Streptococcal and Staphylococcal Infections*. Report of a WHO Expert Committee. Geneva, WHO, 1968. (Technical Report Series 394.)

TETANUS

(037)

(771.3) Neonatal

Synonyms: Trismus, lockjaw.

Etiology: *Clostridium tetani*; the pathology is produced by the neurotoxin of the infectious agent, since the bacterium does not invade the animal body.

Geographic Distribution: Worldwide. The etiologic agent is a soil microorganism that can also be found in the feces of animals and man. The spores of *C. tetani* are found primarily in cultivated land, rich in organic matter, or in pastures. The disease occurs more frequently in the tropics than in temperate or cold climates.

Occurrence in Man: It is estimated that tetanus causes 500,000 deaths annually worldwide, mostly in newborn children. The incidence of the disease in industrialized countries is low; in developing countries it still constitutes a public health problem. In the decade 1951-1960, the mortality rate from tetanus was 0.16 per 100,000 inhabitants in the United States and Canada, and 8.50 per 100,000 in Latin

America excluding Argentina and Brazil. Residents of rural areas are more likely to be exposed than those of cities. Fatality is high in spite of improved therapy.

A study carried out in Paraguay demonstrated that tetanus is more frequent in men than in women, and more common in the newborn and children than in adults (Vera Martínez et al., 1976).

In Argentina, the annual rates of incidence for the period 1965-1977 ranged from 1.2 to 1.7 per 100,000 inhabitants (except in 1967 when the rate was 3.1 per 100,000 inhabitants). The disease was more frequent in subtropical or temperate provinces than in the cold Patagonian provinces. Hospital admissions for tetanus in Buenos Aires between 1968 and 1973 averaged higher during the hot months. Tetanus mortality in these municipal hospitals reached 35.8% and was eight times higher in children younger than 15 days than in other age groups (Mazzáfero et al., 1981). Table 3 shows the morbidity distribution by climate for tetanus in Argentina during the period 1967-1977.

Table 3. Distribution of tetanus morbidity according to political division and climate, Argentina, 1967-1977.

Political division and climate	Average number of notified cases per year	Population at middle of reporting period (in thousands)	Rate per 100,000 inhabitants
Subtropical	*165.8*	*4,221*	*3.9*
Catamarca	3.4	175	1.9
Corrientes	19.2	587	3.3
Chaco	38.5	572	6.7
Formosa	14.2	248	5.6
Jujuy	6.7	323	2.1
Misiones	15.3	470	3.3
Salta	20.4	533	3.8
Santiago del Estero	15.7	519	3.0
Tucumán	32.6	794	4.1
Temperate	*217.6*	*19,409*	*1.1*
Federal district	18.5	2,974	0.6
Buenos Aires	111.9	9,289	1.2
Córdora	20.9	2,177	0.9
Entre Ríos	16.5	838	1.9
La Pampa	3.4	177	2.2
La Rioja	0.6	139	0.4
Mendoza	4.5	1,025	0.4
San Juan	3.1	403	0.7
San Luis	1.5	187	0.8
Santa Fe	36.2	2,200	1.6
Cold	*3.7*	*762*	*0.5*
Chubut	0.6	202	0.3
Río Negro	1.3	281	0.4
Neuquén	1.6	170	0.9
Santa Cruz	0.2	94	0.2
Tierra del Fuego	0.0	15	0.0

Source: Bull Pan Am Health Organ 15:328, 1981.

Occurrence in Animals: The disease is infrequent in animals. There are enzootic areas, mainly in the tropics. Horses are the most susceptible species. Cases also occur in sheep and cattle.

The Disease in Man: It is characterized by painful tonic and clonic spasms of the masseter muscle (trismus) and neck muscles, but it frequently affects other areas of the body. Although the average incubation period is 6 days, it may extend up to 3 weeks. If the disease is not complicated by other infections, temperature is normal or only slightly elevated. Reflexes are exaggerated, and rigidity of the abdominal muscles, retention of urine, and constipation are common. The case fatality rate is high, but quite variable from one country to another. In the United States, fatality diminished from 90% in 1947 to 60% in 1969. The disease is much more severe when the incubation period is short and convulsions appear early. The longer, more frequent, and more intense the convulsions become, the worse the prognosis.

The symptomatology of neonatal tetanus is the same as that of the disease in adults; only the infection's portal of entry differs. In newborn children, the infection usually enters through the umbilical stump. At other ages, the route of entry is a wound. Puncture wounds produced by contaminated objects are especially dangerous. Surgical interventions and induced abortions performed without adequate asepsis have given rise to tetanus.

The Disease in Animals: Horses are very susceptible to tetanus and usually acquire it from shoeing nails. They may also contract it from any other wound contaminated with *C. tetani* under anaerobic conditions.

Postpartum cases are seen in cows, especially if the placenta is retained. Cattle have a high rate of neutralizing antibodies against the neurotoxin (tetanospasmin) of *C. tetani*, but the antibody level drops markedly after parturition, leaving the animal very susceptible to the disease. In calves and lambs, tetanus often follows castration, especially when rubber bands are used, since the necrotic tissue left by this operation favors anaerobiosis.

Dehorning, tail docking, and shearing may also give rise to the disease.

Iatrogenic tetanus sometimes occurs after surgical operations and vaccinations.

The incubation period lasts from 2 to 14 days. The symptomatology is similar to that in man. Death occurs in 4 to 10 days.

Source of Infection and Mode of Transmission: The reservoir and source of the infection is soil that contains *C. tetani*. The etiologic agent is found particularly in richly organic cultivated soils. Areas where the exposure risk is very high are referred to as telluric "foci" of *C. tetani*.

The agent is commonly found in horse feces. It has also been found in other species, such as cattle, sheep, dogs, rats, and chickens; similarly, man may harbor *C. tetani* in the intestinal tract.

Transmission is effected through wounds. Scabs or crusts promote multiplication of the etiologic agent. Some cases are due to dog bite. Tetanospasmin is produced after the spores have germinated, that is, by the vegetative form of the bacteria.

Of 2,337 cases studied from 1946 to 1972 in Paraguay, the portal of entry was the umbilical stump in 31.7% of the cases, small wounds in 38.7%, and lesions caused by the removal of the chigoe flea *Tunga penetrans* in 7.7%. The remaining cases resulted from improper asepsis during induced abortion, surgery, burn treatment, or injections (Vera Martínez *et al.*, 1976).

Role of Animals in the Epidemiology of the Disease: Tetanus is a disease common to man and animals, not a zoonosis. Some authors ascribe the role of reservoir to animals (McComb, 1980; American Public Health Association, 1985), but it is more likely that the disease agent derives from the soil, and that it is present in the digestive tract of herbivores and omnivores only transitorily and does not multiply there (Wilson and Miles, 1975; Smith, 1975). Nevertheless, domesticated animals can disseminate toxigenic strains of *C. tetani* by means of their feces, in cultivated as well as uncultivated areas.

Diagnosis: Prior existence of a wound and accompanying symptoms are the bases for diagnosis. Direct microscopic examination of wound material is useful. Given the urgency of diagnosis, the value of culturing *C. tetani* is doubtful. It is not always possible to isolate the etiologic agent from a wound.

Control: In man, given the soil origin of the infection, the only rational means of control is active immunization with toxoid. Children 2 to 3 months of age should receive two or three doses of the toxoid in DPT vaccine (diphtheria, pertussis, tetanus) at intervals of 1 month to 6 weeks. They should then receive a booster, preferably administered 18 months after the last dose. An initial series of three doses induces protective titers of antitoxin for 5 to 13 years in 90% of those vaccinated. Booster shots ensure higher titers of the antitoxin and probably confer immunity throughout a woman's childbearing years (Halsey *et al.*, 1983). Periodic boosters of tetanus toxoid every 10 years are recommended in areas with a high prevalence of tetanus, principally for the population groups most exposed to risk. The effectiveness of the toxoid was confirmed during World War II. United States soldiers who were vaccinated with three doses of tetanus toxoid experienced one case of tetanus among 455,803 wounded, while in the unvaccinated Japanese army the incidence was 10 cases per 100,000 wounded soldiers. Mothers are vaccinated to prevent neonatal tetanus. Primary immunization of pregnant women consists of three doses of toxoid given 4 to 6 weeks apart, starting in the fourth month of pregnancy (Tavares, 1982).

Passive immunization with antitoxin should be reserved for persons with no previous active immunization who must undergo surgical operations, as well as for women after abortion or birth and for their newborn children in high-risk areas. The use of human antitoxin serum is preferable, but if unavailable, horse or bovine hyperimmune serum can be used after the patient is tested for a possible allergic reaction to the serum.

Wounds should be cleaned and, if necessary, debrided. Persons who have previously received toxoid should be given a booster. Unimmunized persons with a high-risk wound should be given tetanus antitoxin.

Control procedures in animals are similar. Horses in particular should be vaccinated with toxoid; two doses given 1 to 2 months apart are sufficient. Operations such as dehorning, castration, and tail docking should be done in the most aseptic conditions possible, and antiseptics should be applied to surgical wounds.

Lambs in the first month of life can become passively immunized when the ewe is vaccinated with two doses of aluminum phosphate–adsorbed toxoid. The first injection should be administered 8 weeks and the second 3 or 4 weeks before the birth (Cameron *et al.*, 1983).

Bibliography

American Public Health Association. *Control of Communicable Diseases in Man*, 14th ed. (Ed. by A. S. Benenson). Washington, D.C., APHA, 1985.

Arnold, R. B., T. I. Soewarso, and A. Karyadi. Mortality from neonatal tetanus in Indonesia: results of two surveys. *Bull WHO* 64:259-262, 1986.

Bytchenko, B. Geographical distribution of tetanus in the world, 1951-1960. *Bull WHO* 34:71-104, 1966.

Cameron, C. M., B. J. Van Biljon, W. J. S. Botha, and P. C. Knoetze. Comparison of oil adjuvant and aluminum phosphate-adsorbed toxoid for the passive immunization of lambs against tetanus. *Onderstepoort J Vet Res* 50:229-231, 1983.

Centers for Disease Control of the USA. Tetanus—United States, 1982-1984. *Morb Mortal Wkly Rep* 34:602, 607-611, 1985.

Centers for Disease Control of the USA. Tetanus—United States, 1985-1986. *Morb Mortal Wky Rep* 36:477-481, 1987.

Cvjetanović, B. Epidemiology of Tetanus Viewed from a Practical Public Health Angle. *In: Third International Conference on Tetanus*. São Paulo, Brazil, 17-22 August 1970. Washington, D.C., Pan American Health Organization, 1972. (Scientific Publication 253.)

Halsey, M. A., and C. A. de Quadros. *Recent Advances in Immunization*. Washington, D.C., Pan American Health Organization, 1983. (Scientific Publication 451.)

Matzkin, H., and S. Regev. Naturally acquired immunity to tetanus toxin in an isolated community. *Infect Immun* 48:267-268, 1985.

Mazzáfero, V. E., M. Boyer, and A. Moncayo. The distribution of tetanus in Argentina. *Bull Pan Am Health Organ* 15:327-332, 1981.

McComb, J. A. Tetanus (Lockjaw). *In*: Stoenner, H., W. Kaplan, and M. Torten (Section Eds.), *CRC Handbook Series in Zoonoses*, Section A, vol. 2. Boca Raton, Florida, CRC Press, 1980.

Rosen, M. H. Clostridial infections and intoxications. *In*: Hubbert, W. T., W. F. McCulloch, and P. R. Schnurrenberger (Eds.), *Diseases Transmitted from Animals to Man*, 6th ed. Springfield, Illinois, Thomas, 1975.

Rosen, H. M. Diseases caused by clostridia. *In*: Beeson, P. B., W. McDermott, and J. B. Wyngaarden (Eds.), *Cecil Textbook of Medicine*, 15th ed. Philadelphia and London, Saunders, 1979.

Smith, J. W. G. Toxoides diftérico y tetánico. *Bol Of Sanit Panam* 74:152-165, 1973.

Smith, L. D. Clostridial diseases of animals. *Adv Vet Sci* 3:465-524, 1957.

Smith, L. D. *The Pathogenic Anaerobic Bacteria*, 2nd ed. Springfield, Illinois, Thomas, 1975.

Spaeth, R. Tetanus. *In*: Top, F. H., Sr., and P. F. Wehrle (Eds.), *Communicable and Infectious Diseases*, 7th ed. St. Louis, Missouri, Mosby, 1972.

Tavares, W. Profilaxis do tetano. Fundamentos e crítica de sua realização. *Rev Assoc Med Brasil* 28:10-14, 1982.

Vera Martínez, A., C. M. Ramírez Boettner, V. M. Salinas, and R. Zárate. Tétanos: Estudio clínico y epidemiológico de 2.337 casos. *Bol Of Sanit Panam* 80:323-332, 1976.

Wilson, G. S., and A. Miles. *Topley and Wilson's Principles of Bacteriology, Virology and Immunity*, Vol. 2, 6th ed. Baltimore, Williams and Wilkins, 1975.

World Health Organization. Guidelines for the prevention of tetanus. *WHO Chron* 30:201-203, 1976.

World Health Organization. Tetanus. *Wkly Epidemiol Rec* 60:287-288, 1985.

TICK-BORNE RELAPSING FEVER

(087.1)

Synonyms: Endemic relapsing fever, spirochetosis, spirochetal fever, recurrent typhus, borreliasis, borreliosis.

Etiology: Spirochetes of the genus *Borrelia* (syn. *Spirillum, Spirochaeta, Spironema*). Given the specificity between the tick species and the *Borrelia* strain it harbors, classification of the etiologic agent according to its vector has been proposed. Thus, the agent transmitted by *Ornithodoros hermsi* would be named *Borrelia hermsii*, the one found in *O. brasiliensis* would be *B. brasiliensis*, etc. However, not all researchers agree with this taxonomy. Some maintain that all the strains adapted to different *Ornithodoros* species are variants of a single species, *Borrelia recurrentis*, the agent of epidemic relapsing fever, transmitted by lice.

Geographic Distribution: Natural foci of *Borrelia* transmissible to man are found worldwide, with the exception of Australia, New Zealand, and Oceania.

Occurrence in Man: The incidence is low. Man contracts the infection only upon entering the natural foci where infected *Ornithodoros* are found. In some regions of Africa, the vector *O. moubata* has become established in dwellings where it lives in dirt floors. In Latin America, *O. rudis* (*O. venezuelensis*) and *O. turicata* also have an affinity for dwellings.

In 1969, the number of cases in South America was 278, with one death. In 1976, 15 cases were reported in the United States of America. Sporadic cases occur in the western states of that country, in Canada (British Columbia), Mexico, Guatemala, Panama, Colombia, Venezuela, Ecuador, and Argentina.

Even though endemic relapsing fever is usually sporadic, at times group outbreaks occur. In 1973, there was an outbreak of 62 cases (16 confirmed and 46 clinically diagnosed) among tourists at the Grand Canyon in Arizona who were lodged in rustic wooden cabins infested by rodents and their ticks. In 1976, an outbreak occurred under similar circumstances, with six cases among 11 tourists in California (Harwood and James, 1979).

Occurrence in Animals: In natural foci, many wild animal species are infected, among them armadillos, opossums, weasels, tree squirrels, bats, and mice. The etiologic agent has also been isolated from horses and cattle.

The Disease in Man: Epidemic relapsing fever (transmitted by lice) and endemic relapsing fever (transmitted by ticks) have similar clinical pictures. The average incubation period is about 7 days after the tick bite, but may vary from 2 to 10 days. The disease is characterized by an initial pyrexia that lasts 3 to 4 days and begins and disappears suddenly. The fever, which may reach 41°C, is accompanied by chills, profuse sweating, vertigo, cephalalgia, myalgias, and vomiting. At times, erythemas, petechiae, epistaxis, and jaundice of varying degrees of severity may be observed. After some days without fever, the attacks of fever recur several times, lasting longer than in the first episode. Periodic recurrences are attributed to antigenic or mutagenic changes in the borreliae, against which the patient cannot develop immunity. Endemic relapsing fever is fatal in 2 to 5% of the cases.

The Disease in Animals: Little is known about the natural course of infection and its clinical manifestations in wild animals. As with many other reservoirs of infectious agents in natural foci, the hosts and borreliae are probably well adapted to each other, and the latter likely have little or no pathogenic effect on their hosts.

Borreliasis (spirochetosis) of fowl is a serious disease in geese, ducks, and chickens caused by *B. anserina* and transmitted by *Argas persicus* and *A. miniatus*. The bovine infection in South Africa produced by *B. theileri* and transmitted by *Margaropus decoloratus* and *Rhipicephalus evertsi* results in a benign disease. These borreliases affect only animals and are not transmitted to man.

Source of Infection and Mode of Transmission (Figure 18): The borreliae that cause endemic relapsing fever have as their reservoir wild animals and ticks of the genus *Ornithodoros*; in addition, the latter are vectors of the infection. These ticks are xerophilic argasids that are long-lived and very resistant to desiccation and long

Figure 18. Tick-borne relapsing fever. Mode of transmission.

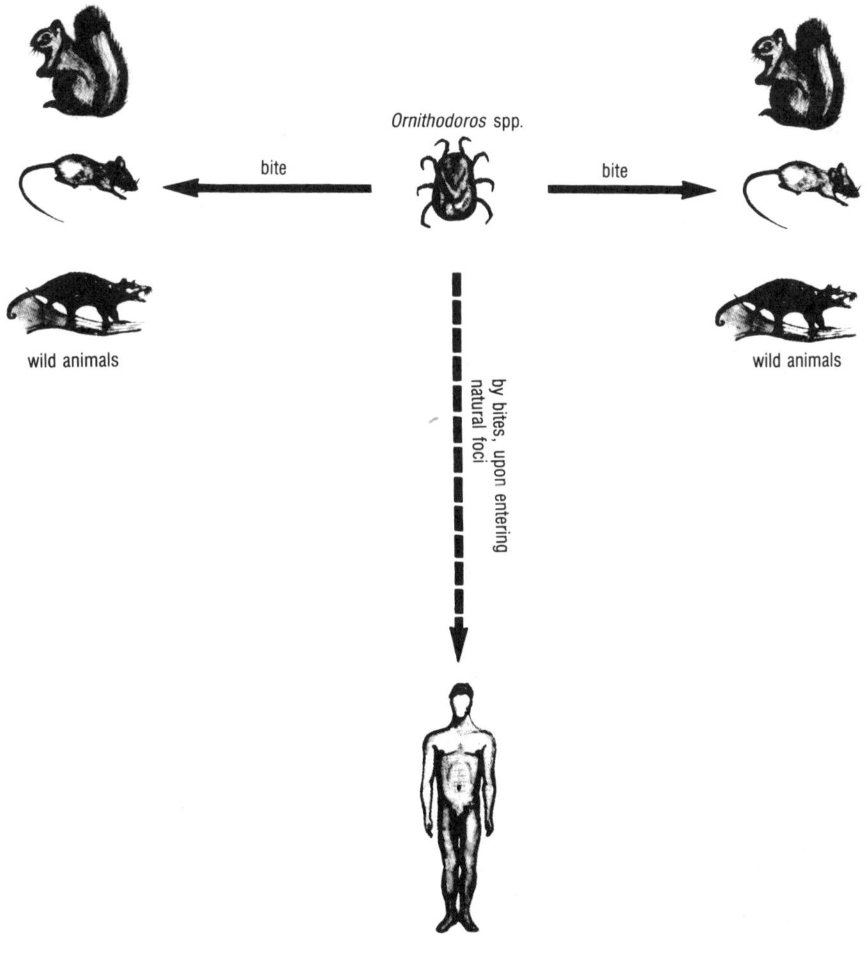

periods of fasting in environments of low humidity and high temperature. Borreliae survive in the ticks a long time. In different species of *Ornithodoros,* transovarial transmission varies from less than 1 to 100%. In the Western Hemisphere the most important vectors of *Borrelia* are *O. hermsi, O. turicata, O. rudis* (*O. venezuelensis*), and possibly *O. talaje.* The continuous circulation of borreliae in nature is assured by the ticks' adaptations and their habit of feeding on infected wild animals. *O. hermsi* lives at altitudes of over 1,000 meters, feeds on squirrel blood, and can be found in rodent burrows and wooden huts. *O. turicata* attacks sheep and goats, among other animals, and infests hides, rodent and snake burrows, and pigsties.

Role of Animals in the Epidemiology of the Disease: Several species of wild animals constitute the reservoir of the etiologic agent. The relative importance of ticks and wild animals as reservoirs is debated, but both undoubtedly play important roles in maintaining the infection in nature. An exception is infection by *B. duttoni* in Africa, which has not been found in animals and is transmitted directly to man by the tick *O. moubata.*

Diagnosis: Diagnosis is based on demonstrating the presence of the etiologic agent in the patient's blood by dark-field microscopy using fresh smears or films stained by the Giemsa or Wright techniques, or by inoculation in mice. The number of borreliae diminishes or disappears at the end of a fever attack, and therefore intraperitoneal inoculation in young mice and examination of their blood 24 to 72 hours after inoculation is advisable.

Control: Control measures are difficult to apply and are not practical, since cases in the Western Hemisphere are rare and usually widely dispersed. The principal means of prevention is avoiding the bite of ticks living in caves, burrows of rodents and other animals, or primitive huts.

Human dwellings should be built to keep out the hosts (rodents or others) of *Ornithodoros.* Similarly, wood storage within or near buildings should be avoided. Persons entering natural foci should examine themselves for ticks periodically, in addition to using protective footwear and clothing. Repellents provide partial protection; dimethyl phthalate is the most highly recommended.

Bibliography

Bruner, D. W., and J. H. Gillespie. *Hagan's Infectious Diseases of Domestic Animals.* Ithaca, New York, Cornell University Press, 1973.

Coates, J. B., B. C. Hoff, and P. M. Hoff (Eds.), *Preventive Medicine in World War II. Vol. VII. Communicable Diseases: Arthropod-borne Diseases Other Than Malaria.* Washington, D.C., Department of the Army, 1964.

Felsenfeld, O. *Borreliae,* human relapsing fever, and parasite-vector-host relationships. *Bacteriol Rev* 29:46-74, 1965.

Francis, B. J., and R. S. Thompson. Relapsing fever. *In*: Hoeprich, P. D. (Ed.), *Infectious Diseases.* Hagerstown, Maryland, Harper and Row, 1972.

Geigy, R. Relapsing fevers. *In*: Weinmann, D., and M. Ristic (Eds.), *Infectious Blood Diseases of Man and Animals, Vol. 2.* New York and London, Academic Press, 1968.

Harwood, K. F., and M. T. James. *Entomology in Human and Animal Health.* New York, MacMillan, 1979.

Jellison, W. J. The endemic relapsing fevers. *In*: Hubbert, W. T., W. F. McCulloch, and P. R. Schnurrenberger (Eds.), *Diseases Transmitted from Animals to Man*, 6th ed. Springfield, Illinois, Thomas, 1975.

Pan American Health Organization. *Reported Cases of Notifiable Diseases in the Americas, 1969*. Washington, D.C., PAHO, 1972. (Scientific Publication 247.)

TULAREMIA

(021)

Synonyms: Francis' disease, deer-fly fever, rabbit fever, Ohara's disease.

Etiology: *Francisella tularensis*, a highly pleomorphic, gram-positive, nonmotile bacillus that can survive several weeks in the external environment.

It has been proposed that *F. tularensis* be subdivided into three subspecies: *F. tularensis* ssp. *tularensis* (Jellison type A), *holarctica* (Jellison type B), and *mediasiatica* (Olsufjev and Meshcheryakova, 1983). Classification into subspecies is not based on antigenic differences, but instead on characteristics of the agent's biochemistry, ecology, virulence, and nosography.

Geographic Distribution: Natural foci of infection are found in the Northern Hemisphere. In the Americas, the disease has been confirmed in Canada, the United States, and Mexico. It is found in most European countries, Tunisia, Turkey, Israel, Iran, China, and Japan. There are extensive areas with natural foci in the USSR.

F. tularensis ssp. *tularensis* (Jellison type A) predominates in North America and causes 90% of human cases in that part of the world. The principal source of infection by this subspecies is lagomorphs, mainly those of the genus *Sylvilagus*. The subspecies *holarctica* (Jellison type B) causes 5 to 10% of human cases; its principal hosts are rodents. Subspecies *tularensis* is more virulent than *holarctica* (Bell and Reilly, 1981).

Subspecies *holarctica* is found in western and northern Europe, Siberia, the Far East, some parts of central Europe, and, less frequently, in North America. A special biotype of this subspecies (biovar *japonica*) is found in Japan. This subspecies exists in natural foci among the Rodentia and Lagomorpha. Subspecies *mediasiatica* is found in the central Asiatic region of the USSR, where natural foci exist among hares of the genus *Lepus* and rodents of the subfamily Gerbilinae. This biotype, like *holarctica*, is moderately virulent (Olsufjev and Meshcheryakova, 1983).

Occurrence in Man: It is not an internationally notifiable disease and its global incidence is hard to establish. The countries that possess the best data are the United States and the USSR. In both, the number of cases has apparently declined sharply. In the USSR, where in the decade of the 1940s about 100,000 cases were reported annually, the incidence has diminished to a few hundred cases per year; in the United States, the average number of annual cases has declined from 1,184 in the 1940s to 274 between 1960 and 1969.

In the 10-year period 1972-1981, the number of cases in the United States ranged from 129 to 288 per year (Sanford, 1983). In Canada there were 31 cases between 1975 and 1979 (Akerman and Embil, 1982).

Occurrence in Animals: The disease affects a great number of vertebrates (more than 100 species of wild and domestic animals) and invertebrates (also more than 100 species). The natural infection has been found in ticks, mosquitoes, horseflies, fleas, and lice that parasitize lagomorphs and rodents.

Epizootic outbreaks have been described in sheep, commercially bred fur-bearers (mink, beaver, and fox), and wild rodents and lagomorphs.

The Disease in Man: It is seen most commonly as sporadic cases, but epidemic outbreaks have occurred in the United States and the USSR.

The incubation period usually lasts from 3 to 5 days, but may vary between 1 and 10 days. Several clinical forms of the disease are known; they are determined principally by the agent's route of entry. In all its forms, the disease is of sudden onset, with rising and falling fever, chills, asthenia, joint and muscle pain, cephalalgia, and vomiting. The most common clinical form is ulceroglandular, which in the Western Hemisphere accounts for 85% of all cases. A local lesion is seen at the site of entry (an arthropod bite, or a scratch or cut inflicted by contaminated nails or knife), which progresses to a necrotic ulceration accompanied by swelling of the nearby lymph node. The node frequently suppurates, ulcerates, and becomes sclerotic. In untreated cases, the disease course lasts 3 to 5 weeks and convalescence takes several weeks to months with intermittent attacks of fever. A variety of this form is the glandular, in which there is no primary lesion; it is the most prevalent type in Japan. The oculoglandular form develops when contaminated material comes in contact with the conjunctiva. The primary lesion localizes on the lower eyelid and consists of an ulcerated papule; at the same time, the regional lymph nodes swell. The primary pulmonary form is caused by aerosols, affects rural and laboratory workers, and produces pneumonia in one or both lungs. An estimated 30% of all tularemia patients, regardless of the infection's route of entry, contract bronchopneumonia. The typhoidal form is uncommon; it is caused by ingestion of contaminated foods—usually infected wild rabbit meat—or contaminated water. The symptoms are gastroenteritis, fever, and toxemia; ulcerative lesions are found in the mucosa of the mouth, pharynx, and intestines, sometimes accompanied by swollen cervical, pharyngeal, and mesenteric lymph glands. If not treated promptly, the disease course may be short and fatal. In the United States, the fatality rate for the pulmonary and typhoidal forms is from 40 to 60%. Before the existence of antibiotics, the fatality rate for all cases of tularemia in the United States was close to 7%. The fatality rate outside of the Americas has rarely exceeded 1%. This difference is attributed to the greater virulence of the tick-transmitted strains (subspecies *tularensis*) of *F. tularensis* in the United States. Untreated cutaneous infections (ulceroglandular form) in the USSR are fatal for less than 0.5% of the patients (subspecies *holarctica*).

The results of serologic and skin sensitivity tests carried out among exposed groups show that inapparent infections are common.

The Disease in Animals: It has been demonstrated experimentally that susceptibility to *F. tularensis* varies in different species of wild animals. Three groups have been established based on the infecting dose and the lethal dose. Group 1, the most susceptible, contains most species of rodents and lagomorphs, which generally suffer a fatal septicemic disease. Group 2 is composed of some other species of mammals and of birds, which, though highly susceptible to the infection, rarely die from it. Group 3 consists of carnivores, which are susceptible but require high doses to become infected, rarely develop bacteremia, and only occasionally manifest overt disease.

Group 1 animals are a source of infection for arthropods, other animals, man, and the environment. The clinical picture in these animals is not well known, since they are usually found dead or dying. Experimentally inoculated hares show weakness, fever, ulcers, abscesses at the inoculation site, and swelling of regional lymph nodes. Death ensues in 8 to 14 days. The lesions resemble those of plague and pseudotuberculosis, with caseous lymph nodes and grayish white foci in the spleen.

High-mortality outbreaks have occurred in sheep in enzootic areas of Canada, the United States, and the USSR. In addition to causing economic losses, tularemia in sheep is a source of infection for man. In the United States, the infection is transmitted by the tick *Dermacentor andersoni*, which during outbreaks is found in great numbers at the base of the sheep's ears and on the neck. Sick animals separate themselves from the flock and manifest fever, rigid gait, diarrhea, frequent urination, and difficulty in breathing. Most deaths occur among young animals. Pregnant ewes may abort. Reactions to serologic tests indicate that many animals have an inapparent infection. Sheep can be classified in group 2 based on their susceptibility to the infection. Autopsy reveals infarcts of the regional lymph nodes, mainly those of the head and neck, as well as pneumonic foci. In this species, tularemia is a seasonal disease, coinciding with tick infestations.

Source of Infection and Mode of Transmission (Figure 19): In natural foci the infection circulates among wild vertebrates, independently of man and domestic animals. Ticks are biological vectors of *F. tularensis*; not only do they transmit the etiologic agent from animal to animal, but they also constitute an important interepizootic reservoir. Each enzootic region has one or more species of vertebrate animals and of ticks that play the primary role in transmitting and maintaining the infection in nature. It is a matter of debate whether very susceptible lagomorphs and rodents (group 1) are true reservoirs or only amplifiers and the main source of infection for man. Less susceptible animals (group 2), together with ticks, are thought to be important reservoirs.

Domestic animals, such as sheep and cats, are accidental hosts, but they may also constitute sources of infection for man.

Humans contract the infection upon entering natural foci of tularemia. Sources of infection and modes of transmission of the causal agent are many. In North America, the animals that most frequently serve as the source of infection are wild rabbits (*Sylvilagus* spp.), hares (*Lepus californicus*), beavers (*Castor canadensis*), muskrats (*Ondatra zibethicus*), microtine mice (*Microtus* spp.), and sheep. The subspecies *tularensis* is generally transmitted by wild rabbits or their ticks (*Ixodes*, *Dermacentor*). The subspecies *holarctica* is more common among rodents. In many enzootic areas the principal route of penetration is through the skin (by means of hematophagous arthropods, scratches, or knife cuts). Another portal of entry is the

Figure 19. Tularemia. Mode of transmission in the Americas.

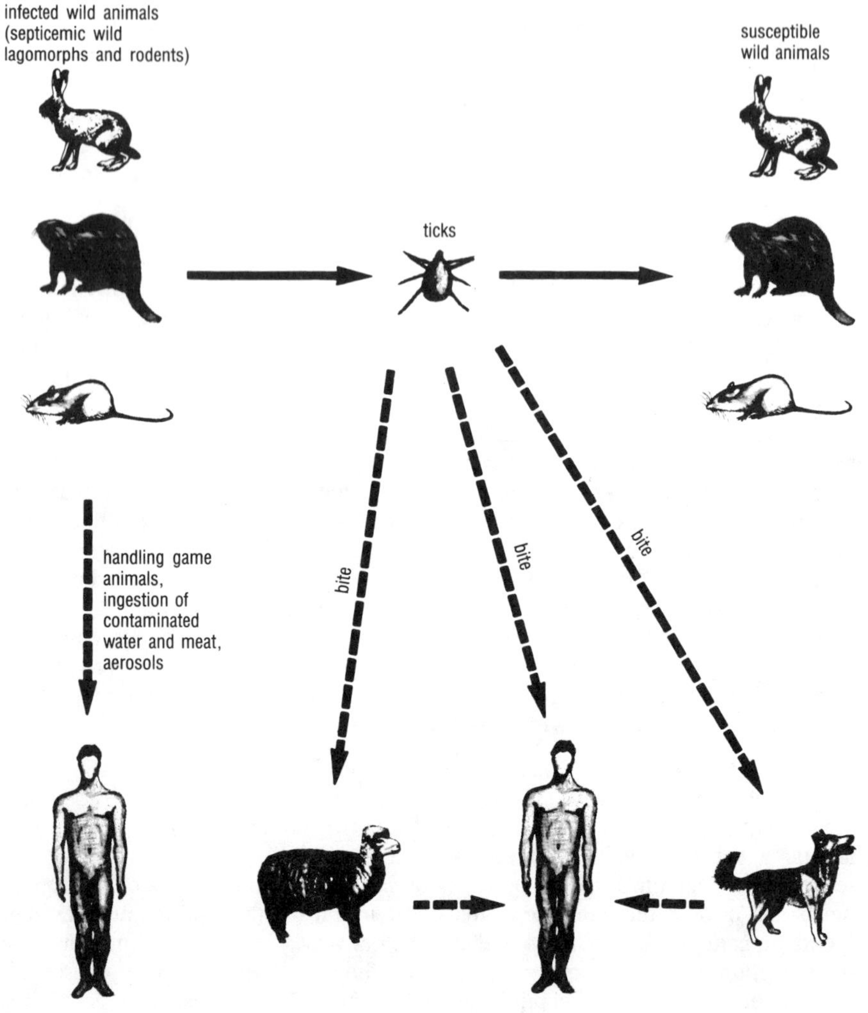

conjunctiva, which can be contaminated by material splashed into the eyes or, in the case of hunters or sheep shearers, by hands soiled from handling sick animals. Infection via the oral route occurs as a result of ingesting water contaminated by dead animals or their urine and feces, or by eating improperly cooked meat of lagomorphs and other infected animals. In addition, the disease can be contracted through the respiratory system by inhaling aerosols contaminated in the laboratory or dust from fodder, grain, or wool contaminated with rodent excreta.

Cases of human infection have been caused by scratches or bites from apparently healthy cats. It is assumed that these animals had recently hunted and captured sick rodents. Another case occurred in a person exposed to a cat with an ulcer (Centers for Disease Control of the USA, 1982). The disease was also contracted by a

Canadian zoo veterinarian who was bitten on the finger when treating a sick primate (*Saguinus nigricollis*). In this zoo, four nonhuman primates in adjacent cages died from tularemia, possibly transmitted by fleas from squirrels that often came near the cages. *F. tularensis* was isolated from one of the squirrels. The primate responsible for infecting the veterinarian had sialorrhea, ocular and nasal discharges, and ulcers on the tongue (Nayar *et al.*, 1979).

The highest incidence of cases occurs in the summer, when ticks are most active. Hunters are an especially vulnerable group, and the number of human cases increases in hunting season.

Role of Animals in the Epidemiology of the Disease: Human-to-human transmission is exceptional. Tularemia is a zoonosis transmitted to man—an accidental host—by contact with wild or domestic animals (of the latter, usually sheep), by a contaminated environment, or by vectors such as ticks, horseflies, and mosquitoes.

Diagnosis: In man, clinical diagnosis is based on the symptomatology and prior contact with a likely source of infection. Laboratory confirmation is based on a) isolation of the etiologic agent from the patient's local lesion, lymph nodes, or sputum by means of direct culture or inoculation into laboratory animals; b) the immunofluorescence test on exudates, sputum, and other contaminated materials; c) the skin test with hyperimmune goat serum, which gives immediate hypersensitivity reactions, and with bacterial allergen, which gives delayed hypersensitivity reactions (these reagents can give a diagnosis during the first week of illness); and d) serologic tests, the most commonly used being agglutination and hemagglutination. More recently, an enzyme-linked immunosorbent assay (ELISA) test with sonicated antigen has been perfected (Viljanem *et al.*, 1983). This test has the advantage of permitting an early diagnosis, which is important for treatment (streptomycin). Antibodies appear in the second or third week of the disease and may persist for years. Cross-agglutination with *Brucella* antigen can occur, but at a lower level than with the homologous antigen. Absorption of the patient's serum with *Brucella* antigen removes all doubt.

In the case of sheep, laboratory confirmation is obtained by isolating the causal agent or by serologic tests.

Control: To prevent the disease in man, general and individual protective measures may be taken. Those of a general nature consist of reducing the source of infection, controlling vectors, changing the environment, and educating the public. Except for the last one, these control measures are costly and difficult to apply. In the USSR, where tularemia was an important public health problem, anti-tularemia institutes have been established in epizootic regions to carry out these control activities.

An important protective measure consists of immunizing individuals, populations, and occupational groups exposed to risk with attenuated live vaccine. In the USSR, the drastic reduction achieved in human morbidity is attributed to this single activity. Other protective measures consist of using repellents and protective clothing to avoid tick infestation and bites of other arthropods, promptly removing ticks from the body, using gloves to handle and skin wild animals, avoiding consumption of untreated water in areas where contamination by *F. tularensis* is suspected, and thoroughly cooking wild animal meat in enzootic areas.

Control of the infection in sheep involves applying tickicides by spray or dip, and administering antibiotics (streptomycin, tetracyclines) in case of an outbreak.

Bibliography

Akerman, M. B., and J. A. Embil. Antibodies to *Francisella tularensis* in the snowshoe hare (*Lepus americanus struthopus*) populations of Nova Scotia and Prince Edward Island and in the moose (*Alces alces americana* Clinton) population of Nova Scotia. *Can J Microbiol* 28:403-405, 1982.

Arata, A., M. Chamsa, A. Farhang-Azad, I. Meščerjakova, V. Neronov, and S. Saidi. First detection of tularemia in domestic and wild mammals in Iran. *Bull WHO* 49:597-603, 1973.

American Public Health Association. *Control of Communicable Diseases in Man*, 14th ed. (Ed. by A. S. Benenson). Washington, D.C., APHA, 1985.

Bell, J. F., and J. R. Reilly. Tularemia. *In*: J. W. Davis, L. H. Karstad, and D. O. Trainer (Eds.), *Infectious Diseases of Wild Mammals*, 2nd ed. Ames, Iowa State University Press, 1981.

Centers for Disease Control of the USA. Tularemia associated with domestic cats—Georgia, New Mexico. *Morb Mortal Wkly Rep* 31:39-41, 1982.

Frank, F. W., and W. A. Meinershagen. Tularemia epizootic in sheep. *Vet Med* 56:374-378, 1961.

Gelman, A. C. Tularemia. *In*: May, J. M. (Ed.), *Studies in Disease Ecology*. New York, Hafner, 1961.

Hornick, R. B. Tularemia. *In*: Hoeprich, P. D. (Ed.), *Infectious Diseases*. Hagerstown, Maryland, Harper and Row, 1972.

Marsh, H. *Newsom's Sheep Diseases*, 2nd ed. Baltimore, Maryland, Williams and Wilkins, 1958.

Meyer, K. F. *Pasteurella* and *Francisella*. *In*: Dubos, R. J., and J. G. Hirsch (Eds.), *Bacterial and Mycotic Infections of Man*, 4th ed. Philadelphia and Montreal, Lippincott, 1965.

Nayar, G. P. S., G. J. Crawshaw, and J. L. Neufeld. Tularemia in a group of non-human primates. *J Am Vet Med Assoc* 175:962-963, 1979.

Olsen, P. F. Tularemia. *In*: Hubbert, W. T., W. F. McCulloch, and P. R. Schnurrenberger (Eds.), *Diseases Transmitted from Animals to Man*, 6th ed. Springfield, Illinois, Thomas, 1975.

Olsufjev, N. G., and I. S. Meshcheryakova. Subspecific taxonomy of *Francisella tularensis* McCoy and Chapin, 1912. *Int J Syst Bacteriol* 33:872-874, 1983.

Pavlosky, E. N. *Natural Nidality of Transmissible Diseases*. Urbana, University of Illinois Press, 1966.

Reilly, J. R. Tularemia. *In*: Davis, J. W., L. Karstad, and D. O. Trainer (Eds.), *Infectious Diseases of Wild Mammals*. Ames, Iowa State University Press, 1970.

Sanford, J. P. Tularemia. *JAMA* 250:3325-3326, 1983.

Syrjälä, H., P. Koskela, T. Ripatti, A. Salmimen, and E. Herva. Agglutination and ELISA methods in the diagnosis of tularemia in different clinical forms and severities of the disease. *J Infect Dis* 153:142-145, 1986.

Thorpe, B. D., R. W. Sidwell, D. E. Johnson, K. L. Smart, and D. D. Parker. Tularemia in the wildlife and livestock of the Great Salt Lake Desert Region, 1951 through 1964. *Am J Trop Med Hyg* 14:622-637, 1965.

Tiggert, W. D. Soviet viable *Pasteurella tularensis* vaccines. A review of selected articles. *Bacteriol Rev* 26:354-373, 1962.

Viljanem, M. K., T. Nurmi, and A. Salminen. Enzyme-linked immunosorbent assay (ELISA) with bacterial sonicate antigen for IgM, IgA, and IgG antibodies to *Francisella tularensis*: comparison with bacterial agglutination test and ELISA with lipopolysaccharide antigen. *J Infect Dis* 148:715-720, 1983.

Woodward, T. E. Tularemia. *In*: Beeson, P. B., W. McDermott, and J. B. Wyngaarden (Eds.), *Cecil Textbook of Medicine*, 15th ed. Philadelphia and London, Saunders, 1979.

Zidon, J. Tularemia. *In*: Van der Hoeden, J. (Ed.), *Zoonoses*. Amsterdam, Netherlands, Elsevier, 1964.

ZOONOTIC TUBERCULOSIS

(010)
(018)

Etiology: The etiologic agents of mammalian tuberculosis are *Mycobacterium tuberculosis* (the main cause of human tuberculosis), *M. bovis* (the agent of bovine tuberculosis), and *M. africanum* (which causes human tuberculosis in tropical Africa). This last species has characteristics intermediate between those of *M. tuberculosis* and *M. bovis*.

The principal agent of zoonotic tuberculosis is *M. bovis*. (Avian tuberculosis is discussed under "Diseases Caused by Nontuberculous Mycobacteria.")

Many authors refer to these bacteria as a single species (*M. tuberculosis*) with human and bovine variants.

Geographic Distribution: Worldwide, with great variations between regions and countries.

Occurrence in Man: The prevalence of human tuberculosis of animal origin has diminished in countries where mandatory pasteurization of milk has been implemented and where successful campaigns of control and eradication of the bovine infection have been carried out. The British Isles—where infection due to *M. bovis* presently has a low incidence and is limited to the elderly—were at one time the most affected area owing to consumption of raw milk. However, in spite of the great reduction in rates of human infection by bovine strains in Great Britain, tuberculosis originated by these strains continues to occur. From 1977 to 1979 in the southeast of England, isolations from 5,021 tuberculosis patients revealed 63 patients (1.25%) infected with "classic bovine strains" (*M. bovis*), 53 of which were from Europeans and 10 from immigrants. Of these cases, 27 (42.86%) had a pulmonary localization and 36 (57.14%) were extrapulmonary tuberculosis. There was a marked difference in the frequency of renal tuberculosis caused by *M. bovis* (23.8%) and that caused by *M. tuberculosis* (8.2%). In commenting on these results, the authors (Collins *et al.*, 1981) suggested the possibility of human-to-human transmission, based on the facts that bovine TB had practically disappeared from Great Britain, that milk is pasteurized, and that some cases occurred in young people. In the Netherlands, where bovine tuberculosis had been declared eradicated, there were 125 human infections caused by *M. bovis* from 1972 to 1975 (Schonfeld, 1982). More than 80% of the patients were born in the era when transmission of *M. bovis* via milk was still possible. The five patients younger than 20 years, who were born after eradication of the bovine infection, were presumed to have contracted the infection outside the Netherlands. Interhuman transmission is still a matter of controversy, but it is undeniable that eradication campaigns against bovine TB have drastically reduced the incidence of human disease of this origin from its former level; for example, in Great Britain in 1945, 5% of all fatal tuberculosis cases and 30% of cases of the disease in children under 5 years old were due to bovine strains (Collins and Granges, 1983).

In countries where milk is routinely boiled, such as those of Latin America, the incidence of infection by *M. bovis* has always been low. Nevertheless, pulmonary as well as extrapulmonary forms of human tuberculosis of animal origin continue to be a problem in areas where the prevalence of infection in cattle is high, because not all milk consumed is boiled, many products are prepared from unpasteurized milk, and, in addition, cases of infection are contracted via aerosols. In Peru (Fernández Salazar *et al.*, 1983), a study of 853 strains of pulmonary tuberculosis identified 38 (4.45%) as *M. bovis*. Several laboratories in Argentina studied a total of 7,195 strains, primarily between 1978 and 1981. Most of the strains were isolated from adult pulmonary patients, and 82 (1.1%) of them were classified as *M. bovis* (Argentine National Commission on Zoonoses, 1982).

Occurrence in Animals: In industrialized countries, bovine tuberculosis has been eradicated or is in an advanced stage of control, while in the majority of developing countries the situation has not improved; in some cases, the disease's prevalence is on the rise. Almost all Western European countries report a prevalence of bovine infection lower than 0.1%. In the Western Hemisphere, Canada and the United States have reduced the infection rate to very low levels. In the latter country in 1969, 0.06% of 4.5 million cattle examined reacted to tuberculin (most of the reactors showed no evident lesions when slaughtered). Of Latin American countries, only Cuba and Venezuela have national control programs. The rate of infection is very low in several Central American and Caribbean nations. The highest infection rates are found in the milk-producing regions surrounding large cities in South America. In South American countries where hogs are fed unpasteurized milk products, the infection rate in swine is similar to or even higher than in cattle, as judged by records of confiscations at slaughterhouses.

Bovine tuberculosis is important not only as a source of human infection, but also as a cause of economic losses.

The Disease in Man: *M. bovis* can cause the same clinical forms and pathologic lesions as *M. tuberculosis* (the human tuberculosis agent). Historically, the most prevalent forms caused by *M. bovis* were extrapulmonary, and children were among those most affected. The reason for extrapulmonary localization of the bovine bacillus is not that it has an affinity for other tissues, but that it is most commonly transmitted by consumption of raw milk or raw milk products. Thus, in those countries where the prevalence of bovine tuberculosis was high and raw milk was consumed, many cases of extrapulmonary tuberculosis—such as cervical adenitis, genitourinary infections, tuberculosis of the bones and joints, and meningitis—used to be caused by *M. bovis*. According to data on typing of tuberculosis bacilli in the British Isles prior to control of the bovine infection, 50% or more of cervical adenitis cases were caused by *M. bovis*. Pulmonary tuberculosis caused by the bovine bacillus occurs less frequently, but its incidence is significant in occupational groups in contact with infected cattle or their carcasses, particularly in countries where animals are kept in barns. This form cannot be distinguished clinically or radiologically from the disease caused by *M. tuberculosis*. Transmission is by aerosol droplets micromillimeters in diameter. In countries where incidence of the human infection caused by *M. tuberculosis* has declined and the bovine infection has not been controlled, it is believed that *M. bovis* could assume a principal role in human pulmonary tuberculosis. Even though Denmark was declared free of bovine tuberculosis in 1952, between 1959 and 1963 127 cases of human infection by *M. bovis*, 58% of which were pulmonary tuberculosis, were detected in the middle-aged and elderly.

In countries where control of bovine tuberculosis is advanced, human cases caused by *M. bovis* are observed mainly in the elderly, who were exposed to the pathogenic agent in their youth or childhood.

Interhuman transmission of *M. bovis* is possible, but few cases have been satisfactorily confirmed. As is the case with most zoonoses, man is generally an accidental host of *M. bovis* and human infection depends on the animal source. Since *M. tuberculosis* and *M. bovis* are very similar in their pathologic effect on man, it is not understood why large-scale interhuman transmission of the bovine infection does not occur. A possible explanation is that pulmonary patients infected by *M. bovis* eliminate fewer bacilli in their sputum than do those infected by *M. tuberculosis* (Griffith, 1937).

The Latin American population has been assumed to be protected from infection by the bovine bacillus by the widespread custom of boiling milk. Undoubtedly, if this practice were not followed, the rate of human infection by *M. bovis* would be much higher, considering the infection's wide distribution and the rate of infection in dairy cattle in many Latin American countries. However, some people in rural areas do drink raw milk and frequently consume products (cream, butter, soft cheese) made at home from raw milk. In Latin America and in other parts of the world, children are the main victims, as indicated by typing data from Brazil, Mexico, and Peru. These data also confirm that there are children who are fed milk or milk products that are not heat-treated.

Although it is not customary to house cattle in barns in Latin America, cases of pulmonary tuberculosis caused by *M. bovis* have been recorded, with rural laborers and employees of abattoirs and locker plants being the most exposed groups. In Argentina, the bovine bacillus was isolated from 8% of 85 pulmonary patients from rural areas, while only one case due to *M. bovis* was found among 55 patients in the capital.

People suffering from pulmonary tuberculosis of bovine origin can, in turn, retransmit the infection to cattle. This occurrence is particularly evident in herds from which tuberculosis has been eradicated that later become reinfected, the source of exposure often being a ranchhand with *M. bovis* tuberculosis. Such episodes have occurred in the United States and in several European countries. Between 1943 and 1952, 128 herds containing more than 1,000 head of cattle were reinfected in Denmark by 107 individuals with tuberculosis. Similar occurrences continued in the same country until 1960 in spite of advances made in the eradication of bovine tuberculosis. In regions where bovine tuberculosis has been eradicated, cattle cease being a source for human infection, but man may continue for years to be a potential source of infection for cattle.

Persons with pulmonary or genitourinary tuberculosis due to the specific human type (*M. tuberculosis*) can temporarily infect and sensitize cattle. Cattle are very resistant to *M. tuberculosis*; the agent does not cause a progressive tuberculosis in these animals, but the bacillus can survive for some time in their tissues, especially the lymph nodes, thus sensitizing the animal to mammalian tuberculin and complicating interpretation of the diagnostic test. Sensitization can persist for 6 to 8 months after the human source of infection is removed. Very occasionally, elimination of *M. tuberculosis* in milk has been confirmed, but tuberculous lesions of the udder were not present. Man can transmit the human bacillus to several animal species, principally monkeys and dogs, in which it produces a progressive tuberculosis.

In many countries, direct or indirect exposure of man to bovine tuberculosis is an important source of sensitization to tuberculin. There is a relationship between the prevalence of bovine tuberculosis and the rate of reactors to tuberculin in the human population. Statistical data indicate that a third of the sensitized population in Denmark between the ages of 30 and 35 owes its tuberculin sensitization to infection with *M. bovis*. The same study suggests that the risk of developing pulmonary tuberculosis later is much smaller among those sensitized by the bovine bacillus, perhaps because *M. bovis* infection is contracted principally through the digestive tract and not via aerosols. Another interesting conclusion is that less calcification occurs in pulmonary tuberculosis resulting from *M. bovis* than in the *M. tuberculosis* type.

The Disease in Animals: Many mammalian species are susceptible to the agents of tuberculosis. Bovine tuberculosis is the most important from the economic point of view and as a zoonosis. Tuberculosis in swine also causes substantial economic losses.

CATTLE: The principal etiologic agent for cattle is *M. bovis*. As in man, the bacillus enters the body mainly by inhalation. The intestinal tract is an important route of infection in calves that are nursed on contaminated milk. The most common clinical and pathologic form is pulmonary tuberculosis. The causal agent enters the lungs and multiplies there, forming the primary focus; this is accompanied by tuberculous lesions in the bronchial lymph nodes of the same side, thus producing the primary complex. These lesions can remain latent or develop further, depending on the interaction between the agent and the host's body. If the animal's resistance to the tuberculosis bacilli breaks down, the infection will spread to other organs via the lymph or blood vessels, giving rise to early generalization of the infection. If the immune system is not competent to destroy the bacilli, they will cause tubercles to form in organs and tissues where they lodge. New foci are produced, principally in the lungs, kidneys, liver, spleen, and their associated lymph nodes. Dissemination may give rise to acute miliary tuberculosis.

In most cases, tuberculosis has a chronic course, with effects limited to the lungs. The disease process is slow and may remain clinically inapparent for a long time. In fact, some animals spend their entire useful lives without any evident symptomatology, though they constitute a potential threat for the rest of the herd. Other animals develop chronic bronchopneumonia, accompanied by coughing, weight loss, and reduced milk production. In advanced cases, when the lungs are largely destroyed, there is pronounced dyspnea.

Pearl disease, a tuberculous peritonitis or pleurisy, is another form sometimes observed in infected herds in countries with no tuberculosis control program.

It is estimated that about 5% of tuberculous cows, especially in advanced cases, have tuberculous lesions of the uterus or tuberculous metritis, and that 1 to 2% have tuberculous mastitis. This clinical form not only has public health repercussions, but also serves as a source of infection for calves nursed naturally or artificially. One of the main signs of tuberculosis acquired by the oral route is swelling of the retropharyngeal lymph nodes. In calves, the primary lesion is usually located in the mesenteric lymph nodes and the intestinal mucosa is not affected.

The disease appears more frequently in older animals because it is chronic in character and because the passage of time allows more opportunity for exposure to the infection. The infection is more prevalent among dairy cattle than among beef cattle, not only because their useful economic life is longer, but because dairy cattle are in closer contact with one another when gathered for milking or when housed in dairy sheds.

Cattle are resistant to *M. avium* and rarely suffer progressive tuberculosis due to this agent. Nevertheless, *M. avium* is important in control programs because cattle can become paraspecifically sensitized to mammalian tuberculin, leading to difficulties in diagnosis. *M. avium* infects cattle through the digestive tract. When lesions are present, they are generally limited to the intestinal and mesenteric lymph nodes. However, lesions can occasionally be found in the lungs and regional lymph nodes but not in other tissues, indicating that the route of entry may sometimes be the respiratory tract. Lesions tend to heal spontaneously. Bovine-to-bovine transmission of *M. avium* infection does not occur (see also "Diseases Caused by Nontuberculous Mycobacteria").

Cattle are very resistant to *M. tuberculosis* and rarely develop anatomicopathologic lesions due to this agent. In several countries, *M. tuberculosis* has been isolated from the lymph nodes of some positive reactors to tuberculin that showed no lesions in postmortem examination. Again in this instance, the infection's importance lies in sensitizing these animals to tuberculin.

An experiment comparing the pathogenicity of *M. africanum*, *M. bovis*, and *M. tuberculosis* for calves inoculated intravenously showed that *M. africanum* (at least the strain used in the experiment) was as pathogenic for calves as *M. bovis* (Kantor et al., 1979).

SWINE: This species is susceptible to the following agents: *M. bovis*, *M. avium-intracellulare*, and *M. tuberculosis*. *M. bovis* is the most pathogenic and invasive for swine and is the cause of most cases of generalized tuberculosis.

The principal route of infection is the digestive tract by consumption of milk or milk products, kitchen and abattoir scraps, and excreta from tuberculous fowl and cattle. The primary infection complex is found in the oropharynx and the submaxillary lymph nodes, or in the intestine and the mesenteric lymph nodes. The lesions are usually confined to this primary complex. Chronic lesions are not found in single organs, as they often are in cattle. Prevalence is lower in young animals than in adults, but the former show a greater tendency toward generalization of the infection. Programs for the eradication of bovine tuberculosis directly help reduce the infection rate among swine. In the United States in 1924, tuberculous lesions were found in 15.2% of hogs butchered, while in 1970 they were found in only 1.09%. The total number of confiscations owing to generalized tuberculosis was reduced even more drastically. In some Latin American countries, *M. bovis* is the cause of 80 to 90% of tuberculous lesions in swine. The relative proportions of *M. bovis* to *M. avium-intracellulare* as the cause of swine tuberculosis are reversed when *M. bovis* infection is controlled in cattle, as it has been in several European countries and the United States.

M. avium-intracellulare usually causes adenitis of the digestive tract and, more rarely, a generalized disease (see also "Diseases Caused by Nontuberculous Mycobacteria").

Swine are also susceptible to the human bacillus (*M. tuberculosis*), which produces an infection of the lymph nodes that drain the digestive system, and can also very rarely cause generalized tuberculosis. The main sources of infection are kitchen scraps and leftovers from tuberculosis sanatoriums. This infection has been confirmed in several countries in the Americas, Europe, and Africa.

Swine-to-swine transmission probably does not occur or, if it does, is insignificant. Intestinal lesions are hyperplastic, and ulcers that would cause the agent to be shed are not observed.

SHEEP AND GOATS: Tuberculosis in sheep is generally rare and sporadic. In the few cases described before 1970, the most important agent was *M. avium* and the second was *M. bovis*. Only two cases involved *M. tuberculosis*. In recent research in New Zealand stemming from a program to eradicate bovine tuberculosis, multiple cases of infection by *M. bovis* were confirmed among sheep sharing the same pasture with infected cattle. In one area, 597 sheep were given the tuberculin test on the inner thigh and 108 (18%) reactors were discovered. Lesions, mostly in the lymph nodes, were found in 43 (61%) out of 70 necropsies. The lungs were affected in eight sheep (Davidson *et al.*, 1981). A similar result was observed in another region of New Zealand, on land where the prevalence of TB in cattle and opossums (*Trichosurus vulpecula*) was high. The tuberculin test yielded positive results in 11% of the sheep, and was judged to have a sensitivity of 81.6% and a specificity of 99.6% (Cordes *et al.*, 1981).

Prevalence in goats seems to be low. In countries with advanced programs to eradicate bovine tuberculosis, the infection in goats is monitored, since this species is not only susceptible to *M. bovis*, but frequently suffers from pulmonary tuberculosis and is able to reinfect cattle. Nannies also suffer from tuberculous mastitis and their milk may constitute a danger to the consumer. In addition to *M. bovis*, goats are also susceptible to *M. avium* and *M. tuberculosis*, and the latter agent sometimes causes generalized processes. Little is known about the disease's occurrence in goats in Latin America, since these animals are usually not slaughtered commercially.

HORSES: Tuberculosis is infrequent in horses. In countries where the incidence of bovine infection is high, the principal agent of the disease in horses is *M. bovis*. The infection's predominant portal of entry is the digestive system. Lesions are generally confined to the lymph nodes of the digestive tract, where they produce a tissue reaction that resembles tumors. Some cases of generalized infection, caused by both *M. bovis* and *M. avium*, have been described. Often, no lesions are found in infections produced by *M. avium*. In Germany, the avian bacillus was isolated from 30% of 208 horses with no apparent lesions.

M. tuberculosis is seldom isolated from horses. In a study carried out some time ago, only 13 of 241 typed strains corresponded to the human bacillus (Francis, 1958).

The disease is very rare in asses and mules.

It is interesting to note that horses are hypersensitive to tuberculin, and thus the allergenic test does not give reliable results.

CATS AND DOGS: Dogs are very resistant to experimental tuberculosis infection. Recorded cases in this species are probably due to massive and repeated exposure brought about by living with human patients or eating contaminated food many times. Infection may be produced by aerosols, or by ingestion of sputa, milk, and viscera. Almost 75% of the cases are due to the human bacillus and the rest to the bovine. The clinical picture is not characteristic. The only symptoms found in eight tuberculous dogs in New York City were anorexia, weight loss, lethargy, vomiting, and leukocytosis. Radiology revealed pleural pericardial effusion, ascites, and hepatomegaly. Granulomatous lesions in soft tissues were similar to those observed in neoplasias (Liu et al., 1980). Infection mainly localizes in the lungs or mesenteric lymph nodes; intestinal ulcers and renal lesions are sometimes found as well. Consequently, dogs can shed bacilli by coughing as well as in the saliva, feces, and urine. It has also been demonstrated that the etiologic agent can be present in the pharynx and feces of dogs living in the same house with tuberculous patients even when the animals show no tuberculous lesions. Although few cases of transmission from dog to man have been confirmed, a tuberculous dog (or even an apparently healthy animal living with a tuberculous patient) certainly represents a potential risk and should be destroyed. A dog infected with *M. bovis* can, in turn, be a potential source of reinfection for cattle.

Cats also have a great natural resistance to tuberculous lesions. *M. bovis* is the most common pathogen in cats, and has been isolated in 90% of the cases. The agent gains entry via the digestive tract when milk or viscera containing tuberculosis bacilli is consumed. Cat-to-cat transmission of *M. bovis* in a scientific institution in Australia has recently been described (Issac et al., 1983). In countries where bovine tuberculosis has been brought under control, infection in cats is rare, and the few recorded cases have been caused by *M. tuberculosis* and occasionally *M. avium-intracellulare*. Destructive lesions are found occasionally; pneumonitis and tuberculosis of the skin are frequent. Several cases of reinfection of cattle herds by tuberculous cats have been described.

WILD ANIMALS: Animals living in the wild, far from man and domestic animals, generally do not contract tuberculosis. On the other hand, captive animals in zoos, on pelt farms, in laboratories, and in family homes may be exposed to infection. Monkeys are susceptible to both *M. tuberculosis* and *M. bovis*. Almost 70% of the isolations from these animals are strains of the human bacillus and the rest are the bovine type. The disease is contracted via the respiratory or digestive route. The infection can be propagated from monkey to monkey and constitutes a grave problem for colonies kept in scientific institutions and zoos. In turn, these animals can retransmit the infection to man. It is not unusual to find tuberculous pet monkeys; they may become infected before their acquisition or by contact with a family member. In France, infection due to *M. africanum* has been described in three chimpanzees and a *Cercopithecus* monkey. Three of these animals belonged to a scientific center and one of the chimpanzees to a zoo. Since *M. africanum* has properties intermediate between those of *M. bovis* and *M. tuberculosis*, it is possible that infection by *M. africanum* was not described earlier in primates because strains isolated previously were misidentified. It still has not been determined whether the infection was transmitted to the primates by man or acquired in their natural forest habitat (Thorel, 1980).

Outbreaks have been described in farmed fur-bearing animals, such as mink and silver foxes; the source of infection was meat or viscera of cattle or of tuberculous fowl. Tuberculosis has been found in wild species of ungulates and carnivores on several nature preserves, and the infection has been confirmed in several animal species in zoos in Latin America and other parts of the world.

In the southwest of England, reinfection of cattle herds has been attributed to the high rate of *M. bovis* infection found in badgers (*Meles meles*). When the badger population was eliminated from certain areas and prevented from repopulating them, transmission to cattle was halted, thus proving the causal relationship between infection in these species (Wilesmith, 1983). A similar relationship was found between infection in a species of opossum (*Trichosurus vulpecula*) and cattle in New Zealand.

Source of Infection and Mode of Transmission (Figure 20): The principal reservoir of *M. bovis* is cattle, which can transmit the infection to many mammalian species, including man. Man contracts the infection primarily by ingesting the agent in raw milk and milk products, and secondarily by inhaling it.

Tuberculosis is transmitted between cattle mainly via aerosols. The digestive route is important before weaning takes place.

Tuberculosis in swine, goats, and sheep has as its principal source of infection cattle, fowl, and at times man. Swine are infected enterogenously, and retransmission to other swine, to other species, and to man is thought to be rare. Goats can constitute a source of infection for man and for cattle.

Dogs often contract the infection from humans and less frequently from cattle. They may in turn retransmit it to man and cattle. Dogs become infected via the

Figure 20. Tuberculosis (*Mycobacterium bovis*). Mode of transmission.

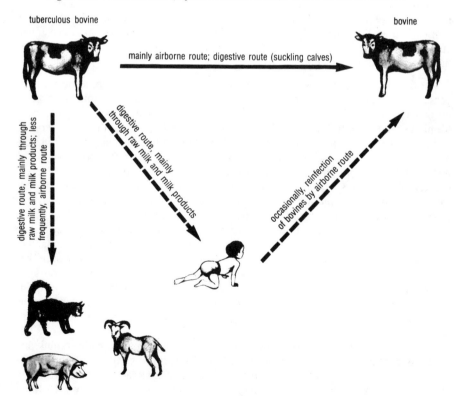

digestive and respiratory tracts. The principal source of infection for cats is cattle and, to a lesser degree, man. The portal of entry is mainly oral. At times cats can be a source of infection for cattle and humans.

Among wild animals in captivity, monkeys are particularly interesting because of their susceptibility to *M. tuberculosis* and *M. bovis*. They contract the infection from man by inhaling the agent. Tuberculous nonhuman primates constitute a health risk for humans.

Role of Animals in the Epidemiology of the Disease: Human-to-human transmission of animal tuberculosis is exceptional. The infection depends on an animal source.

Diagnosis: Since the human infections caused by *M. tuberculosis* and *M. bovis* are clinically and radiologically indistinguishable, diagnosis can only be achieved by isolating and typing the etiologic agent. In this regard, it should be noted that *M. bovis* grows poorly in glycerin-containing culture media, such as Lowenstein-Jensen, that are used for culturing *M. tuberculosis*.

For routine diagnosis of tuberculosis in cattle the only available method is the tuberculin test. The most appropriate tuberculin is the purified protein derivative (PPD), since it is specific and not very costly to produce. It has been made from both human and bovine strains, but research in recent years has shown that tuberculin produced with a strain of *M. bovis* is more specific. In most countries only a mammalian tuberculin is used in eradication campaigns, and the comparative test (simultaneous application of mammalian and avian tuberculin) is reserved for problem herds in which paraspecific sensitization is suspected. The test is carried out by intradermal inoculation of 0.1 ml of tuberculin into the skin of the caudal fold or the wide part of the neck, depending on standards established in the country. It should be borne in mind that the skin of the neck is much more sensitive than that of the caudal fold. The number of tuberculin units injected varies from 2,000 to 10,000 IU in different countries. In general, the test will be more sensitive but less specific when larger doses are used. The effectiveness of the test depends not only on the tuberculin and its correct application, but also on the response capability of the infected animal. Some herds include anergic animals, generally old cows with advanced tuberculosis. Clinical examinations and knowledge of the herd's history can help ensure complete diagnosis.

The tuberculin test may also be applied to goats, sheep, and swine with satisfactory results. In swine, the preferred inoculation site is the base of the ear, with 2,000 IU of mammalian and avian tuberculin; in goats and sheep the tuberculin can be applied to the eyelid, the fold of the tail, or the inner thigh.

The tuberculin test is unsatisfactory for horses, dogs, and cats. Some research has suggested that the test using BCG might give better results in dogs. For monkeys the intrapalpebral test is recommended, as well as radiography in advanced cases.

Control: Prevention of human infection by *M. bovis* consists of the pasteurization of milk, vaccination with BCG, and, above all, control and eradication of bovine tuberculosis.

The only rational approach to reducing and eliminating losses produced by the infection in cattle and preventing human cases caused by *M. bovis* consists of establishment of a control and eradication program for bovine tuberculosis. Eradication campaigns are usually carried out by administering tuberculin tests repeatedly until all infected animals are discovered, and eliminating reactors from the herd.

This method has given excellent results in all countries that have undertaken eradication campaigns. At present, many developed countries are free or practically free of bovine tuberculosis. In developing countries, the inability of governments to compensate owners for the destruction of reactors hinders establishment of eradication programs and makes it necessary to find other incentives, such as a surcharge on milk. Campaigns should be begun in regions of low prevalence, where replacing reacting animals is easier, and later extended to areas of higher prevalence. The success of a program depends on the cooperation of the meat inspection agencies in order that tuberculosis-free herds are correctly certified, activities evaluated, and appropriate epidemiologic surveillance maintained. The cooperation of health services is also important to prevent persons with tuberculosis from working with animals and either infecting or sensitizing them.

Controlling tuberculosis caused by *M. bovis* in its principal reservoir, cattle, is the best method of preventing transmission to other species, including man.

Bibliography

Argentine National Commission on Zoonoses, Subcommission on Bovine Tuberculosis. *La tuberculosis bovina en la República Argentina*. Buenos Aires, Pan American Zoonoses Center, 1982.

Burganova, B., and M. Nagoyova. Tuberculosis caused by *Mycobacterium bovis* in the human population of the USSR in 1979-1983. *Stud Pneumol Phtiseol Cech* 45:342-349, 1985.

Centrángolo, A., L. S. de Marchesini, C. Isola, I. N. de Kantor, and M. Di Lonardo. El *Mycobacterium bovis* como causa de tuberculosis humana. *Actas 13er Congreso Argentino de Tisiología*. Mar del Plata, 1973.

Collins, C. H., M. D. Yates, and J. M. Granges. A study of bovine strains of *Mycobacterium tuberculosis* isolated from humans in South-east England, 1977-1979. *Tubercle* 62:113-116, 1981.

Collins, C. H., and J. M. Granges. The bovine tubercle bacillus. *J Appl Bacteriol* 55:13-29, 1983.

Cordes, D. O., J. A. Bullians, D. E. Lake, and M. E. Carter. Observations on tuberculosis caused by *Mycobacterium bovis* in sheep. *NZ Vet J* 29:60-62, 1981.

Daniel, T. M., G. L. de Murillo, J. A. Sawyer, A. M. Griffin, E. Pinto, S. M. Debanne, P. Espinoza, and E. Cespedes. Field evaluation of enzyme-linked immunosorbent assay for the serodiagnosis of tuberculosis. *Am Rev Respir Dis* 134:662-665, 1986.

Davidson, R. M., M. R. Alley, and N. S. Beatson. Tuberculosis in a flock of sheep. *NZ Vet J* 29:1-2, 1981.

Feldman, W. H. Tuberculosis. *In*: Hull, T. G. (Ed.), *Diseases Transmitted from Animals to Man*, 5th ed. Springfield, Illinois, Thomas, 1963.

Fernández Salazar, M., V. Gómez Pando, and L. Domínguez Paredes. *Mycobacterium bovis* en la patología humana en el Perú. *Bol Inf Colegio Med Vet Perú* 14:16-18, 1983.

Francis, J. *Tuberculosis in Animals and Man. A Study in Comparative Pathology*. London, Cassel, 1958.

Francis, J., C. L. Choi, and A. H. Frost. The diagnosis of tuberculosis in cattle with special reference to bovine PPD tuberculin. *Aust Vet J* 49:246-251, 1973.

García Carrillo, C., and B. Szyfres. *La tuberculosis animal en las Américas y su transmisión al hombre*. Rome, Food and Agriculture Organization of the United Nations, 1963.

Gee, R. W. Bovine tuberculosis eradication in Australia. *Rev Sci Tech Off Int Epizoot* 5:789-793, 1986.

Griffith, A. S. Bovine tuberculosis in man. *Tubercle* 18:528-543, 1937. Cited in Collins and Granges, 1983.

Hawthorne, V. M., and I. M. Lauder. Tuberculosis in man, dog and cat. *Am Rev Respir Dis* 85:858-869, 1962.

Horsburgh, C. R., U. G. Mason III, D. C. Farhi, and M. D. Iseman. Disseminated infection with *Mycobacterium avium-intracellulare*. A report of 13 cases and a review of the literature. *Medicine* 64, 1985.

Huitema, H. Development of a comparative test with equal concentrations of avian and bovine PPD tuberculin for cattle. *Tijdschr Diergeneeskd* 98:396-407, 1973.

Isaac, J., J. Whitehead, J. W. Adams, M. D. Barton, and P. Coloe. An outbreak of *Mycobacterium bovis* infection in cats in an animal house. *Aust Vet J* 60:243-245, 1983.

Kantor, I. N. de, N. Marchevsky, and L. W. Lesslie. Respuesta al PPD en pacientes tuberculosos afectados por *M. tuberculosis* y por *M. bovis*. *Medicina (B Aires)* 36:127-130, 1976.

Kantor, I. N. de, J. Pereira, J. Miquet, and R. Rovére. Pouvoir pathogéne experimental de *Mycobacterium africanum* pour les bovins. *Bull Acad Vet Fr* 52:499-503, 1979.

Kantor, I. N. de, and A. Bernardelli. Identificación preliminar de micobacterias aisladas en muestras de origen humano o animal. *Rev Med Vet (B Aires)* 68:86-90, 1987.

Karlson, A. G. Tuberculosis. *In*: Dunne, H. W. (Ed.), *Diseases of Swine*, 3rd ed. Ames, Iowa State University Press, 1970.

Kleeberg. H. H. Tuberculosis and other mycobacterioses. *In*: Hubbert, W. T., W. F. McCulloch, and P. R. Schnurrenberger (Eds.), *Diseases Transmitted from Animals to Man*, 6th ed. Springfield, Illinois, Thomas, 1975.

Konyha, L. D., and J. P. Kreier. The significance of tuberculin tests in the horse. *Am Rev Respir Dis* 103:91-99, 1971.

Liu, S., I. Weitzman, and G. G. Johnson. Canine tuberculosis. *J Am Vet Med Assoc* 177:164-167, 1980.

Magnus, K. Epidemiological basis of tuberculosis eradication. 3. Risk of pulmonary tuberculosis after human and bovine infection. *Bull WHO* 35:483-508, 1966.

Magnus, K. Epidemiological basis of tuberculosis eradication. 5. Frequency of pulmonary calcification after human and bovine infections. *Bull WHO* 36:703-718, 1967.

Matthias, D. Vergleichende Pathologie der Tuberkulose der Tiere. *In*: Meissner, G., and A. Schmiedel (Eds.), *Mykobakterien und Mykobakterielle Krankheiten*, Teil VII. Jena, German Democratic Republic, Fischer, 1970.

Myers, J. A., and J. H. Steele. *Bovine Tuberculosis Control in Man and Animals*. St. Louis, Missouri, Green, 1969.

Pan American Health Organization. *First International Seminar on Bovine Tuberculosis for the Americas*. Santiago, Chile, 21-25 September 1970. Washington, D.C., PAHO, 1972. (Scientific Publication 258.)

Patterson, A. B., J. T. Stamp, and J. N. Ritchie. Tuberculosis. *In*: Estableforth, A. W., and I. A. Galloway (Eds.), *Infectious Diseases of Animals*. London, Butterworths, 1959.

Roswurm, J. D., and L. K. Konyha. The comparative-cervical tuberculin test as an aid to diagnosing bovine turberculosis. *Proc Annu Meet US Anim Health Assoc* 77:368-389, 1973.

Ruch, T. C. *Diseases of Laboratory Primates*. Philadelphia and London, Saunders, 1959.

Schliesser, T. Epidemiologie der Tuberkulose der Tiere. *In*: Meissner, G., and A. Schmiedel (Eds.), *Mykobakterien und Mykobakterielle Krankheiten*, Teil VII. Jena, German Democratic Republic, Fischer, 1970.

Schmiedel, A. Erkrankungen der Menschen durch *Mycobacterium bovis*. *In*: Meissner, G., and A. Schmiedel (Eds.), *Mykobakterien und Mykobakterielle Krankheiten*, Teil VII. Jena, German Democratic Republic, Fischer, 1970.

Schonfeld, J. K. Human-to-human spread of infection by *Mycobacterium bovis*. *Tubercle* 63:143-144, 1982.

Sjorgen, I., and I. Sutherland. Studies of tuberculosis in man in relation to infection in cattle. *Tubercle* 56:113-127, 1974.

Tarara, R., M. A. Suleman, R. Sapolsky, M. J. Wabomba, and J. G. Else. Tuberculosis in wild olive baboons, *Papio cynocephalus anubis* (Lesson), in Kenya. *J Wildl Dis* 21:137-140, 1985.

Thorel, M. F. Isolation of *Mycobacterium africanum* from monkeys. *Tubercle* 61:101-104, 1980.

Vestal, A. L. *Procedures for the isolation of Mycobacteria.* Atlanta, Georgia, Centers for Disease Control of the USA, 1969. (Public Health Publication 1995.)

Wiessmann, J. Die Rindertuberkulose beim Menschen und ihre epidemiologische Bedentung fur die Veterinarmedizin. *Schweiz Arch Tierheilkd* 102:467-471, 1960.

Wilesmith, J. W. Epidemiological features of bovine tuberculosis in cattle herds in Great Britain. *J Hyg (Camb)* 90:159-176, 1983.

Winkler, W. G., and N. B. Gale. Tuberculosis. *In*: Davis, J. W., L. H. Karstad, and D. O. Trainer (Eds.), *Infectious Diseases of Wild Mammals.* Ames, Iowa State University Press, 1970.

World Health Organization. *Joint FAO/WHO Expert Committee on Zoonoses.* Third Report. Geneva, WHO, 1967. (Technical Report Series 378.)

SUMMARY OF BACTERIAL ZOONOSES

The following is a summary of bacterial zoonoses adapted from the report of a World Health Organization Expert Committee, with the participation of the Food and Agriculture Organization (*Bacterial and Viral Zoonoses*, Geneva, WHO, Technical Report Series 682, 1982). It presents a synopsis of the principal characteristics of these diseases and serves as a quick reference on this subject.

The table provides an easy-to-use guide to bacterial zoonoses. The most important zoonoses are described individually and more completely, while the lesser ones are summarized more briefly. As a convenience to the reader, diseases of special significance are designated with a black dot (•); these diseases constitute a danger because they are associated with epidemics or because they cause high rates of morbidity and/or mortality; some of them are of interest because they have recently begun to pose problems.

Each of the entries for a given disease provides up-to-date information, including the name and distinctive characteristics of the etiologic agent, its main reservoirs, a brief description of the epidemiology, a summary of the clinical picture, and diagnosis and control methods. The table has been prepared in a manner designed to facilitate its use as a quick and simple reference for public health officials and laboratories as well as for professors and students of medicine and veterinary medicine. Although details have not been included in the table, it provides a wide range of information that is sufficient to give a balanced overview of knowledge presently available on zoonoses, in a simple and succinct form.

The headings of the different columns in the table are as follows:

Causative agent: Name of the bacterium or virus, with a brief description of its characteristics.

Disease: Common name of the clinical disease, and synonyms.

Reservoir: Vertebrate or invertebrate animals in which the etiologic agent completes its cycle of infection in nature; these animals serve as a source of transmission to other hosts.

Epizootiology/epidemiology: Sources of infection, modes of transmission, and portals of entry of the pathogenic agents (in man); any other important epidemiologic characteristic is also mentioned.

Principal animals: Vertebrates usually infected in nature; this list is separate from the "reservoir" list when different or unusual hosts exist in nature.

Persons at risk: Classified by professional and social group. These groups are defined as follows:

GROUP I (*Agriculture*): Farmers or other people in close contact with livestock and their products.

GROUP II (*Animal-product processing and manufacture*): All personnel of abattoirs and of plants processing animal products or by-products.

GROUP III (*Forestry, outdoors*): Persons frequenting wild habitats for professional or recreational reasons.

GROUP IV (*Recreation*): Persons in contact with pets or wild animals in the urban environment.

GROUP V (*Clinics, laboratories*): Health care personnel who attend patients, and health workers (including laboratory personnel) who handle specimens, corpses, or organs.

GROUP VI (*Epidemiology*): Public health professionals who do field research.

GROUP VII (*Emergency*): People affected by catastrophes, refugees, or people temporarily living in crowded or highly stressful situations.

Occurrence: Places where the disease has been observed to occur naturally.

Clinical form: The most noticeable clinical symptoms in naturally infected animals and in man, especially those important for diagnosis.

Diagnosis: Indicated laboratory tests; clinical diagnostic tests (when they are characteristic).

Control: Appropriate methods to prevent transmission; protective and therapeutic measures.

BACTERIAL ZOONOSES

Causative agent	Disease	R = Reservoir E = Epizootiology/ epidemiology PA = Principal animals PR = Persons at risk	O = Occurrence CA = Clinical form: animals CM = Clinical form: man	D = Diagnosis C = Control
Bacillus anthracis Gram-positive, aerobic bacillus; forms highly resistant, long-lived spores.	● Anthrax (woolsorters' disease (pulmonary); malignant pustule (cutaneous))	R. A complex of animals and their environment polluted with spores that survive for many years. E. Animal products, especially fertilizers, animal proteins, wool, hair, hides, leather, and soil or water containing spores. Direct contact or inhalation of spores. A laboratory hazard. PA. Herbivores and pigs. PR. Groups I, II, and V.	O. Worldwide, with endemic and sporadic cases. CA. Severe systemic disease: peracute in cattle, sheep, and goats; less severe in horses; chronic in pigs and dogs. CM. Localized persistent cutaneous pustules; pulmonary and gastrointestinal forms rare.	D. Blood film for characteristic bacteremia; culture; inoculation of laboratory animals; Ascoli precipitation test. C. Proper disposal by deep burial with disinfection or total incineration of unopened carcasses; disinfection of animal products, wool, and hair; dust control in factories; vaccination of animals and high-risk persons; therapy.
Borrelia species (spirochetes)	Tick-borne relapsing fever (Borreliasis, spirochetosis, recurrent typhus, spirochetal fever)	R. Wild animals and *Ornithodoros* ticks. E. *Ornithodoros* species of ticks spread the agent among wild animal hosts. Transovarial transmission in ticks. People exposed to tick bites. PA. Armadillos, opossums, weasels, tree squirrels, bats, mice; reported in horses and cattle. *Borrelia* spp. causing serious disease in geese, turkeys, and chickens are not zoonotic. PR. Groups, I, II, and IV.	O. World-wide except for Australia. Human cases are sporadic. CA. Considered to be inapparent. CM. Initial pyrexia of sudden onset and remission followed by recurrent attacks. Erythema, petechial hemorrhage, and jaundice may accompany recurrences.	E. Dark-field microscopy. Stained blood smears. Inoculation of suckling mice. C. Avoid tick-infested areas or wear protective clothing when entering these areas. Construct homes and maintain premises to keep out host animals. Chemotherapy.

Causative agent	Disease	R = Reservoir E = Epizootiology/epidemiology PA = Principal animals PR = Persons at risk	O = Occurrence CA = Clinical form: animals CM = Clinical form: man	D = Diagnosis C = Control
Brucella abortus (8 biotypes) *Brucella melitensis* (3 biotypes) *Brucella suis* (4 biotypes) *Brucella canis* Gram-negative, short rod-shaped bacterium; fastidious in culture.	● Brucellosis	R/PA. Cattle, sheep, goats, pigs, dogs, horses, camels, buffaloes, bison, deer, reindeer. E. Fetal membranes, aborted fetuses. Transmission by raw milk and milk products; inhalation of aerosols. PR. Groups I, II, III, and V.	O. Worldwide, especially in dairy areas, but eradicated from cattle in some countries. CA. Abortion and sterility in female; orchitis and spondylitis in male; lymphadenitis. Epididymitis in rams. Many cases inapparent. Infections chronic. CM. Acute or chronic undulant fever; clinical complications in various organ systems, e.g., lymphadenitis, hepatitis, osteomyelitis.	D. Direct culture. Inoculation of guinea pigs. Serological tests: agglutination, milk-ring test, complement fixation, 2-mercaptoethanol test, Coombs' test and others. C. Pasteurization of milk. Vaccination of cattle, sheep, and goats. Eradication by test and slaughter of infected animals.
Campylobacter fetus subsp. *fetus* and *C. jejuni* Gram-negative, comma- or S-shaped bacteria, thermoduric.	● Campylobacteriosis	R/PA. Cattle, sheep, pigs, dogs, poultry, and shellfish (?). E. Fecal contamination of milk and animal products and water. May survive inadequate heating. Transmitted by ingestion and close contact. PR. Groups I-VI.	O. Probably worldwide as an emerging zoonosis. CA. *C. jejuni*: considered inapparent in cattle; older reports of calf winter dysentery. *C. fetus* subsp. *fetus*: abortion and systemic disease in sheep; suspected hepatitis in poultry. CM. Diarrhea, abdominal cramps, headache, fever.	D. Direct culture of feces, blood, spinal fluid. Serological tests require serotype-specific antigens. C. Personal hygiene. Cleanliness in milk handling. Effective pasteurization of milk; proper cooking of food. Therapy.

196

Causative agent	Disease	R = Reservoir E = Epizootiology/ epidemiology PA = Principal animals PR = Persons at risk	O = Occurrence CA = Clinical form: animals CM = Clinical form: man	D = Diagnosis C = Control
Clostridium botulinum types A–G, toxins preformed in foods. Gram-positive, spore-forming bacilli, anaerobic.	● Botulism (foodborne intox- ication)	R/PA. Complex of environmental contamination and mammals, birds, and fish. E. Growth of organisms in fecal- or soil-contaminated foods stored under anaerobic condi- tions at pH >4.5, allowing toxin production. In infants, toxin may be produced by or- ganisms multiplying in intes- tines. PR. General population.	O. Worldwide CA. Types C and D mostly in ani- mals, A and C in fowl. Neu- rological disease. CM. Mostly types A, B, E, and F. Weakness, oculomotor and other motor cranial nerve pa- ralysis. Death may ensue by respiratory paralysis.	D. Laboratory cultures of foods or feces. Detection of toxin in suspected food or in serum, stomach contents, or feces of patients by animal inoculation. C. Hygienic precautions and regu- latory inspection of industrial kitchens. Proper storage of processed foods. Proper cook- ing of stored foods. Toxin inac- tivated by boiling for 3 min- utes. Therapeutic use of anti- toxins.
Clostridium perfringens type A Gram-positive, spore-forming, anaerobic, rod-shaped bacterium.	*Clostridium perfringens* food poisoning	R. Soil, water, intestinal tracts of animals. E. Fecal- or soil-contaminated food, stored under conditions permitting anaerobic multi- plication of organisms. Ex- posure is by ingestion. Toxin is produced in the intestine. PA. Many domestic and wild ani- mals. PR. General population.	O. Worldwide. CA. Demonstrated experimentally only. CM. Acute gastroenteritis with ab- dominal pain, usually no vomiting.	D. Laboratory culture of remain- ing food. Clinical signs of dis- ease. C. Storage of foods, especially those with meat sauces, above 60°C or below 4°C. Thorough reheating of unrefrigerated foods.

Causative agent	Disease	R = Reservoir E = Epizootiology/ epidemiology PA = Principal animals PR = Persons at risk	O = Occurrence CA = Clinical form: animals CM = Clinical form: man	D = Diagnosis C = Control
Clostridium perfringens type C Gram-positive, spore-forming, anaerobic, rod-shaped bacterium.	Enteritis necroticans (pigbel disease) (a foodborne disease)	R. Ubiquitous in New Guinea soil; intestine of man and pig. E. Disease occurs when large amounts of unhygienically prepared pork are ingested by children, particularly those who eat a lot of sweet potato, which inhibits trypsin. Toxin is produced in the intestine. PA. Pigs. PR. Undernourished children with poor immunity.	O. Common in New Guinea highlands. Not yet looked for elsewhere. CA. No disease in animals. CM. Many clinical forms, but the mild form (with upper abdominal pain, vomiting, and diarrhea followed by constipation) is most common.	D. Culture of feces or intestinal contents. C. Improved pig husbandry; preventing ingestion of pork by undernourished children.
Clostridium tetani Gram-positive, spore-forming, anaerobic, rod-shaped bacterium.	● Tetanus	R. Complex of environmental contamination and animals, especially equines. E. Infection of wounds with spores in soil or dust-contaminated agents. PA. All mammals. Horses (and man) most susceptible; dogs resistant; cats and birds highly resistant. PR. Groups I, II, III, IV, V.	O. Worldwide. Sporadic cases. Episodes especially in subtropical and tropical countries. CA/CM. Toxin produced in wounds causes neurologic effects with painful muscular contractions, paralysis, death.	D. Clinical signs. Direct anaerobic culture of specimens from deep wounds. C. Immunization of children and adults. Prompt wound treatment and injection of antitoxin or booster dose of vaccine (toxoid). Chemotherapy.

Causative agent	Disease	R = Reservoir E = Epizootiology/ epidemiology PA = Principal animals PR = Persons at risk	O = Occurrence CA = Clinical form: animals CM = Clinical form: man	D = Diagnosis C = Control
Erysipelothrix rhusiopathiae Gram-positive, slender, rod-shaped bacterium.	Erysipelas (in animals) Erysipeloid (in man)	R/PA. Complex interaction between environment and animals, especially pigs, turkeys, rodents, fish, and molluscs. E. Contact infection through wound contamination, directly or by means of soil or water. PR. Groups I, II, and III.	O. Worldwide CA. Septicemic disease in pigs, may cause chronic arthritis or cutaneous eruptions. Septicemic disease in turkeys with cyanosis and turgid comb and snood. CM. Skin lesions surrounding contaminated wound, usually on hands and fingers. Erythema, edema, arthritis, pain. Rarely septicemia or endocarditis.	D. Laboratory culture from cutaneous lesions or in animals from blood, joints, or tissues. Mouse inoculation sensitive. C. Vaccination and chemotherapy of pigs and turkeys. Rodent control. Hygienic care of skin abrasions or injuries. Chemotherapy.
Francisella tularensis Gram-negative, bipolar staining, small, rod-shaped bacterium. Two types, A and B, A being more virulent.	Tularemia (rabbit fever, Ohara's disease, deer-fly fever)	R. Wild rodents, lagomorphs, birds, dogs. E. Maintained in nature in tick-animal cycle. Transmitted to livestock and birds by ticks and biting insects. Transmitted to people by ticks, deerflies, mosquitoes, fleas, horseflies, and other arthropods, as well as by contact, ingestion, or inhalation. PA. Wild rodents, lagomorphs, dogs, beavers, birds. Epidemics reported in sheep, minks, and foxes. PR. Groups I, II, and V.	O. Foci in northern hemisphere. CA. Susceptibility varies among species from fatal septicemic disease to inapparent. Caseous lymphadenitis and grayish white splenic foci in fatal cases. Sheep abortions and high mortality, pulmonary foci, and lymphadenitis. CM. Clinical disease varies with portal of entry. Ulceroglandular form with regional lymphadenitis; oculoglandular, pulmonary, and typhoid forms.	D. Clinical signs and history of possible exposure. Laboratory culture, immunofluorescence tests, skin tests, serological tests, inoculation of laboratory animals. Inspection of meat of wild hares killed in endemic foci. C. Rodent and arthropod control. Occupational and personal protection in high-risk areas. Avoid drinking from possibly contaminated streams. Live attenuated vaccine inoculation of populations at risk.

Causative agent	Disease	R = Reservoir E = Epizootiology/ epidemiology PA = Principal animals PR = Persons at risk	O = Occurrence CA = Clinical form: animals CM = Clinical form: man	D = Diagnosis C = Control
Fusobacterium necrophorum Gram-negative, anaerobic, non–spore-forming bacillus. Extremely pleomorphic.	"Necrobacillosis"	R. Cattle, sheep, goats, horses, pigs, and birds. E. Exposure of wounds or abraded skin to infected tissue or to fomites contaminated by infected tissue. PA. Cloven-hoofed animals. PR. Groups I and II.	O. Worldwide. A disease of low incidence in man. CA. Necrotic lesions of interdigital area, coronary bands, and joints. Arthritis. Liver abscesses. CM. Necrotic pustule at site of inoculation; regional lymphadenitis. Rarely a systemic disease with arthritis, pneumonia, internal abscesses.	D. Laboratory culture, inoculation of laboratory animals. C. Personal hygiene. Use of gloves and protective clothing.
Leptospira interrogans Twenty serogroups subdivided into at least 180 serovars, including icterohemorrhagiae, canicola, pomona, hardjo, and grippotyphosa as important pathogens.	• Leptospirosis (Weil's disease, swineherd's disease, swamp fever, mud fever)	R/PA. Rodents, domestic and wild mammals, possibly reptiles. Contaminated soil and water (neutral or alkaline). Serovars linked to preferred hosts. E. Infection from animal to animal and from animal to man by water or food contaminated with infectious urine. Penetrates mucosa or broken skin; rarely by ingestion. Venereal transmission in animals. A laboratory hazard. PR. Groups I-V.	O. Worldwide. Some serovars universal, others regional or local. CA. Variable. Inapparent to an illness causing icterus, bloody diarrhea, uremia, mastitis. Periodic ophthalmia in horses. Carrier state common. CM. Variable. Inapparent to acute febrile illness with fever, conjunctivitis, lymphadenitis, hepatitis and jaundice, nephritis, meningitis.	D. Clinical signs, direct examination of specimens by dark-field microscopy. Direct culture from blood (acute phase) or urine (convalescence). Guinea pig or hamster inoculation and serum agglutination test. C. Occupational protection for persons at risk, e.g., protective clothing. Animal and human vaccines used in some countries. Avoid swimming in contaminated water. Rodent control. Drainage of wet areas. Vaccination available for animals affords clinical protection but does not prevent infection.

Causative agent	Disease	R = Reservoir E = Epizootiology/ epidemiology PA = Principal animals PR = Persons at risk	O = Occurrence CA = Clinical form: animals CM = Clinical form: man	D = Diagnosis C = Control
Listeria monocytogenes Gram-positive, very pleomorphic, rod-shaped bacteria. Many show clubbing. Seven serogroups, of which 1 and 4 are most common.	Listeriosis (mononucleosis)	R. Presumed complex interaction of contaminated soil, leaf litter, sewage, or silage above pH 4.5, and infected animals. E. Organism grows saprophytically in uncultivated soil, leaf litter, bird droppings, silage, sewage, animal manure. Present in tissues and feces of infected animals; may pass through animals' digestive tracts. Exposure oral or by inhalation, and possibly venereal. Transmission intrauterine or during birth. Sporadic in both animals and man. PA. Sheep, goats, cattle, chickens, turkeys, wild birds. Rare in pigs and dogs. PR. General population.	O. Worldwide. Apparently more common in temperate zones than in tropics. CA. Meningoencephalitis, abortion; septicemia in young. In poultry septicemia with degenerative lesions, meningoencephalitis. CM. Inapparent to influenzalike to meningitis or meningoencephalitis. Abortion, or infant is born with septicemia. Neonatal meningitis may lead to hydrocephalus.	D. Isolation of organisms by direct culture. Storage of brain specimens at 4°C for 2 weeks increases the isolations. Inoculation of mice. Serological tests cross-react with enterococci and staphylococci. C. Hygiene, especially for pregnant women. Antibiotic therapy. Rodent control. Proper handling of silage. Pasteurization of milk.
Mycobacterium tuberculosis *Mycobacterium bovis* Acid-fast, slender bacilli. *M. tuberculosis* stains beaded.	● Tuberculosis[a]	R/PA. Man and domestic animals—cattle, sheep, goats, pigs, cats, dogs—and wild animals. E. Transmission among animals by respiratory droplets or fecal-orally. Infected dams may also transmit to offspring by milk. Transmission to people usually through milk or respiratory exposure, but may be through meat. PR. Groups I, II, IV, and V.	O. Worldwide, with great regional variation. In cattle, eradicated from some areas. CA. Pulmonary disease, tuberculosis lesions in lymph nodes, miliary lesions of internal organs. Usually very chronic, inapparent infection. CM. *M. bovis* may cause pulmonary disease, cervical adenitis, genitourinary disease, bone and joint disease, or meningitis.	E. Intradermal tuberculin tests used in animals and people. Radiography used in human patients. Culture and identification. C. Elimination of sick and tuberculin-reacting livestock. Eliminate infected pets. Keep infected people away from pigs, dogs, and cattle. BCG vaccine and chemotherapy used in man only.

[a] Disease in man caused by numerous other mycobacteria (such as *M. avium*) should not be called tuberculosis; for example, pulmonary disease, lymphadenitis, or granulomatous lesions caused by *M. avium* are rare, although infected poultry and fowl constitute a reservoir.

Causative agent	Disease	R = Reservoir E = Epizootiology/ epidemiology PA = Principal animals PR = Persons at risk	O = Occurrence CA = Clinical form: animals CM = Clinical form: man	D = Diagnosis C = Control
Pasteurella multocida, serogroups A, B, D, E. Gram-negative, small ovoid, rod-shaped bacteria, commonly bipolar staining.	Pasteurellosis	R. Man and many wild and domestic animals harboring the agent in the respiratory tract and mouth. E. Infections of man mostly by bites or scratches, especially from dogs and cats, or may be secondary to tooth extraction or oral infections. PA. Wild and domestic animals and birds, with or without clinical symptoms. PR. Groups III and IV.	O. Worldwide, but only sporadic clinical cases in man. Organism frequently isolated from animals and man. CA. Inapparent to acute septicemic disease. Carrier animals develop disease under stress. Respiratory disease, hemorrhagic septicemia with high mortality, mastitis. CM. Local cellulitis and inflammation of infected bites or scratches. Occasionally respiratory disease, tonsillitis, alveolitis; rarely septicemia.	D. Direct culture of exudate or tissue. In fowl, usually blood culture. Direct staining of blood. C. Prevention of bites by dogs and cats. Prompt treatment of bite wounds.
Pseudomonas mallei Gram-negative, long, slender, rod-shaped bacterium. Growth is slow in laboratory culture.	Glanders (malleus, farcy)	R. Asses, mules, horses. E. Contact with nasal secretions and exudates of infected animals; more rarely by ingestion of meat or by inhalation of aerosols from laboratory cultures. PA. Horses, asses, mules; occasionally carnivores ingesting infected meat. PR. Groups I-V.	O. Mostly eradicated, but endemic areas remain in East Africa, Asia, and South America. CA. Usually acute in asses and mules. In horses, usually chronic with nodules or pulmonary foci; necrotic ulcers of nostrils, pharynx, trachea; deep or superficial skin nodules or ulcers; and lymphadenitis. CM. Nodules and ulcers of nares, larynx, trachea, bronchi, and lungs; usually of skin at site of entry. Usually chronic.	D. Direct culture of nasal secretions and inoculation of hamsters. Intradermopalpebral mallein testing. C. Legislation to eliminate positive-reactor solipeds. Chemotherapy in human cases.

Causative agent	Disease	R = Reservoir E = Epizootiology/ epidemiology PA = Principal animals PR = Persons at risk	O = Occurrence CA = Clinical form: animals CM = Clinical form: man	D = Diagnosis C = Control
Pseudomonas pseudomallei Gram-negative, usually bipolar-staining, rod-shaped bacterium.	Melioidosis (Whitmore's disease)	R/PA. Rodents and most other mammals. Nonhuman primates. Surface water and soil, e.g., rice fields and oil-palm plantations. E. Organism lives in soil and water, and is transmitted to people through abraded skin. Infected animals and people may transport it. Most cases in rainy seasons. PR. Group I.	O. Tropical and subtropical areas. Rare but occasional episodes reported from Southeast Asia and tropical America. CA. Sheep: abscesses in viscera, joints, and lymph nodes; polyarthritis, coughing, nervous signs. Pigs: coughing and arthritis. CM. Fever, pneumonia, gastroenteritis; there may be visceral abscesses. In chronic cases, necrotic and granulomatous lesions of bones or soft tissues.	D. Direct culture. Inoculation of young hamsters. Hemagglutination test. C. Protective clothing, especially boots for workers at risk. Drainage of low-lying areas may be appropriate during outbreaks.
Salmonella About 2000 serotypes, variously named and with various host specificities, including more than 300 serotypes of *Salmonella arizonae*. Gram-negative, short, rod-shaped bacteria.	● Salmonellosis (foodborne disease)	R/PA. Complex of environmental contamination and infected humans, mammals, reptiles, and birds. E. Complex cycles of infection between man and animals via feces, sewage, and effluents contaminating drinking water and foods such as raw milk, frozen poultry, egg products, sausage, meat, and meat products. Arthropods may carry them mechanically. Transmitted by ingestion or by direct contact in hospitals. PR. Groups I-VI.	O. Worldwide. Regional variations in serotypes. CA. Wide clinical disease range. Septicemia and severe enteritis most common in the young. Infections in older animals manifested as enteritis, abortion, or are inapparent. Inapparent in turtles. CM. Zoonotic serotypes usually cause abdominal pains, nausea, vomiting, and diarrhea. Generalized infection occasional.	D. Direct culture and serotyping and/or phage-typing. C. Interrupt spread of infection through food chains by human-effluent treatment and proper disposal of animal wastes. Proper hygiene during slaughter, processing, handling, and cooking of foods of animal origin. Pasteurization of milk. Elimination of sources of infection. Proper use of antibiotic therapy to control the carrier state and prevent spread of antibiotic-resistant stains.

203

Causative agent	Disease	R = Reservoir E = Epizootiology/epidemiology PA = Principal animals PR = Persons at risk	O = Occurrence CA = Clinical form: animals CM = Clinical form: man	D = Diagnosis C = Control
Shigella dysenteriae *Shigella flexneri* *Shigella boydii* *Shigella sonnei* Gram-negative, short bacilli. The four species are divided into serotypes.	Shigellosis (bacillary dysentery) (foodborne disease)	R. Man and captive nonhuman primates. Dogs may be short-term shedders. E. Most infections are fecal-oral, from man to man, directly or indirectly via fomites. Can be transmitted by mechanical vectors such as flies. Transmission to nonhuman primates and other animals is usually from man. PA. Monkeys transmit the infection rapidly in captivity but do not maintain it in nature. Reported in dogs, horses, bats, and rattlesnakes. PR. Groups IV and V.	O. Worldwide as a human disease. Animal involvement is aberrant. CA. Abdominal pains, diarrhea, dehydration in nonhuman primates. Inapparent in other animals. CM. Fever; abdominal pains; mucoid, bloody diarrhea; dehydration.	D. Laboratory culture and serologic typing. C. Strict personal and environmental hygiene. Proper water supply and sewage disposal. Food protection. Education and supervision of food handlers. Fly control.
Staphylococcus aureus Gram-positive cocci, coagulase-positive, hemolytic. Many strains resistant to a variety of antibiotics.	Staphylococcal disease	R/PA. Variety of mammals, including man. Cattle and pets, as well as livestock and people receiving antibiotics. E. Transmitted from suppurative lesions or mastitis by direct contact, fomites, aerosols, or milk. Resistant to environmental inactivation. Interspecies transmission uncommon. PR. Groups I, II, and IV. Greatest risk in neonates, new mothers, debilitated and surgical patients, and patients receiving antibiotics or steroids.	O. Worldwide. Greatest hazard where human and animal infections are antibiotic-resistant. CA. Predominantly subclinical. Suppurative lesions in skin, lungs, mammary glands, rarely septicemia. CM. Predominantly subclinical. Suppurative impetigo, furuncles or boils, pneumonia, mastitis, osteomyelitis, or endocarditis. Wound infection, rarely septicemia. Toxic epidermal necrosis of infants.	D. Laboratory culture; phage-typing and antibiograms of epidemiological use. Clinical syndrome. C. Personal hygiene, especially for high-risk persons. Proper use of antibiotics in animals and man. Proper disinfection of contaminated materials; strict asepsis in surgery.

Causative agent	Disease	R = Reservoir E = Epizootiology/epidemiology PA = Principal animals PR = Persons at risk	O = Occurrence CA = Clinical form: animals CM = Clinical form: man	D = Diagnosis C = Control
Staphylococcus aureus toxins Gram-positive cocci; major toxins A–E. Nearly all enterotoxigenic strains are coagulase-positive. Toxins preformed in foods are heat resistant.	Staphylococcal food poisoning (staphylococcal enterotoxicosis)	R/PA. Man, especially nasal or skin carriers. Cattle and dogs may carry human or animal strains. E. Human carriers may infect cattle or animal products. Organisms multiply and produce toxins in foods which stand at warm temperatures for over 2 hours. Transmitted by ingestion. Purulent infections and staphylococcal mastitis in animals may be sources of organisms. PR. General population.	O. Worldwide. CA. Not recognized as enterotoxicosis in nature in animals. Experimentally, monkeys, dogs, and cats develop diarrhea. CM. Abdominal cramps, explosive diarrhea, nausea, and vomiting.	D. Clinical signs, culture and serologic detection of toxin in culture filtrate or in food extract C. Education and application of personal hygiene in handling and processing of food. Adequate and rapid refrigeration of foods of animal origin or maintenance at >60°C.
Streptobacillus moniliformis Gram-negative, curved bacterium. "*Spirillum minus*" Spiral bacterium.	"Rat-bite fever" (Haverhill fever, Sodoku, streptobacillosis, spirillosis)	R/PA. Rats, wild rats, and other rodents may be nasopharyngeal carriers. *S. moniliformis* also infects other animals, including turkeys. E. Rats are subclinical carriers. Infected saliva transmission by bites. Milk contamination by rats reported. PR. General population.	O. Worldwide; human cases sporadic only. CA. Usually inapparent in rats. *S. moniliformis* has caused lesions on gums of rats, polyarthritis and gangrene in mice, cervical suppurative lymphadenitis in guinea pigs, arthritis in turkeys. "*S. minus*" infection is inapparent. CM. *S. moniliformis* causes an influenzalike onset, then rash, arthralgia and polyarthritis, myalgia, and rarely endocarditis. "*S. minus*" causes recurrent fever and rash.	D. Direct culture of *S. moniliformis*; difficult to culture "*S. minus*." Dark-field microscopy. Serum agglutination test. Inoculation of mice. C. Rat control and avoidance of rat bites. Protective clothing, e.g., boots. Pasteurization of milk. Protect laboratory animals from exposure.

205

Causative agent	Disease	R = Reservoir E = Epizootiology/epidemiology PA = Principal animals PR = Persons at risk	O = Occurrence CA = Clinical form: animals CM = Clinical form: man	D = Diagnosis C = Control
Streptococcus pyogenes (Lancefield group A) Other *Streptococcus* spp. (Lancefield groups B, C, D, F, and G) Gram-positive cocci, beta-hemolytic; 14 Lancefield groups, A-H and K-P. Group A most common in man; B, C, D, F, and G sporadic. Groups B, C, and E most common in animals.	Streptococcal disease	R. Principal reservoir of Group A is man, rarely milk-producing cows. Many animals are infected with other groups. E. Usually transmitted from the throats of infected patients directly or via fomites. Cows may become infected from patients and shed the organism in milk. PA. Cattle, horses, pigs, and other animals. PR. General population.	O. Worldwide. CA. Group A udder infections are inapparent. Other groups cause mastitis, strangles, abortions, metritis, and sometimes septicemia. CM. Group A causes sore throat, scarlet fever, puerperal fever, erysipelas, ulcerative endocarditis, glomerulonephritis, and rheumatic fever. Other groups may cause similar symptoms.	D. Cultures from patients and suspected sources. Serotyping of isolates. C. Personal hygiene and disinfection. Milk hygiene, mastitis control, pasteurization. Chemotherapy.
Vibrio parahaemolyticus Gram-negative, curved bacterium; Kanagawa-positive strains are associated with disease in man.	● Disease caused by *Vibrio parahaemolyticus* (foodborne disease)	R/PA. Sea water, marine fish, and shellfish. E. Organisms ingested with inadequately cooked, contaminated, or infected seafoods. Cross contamination in the kitchen. PR. Group III.	O. Worldwide, particularly in coastal areas. CA. Inapparent. CM. Acute gastroenteritis with vomiting and diarrhea.	D. Laboratory culture of remaining food and feces of patients. Serotyping, Kanagawa test (hemolysis). C. Hygiene in handling seafoods. Adequate cooking before eating.

206

Causative agent	Disease	R = Reservoir E = Epizootiology/epidemiology PA = Principal animals PR = Persons at risk	O = Occurrence CA = Clinical form: animals CM = Clinical form: man	D = Diagnosis C = Control
Yersinia enterocolitica *Yersinia pseudotuberculosis* ssp. *pseudotuberculosis* Gram-negative, small rod-shaped bacteria, serologically cross-react with *Brucella*. Of six groups of *Y. enterocolitica*, only serotypes O3 and O9 are important in zoonoses.	Yersiniosis (diseases other than plague)	R. Wild rodents; pigs, especially for *Y. enterocolitica*; sometimes birds. *Y. enterocolitica* may multiply in meat at refrigerator temperatures. E. Not yet fully defined for *Y. enterocolitica*. Most important in transmission to man are pigs, sometimes wild rodents; role of other animals uncertain. Exposure is probably by ingestion. Dogs and cats are important in transmission of *Y. pseudotuberculosis* to man. PA. *Y. enterocolitica*: in domestic mammals, guinea pigs, hares, and monkeys. *Y. pseudotuberculosis*: in wild rodents, fowl, colonies of laboratory animals, and birds. PR. Groups I-V.	O. *Y. pseudotuberculosis* probably occurs worldwide in wild animals; sporadic in domestic animals. *Y. enterocolitica* is under study in the USA and northern Europe; world distribution is not elucidated. CA. Probably inapparent or diarrhea. Septicemia reported in young animals. CM. Acute ileitis, splenic and colonic abscesses, peritonitis, coleocystitis, occasionally resembling appendicitis; rarely septicemia, reactive arthritis, and diarrhea of varying severity.	D. Laboratory culture of feces by the cold enrichment technique. Serotyping crosses with *Brucella*. C. Hygiene to protect water and food from contamination. Freezing and proper handling and cooking of meat. Rodent and bird control. Control of *Y. pseudotuberculosis* is difficult owing to the large number of animal reservoirs.

Causative agent	Disease	R = Reservoir E = Epizootiology/ epidemiology PA = Principal animals PR = Persons at risk	O = Occurrence CA = Clinical form: animals CM = Clinical form: man	D = Diagnosis C = Control
Yersinia pseudotuberculosis ssp. *pestis* Gram-negative, bipolar staining, rod-shaped bacterium. Three biological variants: orientalis, antiqua, mediaevalis.	● Plague (pest, black death, bubonic plague, pneumonic plague, sylvatic plague)	R. Rodents and their fleas, especially *Xenopsylla cheopis* and *X. brasiliensis*; man. E. Generally, local rodents of low susceptibility maintain the infection. Highly susceptible species play a transmission role. Fleas become infected from rodents or carry the microbe mechanically. Exposure by flea bites. Inhalation exposure from man to man in pneumonic or tonsillar infections. A laboratory hazard. PA. At least 230 species of wild rodents worldwide. Synanthropic rats very susceptible. Dogs are quite resistant but may transmit to fleas. Cases in cats are increasingly reported, with possibility of pneumonic transmission to man. Camel cases also reported. PR. Groups III, IV, V, and VII.	O. Natural foci of sylvatic plague on all continents except Australia and New Zealand. CA. Animal disease similar to that in man. Inapparent or mild in resistant species. CM. Septicemic disease varying in severity. Bubonic, septicemic, and pneumonic forms. Tonsillar infections may be inapparent.	D. Direct cultures; inoculation of guinea pigs or mice. Immunofluorescent microscopic test. Direct examination of stained exudate from buboes. Early diagnosis is essential to prevent large outbreaks. C. Use of effective insecticides prior to rodenticiding. Rodent control. Vaccination of high-risk groups. Isolation and treatment of patients. International health regulations are applicable.

Part II

MYCOSES

ADIASPIROMYCOSIS

(117.9)

Synonyms: Adiaspirosis, haplomycosis, haplosporangiosis.

Etiology: *Emmonsia crescens* and *E. parva*, saprophytic soil fungi that characteristically form large spherules (adiaspores) in the lungs. In the tissular phase the fungus does not multiply. *E. crescens* is the most common agent in man and animals. *E. parva* occurs only in animals and forms smaller spherules than *E. crescens*.

Geographic Distribution: Worldwide. In the Americas, the infection has been confirmed in Canada, the United States, Honduras, Guatemala, Venezuela, and Argentina.

Occurrence in Man: Rare.

Occurrence in Animals: Frequent in small wild mammals. The disease has been confirmed in at least 124 mammalian species or subspecies (Leighton and Wobeser, 1978).

The Disease in Man and Animals: The only clinically significant form, in man as well as in animals, is pulmonary adiaspiromycosis. The few human cases have been diagnosed from biopsy or autopsy specimens. The fungus causes light gray to yellowish lesions in the lungs, without greatly affecting the general state of the animal's health. The number of spherules (adiaspores) in the lung tissue depends on the number of conidia (spores) inhaled. In the lungs, the fungus increases greatly in size (adiaspores of 4 microns can reach 500 microns or larger). The etiologic agent may also be found in other organs, though rarely; only two cases of human cutaneous adiaspiromycosis are known.

Source of Infection and Mode of Transmission: The great preponderance of pulmonary localizations indicates that the infection is contracted by inhalation. *E. crescens* has been isolated from the soil. Differences in the infection rates found in three very similar species of squirrels indicate that the fungus may be present in specific habitats (Leighton and Wobeser, 1978), possibly linked to the root microflora of certain plants. Other authors (cit. by Mason and Gauhwin, 1982) suggest that hunter-prey interactions affect its distribution: Upon ingesting infected animals, carnivores eliminate adiaspores in their feces, where the spores germinate and develop. This phenomenon was demonstrated in cats, in a mustelid (*Mustela nivalis*), and also in birds of prey. Thus, predators would play a role in disseminating the etiologic agent.

Diagnosis: Diagnosis may be made by observation of spherules in lung tissue, by stained histologic preparations, and by culture and inoculation into laboratory animals. The most effective method for detecting adiaspores in the lungs of animals is tissue digestion with a 2% sodium hydroxide solution (Leighton and Wobeser, 1978).

Bibliography

Ainsworth, G. C., and P. K. C. Austwick. *Fungal Diseases of Animals*, 2nd ed. Farnham Royal, Slough, England, Commonwealth Agricultural Bureau, 1973.

Alfassam, M. A., R. Bhatnagar, L. E. Lillie, and L. Roy. Adiaspiromycosis in striped skunks in Alberta, Canada. *J Wildl Dis* 22:13-18, 1986.

Cueva, J. A., and M. D. Little. *Emmonsia crescens* infection (adiaspiromycosis) in man in Honduras. *Am J Trop Med Hyg* 20:282-287, 1971.

Jellison, W. L. Adiaspiromycosis. *In*: Davis, J. W., L. H. Karstad, and D. O. Trainer (Eds.), *Infectious Diseases of Wild Mammals*. Ames, Iowa State University Press, 1970.

Leighton, F. A., and G. Wobeser. The prevalence of adiaspiromycosis in three sympatric species of ground squirrels. *J Wildl Dis* 14:362-365, 1978.

Mason, R. W., and M. Gauhwin. Adiaspiromycosis in South Australian hairy-nosed wombats (*Lasiorhinus latifrons*). *J Wildl Dis* 18:3-8, 1982.

Salfelder, K. New and uncommon opportunistic fungal infections. *In: Proceedings, Third International Conference on the Mycoses*. Washington, D.C., Pan American Health Organization, 1975. (Scientific Publication 304.)

ALGAL INFECTION

(686.9)

Etiology: In recent years mycologists have called attention to infections in man and animals produced by achlorophyllous unicellular algae of the genus *Prototheca* and, more recently, to infections by green algae similar to those of the genus *Chlorella*.

Protothecosis is an infection caused by the achlorophyllous algae *Prototheca wickerhamii* and *P. zopfii*. These algae reproduce asexually; hyaline cells, called sporangia when mature, produce from two to 20 endospores in their interior. The parent cell ruptures and frees the endospores, which enlarge and, upon maturing, repeat the reproductive cycle. The cells are round or oval, and from 2 to 16 microns in diameter. The taxonomic position of *Prototheca* is still uncertain, and some researchers question whether they are true alae or are fungi (Kaplan, 1978).

Geographic Distribution: The agents are distributed worldwide.

Occurrence in Man: Just over 30 cases of human protothecosis have been described, 60% of them in males. With the exception of one case due to *P. zopfii*, the causal agent in all other cases in which the species was identified has been *P. wickerhamii*. Recently, an infection caused by green algae has been described (Jones, 1983).

Occurrence in Animals: Protothecosis occurs in many animal species, but above all in cattle and dogs. Numerous isolations have been recorded (McDonald *et al.*, 1984). Most infections are due to *P. zopfii*. Occurrence is sporadic. Nevertheless, 23 infected animals were found in one dairy herd of 90 cows.

To date, 16 cases of infection by unicellular green algae are known, 12 in cattle and four in sheep.

The Disease in Man: The incubation period is unknown. Protothecosis manifests itself in two principal clinical forms (Kaplan, 1978). One is progressive ulcerative or verrucous lesions of the cutaneous and subcutaneous tissue on exposed skin. The other is chronic olecranon bursitis, with swelling and pain. In one case of dissemination, intraperitoneal and facial nodules were observed.

The Disease in Animals: The predominant form of protothecosis in cattle is mastitis, which at times may affect all four quarters of the udder. Temperature and appetite remain normal. Milk production in the affected quarter diminishes, and small clots may be found in the milk. The disease was reproduced experimentally using a small number of *P. zopfii* (McDonald *et al.*, 1984).

Protothecosis in dogs is usually a systemic disease, with dissemination of the infection to many internal organs. The severity of the disease varies with the organs affected. Debility and weight loss have been observed in all disseminated cases (Kaplan, 1978).

Infection caused by green algae in cattle and sheep is found post-mortem. Green-colored lesions were observed in the retropharyngeal and mandibular lymph nodes in cattle (Rogers *et al.*, 1980). In sheep, green-colored lesions were found in the lungs, liver, and kidneys (Kaplan *et al.*, 1983).

Source of Infection and Mode of Transmission: *Prototheca* spp. and green algae are saprophytes found in nature, principally in stagnant or slow-moving water. Man acquires the infection, possibly through skin lesions, when he comes into contact with contaminated water or other habitats of these agents. The profusion of the agents in the environment and the few human cases described indicate that they are not very virulent and that lowered host resistance is required for them to act as pathogens. In fact, five of nine patients with cutaneous or subcutaneous protothecosis had a preexisting or intercurrent disease. Similarly, seven of eight patients with the olecranon bursitis form had previously sustained a trauma to the elbow (Kaplan, 1978).

Cattle contract mastitis caused by *Prototheca zopfii* by contact with the alga in its natural environment, and the portal of entry is probably the teat. Little is known of predisposing conditions in dogs, which almost always manifest systemic protothecosis.

In cattle, the lymph nodes that are affected by green algae (retropharyngeal and mandibular) indicate that the infection is possibly contracted by ingestion of contaminated water. The few cases described in cattle and sheep suggest that these species are not very susceptible to green algal infection.

Diagnosis: Special stains such as Gomori, Gridley, and PAS (periodic acid–Schiff) applied to histologic sections from affected tissues permit detection of protothecas in all developmental stages. To determine the species, cultures or the immunofluorescence test with species-specific reagents must be used. The immunofluorescence technique can be used for cultures as well as for biopsy specimens stained with hematoxylin-eosin, but not for those stained with the methods mentioned above.

Green algae maintain their color in cultures and in fresh preparations.

Control: None.

Bibliography

Jones, J. W., H. W. McFadden, F. W. Chandler, W. Kaplan, and D. H. Conner. Green algal infection in a human. *Am J Clin Pathol* 80:102-107, 1983.

Kaplan, W. Prototothecosis and infections caused by morphologically similar green algae. *In*: *Proceedings, Fourth International Congress on Mycoses*. Washington, D.C., Pan American Health Organization, 1978. (Scientific Publication 356.)

Kaplan, W., F. W. Chandler, C. Choudary, and P. K. Ramachandran. Disseminated unicellular green algal infection in two sheep in India. *Am J Trop Med Hyg* 32:405-411, 1983.

McDonald, J. S., J. L. Richard, and N. F. Cheville. Natural and experimental bovine intramammary infection with *Prototheca zopfii*. *Am J Vet Res* 45:592-595, 1984.

Rogers, R. J., M. D. Connole, J. Norton, A. Thomas, P. W. Ladds, and J. Dickson. Lymphadenitis of cattle due to infection with green algae. *J Comp Pathol* 90:1-9, 1980.

ASPERGILLOSIS

(117.3)

Synonyms: Pneumonomycosis, aspergillomycosis, bronchomycosis (in animals).

Etiology: *Aspergillus fumigatus* and occasionally other species of the genus *Aspergillus*, such as *A. flavus*, *A. nidulans*, *A. niger*, and *A. terreus*. These saprophytic fungi are common components of the soil microflora; they play an important role in the decomposition of organic matter.

Geographic Distribution: The fungus is ubiquitous and has a worldwide distribution. The disease has no particular distribution.

Occurrence in Man: Aspergillosis occurs sporadically and is uncommon. Its incidence, like that of other opportunistic mycoses[1] (candidiasis, zygomycosis), is increasing because of the growing use of antibiotics, antimetabolites and corticosteroids. It is frequently associated with advanced cases of cancer.

Occurrence in Animals: Sporadic cases have been described in many species of mammals and birds, domestic as well as wild. The disease in fowl and cattle (mycotic abortions) has some economic importance. The incidence is low in adult domestic fowl, but outbreaks in chicks and poults can cause considerable losses on some farms.

The Disease in Man: Aspergillosis establishes itself in patients debilitated by chronic diseases (such as diabetes, cancer, tuberculosis, deep mycoses) and diseases of the immune system, as well as in those treated over a prolonged period with antibiotics, antimetabolites, and corticosteroids. Persons occupationally exposed for

---

[1] Mycoses that attack debilitated persons or those treated over a long period with antibiotics, antimetabolites, or corticosteroids.

long periods to materials contaminated by fungus spores (grain, hay, cotton, wool, and others) run a greater risk.

Two clinical forms of the disease are distinguished: localized and invasive. Aspergillosis is essentially a respiratory tract infection. The fungus can cause a type of bronchopneumonia, with the symptom complex common to this syndrome. The incubation period is still not well known, but it is thought to be several weeks. In the invasive form, which is usually serious, the infection may disseminate and affect any organ; it often localizes in the thyroid, brain, or myocardium. The fungus also commonly colonizes the paranasal sinuses and the eye sockets. Another form is the fungus ball or aspergilloma, which occurs when the fungus colonizes respiratory cavities caused by other preexisting diseases (bronchitis, bronchiectasis, tuberculosis). This form is relatively benign, but it occasionally produces hemoptysis.

"Allergic aspergillosis" is caused by hypersensitivity to inhaled fungus conidia; strictly speaking, it is not an infection. Otomycosis is often caused by *A. niger*.

In Mexico, aspergillosis lesions were found in 1.2% of more than 2,000 randomly selected autopsies carried out in a general hospital (González-Mendoza, 1970).

The Disease in Animals: Aspergillosis occurs sporadically in many animal species, principally affecting the respiratory system. The following discussion deals only with the disease in cattle and fowl.

CATTLE: It is estimated that 75% of mycotic abortions are due to *Aspergillus*, particularly *A. fumigatus*, and 10 to 15% to fungi of the order Mucorales. As brucellosis, campylobacteriosis, and trichomoniasis are brought under control, the relative role of fungi as a cause of abortions grows. Mycotic abortion is seen mainly in stabled animals; for this reason it occurs most frequently in cold or temperate countries in winter. Generally, only one or two females in a herd abort.

The pathogenesis of the disease is not well known. It is thought that the fungus first localizes in the lungs or the digestive tract, where it multiplies, before invading the placenta via the bloodstream and causing placentitis. Most abortions occur in the last three months of pregnancy. The cotyledons swell and assume a brownish gray color. In serious cases, the placenta becomes wrinkled and leathery. The fungus may also invade the fetus, causing dermatitis and bronchopneumonia. Retention of the placenta is common. Other forms of the infection are the pulmonary form, due mainly to *A. fumigatus*, and skin aspergillomas, caused by *A. terreus* (Schmitt, 1981).

FOWL: Outbreaks of acute aspergillosis occur in chicks and young turkeys, sometimes causing considerable losses. Symptoms include fever, loss of appetite, difficulty in breathing, diarrhea, and emaciation. In chronic aspergillosis, which appears sporadically in adult birds, the clinical picture is varied and depends on the localization. Affected birds can survive a long time in a state of general debilitation. Yellowish granulomas of 1 to 3 mm (or larger if the process is chronic) are found in the lungs. Plaques develop in the air sacks and may gradually cover the entire lining; the same lesions or a mucoid exudate are found in the bronchial tubes and the trachea. Granulomatous lesions are also found frequently in different organs, in the form of either nodules or plaques.

Source of Infection and Mode of Transmission: The reservoir is the soil. The infecting element is the conidia (exospores) of the fungus, which are transmitted to man and animals by the airborne route. The causal agent is ubiquitous and can survive in the most varied environmental conditions. In spite of this, the disease is not common in man, which indicates a natural resistance to the infection. This resistance may be broken down by the use of immunosuppressants or by factors that impair the functioning of the immune system. An important source of infection for domestic animals and fowl, as well as for personnel working with them, is fodder and bedding contaminated by the fungus, which liberates conidia upon maturing. Apparently, exposure must be prolonged or massive for the infection to become established.

Role of Animals in the Epidemiology of the Disease: The source of infection is always the environment. The infection is not transmitted from one individual to another (man or animal).

Diagnosis: Because of the ubiquitous nature of the agent, isolation by culture is not a reliable test, since the agent may exist as a contaminant in the environment (laboratory or hospital) or as a saprophyte in the upper respiratory tract. Conclusive diagnosis may be obtained by carrying out a histologic examination using biopsy material and confirming the presence of conidiophores in the preparation. The agent may also be isolated by culture of specimens obtained aseptically from lesions unexposed to the outside environment. The species can only be identified by means of culture. The immunodiffusion test has given very good results in diagnosis of aspergillosis. At least 90% of sera from patients with aspergilloma or invasive aspergillosis produce multiple and intense precipitant bands. Another test that has given very good results is counterimmunoelectrophoresis and more recently enzyme-linked immunosorbent assay (ELISA) (Mishra *et al.*, 1983). In fowl, the presence of the fungus can be established by direct observation or by culturing material from lesions of sacrificed birds.

Control: The ubiquitous nature of the fungus does not permit establishment of practical control measures. Prolonged treatment with antibiotics or corticosteroids should be limited to cases in which such therapy is indispensable. Moldy bedding and fodder should not be handled or used for domestic mammals or fowl.

Bibliography

Ainsworth, G. C., and P. K. C. Austwick. *Fungal Diseases of Animals,* 2nd ed. Farnham Royal, Slough, England, Commonwealth Agricultural Bureau, 1973.

Ajello, L., L. K. Georg, W. Kaplan, and L. Kaufman. *Laboratory Manual for Medical Mycology.* Washington, D.C., U.S. Government Printing Office, 1963. (Public Health Service Publication 994.)

Chute, H. L. Diseases caused by fungi. *In:* Biester, H. E., and L. H. Schwarte (Eds.), *Diseases of Poultry,* 4th ed. Ames, Iowa State University Press, 1959.

Day, M. J., W. J. Penhale, C. E. Eger, S. E. Shaw, M. J. Kabay, W. F. Robinson, C. R. Huxtable, J. N. Mills, and R. S. Wyburn. Disseminated aspergillosis in dogs. *Aust Vet J* 63(2): 55-59, 1986.

González-Mendoza, A. Opportunistic mycoses. *In: Proceedings, International Symposium on Mycoses.* Washington, D.C., Pan American Health Organization, 1970. (Scientific Publication 205.)

Gordon, M. A. Current status of serology for diagnosis and prognostic evaluation of opportunistic fungus infections. *In: Proceedings, Third International Conference on the Mycoses.* Washington, D.C., Pan American Health Organization, 1975. (Scientific Publication 304.)

Mishra, S. K., S. Falkenberg, and N. Masihi. Efficacy of enzyme-linked immunosorbent assay in serodiagnosis of aspergillosis. *J Clin Microbiol* 17:708-710, 1983.

Opal, S. M., A. A. Asp, P. B. Cannady, Jr., P. L. Morse, L. J. Burton, and P. G. Hammer II. Efficacy of infection control measures during a nosocomial outbreak of disseminated aspergillosis associated with hospital construction. *J Infect Dis* 153:634-637, 1986.

Pal, M., and B. S. Mehrotra. Studies on association of *Aspergillus fumigatus* with ocular infections in animals. *Vet Rec* 118:42-44, 1986.

Schmitt, J. A. Mycotic diseases. *In:* Ristic M., and I. McIntyre (Eds.), *Diseases of Cattle in the Tropics.* The Hague, Martinus Nijhoff, 1981.

Utz, J. P. The systemic mycoses. *In:* Wyngaarden J. B., and L. H. Smith, Jr. (Eds.), *Cecil Textbook of Medicine,* 16th ed. Philadelphia, Saunders, 1982.

Winter, A. J. Mycotic abortion. *In:* Faulkner, L. C. (Ed.), *Abortion Diseases of Livestock.* Springfield, Illinois, Thomas, 1968.

BLASTOMYCOSIS

(116.0)

Synonyms: North American blastomycosis, Chicago disease, Gilchrist's disease.

Etiology: *Blastomyces dermatitidis*, a dimorphic fungus existing in mycelial form in cultures and as a budding yeast in the tissues of infected mammals.

Geographic Distribution: The disease has been observed in the United States, eastern Canada, Zaire, Tanzania, South Africa, and Tunisia. Autochthonous cases may have occurred in some Latin American countries.

Occurrence in Man: Sporadic. Most of the cases have been recorded in the United States, where the area of greatest prevalence is the Ohio and Mississippi river valleys. From 1885 to 1968, 1,573 cases occurred in that country (Menges, R., cited in Selby, 1975). The disease is more frequent among males and the highest rate of infection is found in men over 20 years of age.

Occurrence in Animals: Sporadic. Canines are the most affected species, and the greatest concentration of cases is seen in Arkansas (USA). Cases have also been described in cats, a horse, a captive sea lion (*Eumetopias jubata*), and an African lion (*Panthera leo*) in a zoo.

The Disease in Man: The incubation period is not well known; it possibly extends to several weeks or months. Blastomycosis is a chronic disease that principally affects the lungs. The respiratory symptomatology initially resembles influenza; purulent or bloody expectoration, weight loss, and cachexia, in addition to fever and cough, may develop later. If the infection remains localized, it can become asymptomatic. When it disseminates, it can cause subcutaneous abscesses as well as localized infections in several organs. Death frequently results in cases of untreated disseminated infection. The cutaneous form is commonly secondary to the pulmonary and is characterized by an irregular-shaped, scabby ulcer that has raised borders and contains minute abscesses. Lesions develop on exposed parts of the body.

The Disease in Animals: The highest incidence is observed in dogs around 2 years of age. The symptoms consist of weight loss, chronic cough, dyspnea, cutaneous abscesses, fever, anorexia, and sometimes blindness. The lesions localize in the lungs, lymph nodes, eyes, skin, and joints and bones. Of 47 clinical cases recently described, 72% occurred in large males. There were lesions of the respiratory tract in 85% of the cases (Legendre *et al.*, 1981).

Source of Infection and Mode of Transmission: The reservoir is environmental, probably the soil, but the ecologic biotope has not been determined. Transmission to man and to animals is effected by aerosols; the fungal conidia are the infecting element.

Persons at highest risk are those having the most contact with the soil. Dogs most frequently infected are sporting and hunting breeds.

Role of Animals in the Epidemiology of the Disease: None. It is a disease common to man and animals. Cases of transmission from individual to individual (man or animal) are not known.

Diagnosis: Diagnosis is based on direct microscopic examination of sputum and material from lesions, on isolation of the agent in culture media, and on examination of histologic preparations. *B. dermatitidis* grows well in Sabouraud's culture medium or other adequate media; it is most distinctive in its sprouting yeast form, and therefore the inoculated medium should be incubated at 37°C, since at ambient temperature the mycelial form of the fungus is obtained. *B. dermatitidis* in its yeast form (in tissues or cultures at 37°C) is characterized by a single bud attached to the parent cell by a wide base, from which it detaches when it has reached a size similar to the parent cell. In contrast, *Paracoccidioides brasiliensis*, the agent of paracoccidioidomycosis ("South American blastomycosis"), has multiple buds in the yeast phase.

Serologic tests in use are complement fixation and gel immunodiffusion; the latter gives better results. It should be borne in mind that cross-reactions with *Histoplasma* and *Coccidioides* may occur. At present, the intradermal test is considered to have no diagnostic value.

Control: As long as the ecologic biotope remains poorly defined, practical prevention methods cannot be established.

Bibliography

Ajello, L. Comparative ecology of respiratory mycotic disease agents. *Bacteriol Rev* 31:6-24, 1967.

American Public Health Association. *Control of Communicable Diseases in Man*, 14th ed. (Ed. by A. S. Benenson). Washington, D.C., APHA, 1985.

Drutz, D. J. The Mycoses. *In*: Wyngaarden, J. B., and L. H. Smith, Jr. (Eds.), *Cecil Textbook of Medicine*, 16th ed. Philadelphia, Saunders, 1982.

Kaplan, W. Epidemiology of the principal systemic mycoses of man and lower animals and the ecology of their etiologic agents. *J Am Vet Med Assoc* 163:1043-1047, 1973.

Kaufman, L. Current status of immunology for diagnosis and prognostic evaluation of blastomycosis, coccidioidomycosis, and paracoccidioidomycosis. *In*: *Proceedings, Third*

International Conference on the Mycoses. Washington, D.C., Pan American Health Organization, 1975. (Scientific Publication 304.)

Legendre, A. M., M. Walker, N. Buyukmihci, and R. Stevens. Canine blastomycoses: a review of 47 clinical cases. *J Am Vet Med Assoc* 178:1163-1168, 1981.

Menges, R. W. Blastomycosis in animals. *Vet Med* 55:45-54, 1960.

Selby, L. A. Blastomycosis. *In*: Hubbert, W. T., W. F. McCulloch, and P. R. Schnurrenberger (Eds.), *Diseases Transmitted from Animals to Man*, 6th ed. Springfield, Illinois, Thomas, 1975.

Thiel, R. P., L. D. Mech, G. R. Ruth, J. R. Archer, and L. Kaufman. Blastomycosis in wild wolves. *J Wildl Dis* 23:324-327, 1987.

CANDIDIASIS

(112)

Synonyms: Moniliasis, candidosis, thrush.

Etiology: *Candida albicans* (*Monilia albicans*, *Oidium albicans*), and occasionally other species of *Candida*. This yeast is part of the normal flora of the human and animal digestive system, mucosa, and, to a lesser degree, skin; it is also found in the soil, plants, and fruits. In their normal habitat the candidae grow as budding yeasts, but in infected tissues they can produce hyphae and pseudohyphae.

Geographic Distribution: Worldwide. There are no delimited endemic zones.

Occurrence in Man: It is the most frequent opportunistic mycosis. Its incidence has increased in recent years as a result of prolonged treatments with antibiotics and corticosteroids. Candidiasis is a sporadic disease; epidemics have occurred in nurseries. It is estimated that the disease is responsible for almost a quarter of the deaths due to mycoses. In a general hospital in Mexico, candidiasis lesions were found in 5.4% of randomly selected autopsies (González-Mendoza, 1970).

Occurrence in Animals: The disease has been confirmed in a large number of mammalian and avian species. Moniliasis in chicks and poults, is common and can be economically important. Outbreaks have been described in several parts of the world.

The Disease in Man: *Candida* is found as a commensal in the digestive tract of a high percentage of healthy individuals. One of the most common clinical forms of the disease is mycotic stomatitis, or thrush, which is characterized by white plaques lightly adhering to the oral mucosa, though it is also found in the pharynx and esophagus. Oral moniliasis is more frequent in nursing infants than in adults. "Diaper rash" and cheilitis (perlèche) are frequently caused by *Candida*. In adults, candidiasis is almost always associated with debilitating diseases or conditions, such as diabetes, tuberculosis, syphilis, cancer, obesity, and others. The agent often is responsible for intertrigo of large skin folds, vulvovaginal thrush, and onychia with paronychia (especially in adult women whose work requires frequent immersion of the hands in water).

Although candidiasis is usually limited to mucocutaneous forms, systemic infection can occur by hematogenous dissemination, mainly in weakened patients subjected to prolonged antibiotic treatment. These cases often develop as a result of lesions caused by medical exploration using catheters, the insertion of these instruments in the urethra, or surgical interventions. The localization may be in any organ, but is most frequently in the eyes, kidneys, and bones.

The Disease in Animals: Candidiasis in chicks, poults, and geese is usually seen sporadically. Epidemic outbreaks sometimes occur, mainly in poults, with mortality of 8 to 20%. Avian candidiasis is an infection of the upper digestive system. In young birds it sometimes has a chronic course with nervous symptoms. Nevertheless, the disease is generally asymptomatic and diagnosis is made post-mortem. The most frequent lesion is found in the crop and consists of plaques that resemble curdled milk and adhere lightly to the mucosa. In adult birds candidiasis has a chronic course and causes thickening of the crop wall, on which a yellowish necrotic material accumulates.

Oral candidiasis occurs sporadically in calves, colts, lambs, swine, dogs, laboratory mice, and guinea pigs, and also in zoo animals. On rare occasions *Candida* spp. gives rise to mastitis and abortions in cattle.

Source of Infection and Mode of Transmission: *C. albicans* is found as a component of the normal flora of the digestive system in a high percentage of people and animals. The yeast is also distributed in nature.

In young fowl *C. albicans* is probably a primary etiologic agent, while candidiasis in man is almost always associated with other diseases. Prolonged treatment with antibiotics, cytotoxic agents, and corticosteroids is a predisposing factor. A diet rich in carbohydrates may be another factor facilitating colonization by the agent, in man as well as in animals.

Most infections have an endogenous source. Candidiasis can be transmitted by contact with secretions from the mouth, skin, vagina, and feces of patients or carriers. Mothers with vaginal thrush can infect their offspring during birth.

Role of Animals in the Epidemiology of the Disease: It is a disease common to man and animals. There are no known cases of transmission from animal to animal, but human-to-human transmission has occurred, as in the case of mothers infecting their children during birth.

Diagnosis: Given the ubiquitous nature of the yeast, laboratory diagnosis should be done with extreme care. Direct examination of lesions of the nails, skin (in potassium hydroxide), or mucous membranes (in lactophenol-cotton blue), or microscopic examination of Gram-stained films is diagnostically significant if large numbers of the microorganisms are found. The examination should be carried out with fresh specimens. The presence in lesions of the budding yeast form together with hyphae or pseudohyphae has diagnostic value. Isolation of the agent from blood, pleural or peritoneal fluid, cerebrospinal fluid, or biopsy material obtained aseptically from closed localized foci permits diagnosis of disseminated candidiasis. Nevertheless, it should be borne in mind that fungemia can be only transient and not indicate a systemic infection. At present, a labeled anti-*C. albicans* globulin exists for immunofluorescence testing of smears of pathologic or cultured materials.

The most widely used serologic test for diagnosis of systemic candidiasis is immunodiffusion or double diffusion in Ouchterlony's agar gel, which experience has indicated is highly sensitive and specific. The immunoelectrophoresis test gives good correlation with the immunodiffusion test, and the results can be obtained in just 2 hours. Notwithstanding, serologic diagnosis of systemic candidiasis presents serious difficulties and a rise in patients' titers should be confirmed. Tube agglutination, indirect immunofluorescence, and indirect hemagglutination are also very useful tests if the antibody level detected is above that prevalent in the normal population. The predominant or only antibodies in healthy persons are IgM; on the other hand, systemic candidiasis causes an initial rapid rise of IgM and then of IgG immunoglobulins, with a subsequent reduction of IgM and persistence of IgG.

Control: Neonatal thrush can be prevented by treating the mother's vaginal candidiasis with nystatin during the final trimester. This antimycotic antibiotic can also be used in patients undergoing prolonged treatment with broad-spectrum antibiotics. Plastic catheters should be avoided. Generalization of thrush in weakened patients can be stopped by treating the oral lesions. To prevent epidemics in nurseries, patients with oral thrush should be isolated and strict hygiene measures followed. Nutritional deficiencies should be corrected as a preventive measure, since candidiasis is more frequent in those with vitamin deficiencies or inadequate diet (Ajello and Kaplan, 1980).

Recommended control measures in case of a moniliasis outbreak among fowl include destroying all sick birds and administering copper sulphate (1:2,000) in the drinking water and nystatin (110 mg/kg) in the feed.

Bibliography

Ainsworth, G. C., and P. K. C. Austwick. *Fungal Diseases of Animals*, 2nd ed. Farnham Royal, Slough, England, Commonwealth Agricultural Bureau, 1973.

Ajello, L., and W. Kaplan. Systemic mycoses. *In*: Stoenner, H., W. Kaplan, and M. Torten (Section Eds.), *CRC Handbook Series in Zoonoses*. Section A, vol. 2. Boca Raton, Florida, CRC Press, 1980.

American Public Health Association. *Control of Communicable Diseases in Man*, 14th ed. (Ed. by A. S. Benenson). Washington, D.C., APHA, 1985.

Anderson, K. L. Pathogenic yeasts. *In*: Hubbert, W. T., W. F. McCulloch, and P. R. Schnurrenberger (Eds.), *Diseases Transmitted from Animals to Man*, 6th ed. Springfield, Illinois, Thomas, 1975.

Carter, G. R. *Diagnostic Procedures in Veterinary Microbiology*, 2nd ed. Springfield, Illinois, Thomas, 1973.

Gonzáles-Mendoza, A. Opportunistic mycoses. *In*: *Proceedings, International Symposium on Mycoses*. Washington, D.C., Pan American Health Organization, 1970. (Scientific Publication 205.)

Gordon, M. A. Current status of serology for diagnosis and prognostic evaluation of opportunistic fungus infections. *In*: *Proceedings, Third International Conference on the Mycoses*. Washington, D.C., Pan American Health Organization, 1975. (Scientific Publication 304.)

Negroni, P. *Micosis cutáneas y viscerales*, 5th ed. Buenos Aires, López, 1972.

Soltys, M. A. *Bacteria and Fungi Pathogenic to Man and Animals*. London, Baillière, Tindall and Cox, 1963.

COCCIDIOIDOMYCOSIS

(114)

Synonyms: Posada's disease, San Joaquin Valley fever, desert fever, valley fever, desert rheumatism, coccidioidal granuloma.

Etiology: *Coccidioides immitis*, a diphasic fungus that exists in the mycelial phase when it is a soil saprophyte, and in the spherule phase in organic tissues and fluids.

The life cycle of *C. immitis* is unique among pathogenic fungi. The fungus occurs in one phase in the natural environment, that is, the soil of semiarid regions, and in another when it is parasitic in the mammalian host. *C. immitis* develops as a mycelium in the soil (a mass of filamentous hyphae that make up the fungus). The cycle begins with the arthroconidium, or arthrospore (a spore formed in the hyphae), which in an appropriate medium germinates and forms a branching, septate mycelium. When the mycelium fragments, it releases arthroconidia, 2 to 5 microns in size, into the air. The parasitic phase begins with inhalation of arthroconidia by man and animals. Arthroconidia enlarge into spherules of 10 to 80 microns in diameter. The cytoplasm of the spherule divides to produce hundreds of endospores which, when freed, disperse into the surrounding tissue and give rise to new spherules. The parasitic cycle lasts from 4 to 6 days (Drutz and Huppert, 1983).

Geographic Distribution: Limited to the Americas. The fungus is found in arid and semiarid zones of the southwestern United States, northwestern Mexico, Guatemala, Honduras, Colombia, Venezuela, Paraguay, Argentina, and probably Bolivia. The endemic area in Latin America is estimated to cover 1.5 million km^2, more than 1 million km^2 of which is in Mexico (Borelli, 1970).

Occurrence in Man: In some endemic areas the rate of infection seems to be high. It is estimated that almost 100% of the population of some hyperendemic zones in the United States may contract the infection over the span of a few years (Fiese, M. J., cited in Ajello, 1970). From 25,000 to 100,000 cases per year are thought to occur in the USA. Approximately 20% of the cases show up in persons who live outside endemic areas and become infected while visiting them (Drutz and Huppert, 1983). The rate of reactors to the skin test varies from 5% to more than 50% of the population in different endemic areas. Data regarding South America are fragmentary, but the rate of infection appears to be lower in this region.

Extrapulmonary dissemination is more frequent in men than in women and more frequent among blacks than among whites.

Occurrence in Animals: Natural infection has been found in many species of mammals. Infection is very frequent in cattle and dogs in endemic areas. Veterinary inspection has discovered coccidioidomycosis lesions in 5 to 20% of bovines sacrificed in abattoirs in central Arizona (USA). Several million cattle are thought to be infected in endemic zones of the southwestern USA. Infection has also been demonstrated in sheep, horses, swine, and wild rodents.

Several studies have been carried out on animals in the endemic region of Mexico. In the state of Sinaloa, sera of 100 hogs and 200 cattle were examined by immunoelectrophoresis, and 12% and 13%, respectively, were found to be reactors (Velasco Castrejón and Campos Nieto, 1979). In the state of Sonora, when the intradermal test using coccidioidin was applied to 459 cattle, 6.75% tested positive. Another investigation, in which granulomatous lesions discovered in 3,032 sacrificed cattle were studied histologically, found that the lesions in 77 (44%) of 175 animals confiscated for tuberculosis were actually caused by *C. immitis*, indicating a rate of infection of 2.5% in all the animals (Cervantes *et al.*, 1978).

The Disease in Man: The incubation period lasts from 1 to 4 weeks. An estimated 60% of infections occur asymptomatically and are only recognizable by the intradermal test. The remaining 40% result in a respiratory disease with acute symptomatology similar to that of influenza, and generally pass without sequelae. About 5% of primary infections develop either an erythema multiforme or an erythema nodosum arthralgia. When the respiratory infection does have sequelae, these consist of fibrotic or cavernous lesions of the lungs. In some patients pneumonia can persist for 6 to 8 weeks, with fever, chest pain, cough, and prostration (persistent coccidioidal pneumonia). Mortality in these cases is high in immunocompromised patients. Another disease form is the chronic, which can be confused with tuberculosis (Drutz, 1982).

Extrapulmonary dissemination generally occurs following the primary disease, and thoracic radiography may or may not show abnormalities. The most common localization is in the cutaneous and subcutaneous tissues. Osteomyelitis occurs in 10 to 50% of disseminated cases and may affect one or more of the bones. Meningitis cases are frequent (33 to 50% of these patients) and are generally fatal within 2 years. Other manifestations are thyroiditis, tenosynovitis, and prostatitis (Drutz, 1982). Clinical coccidioidomycosis is more frequent among migrant workers and soldiers transferred to endemic zones.

The Disease in Animals: The infection in cattle is asymptomatic. Lesions are usually limited to the bronchial and mediastinal lymph nodes. On rare occasions, small granulomatous lesions are found in the lungs and the submaxillary and retropharyngeal lymph nodes.

The disease in dogs is similar to that in man.

Source of Infection and Mode of Transmission: *C. immitis* is a soil saprophyte in arid and semiarid regions. Its distribution in endemic zones is not uniform. The infection is contracted by man and animals via inhalation of wind-borne arthrospores of the fungus; it occurs more frequently after dust storms. In the laboratory the infection can be contracted by inhalation of the spores originating from fungal cultures.

Role of Animals in the Epidemiology of the Disease: The soil is the common source of infection for man and animals. The fungus is not transmitted from one individual to another.

Diagnosis: Diagnosis is based on confirmation of the fungus's presence by means of direct microscopic examination that reveals spherules with endospores in the sputum, pus, pleural fluid, or gastric juices (treated with a 10% solution of potassium hydroxide); culture of clinical material; intratesticular inoculation of guinea pigs; or histopathology.

The skin test using coccidioidin or spherulin (considered to be more sensitive) is of great value in epidemiologic studies. It is applied in the same way as tuberculin. The test should be read at 24 and 48 hours; a reaction of 5 mm or more is considered positive. This test is useful for delimiting endemic areas. Infection by *C. immitis* may yield cross-reactions with other fungal antigens, especially histoplasmin. In clinical diagnosis, a positive test result is only significant if the the patient showed no reaction at the beginning of the illness. In a comparative study between coccidioidin (prepared with the mycelial phase fungus) and spherulin (prepared with the parasitic phase) in patients with coccidioidomycosis, one preparation could not be shown superior to the other for diagnosis. Both preparations elicited positive reactions in 43% of the patients, another 43% reacted negatively to both, and 14% gave contradictory results. The lack of reaction in a high proportion of patients may be due to defects of the immune system, especially in cases of advanced disease (Gifford and Catanzaro, 1981). Serologic tests in use are complement fixation (CF), precipitation, immunodiffusion, and latex agglutination. Combining immunobiologic tests provides useful information for both diagnosis and prognosis. In the first 2 weeks of the disease, IgM antibodies predominate, as can be demonstrated by the tube precipitation, latex agglutination, and immunodiffusion tests. IgG antibodies appear somewhat later and may be detected by CF or immunodiffusion. A persistent, high CF titer with loss of reactivity to the skin test indicates dissemination of the infection. Antibodies can be detected with the CF test in 75 to 95% of cases of meningitis (Drutz, 1982). Radioimmunoassay is useful for diagnosis and prognosis of the pulmonary disease. As patients improve, the test titer decreases (Catanzaro and Flataner, 1983).

Control: It is recommended that persons from nonendemic areas not work in endemic areas, since they lack immunity against coccidioidomycosis. In the United States, dust control methods (paving roads, seeding lawns, sprinkling dust with oil) have been used successfully for protection of military personnel.

Persons at risk of contracting disseminated coccidioidomycosis (pregnant women, immunocompromised patients) should be advised to avoid endemic zones. Trials of a vaccine made from formalin-inactivated spherules are being carried out in Arizona and California. Animal tests have demonstrated that the vaccine does not prevent the infection, but does arrest its progress and prevent dissemination (Drutz and Huppert, 1983). Treatment with ketoconazole may be useful to prevent dissemination in high-risk patients with primary coccidioidomycosis.

Bibliography

Ajello, L. Comparative ecology of respiratory mycotic disease agents. *Bacteriol Rev* 31:6-24, 1967.

Ajello, L. The medical mycological iceberg. *In: Proceedings, International Symposium on Mycoses*. Washington, D.C., Pan American Health Organization, 1970. (Scientific Publication 205.)

Ajello, L., L. K. Georg, W. Kaplan, and L. Kaufman. *Laboratory Manual for Medical Mycology*. Washington, D.C., U.S. Government Printing Office, 1963. (Public Health Service Publication 994.)

American Public Health Association. *Control of Communicable Diseases in Man*, 14th ed. (Ed. by A. S. Benenson). Washington, D.C., APHA, 1985.

Borelli, D. Prevalence of systemic mycoses in Latin America. *In: Proceedings, International Symposium on Mycoses*. Washington, D.C., Pan American Health Organization, 1970. (Scientific Publication 205.)

Bylund, D. J., J. J. Nanfro, and W. L. Marsh, Jr. Coccidioidomycosis of the female genital tract. *Arch Pathol Lab Med* 110:232-235, 1986.

Catanzaro, A., and F. Flataner. Detection of serum antibodies in coccidioidomycosis by solid-phase radioimmunoassay. *J Infect Dis* 147:32-39, 1983.

Cervantes, R. A., A. J. Solózano, and C.B.J. Pijoan. Presencia de coccidioidomicosis en bovinos de Estado de Sonora. *Rev Lat-Am Microbiol* 20:247-249, 1978.

Davis, J. W. Coccidioidomycosis. *In*: Davis, J. W., L. H. Karstad, and D. O. Trainer (Eds.), *Infectious Diseases of Wild Mammals*. Ames, Iowa State University Press, 1970.

Drutz, D. J. The mycoses. *In*: Wyngaarden, J. B., and L. H. Smith, Jr. (Eds.), *Cecil Textbook of Medicine*, 16th ed. Philadelphia, Saunders, 1982.

Drutz, D. J., and M. Huppert. Coccidioidomycosis: Factors affecting the host-parasite interaction. *J Infect Dis* 147:372-390, 1983.

Gifford, J., and A. Catanzaro. A comparison of coccidioidin and spherulin skin testing in the diagnosis of coccidioidomycosis. *Am Rev Respir Dis* 124:440-444, 1981.

Huntington, R. W., Jr. Coccidioidomycosis—a great imitator disease. *Arch Pathol Lab Med* 110:182, 1986.

Maddy, K. T. Coccidioidomycosis. *Adv Vet Sci* 6:251-286, 1960.

Negroni, K. T. *Micosis cutáneas y viscerales*, 5th ed. Buenos Aires, López, 1972.

Velasco Castrejón, O., and E. Campos Nieto. Estudio serológico de la coccidioidomicosis bovina y porcina del Estado de Sinaloa (México). *Rev Lat-Am Microbiol* 21:99, 1979.

CRYPTOCOCCOSIS

(117.5)

Synonyms: Torulosis, European blastomycosis, Busse-Buschke's disease.

Etiology: *Cryptococcus neoformans* (*Saccharomyces neoformans*, *Torulopsis neoformans*, *Torula histolytica*), a saprophytic yeast growing in certain soils. The agent has a spheroid or ovoid shape, is encapsulated, ranges from 4 to 7 microns in diameter, and is gram-positive. It reproduces by means of buds attached by a delicate base to the parent cell. Recent studies have shown that *C. neoformans* also has a sexual form and is a basidiomycete.

C. neoformans is subdivided into four serotypes (A, B, C, and D) on the basis of capsular polysaccharide antigens; this division is of epidemiologic interest. In turn, the serotypes are categorized into two varieties: *C. neoformans* var. *neoformans* (serotypes A and D) and *C. neoformans* var. *gatti* (types B and C).

Geographic Distribution: Worldwide. In the Americas the disease has been confirmed in Argentina, Brazil, Colombia, Venezuela, Mexico, the United States, and Canada (countries in which five or more cases have been recorded). Serotype A is the most prevalent worldwide; type D is common in some European countries (Denmark, Italy, Switzerland), but infrequent in the USA. On the other hand, serotypes B and C are more localized; they are recognized as disease agents mainly in southern California, southeastern Oklahoma, and some other areas of the United States, as well as in Asia (Kaplan *et al.*, 1981; Fromtling *et al.*, 1982).

Occurrence in Man: Cases are sporadic, with a higher incidence in men than in women. From 1965 to 1977, 1,264 cases of cryptococcosis were documented in the United States. Of 848 confirmed cases between 1973 and 1977, 608 patients had meningitis and 240 had extrameningeal localizations. These data indicate a great increase in comparison with previous periods (Kaufman and Blumer, 1978). From 1974 to 1980, 85 cases occurred in Malaysia, the majority among the Chinese ethnic group (Pathmanathan and Soo-Hoo, 1982). In the United States and Europe, cryptococcosis occurs mainly in patients with immune system defects, especially AIDS. In Malaysia, however, only 14% of the patients studied were in this category. Epidemiologic investigations based on skin tests indicate that many people exposed to the agent do not manifest disease symptoms.

Occurrence in Animals: Rare, sporadic cases. Some epizootic outbreaks of cryptococcal mastitis have been described in cows.

The Disease in Man: The great majority of cases are meningitis or meningoencephalitis. This form is preceded by a pulmonary infection. The primary pulmonary infection may either resolve spontaneously, give rise to a granulomatous mass ("cryptococcoma"), or disseminate hematogenously. The pulmonary form manifests itself with fever, cough, chest pain, and hemoptysis. Radiography shows single or multiple nodules or large cryptococcomas. The course is usually chronic. When dissemination from the original pulmonary focus occurs, the infection localizes mainly in the meninges and can spread to the brain. Other localizations occur in the skin, mucosa, and bones, as well as in other organs. Cutaneous localization is characterized by the formation of papules and abscesses with later ulceration. The most salient symptoms of the meningeal form are headache, stiffness of the neck, and visual disturbances. Other symptoms may include confusion, personality changes, agitation, and lethargy. Cryptococcal meningitis is almost always fatal if not treated adequately (amphotericin B and flucytosine simultaneously) (Drutz, 1982). Asymptomatic meningitis sometimes occurs when there are other localizations; it can be discovered by lumbar puncture and culture of cerebrospinal fluid (Liss and Rimland, 1981).

Cryptococcosis often appears in patients weakened by other diseases (disorders of the reticuloendothelial system, especially Hodgkin's disease) and by corticosteroid treatment. The incubation period is unknown. Pulmonary lesions may precede cerebral lesions by months or years. In the United States it is estimated that 100 deaths occur annually from cryptococcosis.

The Disease in Animals: The disease has been recognized in cattle, horses, sheep, goats, dogs, cats, nonhuman primates, and several species of wild animals (in zoos), but not in birds. The disseminated form is the most commonly diagnosed in cats and dogs. Of 21 canine cases with a clinical history, 13 manifested the meningeal form, four the nasal form, two osteoarticular disease, and the rest lesions in other organs. Six cases reported from Australia were all of the meningeal form (Sutton, 1981). Likewise, the main form diagnosed in cats is disease of the central nervous system, with granuloma in the eyes and nasal passages; the cutaneous form has also been diagnosed. Tumors with myxomatous consistency have also been observed in the nose and lungs of some species. Several outbreaks of mastitis in cows have been confirmed; the disease caused visible udder abnormality or changes in the milk.

Source of Infection and Mode of Transmission: Serotypes A and D (*C. neoformans* var. *neoformans*) are ubiquitous and have been isolated from several sources in the environment, such as soil, certain plants, bird feces, raw milk, and fruit juices. The causal agent is very commonly found in pigeon roosts and in soil contaminated by pigeon feces. The creatinine in pigeon fecal material serves as a source of nitrogen for *C. neoformans*, favoring its development and prolonging its survival in the soil. Pigeons do not become ill with cryptococcosis. Serotypes B and C (*C. neoformans* var. *gatti*) are seldom isolated from the external environment and almost nothing is known about their ecologic biotope. Man and animals become infected via the respiratory route by inhaling dust containing the causal agent; *C. neoformans*, which has no capsule in nature, becomes encapsulated in the lungs, allowing it to resist phagocytosis. Although researchers agree that the infection is contracted by inhalation, the infecting element is still debated. According to some, it is the yeast form of the agent, and according to others, it is the basidiospores of the agent's sexual phase. It has been pointed out that the yeast form is too large (4 to 7 microns) to enter the alveoli, while basidiospores measure only about 2 microns in diameter (Cohen, 1982).

Role of Animals in the Epidemiology of the Disease: No cases are known in which the disease was transmitted from animal to animal, from animal to man, or from man to man.

Diagnosis: Diagnosis can be made by microscopic observation of encapsulated *C. neoformans* in tissues and body fluids, and can be confirmed by culture. Serotyping is now facilitated by the use of culture media to differentiate serotypes A and D from B and C (Salkind and Hurd, 1982; Kwon-Chung *et al.*, 1982). For the same purpose, the direct immunofluorescence test can be used for cultures and for some histologic preparations (Kaplan *et al.*, 1981).

As the etiologic agent multiplies in the human host, the capsular polysaccharide of *C. neoformans* neutralizes antibodies. Excess antibodies can be detected in blood and urine as well as in the cerebrospinal fluid in cases in which the central nervous system is affected. Cases coming to the attention of a physician often are already very advanced; consequently, better results are obtained if the examination is directed toward detecting the specific antigen rather than the antibodies. The plate latex agglutination test with particles sensitized by anticryptococcal globulin is used to detect the cryptococcal antigen. ELISA is available to detect the capsular polysaccharide antigen of the etiologic agent; this test is much more sensitive than latex agglutination and permits an earlier diagnosis (Scott *et al.*, 1980).

Control: Control of pigeon populations might prevent some cases. Man should avoid exposure to accumulations of pigeon excrement in roosts, nests, and on window sills and other perches.

Bibliography

Ainsworth, G. C., and P. K. C. Austwick. *Fungal Diseases of Animals*, 2nd ed. Farnham Royal, Slough, England, Commonwealth Agricultural Bureau, 1973.

American Public Health Association. *Control of Communicable Diseases in Man*, 14th ed. (Ed. by A. S. Benenson). Washington, D.C., APHA, 1985.

Cohen, J. The pathogenesis of cryptococcosis. *J Infect* 5:109-116, 1982.

Drutz, D. J. The mycoses. *In*: Wyngaarden, J. B., and L. H. Smith, Jr. (Eds.), *Cecil Textbook of Medicine*, 16th ed. Philadelphia, Saunders, 1982.

Fromtling, R. A., S. Shadomy, H. J. Shadomy, and W. E. Dismukes. Serotypes B/C *Cryptococcus neoformans* isolated from patients in nonendemic areas. *J Clin Microbiol* 16:408-410, 1982.

Gordon, M. A. Current status of serology for diagnosis and prognostic evaluation of opportunistic fungus infections. *In: Proceedings, Third International Conference on the Mycoses.* Washington, D.C., Pan American Health Organization, 1975. (Scientific Publication 304.)

Kaplan, W., S. L. Bragg, S. Crane, and D. G. Ahearn. Serotyping *Cryptococcus neoformans* by immunofluorescence. *J Clin Microbiol* 14:313-317, 1981.

Kaufman, L., and S. Blumer. Cryptococcosis: the awakening giant. *In: Proceedings, Fourth International Conference on Mycoses.* Washington, D.C., Pan American Health Organization, 1978. (Scientific Publication 356.)

Kwon-Chung, K. J., I. Polacheck, and J. E. Bennett. Improved diagnostic medium for separation of *Cryptococcus neoformans* var. *neoformans* (serotypes A and D) and *Cryptococcus neoformans* var. *gatti* (serotypes B and C). *J Clin Microbiol* 15:535-537, 1982.

Liss, H. P., and D. Rimland. Asymptomatic cryptococcal meningitis. *Am Rev Respir Dis* 124:88-89, 1981.

Muchmore, H. G., F. G. Felton, S. B. Salvin, and E. R. Rhoades. Ecology and epidemiology of cryptococcosis. *In: Proceedings, International Symposium on Mycoses.* Washington, D.C., Pan American Health Organization, 1970. (Scientific Publication 205.)

Negroni, P. *Micosis cutáneas y viscerales*, 5th ed. Buenos Aires, López, 1972.

Pathmanathan, R., and T. S. Soo-Hoo. Cryptococcosis in the University Hospital Kuala Lumpur and review of published cases. *Trans R Soc Trop Med Hyg* 76:21-24, 1982.

Salkind, I. F., and N. J. Hurd. New medium for differentiation of *Cryptococcus neoformans* serotype pairs. *J Clin Microbiol* 15:169-171, 1982.

Scott, E. N., H. G. Muchmore, and F. G. Felton. Comparison of enzyme immunoassay and latex agglutination methods for detection of *Cryptococcus neoformans* antigen. *Am J Clin Pathol* 73:790-794, 1980.

Staib, F. Sampling and isolation of *Cryptococcus neoformans* from indoor air with the aid of the Reuter Centrifugal Sampler (RCS) and guizotia abyssinica creatinine agar. A contribution to the mycological-epidemiological control of *C. neoformans* in the fecal matter of caged birds. *Zentralbl Bakteriol Mikrobiol Hyg* [B]180(5-6):567-575, 1985.

Sutton, R. H. Cryptococcosis in dogs: a report on 6 cases. *Aust Vet J* 57:558-564, 1981.

DERMATOPHYTOSIS

(110)

Synonyms: Tinea, dermatomycosis, ringworm.

Etiology: Several species of *Microsporum* and *Trichophyton* and the species *Epidermophyton floccosum*. From the ecologic and epidemiologic standpoints, three groups of species are distinguished according to their reservoirs: anthropophilic, zoophilic, and geophilic. This discussion will consider only zoophilic species transmissible to man.

Dermatophytes were considered to be imperfect fungi (Fungi Imperfecti or Deuteromycetes). However, several species have been shown to reproduce sexually, and they are now classified as Ascomycetes.

Geographic Distribution: Among the zoophilic species, *M. canis*, *T. verrucosum*, *T. equinum*, and *T. mentagrophytes* are distributed worldwide. Other species, such as *T. erinacei*, have a limited distribution (New Zealand, Great Britain, France, and Italy).

Occurrence in Man: Dermatophytic infections are common, but their exact prevalence is not known. The disease is not notifiable and, moreover, many persons with mild cases do not consult a physician; most data originate from dermatologists, mycology laboratories, and epidemiologic investigations. The economically advanced countries have witnessed a marked reduction in the incidence of some anthropophilic dermatophyte infections, such as epidemic outbreaks of tinea capitis caused by *M. audouinii*. In these countries, zoophilic dermatophytes are at present much more important. *M. canis*, *T. verrucosum*, and *T. mentagrophytes* are the most important zoophilic species in human infection. Other zoophilic species are *M. equinum*, *M. distortum*, *T. equinum*, and *T. gallinae*. All these species are transmissible to man in different areas and with varying frequencies (Padhye, 1980).

In Peru, zoophilic species are probably responsible for 21% of human dermatomycoses (Gómez Pando and Matos Díaz, 1982). A study carried out in India found *T. verrucosum* and *T. mentagrophytes* var. *mentagrophytes* in 56 (38.6%) of 145 isolations from man and in 50 (53.8%) of 93 human cases in the rural area (Chatterjee *et al.*, 1980).

On a rabbit farm in Hungary, where all of the 5,500 animals became infected with *T. mentagrophytes* var. *mentagrophytes* (var. *granulosum*) in the course of 6 months, there were 38 human cases among the personnel and their families (Szili and Kohalmi, 1981).

Occurrence in Animals: Epidemiologic studies in recent years have demonstrated that dermatophytic infection in animals is very common. Tinea occurs more frequently in stabled animals than in those kept in open pasture for the entire year.

Infection by *M. canis* occurs very frequently in cats and dogs, often asymptomatically. In Lima, Peru, and environs, *M. canis* was found in 12 (15%) of 79 cats without apparent lesions, and *T. mentagrophytes* in eight (10%). *M. canis* was isolated from 17 (3.9%) of 432 samples from dogs, and *T. mentagrophytes* from 22 (5%) (Gómez Pando and Matos Díaz, 1982).

The Disease in Man: Dermatophytosis or tinea is a superficial infection of the keratinized parts of the body (skin, hair, and nails). As a general rule, zoophilic and geophilic dermatophytes produce more acute inflammatory lesions than the anthropophilic species, which are parasites better adapted to man. Species belonging to *Microsporum* cause most of the cases of tinea capitis and tinea corporis, but they are rarely responsible for infection of nails (onychosis) or skin folds (intertrigo). However, *Trichophyton* species can invade the skin of any part of the body.

There are two varieties of *T. mentagrophytes*: an anthropophilic variety (var. *interdigitale*) that is relatively nonvirulent for man and localizes on the feet (athlete's foot), and a zoophilic type (morphologically granular) that causes a very inflammatory dermatophytosis on different areas of the human body. The zoophilic variety is commonly found in rodents, cats, dogs, and other animals. Transmission to man probably occurs by means of contamination of his habitat with hair from infected animals. Several epidemic outbreaks of inflammatory dermatophytosis on various parts of the body were caused by *T. mentagrophytes* var. *mentagrophytes* (var. *granulosum*) among US troops in Vietnam. About one-quarter of the rats trapped close to the military camps were infected with strains of the same variety of fungus. Among inhabitants of the region, the infection was observed only in children, suggesting that adults had acquired immunity by way of infections contracted during childhood.

At present, *M. canis* is one of the principal etiologic agents of tinea, and in many countries it has replaced the anthropophilic species *M. audouinii* as a cause of tinea capitis. In South America, *M. canis* is the most common of the microspora.

The incubation period of the disease lasts from 1 to 2 weeks. Infection of the scalp is most frequent between the ages of 4 and 11 years, and has a higher incidence among males. The disease begins with a small papule, the hair becomes brittle, and the infection spreads peripherally, leaving scaly, bald patches. Suppurative lesions (kerions) are frequent when the fungus is of animal origin. Tinea caused by *M. canis* heals spontaneously during puberty.

Suppurative tinea barbae, which affects rural dwellers, is due to *T. mentagrophytes* of animal origin. However, in the United States dry tinea barbae is caused by *T. mentagrophytes* of human origin and by *T. rubrum* (Silva-Hunter *et al.*, 1981).

Tinea corporis is characterized by flat lesions that tend to be annular. They contain microvesicles or are scaly, and the borders are reddish and sometimes raised.

Tinea corporis in children is usually an extension of tinea capitis to the face and is due to *M. canis* and *M. audouinii*. Active lesions may also appear on the wrists and neck of mothers or young adults who have been in contact with an infected child. Tinea corporis in adults appears mainly on the extremities and trunk, is chronic in nature, and is generally the result of infection by the anthropophilic dermatophyte *T. rubrum* (Silva-Hunter *et al.*, 1981).

Tinea pedis (athlete's foot), which is increasing in incidence worldwide, is due to anthropophilic species of *Trichophyton* and, to a lesser extent, to *Epidermophyton floccosum* (also anthropophilic).

The Disease in Animals: The most important species to be considered as reservoirs of dermatophytes transmissible to man are cats, dogs, cattle, and rodents.

CATS AND DOGS: The most important etiologic agent in these animals is *M. canis*. This species of dermatophyte is very well adapted to cats, and approximately 90% of infected animals manifest no apparent lesion. When lesions do occur they appear primarily on the face and paws.

In dogs, lesions are common and evident. They can occur on any part of the body in the form of tinea circinata (ringworm).

Dogs and cats can also be infected by other dermatophytes, especially *T. mentagrophytes*.

CATTLE: The main etiologic agent of tinea in cattle is *T. verrucosum* (*T. faviforme, T. ochraceum, T. album, T. discoides*). The disease is most frequent in countries where animals are stabled during the winter, and its incidence is greater in calves than in adults. Lesions may be as small as 1 cm in diameter or cover extensive areas. They are most frequently located on the face and neck, but in some instances can be found on other parts of the body, such as the flanks and legs. At the onset, tinea is characterized by grayish white, dry areas containing a few brittle hairs; the lesion then increases in thickness and resembles a light brown scab.

HORSES: Dermatophytosis in horses is caused by *T. equinum* and *M. equinum*; the latter is infrequent in the Americas. Lesions are usually localized in places where the harness causes friction. They are dry, bald, covered with scales, and the skin is thickened.

RODENTS: Tinea favus of mice, caused by *T. mentagrophytes* var. *quinckeanum*, is widely distributed throughout the world and is transmissible to domestic animals and to man. The lesion is white and scabby and is localized on the head or trunk. *T. mentagrophytes* var. *mentagrophytes* is another dermatophyte common to rodents. Laboratory mice and guinea pigs are infected mostly by *T. mentagrophytes*, but may not have noticeable lesions. The agent's presence is often detected only when humans contract the infection. It is also transmissible to dogs.

SHEEP AND GOATS: Tinea is not common in these species. Lesions localize on the head and face. The most frequently found agent is *T. verrucosum*.

SWINE: The most common agent of swine tinea is *M. nanum*. The infection has been confirmed in Canada, the United States, Mexico, Cuba, Kenya, and Australasia. This dermatophyte has been isolated from only a few human cases. The lesion is characterized by a wrinkled area covered with a thin, brown scab that easily becomes detached. *M. nanum* lives as a soil saprophyte in areas where swine are raised, and it is classified as geophilic.

FOWL: Tinea favus in chickens occurs sporadically throughout the world and is transmissible to man. Its agent is *T. gallinae*.

Source of Infection and Mode of Transmission: The natural reservoirs of zoophilic dermatophytes are animals. Transmission to man occurs by direct contact with an infected animal (sick or carrier) or indirectly by means of spores on hair and dermal scales shed by the animal. Dermatophytes remain viable in shed epithelium for many months and even years. The same animal can infect several persons in a family, but a zoophilic dermatophyte is rarely spread from person to person and does not cause epidemic tinea, as do anthropophilic dermatophytes. Cases of human-to-human transmission of *M. canis* have been observed, but the agent loses its infectiveness for man after a few intermediaries (Padhye, 1980). *T. verrucosum*, which has cattle as its principal reservoir, is found in infections in rural populations, while infection due to *M. canis* is transmitted by cats and dogs to both city and country dwellers. Infection due to *T. mentagrophytes* var. *mentagrophytes* (var. *granulosum*) and *T. mentagrophytes* var. *quinckeanum* is transmitted indirectly by rodents to man by means of residues of shed epithelium in the environment. Cats and dogs can also be infected by these dermatophytes, either via the same route or by direct contact when hunting rodents, and in turn can transmit the infection to man.

Animal-to-animal transmission occurs by the same routes. Crowding and reduced resistance to disease influence the incidence of the infection.

Role of Animals in the Epidemiology of the Disease: Animals are the reservoir of zoophilic dermatophytes and the source of infection for man. As in other zoonoses, human-to-human transmission is rare. Transmission of anthropophilic dermatophytes from man to animals is also rare.

The dermatophyte *M. gypseum* is the causal agent of sporadic cases of tinea in man and animals. Its reservoir is the soil (geophilic).

Diagnosis: Clinical diagnosis can be confirmed by the following methods: a) microscopic examination of hair and scales from lesions (this method provides a diagnosis at the genus level since in infection due to *Microsporum*, the spores surround the hair shaft in an irregular mosaic, while in infection caused by *Tri-chophyton*, the spores are arranged in chains); b) the use of filtered ultraviolet light (Wood's light), under which the spores of *Microsporum* exhibit a bright, bluish green fluorescence; and c) isolation in culture media, the only method that permits identification of the species.

Control: Prevention of human dermatophytoses caused by zoophilic strains should be based on control of the infection in animals, but this is difficult to accomplish. Avoiding contact with obviously sick animals can prevent a certain proportion of human cases. These animals should be isolated and treated with topical fungicides (antimycotics) and/or griseofulvin administered orally. Remains of hair and scales should be burned and all utensils, rooms, and stables should be disinfected. Apparently healthy cats can be examined using Wood's light. Control of the rodent population is a useful measure.

In cold climates, where animals are stabled over long periods of time, der-matophytosis can be a problem in cattle and horses. In the USSR, two vaccines were developed: one for cattle, made from an attenuated strain of *T. verrucosum*, and another for horses, made from *T. equinum*. Both vaccines gave satisfactory results in the prevention of dermatophytosis. In Norway, the vaccine was used on 200,000 cattle with very good results (Aamodt *et al.*, 1982).

Bibliography

Aamodt, O., B. Naess, and O. Sandvik. Vaccination of Norwegian cattle against ring-worm. *Zentralbl Veterinarmed* B29:451-456, 1982.

Ainsworth, G. C., and P. K. C. Austwick. *Fungal Diseases of Animals*, 2nd ed. Farnham Royal, Slough, England, Commonwealth Agricultural Bureau, 1973.

Allen, A. M., and D. Taplin. Epidemiology of cutaneous mycoses in the tropics and subtropics: newer concepts. *In: Proceedings, Third International Conference on the Mycoses.* Washington, D.C., Pan American Health Organization, 1975. (Scientific Publication 304.)

American Public Health Association. *Control of Communicable Diseases in Man*, 14th ed. (Ed. by A. S. Benenson). Washington, D.C., APHA, 1985.

Chatterjee, A., D. Chattopadhyay, D. Bhattacharya, A. K. Dutta, and D. N. Sen Gupta. Some epidemiological aspects of zoophilic dermatophytosis. *Int J Zoonoses* 7:19-33, 1980.

Chmel, L. Epidemiological aspects of zoophilic dermatophytes. *In*: Chmel, L. (Ed.), *Recent Advances in Human and Animal Mycology*. Bratislava, Czechoslovakia, Slovak Acad-emy of Sciences, 1967.

Emmons, C. W. Mycoses of Animals. *Adv Vet Sci* 2:47-63, 1955.

English, M. P. The epidemiology of animal ringworm in man. *Br J Dermatol* 86 (Suppl) 8:78-87, 1972.

Gentles, J. C. Ringworm. *In*: Graham-Jones, O. (Ed.), *Some Diseases of Animals Commu-nicable to Man in Britain*. Oxford, Pergamon Press, 1968.

Georg, L. K. *Animal Ringworm in Public Health, Diagnosis and Nature*. Atlanta, Geor-gia, Centers for Disease Control of the USA, 1960. (Public Health Service Publication 727.)

Gómez Pando, V., and J. Matos Díaz. Dermatofitos: aspectos epidemiológicos. *Bol Inf Colegio Med Vet Perú* 17:16-19, 1982.

Negroni, P. *Micosis cutáneas y viscerales*, 5th ed. Buenos Aires, López, 1972.

Padhye, A. A. Cutaneous mycoses. *In*: Stoenner, J., W. Kaplan, and M. Torten (Section Eds.), *CRC Handbook Series in Zoonoses*. Section A, vol. 2. Boca Raton, Florida, CRC Press, 1980.

Pepin, G., and P. K. C. Austwick. Skin diseases of domestic animals. II. Skin disease, mycological origin. *Vet Rec* 82:208-214, 1968.

Pepin, G. A., and M. Oxenhan. Zoonotic dermatophytosis (ringworm). *Vet Rec* 118:110-111, 1986.

Raubitscheck, F. Fungal diseases. *In*: Van der Hoeden, J. (Ed.), *Zoonoses*. Amsterdam, Netherlands, Elsevier, 1964.

Rebell, G., and D. Taplin. *Dermatophytes: Their Recognition and Identification*. Miami, Florida, University of Miami Press, 1970.

Sarkisov, A. K. New methods of control of dermatomycoses common to animals and man. *In*: Lysenko, A. (Ed.), *Zoonoses Control*, vol. 2. Moscow, Center of International Projects, 1982.

Silva-Hunter, M., I. Weitzman, and S. A. Rosenthal. Cutaneous mycoses (dermatomycoses). *In*: Balows, A., and W. J. Hausler, Jr. (Eds.), *Diagnostic Procedures for Bacterial, Mycotic and Parasitic Infections*, 6th ed. Washington, D.C., American Public Health Association, 1981.

Smith, J. M. B. Superficial and cutaneous mycoses. *In*: Hubbert, W. T., W. F., McCulloch, and P. R. Schnurrenberger (Eds.), *Diseases Transmitted from Animals to Man*, 6th ed. Springfield, Illinois, Thomas, 1975.

Szili, M., and I. Kohalmi. Endemic *Trichophyton mentagrophytes* infection of rabbit origin. *Mykosen* 24:412-420, 1981. *Abstr Rev Med Vet (B Aires)* 64:65, 1983.

Törnquist, M., P. H. Bendixen, and B. Pehrson. Vaccination against ringworm of calves in specialized beef production. *Acta Vet Scand* 26:21-29, 1985.

HISTOPLASMOSIS

(115)

Synonyms: Reticuloendothelial cytomycosis, cavern disease, Darling's disease.

Etiology: *Histoplasma capsulatum*, a dimorphic fungus that has a yeast form in the parasitic phase, but in the saprophytic phase develops a filamentous mycelium producing macroconidia and microconidia. The yeast form may also be grown in the laboratory by culturing the fungus in an enriched medium at 37°C.

Two varieties of the agent are known: *H. capsulatum* var. *capsulatum* and *H. capsulatum* var. *duboisii*; they are indistinguishable in the mycelial phase, but in infected tissues the yeast-form cells of var. *duboisii* are much larger (7-15 microns) than those of var. *capsulatum* (2-5 microns). The tissue reactions they produce are also different.

Geographic Distribution: Distribution of var. *capsulatum* is worldwide, while var. *duboisii* is only known in central Africa, where the other variety also occurs. Distribution of the fungus in the soil is not uniform; some regions are more contaminated than others and microfoci exist where the agent is highly concentrated.

Occurrence in Man: Judging from results of the histoplasmin intradermal test, the rate of infection is very high in endemic areas. It has been estimated that in the United States, where the infection is concentrated in the Missouri, Mississippi, and Ohio river valleys, 30 million people have been infected with *Histoplasma* and about a half million persons become infected each year (Selby, 1975). The disease occurs sporadically or in epidemic outbreaks. Isolated cases often elude diagnosis. In 1980 an outbreak of 138 cases of acute pulmonary disease occurred among lime quarry workers in northern Michigan, which was not considered an endemic area (Waldman *et al.*, 1983). Another outbreak affecting 435 persons occurred on the Indianapolis campus of Indiana University in 1978-1979; in 1980-1981 the disease recurred in an area near the campus, with 51 cases (Schlech *et al.*, 1983). Endemic regions also exist within Latin America. Although prevalence varies from one area to another, it has been postulated that the entire population of Latin America lives within or near areas where the infection can be contracted (Borelli, 1970). In Mexico, all states except two have recorded epidemic outbreaks or isolated cases of the disease. In that country, a study was conducted of 11 outbreaks affecting 75 persons in 1979, with a case fatality rate of 5.3%, and of 12 outbreaks in 1980 that affected 68 individuals. The majority of cases occurred among persons who for occupational, educational, or recreational reasons visited caves, abandoned mines, and tunnels in which bat droppings had accumulated. More than 2,000 large mines have had to be abandoned because of high concentrations of *H. capsulatum* resulting from the presence of large bat colonies (Pan American Health Organization, 1981). Endemic areas also exist in Guatemala, Venezuela, and Peru (Ajello and Kaplan, 1980).

Although the infection is common, the clinical disease is much less so. Radiography revealed pulmonary calcifications in a high proportion (approximately 25%) of persons reacting to histoplasmin. Around 90% of persons with a positive reaction to the histoplasmin hypersensitivity skin test are clinically healthy.

Occurrence in Animals: Many species of domestic and wild animals are susceptible to the infection. Surveys employing the histoplasmin test have demonstrated that the infection is frequent in cattle, sheep, and horses in endemic areas. Dogs are the animal species in which the infection is most often clinically apparent.

The Disease in Man: Most cases are asymptomatic. The incubation period is from 5 to 18 days. Three basic clinical forms are distinguished: acute pulmonary, chronic cavitary pulmonary, and disseminated. The acute pulmonary form, which is the most frequent, resembles influenza and produces febrile symptoms that may last from 1 day to several weeks. Erythema nodosum or multiforme, diffuse eruption, and arthralgia may be present. This form often escapes notice. In mild cases recovery takes place without treatment, and may or may not leave calcification in the lungs. The chronic form is seen mainly in persons over 40 years of age, predominantly males and almost always individuals with a history of prior pulmonary disease; it is clinically similar to pulmonary tuberculosis, causing cavitation. The course may vary from months to years, and in many cases there may be spontaneous recovery. The disseminated form is more serious and is seen mainly in the very young or the elderly, in whom it may take an acute or chronic course. The acute course develops principally among nursing babies and small children, and is characterized by varying degrees of hepatosplenomegaly, fever, and prostration. It is often confused with miliary tuberculosis and, if untreated, is highly fatal. The symptomatology of the chronic disseminated form depends on the localization of the fungus (pneumonia, hepatitis, endocarditis, etc.). These cases frequently include ulceration of the mucosa and hepatosplenomegaly. This form appears primarily in adults; patients may survive many years, but the disease is usually fatal if untreated.

In the period 1952-1963 in the United States, an average of only 68 deaths per year were attributed to histoplasmosis in spite of its high prevalence in endemic areas. These statistics confirm that the disease is usually benign.

African histoplasmosis, due to var. *duboisii*, most frequently causes lesions of the skin, subcutaneous tissue, and bones. Granulomas of the skin manifest themselves as nodules or ulcerous or eczematous lesions. Abscesses can be observed in subcutaneous tissues. Histoplasmosis of the bone gives rise to isolated or multiple lesions that at times pass asymptomatically (Manson-Bahr and Apted, 1982). When the disease is progressive and serious, giant cell granulomas may form in many internal organs.

The Disease in Animals: Dogs are the species most frequently manifesting clinical symptoms, but, as in man, most infections in dogs are asymptomatic. The primary respiratory form almost always heals by encapsulation and calcification. In cases of dissemination, the dog loses weight and has persistent diarrhea, ascites, and a chronic cough; hepatosplenomegaly and lymphadenopathy may also be observed.

H. capsulatum has also been isolated from the intestinal contents and several organs of bats. High rates of reactors have been found in different domestic species (cattle, horses, sheep) in endemic areas, and the agent has been isolated from lymph nodes of dogs and cats, from a wild rodent (*Proechimys guyanensis*), and from a sloth in Brazil. Birds are not susceptible to histoplasmosis, perhaps because their high body temperature does not allow the fungus to develop.

Source of Infection and Mode of Transmission: The reservoir of the agent is the soil, where it lives as a saprophyte. Its distribution in the soil is uneven and depends on many factors, such as temperature, humidity, and others as yet undetermined. Microfoci that have given rise to sporadic cases and to epidemic outbreaks have generally been associated with soils in which the excreta of bats or certain species of birds have accumulated over time. These excreta apparently permit the fungus to compete with other soil microorganisms, thereby assuring its survival. In contrast to birds, which are not infected by *H. capsulatum* and whose role in the epidemiology is limited to the enabling function of their excreta, certain bats, especially colonial species, do become infected and eliminate the fungus in their droppings, thus contributing to its dissemination. The infection occurs frequently in humans visiting caves, tunnels, and abandoned mines where there are large populations of bats and a large accumulation of guano. Most of the cases in Mexico were due to exposure to bat droppings; the cases occurred among explorers, tourists, spelunkers, geologists, biologists, and others entering caves and similar places for work or study.

Man and animals acquire the infection from the same source (the soil) by the respiratory route. Microconidia of the fungus constitute the infecting element. The infection usually develops when natural foci are disturbed by activities that disperse the etiologic agent, such as bulldozing, cleaning or demolishing rural structures (especially chicken houses), visiting bat caves, and other activities.

Histoplasmosis is found predominantly in rural areas, but has also produced outbreaks among urban inhabitants, particularly construction workers. This was the case in the epidemics that occurred on the Indianapolis campus of Indiana University, where multiple human cases developed following excavations and demolition of old structures (see Occurrence in Man).

In dogs, the disease occurs most frequently among working and sporting breeds.

Role of Animals in the Epidemiology of the Disease: Both man and animals are accidental hosts of the etiologic agent and do not play a role in maintaining or transmitting the infection. Only certain bat species play an active role in disseminating the infection, in addition to contributing to its development by means of their accumulated droppings. Nevertheless, more studies are needed to evaluate the role of bats in the dispersal of the agent from one roost to another, as well as to determine the susceptibility of different species to histoplasmosis (Hoff and Bigler, 1981).

Diagnosis: Laboratory diagnosis can be accomplished by microscopic examination of stained smears; immunofluorescence using clinical specimens such as sputum, ulcer exudate, and others; isolation in culture media; inoculation of mice; and examination of histopathologic sections (bone marrow, lung, liver, and spleen).

The histoplasmin test is applied in a manner similar to the tuberculin test and is read after 24 and 48 hours. Sensitivity is established from 1 to 2 months after infection and lasts many years. This test is of great value for epidemiologic research; nevertheless, it has only limited utility in clinical diagnosis. It is advisable to apply the test in conjunction with the coccidioidin and blastomycin tests because of cross-reactions. A negative test result in a patient may indicate that the infection is recent or that the disease has a different etiology.

Serologic tests (complement fixation, precipitation, latex agglutination) are a great aid to diagnosis. Tests for blastomycosis and coccidioidomycosis should be applied simultaneously. It should be borne in mind that the histoplasmin test can give rise to antibodies; therefore, a blood sample should be obtained at the same time the test is given.

Control: The principal method of protection consists of reducing people's exposure to dust by spraying a 3% formalin solution on the ground when cleaning chicken coops or other places that may be contaminated. Use of protective masks is recommended. Control of the agent in natural foci is difficult. During one outbreak it was possible to eradicate the fungus from its natural focus by spraying the soil with formalin.

Bibliography

Ajello, L. Comparative ecology of respiratory mycotic disease agents. *Bacteriol Rev* 31:6-24, 1967.

Ajello, L., and W. Kaplan. Systemic mycoses. *In*: Stoenner, H., W. Kaplan, and M. Torten (Section Eds.), *CRC Handbook Series in Zoonoses*. Section A, vol. 2. Boca Raton, Florida, CRC Press, 1980.

American Public Health Association. *Control of Communicable Diseases in Man*, 14th ed. (Ed. by A. S. Benenson). Washington, D.C., APHA, 1985.

Borelli, D. Prevalence of systemic mycoses in Latin America. *In*: *Proceedings, International Symposium on Mycoses*. Washington, D.C., Pan American Health Organization, 1970. (Scientific Publication 205.)

Hoff, G. L., and W. J. Bigler. The role of bats in the propagation and spread of histoplasmosis: a review. *J Wildl Dis* 17:191-196, 1981.

Kaplan, W. Epidemiology of the principal systemic mycoses of man and lower animals and the ecology of their etiologic agents. *J Am Vet Med Assoc* 163:1043-1047, 1973.

Manson-Bahr, P. E. C., and F. I. C. Apted. *Manson's Tropical Diseases*, 18th ed. London, Baillière Tindall, 1982.

Menges, R. W., R. T. Habermann, L. A. Selby, H. R. Ellis, R. F. Behlow, and C. D. Smith. A review and recent findings of histoplasmosis in animals. *Vet Med* 58:334-338, 1963.

Negroni, P. *Histoplasmosis; Diagnosis and Treatment*. Springfield, Illinois, Thomas, 1965.

Negroni, P. *Micosis cutáneas y viscerales*, 5th ed. Buenos Aires, López, 1972.

Pan American Health Organization. Histoplasmosis in Mexico, 1979-1980. *Epidemiol Bull* 2:12-13, 1981.

Sanger, V. L. Histoplasmosis. *In*: Davis, J. W., L. H. Karstad, and D. O. Trainer (Eds.), *Infectious Diseases of Wild Mammals*. Ames, Iowa State University Press, 1970.

Schlech, W. F., L. J. Wheat, J. L. Ho, M. L. V. French, R. J. Weeks, R. B. Kohler, C. E. Deane, H. E. Eitzen, and J. D. Band. Recurrent urban histoplasmosis, Indianapolis, Indiana, 1980-1981. *Am J Epidemiol* 118:301-302, 1983.

Selby, L. A. Histoplasmosis. *In*: Hubbert, W. T., W. F. McCulloch, and P. R. Schnurren-berger (Eds.), *Diseases Transmitted from Animals to Man*, 6th ed. Springfield, Illinois, Thomas, 1975.

Sweany, H. C. (Ed.). *Histoplasmosis*. Springfield, Illinois, Thomas, 1960.

Waldman, R. J., A. C. England, R. Tauxe, T. Kline, R. J. Weeks, L. A. Ajello, L. Kaufman, B. Wentworth, and D. W. Fraser. A winter outbreak of acute histoplasmosis in northern Michigan. *Am J Epidemiol* 117:68-75, 1983.

MADUROMYCOSIS

(117.4)

Synonyms: Madura foot, maduromycotic mycetoma, eumycotic mycetoma, actinomycetoma.

Etiology: Maduromycosis (mycetoma) is caused by many species of fungi (eumycetoma) or by bacterial agents (actinomycetoma). The principal agents of eumycetoma are *Madurella mycetomatis*, *M. grisea*, *Leptosphaeria senegalensis* (all producing black granules), *Pseudoallescheria* (*Petriellidium*, *Allescheria*) *boydii*, and several species of *Acremonium* (white or yellow granules). Actinomycetoma are caused by *Nocardia brasiliensis* and *N. asteroides*, *Streptomyces somaliensis*, *Actinomadura madurae*, and *A. pelletierii*. The principal agents of animal mycetomas are *P. boydii* and *Curvularia geniculata*.

Both the fungi and the actinomycetes are soil saprophytes that accidentally enter the hosts' tissues, where they form granules (colonies). Eumycetoma granules contain thick hyphae; in contrast, actinomycetoma granules contain fine filaments.

Geographic Distribution: The agents of maduromycosis are distributed worldwide but are most abundant in the tropics.

Occurrence in Man: Infrequent. It is more common in tropical and subtropical zones, especially where people go barefoot.

Most cases occur in Africa. In Sudan, 1,231 patients required hospitalization in a 2½-year period. Maduromycosis is endemic in many areas of India. In the Americas, it occurs most frequently in Mexico and Central America (mainly caused by *Nocardia brasiliensis*) (Manson-Bahr and Apted, 1982). From 1944 to 1978, 154 cases were observed in São Paulo, Brazil, of which 73.4% were actinomycetomas and 26.6% eumycetomas.

Mycetomas occur mainly in males from rural areas.

Occurrence in Animals: Rare.

The Disease in Man: Maduromycosis is a slowly developing, chronic infection that localizes most frequently on the foot or the lower leg, occasionally on a hand, and rarely on another part of the body. The incubation period is several months from the time of inoculation. The lesion may begin as a papule, nodule, or abscess. The mycetoma spreads to deep tissue and the foot (or hand) can swell to two or three times its normal size. Numerous, small abscesses form, as well as fistulous tracks in the subcutaneous tissue that branch out to the tendons and may even reach the bones. Pus discharged to the surface contains characteristic granules (microcolonies) that may be white or another color depending on the causal agent. There is no loss of sensibility in the skin and, in general, the patient experiences no pain. Actinomycetomas almost always respond to antibacterial antibiotics (penicillin, streptomycin, co-trimoxazole), but eumycetomas are quite resistant (ketoconazole, mycanzole) and often lead to amputation.

The Disease in Animals: Almost all confirmed cases have occurred in the United States. Eumycetomas described in animals (dogs, cats, horses) were localized in the feet, lymph nodes, abdominal cavity, and other regions of the body. Except for the case of mycetoma caused by *P. boydii* in a dog, other cases have been due to fungi different from those responsible for eumycetoma in man.

Source of Infection and Mode of Transmission: The etiologic agents of this disease are saprophytes in the soil and vegetation. The fungus is introduced into subcutaneous tissue through wounds. Contaminated thorns or splinters can be the immediate source of infection.

Role of Animals in the Epidemiology of the Disease: None.

Diagnosis: Microscopic examination of pus or material from curettage or biopsy can distinguish granules of eumycetoma from those of actinomycetoma (nocardiosis). Isolation by culture is necessary to identify the agent. To ensure proper treatment, the agent's sensitivity to different medications must be determined.

In a study done in Sudan, specific diagnosis was achieved for 78% of the specimens by using histologic methods, and for 82% of the cases by immunodiffusion (Mahgoub, 1975). The choice of strains for the serologic test is very important.

Control: Humans can avoid becoming infected by wearing shoes.

Bibliography

American Public Health Association. *Control of Communicable Diseases in Man*, 14th ed. (Ed. by A. S. Benenson). Washington, D.C., APHA, 1985.

Brodey, R. S., H. F. Schryver, M. J. Deubler, W. Kaplan, and L. Ajello. Mycetoma in a dog. *J Am Vet Med Assoc* 151:442-451, 1967.

Conant, N. F. Medical mycology. *In*: Dubos, R. J., and J. G. Hirsch (Eds.), *Bacterial and Clinical Mycology*, 2nd ed. Philadelphia and London, Saunders, 1963.

Conant, N. F. Medical mycology. *In*: Dubos, R. J., and J. G. Hirsch (Eds.), *Bacterial and Mycotic Infections of Man*, 4th ed. Philadelphia, Lippincott, 1965.

Jang, S. S., and J. A. Popp. Eumycotic mycetoma in a dog caused by *Allescheria boydii*. *J Am Vet Med Assoc* 157:1071-1076, 1970.

Mahgoub, E. S. Serologic diagnosis of mycetoma. *In*: *Proceedings, Third International Conference on the Mycoses*. Washington, D.C., Pan American Health Organization, 1975. (Scientific Publication 304.)

Manson-Bahr, P. E. C., and F. I. C. Apted. *Manson's Tropical Diseases*, 18th ed. London, Baillière Tindall, 1982.

Rinaldi, M. G., P. Phillips, J. G. Schwartz, R. E. Winn, G. R. Holt, F. W. Shasets, J. Elrod, G. Nishioka, and T. B. Aufdemorte. Human *Curvularia* infections. Report of five cases and review of the literature. *Diagn Microbiol Infect Dis* 6:27-39, 1987.

Segretain, G., and F. Mariat. Mycetoma. *In*: Warren, K. S., and A. A. F. Mahmoud (Eds.), *Tropical and Geographical Medicine*, New York, McGraw-Hill Book Company, 1984.

RHINOSPORIDIOSIS

(117.0)

Etiology: *Rhinosporidium seeberi*, a fungus that in the tissues forms sporangia containing a large number of sporangiospores. The fungus has not been cultured.

Geographic Distribution (Map 1): The disease has been confirmed in the Americas, Asia (endemic zones in India and Sri Lanka), Africa, and Europe.

Occurrence in Man and Animals: The disease has a very low incidence throughout the world. Up to 1970, data from Latin America show 108 cases in humans and 45 in animals; most of the human cases occurred in Paraguay (56), Brazil (13), and Venezuela (13) (Mayorga, 1970). According to more recent data, more than 50 cases have occurred in Venezuela, mainly in the states of Barinas and Portuguesa. The disease has also been confirmed in Cuba and Argentina. In the United States, 13 cases have been recorded (Sauerteig, 1980). Recently, five cases were described in Trinidad (Raju and Jamalabadi, 1983); four of these affected the conjunctiva. Most of the cases in Africa were recorded in Uganda. Some 1,000 cases have occurred in India and Sri Lanka, and 72 occurred in Iran over a 30-year period.

The disease is seen mostly in children and young people, predominantly in males (Mohapatra, 1984).

The Disease in Man and Animals: Rhinosporidiosis is characterized by pedunculated or sessile polyps on the mucous membranes, especially of the nose and eyes. The polyps are soft, lobular, and reddish in color with small white spots (the sporangia). The excrescences are not painful, but they bleed easily. In man, these granulomatous formations can also be found in the pharynx, larynx, ear, vagina, penis, rectum, and on the skin. Cases of dissemination to internal organs are rare.

Source of Infection and Mode of Transmission: The natural habitat of the agent is not known. It is suspected that the infection enters the body with soil particles through lesions of the mucous membranes. In India and Sri Lanka, where most cases have been recorded, the source of infection has been associated with stagnant

Map 1. Distribution of notified cases of rhinosporidiosis.

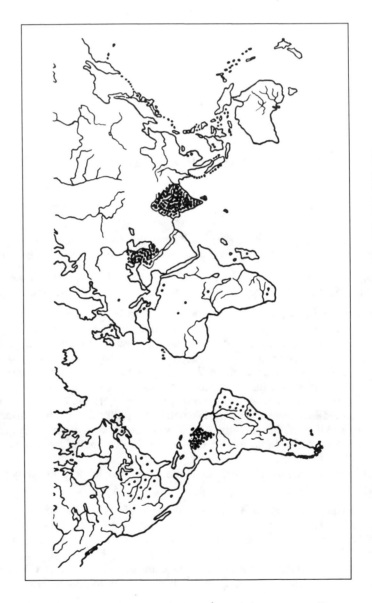

Source: Proceedings, Fifth International Conference on the Mycoses. PAHO, 1980. (Sci. Publ. 396).

waters, but it has not yet been possible to demonstrate the presence of the fungus in such waters or in aquatic animals.

Role of Animals in the Epidemiology of the Disease: Rhinosporidiosis is a disease common to man and animals, contracted from an as yet unknown environmental source. It is not transmitted from one individual to another.

Diagnosis: Since the fungus cannot be cultured, diagnosis depends on the clinical appearance of the lesions and demonstration of the agent's presence in tissues. Best results are obtained using stained histopathologic preparations.

Control: No practical control measures are available.

Bibliography

Ajello, L., L. K. Georg, W. Kaplan, and L. Kaufman. *Laboratory Manual for Medical Mycology.* Washington, D.C., U.S. Government Printing Office, 1963. (Public Health Service Publication 994.)

Jimenez, J. F., J. B. Cornelius, and E. S. Gloster. Canine rhinosporidiosis in Arkansas. *Lab Anim Sci* 36:54-55, 1986.

Mayorga, R. Prevalence of subcutaneous mycoses in Latin America. *In: Proceedings, International Symposium on Mycoses.* Washington, D.C., Pan American Health Organization, 1970. (Scientific Publication 205.)

Mahapatra, L. N. Rhinosporidiosis. *In:* Warren, K. S., and A. A. F. Mahmoud (Eds.), *Tropical and Geographical Medicine.* New York, McGraw-Hill Book Company, 1984.

Negroni, P. *Micosis cutáneas y viscerales*, 5th ed. Buenos Aires, López, 1972.

Raju, G. C., and M. H. Jamalabadi. Rhinosporidiosis in Trinidad. *Trop Geogr Med* 35:257-258, 1983.

Sauerteig, E. Rhinosporidiosis in Barinas, Venezuela. *In: Proceedings, Fifth International Conference on the Mycoses.* Washington, D.C., Pan American Health Organization, 1980. (Scientific Publication 396.)

Utz, J. P. The mycoses. *In:* Beeson, P. B., W. McDermott, and J. B. Wyngaarden (Eds.), *Cecil Textbook of Medicine*, 15th ed. Philadelphia and London, Saunders, 1979.

SPOROTRICHOSIS

(117.1)

Etiology: *Sporothrix schenckii* (*Sporotrichum schenckii*, *Sporotrichum beurmanni*), a saprophytic fungus that lives in soil, plants, and decaying vegetation.

S. schenckii is a dimorphic fungus that occurs in a mycelial form in nature and a yeast form in infected animal tissues or on enriched culture media (such as blood agar) at 37°C. The latter form generally produces multiple buds and occasionally a single bud.

Geographic Distribution: Worldwide.

Occurrence in Man: Sporadic; its frequency varies from region to region. The disease has been confirmed in all Latin American countries with the exceptions of Chile, Bolivia, and Nicaragua. It is more frequent in Brazil, Mexico, Central America, Zimbabwe, and South Africa than in other countries. Even though this disease is relatively rare, an epidemic affecting 3,000 workers was recorded in South African gold mines. A group of cases also occurred in the United States among forestry workers who contracted the disease while planting pine trees, and another among students who came into contact with contaminated bricks (Mitchell, 1983). In the area around Ayerza Lagoon in Guatemala, 53 cases were seen between 1971 and 1975 (Mayorga *et al.*, 1979). Results of skin hypersensitivity tests using antigens of *S. schenckii* and *Ceratocystis stenoceras* (a closely related species) indicated that asymptomatic infection is probably frequent in occupational groups that work with plants. The study done in the Ayerza Lagoon region (Mayorga *et al.*, 1979), found cutaneous hypersensitivity among local inhabitants at least 10 times higher than among residents of Guatemala City. In a study carried out in Brazil among exposed and unexposed urban and rural occupational groups, the results were similar (Lima and Pereira, Jr., 1981).

The disease is more prevalent in males than in females.

Occurrence in Animals: Occasional. The horse is the most frequently affected species. Cases have been recorded in dogs, cats, rodents, cattle, swine, camels, birds, and wild animals.

The Disease in Man: The incubation period can vary from 3 weeks to 3 months. The most common clinical form is cutaneolymphatic; it begins with a nodule or pustule at the point where broken skin allowed inoculation. The primary lesion is usually located on exposed extremities. The infection may remain confined to the entry site or may eventually spread and produce subcutaneous nodules along the enlarged lymph ducts. These nodules may ulcerate, and a gray or yellowish pus appears. The patient's general state of health is usually not affected.

Vegetative and verrucous dermal forms are also observed. Disseminated forms, which are rare, may give rise to localizations in different organs, especially the bones and joints, as well as in the mouth, nose, kidneys, or the subcutaneous tissue over large areas of the body. Some researchers have concluded that dissemination occurs via the bloodstream or the lymphatic system from the inoculation site on the skin, while others believe that a primary focus in the lungs is involved.

Pulmonary sporotrichosis results from inhalation of the fungus. Its course may be acute, but in general it is chronic and can be confused with tuberculosis.

Because of their occupation, farmers, gardeners, and floriculturists are the persons most exposed to the infection.

The Disease in Animals: The disease in horses and mules is similar to that in man; it must be differentiated from epizootic lymphangitis caused by *Histoplasma farciminosum* (*Cryptococcus farciminosum*). The skin covering the spherical nodules becomes moist, the hair falls out, and a scab forms. The ulcers heal slowly and leave a bald scar. The affected extremity swells owing to lymphatic stasis. No cases of dissemination have been described in horses.

The disease in dogs may take the cutaneolymphatic form, but it frequently affects the bones, liver, and lungs.

Source of Infection and Mode of Transmission: The reservoirs of the fungus are soil and plants. Man and animals almost always become infected through a cutaneous lesion. The infection can be contracted from handling moss, wood splinters, firewood, or dead vegetation on which the fungus has developed. The source of infection in the Transvaal, South Africa, epidemic was timbers in the gold mines on which *S. schenckii* was growing. Nevertheless, the source of infection is not always easily recognizable. Out of the 53 cases of sporotrichosis that occurred in the Ayerza Lagoon area in Guatemala, 24 (45.3%) patients attributed the wound and subsequent ulceration to handling fish, 6 (11.3%) attributed it to wood splinters, and 20 (37.7%) could not remember any trauma. An attempt to isolate *S. schenckii* from 58 environmental samples gave negative results (Mayorga *et al.*, 1979).

Inhalation provides another route of entry for the fungus and is responsible for the small number of pulmonary sporotrichosis cases that have been recorded.

Role of Animals in the Epidemiology of the Disease: Although some cases of animal-to-man transmission have been described, animals are thought to play no role in the epidemiology of the infection. Sporotrichosis is a disease common to man and animals.

Diagnosis: Diagnosis can be confirmed by culture and identification of the fungus. Indirect immunofluorescence is the preferred serologic test because of its sensitivity; other useful tests are latex agglutination and tube agglutination. Serologic tests are especially important in diagnosing disseminated sporotrichosis.

Control: It is recommended that wood be treated with fungicides in industries where cases occur.

Bibliography

Ainsworth, G. C., and P. K. C. Austwick. *Fungal Diseases of Animals*, 2nd ed. Farnham Royal, Slough, England, Commonwealth Agricultural Bureau, 1973.

American Public Health Association. *Control of Communicable Diseases in Man*, 14th ed. (Ed. by A. S. Benenson). Washington, D.C., APHA, 1985.

Bruner, D. W., and J. H. Gillespie. *Hagan's Infectious Diseases of Domestic Animals*, 6th ed. Ithaca, New York, Cornell University Press, 1973.

Dunstan, R. W., K. A. Reimann, and R. F. Langham. Feline sporotrichosis. Zoonosis update. *J Am Vet Med Assoc* 189:880-883, 1986.

Lima, L. B., and A. C. Pereira, Jr. Esporotricose-Inquerito epidemiológico. Importancia como doença profissional. *An Bras Dermatol* 56:243-248, 1981.

Mackinon, J. E. Ecology and epidemiology of sporotrichosis. *In: Proceedings, International Symposium on Mycoses*. Washington, D.C., Pan American Health Organization, 1970. (Scientific Publication 205.)

Mayorga, R., A. Cáceres, C. Toriello, G. Gutiérrez, O. Alvarez, M. E. Ramírez, and F. Mariat. Investigación de una zona endémica en la región de la laguna de Ayerza, Guatemala. *Bol Of Sanit Panam* 87:20-34, 1979.

Mitchell, T. G. Subcutaneous Mycoses. *In*: Joklik, W. K., H. P. Willet, and D. B. Amos (Eds.), *Zinsser Microbiology*, 18th ed. Norwalk, Connecticut, Appleton-Century-Crofts, 1984.

Negroni, B. *Micosis cutáneas y viscerales*, 5th ed. Buenos Aires, López, 1972.

Richard, J. L. Sporotrichosis. *In*: Hubbert, W. T., W. F. McCulloch, and P. R. Schnurrenberger (Eds.), *Diseases Transmitted from Animals to Man*, 6th ed. Springfield, Illinois, Thomas, 1975.

ZYGOMYCOSIS

(117.7)

Synonyms: Phycomycosis, mucormycosis, entomophthoromycosis.

Etiology: Zygomycosis denotes a group of diseases caused by several genera and species of fungi belonging to the class Zygomycetes, orders Entomophthorales and Mucorales. Consequently, the etiologic agents are numerous; the principal ones are mentioned below in connection with the different diseases they cause, which can be subdivided into entomophthoromycoses and mucormycoses (Council for International Organizations of Medical Sciences [CIOMS], 1982).

Geographical Distribution: Worldwide.

Occurrence in Man: Sporadic cases are seen, principally in patients debilitated by other diseases. At present, the incidence of zygomycosis is increasing because of the longer survival of diabetics and the growing number of immunosuppressed patients. Entomophthoromycoses occur mainly in the tropics. Of 170 cases due to *Basidiobolus ranarum* (*B. haptosporus*) described up to 1975, 112 occurred in Africa, and an additional 75 cases in Uganda became known later (Kelly *et al.*, 1980). This disease also occurs in Southeast Asia, and some cases have appeared in Latin America and the United States. Entomophthoromycoses caused by fungi of the genus *Conidiobolus* also occur in the tropics and are more common in males (CIOMS, 1982). Mucormycoses (phycomycoses) do not have a definite geographic distribution.

Occurrence in Animals: It occurs sporadically in many species of domestic and wild mammals, birds, reptiles, amphibians, and fish.

The Disease in Man: The agents of mucormycoses are potential pathogens that are classified as opportunistic, since they invade tissues of patients weakened by other diseases or treated for a long time with antibiotics or corticosteroids. About 40% of the cases have been associated with diabetes mellitus. By contrast, in Africa and Asia entomophthoromycoses occur in individuals without histories of preexisting illness (Bittencourt *et al.*, 1982).

Entomophthoromycoses caused by *Basidiobolus ranarum* (*B. haptosporus*) are characterized by the formation of granulomas with eosinophilic infiltration of subcutaneous tissues. In general, the buttock or thigh is the affected region, with a hard swelling of the subcutaneous tissue and a sharp demarcation of the healthy part. The disease is usually benign, but it can occasionally be invasive and result in death (Greenham, 1979; Kelly *et al.*, 1980).

Entomophthoromycoses due to *Conidiobolus coronatus* and *C. incongruens* usually begin in the inferior nasal concha and invade the subcutaneous facial tissues and the paranasal sinuses. Lesions of the pericardium, mediastinum, and lungs have also been described (CIOMS, 1982).

Mucormycoses are caused by fungi of the genera *Absidia*, *Mucor*, *Rhizopus*, *Cunninghamella*, and *Rhizomucor*. The infection begins in the nasal mucosa and the paranasal sinuses, where the fungi may multiply rapidly and spread to the eye sockets, meninges, and brain. The clinical forms caused by these fungi are rhinocerebral, pulmonary, gastrointestinal, disseminated, and subcutaneous mucormycoses. The rhinocerebral form appears mainly in patients with diabetes mellitus and is quickly fatal. Patients with a malignant blood disease and those receiving immunosuppressants primarily suffer from pulmonary and disseminated mucormycoses and less frequently from the rhinocerebral form. The gastrointestinal form has occurred in a few cases in malnourished children. The cutaneous and subcutaneous forms can occur as a consequence of deep burns, injections, and application of contaminated bandages. Mucormycoses are characterized by vascular occlusion with fungal hyphae, thrombosis, and necrosis.

The Disease in Animals: Zygomycosis in animals is usually found during necropsy or postmortem inspection in abattoirs. Few cases are confirmed by isolation and identification of the causal agent. Lesions are granulomatous or ulcerative. Zygomycosis in cattle, sheep, and goats usually appears as ulcers of the abomasum. These fungi are an important cause of mycotic abortions in some countries. In Great Britain they account for 32% of abortions caused by fungi, and in New Zealand for 75%.

In horses, zygomycosis takes the form of a chronic, localized disease that causes the formation of cutaneous granulomas on the extremities. In India, Indonesia, Brazil, Australia, France, and the United States, cases of the subcutaneous form caused by *Hyphomyces destruens* have occurred. A clinical study carried out in tropical Australia of 266 cases of zygomycosis found that 76.6% were attributable to *H. destruens*, 18% to *Basidiobolus ranarum* (*B. haptosporus*), and 5.3% to *Conidiobolus coronatus*. Horses infected by *H. destruens* presented large granulomatous, coralliform masses containing necrotic cells and hyphae. The lesions were usually located on the extremities and the venter. *H. destruens* is found mainly in a wet habitat and lesions appear in the rainy season. The disease due to *B. ranarum* is clinically similar to that caused by *H. destruens*; lesions are found most often on the trunk and face. On the other hand, lesions caused by *C. coronatus* are located in the nasal region (Miller and Campbell, 1982). Pulmonary infection, disease of the guttural pouch, systemic infection, and some mycotic abortions have also been described in horses.

Zygomycosis in swine produces a gastric ulceration.

In dogs and cats, the disease usually affects the gastrointestinal tract, and mortality is very high. Lesions of the stomach or small intestine are accompanied by vomiting, and lesions in the colon by diarrhea and tenesmus (Ader, 1979).

Source of Infection and Mode of Transmission: Zygomycetes are ubiquitous saprophytes that produce a large number of spores; they are common inhabitants of decomposing organic material and the gastrointestinal tract of reptiles and amphibians. Man contracts the infection by inhalation, ingestion, inoculation, and contamination of the skin with spores. The common route of entry is the nose, by inhalation of spores. Debilitating diseases, such as diabetes mellitus, and prolonged treatment with immunosuppressants and antibiotics are important causal factors of mucormycoses. Subcutaneous entomophthormycoses due to *Basidiobolus* develop as a result of direct inoculation by thorns.

The digestive route seems to be more important than the respiratory in domestic animals. In horses, direct exposure of the skin (abrasions, wounds) to fungi provides the portal of entry for infections caused by *Hyphomyces destruens*.

Role of Animals in the Epidemiology of the Disease: Man and animals contract the infection from a common source in the environment. The infection is not transmitted from one individual to another (man or animal).

Diagnosis: Diagnosis is based on confirmation of the agents' presence in scrapings or biopsies of lesions by means of direct microscopic observation or by culture. Zygomycetes in tissue can be identified by their large nonseptate hyphae. The species of fungus can only be determined by culture and spore identification (Ader, 1979).

Control: Human zygomycosis can be prevented in many cases by proper treatment of metabolic disorders, especially diabetes mellitus. Prolonged antibiotic and corticosteroid treatment should be confined to those cases in which it is absolutely necessary. Animals should not be allowed to consume moldy fodder.

Bibliography

Ader, P. L. Phycomycosis in fifteen dogs and two cats. *J Am Vet Med Assoc* 174:1216-1223, 1979.

Ainsworth, G. C., and P. K. C. Austwick. *Fungal Diseases of Animals*, 2nd ed. Farnham Royal, Slough, England, Commonwealth Agricultural Bureau, 1973.

Ajello, L., L. K. Georg, W. Kaplan, and L. Kaufman. *Laboratory Manual for Medical Mycology*. Washington, D.C., U.S. Government Printing Office, 1963. (Public Health Service Publication 994.)

Bittencourt, A. L., G. Serra, M. Sadigursky, M. G. S. Araujo, M. C. S. Campos, and L. C. M. Sampaio. Subcutaneous zygomycosis caused by *Basidiobolus haptosporus*: presentation of a case mimicking Burkitt's lymphoma. *Am J Trop Med Hyg* 31:370-373, 1982.

Carter, G. R. *Diagnostic Procedures in Veterinary Microbiology*, 2nd ed., Springfield, Illinois, Thomas, 1973.

Council for International Organizations of Medical Sciences. *International Nomenclature of Diseases*, Vol. 2: Infectious Diseases, Part 2: Mycoses. Geneva, CIOMS, 1982.

González-Mendoza, A. Opportunistic mycoses. *In*: *Proceedings, International Symposium on Mycoses*. Washington, D.C., Pan American Health Organization, 1970. (Scientific Publication 205.)

Greenham, R. Subcutaneous phycomycosis: not always benign. *Lancet* 1:97-98, 1979.

Kelly, S., N. Gill, and M. S. R. Hutt. Subcutaneous phycomycosis in Sierra Leone. *Trans R Soc Trop Med Hyg* 74:396-397, 1980.

Miller, R. I., and R. S. F. Campbell. Clinical observations on equine phycomycosis. *Aust Vet J* 58:221-226, 1982.

Richard, J. L. Phycomycoses. *In*: Hubbert, W. T., W. F. McCulloch, and P. R. Schnurrenberger (Eds.), *Diseases Transmitted from Animals to Man*, 6th ed. Springfield, Illinois, Thomas, 1975.

Sanford, S. E., G. K. Josephson, and F. H. Waters. Submandibular and disseminated zygomycosis (mucormycosis) in feeder pigs. *J Am Vet Med Assoc* 186:171-174, 1985.

Soltys, M. A. *Bacteria and Fungi Pathogenic to Man and Animals*. London, Baillière, Tindall and Cox, 1963.

Part III

CHLAMYDIOSES
AND RICKETTSIOSES

ASIAN IXODO-RICKETTSIOSIS

(082.2)

Synonyms: North Asian tick rickettsiosis, Siberian tick typhus.

Etiology: *Rickettsia siberica* (*Dermacentroxenus sibericus*). This agent belongs to the group of rickettsiae that produce spotted fever.

Geographic Distribution: Siberia, various islands in the Sea of Japan, Mongolian People's Republic, various asiatic republics of the Soviet Union (Armenia, Kirghizia, Kazakhstan). *R. siberica* has also been isolated from ticks in Czechoslovakia and Pakistan.

Occurrence in Man: Sporadic. Occurs mostly in farmers, hunters, forestry workers, and persons entering the natural foci of the disease. In urban areas, the infection can be transmitted by ticks carried from natural foci by domestic animals, with firewood, or by other means.

Occurrence in Animals: The etiologic agent has been isolated from a large variety of wild rodent species that live in natural foci, as well as from the domestic mouse and the European hare.

The Disease in Man: It is an acute, febrile, and benign disease, clinically similar to Boutonneuse fever (see Boutonneuse Fever).

The Disease in Animals: No information is available on the natural course of the disease in wild rodents or in other species from which the rickettsia has been isolated; it is probably asymptomatic.

Source of Infection and Mode of Transmission: Man contracts the infection through tick bites. The main vectors are ticks of the genera *Dermacentor* and *Haemaphysalis*. The survival of the etiologic agent in ticks during hibernation, transovarial transmission from one generation of arthropods to the next, and infection of a variety of small mammal species ensures a continuous circulation of the rickettsiae in natural foci.

At the end of hibernation and before egg laying, the ticks attach themselves to large mammals (domestic and wild animals) and accidentally to man when he enters the habitat. The highest incidence of the disease in man thus occurs in spring, coinciding with the period of greatest adult tick activity. Generally, it is adult ticks that attack man, but larvae and nymphs of *Dermacentor nuttalli* and *Haemaphysalis concinna* may also. Larvae and nymphs usually feed on small mammals, mainly rodents, assuring an additional reservoir and source of infection. In autumn, adult ticks of a new generation occasionally attach themselves to man and produce cases of the disease.

Role of Animals in the Epidemiology of the Disease: Man is an accidental host. The reservoir is made up of wild rodents and ticks, the latter having the principal role in maintaining and transmitting the infection. Transovarial and transstadial transmission of *R. siberica* has been observed in *D. marginatus* through at least 5 years (Harwood and James, 1979). Domestic animals (cattle, horses, dogs) serve as main hosts for the adult vectors.

Diagnosis: As with other spotted fevers, laboratory confirmation can be obtained by means of serologic tests (Weil-Felix with *Proteus* OX-19, complement fixation, micro-immunofluorescence) and by isolation via inoculation in laboratory animals (guinea pigs, rats, hamsters).

Control: Control measures are directed against the vectors and include the use of tickicides on domestic animals and in their environment and reduction of rodent populations, since rodents are the main hosts for tick larvae and nymphs. For individual protection, protective clothing and repellents are recommended.

Bibliography

Bosler, E. M., J. L. Coleman, J. L. Benach, D. A. Massey, J. P. Hanrahan, W. Burgdorfer, and A. G. Barbour. Natural distribution of the *Ixodus dammini* spirochete. *Science* 220:321-322, 1983.

Burgdorfer, W. North Asian tick typhus. *In*: Hubbert, W. T., W. F. McCulloch, and P. R. Schnurrenberger (Eds.), *Diseases Transmitted from Animals to Man*, 6th ed. Springfield, Illinois, Thomas, 1975.

Harwood, R. F., and M. T. James. *Entomology in Human and Animal Health*, 7th ed. New York, Macmillan, 1979.

Zdrodovskii, P. F., and H. M. Golinevich. *The Rickettsial Diseases*. Oxford, Pergamon Press, 1960.

AVIAN CHLAMYDIOSIS

(073)

Synonyms: Psittacosis (in birds of the family Psittacidae), ornithosis (in other birds).

Etiology: The genus *Chlamydia* contains two species: *Chlamydia trachomatis,* a human pathogen, and *C. psittaci,* a pathogen of birds and mammals that is transmitted to man. Chlamydiae are intracellular microorganisms with a unique reproductive cycle that includes two phases, only one of which is infectious. This cycle and other metabolic and structural characteristics of chlamydiae distinguish them from bacteria and even more so from rickettsiae and viruses.

The infectious stage is the elementary body, which is engulfed when it comes in contact with a susceptible cell. After 6 to 8 hours the elementary body reorganizes into a noninfectious reticulate body which divides by binary fission. After 18 to 24 hours, some of the reticulate bodies undergo another reorganization, condensing and changing into elementary bodies of about 0.4 micron in diameter. Consequently, the intracellular inclusion bodies contain the larger reticulate bodies (about 0.8 micron) and the elementary bodies (about 0.4 micron). When the host cell disintegrates, the elementary bodies are released and reinitiate the cycle of infection.

Geographic Distribution: Worldwide.

Occurrence in Man: Generally sporadic. Between 1929 and 1930 a pandemic affected 12 countries, causing about 1,000 cases and 200 to 300 deaths. The outbreaks were due to the importation of psittacines from South America (Schachter, 1975). In recent years, outbreaks have occurred among workers in turkey processing plants. In the United States, in 1974 four outbreaks took place in Texas, in 1976 an outbreak affected 28 of 98 employees in a Nebraska plant, and in 1981 in Ohio 27 of 80 workers became ill (Centers for Disease Control, USA, 1982). Likewise, 21 people are believed to have been affected in an outbreak associated with the necropsy of turkeys in 1978 at the Veterinary School of New York (Filstein *et al.*, 1981). In the same country at present, infection by *C. psittaci* is largely an occupational disease related to working with turkeys, as in central and eastern Europe it is associated with ducks. Many sporadic cases are not diagnosed at all or are attributed to other diseases. Information from developing countries is scarce.

Occurrence in Animals: Natural infection caused by chlamydiae has been found in 130 species of domestic and wild birds, more than half of which belong to the family Psittacidae. For practical purposes, all avian species can be considered potential reservoirs of chlamydiae. The disease is very common in psittacines, fringillids, and pigeons as well as in ducks, turkeys, and poultry. The infection rate is generally lower in wild birds than in domestic fowl. *C. psittaci* was isolated from 20% of 287 dead pet birds in Florida, USA, 250 of which were psittaciforms (Schwartz and Fraser, 1982). In Japan, in a similar study of dying and dead birds, *C. psittaci* was isolated from 19 (24.7%) of 77 psittaciform birds and from 12 (26.1%) of 46 passeriforms (Hirai *et al.*, 1983). Of 716 wild pigeons in residential areas of Japan, the agent was isolated from only 6 (0.8%), but 37% of 568 had antibodies in the complement fixation test (Fukushi *et al.*, 1983). Moreover, *C. psittaci* parasitizes many species of domestic and wild mammals.

The Disease in Man: The incubation period is usually 1 to 2 weeks, but sometimes longer. Many infections pass asymptomatically, while others show symptoms which vary in severity. Mild forms of psittacosis may be confused with common respiratory illnesses and often go unnoticed. The disease can have a sudden onset with fever, chills, sweating, muscle aches, anorexia, and headache. There are also cases in which the onset is insidious. Symptoms last from 7 to 10 days. In cases producing atypical pneumonia, early radiographs show infiltrations and, less frequently, areas of consolidation in the lower part of the lungs that may develop into bronchopneumonia. Initially, there may be a dry cough; later, some expectoration occurs of a mucoid sputum that becomes mucopurulent. The most serious form of the disease occurs in persons over 50 years old and includes hepatosplenomegaly, vomiting, diarrhea, constipation, insomnia, disorientation, mental depression, and even delirium.

Early treatment (tetracyclines) is important to shorten the illness and avoid complications. The case fatality rate is less than 1% when patients receive appropriate treatment.

The Disease in Animals: Most infections in birds are latent and inapparent. In general, birds develop the disease when their overall resistance is diminished due to stress factors (crowding, concurrent infections, unhygienic conditions, nutritional deficiencies, prolonged transport, and other factors). Outbreaks have been observed in establishments selling pet birds such as parrots and parakeets or, more frequently, during shipment of these animals. Outbreaks of the disease have also occurred in pigeons, ducks, and turkeys. The symptomatology is not characteristic and consists of fever, diarrhea, anorexia, emaciation, and respiratory distress. Conjunctivitis is common, varying in severity from simple conjunctival congestion to necrotic obstruction of the orbit. Postmortem examination reveals inflamed pleura covered with a fibrinous exudate, lungs with edematous or hyperemic areas, and an enlarged and striated liver. Splenomegaly is common in psittacine birds, as are epicarditis and myocarditis in turkeys. In poultry, however, the infection is almost always inapparent.

C. psittaci causes a variety of diseases in mammals, such as enzootic abortion in sheep, epizootic abortion in cattle, conjunctivitis in guinea pigs, pneumonitis in cats and other species, encephalomyelitis in cattle, and polyarthritis in lambs and calves.

The relationship between strains of *C. psittaci* from fowl and those from domestic mammals is not well known. Parenteral inoculation of chlamydiae from ovine polyarthritis has reproduced the disease in turkeys; likewise, chlamydiae associated with ovine enzootic abortion were fatal to sparrows and caused infection in pigeons. Nevertheless, oral administration of chlamydiae from domestic mammals to various species of wild fowl produced neither observable seroconversion nor elimination of the agent in the feces (Johnson and Grimes, 1983). In general, fowl strains are thought to be species-specific and not communicable to domestic mammals and vice versa.

Source of Infection and Mode of Transmission (Figure 21): The natural reservoirs of *C. psittaci* are wild and domestic birds. Mammalian chlamydiae (except *C. trachomatis,* which is found in humans and is the agent of mouse pneumonitis) also belong to the species *C. psittaci.* Notwithstanding, the mammalian strains of *C. psittaci* are rarely pathogenic to man and only a few cases of human infection from this source are known, contracted in the laboratory or by natural exposure (Schachter and Dawson, 1979).

Man contracts the infection from fowl by inhaling the airborne agent in contaminated environments. In some regions, ducks or turkeys are the principal source of infection; in others, psittacines and pigeons. Chlamydiosis of avian origin is largely an occupational disease of workers in turkey processing plants, as well as duck and geese pluckers, pigeon breeders, and employees in shops trading in exotic and other pet birds. In Czechoslovakia and the German Democratic Republic, over 1,000 cases of infection (one-third with clinical disease) occurred in workers engaged in plucking ducks and geese.

In birds, the infection is primarily gastrointestinal, and diarrhea is a common symptom. Since the agent is shed through the feces, birds with diarrhea contaminate the environment (including their plumage) with large numbers of chlamydiae. As the fecal matter dries, it releases the agent into the air. Strains isolated from different birds vary greatly in virulence; this fact along with exposure to differing doses of the agent could explain the wide range of severity of the disease in man.

Transmission between birds occurs by inhalation of chlamydiae and also by their ingestion (coprophagia, cannibalism). The source of infection for domestic birds such as turkeys, ducks, geese, and sometimes chickens is probably wild fowl, which constitute an ample reservoir of the infective agent. Migratory birds can give rise to new foci of infection (Grimes, 1978). Neither transovarial transmission, which has been confirmed in ducks, nor mechanical transmission by arthropod vectors is considered important.

Figure 21. Avian chlamydiosis (psittacosis, ornithosis). Transmission cycle.

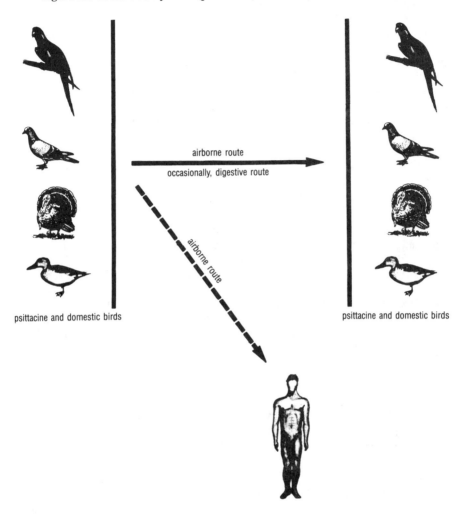

Role of Animals in the Epidemiology of the Disease: Human infection with *C. psittaci* is a zoonosis and, as in most of these diseases, man is an accidental host. Human-to-human transmission of the infection is rare and has only been observed in some cases of nurses who cared for patients with psittacosis.

Diagnosis: Diagnosis can be confirmed by means of serologic tests, especially the complement fixation (CF) test. A titer is considered diagnostically significant if it shows a four-fold increase between the onset of the disease and convalescence, based on two serum samples. When only one serum sample is available, results must be interpreted carefully, since *C. psittaci* gives cross-reactions with *C. trachomatis*, the chlamydiae from humans. Diagnosis can also be confirmed by isolating the agent from sputum or blood taken during the febrile period and inoculating embryonated eggs, mice, or tissue cultures. Several passages may be necessary. Early treatment of the patient with tetracyclines may interfere with the isolation of the agent, as well as with the formation of antibodies.

The complement fixation test can be used in psittacines, both to diagnose the clinical disease and to detect latent infections, and in pigeons to diagnose recent infections. The ELISA method, recently developed, is considered superior in sensitivity and specificity to CF for pigeon sera and permits identification of carriers having only IgM antibodies, not detectable by CF (Schmeer, 1983). The indirect complement fixation test is used for turkeys, ducks, and pheasants.

When attempting to isolate the agent, samples from various origins, such as spleen, liver, and intestinal contents, should be used at the same time.

A quick preliminary diagnosis can be obtained with smears of serous membrane exudates, spleen, liver, or lung tissue stained by the Macchiavello, Giménez, or Giemsa methods.

Isolation of the agent from man or animals should only be done in laboratories observing the highest safety standards.

Control: Because of the large number of hosts, including free-ranging fowl, eradication of the disease is not feasible. There are no effective vaccines for control of the disease. The control method that has given the best results is chemo-prophylaxis with tetracyclines in birds. Psittacines and other birds are treated with 0.5% chlortetracycline in their feed for 45 days prior to shipment or after arrival at their destination. Mass treatment has also been carried out on turkey-raising farms. Epidemiologic surveillance using serologic methods is necessary to identify infected flocks, which are then placed under quarantine and treated with tetracyclines for a period of 3 to 4 weeks.

Bibliography

Arnstein, P., B. Eddie, and K. F. Meyer. Control of psittacosis by group chemotherapy of infected parrots. *Am J Vet Res* 29:2213-2227, 1968.

Bevan, B. J., and C. D. Bracewell. Chlamydiosis in birds in Great Britain. 2. Isolation of *Chlamydia psittaci* from birds sampled between 1976 and 1984. *J Hyg (Camb)* 96:453-458, 1986.

Centers for Disease Control of the USA. Follow up on turkey-associated psittacosis. *Morb Mortal Wkly Rep* 23:309-310, 1974.

Centers for Disease Control of the USA. Psittacosis associated with turkey processing—Ohio. *Morb Mortal Wkly Rep* 30:638-640, 1982.

Filstein, M. R., A. B. Ley, M. S. Vernon, K. A. Gaffney, and L. T. Glickman. Epidemic of psittacosis in a college of veterinary medicine. *J Am Vet Med Assoc* 179:559-572, 1981.

Fukushi, H., K. Itoh, Y. Ogawa, Y. Hayashi, M. Kuzuya, K. Hirai, and S. Shimakura. Isolation and serological survey of *Chlamydia psittaci* in feral pigeons from Japan. *Jpn J Vet Sci* 45:847-848, 1983.

Grimes, J. E. Transmission of chlamydiae from grackles to turkeys. *Avian Dis* 22:308-311, 1978.

Hirai, K., K. Itoh, T. Yamashita, H. Fukushi, Y. Hayashi, M. Kuzuya, S. Shimakura, A. Hashimoto, and K. Akiyama. Prevalence of *Chlamydia psittaci* in pet birds maintained in public places or in close human contact. *Jpn J Vet Sci* 45:843-845, 1983.

Johnson, F. W. A., B. A. Matheson, H. Williams, A. G. Laing, V. Jandial, R. Davidson-Lamb, G. J. Halliday, D. Hobson, S. Y. Wong, K. M. Hadley, M. A. J. Moffat, and R. Postlethwaite. Abortion due to infection with *Chlamydia psittaci* in a sheep farmer's wife. *Br Med J* 290, 1985.

Johnson, M. C., and J. E. Grimes. Resistance of wild birds to infection by *Chlamydia psittaci* of mammalian origin. *J Infect Dis* 147:162, 1983.

Meyer, K. F. Ornithosis. *In*: Biester, H. E., and L. H. Schwarte (Eds.), *Diseases of Poultry*, 5th ed. Ames, Iowa State University Press, 1965.

Meyer, K. F. Psittacosis—Lymphogranuloma venereum agents. *In*: Horsfall, F. I., and I. Tamm (Eds.), *Viral and Rickettsial Infection of Man*, 4th ed. Philadelphia, Lippincott, 1965.

Page, L. A., W. T. Derieux, and R. C. Cutlip. An epornitic of fatal chlamydiosis (ornithosis) in South Carolina turkeys. *J Am Vet Med Assoc* 166:175-178, 1985.

Schachter, J. Psittacosis (Ornithosis, feline pneumonitis and other infections with *Chlamydia psittaci*). *In*: Hubbert, W. T., W. F. McCulloch, and P. R. Schnurrenberger (Eds.), *Diseases Transmitted from Animals to Man*, 6th ed. Springfield, Illinois, Thomas, 1975.

Schachter, J., H. B. Oster, and K. F. Meyer. Human infection with the agent of feline pneumonitis. *Lancet* 1:1063-1065, 1969.

Schachter, J., and C. R. Dawson. Psittacosis—Lymphogranuloma venereum agents/TRIC agents. *In*: Lennette, E. H., and N. J. Schmidt (Eds.), *Diagnostic Procedures for Viral and Chlamydial Infections*, 5th ed. Washington, D. C., American Public Health Association, 1979.

Schmeer, N. Enzymimmuntest zum Nachweis von IgG- und IgM-Antikorpern gegen *Chlamydia psittaci* bei der Taube. *Zentralbl Veterinarmed [B]* 30:356-370, 1983.

Schwartz, J. C., and W. Fraser. *Chlamydia psittaci* in companion birds examined in Florida. *Avian Dis* 26:211-213, 1982.

South, M., T. G. Wreghitt, and E. D. Caul. Stevens-Johnson syndrome associated with psittacosis. *J Infect* 11:173, 1985.

Spalatin, J., and J. O. Iversen. Epizootic chlamydiosis of muskrats and snowshoe hares. *In*: Davis, J. W., L. H. Karstad, and D. O. Trainer (Eds.), *Infectious Diseases of Wild Mammals*. Ames, Iowa State University Press, 1970.

Storz, J. Comparative studies on EBA and EAE, abortion diseases of cattle and sheep resulting from infection with psittacosis agents. *In*: Faulkner, L. C. (Ed.), *Abortion Diseases of Livestock*. Springfield, Illinois, Thomas, 1968.

Storz, J. *Chlamydia and Chlamydia Induced Diseases*. Springfield, Illinois, Thomas, 1971.

BOUTONNEUSE FEVER

(082.1)

Synonyms: Marseilles fever, Mediterranean exanthematic fever, South African tick typhus, Kenya tick typhus, Kenya fever, Indian tick typhus, Conor and Bruch's disease.

Etiology: *Rickettsia conorii* (*Dermacentroxenus conorii*). This microorganism belongs to the group of rickettsiae that produce spotted fever.

Geographic Distribution: The disease occurs in much of Africa; areas of Europe and the Middle East adjacent to the Mediterranean, Black, and Caspian seas; India; and Southeast Asia.

Occurrence in Man: Sporadic. It is the most common rickettsial disease in South Africa. In Talavera de la Reina, an endemic area in Spain, 85 cases were diagnosed in 1982 (Ministry of Health and Consumption, 1983). Most of the cases in the Mediterranean basin occur in summer when ticks are most active.

Occurrence in Animals: In some areas, such as Kenya, serologic studies have revealed a high proportion of reactors in some species of wild rodents (Heisch *et al.*, 1962). *R. conorii* has been isolated from several species of rodents in South Africa and Kenya. Antibodies for rickettsiae of the spotted fever group were found in a small number of serum samples from sheep and goats in Ethiopia (Philip *et al.*, 1966), as well as in nonhuman primates from the Kruger Reserve in South Africa (Kaschula *et al.*, 1978).

The Disease in Man: Boutonneuse fever is a benign variety within the spotted fever group. It is characterized by a primary lesion at the site where the tick was attached. The lesion consists of a small reddish ulcer covered by a small black scab ("tache noir"), which may last throughout the course of the illness. Regional lymphadenitis is often seen. The fever appears 5 to 7 days after the tick bite and is accompanied by severe cephalalgia and muscular and joint pains. A generalized eruption, at first macular and then maculopapular, appears the fourth or fifth day of the fever and lasts approximately 1 week. Mortality is low.

The Disease in Animals: Dogs infested with *Rhipicephalus sanguineus,* the principal vector in the Mediterranean region, may have rickettsemia but show no clinical infection. Elsewhere, in wild rodents from which the agent has been isolated, the natural course of infection is unknown, but it is probably asymptomatic.

Source of Infection and Mode of Transmission: The vector of the infection in the Mediterranean, Caspian, and Black Sea basins is the brown dog tick, *R. sanguineus*. This tick is responsible for the focal nature of boutonneuse fever. All the human cases in this region correspond to the distribution of *R. sanguineus*. The tick completes its entire life cycle near human dwellings. *R. sanguineus* always prefers a dog as its host and only occasionally bites man, which could explain the limited number of human cases in spite of the abundance of infected ticks. The causal agent is transmitted transovarially from generation to generation of canine tick, so this arthropod serves as both vector and reservoir. The dog and its ticks constitute the principal source of infection for man; the natural reservoir is wild rodents and their ticks. In South Africa, the dog ticks *Haemaphysalis leachi* and *R. sanguineus* are likewise the principal vectors of human infection. The agent has been isolated from many other tick species in their natural habitat and they are probably involved in its primary life cycle in the wild. Studies carried out in Kenya and Malaysia confirm that the agent circulates between small wild animals and ticks in a basic cycle in natural foci.

Role of Animals in the Epidemiology of the Disease: Man is an accidental host. The infection is maintained in nature by wild rodents and their ticks. Dogs play a very important role by carrying infected ticks to the human environment.

Diagnosis: Laboratory confirmation is accomplished primarily by serologic tests. A quick presumptive diagnosis can be obtained with the Weil-Felix test and later can be confirmed by the complement fixation or microagglutination test, using washed type-specific antigens. Specific anti-IgM and anti-IgG sera should be used in the immunofluorescence test to distinguish recent infections from past ones (Edlinger, 1979).

Control: Control measures are directed against the vector and consist of the use of tickicides on dogs and in their environment.

Bibliography

American Public Health Association. *Control of Communicable Diseases in Man*, 14th ed. (Ed. by A.S. Benenson). Washington, D.C., APHA, 1985.

Burgdorfer, W. Boutonneuse fever. *In*: Hubbert, W. T., W. F. McCulloch, and P. R. Schnurrenberger (Eds.), *Diseases Transmitted from Animals to Man*, 6th ed, Springfield, Illinois, Thomas, 1975.

Edlinger, E. Serological diagnosis of Mediterranean spotted fever. *Ann Microbiol (Inst Pasteur)* 130A:203-211, 1979.

Heisch, R. B., W. E. Grainger, A. E. C. Harvey, and G. Lister. Feral aspects of rickettsial infections in Kenya. *Trans R Soc Trop Med Hyg* 56:272-282, 1962.

Kaschula, V. R., A. F. Van Dellen, and V. De Vos. Some infectious diseases of wild vervet monkeys (*Cercopithecus aetiops pygertythrus*) in South Africa. *J S Afr Vet Assoc* 49:223-227, 1978.

Ministry of Health and Consumption of Spain. Vigilancia de la fiebre exantemática mediterránea. *Bol Epidemiol Sem (España)* nl. 588:137-138, 1983.

Phillip, C. B., H. Hoogstraal, R. Reiss-Gutfreund, and C. M. Clifford. Evidence of rickettsial disease agents in ticks from Ethiopian cattle. *Bull WHO* 35:127-131, 1966.

Raoult, D., B. Toga, S. Dunan, B. Davoust, and M. Quilici. Mediterranean spotted fever in the South of France: serosurvey of dogs. *Trop Geogr Med* 37:258-260, 1985.

Tringali, C., V. Intonazzo, A. M. Perna, S. Mansuetto, G. Vitale, and D. H. Walker. Epidemiology of boutonneuse fever in Western Sicily: distribution and prevalence of spotted fever group rickettsial infection in dog ticks. (*Rhipicephalus sanguineus*). *Am J Epidemiol* 123:721-727, 1986.

Zdrodovskii, P. F., and H. M. Golinevich. *The Rickettsial Diseases*. Oxford, Pergamon Press, 1960.

FLEA-BORNE TYPHUS

(081.0)

Synonyms: Murine typhus, endemic typhus, urban typhus.

Etiology: *Rickettsia typhi* (*R. mooseri*), which belongs to the same group as *R. prowazekii*, the agent for epidemic louse-borne typhus, and *R. canada* (not pathogenic to man), isolated from the tick *Haemaphysalis leporispalustris*.

Geographic Distribution: Endemic areas are recognized worldwide.

Occurrence in Man: Sporadic. From 1963 to 1967, an annual average of 241 cases was recorded in the Americas. Countries that reported cases during this period were Argentina, Brazil, Chile, Colombia (over one-third of the total), Costa Rica, Ecuador, Mexico, Peru, the United States, and Venezuela. In the United States, about 42,000 cases occurred during the period 1931-1946; after 1946 the incidence began to decline, and since 1961 fewer than 50 cases per year have been recorded (Burgdorfer, 1975). The occurrence of the disease is associated with rat infestation. In Kuwait, there were 254 cases between April and August of 1978, mostly among people of the lowest socioeconomic class, 80% of whose dwellings were rat-infested (Al-Awadi *et al.*, 1982).

The incidence is greatest in summer and fall when rat fleas are more active.

Occurrence in Animals: The most important reservoirs of infection are the domestic rats *Rattus norvegicus* and *R. rattus*. The main vector is the eastern rat flea, *Xenopsylla cheopis*. The basic transmission cycle of the infection is rat-flea-rat and, accidentally, rat-flea-man. Many other species of wild and domestic animals as well as some of their ectoparasites have been found to be naturally infected or experimentally susceptible, but their role in the epidemiology of endemic typhus does not appear to be important. Nevertheless, there may be independent cycles of the agent in addition to the basic cycle. Such would be the case of the natural infection found in the opossum *Didelphis marsupialis* and the flea *Ctenocephalides felis,* which frequently parasitizes this marsupial in suburban and rural southern California. In this area, the classic vector *X. cheopis* is absent and rats are serologically negative.

The infection rate in rats varies greatly in the different enzootic foci.

The Disease in Man: The incubation period is from 6 to 14 days. The disease has a similar symptomatology to that of epidemic louse-borne typhus, but its course is shorter and more benign. It begins with fever, severe cephalalgia, and generalized pains. Five or 6 days later, a macular eruption appears, at first on the trunk and then on the extremities, but it does not affect the palms of the hands, the soles of the feet, or the face. The symptomatology also includes coughing, nervousness, nausea, and vomiting. Complications are rare. In untreated patients, convalescence can last several months. Case fatality is less than 2%.

The Disease in Animals: Rickettsemia occurs in rats during the first week of infection. The agent remains viable for long periods in the brain and other organs. The infection is asymptomatic.

Source of Infection and Mode of Transmission (Figure 22): The most important reservoir of *R. typhi* is the rat and the main vector is the flea *X. cheopis*. Fleas are infected by feeding on a host that is in the rickettsemial period. The agent multiplies in the intestine and Malpighian tubules without causing apparent damage to the flea. The vector eliminates *R. typhi* in its feces throughout its lifetime, but not in its saliva. *X. cheopis* does not transmit the infection to its progeny, and the new generations of fleas only become infected by feeding on rickettsemic hosts. Infection in other species of fleas follows the same pattern.

The infection is transmitted from rat to rat by means of the flea *X. cheopis* and the louse *Polyplax spinulosa*. The agent can survive for lengthy periods in flea feces, and infection can occur in contaminated rodent burrows through the mucous membranes of the conjunctiva or mouth, or by inhalation of the agent.

Man is infected when the rat flea (or possibly another flea, such as *Ctenocephalides felis*) bites him and defecates on his skin. By scratching, he introduces the contaminated fecal material through the bite or other skin abrasion. It

Figure 22. Flea-borne typhus (*Rickettsia typhi*). Transmission cycle.

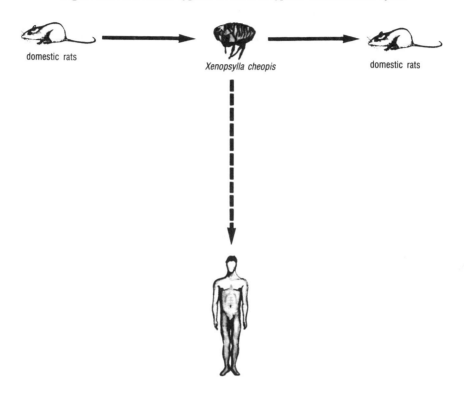

domestic rats

Xenopsylla cheopis

domestic rats

is also probable that man can acquire the infection by other routes such as through the conjunctiva or by inhalation. These modes of transmission are, nevertheless, of little importance.

The incidence of the disease in man is determined by the level of enzootic occurrence among rats and the degree of human contact with these animals and their fleas. Although the disease used to occur primarily in rat-infested buildings in urban areas, it has now spread to rural areas.

Role of Animals in the Epidemiology of the Disease: The infection is not transmitted from person to person. It is a rat infection that is accidentally transmitted to man by fleas.

Diagnosis: The agent can be isolated by inoculating blood of a febrile patient into male guinea pigs and embryonated eggs. In guinea pigs, the infection causes the Neill-Mooser reaction (adhesions of the tunica vaginalis testis that do not allow the testicles to reenter the abdomen). This reaction occurs with the murine typhus agent as well as with those of the spotted fever group.

The seroconversion detected by the Weil-Felix test is useful for a preliminary diagnosis. The complement fixation test (CF) is the most commonly used. The antibodies for this test appear towards the end of the second week of illness and reach their maximum in the two following weeks, declining slowly thereafter (Elisberg and Bozeman, 1979). Use of the easily administered microagglutination test permits an earlier diagnosis and avoids the inconvenience of anticomplementary sera, which exists with the CF. Group specificity is good, although in human patients (but not in rodents) it is difficult to distinguish murine typhus from epidemic typhus. The immunofluorescence test is also useful and it can be adapted to distinguish IgM and IgG antibodies (Wisseman, 1982).

The use of washed species-specific antigens in the complement fixation test permits differentiation between murine typhus and epidemic typhus.

Control: Control measures should be directed first against the vector and later against rodents. To decrease the number of fleas among rats, residual action insecticides (DDT or other compounds) should be applied to rat pathways, nests, and holes. Once the flea population has been reduced, the rat population can be controlled using rodenticides. Environmental sanitation measures should also be taken, such as eliminating rat hiding places and possible food sources, and rat-proofing buildings.

Bibliography

Adams, W. H., R. W. Emmons, and J. E. Porooks. The changing ecology of murine (endemic) typhus in southern California. *Am J Trop Med Hyg* 19:311-318, 1970.

Al-Awadi, A. R., N. Al-Kazemi, G. Ezzat, A. J. Saah, C. Shepard, T. Zaghloul, and B. Gherdian. Murine typhus in Kuwait in 1978. *Bull WHO* 60:283-289, 1982.

American Public Health Association. *Control of Communicable Diseases in Man,* 14th ed. (Ed. by A.S. Benenson). Washington, D.C., APHA, 1985.

Burgdorfer, W. Murine (flea-borne) typhus fever. *In*: Hubbert, W. T., W. F. McCulloch, and P. R. Schnurrenberger (Eds.), *Diseases Transmitted from Animals to Man,* 6th ed. Springfield, Illinois, Thomas, 1975.

Elisberg, B. L., and F. M. Bozeman. Rickettsiae. *In*: Lennette, E. H., and N. J. Schmidt (Eds.), *Diagnostic Procedures for Viral and Rickettsial Infections,* 4th ed. New York, American Public Health Association, 1969.

Elisberg, B. L., and F. M. Bozeman. The rickettsiae. *In*: Lennette, E. H., and N. J. Schmidt (Eds.), *Diagnostic Procedures for Viral, Rickettsial and Chlamydial Infections,* 5th ed. Washington, D.C., American Public Health Association, 1979.

Pan American Health Organization. *Reported Cases of Notifiable Diseases in the Americas,* 1967. Washington, D.C., PAHO, 1970. (Scientific Publication 199.)

Snyder, J. C. The typhus group. *In*: Beeson, P. B., W. McDermott, and J. B. Wyngaarden (Eds.), *Cecil Textbook of Medicine,* 15th ed. Philadelphia and London, Saunders, 1979.

Tselentis, Y., E. Edlinger, G. Alexious, D. Chrysantis, and A. Levendis. An endemic focus of murine typhus in Europe. *J Infect* 13:91-92, 1986.

Wisseman, C. L., Jr. Rickettsial diseases. *In*: Wyngaarden, J. B., and L. H. Smith, Jr. (Eds.), *Cecil Textbook of Medicine,* 16th ed. Philadelphia, Saunders, 1982.

Zdrodovskii, P. E., and H. M. Golinevich. *The Rickettsial Diseases.* Oxford, Pergamon Press, 1960.

Q FEVER

(083.0)

Synonyms: Pneumorickettsiosis, Balkan influenza, coxiellosis, abattoir fever, Australian Q fever, hiberno-vernal bronchopneumonia, nine-mile fever.

Etiology: *Coxiella burnetii* (*Rickettsia burnetii*), which differs from other rickettsiac in its filterability and its high resistance to physical and chemical agents (it is more resistant than the majority of nonsporogenic microorganisms). Moreover, it does not produce agglutinins for the Weil-Felix test, does not cause cutaneous rashes in man, and can be transmitted without the involvement of vectors.

Two antigenic phases (I and II), similar to the S to R variation of salmonellae or brucellae, are recognized. *C. burnetii* is found in phase I in the bodies of its host animals and ticks, but converts to the avirulent phase II after several passes through embryonated eggs (yolk sac). This antigenic variation is important in diagnosis.

Geographic Distribution: Worldwide. The infection is endemic in many areas and has been found in at least 50 countries. The northernmost countries of Europe are said to be free of Q fever and the diagnosed cases there are thought to be patients who acquired the infection outside their country (Lumio *et al.*, 1981).

Occurrence in Man: Q fever appears as outbreaks or sporadic cases. Human infection is often asymptomatic. When clinical symptoms are evident, the illness can be confused with other febrile diseases. For this reason, sporadic cases often go undiagnosed and the true incidence of the disease is unknown. Clinical identification of Q fever as well as other rickettsioses and bacterioses is jeopardized by the indiscriminate use of antibiotics in febrile patients. In Australia, considered an endemic area, about 2,000 confirmed cases occurred between 1979 and 1980 (Hunt *et al.*, 1983). There have been epidemic outbreaks in abattoirs and wool-processing plants. In Uruguay, a large epidemic outbreak occurred in 1976 in a meat-packing plant where, in the course of 1 month, 310 individuals out of 630 workers and veterinary inspection personnel became ill. Cases were most concentrated among workers involved in bone-milling and collection of animal wastes such as placentas, fetuses, and viscera. The outbreak was attributed to aerosols that probably originated from placentas and amniotic fluids. In different parts of the world, epidemic outbreaks continue to occur among slaughterhouse workers. Such episodes include outbreaks in Australia, where 110 workers in a rural goat-slaughterhouse were affected (Buckley, 1980), and in Romania, where 149 workers in a municipal slaughterhouse contracted the infection (Blidaru *et al.*, 1982). Ranchhands and other workers on farms raising cattle, sheep, and goats form another occupational group at high risk. On a dairy cooperative in Romania, an outbreak during the calving season affected 45 people. The source of infection was traced to cows acquired from various places to form a new dairy unit (Blidaru *et al.*, 1980). Of relatively recent epidemiologic concern are outbreaks of Q fever in scientific institutions that use sheep as models for the study of human diseases. Outbreaks occurred in two universities in 1969 and 1971 and, more recently, four similar outbreaks were recorded which affected many people, the majority of whom did not work directly with animals (Spinelli *et al.*, 1981; Meiklejohn *et al.*, 1981; Hall *et al.*, 1982). There was also an outbreak in a human pathology institute at a German university immediately following an autopsy on a patient. All the people who took part in the autopsy became ill, as did seven other individuals who worked in different buildings (Gerth *et al.*, 1982). During World War II, numerous epidemics (Balkan influenza) of greater or lesser extent were recorded in southern and southeastern Europe among both German and Allied troops. Important epidemics have also taken place in the postwar years in the civilian population of Germany, with 2,000 confirmed cases, and in Italy, where an estimated 20,000 cases occurred in a 2-year period (Babudieri, 1959).

Occurrence in Animals: The infection has been found in almost all species of domestic animals and many wild animals, including birds. In India, the agent was also isolated from amphibians (Kumar and Yadav, 1981) and a python. From the public health standpoint, the most important species are cattle, sheep, and goats, which serve as the source of human infection.

Serologic studies carried out in several endemic areas have demonstrated significant numbers of reactors among cattle, goats, and sheep. In a seroepidemiologic study in Colombia, 57% of 482 dairy cows had antibodies according to the complement fixation test (Lorbacher and Suárez, 1975). In California, USA, 2,097 sheep and 1,475 goats from various sources were examined serologically, with results of 24% and 57% reactors, respectively, in these two species (Ruppaner *et al.*, 1982). Serologic studies in France found the prevalence of reactors in some provinces to be 15% for cattle and 20% for sheep and goats.

Antibodies for *C. burnetii* are also commonly found in wild animals. According to results of microagglutination tests, 3% of 759 rodents belonging to 15 different species were seropositive and 20% of 583 wild birds were reactive (Riemann *et al.*, 1979). In India, 1.2% of 342 birds and 14.3% of 91 wild terrestrial animals were reactive (Yadav and Sethi, 1980).

The Disease in Man: The incubation period is from 2 weeks to 1 month. The disease has a sudden onset, with fever, chills, profuse sweating, malaise, anorexia, myalgia, and sometimes nausea and vomiting. The fever is remittent and generally lasts between 9 and 14 days. A prominent symptom of the disease is severe cephalalgia, and retro-ocular pain is common. In approximately half of the patients, X-ray examination reveals pneumonitis, which manifests itself clinically in the form of mild cough, scanty expectoration, and sometimes thoracic pain. About 50% of the patients have gastrointestinal disorders (nausea, vomiting, diarrhea). In contrast to the other rickettsioses, no cutaneous eruption is seen in Q fever. The severity of the disease varies, but it is benign in most cases. Q fever rarely attacks children under 10 years old. The disease is more serious in people over 40. Mortality is less than 1%. When the disease takes a chronic course, it primarily affects the cardiovascular system. In Great Britain, out of 839 confirmed cases of Q fever, 92 (11%) had endocarditis and 10 had liver complications (Palmer and Young, 1982). Nevertheless, outside of Great Britain and Australia, endocarditis has been diagnosed only in isolated cases. Many human infections are mild and inapparent and thus go undetected.

The Disease in Animals: As a general rule, the infection in domestic animals is clinically inapparent. In ruminants, after invasion of the bloodstream, *C. burnetii* becomes localized in the mammary glands, the supramammary lymph nodes, and the placenta. Many cows get rid of the infection after a few months, but others become carriers, with the agent localized in the mammary glands and eliminated throughout many lactation periods. During calving, a large number of rickettsiae are eliminated with the placenta and, to a lesser extent, with the amniotic fluid, feces, and urine. The high resistance of the agent to environmental factors ensures its survival and, thus, permits it to infect new susceptible animals and man. The activation of the infection during calving, with massive elimination of the agent in various secretions and excretions, explains why many sporadic outbreaks in man coincide with that period.

As a general rule, neither milk production nor the development of the fetus or newborn animal is affected by the infection.

An epizootic of abortions related to Q fever occurred among sheep and goats in Cyprus during the hostilities there in 1974. Twenty-one outbreaks of abortions among these animals were recorded, all in the southeastern part of the country. At the same time, 78 cases of Q fever were reported among the British soldiers. It is very likely that the large accumulation of livestock in this part of the island together with the lack of adequate feed may have been contributory factors to the abortions (Crowther and Spicer, 1976). In the United States, abortion in domestic animals is rarely associated with infection by *C. burnetii*, and even milk cows with heavily infected placentas have given birth to healthy calves. In Europe, on the other hand, especially in France, this agent is thought to be responsible for 2 to 7% of abortions in cattle and a similar rate in sheep. Up to now, there is no explanation for this difference between the United States and Europe.

Little is known of the natural course of the infection in wild animals.

Source of Infection and Mode of Transmission (Figures 23 and 24): Two cycles of the infection can be distinguished in nature: one in domestic animals (mainly cattle, sheep, and goats) and the other in natural foci where the agent circulates between wild animals and their ectoparasites, especially ticks.

Many species of wild animals, among them marsupials, rodents, and lagomorphs, have been found to be infected. The natural infection has also been verified in more than 40 species of ticks (of the families Ixodidae and Argasidae), as well as in other arthropods that feed on animals. Not all tick species—even if they are infected—can function as vectors and transmit the infection to vertebrates.

The relationship between the two cycles (that in the natural foci and that in domestic animals) has not been well studied. There are indications that domestic animals may contract the infection through infected ticks from these foci. Nevertheless, the infection of domestic animals does not depend on this mechanism, since Q fever can perpetuate itself independently of the natural foci. The most common mode of transmission of the infection between domestic animals is by the inhalation of aerosols from placental material and amniotic fluid. The agent can be transported for some distance by dust particles.

Due to its high resistance to environmental factors, the agent can be isolated from the soil up to 6 months after infected animals have been removed from an area. New foci of infection are produced when an infected animal is introduced into a clean herd.

The main sources of human infection are domestic animals and their contaminated products. The principal mode of transmission is by aerosols. People most affected are those who, because of occupation or residence, are in close contact with infected animals or their products, such as hides and wool. Although the agent is eliminated through milk (and pasteurization at the usual temperatures does not inactivate it very effectively), very few cases of human infection stemming from consumption of contaminated milk have been recorded. It would appear that man can be infected through the digestive tract, but infection by that route is rarely clinically apparent, possibly owing to the high titer of antibodies in milk.

The causal agent, because of its high resistance, can be transported large distances in inert material. In Switzerland, an outbreak of 19 cases was recorded in factory workers who handled contaminated straw used in the packaging of a machine shipped from the United States (Stoker, 1955).

Man can acquire the infection by entering a natural focus and being bitten by an infected tick, but these cases are rare.

Role of Animals in the Epidemiology of the Disease: Human-to-human transmission is rare. Nevertheless, such an outbreak involving 38 cases was reported from a hospital in Frankfurt, West Germany. The outbreak derived from a member of the staff who was working with *C. burnetii,* and the microorganism was isolated from his sputum. A similar episode originating in an autopsy room has been recorded.

As a general rule, however, man acquires the infection from domestic animals. Q fever is a zoonosis.

Figure 23. Q fever. Transmission—wildlife cycle.

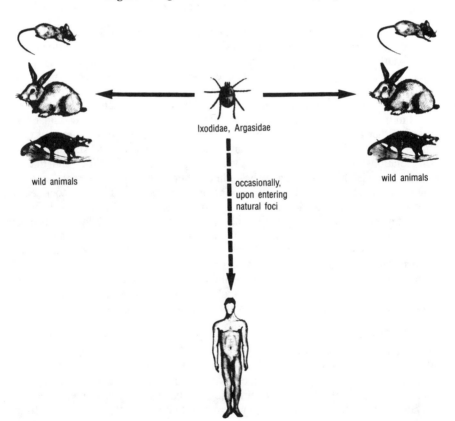

wild animals

Ixodidae, Argasidae

occasionally, upon entering natural foci

wild animals

Figure 24. Q fever. Transmission—domestic cycle.

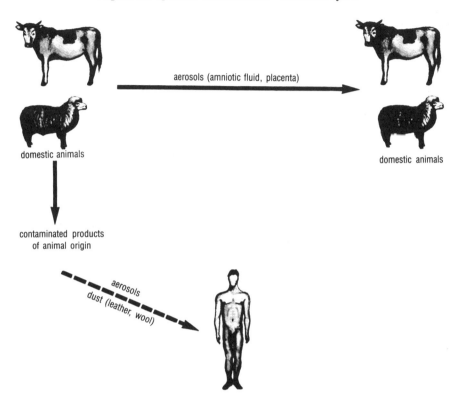

aerosols (amniotic fluid, placenta)

domestic animals

domestic animals

contaminated products
of animal origin

aerosols
dust (leather, wool)

Diagnosis: There are relatively few laboratories equipped with adequate installations and equipment to permit safe isolation of *C. burnetii*. For this reason, diagnosis by serologic tests is preferable. The Weil-Felix test is not applicable for infections caused by *C. burnetii*. The complement fixation test is the most widely used; diagnosis is based on the difference in titers between a sample obtained during the acute period of the disease and another obtained during convalescence. Variations in the phase of the agent must be borne in mind when carrying out these serologic tests. Recently isolated strains of *C. burnetii* or strains maintained by passage in laboratory animals are usually in phase I; after a variable number of passages in embryonated eggs, strains convert to phase II. The complement fixation test (CF) with antigens in phase II will detect the infection in about 65% of patients in the second week of the illness and in about 90% around the fourth week. When there are no complications, patients rarely react to the CF test using phase I antigens. In cases of endocarditis, on the other hand, the phase I titers are high, making this test useful to detect possible complications during convalescence. Various agglutination tests are available (standard agglutination, microagglutination, agglutination-resuspension, capillary test). In about 50% of patients, the presence of agglutinins can be detected at the end of the first week of the disease and in 92% during the second week. The Luoto capillary agglutination test, which uses phase I antigen stained with hematoxylin, is especially useful for epizootiologic studies since it can be used for milk samples. Indirect immunofluorescence and precipita-tion radioimmunoassay can also be used. When serum from the acute period of the illness is not available to test for seroconversion by comparison with serum obtained during convalescence, the indirect immunofluorescence test for IgM antibodies with phase I and II antigens can be useful. In an experiment carried out in Australia, all Q fever patients had a positive reaction about 2 weeks after the onset of the disease and thus the diagnosis was accomplished using only one serum sample (Hunt *et al.*, 1983).

The agent can be isolated from febrile blood and sometimes from sputum and urine in humans, as well as from milk, placentas, and amniotic fluid from animals; these materials are inoculated into laboratory animals, such as guinea pigs and mice, or embryonated eggs. As noted before, isolation work should only be attempted in high-safety laboratories.

Control: To protect occupational groups exposed to high risk, such as laboratory and slaughterhouse workers, wool workers, and cattlemen, a formalin-inactivated vaccine (*C. burnetii*, phase I) has been developed. Recently, this vaccine has been tested on volunteers with good results (Ascher *et al.*, 1983), but it is still unavailable outside Q fever research laboratories. Another promising vaccine is one without microbial cells (acellular or "soluble vaccine"), developed in Romania.

In enzootic regions milk should be boiled.

Direct measures to prevent infection of the animal reservoir (domestic animals) are difficult to apply because Q fever does not cause definite economic losses and cattlemen generally are unwilling to make the economic investment necessary for prophylaxis. When practicable, vaccination, separation of cows from the remainder of the herd prior to calving, and destruction of placentas and fetal membranes by incineration or burying are recommended.

Bibliography

Adesiyun, A. A., A. G. Jagun, J. K. P. Kwaga, and L. B. Tekdek. Shedding of *Coxiella burnetii* in milk by Nigerian dairy and dual purposes cows. *Int J Zoonoses* 12:1-5, 1985.

Ascher, M. S., M. A. Berman, and R. Ruppaner. Initial clinical and immunological evaluation of a new phase I Q fever vaccine and skin test in humans. *J Infect Dis* 148:214-222, 1983.

Babudieri, B. Q fever: a zoonosis *Adv Vet Sci* 5:810-812, 1959.

Bell, J. F. Q (Query) fever. *In*: Davis, J. W., L. H. Karstad, and D. O. Trainer (Eds.), *Infectious Diseases of Wild Mammals*. Ames, Iowa State University Press, 1970.

Blidaru, I., C. Petrescu, M. Stan, I. Radu, D. Luta, N. Lamba, C. Bordeianu, M. Constantinescu, and M. Purnichescu. (Clinico-epidemiological considerations on an out-break of Q fever in the Arges region). *Bacteriol Virusol Parazitol Epidemiol* 25:171-174, 1980.

Blidaru, I., N. Lamba, C. Petrescu, C. Drumea, M. Ghica, G. Matescu, M. Plesanu, M. Purnichescu, and A. Pavel. Episod de febra Q intr-un abator municipal. *Bacteriol Virusol Parazitol Epidemiol* 27:179-184, 1982.

Buckley, B. Q fever epidemic in Victorian general practice. *Med J Aust* 1:593-595, 1980.

Burgdorfer, W. Q fever. *In*: Hubbert, W. T., W. F. McCulloch, and P. R. Schnurrenberger (Eds.), *Diseases Transmitted from Animals to Man*, 6th ed. Springfield, Illinois, Thomas, 1975.

Crowther, R. W., and A. J. Spicer. Abortion in sheep and goats in Cyprus caused by *Coxiella burnetii*. *Vet Rec* 99:29-30, 1976.

Evenchik, Z. Q fever. *In*: Van der Hoeden, J. (Ed.), *Zoonoses*. Amsterdam, Netherlands, Elsevier, 1964.

Fiset, P., and R. A. Ormsbee. The antibody response to antigens of *Coxiella burnetii*. *Zentralbl Bakteriol [Orig]* 206:321-329, 1968.

Gerth, H. J., U. Leidig, and T. Riemenschneider. Q fever epidemic in an institute of human pathology. *Dtsch Med Wochenschr* 107:1391-1395, 1982.

Giroud, P., and M. Capponi. *La Fièvre Q ou Maladie de Derrick et Burnet*. Paris, Flammarion, 1966.

Hall, C. J., S. J. Richmond, E. O. Caul, H. H. Pierce, and I. A. Silver. Laboratory outbreak of Q fever acquired from sheep. *Lancet* 1:1004-1006, 1982.

Hunt, J. G., P. R. Field, and A. M. Murphy. Immunoglobulin response to *Coxiella burnetii* (Q fever): single-serum diagnosis of acute infection, using an immunofluorescence technique. *Infect Immun* 29:977-981, 1983.

Kosatsky, T. Household outbreak of Q-fever pneumonia related to a parturient cat, *Lancet* 2, 1984.

Kumar, S., and M. P. Yadav. Note on coxiellosis (*Coxiella burnetii*) infection in amphibians. *Indian J Anim Sci* 51:390-391, 1981.

Ley, H. L. Q fever. *In*: Beeson, P. B., W. McDermott, and J. B. Wyngaarden (Eds.), *Cecil Textbook of Medicine*, 15th ed. Philadelphia and London, Saunders, 1979.

Lorbacher, H., and J. B. Suárez. Fiebre Q en Antioquia. *Antioquia Méd* 25:37-42, 1975.

Lumio, J., K. Penttinem, and T. Pattersson. Q fever in Finland: clinical, immunological and epidemiological findings. *Scand J Infect Dis* 13:17-21, 1981.

Meiklejohn, G., L. G. Reimer, P. S. Graves, and C. Helmick. Cryptic epidemic of Q fever in a medical school. *J Infect Dis* 144:107-113, 1981.

Ormsbee, R. A., E. J. Bell, D. B. Lackman, and G. Tallent. The influence of phase on the protective potency of Q fever vaccine. *J Immunol* 92:404-412, 1964.

Ormsbee, R. A. Q fever rickettsia. *In*: Horsfall, F. L., and I. Tamm (Eds.), *Viral and Rickettsial Infections of Man*, 4th ed. Philadelphia, Lippincott, 1965.

Palmer, S. R., and S. E. Young. Q fever endocarditis in England and Wales, 1975-81. *Lancet* 2:1448-1449, 1982.

Quignard, H., M. F. Geral, J. L. Pellerin, A. Milon, and R. Lautie. La fièvre Q chez les petits ruminants. Enquête épidémiologique dans la région Midi-pyrenées. *Rev Méd Vét* 133:413-422, 1982.

Riemann, H. P., D. E. Behymer, C. E. Franti, C. Crabb, and R. G. Schwab. Survey of Q fever agglutinins in birds and small rodents in Northern California, 1975-1976. *J Wildl Dis* 15:515-523, 1979.

Roges, G., and E. Edlinger. Immunoenzymatic test for Q fever. *Diagn Microbiol Infect Dis* 4:125-132, 1986.

Ruppanner, R., D. Brooks, C. E. Franti, D. E. Behymer, D. Morrish, and J. S. Spinelli. Q fever hazards from sheep and goats used in research. *Arch Environ Health* 37:103-110, 1982.

Somma-Moreira, R. E., R. M. Caffarena, G. Pérez, S. Somma-Saldias, and M. Monteiro. Fiebre Q en el Uruguay. Unpublished.

Spinelli, J. S., M. S. Ascher, D. L. Brooks, S. K. Dritz, H. A. Lewis, R. H. Morrish, and R. L. Ruppanner. Q fever crisis in San Francisco: controlling a sheep zoonosis in a lab animal facility. *Lab Anim* 10:24-27, 1981.

Stoker, M. G. P., and B. P. Marmion. The spread of Q fever from animals to man. The natural history of rickettsial disease. *Bull WHO* 13:781-806, 1955.

Yadav, M. P., and M. S. Sethi. A study of the reservoir status of Q fever in avifauna, wild mammals and poikilotherms in Uttar Pradesh (India). *Int J Zoonoses* 7:85-89, 1980.

Zdrodovskii, P. F., and H. M. Golinevich. *The Rickettsial Diseases*. Oxford, Pergamon Press, 1960.

QUEENSLAND TICK TYPHUS

(082.3)

Etiology: *Rickettsia australis,* a member of the group of rickettsiae that produce spotted fever.

Geographic Distribution: Limited to Queensland, Australia.

Occurrence in Man: Sporadic.

Occurrence in Animals: A serologic study of wild animals in an area of Queensland revealed reactors among various species of marsupials and rodents.

The Disease in Man: *R. australis* produces a benign macular disease similar to Boutonneuse fever and Asian ixodo-rickettsiosis. An eschar is frequently seen at the site where the tick (larva or adult) was attached, and painful regional adenopathy is also observed. The eruption, which appears in the first week of the disease, disappears soon after the fever.

The Disease in Animals: The natural course of the infection in marsupials and rodents is not known.

Source of Infection and Mode of Transmission: The natural history of *R. australis* is not yet well understood. In a focus in southeastern Queensland, *R. australis* was isolated from two species of ticks, *Ixodes holocyclus* and *I. tasmani.* The infection in man has been associated for a long time with the bite of *I. holocyclus,* a species that feeds on a large variety of vertebrate animals and often bites man.

Diagnosis: The disease must be distinguished from scrub typhus (*R. tsutsugamushi*) and from endemic murine (flea-borne) typhus (*R. typhi*), which also exist in Queensland.

R. australis can be isolated by inoculating the blood of febrile patients into suckling guinea pigs and mice. The sera of convalescent mice, inoculated with material containing *R. australis,* have species-specific antibodies that can be distinguished by the complement fixation test from antibodies to other rickettsial antigens of the spotted fever group. The Weil-Felix test with *Proteus* OX-19 gives high titers with sera from patients infected by *R. australis,* while sera from patients with scrub typhus react only with *Proteus* OX-K.

Control: Control measures are similar to those used against infections caused by other rickettsiae of the spotted fever group.

Bibliography

Burgdorfer, W. Queensland tick typhus. *In*: Hubbert, W. T., W. F. McCulloch, and P. R. Schnurrenberger (Eds.), *Diseases Transmitted from Animals to Man,* 6th ed. Springfield, Illinois, Thomas, 1975.

Pickens, E. G., E. J. Bell, D. B. Lackman, and W. Burgdorfer. Use of mouse serum in identification and serologic classification of *Rickettsia akari* and *Rickettsia australis. J Immunol* 94:883-899, 1965.

RICKETTSIALPOX

(083.2)

Synonyms: Vesicular rickettsiosis, gamaso-rickettsiosis varicelliformis.

Etiology: *Rickettsia akari* (*Dermacentroxenus murinus*). This microorganism belongs to the group of rickettsiae that produce spotted fever.

Geographic Distribution: The disease has been found in New York and other cities of the United States; a similar or identical disease has been observed in the Soviet Union. On the basis of clinical observations, it is suspected that this rickettsiosis occurs among natives of equatorial Africa and in South Africa (where there is also serologic evidence). On the basis of a serologic study carried out in Central America, it is suspected that the disease could have occurred in Costa Rica. *R. akari* was isolated from a vole (*Microtus*) in Korea.

Occurrence in Man: Occasional. After the disease was discovered in New York in 1946, some 180 cases were recorded annually for a period of time, after which the incidence decreased. Since 1969, no cases have been reported in the United States. A large reduction in the incidence of the disease has also occurred in the Ukraine (USSR), where the infection was widespread in the Donets Basin.

Occurrence in Animals: The natural hosts of *R. akari* are the house mouse (*Mus musculus*) and the rat (*Rattus* spp.). The infection is transmitted by a mite, *Liponyssoides sanguineus* (*Allodermanyssus sanguineus*). The frequency of the infection in rodents is not known.

The Disease in Man: The course of the disease is benign. It is characterized by an initial cutaneous lesion at the site of the mite bite and fever lasting about a week, accompanied by a varicelliform eruption. Symptoms appear 10 to 24 days after the patient is bitten by the mite *L. sanguineus*. The initial cutaneous lesion appears approximately 1 week before the fever in the form of a small papule that forms a central vesicle, then a dark scab. It leaves a small scar. The febrile period is characterized by chills, profuse sweating, intermittent fever, cephalalgia, and myalgia. Between the first and fourth days of fever, a maculopapular eruption occurs. It becomes maculovesicular and disappears after 1 week without leaving scars. The eruption is not painful. It may appear on many parts of the body, but does not affect the palms of the hands or soles of the feet.

The Disease in Animals: The natural course of the infection in mice or other rodents is not known. Laboratory mice are very susceptible to experimental infection. Intranasal inoculation causes a pneumonia that is often fatal, while intraperitoneal inoculation causes peritonitis with a sanguinolent exudate, lymphadenitis, and splenomegaly. Death occurs between 9 and 18 days after inoculation. The strains of *R. akari* vary in their virulence.

Source of Infection and Mode of Transmission (Figure 25): The main reservoir consists of house mice, but a wildlife cycle is also possible, as can be inferred from the isolation of the agent from a wild rodent in Korea and the suspected occurrence of the disease in the "bushveld" (level, steppelike grassland with abundant shrubs and thorny vegetation) of South Africa.

Figure 25. Rickettsialpox (*Rickettsia akari*). Transmission cycle.

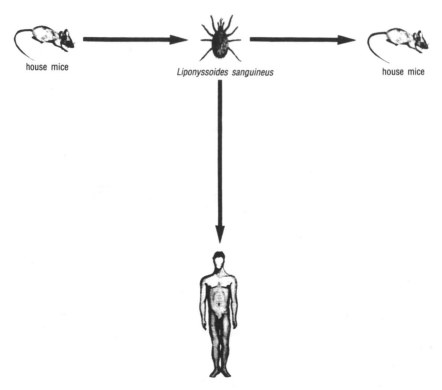

house mice

Liponyssoides sanguineus

house mice

Both in the United States and in the Soviet Union human rickettsialpox has occurred in rodent-infested dwellings in urban areas. The etiologic agent is transmitted by the mite *Liponyssoides sanguineus* from one mouse to another and accidentally to man. It has been shown that *R. akari* can be transmitted transovarially, and it is likely that mites are the main reservoir of the agent. Thus, *L. sanguineus* would not only be the vector of the infection, but would also serve as the reservoir. House mice are the preferred host for the mite, but it also feeds on rats and other rodents. *L. sanguineus* is not found permanently on the host, visiting it only for an hour or two to feed. Replete nymphs and adult mites can be found in large numbers in buildings located near rodent paths and nests (Harwood and James, 1979; Bell, 1981).

Role of Animals in the Epidemiology of the Disease: The infection is perpetuated by rodents and by the mite *L. sanguineus,* man being an accidental victim.

Diagnosis: Laboratory confirmation is accomplished by isolating the agent from blood taken during the febrile period and mouse inoculation. The complement fixation test using paired serum samples obtained in the acute phase of the disease and 3 to 4 weeks later can also be employed. The Weil-Felix agglutination test is not useful for diagnosis.

Control: Control measures are directed against the vector and rodents. They consist of the use of acaricides and then rodenticides in the infested environment, as well as elimination of havens for mice and rats in buildings through proper use of incinerators for garbage disposal.

Bibliography

Bell, J. F. Tick-borne fever and rickettsialpox. *In:* Davis, J. W., L. H. Karstad, and D. O. Trainer (Eds.), *Infectious Diseases of Wild Mammals,* 2nd ed. Ames, Iowa State University Press, 1981.

Burgdorfer, W. Rickettsialpox. *In:* Hubbert, W. T., W. F. McCulloch, and P. R. Schnurrenberger (Eds.), *Diseases Transmitted from Animals to Man,* 6th ed. Springfield, Illinois, Thomas, 1975.

Fuentes, L., A. Calderon, and L. Hun. Isolation and identification of *Rickettsia rickettsii* from the rabbit tick (*Haemaphysalis leporis palustris*) in the Atlantic zone of Costa Rica. *Am J Trop Med Hyg* 34, 1985.

Harwood, R. F., and M. T. James. *Entomology in Human and Animal Health,* 7th ed. New York, Macmillan, 1979.

Ley, H. L., Jr. Rickettsialpox. *In:* Beeson, P. B., W. McDermott, and J. B. Wyngaarden (Eds.), *Cecil Textbook of Medicine,* 15th ed. Philadelphia and London, Saunders, 1979.

Woodward, T. E., and E. B. Jackson. Spotted Fever Rickettsiae. *In:* Horsfall, F. L., and I. Tamm (Eds.), *Viral and Rickettsial Infections of Man,* 4th ed. Philadelphia, Lippincott, 1965.

Zdrodovskii, P. F., and E. H. Golinevich. *The Rickettsial Diseases.* Oxford, Pergamon Press, 1960.

ROCKY MOUNTAIN SPOTTED FEVER

(082.0)

Synonyms: Spotted fever, petechial fever, macular fever (Brazil), tick-borne typhus, New World spotted fever, Choix fever, pinta fever (Mexico).

Etiology: *Rickettsia rickettsii* (*Dermacentroxenus rickettsii*). This microorganism is the prototype of the group of rickettsiae that produce spotted fever.

Geographic Distribution: The disease has been confirmed in Canada (western), the United States, Mexico (western and central), Costa Rica, Panama, Colombia, and Brazil (São Paulo, Minas Gerais, Rio de Janeiro). In the United States it occurs everywhere except Maine, New Hampshire, Alaska, and Hawaii.

Occurrence in Man: Sporadic. In the United States, where the disease is under epidemiologic surveillance, an annual average of 528 cases was recorded from 1970 to 1973; in the decade of the 1970s an increase in cases was observed. During the period from 1977 to 1980, 4,411 cases were recorded, with an annual average of 1,103. The highest incidence was found in the southeastern states. The rate for the whole country was 5.2 cases per million inhabitants. Cases are seen most commonly between mid-April and mid-September, more frequently among children and young adults, and predominantly among males (Bernard *et al.*, 1982). Recent data are not available on the incidence of the disease in Latin America.

Occurrence in Animals: The etiologic agent has been isolated from dogs, opossums, and wild rabbits (*Sylvilagus* spp.) in Brazil. In the endemic areas of the United States, *R. rickettsii* has been isolated from many species of wild rodents, rabbits, opossums, and dogs. Many animal species, especially rodents, have been shown experimentally to suffer from a prolonged, high-titer rickettsemia.

Serologic studies in the United States confirmed that many species of mammals and wild birds have antibodies for *R. rickettsii*. Since dogs infested by the tick *Dermacentor variabilis* are an important link in transmission of the infection to man, it is of interest to find out their degree of exposure to infected ticks. Several serologic studies have demonstrated a high incidence of reactors among dogs in endemic areas. The highest rate of seroreactivity was obtained in Columbus, Ohio, where 45.2% of 73 dogs examined by means of microimmunofluorescence tested positive (Smith *et al.*, 1983).

The Disease in Man: Clinical symptoms appear 2 to 14 days after the tick bite. The disease has a sudden onset and is characterized by fever, chills, cephalalgia, and pain in the muscles, joints, and bones. Fever of about 40°C lasts until the end of the second week of illness. A generalized macular eruption, which at first resembles measles but often becomes petechial, appears between the third and sixth day after the onset of fever. Towards the end of the first week, the nervous system may be affected, with symptoms such as agitation, insomnia, delirium, and coma. During the second week of the disease, circulatory and pulmonary complications can occur. In patients who receive treatment (tetracyclines, chloramphenicol) convalescence can be short, but the disease lasts weeks or months in untreated patients. The fatality rate from the disease in the United States is 4.5% (Bernard *et al.*, 1982).

The Disease in Animals: The infection is inapparent in the majority of its natural hosts. Dogs infected experimentally or naturally may show clinical symptoms. Of four dogs diagnosed serologically, three had high fever, abdominal pain, depression, and anorexia. Two of them also displayed lethargy and nystagmus, and the third, conjunctivitis and petechiae in the mouth. The fourth dog did not show any clinical symptoms. It is possible that dogs in endemic areas are exposed to *R. rickettsii* at an early age and that maternal antibodies protect them from a severe form of the disease. Upon later reexposure, they may become actively immune and able to resist an infection with clinical manifestations (Lissman and Benarch, 1980). As dogs have more exposure to ticks than man does, they can serve as an indicator of the prevalence and location of the disease foci (Feng *et al.*, 1979).

Source of Infection and Mode of Transmission (Figures 26 and 27): The natural reservoir is a complex of ticks of the family Ixodidae and small wild mammals. In the United States, *Dermacentor andersoni* in the Rocky Mountain region and the dog tick *D. variabilis* in the east and southeast serve as the main vectors (and reservoirs). Currently, *D. variabilis* is much more important as a vector since the majority of human cases occur in the eastern region. In the endemic areas of Latin America the principal vector is *Amblyomma cajennense*. This tick bites man at any stage in its development, while *D. andersoni* and *D. variabilis* do so only as adults. In Mexico *Rhipicephalus sanguineus*, the brown dog tick, is also a vector.

Figure 26. Rocky Mountain spotted fever. Transmission cycle in the United States.

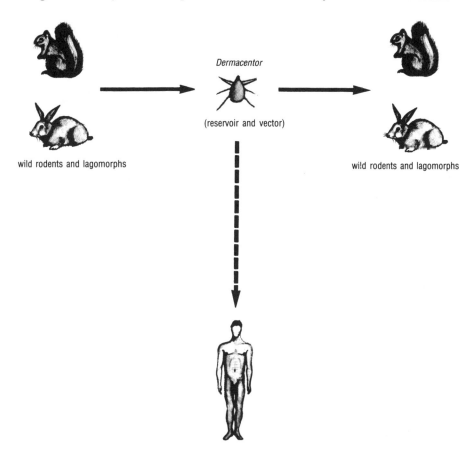

The main reservoirs of *R. rickettsii* are small wild rodents. The infective agent circulates in natural foci by means of ticks, which become infected from feeding on rickettsemic rodents and transmit the agent to other susceptible animals. Wild rabbits (*Sylvilagus* spp.) were thought to be a primary reservoir, but doubts exist about their efficiency in transmitting the infection to ticks (Burgdorfer *et al.,* 1980). Ticks play an important role, not only as biological vectors but also as reservoirs, because they can transmit *R. rickettsii* vertically to their offspring by transovarial transmission.

The rate of infected ticks, even in endemic areas, is low and varies from year to year. Nevertheless, the infection may be maintained in nature by transovarial transmission alone. In this situation, ticks would be the main reservoir of the infection and the animals to which the ticks attach would serve only to feed them.

The role of other animals as natural reservoirs capable of maintaining the infection has not been verified. Dogs play a very important role in the disease's epidemiology by carrying infected ticks to the human environment, but it is doubtful that dogs can infect ticks under natural conditions.

Figure 27. Rocky Mountain spotted fever. Transmission cycle in Latin America.

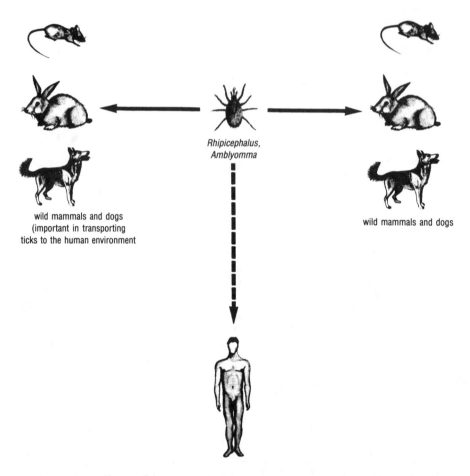

wild mammals and dogs
(important in transporting
ticks to the human environment

*Rhipicephalus,
Amblyomma*

wild mammals and dogs

NOTE: Transovarial transmission of *Rickettsia rickettsii* in ticks may possibly perpetuate the infection by itself.

Man becomes infected when a tick bites and remains attached to the body for at least 10 to 20 hours, allowing "reactivation" of the rickettsiae (passing from an avirulent to a virulent stage) to occur. Less frequently, rickettsiae in tick feces or tissues penetrate through broken skin when the tick is destroyed during its removal.

Man contracts the infection either by going into tick-infested areas or through contact with ticks carried by dogs to suburban homes. The human infection is seasonal, coinciding with annual periods of greatest tick activity.

Role of Animals in the Epidemiology of the Disease: Man is an accidental host. The basic cycle in the wild develops between small rodents and their ticks. Dogs are an important link in transmission of the infection to man by carrying vector ticks such as *D. variabilis, Amblyomma cajennense,* and *Rhipicephalus sanguineus* to his environment.

Diagnosis: Laboratory confirmation of the clinical diagnosis is accomplished by isolating *R. rickettsii* from the blood of the patient during the first week of fever and inoculating a blood clot suspension into male guinea pigs or embryonated eggs. Four to 6 days after inoculation of the guinea pigs, stained films of the tunica vaginalis testis can be examined microscopically. Although rickettsial isolation is the most reliable test, it should be carried out only in laboratories specially equipped for this procedure, owing to the risk of environmental contamination. An early presumptive diagnosis is possible using the Weil-Felix test (*Proteus* OX-19 or OX-2) if the titer shows a four-fold increase or is equal to or greater than 1:320. Diagnosis can be verified serologically with more specific and sensitive tests such as complement fixation, immunofluorescence, hemagglutination, latex agglutination, or microagglutination (Bernard *et al.*, 1982). The recently developed ELISA test for IgM or IgG antibodies could serve as an excellent tool in seroepidemiology and perhaps also for diagnosis. The value of serologic tests for diagnosis is limited by the fact that seroconversion is not observed until 6 days after the onset of the disease (Clements *et al.*, 1983a).

Control: Control measures include the application of tickicides in limited areas to exterminate or reduce the vector population, use of protective clothing and chemical repellents (diethyltoluamide, dimethylphthalate) for individual protection, inspection of clothing twice a day to get rid of unattached ticks, and careful removal of attached ticks. Vaccines to protect people at high risk of exposure (laboratory workers, ecologists) have not had satisfactory results. An improved vaccine, cultured in chicken embryo fibroblasts, inactivated in formalin, and purified, has been tested on volunteers. The vaccine provided only partial protection (25% efficacy), but the volunteers who did become ill had a milder disease (Clements *et al.*, 1983b). It is also important to apply residual tickicides to dogs, kennels, and dwellings at 2-week intervals.

Bibliography

American Public Health Association. *Control of Communicable Diseases in Man,* 14th ed. (Ed. by A.S. Benenson). Washington, D. C., APHA, 1985.

Bernard, K. W., C. G. Helmick, J. E. Kaplan, and W. G. Winkler. Surveillance of Rocky Mountain spotted fever in the United States, 1978-1980. *J Infect Dis* 146:297-299, 1982.

Bier, O. *Bacteriología e inmunología,* 12th ed. São Paulo, Brazil, Melhoramentos, 1965.

Burgdorfer, W. Rocky Mountain spotted fever. *In*: Hubbert, W. T., W. F. McCulloch, and P. R. Schnurrenberger (Eds.), *Diseases Transmitted from Animals to Man,* 6th ed. Springfield, Illinois, Thomas, 1975.

Burgdorfer, W., K. T. Friedhoff, and J. L. Lancaster. Natural history of tick-borne spotted fever in the USA. Susceptibility of small mammals to virulent *Rickettsia rickettsii. Bull WHO* 35:149-153, 1966.

Burgdorfer, W., J. C. Cooney, A. J. Mavros, W. L. Jellison, and C. Maser. The role of cottontail rabbits (*Sylvilagus* spp.) in the ecology of *Rickettsia rickettsii* in the United States. *Am J Trop Med Hyg* 29:686-690, 1980

Centers for Disease Control of the USA. Rocky Mountain spotted fever—United States, 1986. *Morb Mortal Wkly Rep* 36:314-315, 1987.

Clements, M. L., J. S. Dumler, P. Fiset, C. L. Wisseman, Jr., M. J. Snyder, and M. M. Levine. Serodiagnosis of Rocky Mountain spotted fever: comparison of IgM and IgG enzyme-linked immunosorbent assays and indirect fluorescent antibody test. *J Infect Dis* 148:876-880, 1983a.

Clements, M. L., C. L. Wisseman, Jr., T. E. Woodward, P. Fiset, J. S. Dumler, W. McNamee, R. E. Black, J. Rooney, T. P. Hughes, and M. M. Levine. Reactogenicity, immunogenicity, and efficacy of a chick embryo cell-derived vaccine for Rocky Mountain spotted fever. *J Infect Dis* 148:922-930, 1983b

Feng, W. C., E. S. Murray, G. E. Rosenberg, J. M. Spielman, and J. L. Waner. Natural infection of dogs on Cape Cod with *Rickettsia rickettsii*. *J Clin Microbiol* 10:322-325, 1979.

Fuentes, L. Ecological study of Rocky Mountain spotted fever in Costa Rica. *Am J Trop Med Hyg* 35:192-196, 1986.

Hattwick, M. A. W., H. Retailliau, R. J. O'Brien, M. Slutzker, R. E. Fontaine, and B. Hanson. Fatal Rocky Mountain spotted fever. *JAMA* 240:1499-1503, 1987.

Kaplan, J. E., and L. B. Schonberger. The sensitivity of various serologic tests in the diagnosis of Rocky Mountain spotted fever. *Am J Trop Med Hyg* 35:840-844, 1986.

Kenyon, R. H., L. St. C. Sammons, and C. E. Pedersen, Jr. Comparison of three Rocky Mountain spotted fever vaccines. *J Clin Microbiol* 2:300-304, 1975.

Ley H. L. Rocky Mountain spotted fever. *In*: Beeson, P. B., W. McDermott, and J. B. Wyngaarden (Eds.), *Cecil Textbook of Medicine,* 15th ed. Philadelphia and London, Saunders, 1979.

Lissman, B. A., and J. L. Benach. Rocky Mountain spotted fever in dogs. *J Am Vet Med Assoc* 176:994-995, 1980.

Murray, E. S. The spotted fevers. *In*: Hoeprich, P. D. (Ed.), *Infectious Diseases.* Hagerstown, Maryland, Harper and Row, 1972.

Smith, R. C., J. C. Gordon, S. W. Gordon, and R. N. Philip. Rocky Mountain spotted fever in an urban canine population. *J Am Vet Med Assoc* 183:1451-1453, 1983.

Wolff, J. W. Tick-borne rickettsioses. *In*: Van der Hoeden, J. (Ed.), *Zoonoses*. Amsterdam, Netherlands, Elsevier, 1964.

Woodward, T. E., and E. B. Jackson. Spotted fever rickettsiae. *In*: Horsfall, F. L., and I. Tamm (Eds.), *Viral and Rickettsial Infections of Man,* 4th ed. Philadelphia, Lippincott, 1965.

SCRUB TYPHUS

(081.2)

Synonyms: Tsutsugamushi disease, mite-borne typhus fever, tropical typhus, and various local names.

Etiology: *Rickettsia tsutsugamushi* (*R. orientalis*). There is a marked antigenic heterogeneity among different strains of the agent. Eight antigenic prototypes are recognized and it is possible that more exist. Immunity to the homologous strain is prolonged, but it is only transitory against heterologous strains. In an endemic area where several serotypes coexist, one may predominate (Shirai and Wisseman, 1975). Of 168 isolations obtained from various species of *Leptotrombidium* mites in Malaysia, 68.5% contained only one type, with Karp prototype predominating (Shirai *et al.,* 1981). The different strains of *Rickettsia tsutsugamushi* vary in their virulence.

Geographic Distribution: East and Southeast Asia, India, Pakistan, islands of the eastern Pacific, and northern Australia. In these areas the infection occurs under the most varied ecologic conditions (primary forest, semidesert, mountainous desert, and alpine meadows of the Himalayas). Distribution is not uniform and depends on the presence of the agent and the vector-reservoir complex, consisting of trombiculid mites and small mammals (especially rodents) which form "ecologic islands of infection."

Occurrence in Man: During World War II, scrub typhus constituted a problem of considerable importance for both Allied and Japanese forces in the southwestern Pacific and in the China-Burma-India field of operations. It is estimated that some 18,000 cases occurred among Allied troops. Mortality in various outbreaks varied from 0.6 to 35.3%, depending on the geographic area. The disease continues to be a public health problem in some endemic areas. In most cases it occurs sporadically. The incidence of clinical cases in Malaysia between 1967 and 1974 was very low, with an average of 55 patients per year. Nevertheless, the incidence of the disease is thought to be higher. In a study carried out in two communities of peninsular Malaysia, the incidence per month was calculated at 3.9% in one and 3.2% in the other. The lack of adequate laboratories in rural areas precludes differentiation between scrub typhus and other febrile diseases (Brown *et al.*, 1978).

The rate of serologic reactors can be very high in areas of great endemicity. In a study of a village in Thailand, 77% of the adults were reactive according to the indirect immunofluorescence test. Similar results were found in Malaysia, especially among jungle aborigines, and much lower rates among village inhabitants. It is probable that inhabitants of endemic areas are continuously exposed to the infection.

Occurrence in Animals: The natural infection has been found in many mammal species; of special interest are rats (*Rattus* spp.) and, in some regions, voles and field mice (*Microtus* spp., *Apodemus* spp.) as well as arboreal shrews. The species of infected mammals vary according to the zoogeographic region where the natural foci of infection are found.

The Disease in Man: One to 3 weeks after being bitten by a mite of the genus *Leptotrombidium* the patient develops fever, headache, conjunctival congestion, and generalized aches and lymphadenopathy. Interstitial pneumonitis is common. A skin ulceration with a black scab at the site of the bite is often found among patients of the Caucasian race and rarely among Asian patients. At the end of the first week of fever, a macular eruption occurs; it may last just a few hours or become a dark purple maculopapular eruption that lasts 1 week. Convalescence is long. The severity of the disease depends on the infecting strain and above all on the dose received; thus, within these parameters, the clinical picture can vary from very mild to very severe. In untreated patients pulmonary, encephalic, or cardiac complications may occur, often with fatal results. The basic pathologic lesions, as in other rickettsioses, are found in the smaller blood vessels. The case fatality rate can vary from 0 to 30% (Wisseman, Jr., 1982).

The Disease in Animals: In natural hosts, the infection is inapparent or relatively mild.

Source of Infection and Mode of Transmission (Figure 28): The most important vectors of *R. tsutsugamushi* are several mite species of the genus *Leptotrombidium*. The most important are *L. akamushi, L. deliense, L. fletcheri, L. arenicola,*

Figure 28. Scrub typhus (*Rickettsia tsutsugamushi*). Transmission cycle.

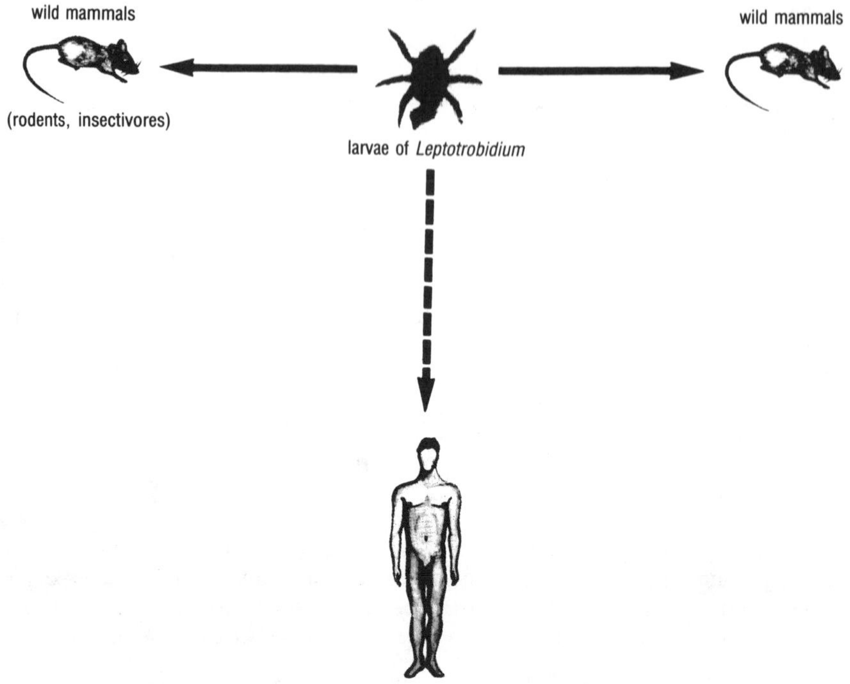

L. pallidum, and *L. pavlovsky.* The vector species is different in different eco-systems. Thus, for example, *L. akamushi* inhabits partially cultivated fields in Japan which flood in spring and early summer, while *L. deliense* is more often encountered in jungles. The mites are often found in very circumscribed foci (little pockets or islands) in scrub vegetation areas, hence the name of the disease. Only the larvae of these mites attach themselves to vertebrate hosts for feeding and in doing so transmit the infection. In other developmental phases (egg, nymph, and adult), the mite lives in the surface layers of the soil. *Leptotrombidium* serves not only as vector but also as an important reservoir since transovarial transmission of the agent, which per-petuates the infection from one generation to the next, has been confirmed in these mites. Wild vertebrates form an additional reservoir. Their principal role, however, is as a source of food for the mites.

The mite larvae transmit the infection to wild vertebrates (rodents, insectivores) and accidentally to man. Man is infected when, for reasons of work or recreation, he enters the natural foci of infection. The highest incidence was found among soldiers during military operations and among farmers who enter the agent's ecologic areas.

It is suspected that some bird species that are frequently parasitized by larvae of trombiculid mites could serve to transport these larvae and give rise to new infection foci.

Role of Animals in the Epidemiology of the Disease: Man is only an accidental host of *R. tsutsugamushi*. In natural foci the infection circulates among small mammals by means of the trombiculid vector. Nevertheless, these animals may not be indispensable for maintaining the infection in nature, since the mites seem to be able to do so by themselves.

Diagnosis: A presumptive diagnosis can be obtained with the Weil-Felix test using *Proteus* OX-K as antigen, based on an increase in the titer during the disease course. However, this method is limited in sensitivity and gives a significant number of false negative results. Indirect immunofluorescence is the indicated serologic test, as it is more specific and sensitive. The etiologic agent can be isolated from the blood by mouse inoculation.

Control: Control measures consist of the application of residual acaricides, such as dieldrin or lindane, in areas where agricultural work or military operations are carried out. Individual protection can be achieved by using clothing impregnated with acaricides (benzyl benzoate) in conjunction with repellents.

In military camps established in endemic areas, burning of surrounding vegetation or the use of defoliants and herbicides may be indicated.

No effective vaccine is available, primarily due to the antigenic heterogeneity of the different strains of the agent.

Chemoprophylaxis based on a dose of 200 mg of doxycycline per week was shown to be effective in a study of 1,125 soldiers who were sent to Pescadores Island, Taiwan, a hyperendemic area (Olson *et al.*, 1980).

Bibliography

Brown, G. W., D. M. Robinson, and D. L. Huxsoll. Serological evidence for a high incidence of transmission of *Rickettsia tsutsugamushi* in two Orang Asli settlements in peninsular Malaysia. *Am J Trop Med Hyg* 27:121-124, 1978.

Burgdorfer, W. Scrub typhus. *In*: Hubbert, W. T., W. F. McCulloch, and P. R. Schnurren-berger (Eds.), *Diseases Transmitted from Animals to Man,* 6th ed. Springfield, Illinois, Thomas, 1975.

Ley, J. L. Scrub typhus. *In*: Beeson, P. B., W. McDermott, and J. E. Wyngaarden (Eds.), *Cecil Textbook of Medicine,* 15th ed. Philadelphia and London, Saunders, 1979.

Olson, J. G., A. L. Bourgeois, R. C. Y. Fang, J. C. Coolbaugh, and D. T. Dennis. Prevention of scrub typhus. Prophylactic administration of doxycycline in a randomized double blind trial. *Am J Trop Med Hyg* 29:989-997, 1980.

Smadel, J. E., and B. L. Elisberg. Scrub typhus rickettsia. *In*: Horsfall, F. L., and I. Tamm (Eds.), *Viral and Rickettsial Infections of Man,* 4th ed. Philadelphia, Lippincott, 1965.

Shirai, A., and C. L. Wisseman. Serologic classification of scrub typhus isolates from Pakistan. *Am J Trop Med Hyg* 24:145-153, 1975.

Shirai, A., A. L. Dohany, S. Ram, G. L. Chiang, and D. L. Huxsoll. Serological classification of *Rickettsia tsutsugamushi* organisms found in chiggers (Acarina: Trom-biculidae) collected in peninsular Malaysia. *Trans R Soc Trop Med Hyg* 75:580-582, 1981.

Traub, R., and C. L. Wisseman, Jr. Ecological considerations in scrub typhus. *Bull WHO* 39:209-237, 1968.

Wisseman, C. L., Jr. Scrub typhus. *In*: Wyngaarden, J. B., and L. H. Smith, Jr. (Eds.), *Cecil Textbook of Medicine,* 16th ed. Philadelphia, Saunders, 1982.

Zdrodovskii, P. F., and H. M. Golinevich. *The Rickettsial Diseases*. Oxford, Pergamon Press, 1960.

ZOONOTIC TYPHUS CAUSED BY *RICKETTSIA PROWAZEKII*

(080)

Until a few years ago, epidemic or classic typhus was considered an exclusively human infection, transmitted by means of the body louse (Pediculus humanus humanus). *With the exception of man, no other reservoir for the etiologic agent,* Rickettsia prowazekii, *was known. Nevertheless, research carried out in recent years in the United States has proven that in that country an ample reservoir of* R. prowazekii *exists in nature, independent of man.*

Synonym: *R. prowazekii* wild typhus.

Etiology: *Rickettsia prowazekii;* it was isolated from the eastern flying squirrel, *Glaucomys volans volans*, in Florida, USA. This rickettsia is not distinguishable antigenically or by the toxin neutralization test from the classic strains of the etiological agent of epidemic louse-borne typhus (Bozeman *et al.*, 1975).

Geographic Distribution: The agent has been isolated from flying squirrels or their ectoparasites only in Virginia and Florida, USA. Nevertheless, indications are that the distribution is wider, judging from the points of origin of human cases. The distribution of the natural host, the flying squirrel, encompasses the whole eastern part of the United States, north to southern Canada (McDade *et al.*, 1980).

Occurrence in Man: Sporadic. From 1976 to 1979, 1,575 sera were examined for diagnosis of rickettsial diseases at the Centers for Disease Control in Atlanta. Of these sera, 85.7% were negative to all rickettsial antigens, 14% were positive for various rickettsial diseases, and 8 (3.5% of the 226 positives) were positive for *R. prowazekii*. Five of the patients were from Georgia and the other three were from Tennessee, Pennsylvania, and Massachusetts. These patients were not parasitized by lice nor did any of their contacts become ill, and therefore the classic transmission cycle of man-louse-man did not apply. Two of the patients reported having had contact with flying squirrels (McDade *et al.*, 1980). Between July 1977 and January 1980, seven more sporadic cases were diagnosed in Virginia, West Virginia, and North Carolina, which also were not associated with human lice (Duma *et al.*, 1981).

The disease occurs in winter.

Occurrence in Animals: From 1972 to 1975, 557 flying squirrels, captured in Virginia, Maryland, and Florida, were studied serologically; 54.2% were positive. Most seroconversions in these animals were observed in autumn and early winter, the season of maximum abundance of ectoparasites on squirrels. The infection spreads rapidly among the young animals in autumn when they crowd into their nests. No other infected animal species were found in these habitats (Sonenshine *et al.*, 1978).

The Disease in Man: The disease has a sudden onset, with fever, cephalalgia, myalgia, and exanthema. Except in some severe cases, the disease appears more benign than classic epidemic louse-borne typhus (Duma *et al.*, 1981). Some patients also suffer nausea, vomiting, and diarrhea. Exanthema was present in four out of eight cases in one group of patients. The disease lasted 2 to 3 weeks in patients who did not receive appropriate treatment. It was shorter in those who received treatment (tetracyclines or chloramphenicol) (McDade *et al.*, 1980).

The Disease in Animals: The natural course of the infection in flying squirrels is not known. Animals inoculated intraperitoneally with high doses of the agent died on the seventh day.

Rickettsemia in experimentally infected animals lasts 2 or 3 weeks.

Source of Infection and Mode of Transmission: The last outbreak of epidemic louse-borne typhus in the United States was in 1922. One proven case in 1950 was contracted outside the country, and recrudescent typhus (Brill-Zinsser disease) has been observed only in survivors of concentration camps or in immigrants from eastern Europe (McDade *et al.*, 1980).

Recent cases of human infection by *R. prowazekii* are zoonotic in character, as opposed to the classic epidemic louse-borne typhus.

The reservoir (probably unique) of wild typhus is the flying squirrel, *Glaucomys volans volans,* which shows a high rate of infection and a rickettsemia lasting several weeks. Experiments have demonstrated that infection among these animals is not transmitted by cohabitation and that, out of the many ectoparasites infesting them, the louse *Neohaematopinus sciuropteri* is the vector responsible for transmission. The mode of transmission to man is still not well known. The squirrel louse, *N. sciuropteri,* does not feed on man. The squirrel flea (*Orchopeas howardii*) becomes infected but cannot transmit the infection to susceptible squirrels. It is possible that this flea, which bites man, may transmit the infection to him if it is crushed on broken skin, or that man may become infected by aerosols originating from the feces of squirrel lice, especially during the most intense epizootic periods (Bozeman *et al.*, 1981).

Most of the cases described so far have occurred among rural inhabitants, some of whom stated that they had had contact with flying squirrels. The season (November to March) when the human cases occurred coincides with the period of greatest transmission among squirrels.

Diagnosis: Up to now, the diagnosis of human cases has been carried out by laboratory tests such as complement fixation, indirect immunofluorescence, toxin neutralization, and cross-absorption.

Control: The small number of confirmed human cases does not justify any special measures.

Bibliography

Bozeman, F. M., S. A. Masiello, M. S. Williams, and B. L. Elisberg. Epidemic typhus rickettsiae isolated from flying squirrels. *Nature* 255:545-547, 1975.

Bozeman, F. M., D. E. Sonenshine, M. S. Williams, D. P. Chadwick, D. M. Lauer, and B. L. Elisberg. Experimental infection of ectoparasite arthropods with *Rickettsia prowazekii* (GrF-16 strain) and transmission to flying squirrels. *Am J Trop Med Hyg* 30:253-263, 1981.

Duma, R. I., D. E. Sonenshine, F. M. Bozeman, J. M. Yeazey, Jr., R. L. Elisberg, D. P. Chadwick, N. I. Stocks, T. M. McGill, G. B. Miller, Jr., and J. N. McCormack. Epidemic typhus in the United States associated with flying squirrels. *JAMA* 245:2318-2323, 1981.

McDade, J. E., C. C. Shepard, M. A. Redus, V. F. Newhouse, and J. D. Smith. Evidence of *Rickettsia prowazekii* infections in the United States. *Am J Trop Med Hyg* 29:277-284, 1980.

Sonenshine, D. E., F. M. Bozeman, M. S. Williams, S. A. Masiello, D. P. Chadwick, N. I. Stocks, D. M. Lauer, and B. L. Elisberg. Epizootiology of epidemic typhus *(Rickettsia prowazekii)* in flying squirrels. *Am J Trop Med Hyg* 27:339-349, 1978.

SUMMARY OF RICKETTSIAL AND CHLAMYDIAL ZOONOSES[1]

Causative agent	Disease	R = Reservoir E = Epizootiology/ epidemiology PA = Principal animals PR = Persons at risk	O = Occurrence CA = Clinical form: animals CM = Clinical form: man	D = Diagnosis C = Control
Coxiella burnetti Tiny coccoid organisms, growing intracellularly as obligate parasites; very resistant in the environment.	● Q fever (pneumorickettsiosis, Balkan influenza, coxiellosis, abbatoir fever)	R. Two reservoirs: (a) wild animals and ticks; (b) cattle, sheep, and goats. E. One cycle involves wild animals and ticks; ticks may transmit to domestic animals through their feces. Infected animals initiate transmission to man by inhalation of contaminated dust. Man also infected by direct contact with infected and especially aborting animals or their products, especially milk. PA. Cattle, sheep, and goats; wild animals and ticks. PR. Groups I, II, and V.	O. Worldwide CA. In cattle, infection localizes subclinically in the udder. Infection of the placenta may cause abortion. Abortion also occurs in sheep. CM. Varies from subclinical to recurrent fever and headaches leading to pneumonia.	D. Microagglutination, immunofluorescence, and complement fixation tests. Luoto capillary agglutination test on milk. Isolation of *Coxiella* by inoculation of guinea pigs or mice. C. Formalin-inactivated vaccine for high-risk groups available in some countries. High-temperature pasteurization of milk is required. Milk may be boiled in enzootic areas. Special care needed for laboratory safety. Chemotherapy with tetracyclines.
Rickettsia akari Organism belongs to the spotted fever group of rickettsiae.	Rickettsialpox (vesicular rickettsiosis)	R/PA. Domestic mice and rats; possibly wild rodents. E. The infection is perpetuated by rodents and by the mite *Allodermanyssus sanguineus*, man being an accidental victim.	O. USA, USSR, equatorial and South Africa, Korean peninsula. CA. No information available. CM Benign course with fever and cutaneous lesions.	D. Mouse inoculation with blood from febrile patient; complement fixation test. C. Use of acaricides and rodenticides; elimination of mice and rat burrows from buildings.
Rickettsia conorii Organism belongs to the spotted fever group of rickettsiae.	Boutonneuse fever (Kenya typhus, South African tick typhus, Indian typhus, Marseilles fever, Mediterranean tick fever)	R. Wild rodents and ticks. E. Cycle in wild animals not defined. Dogs carry ticks, especially *Rhipicephalus sanguineus*, into the human environment and man may become an accidental host.	O. Africa, Europe, Middle East, and Southeast Asia. CA. Clinical disease not described in animals. CM. Benign fever. Local lesions and lymphadenitis. Generalized maculopapular eruption later. Mortality low.	D. Complement fixation test, Weil-Felix test. C. Control vectors in the environment. Use of acaricides on dogs.

[1] See introduction to Summary of Bacterial Zoonoses.

Causative agent	Disease	R = Reservoir E = Epizootiology/ epidemiology PA = Principal animals PR = Persons at risk	O = Occurrence CA = Clinical form: animals CM = Clinical form: man	D = Diagnosis C = Control
Rickettsia rickettsii Prototype organism of the spotted fever group of rickettsiae.	● Rocky Mountain spotted fever	R/PA. A complex of ticks of family Ixodidae and small wild mammals; also domestic dogs. E. Cycle of infection in wild mammals and several species of ticks of family Ixodidae. Domestic dogs may convey the ticks to the human environment. Ticks must be attached to the body for several hours before the rickettsiae are activated and transmitted through bites. Man is an accidental host.	O. North, Central, and South America in endemic foci. CA. Usually inapparent. May be a febrile disease in puppies. CM. Fever; muscle and joint pains with generalized macular hemorrhagic eruption. Nervous symptoms and pulmonary complications give a high mortality.	D. Isolate agent by inoculation of male guinea pigs or embryonated eggs. Weil-Felix, complement fixation, and indirect immunofluorescence tests. C. Control ticks. Use protective clothing and repellents. Protect high-risk personnel with vaccine; acaricides on dogs, in kennels, etc. Special care in laboratory safety. Antibiotic therapy.
Rickettsia siberica Organism belongs to the spotted fever group of rickettsiae.	"Siberian tick typhus" (North Asian tick-borne rickettsiosis, Asian ixodo-rickettsiosis, North Asian tick fever)	R. Wild rodents and ticks. E. Cycles of infection between wild rodents and ticks, especially of *Dermacentor* and *Haemaphysalis* spp. Man is an accidental host, by exposure to tick bites or contact with tick-contaminated fomites. PA. Wild rodents and ticks. Also cattle, horses, and dogs. PR. Groups I and III.	O. Siberia, Eastern USSR, and Mongolia; similar disease in Japan, Pakistan, and Czechoslovakia. CA. No information is available. CM. Benign acute fever; occurrence is sporadic.	D. Serological tests, including Weil-Felix test. Isolation in laboratory animals. C. Tick control on domestic animals. Rodent control. Protective clothing and repellents for individual protection.
Rickettsia tsutsugamushi Antigenic heterogeneity among strains.	Scrub typhus (Tsutsugamushi disease, mite-borne typhus fever)	R. Mites, especially *Leptotrombidium* (*Trombicula*) *akamushi*, *L. deliense*, *L. fletcheri*, *L. arenicola*, *L. pallidum*, and *L. pavlovsky* and insectivorous mammals. E. Cycles of infection between mites and wild animals. Man is infected accidentally on entering the natural foci of infection. PA. Wild insectivorous mammals, wild rodents. Birds may transport the mites. PR. Groups I and III.	O. East and Southeast Asia. North Australia. CA. In nature, the infection is inapparent or a mild disease. CM. Fever, generalized lymphadenopathy. Macular eruption. If untreated, pulmonary, encephalic, and cardiac complications may result in death.	D. Isolation of agent by mouse inoculation. Weil-Felix test. Complement fixation test. C. Use acaricides and repellents where there are special risks. Burn vegetation around camps, etc. Antibiotic therapy.

Causative agent	Disease	R = Reservoir E = Epizootiology/ epidemiology PA = Principal animals PR = Persons at risk	O = Occurrence CA = Clinical form: animals CM = Clinical form: man	D = Diagnosis C = Control
Rickettsia typhi Organism belongs to the typhus group of rickettsiae.	● Flea-borne typhus (murine typhus, endemic typhus)	R. Synanthropic rats, especially *Rattus rattus* and *R. norvegicus*; also opossums. E. Primary cycles in rats and *Xenopsylla cheopis* fleas; also opossums and *Ctenocephalides felis* fleas. Enters man through flea's feces, especially from scratching after being bitten. No man-to-man transmission. PA. Rats, opossums, and perhaps other animals. PR. General public, especially group VII.	O. Worldwide, prominent endemic foci. CA. No recognized clinical disease in animals. CM. Fever, headache, macular eruptions; complications rare with low mortality.	D. Isolation by inoculation of guinea pigs or embryonated eggs. Complement fixation, immunofluorescence, and Weil-Felix serological tests. C. Control of fleas and rats. Environmental sanitation measures.
Chlamydia psittaci	● Ornithosis/ Psittacosis	R/PA. Wild and domestic birds, especially of families Psittacidae and Columbidae. E. Feces of infected birds spread the agent. Dried feces are infective for both birds and man. Man is sporadically infected as an accidental host and rarely transmits infection. Transmission is by inhalation. PR. Groups I–VI.	O. Worldwide. CA. Mostly subclinical. Mild to severe respiratory and enteric signs. with stress-associated recurrences. Conjunctivitis. CM. Mostly subclinical or mild respiratory symptoms, often more severe than in birds. Atypical pneumonia and more severe symptoms in the elderly.	D. Serological tests, especially complement fixation and indirect complement fixation tests. Enlarged spleens in birds. Examine smears of the exudate for the agent. Isolation in embryonated eggs and cell culture. C. Special precautions and surveillance for workers in poultry processing plants. Tetracycline therapy of patients. Tetracycline treatment before, during, and following transport of birds; quarantine of imported birds. Special care with regard to exotic birds as pets.

285

Part IV

VIROSES

ARGENTINE HEMORRHAGIC FEVER

(078.7)

Synonyms: Junín disease, mal de rastrojos, O'Higgins disease, northwestern Buenos Aires hemorrhagic virosis, endemic-epidemic hemorrhagic virosis.

Etiology: Junín virus, an RNA virus of the genus *Arenavirus*, family Arenaviridae. Junín virus belongs to the Tacaribe complex (New World arenaviruses), which is composed of nine viruses (Junín, Tacaribe, Machupo, Ampari, Tamiami, Pichindé, Paraná, Latino, and Flexal). Only Junín and Machupo are human pathogenic agents under natural conditions (Weissenbacher and Damonte, 1983), but laboratory infections have occurred with the Pichindé and Tacaribe viruses (Johnson, 1981).

Geographic Distribution and Occurrence (Map 2; Figures 29 and 30): Argentine hemorrhagic fever (AHF) occurs widely in that country's moist pampas area, which is devoted primarily to the cultivation of corn and other grains. The endemic area measures about 100,000 km², contains somewhat more than 1 million inhabitants, and includes the northwest portion of Buenos Aires Province, the southeast and southern portions of Córdoba and Santa Fé Provinces, respectively, and the eastern portion of La Pampa Province. Recent studies have shown that the virus is active outside the known endemic areas; it was isolated from the field mouse *Akodon azarae*, and antibodies were found in two of 449 inhabitants of Pila, southwest of Buenos Aires, where the disease in man has not been confirmed (Weissenbacher *et al.*, 1983a). The first epidemics occurred in 1953 and 1954; the etiologic agent was isolated for the first time in 1958. Since then there have been annual epidemics of varying intensity. Over a 23-year period (1958 to 1980), more than 18,000 clinically confirmed cases of Argentine hemorrhagic fever were reported in the country, with a 10 to 15% fatality rate in untreated cases. Figure 29 shows the annual distribution of cases over this period. The number of cases has peaked every two or three years, with the 1964 epidemic being the largest. From 1977 to 1980 a reduction in the number of cases was observed (from 989 in 1977 to 161 in 1980) (Pan American Health Organization, 1982). The 3-year period from 1981 to 1983 had an average of 302 cases per year (Argentine Ministry of Health and Social Action, 1981-1983). In a study carried out in two rural populations where AHF had been occurring for 14 years, neutralizing antibodies were found in about 12% of the inhabitants, of which 7.6% and 9.7% were due to clinical infection and 4.4% and 1.9% were due to subclinical infection in the two areas (Weissenbacher *et al.*, 1983b).

The disease mostly affects the rural population and particularly farm workers, many of whom are migrant workers employed in the harvest of corn and other grains. This explains why the incidence is greatest in adult males.

Most cases occur between April and July, generally with a peak in May. The seasonal distribution coincides with an increase both in farm work and in contact with reservoir rodents, whose population density is significantly greater during that period of the year.

The Disease in Man: The incubation period is from 10 to 16 days. The symptomatology is similar to that of Bolivian hemorrhagic fever. The disease has an

Map 2. Progressive extension of the endemoepidemic area of Argentine hemorragic fever, 1958-1977.

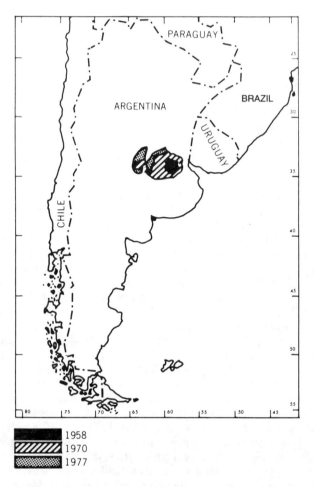

1958
1970
1977

Source: PAHO Epidemiol Bull 1(5):8, 1980

insidious onset, and its clinical manifestations are fever, malaise, chills, fatigue, dizziness, cephalalgia, and dorsalgia. Most patients show conjunctival congestion, retro-ocular pain, epigastralgia, halitosis, nausea, vomiting, and constipation or diarrhea. Other symptoms are accentuation of the vascular network in the soft palate, axillary and inguinal adenopathies, petechiae on the skin and the palate, and a congestive halo on the gums. Leukopenia, thrombocytopenia, albuminuria, and cylindruria are always present. The fever lasts for 5 to 8 days. After the fourth day epistaxis, gingival hemorrhages, mental dullness, unsteady gait, hypotension (75% of the patients), bradycardia, muscular hypotonia, and osteotendinous hyporeflexia appear.

Figure 29. Total number of notified cases per year of clinically diagnosed hemorrhagic fever, Argentina, 1958-1980.

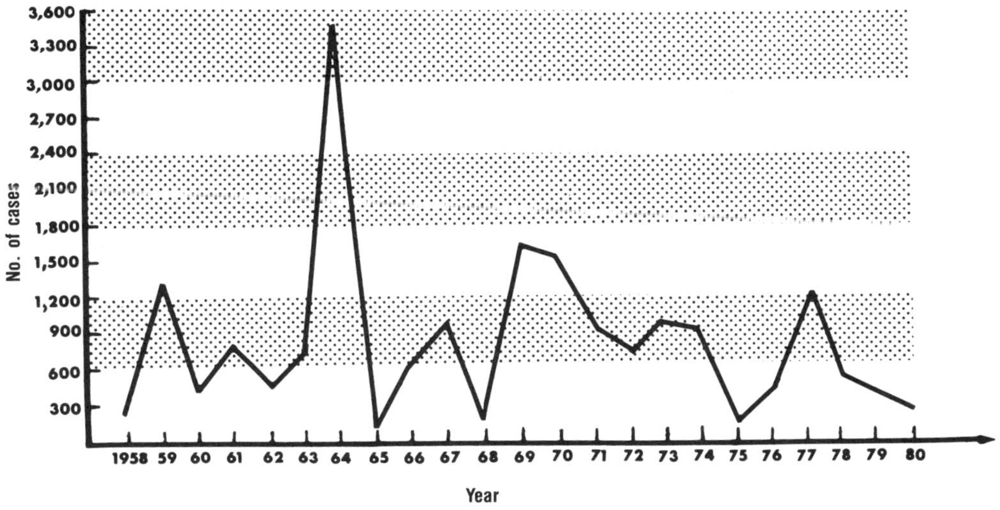

Source: *PAHO Epidemiol Bull* 3(2), 1982.

Mild forms of the disease last about 6 days. The serious hemorrhagic forms include hematemesis and melena in addition to epitaxis and gingival hemorrhages, which are prominent. When neurologic symptomatology predominates, the patient manifests muscular tremors of the tongue and hands, confusion or excitation, and sometimes tonic-clonic convulsive seizures. Forms intermediate between mild and serious are the most common (about 60% of patients). Convalescence lasts several weeks and, with a few exceptions, leaves no sequelae. Some patients, after an apparent recovery, develop a cerebellar syndrome that heals after a few days without sequelae. Of 130 patients with laboratory-confirmed diagnosis, 12 (9%) died (Argentine Ministry of Social Welfare, 1974).

The Disease in Animals: Rodents are the reservoir for maintenance of the Junín virus in nature, as is true for other arenavirus infections (with the exception of the Tacaribe virus whose reservoir is bats). The main hosts for the Junín virus are cricetid rodents: *Calomys musculinus*, *C. laucha*, and *Akodon azarae*. Experimental inoculation of *C. musculinus* and *C. laucha*, using field strains of the Junín virus, demonstrated that infection in these animals occurred asymptomatically, regardless of the age of the animal, the route of infection, or the amount of virus administered (Sabattini *et al.*, 1977). Experimental infection of *Akodon* produces symptomatology only when the animal is inoculated during the first week of life (Weissenbacher and Damonte, 1983).

Source of Infection and Mode of Transmission (Figure 31): Within the endemic region the risk of infection is not uniform. Between 1965 and 1974, 8,728 cases were reported; of these, 3,075 (35%) originated in Pergamino, Buenos Aires Province. Most of the 3,075 people contracted the infection in that district, which represents a very small area of the whole region affected by hemorrhagic fever. The

**Figure 30. Monthly distribution of total notified cases of hemorrhagic
fever, Argentina, 1978-1980.**

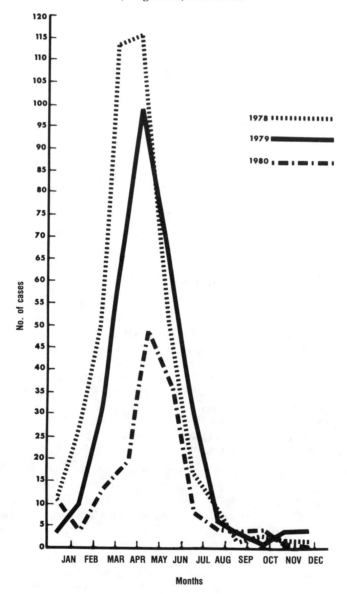

Source: PAHO Epidemiol Bull 3(2), 1982.

disease is more prevalent in males than in females (4:1) and appears among workers
in rural areas. Its seasonality is due to variations in the size of rodent populations
and variable amounts of exposure of workers to the predominant rodents. In 1977 a

Figure 31. Argentine hemorrhagic fever. Probable cycle of the Junín virus.

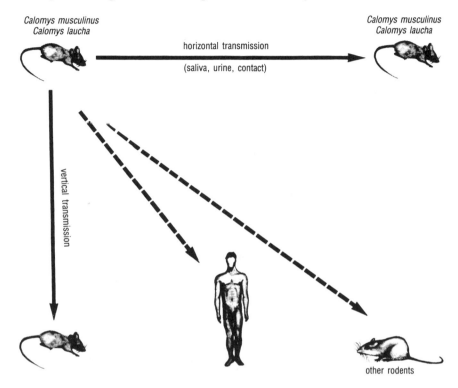

large outbreak occurred in that same area, and during the period from April to June more than 300 cases were reported (Bond, 1977).

More intense epidemics coincide with increases in the density of rodents in endemic areas. Similarly, there is a parallel relationship between the epidemic curve and the annual variation in rodent population size. Maximum incidence occurs in autumn (April-June), and this corresponds to the time of highest rodent populations, while the decrease in human cases in winter coincides with the obvious reduction in the population of these animals.

The Junín virus has been isolated from several species of cricetids, such as *Akodon azarae*, *A. obscurus*, *Calomys musculinus*, *C. laucha*, and *Oryzomys nigripes*. The primary habitat of these rodents is the abundant tall brush along fences in cultivated fields, roadsides, stream banks, and railroad tracks. The reactions of different species of rodents to Junín virus are distinct and may serve as indicators of their relative importance in maintenance of the agent in nature. Persistent viremia has been found in specimens of *C. musculinus* that have been captured and then recaptured two or three times at intervals of up to 55 days; they have also been found to eliminate the virus in their urine under natural conditions. Experimental inoculation of newborn animals has confirmed that this rodent, without manifesting clinical symptoms, suffers from a chronic infection with persistent viremia and eliminates the virus through buccopharyngeal secretions and urine. Infection of adult animals leads to shorter-term viremia and viruria, in the presence of complement-fixing antibodies. Very similar findings were made with respect to *C. callosus*, which is considered the main reservoir of Machupo virus, the agent of Bolivian hemorrhagic fever. In addition, it has been demonstrated that infection in *C. musculinus* is transmitted both vertically and horizontally (Sabattini *et al.*, 1977), and, although the population of this cricetid decreases enormously in winter, the virus can survive in nature because of the persistent viremia characteristic of this species. Trapping carried out in endemic areas of Córdoba Province revealed not only that *C. musculinus* is the most abundant rodent, but also that the rate of virus isolations was very high. Virus was also isolated from four out of 40 captured *Akodon*, but their scant numbers in cultivated fields would indicate that this rodent plays a limited role in the epidemiology of AHF (Sabattini, 1977).

It has been suggested that the emergence and later expansion of AHF were due to changes in the environment caused by cultivation of grains that favor the *Calomys* population (Villafañe *et al.*, 1977).

The type of crop in cultivation is important in the ecology of the virus. The rodent density is lower in soybean fields, especially for cricetids of the genus *Calomys*, compared with corn and sunflower fields. In areas where soybean fields increased, the number of cases of AHF decreased (Kravetz *et al.*, 1981, cit. in Weissenbacher and Damonte, 1983).

Although the virus has been isolated from mites that parasitize rodents, it has not been demonstrated that they can transmit the virus; currently, no role is ascribed to them in the ecology of the virus or the epidemiology of the disease. Isolation of the virus from oral swabs and from urine of *Calomys* indicates that these secretions constitute the main sources of virus infection for other members of the same species and probably for other species of rodents with which the *Calomys* come in contact. In fact, transmission of the disease from mother to litter and between animals placed in the same cage has been confirmed. The important role played by *Calomys* in the natural cycle of the virus is evident.

Man becomes infected by contact with infected rodents and their excreta. The penetration route of the virus in man could be through skin lesions, by ingestion, or by aerosols that enter through the conjunctiva and nasal or oral mucosa. These means of entry have been confirmed experimentally. Transmission between humans is exceptional, but precautions should be taken, since virus has been isolated from pharyngeal swabs and from urine of patients. As in the case of Bolivian hemorrhagic fever, infection may occur by close contact, since viremic patients can experience hemorrhages and virus can sometimes be isolated from the mouth and urine.

Diagnosis: At one time, AHF was called "rubber stamp disease," as it was considered easy to diagnose by its signs and symptoms. Nevertheless, recent studies prove that only about 60% of the cases can be correctly diagnosed by clinical examination. Until 1965, virologic diagnosis of the disease had only been attempted in a few identified cases. From 1965 to 1974, diagnosis was confirmed virologically in 64% of the reported cases. Specific diagnosis can be carried out by isolation of virus and by serologic tests with blood samples obtained in the acute and convalescent phases. Virus can be successfully isolated from blood of febrile patients or autopsy material inoculated intracerebrally into suckling mice, and intraperitoneally or intramuscularly in guinea pigs. The virus can be isolated also by culturing the patient's blood in monolayer VERO cells and finding viral antigen by immunoperoxidase staining (Lascano *et al.*, 1981); this procedure takes much less time (2 to 8 days) than inoculation of laboratory animals. The serologic tests most often used are complement fixation (CF), neutralization (N), and indirect immunofluorescence (IIF). CF is the least sensitive and the antibodies it detects appear late and disappear rapidly. N is the most specific test and detects antibodies 3 to 4 weeks after onset of disease. IIF gives the earliest and fastest results, and is economical and simple (Samoilovich *et al.*, 1983). In 50 persons who had AHF between 1 and 14 years earlier, IIF detected antibodies in 88%, N in 96%, and CF in only 30% (Damilano *et al.*, 1983).

Recently, the ELISA test for arenaviruses, including the antigen for Junín virus, has been described (Ivanov *et al.*, 1981).

Control: An epidemic of Machupo virus hemorrhagic fever in an urban environment in Bolivia was demonstrated to be controllable by controlling rodents. However, in agricultural areas of Argentina application of this measure would be very difficult and costly. Hope centers on the development of a safe and effective vaccine. Attempts to obtain an inactivated vaccine seem to have been abandoned, and greater effort is being dedicated to development of attenuated live vaccines. Currently, several vaccines with attenuated strains ($XJC1_3$, XJO, Candid 1) are in the experimental phase and are being tested on laboratory animals. The $XJC1_3$ strain vaccine was administered to 636 volunteers. It induced subclinical infection or mild clinical manifestations, and neutralizing antibodies that lasted 7 to 9 years in 90% of the individuals. When the strain is inoculated intracerebrally in guinea pigs and the monkey *Cebus* spp., neurovirulence results. In the marmoset *Callithrix jacchus*, considered to be a useful animal model for AHF, the strain gave good protection (Weissenbacher and Damonte, 1983).

The vaccine with attenuated strain Candid 1 holds the greatest promise in the short term as the "safe and effective vaccine." Tests carried out in laboratory animals showed high titers of seroconversion, very good protection against virulent strains, and no neurovirulence in monkeys. When it was recently used on human volunteers, this vaccine produced no complications of any kind and induced satisfactory seroconversion (Barrera Oro, 1986).

In addition to the attenuated strains of the Junín virus, Tacaribe virus, which is antigenically closely related, is being studied for use in vaccines. Tests on guinea pigs and *C. jacchus* demonstrated that this virus confers good protection against virulent strains without producing clinical or hematologic alterations, and without persisting in the organs of the primates (Weissenbacher and Damonte, 1983).

Bibliography

Andrewes, C., and H. I. G. Pereira. *Viruses of Vertebrates*, 3rd ed. Baltimore, Maryland, Williams and Wilkins, 1972.

Argentine Ministry of Social Welfare. Bureau of Public Health. *Bol Epidemiol Nac*, 1971-1974.

Argentine Ministry of Health and Social Action. *Bol Epidemiol Nac*, vol. 12-14, 1981-1983.

Barrera Oro, J. Personal communication, March 1986.

Bond, J. O. Hemorrhagic fever in Latin America. Paper presented at the Sixteenth Meeting of the PAHO Advisory Committee on Medical Research. Washington, D.C., Pan American Health Organization, 1977.

Casals, J. Arenaviruses. *In*: A. S. Evans (Ed.), *Viral Infections of Humans. Epidemiology and Control*. New York, Plenum, 1976.

Coto, C. E. Junín virus. *Progr Med Virol* 18:127-142, 1974.

Damilano de, A. J., S. C. Levis, A. M. Ambrosio, D. A. Enria, and J. I. Maiztegui. Diagnóstico serológico de infección por virus Junín por fijación del complemento, immunofluorescencia y neutralización. *In: Primer Congreso Argentino de Virología*. Buenos Aires, 1-5 August 1983.

Guerrero, L. B. de. Ensayo de vacunación. Mesa redonda. Fiebre hemorrágica argentina: aspectos immunológicos. *Rev Asoc Argent Microbiol* 5:163-164, 1973.

Ivanov, A. P., V. N. Bashkirtsev, and E. A. Tkachenko. Enzyme-linked immunosorbent assay for detection of arenaviruses. *Arch Virol* 67:71-74, 1981.

Johnson, K. M., S. B. Halstead, and S. N. Cohen. Hemorrhagic fevers of southeast Asia and South America. *Progr Med Virol* 9:105-158, 1967.

Johnson, K. M., P. A. Webb, and G. Justines. Biology of Tacaribe-complex viruses. *In*: Lehman-Grube, F. (Ed.), *Lymphocytic Choriomeningitis Virus and Other Arenaviruses*. Heidelberg, Springer, 1973.

Johnson, K. M. Arenaviruses: Diagnosis of infection in wild rodents. *In*: Kurstak, E., and C. Kurstak (Eds.), *Comparative Diagnosis of Viral Diseases*, vol. 4. New York, Academic Press, 1981.

Lascano, E. F., M. I. Berria, and N. Candurra. Diagnosis of Junín virus in cell culture by immunoperoxidase staining. *Arch Virol* 70:79-82, 1981.

Lord, R. D., A. M. Vilches, J. I. Maiztegui, E. C. Hall, and C. A. Soldini. Frequency of rodents in habitats near Pergamino, Argentina, as related to Junín virus. *Am J Trop Med Hyg* 20:338-342, 1971.

Maiztegui, J. I. Epidemiología de la fiebre hemorrágica argentina. *In*: Bacigalupo, J. C., and E. R. Castro (Eds.), *Conferencias, Simposios y Plenario. V Congreso Latinoamericano de Microbiología*. Montevideo, Uruguayan Microbiology Society, 1971.

Mettler, N. E. *Fiebre hemorrágica argentina: conocimientos actuales*. Washington, D.C., Pan American Health Organization, 1970. (Scientific Publication 183.)

Pan American Health Organization. Argentine hemorrhagic fever. *Epidemiol Bull* 3(2):1-3, 1982.

Ruggiero, H. R., A. S. Parodi, H. A. Ruggiero, F. A. Cintora, C. Magnoni, and H. Milani. *Síntesis médica sobre la fiebre hemorrágica argentina*, 2nd ed. Buenos Aires, Ministry of Social Welfare, 1969.

Sabattini, M.S. *In*: Bacigalupo, J. C., and E. R. Castro (Eds.). *Conferencias, Simposios y Plenario. V Congreso Latinoamericano de Microbiología*. Montevideo, Uruguayan Microbiology Society, 1971.

Sabattini, M. S., and J. I. Maiztegui. Fiebre hemorrágica argentina. *Medicina* 30(Supl 1):111-128, 1970.

Sabattini, M. S., L. E. Gonzales de Rios, G. Díaz, and V. R. Vega. Infección natural y experimental de roedores con virus Junín. *Medicina (B Aires)* 37(Supl 3):149-161, 1977.

Samoilovich, S. R., G. Carballal, M. J. Frigerio, and M. C. Weissenbacher. Detección de infecciones de laboratorio por virus Junín utilizando comparativamente las técnicas de neutralización e immunofluorescencia. *Rev Argent Microbiol* 15:113-118, 1983.

Schwartz, E. R., O. G. Mando, J. I. Maiztegui, and A. M. Vilches. Síntomas y signos iniciales de mayor valor diagnóstico en la fiebre hemorrágica argentina. *Medicina (B Aires)* 30(Supl 1):8-14, 1970.

Vilches, A. M. Ecología y control de la fiebre hemorrágica argentina. *In*: Bacigalupo, J. C., and E. R. Castro (Eds.), *Conferencias, Simposios y Plenario. V Congreso Latinoamericano de Microbiología*. Montevideo, Uruguayan Microbiology Society, 1971.

Villafañe, G. de, F. O. Kravetz, O. Donado, R. Percich, L. Knecher, M. P. Torres, and N. Fernández. Dinámica de las comunidades de roedores en agro-ecosistemas pampásicos. *Medicina (B Aires)* 37(Supl 3):128-140, 1977.

Weissenbacher, M. C., C. E. Coto, M. Calello, M. J. Frigerio, and E. Damonte.

Protección experimental contra virus Junín por inoculación de virus Tacaribe. *Medicina* (*B Aires*) 37(Supl 3):237-243, 1977.

Weissenbacher, M. C., and E. B. Damonte. Fiebre hemorrágica argentina. *Adel Microbiol Enferm Infecc* (*B Aires*) 2:119-171, 1983.

Weissenbacher, M. C, M. Calello, G. Carballal, N. Planes, and F. Kravetz. Actividad del virus Junín en áreas no endémicas: su aislamiento en roedores y detección de anticuerpos en humanos. *In: Primer Congreso Argentino de Virología.* Buenos Aires, 1-5 August 1983.

Weissenbacher, M. C., M. S. Sabattini, M. M. Avila, F. M. Sangiorgio, M. R. F. de Sensi, M. S. Contigiani, S. del C. Levis, and J. I. Maiztegui. Junín virus activity in two rural populations of the Argentine hemorrhagic fever (AHF) endemic area. *J Med Virol* 12:273-280, 1983.

BOLIVIAN HEMORRHAGIC FEVER

(078.7)

Synonym: Black typhus.

Etiology: Machupo virus, an RNA virus, genus *Arenavirus*, family Arenaviridae; this virus belongs to the Tacaribe complex (see Argentine Hemorrhagic Fever).

Geographic Distribution: Known endemic foci are found in the provinces of Mamoré, Iténez, and Yacuma, Beni Department, Bolivia.

Occurrence: Bolivian hemorrhagic fever (BHF) was recognized clinically in 1959, and in the provinces of Mamoré and Iténez annual outbreaks occurred until 1964. It is estimated that in this period 1,100 persons contracted the illness (out of a population of 4,000 to 5,000), 260 of whom died (24%). Until 1962, the disease occurred in many small foci in rural areas, but during that year there was an outbreak in the village of El Mojón on the Orobayaya, whose 600 inhabitants abandoned the town in fear. The worst epidemic (650 cases and 122 deaths) occurred between 1963 and 1964 in San Joaquín, capital of Mamoré Province, a town with approximately 2,500 inhabitants (Bolivian Hemorrhagic Fever Research Commission, 1975). Human-to-human transmission was not observed during these epidemics. Nevertheless, in 1963 two cases occurred in a hospital in Panama where two United States researchers had been taken after they became ill in Bolivia. Following an extensive outbreak in 1962-1963, the disease disappeared until 1968 when six cases, all of them fatal, were reported from the northern region near Magdalena in Iténez Province. In 1969, nine more cases were recognized in the same area. In 1971, an outbreak of significant epidemiologic interest occurred in a hospital in Cochabamba, which is located outside the endemic area of the disease. This nosocomial outbreak, which brought to mind similar episodes of Lassa fever, involved six cases, five of them fatal. The index case was a nursing student who visited the village of Fortaleza, Beni, where the infection had not yet been recognized. The student fell ill and was later hospitalized in Cochabamba. Four secondary cases occurred among her contacts in the hospital. A tertiary case also ensued in a pathologist who cut his finger when performing an autopsy on one of the victims of the disease. In the second half of 1971 another four cases were reported in Yacuma Province, also located in the extreme north. Between December 1974 and January 1975 there were four cases with two deaths in the locality of El Recuerdo, Mamoré Province.

Epidemic outbreaks are related to a great abundance of *Calomys* rodents and to the rate of infection in these cricetids (up to 35%). Conversely, where human cases are absent, population density of the rodents and their rate of infection are low (Johnson *et al.*, 1978).

Although no human cases have been reported since 1975, the virus is still active in the reservoir, *Calomys callosus*. In May 1977, a continuing study noted a high proportion of rodents with splenomegaly in the province of Iténez, near the Brazil frontier, and more recently in the province of Cercado de Beni (Pan American Health Organization, 1982). Currently, virologic studies are being carried out to determine if those findings represent a new focus of the enzootic disease.

Most cases occurred in the dry season from April to September.

The Disease in Man: The incubation period is about 2 weeks. Onset of BHF is insidious. The symptomatology is similar to that of Argentine hemorrhagic fever. All of the patients have sustained pyrexia (38-41°C) for at least 5 days. Almost invariably they suffer from myalgia, conjunctivitis, and cephalalgia; cutaneous hyperesthesia and gastrointestinal symptoms are also common. A variable proportion of patients (30% or more) experience hemorrhages between the fourth and sixth days of the disease. Petechiae of the oral mucosa and hemorrhage of the gums, nose, stomach, intestine, and sometimes the uterus are common. In general, the loss of blood is not great. Hypotension occurs between the sixth and tenth days following onset of the disease in approximately 50% of the patients. In some of these patients hypotension is transitory, while in others it leads to hypovolemic shock and death. A high proportion of cases (30 to 50%) show symptoms of central nervous system involvement, with tremors of the tongue and extremities and, sometimes, convulsions and coma. Leukopenia is a regular sign and is especially pronounced between the fifth and ninth days of the disease. Hemoconcentration and proteinuria are also common. Convalescence is lengthy, and temporary hair loss and transverse furrows in fingernails and toenails frequently occur. Among the pathologic findings are generalized adenopathy and focal hemorrhages in the gastric and intestinal mucosa, lungs, and brain.

The Disease in Animals: The virus has been isolated only from the cricetid rodent *Calomys callosus*. The infection in this species does not produce acute disease. Newborn rodents infected experimentally suffer chronic hemolytic anemia with splenomegaly and growth retardation. Females with chronic infection abort. In field studies a positive correlation was found between splenomegaly and the rate of virus isolations (Johnson, 1981).

Source of Infection and Mode of Transmission (Figure 32): The disease foci are found in the Mojos plains, an extensive flat area where the vegetation consists primarily of open pasture land and savannas (in the higher areas) mixed with "islands" of semideciduous jungle vegetation. In general, the farming communities are located around the wooded areas. In the localities where epidemics occur, the spiny rat *Proechimys guyannensis* and the cricetid rodent *C. callosus* are always found. The Machupo virus has been isolated from 24% of the 122 specimens of *C.*

Figure 32. Bolivian hemorrhagic fever (Machupo virus). Transmission cycle.

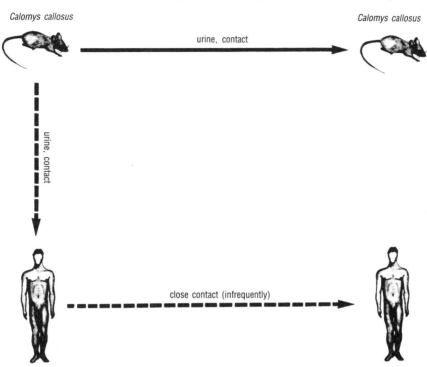

callosus examined, but not from *Proechimys* or other rodents. Based on this finding, as well as experimental evidence, no doubts exist that *C. callosus* is the reservoir for maintenance of the virus in nature. Chronic infection of that host and its shedding of the virus through excretions and secretions assure the persistence of the agent in the cricetid population. The preferred habitat of *Calomys* is savannas and fallow fields, but they are also attracted to houses by food and then proliferate there, as was the case during the San Joaquín epidemic. It is believed that the great population increase of *Calomys* in this village was due to a decrease in the number of cats since 1959, as a result of mortality from DDT used in the antimalaria campaign. Absence of their natural enemy and the abundance of food in houses are thought to have been factors in the migration of *Calomys* from their natural habitat.

Observations made during the San Joaquín epidemic indicated that the virus was being transmitted in or around the houses. The successful control of that epidemic by means of a *Calomys* extermination campaign confirms the predominant role played by that rodent in the epidemiology of the disease. During the antirodent campaign, Machupo virus was isolated from 13 out of 17 captured *Calomys* and, even more significant, the agent was found in the urine of five out of nine specimens examined.

In the search for a vector, attempts have been made to isolate the virus from arthropods. More than 25,000 specimens, especially rodent ectoparasites, were processed with negative results. This finding reinforces the idea that the source of infection is virus in the urine of infected rodents (Johnson, 1975).

The establishment of a breeding unit for *C. callosus* at the Meso-American Research Unit (MARU) in Panama has contributed greatly to a better knowledge of the natural history of BHF. The rodent can be infected experimentally through oral and nasal mucosa and by cohabitation in the same cage. When *Calomys* 9 or more days old are inoculated with the virus, approximately half the infected animals develop immunotolerance, while the other half remain immunocompetent. The immunotolerant animals experience viremia and eliminate virus in their urine during their entire life, but do not develop neutralizing antibodies. By contrast, immunocompetent animals have neutralizing antibodies but no viremia; however, it is possible, for a variable period of time, to isolate virus from their urine and viscera. In immunocompetent animals the size and weight of the spleen are normal, while in immunotolerant animals the spleen is enlarged three to six times. Animals born of immunotolerant mothers invariably become infected and suffer viremia for life, while those born of immunocompetent mothers are protected passively by the neutralizing antibodies of the mother for about 2 months, after which they become susceptible. The infection is clinically inapparent in adult *Calomys* that are inoculated with the virus. In this sense, their response is different from that of house mice to the lymphocytic choriomeningitis virus. Persistent anemia is seen in immunotolerant animals with chronic viremia.

Man is infected in the field or at home by contact with cricetids or their excreta and secretions, which may contaminate food or water. The Cochabamba episode showed, on the other hand, that close contact with secretions of a sick person can give rise to secondary cases by transmission between humans. In fact, the Machupo virus, or a slight antigenic variant of it, has been isolated from a laryngeal swab, but not from urine, of some patients.

Diagnosis: The Machupo virus can be isolated from the blood of febrile patients and from the spleen of those who have died as a consequence of the disease. The materials are inoculated intracerebrally into suckling hamsters and mice.

Serologic diagnosis can be carried out by means of the complement fixation test (group-specific for the Tacaribe viruses), the plaque neutralization test in VERO cells (type-specific for Machupo), and the indirect immunofluorescence test (group-specific). The tests should be done with paired samples, obtained during the acute and convalescent phases of the disease.

Control: The control campaign in San Joaquín shows that, at least in small cities where *Calomys* develops domestic or peridomestic habits, excellent results can be obtained with measures directed against the rodents. In San Joaquín, some 3,000 *C. callosus* were destroyed in a 60-day period by means of traps and rodenticide baits, resulting in an impressive reduction in the incidence of human cases. These measures are not easy to apply under other ecologic conditions, and thus work is under way to develop a vaccine to protect the exposed population in endemic areas.

Bibliography

Andrewes, C., and H. G. Pereira. *Viruses of Vertebrates*, 3rd ed. Baltimore, Maryland, Williams and Wilkins, 1972.

Bolivian Hemorrhagic Fever Research Commission. Fiebre hemorrágica en Bolivia. *Bol Of Sanit Panam* 58:93-105, 1965.

Bond, J. O. Hemorrhagic fever in Latin America. Paper presented at the Sixteenth Meeting of the PAHO Advisory Committee on Medical Research. Washington, D.C., Pan American Health Organization, 1977.

Casals, J. Arenaviruses. *In*: A. S. Evans (Ed.), *Viral Infections of Humans. Epidemiology and Control*. New York, Plenum, 1976.

Johnson, K. M. Arenaviruses: diagnosis of infection in wild rodents. *In*: Kurstak, E., and C. Kurstak (Eds.), *Comparative Diagnosis of Viral Diseases*. New York, Academic Press, 1981.

Johnson, K. M., R. B. Mackenzie, P. A. Webb, and M. L. Kuns. Chronic infection of rodents by Machupo virus. *Science* 150:1618-1619, 1965.

Johnson, K. M., S. B. Halstead, and S. N. Cohen. Hemorrhagic fevers of southeast Asia and South America: A comparative appraisal. *Progr Med Virol* 9:105-158, 1967.

Johnson, K. M., P. A. Webb, and G. Justines. Biology of Tacaribe-complex viruses. *In*: Lehmann-Grube, F. (Ed.), *Lymphocytic Choriomeningitis Virus and Other Arenaviruses*. Heidelberg, Springer, 1973.

Johnson, K. M., and P. A. Webb. Rodent transmitted hemorrhagic fevers. *In*: Hubbert, W. T., W. F. McCulloch, and P. R. Schnurrenberger (Eds.), *Diseases Transmitted from Animals to Man*, 6th ed. Springfield, Illinois, Thomas, 1975.

Johnson, K. M., P. A. Webb, G. Justines, and F. A. Murphy. Ecology of hemorrhagic fever viruses: Arenavirus biology and the Marburg-Ebola riddle. *In*: *Proceedings, 3rd Munich Symposium on Microbiology*, June 7-8, 1978.

Mackenzie, R. B., H. K. Beye, L. Valverde, and H. Garron. Epidemic hemorrhagic fever in Bolivia. I. A preliminary report of the epidemiologic and clinical findings in a new epidemic area in South America. *Am J Trop Med Hyg* 13:620-625, 1964.

Pan American Health Organization. Bolivian hemorrhagic fever. *Epidemiol Bull* 3(5):15-16, 1982.

Pan American Health Organization. Fiebre hemorrágica. Bolivia. *Inf Epidemiol Sem* 47:264, 1975.

Peters, C. J., P. A. Webb, and K. M. Johnson. Measurement of antibodies to Machupo virus by the indirect fluorescent technique. *Proc Soc Exp Biol Med* 142:526-531, 1973.

Peters, C. J., R. W. Kuehne, R. R. Mercado, R. H. Le Bow, R. O. Spretzel, and P. A. Webb. Hemorrhagic fever in Cochabamba, Bolivia, 1971. *Am J Epidemiol* 99:425-433, 1974.

Symposium on some aspects of hemorrhagic fevers in the Americas. *Am J Trop Med Hyg* 14:789-818, 1965.

BOVINE PAPULAR STOMATITIS

(051.9)

Synonyms: Granular stomatitis, proliferating stomatitis.

Etiology: RNA virus, genus *Parapoxvirus* of the family Poxviridae; the viruses of contagious ecthyma and milkers' nodules (pseudocowpox) belong to the same genus.

Geographic Distribution: Bovine papular stomatitis (BPS) has been observed in Canada, the United States, Mexico, several European countries, Kenya, Nigeria, and Australia, indicating a worldwide distribution.

Occurrence in Man: Very few cases have been confirmed. From 1953 to 1972, 19 cases were described in the United States, Europe, and Australia (Schnurrenberger *et al.*, 1980). Nevertheless, the disease must occur more frequently, as demonstrated by the report of five cases among students and professors at an American veterinary school, who contracted the infection while tube-feeding a bull. The following 2 years, three more isolated cases were discovered as a result of the surveillance established (Bowman *et al.*, 1981). One human case in Mexico was caused by handling experimentally infected cows (Aguilar-Setién *et al.*, 1980). Since the disease is clinically mild, it is likely that neither patient nor physician pays attention to it.

Occurrence in Animals: The incidence of the disease is not well known. A study in a slaughterhouse in Australia estimated that approximately 5% of young cattle had "erosive stomatitis" lesions. On some ranches, the morbidity rate can be high, as was found in one establishment in Mexico where 31 out of 120 calves became ill (Aguilar-Setién *et al.*, 1980). Inapparent infection and the carrier state must be more common than was once thought, as illustrated by the previously mentioned human cases in the American veterinary school (see Occurrence in Man), acquired during the necropsy of animals without apparent lesions (Bowman *et al.*, 1981).

Although the disease may cause developmental delay in calves due to lesions in the mouth, it is generally considered not to have economic repercussions, and its importance arises from its possible confusion with other vesicular diseases.

The Disease in Man: The incubation period is from 3 to 8 days. The lesion is usually on a finger or hand, corresponding to the penetration site of the agent. In general, the lesion consists of a papule or verrucous nodule measuring 3 to 8 mm in diameter, which begins to decrease in size after 2 weeks and disappears in approximately a month. One case presented an erythematous eruption lasting 3 days on an arm, and another case displayed axillary adenopathy and myalgia. Sometimes the papule becomes vesiculated. All of the cases were afebrile.

The lesions in man are similar to those of contagious ecthyma or milkers' nodule (pseudocowpox).

The Disease in Animals: Cattle are the only susceptible species. In the Western Hemisphere the disease was first recognized in 1960 in the United States as a mild disease characterized by proliferative lesions in and around the mouth, unaccompanied by any systemic reaction. In subsequent outbreaks, animals were found with fever, profuse salivation, diarrhea, and teat lesions. More often, the infection is clinically inapparent or causes a mild and benign afebrile disease. It is seen mostly in young cattle and it begins with hyperemic foci measuring 2 to 4 mm in diameter in the nostrils, on the palate, or on the inner surface of the lips. These foci develop rapidly to form papules surrounded by a hyperemic border. Some of these lesions turn into wrinkled papulomatous plaques. The papules may last from 1 day to 3 weeks. During the course of the disease, lesions can be found in various stages of development, ranging from new papules to yellow or reddish-brown spots left by the healed lesions. The disease persists in this way for several months. Morbidity in some affected herds may be very high.

Source of Infection and Mode of Transmission: Cattle are the natural host of the infection. The disease has not been confirmed in other domestic species. The epidemiology of papular stomatitis is still not clear. It is thought that the disease is transmitted by direct and indirect contact. Man contracts the infection from infected cattle. Preexisting skin abrasions and lacerations or an accidental bite when examining an animal's mouth serve as portals of entry for the virus.

Diagnosis: The virus can be isolated in tissue cultures, such as bovine testicle or kidney culture, in which it produces a cytopathic effect. Histopathology and electron microscopy are useful for diagnosis.

Differential diagnosis is important to distinguish BPS from bovine viral diarrhea, vesicular stomatitis, foot-and-mouth disease, bovine plague, bovine infectious rhinotracheitis, and mycotic stomatitis (Tripathy *et al.*, 1981).

Control: Based on current data on the epidemiology of the disease, it is not possible to establish effective control measures. Persons who handle animals with papular stomatitis should take all necessary precautions to avoid contracting the infection.

Bibliography

Aguilar-Setién, A., P. Correa-Girón, E. Hernández-Baumgarten, A. Cruz-Gómez, and P. Hernández-Jauregui. Bovine papular stomatitis. First report of the disease in Mexico. *Cornell Vet* 70:10-18, 1980.

Bowman, K. F., R. T. Barbery, L. J. Swango, and P. R. Schnurrenberger. Cutaneous form of bovine papular stomatitis in man. *JAMA* 246:2813-2818, 1981.

Carson, C. A., and K. M. Kerr. Bovine papular stomatitis with apparent transmission to man. *J Am Vet Med Assoc* 151:183-187, 1967.

Griesemer, R. A., and C. R. Cole. Bovine papular stomatitis. I. Recognition in the United States. *J Am Vet Med Assoc* 137:404-410, 1960.

McEvoy, J. D. S., and B. C. Allan. Isolation of bovine papular stomatitis virus from humans. *Med J Aust* 1:1254-1256, 1972.

Schnurrenberger, P. R., L. J. Swango, G. M. Bowman, and P. J. Luttgen. Bovine papular stomatitis incidence in veterinary students. *Can J Comp Med* 44:239-243, 1980.

Tripathy, D. N., L. E. Hanson, and R. A. Crandall. Poxviruses of veterinary importance: diagnosis of infections. *In*: Kurstak, E., and C. Kurstak (Eds.), *Comparative Diagnosis of Viral Diseases*, vol. 3. New York, Academic Press, 1981.

CALIFORNIA ENCEPHALITIS

(062.5)

Synonym: La Crosse encephalitis.

Etiology: La Crosse (LAC) virus, an RNA virus belonging to the genus *Bunyavirus* of the family Bunyaviridae. The LAC virus, the main etiologic agent of the disease, forms part of the California encephalitis virus complex, which includes several other antigenically related viruses that, with a few exceptions, are not or are only rarely pathogenic for man. Since 1980 researchers have begun to consider the Jamestown Canyon (JC) virus, a member of that complex, to be a human pathogen (Centers for Disease Control of the USA, 1982). On the other hand, no more cases of the original California encephalitis virus have been positively identified since 1945 when three human cases were diagnosed serologically in that state, giving the disease its name. In Canada, four cases of this type of encephalitis were probably caused by the Snowshoe virus (McFarlane *et al.*, 1982). In several European countries, a febrile illness in man is attributed to the Tahyna virus, and in Finland to the Inkoo virus, both of which are included in the same virus group.

Geographic Distribution and Occurrence: The viruses that cause encephalitis in man, especially the LAC virus, are found mainly in the North Central region of the United States, and their distribution extends to the midwestern and eastern states. California encephalitis is second in incidence among the arboviral encephalitides in the United States. As is the case with other arboviruses, the rate of subclinical infection with California viruses is much higher than the rate of clinical cases. From 1960 to 1970, 509 human cases were recorded in the central and eastern states of the United States, the majority in Ohio, Wisconsin, and Minnesota. In 1978, 109 cases were diagnosed in that country (Centers for Disease Control of the USA, 1981). Serologic studies in various parts of the United States have found that between 6 and 60% of rural resident workers had antibodies for the viruses of the California group. It has also been shown that approximately 75% of the Indians in southern Florida have antibodies by the time they reach 50 years of age. The disease occurs in summer.

In several European countries, antibodies have been found in 5 to 60% of the individuals examined by the serum neutralization test. In one study area, 24 of 103 febrile patients had positive serologic reactions to the Tahyna virus.

The Disease in Man: The disease caused by the LAC virus occurs primarily in children and adolescents under 15 years of age. The symptomatology varies from benign aseptic meningitis to severe encephalitis. Nevertheless, it is likely that many cases pass as mild, undifferentiated fevers. Common symptoms of the disease are fever, headache, nausea, vomiting, and stiffness of the neck; in more serious cases lethargy and convulsions are observed. The nervous symptoms generally appear the third day of illness and disappear in one week, although they persist longer in the more severe cases. The La Crosse virus is the only one of the group that is known with certainty to cause human illness in the United States, but the possibility exists that other viruses of the California group possess comparable pathogenic activity, as might be indicated by the cases attributed to Jamestown Canyon and California encephalitis viruses.

In five cases in New York, recently described and presumably due to the
Jamestown Canyon virus, the fatality rate in adults was high. Isolated cases at-
tributed to this same virus were also discovered in Indiana and in Ontario, Canada
(Centers for Disease Control of the USA, 1982).

In Europe, the Tahyna virus has been observed to cause clinical symptoms of
infection, such as pneumonia and pleuritis, acute arthritis, pharyngitis, undifferentiated fevers, and, sometimes, affliction of the central nervous system.

The Disease in Animals: The natural hosts of the LAC virus, such as the
chipmunk (*Tamias striatus*) and arboreal squirrels, develop viremia when infected
experimentally, but the infection is asymptomatic in inoculated adult animals
(Thompson, 1981).

Source of Infection and Mode of Transmission (Figure 33): The La Crosse
virus has been isolated from many species of mosquitoes, but the frequency of
isolation indicates that the main vector is *Aedes triseriatus*, which breeds in holes in
trees or other places where water collects, either in the woods or near houses. The
virus is transmitted by the vector to rodents whose habitat is oak forests. A high rate
of neutralizing antibodies has been found in squirrels (*Tamias striatus*, *Sciurus
carolinensis*, and *S. niger*) and, to a lesser extent, in wild rabbits (*Sylvilagus*

Figure 33. California encephalitis (La Crosse virus). Transmission cycle.

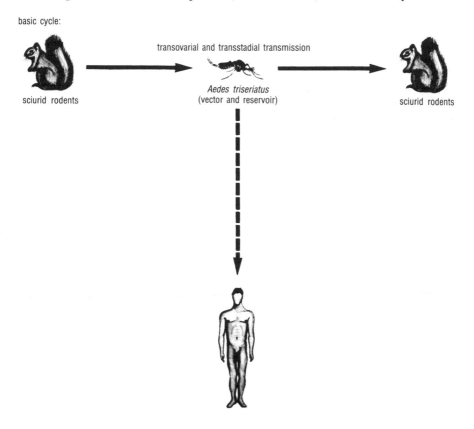

floridanus). The squirrels (*T. striatus* and *S. carolinensis*) develop viremia for 2 to 5 days when inoculated experimentally with La Crosse virus, and *A. triseriatus* that feed on these mammals transmit the infection to suckling mice 15 to 17 days after ingesting the viremic blood.

Recent data have helped clarify the ecology of the La Crosse virus, especially its mechanism for overwintering. The virus has been isolated from larvae of *A. triseriatus*, which indicates that the agent is transmitted transovarially. In addition, the La Crosse virus can be recovered from eggs, larvae, and adults produced from experimentally infected *A. triseriatus*. The F_1 females transmitted the virus by biting suckling mice and squirrels. These experimental findings were recently confirmed by discovery of the virus in eggs and larvae of the vector collected in the field. The LAC virus can also be transmitted sexually in *A. triseriatus*. In conclusion, *A. triseriatus* serves not only as vector but also as reservoir, as it can transmit the infection transovarially for several generations. The virus survives during winter in infected mosquito eggs in diapause (a state of inactivity and greatly reduced metabolism). When summer comes, adult mosquitoes begin feeding on the chipmunk (*T. striatus*) and the gray squirrel (*Sciurus carolinensis*), infecting them with the virus and thus widening the reservoir of the agent. In serologic testing of these rodent species, a high rate of neutralizing antibodies has been found. According to recent studies, the red fox (*Vulpes fulva*) in endemic areas could serve as an amplifying and disseminating host of the LAC virus (Amundson and Yuill, 1981).

In the United States, the period of greatest activity of the LAC virus is from July to the end of September. The human infection occurs primarily in deciduous oak forests during work or recreational activities. The virus is transmitted to man by the bites of the vectors.

The other viruses of the California group have different vectors and hosts, according to the distribution of the virus and the ecologic characteristics of the area. In Europe, the hare is an important reservoir of the Tahyna virus and the vectors are several mosquitoes of the genus *Aedes* (*A. vexans*, *A. caspius*, and others). Antibodies to various viruses of this group have been found in horses, swine, and cattle, and also in deer, but not in birds.

The Jamestown Canyon virus is transmitted in New York by mosquitoes of the group *A. communis*. This vector transmits the infection vertically (transovarially) to its progeny and horizontally to vertebrates, especially white-tailed deer, *Odocoileus virginianus* (Centers for Disease Control of the USA, 1982). The Snowshoe virus has been isolated from *Lepus americanus*, and a high rate of serologic reactors for this type has been found in moose (*Alces alces americana*). The vectors are probably *A. communis* and *A. canadensis* (McClean *et al.*, 1975; McFarlane *et al.*, 1982). The virus was isolated from larvae of *Aedes* spp. mosquitoes in the Yukon Territory, Canada, which proves that the virus survives the extreme winter conditions at those latitudes by means of transovarial transmission (McClean *et al.*, 1975).

Role of Animals in the Epidemiology of the Disease: *Aedes triseriatus* is the main vector of the La Crosse (LAC) virus and also serves as reservoir by virtue of transovarial transmission of the agent. By this mechanism, both the LAC virus and some others of the California complex can survive winter in temperate or even the coldest climates (Snowshoe virus). Vertebrates serve as amplifiers of the virus in summer. These hosts are important in the ecology of the disease, since venereal and transovarial transmission of the virus in mosquitoes is relatively inefficient to ensure the endemicity of California encephalitis in the affected regions (Amundson and Yuill, 1981). Man is an accidental host who contracts the disease in natural foci.

Diagnosis: Laboratory confirmation can be achieved by serologic diagnosis. A four-fold or more increase in titer between serum samples from the acute and convalescent phases of the disease is considered significant. The tests most often used are hemagglutination inhibition (HI), complement fixation (CF), and virus neutralization (VN). The virus neutralization test is the most sensitive and is preferred, but it can only be done in a few laboratories. The CF test detects antibodies later than the other tests, while production of antigens for the HI test presents difficulties. Lately, an indirect immunofluorescence technique has been perfected which is as sensitive as the VN or HI but simpler to perform (Beaty *et al.*, 1982). Isolation of the virus from the blood of a febrile patient is difficult owing to the short duration of viremia. The virus has been isolated from the brain in fatal cases.

Control: Individual prevention measures consist of the use of protective clothing and repellents. Control of *Aedes* in extensive areas is difficult. Repeated and ample application of insecticides within and around camps for children and youth is recommended.

Bibliography

Amundson, T. E., and T. M. Yuill. Natural La Crosse virus infection in the red fox (*Vulpes fulva*), gray fox (*Urocyon cinereoargenteus*), raccoon (*Procyon lotor*) and opossum (*Didelphis virginiana*). *Am J Trop Med Hyg* 30:706-774, 1981.

Andrewes, C., and H. G. Pereira. *Viruses of Vertebrates*, 3rd ed. Baltimore, Maryland, Williams and Wilkins, 1972.

Balfour, H. H., C. K. Edelman, F. E. Cook, W. I. Barton, A. W. Busicky, R. A. Siem, and H. Bauer. Isolates of California encephalitis (La Crosse) virus from field-collected eggs and larvae of *Aedes triseriatus*: Identification of the overwintering site of California encephalitis. *J Infect Dis* 131:712-716, 1975.

Beaty, B. J., J. Casals, K. L. Brown, C. B. Gundersen, D. Nelson, J. T. McPherson, and W. H. Thompson. Indirect fluorescent-antibody technique for serological diagnosis of La Crosse (California) virus infections. *J Clin Microbiol* 15:429-434, 1982.

Berge, T. O. (Ed.). *International Catalogue of Arboviruses*, 2nd ed. Atlanta, Georgia, Centers for Disease Control of the USA, 1975. (DHEW Publ. CDC 75-8301.)

Boromisa, R. D., and P. R. Grimstad. Seroconversion rates to Jamestown Canyon virus among six populations of white-tailed deer (*Odocoileus virginianus*) in Indiana. *J Wildl Dis* 23:23-33, 1987.

Centers for Disease Control of the USA. *Encephalitis Surveillance. Annual Summary 1978*. Atlanta, CDC, 1981.

Centers for Disease Control of the USA. Arboviral encephalitis—United States, 1982. *Morb Mortal Wkly Rep* 31:433-435, 1982.

Centers for Disease Control of the USA. Arboviral infections of the central nervous system—United States, 1986. *Morb Mortal Wkly Rep* 36(27):450-455, 1987.

Chamberlain, R. W. Arbovirus infections of North America. *In*: Sanders, M., and M. Schaeffer (Eds.), *Viruses Affecting Man and Animals*. St. Louis, Missouri, Green, 1971.

Downs, W. G. Arboviruses. *In*: A. S. Evans (Ed.), *Viral Infections of Humans. Epidemiology and Control*. New York, Plenum, 1976.

Dykers, T. I., K. L. Brown, C. B. Gundersen, and B. J. Beaty. Rapid diagnosis of La Crosse encephalitis: detection of specific immunoglobulin M in cerebrospinal fluid. *J Clin Microbiol* 22:740-744, 1985.

Eldridge, B. F., C. H. Calisher, J. L. Fryer, L. Bright, and D. J. Hobbs. Serological evidence of California serogroup virus activity in Oregon. *J Wildl Dis* 23:199-204, 1987.

Grimstad, P. R. California group virus disease. *In*: Monath, T. P. (Ed.), *Epidemiology of Arthropod-Borne Viral Diseases*. Boca Raton, Florida, CRC Press (in press).

Grimstad, P. R., C. H. Calisher, R. N. Harroff, and B. B. Wentworth. Jamestown Canyon virus (California serogroup) is the etiologic agent of widespread infection in Michigan humans. *Am J Trop Med Hyg* 35:376-386, 1986.

Henderson, B. E., and P. H. Coleman. The growing importance of California arboviruses in the etiology of human disease. *Progr Med Virol* 13:405-461, 1971.

McFarlane, B. L., J. E. Embree, J. A. Embil, K. R. Rozee, and H. Artsob. Antibodies to the California group of arboviruses in animal populations of New Brunswick. *Can J Microbiol* 28:200-204, 1982.

McLean, D. M., S. K. A. Bergman, A. P. Gould, P. N. Grass, M. A. Miller, and E. E. Spratt. California encephalitis virus prevalence throughout the Yukon Territory 1971-1974. *Am J Trop Med Hyg* 24:676-684, 1975.

Moulton, D. W., and W. H. Thompson. California group virus infections in small, forest-dwelling mammals of Wisconsin. *Am J Trop Med Hyg* 20:474-482, 1971.

Parkin, W. E. Mosquito-borne arboviruses other than Group A, primarily in the Western Hemisphere. *In*: Hubbert, W. T., W. F. McCulloch, and P. R. Schnurrenberger (Eds.), *Diseases Transmitted from Animals to Man*, 6th ed. Springfield, Illinois, Thomas, 1975.

Thompson, W. H. California group viral infections in the U.S. *In*: Baran, G. W. (Section Ed.), *CRC Handbook Series in Zoonoses*, Section B, vol. 1. Boca Raton, Florida, CRC Press, 1981.

Thompson, W. H., and A. S. Evans. California encephalitis virus studies in Wisconsin. *Am J Epidemiol* 81:230-244, 1965.

Work, T. H. California encephalitis. *In*: Beeson, P. B., W. McDermott, and J. B. Wyngaarden (Eds.), *Cecil Textbook of Medicine*, 15th ed. Philadelphia and London, Saunders, 1979.

Watts, D. M., S. Pantuwatana, G. R. De Foliart, T. M. Yuill, and W. H. Thompson. Transovarial transmission of La Crosse virus (California encephalitis group) in the mosquito *Aedes triseriatus*. *Science* 182:1140-1141, 1973.

Watts, D. M., J. W. Leduc, C. L. Bailey, J. M. Dalrymple, and T. P. Gargan II. Serologic evidence of Jamestown Canyon and Keystone virus infections in vertebrates of the Delmarva peninsula. *Am J Trop Med Hyg* 31:1245-1251, 1982.

CHIKUNGUNYA FEVER

(066.3)

Etiology: RNA genome virus (CHIK) belonging to the genus *Alphavirus* (group A of the arboviruses), family Togaviridae. There is an antigenic relationship between this virus and the Mayaro (see Mayaro Fever), O'nyong-nyong,[1] and Semliki[2] viruses.

Geographic Distribution: The virus is widely distributed in sub-Saharan Africa, Southeast Asia, India, and the Philippines (Tesh, 1982).

Occurrence in Man: The infection is endemic in vast rural areas. Epidemics, many times explosive in nature, also occur in cities when there is a sufficiently large susceptible population. In South Africa, there were annual epidemics in 1975, 1976, and 1977 (Brighton *et al.*, 1983). In Ibadan, Nigeria, an outbreak occurred for the first time in 1969, and isolated cases in children were confirmed both before and after that epidemic. Five years later, there was another epidemic. In both outbreaks, the highest morbidity rate was recorded in children under 5 years of age, which seems to indicate that older age groups have acquired immunity. In the period between the two epidemics, the rate of neutralizing antibodies in children in a pediatric hospital declined significantly (Tomori *et al.*, 1975). In other areas, the interval between urban epidemics can be much longer. The disease is not always recognized and it is often confused with dengue, which is clinically similar. A study carried out in northern Malaysia found that 35% of the inhabitants examined had neutralizing antibodies, although the disease had not been recorded in the country. The high prevalence of reactors suggests that the disease occurred but was not diagnosed correctly (Tesh *et al.*, 1975).

The disease occurs during the rainy season when population density of the vector mosquitoes is greatest.

Occurrence in Animals: Antibodies against the CHIK virus have been found many times in South African primates, such as green monkeys (*Cercopithecus aethiops*) and baboons (*Papio ursinus*). The virus circulates with high titers in both species (McIntosh, 1970). In a serologic study carried out in Kruger National Park in South Africa, antibodies against CHIK were found in nearly 50% of the vervet monkeys (Kaschula *et al.*, 1978). In other regions of Africa, reactors have been found among *Colobus abyssinicus*, chimpanzees, and the baboon *Papio dogueri*, besides the species already mentioned.

---

[1]The O'nyong-nyong (ONN) virus caused one of the most extensive epidemics in Africa from 1959 to 1963, with 2 million persons affected. This virus has been isolated only one other time, in 1978 (Johnson *et al.*, 1981). It produces a clinical picture similar to CHIK fever. The virus is transmitted by *Anopheles funestus* and *A. gambiae*; the former is the more efficient vector. The only known reservoir is man and the virus has not been found in other vertebrates.

[2]Semliki (Semliki Forest) is an alphavirus isolated in Africa from several species of mosquitoes, birds, and mammals. A high proportion of the human population has antibodies against this virus. No disease in man or animals attributable to this infection has been confirmed.

The Disease in Man: For a long time this disease was confused with dengue; isolation of the CHIK virus is relatively recent, dating from 1955.

The incubation period lasts 4 to 7 days. The disease has a sudden onset with fever, chills, cephalalgia, anorexia, lower back pain, and conjunctivitis; adenopathy is frequent. Many patients (60 to 80%) show a morbilliform rash and sometimes purpura on the trunk and extremities. The cutaneous eruption can recur every 3 to 7 days. A prominent symptom, which appears predominantly in adult patients, is arthropathy, and this symptom gives the disease its name (in Swahili, "chikungun-ya" = to walk bent over). Arthropathy is manifested by pain, swelling, and rigidity, especially of the metacarpophalangeal, wrist, elbow, shoulder, knee, ankle, and metatarsal joints (Kennedy *et al.*, 1980).

The arthropathy appears 3 to 6 days after the initial clinical symptoms and in some patients can persist many months or even years (Brighton *et al.*, 1983). In this aspect CHIK fever is similar to Ross River, Mayaro, Sindbis, and O'nyong-nyong fevers (Tesh, 1982).

No deaths due to CHIK fever have been recorded.

The Disease in Animals: Clinically apparent infection has not been confirmed in animals.

Source of Infection and Mode of Transmission: Studies indicate the existence of a wild cycle of the virus, similar to that of yellow fever, between jungle primates and *Aedes africanus* and the *A. furcifer-taylori* group mosquitoes. In the wild primates *Cercopithecus aethiops* and *Papio ursinus*, a high-titer viremia occurs, and transmission of the virus to green monkeys by the mosquitoes has been experimentally confirmed (McIntosh, 1970). Epizootics in monkeys occur when a large part of the population consists of nonimmune individuals, and stop if the proportion of immune monkeys is high. When epizootics occur in monkeys, the human population in areas near the jungle is exposed to the infection.

A study was carried out in an epidemic area in northern Natal, South Africa, over five years (1964-1969). The first year, antibodies were confirmed in a high proportion (54%) of wild primates, including young ones, while at the end of the period serologic reactors could only be found in primates at least 4 years old. After 1964 the virus could not be isolated from mosquitoes, nor could viral activity be confirmed in sentinel monkeys during the later period. It was deduced that some time before the study was initiated, an epizootic occurred among the primates and then died out, with disappearance of the virus. At least in this particular ecosystem, the wild primates were not able to serve as maintenance hosts and the epizootics probably began with virus introduced from other areas more favorable to the perpetuation of the agent (McIntosh, 1970). In light of this study, it would seem that the virus maintains itself only in very special ecosystems and that its ecology has not yet been completely elucidated.

In urban outbreaks, the main vector is *A. aegypti*. It is probable that there is a mosquito-man-mosquito cycle, as high viremia titers in febrile patients have been confirmed. Given that extrinsic incubation in *A. aegypti* is relatively long, the explosive character of some outbreaks is possibly due to mechanical transmission by mosquitoes whose feeding on viremic patients is interrupted and then continued on susceptible persons (Halstead, 1981).

Diagnosis: The virus can be isolated from the blood of febrile patients by intracerebral inoculation of suckling mice or in VERO cells.

Serologic diagnosis, which is most commonly used, is based on proving seroconversion of blood serum secured from the acute and convalescent phases, using the hemagglutination inhibition, neutralization, and complement fixation tests.

If O'nyong-nyong fever also occurs in the same region, difficulties in both identification of the virus and in serologic diagnosis can result, since the viruses are antigenically related. Differentiation is based mainly on higher titers for the homologous sera used in the identification of both viruses, and on higher serum antibody titers for homologous antigens used in serologic diagnosis (Filipe and Pinto, 1973).

Control: Prevention of urban epidemics should center on controlling the vector *A. aegypti*. In Luanda, Angola, where in 1970 simultaneous yellow fever and Chikungunya fever epidemics occurred, it was possible to interrupt both with intense antimosquito measures (Filipe and Pinto, 1973). Nevertheless, eradication of *A. aegypti* in Africa or Asia presents great difficulties. A formalin-inactivated vaccine has given satisfactory experimental results in mice, but is still not available for use on humans (White *et al.*, 1972).

Bibliography

Brighton, S. W., O. W. Prozesky, and A. L. De La Harpe. Chikungunya virus infection. A retrospective study of 107 cases. *S Afr Med J* 63:313-315, 1983.

Filipe, A. R., and M. R. Pinto. Arbovirus studies in Luanda, Angola. 2. Virological and serological studies during an outbreak of dengue-like disease caused by the Chikungunya virus. *Bull WHO* 49:37-40, 1973.

Halstead, S. B. Chikungunya fever. *In*: Beran, G. W. (Section Ed.), *CRC Handbook Series in Zoonoses*. Section B, vol. 1. Boca Raton, Florida, CRC Press, 1981.

Johnson, B. K., A. Gichoco, G. Gitan, N. Patel, G. Ademba, R. Kirui, R. B. Highton, and D. H. Smith. Recovery of O'nyong-nyong virus from *Anopheles funestus* in Western Kenya. *Trans R Soc Trop Med Hyg* 75:239-241, 1981.

Kaschula, V. R., A. F. Van Dellen, and V. de Vosi. Some infectious diseases of wild vervet monkeys (*Cercopithecus aetiops pygerythrus*) in South Africa. *J S Afr Vet Med Assoc* 49:223-227, 1978.

Kennedy, A. C., J. Fleming, and L. Solomon. Chikungunya viral arthropathy: a clinical description. *J Rheumatol* 7:231-236, 1980.

McIntosh, B. M. Antibody against Chikungunya virus in wild primates in Southern Africa. *S Afr J Med Sci* 35:65-74, 1970.

Pavri, K. Disappearance of Chikungunya virus from India and South East Asia. *Trans R Soc Trop Med Hyg* 80:491, 1986.

Tesh, R. B., C. Gajdusek, R. M. Garruto, J. H. Cross, and L. Rosen. The distribution and prevalence of group A arbovirus neutralizing antibodies among human populations in southeast Asia and the Pacific Islands. *Am J Trop Med Hyg* 24:664-675, 1975.

Tesh, R. B. Arthritides caused by mosquito-borne viruses. *Ann Rev Med* 33:31-40, 1982.

Tomori, O., A. Fagbami, and A. Fabiyi. The 1974 epidemic of Chikungunya fever in children in Ibadan. *Trop Geogr Med* 27:413-417, 1975.

White, A., S. Berman, and J. P. Lowenthal. Comparative immunogenicities of Chikungunya vaccines propagated in monkey kidney monolayers and chick embryo suspension cultures. *Appl Microbiol* 23:951-952, 1972.

COLORADO TICK FEVER

(066.1)

Synonym: Mountain fever.

Etiology: RNA genome virus of the genus *Orbivirus*, family Reoviridae.

Geographic Distribution: The distribution of the virus corresponds to the dispersion of its vector, *Dermacentor andersoni*, in the mountainous portion of 11 states in the USA and the provinces of Alberta and British Columbia in Canada.

Occurrence: In the United States 200 to 300 human cases occur annually. The infection always originates in endemic areas and affects both residents and visitors to those localities. The states with the greatest number of patients (more than 80% of cases) are Colorado and Wyoming. From 1970 to 1977 there was an annual average of 174 cases in Colorado (McLean *et al.*, 1981).

No human cases have been recorded in Canada; the virus has been isolated from the vector only (Artsob and Spence, 1979).

The disease occurs in spring and early summer.

The Disease in Man: The incubation period is from 3 to 6 days. In all cases, the patient has been exposed to ticks. Since the bite of *Dermacentor* is not painful, the patient often does not realize that a tick has attached itself, and a search is necessary in order to find it. The onset of the disease is sudden, with fever, chills, cephalalgia, retro-ocular pain, and severe muscular pains. Just over 10% of patients develop a skin rash. The disease is often biphasic and similar to dengue in its symptomatology. The symptoms last about 2 days, disappear for a few days, and then reappear for a slightly longer period than in the first attack. On the fourth or fifth day of fever, leukopenia is seen, with an increase in immature leukocytic forms. The symptoms may worsen progressively in three or four stages. The disease is benign in adults, but in approximately 15% of children under 10 years of age hemorrhagic complications and encephalitis occur. The fatality rate is very low.

The Disease in Animals: The virus has been isolated from various species of squirrels and other rodents and small mammals. Experimental inoculation causes prolonged viremia without clinical symptomatology.

Source of Infection and Mode of Transmission (Figure 34): The disease occurs in spring and early summer during the period of greatest activity of *Dermacentor*. The main reservoirs of the virus are several species of sciurids. A study carried out in Rocky Mountain National Park determined that the most important hosts were the species *Eutamias minimus* and *Spermophilus* (*Citellus*) *lateralis*, which serve as the main source of the virus for the immature stages (larva and nymph) of the main vector, *D. andersoni*. The prevalence of infection in the rodents was constant from April to July, and 5 to 6% had viremia (Bowen *et al.*, 1981). Viremia in these squirrels lasts from 15 to 20 days, with sufficiently high titers to infect the vector. The infection also occurs in other rodent species, but they do not play an important role in maintaining the virus.

The main vector is the tick *D. andersoni*, in which the disease is transmitted from one developmental stage to the next, but not transovarially. The virus is maintained

Figure 34. Colorado tick fever. Virus cycle.

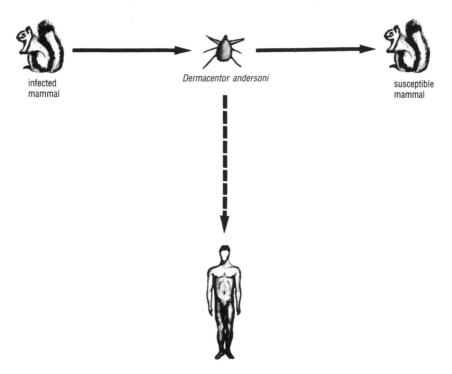

infected mammal

Dermacentor andersoni

susceptible mammal

during winter by nymphs of *D. andersoni*, which feed on and infect small rodents when spring arrives. Experimental studies on the ground squirrel *S. lateralis* indicate that the virus can survive in hibernating rodents (Emmons, 1966); thus the virus may make use of two overwintering mechanisms: persistence in vector nymphs and in the hibernating host.

The infection has been found in other species of ticks, but their role in the ecology of the virus is not clear yet. In areas not infested by *D. andersoni* the virus can circulate among hosts and vectors different from those in endemic areas.

The virus (or a very similar one) has been isolated in California from a jackrabbit (*Lepus californicus*) and a gray squirrel (*Sciurus griseus*) outside the endemic area and in the absence of *D. andersoni* (Lane *et al.*, 1982). Likewise, antibodies against the virus have been found in Ontario, Canada, in a wild hare (*Lepus americanus*), which suggests the circulation of the agent in nature in the eastern part of that country. Nevertheless, no human cases of the disease have been confirmed outside the range of *D. andersoni*.

Man is infected by the bite of adult *D. andersoni* ticks. In certain enzootic areas, at approximately 1,300 meters elevation, infection rates between 14 and 40% have been found in this tick species in the springtime. Viremia in man is very prolonged (up to 110 days after the onset of the disease). A case of transmission between humans as a result of blood transfusion has occurred (Centers for Disease Control of the USA, 1975).

Diagnosis: Clinical diagnosis can be confirmed by isolating the virus from the patient's blood. Best results are obtained by combining the inoculation of blood into suckling mice or hamsters with the immunofluorescence test on the patient's red blood cells.

Diagnosis can also be carried out by means of neutralization, indirect immunofluorescence, and complement fixation tests on serum samples obtained during the acute and convalescent phases to demonstrate an increase in the antibody titer. A fourfold or greater increase in the titer is significant.

Control: Individual prevention measures consist of avoiding tick habitats or using protective clothing or repellents when in such places; examining the body for ticks and removing them before they become attached; or, if a tick is attached, applying an irritant such as tincture of iodine or acetone and removing the arthropod by inserting a needle between the mouth parts.

Bibliography

Andrewes, C., and H. G. Pereira. *Viruses of Vertebrates*, 3rd ed. Baltimore, Maryland, Williams and Wilkins, 1975.

Artsob, H., and L. Spence. Arboviruses in Canada. *In*: Kurstak, E. (Ed.), *Arctic and Tropical Arboviruses*. New York, Academic Press, 1979.

American Public Health Association. *Control of Communicable Diseases in Man*, 14th ed. (Ed. by A. S. Benenson). Washington, D.C., APHA, 1985.

Bowen, G. S., R.G. McLean, R. B. Shriner, D. B. Francy, K. S. Pokorný, J. M. Trimble, R. A. Bolin, A. M. Barnes, C. H. Calisher, and D. J. Muth. The ecology of Colorado tick fever in Rocky Mountain National Park in 1974. II. Infection in small mammals. *Am J Trop Med Hyg* 30:490-496, 1981.

Casals, J., and D. H. Clarke. Arboviruses other than groups A and B. *In*: Horsfall, F. L., and I. Tamm (Eds.), *Viral and Rickettsial Infections of Man*, 4th ed. Philadelphia, Lippincott, 1965.

Centers for Disease Control of the USA. *International Catalogue of Arboviruses*, 2nd ed. (Ed. by T. O. Berge). Atlanta, Georgia, 1975. (DHEW Publ. CDC 75-8301.).

Centers for Disease Control of the USA. Colorado tick fever—Maryland. *Morb Mortal Wkly Rep* 24:219, 1975.

Centers for Disease Control of the USA. Transmission of Colorado tick fever virus by blood transfusion—Montana. *Morb Mortal Wkly Rep* 24:422, 1975.

Downs, W. G. Arboviruses. *In*: Evans, A. S. (Ed.), *Viral Infections of Humans, Epidemiology and Control*. New York, Plenum, 1976.

Emmons, R. W. Colorado tick fever: prolonged viremia in hibernating *Citellus lateralis*. *Am J Trop Med Hyg* 15:428-433, 1966.

Florio, L. Colorado tick fever. *In*: Beeson, P. B., W. McDermott, and J. B. Wyngaarden (Eds.), *Cecil Textbook of Medicine*, 15th ed. Philadelphia, Saunders, 1979.

Lane, R. S., R. W. Emmons, V. Devlin, D. V. Dondero, and B. C. Nelson. Survey for evidence of Colorado tick fever virus outside of the known endemic area in California. *Am J Trop Med Hyg* 31:837-843, 1982.

McLean, R. G., D. B. Francy, G. S. Bowen, R. E. Bailey, C. H. Calisher, and A. M. Barnes. The ecology of Colorado tick fever in Rocky Mountain National Park in 1974. I. Objectives, study design, and summary of principal findings. *Am J Trop Med Hyg* 30:483-489, 1981.

CONTAGIOUS ECTHYMA

(051.2)

Synonyms: Contagious pustular dermatitis, contagious pustular stomatitis, orf.

Etiology: DNA virus of the genus *Parapoxvirus* (Poxviridae family), which also includes the viruses causing milker's nodule (pseudocowpox) and bovine papular stomatitis.

Geographic Distribution: Occurs in all sheep-raising countries.

Occurrence in Man: Rare. In New Zealand, a country with a large sheep-raising industry, an increase in human cases has been noted. Only two cases were recorded in 1975, while the number rose to 143 in 1979, primarily affecting packinghouse workers (Robinson and Balassu, 1981).

Occurrence in Animals: The disease occurs in sheep, goats, alpacas, camels, and sometimes in dogs. There are enzootic areas throughout the world in which the disease appears annually on ranches with a history of infection. The disease has also been detected in several wild species.

A study was carried out in New Zealand to determine the rate of infection among lambs slaughtered at two packinghouses. Of 6,300,000 lambs killed in the course of 3 years, 0.5% had contagious ecthyma lesions, with a peak of 2.2% in the early summer. By extrapolation of the results, it is estimated that there would be 1,250,000 lambs with lesions per year in the country's slaughterhouses (Robinson, 1983).

The Disease in Man: It occurs in persons (herders, veterinarians, butchers, shearers) in close contact with sick animals. The incubation period is from 3 to 7 days. The lesion is usually localized on a finger, hand, or other exposed part of the body that has been in contact with the infecting material. A papular lesion appears at the penetration site of the virus. This lesion turns into a vesicle or pustule that may be accompanied by axillary adenopathy. If no secondary infection occurs, the lesion heals in 2 to 4 weeks. The scab falls off and leaves no scar. Occasionally, a generalized vesiculopapular eruption with pronounced pruritus may develop. Although rare, ocular lesions can also result.

The Disease in Animals: Sheep and goats of any age are susceptible, but the disease is seen primarily in animals under 1 year old since adult animals on infected ranches are generally immune as a result of previous exposure. The incubation period lasts 2 to 3 days. The lesions pass through papular, vesicular, and pustular stages. After about 11 days, thick brown scabs begin to form and persist 1 or 2 weeks. The lesions are localized on the lips, mouth, nostrils, eyelids, and ears. If they are few, the animal does not suffer greatly, but if they are numerous and confluent, the intense pain interferes with eating. Lesions on the teats and udder can also be observed in ewes that are nursing infected lambs.

Morbidity can be very high, but mortality is low and is generally due to complications from secondary infections. One important complication is myiasis caused by larvae of the fly *Cochliomyia hominivorax*.

Source of Infection and Mode of Transmission (Figure 35): The natural hosts of the virus are sheep and goats. During an outbreak the disease may be transmitted by direct contact or indirectly by contaminated objects and installations. The virus is resistant to desiccation and survives in the scabs for many months. The seasonal recurrence of outbreaks, at the time of year when there are susceptible young animals, can result from contamination of pasture with scabs and from contact with infected animals (those with a latent infection, according to some investigators). Rough pasture may injure the epithelium of the mouth, facilitating penetration of the virus and infection.

Man is infected accidentally by contact with animals with contagious ecthyma lesions, and transmission occurs through abrasions or other broken skin. For slaughterhouse workers, another possible source of infection is sheep wool, on which the virus can persist for approximately 1 month after the lesions have disappeared (Robinson, 1983). Personnel who vaccinate lambs with live vaccine are also exposed to the infection.

Figure 35. Contagious ecthyma. Transmission cycle.

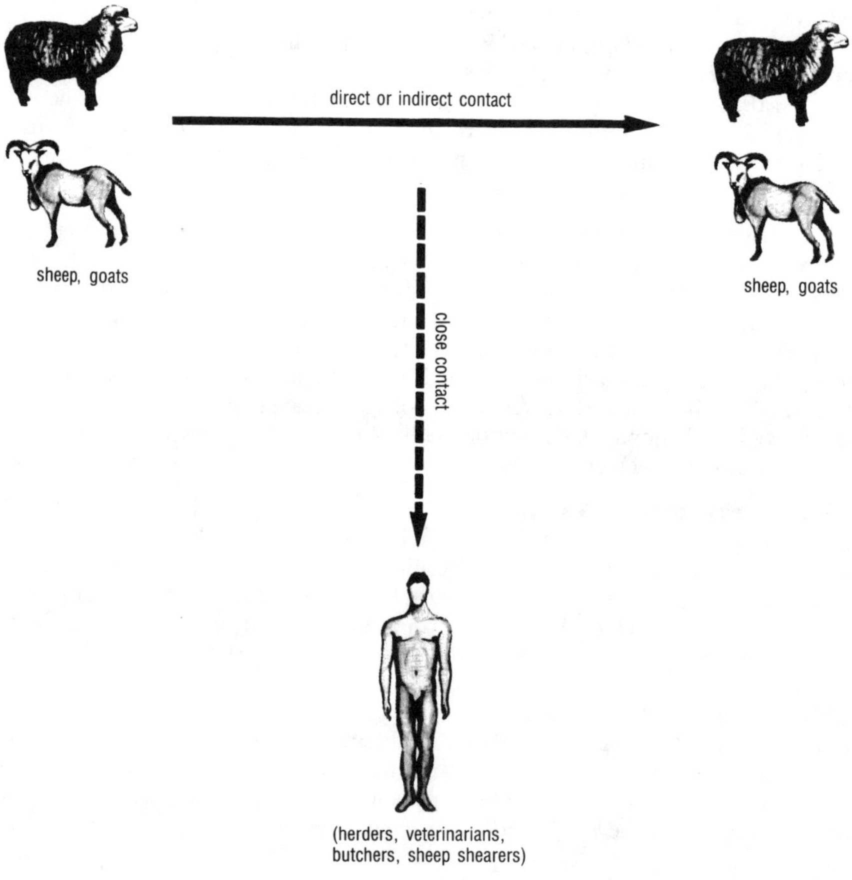

sheep, goats

direct or indirect contact

sheep, goats

close contact

(herders, veterinarians, butchers, sheep shearers)

Role of Animals in the Epidemiology of the Disease: Contagious ecthyma is a zoonosis of low incidence in man.

Diagnosis: Clinical symptomatology in sheep and goats is usually sufficient to establish the diagnosis. In differential diagnosis, sheep-pox (with intense systemic reaction) and ulcerative dermatosis (with ulcers and scabs on the skin of the face, feet, and genital organs) should be taken into account.

In man, laboratory confirmation is important and consists of the following. a) the complement fixation test to show the presence of the viral antigen (using vesicular fluid or a suspension of scabs) or to demonstrate the presence of antibodies (using sera), and b) isolation of the virus in a cell culture (embryonic sheep kidney) and use of the immunofluorescence test. Other tests that are utilized are immunodiffusion in agar gel, virus neutralization, and capillary agglutination.

Control: Control is accomplished by vaccination of lambs on infected farms. The most commonly used vaccine is a suspension of pulverized virulent scabs in a glycerinated solution, and therefore application of such a vaccine should be restricted to flocks with a history of infection. Recent observations in Great Britain indicate that vaccination can be carried out in lambs 1 to 2 days old, the vaccine being applied by scarification in the axilla. A great drawback of the vaccines currently in use is that they perpetuate the infection in the environment (Robinson and Balassu, 1981). Also, vaccination failures can occur and their cause is not well understood (Buddle *et al.*, 1984). Recently, an attenuated cell culture vaccine has been developed in Germany. It is administered subcutaneously and, according to its authors (Mayr *et al.*, 1981), has given good results in laboratory and field tests.

Prevention of the infection in man consists of protecting skin wounds when working with sick animals and using gloves when vaccinating sheep.

Bibliography

Buddle, B. M., R. W. Dellers, and G. G. Schurig. Contagious ecthyma virus-vaccination failures. *Am J Vet Res* 45:263-266, 1984.

Deeking, F. Contagious pustular dermatitis. *In*: Van der Hoeden, J. (Ed.), *Zoonoses*. Amsterdam, Netherlands, Elsevier, 1964.

Ericson, G. A., E. A. Carbrey, and G. A Gustafson. Generalized contagious ecthyma in a sheep rancher. Diagnostic considerations. *J Am Vet Med Assoc* 166:262-263, 1975.

Hanson, L. E. Poxviruses. *In*: Hubbert, W. T., W. F. McCulloch, and P. R. Schnurrenberger (Eds.), *Diseases Transmitted from Animals to Man*, 6th ed. Springfield, Illinois, Thomas, 1975.

Jensen, R. *Diseases of Sheep*. Philadelphia, Lea and Febiger, 1974.

Kerry, J. B., and D. G. Powell. The vaccination of young lambs against contagious pustular dermatitis. *Vet Rec* 88:671-672, 1971.

Mayr, A., M. Herlyn, H. Mahnel, A. Danco, A. Zach, and H. Bostedt. Bekampfung des Ecthyma contagiosum (Pustulardermatitis) der Schafe mit einem neuen Parenteral-Zellkultur-Lebendimpfstoff. *Zentralbl Veterinarmed [B]* 28:535-552, 1981.

Moore, R. M., Jr. Human orf in the United States, 1972. *J Infect Dis* 127:731-732, 1973.

Robinson, A. J. Prevalence of contagious pustular dermatitis (orf) in six million lambs at slaughter: a three year study. *NZ Vet J* 31:161-163, 1983.

Robinson, A. J., and T. C. Balassu. Contagious pustular dermatitis (orf). *Vet Bull* 51:771-782, 1981.

COWPOX

(051.0)

Synonym: Natural cowpox (as distinguished from the disease produced by the vaccinia virus).

Etiology: DNA genome virus, belonging to the genus *Orthopoxvirus*, family Poxviridae. This same genus includes, among others, the smallpox (variola), vaccinia, monkeypox, and whitepox viruses. Antigenically, the agent is closely related to the vaccinia virus, from which it can be distinguished by differentiated complement fixation, agar gel diffusion, and antibody absorption tests. The virus does not cause development of pustules in the chorioallantoic membrane when incubated above 40°C. Viruses very similar to cowpox virus have been isolated recently from zoo animals (Moscow, Berlin, London); they can be distinguished from each other only by a combination of biological tests (Baxby *et al.*, 1979).

Geographic Distribution: Cowpox (CP) virus has been isolated only in Great Britain and some western European countries. The Americas, Australia, and New Zealand are probably free of the disease (Odend'hal, 1983).

Occurrence: Little information is available on the frequency of the disease. CP is recognized only when many cases show up in bovines or when the disease occurs in man. Serologic studies carried out in Great Britain have confirmed that the disease is not enzootic among bovines there, as was previously believed (low titers of antibodies were found in only seven of 1,076 sera examined). CP virus is isolated once or twice a year in Great Britain. It appears to be more frequent in the Netherlands; 17 isolations were obtained in one year from 36 livestock properties in Friesland, which might indicate that CP is enzootic in that area (Baxby, 1977; Baxby and Osborne, 1979).

CP in man is rare in Great Britain and is estimated at one or two cases a year.

Outbreaks caused by a virus related to CP occurred among felines and insectivores in a zoo in Moscow in 1973 and 1974. Concurrently, a female zoo employee became ill (Marennikova *et al.*, 1977). The outbreaks originated from white rats used to feed the wild cats and pumas. Serologic investigations confirmed that 42% of these rats had antibodies against the virus. At the same time, two pox outbreaks produced by a virus related to CP occurred in a colony of white rats; the fatality rate was 30%. Two persons tending the colony developed a cutaneous eruption on their hands, shoulders, knees, and head (Marennikova *et al.*, 1978). An identical virus was isolated in Turkmenistan from wild rodents (*Rhombomys opimus* and *Citellus fulvus*). Viruses similar to CP have also been isolated from zoo or circus animals in the Netherlands, West Germany (elephant pox), and Great Britain (Baxby *et al.*, 1982). In the elephant pox episode in West Germany, several cases of human infection occurred. In recent years, domestic cats have been found affected by pox due to a virus similar to CP (Hoare *et al.*, 1984).

The Disease in Man and Cattle: In bovines the disease begins with mild fever, after an incubation period of 3 to 6 days. Papules that progress to vesicles and then to pustules are observed on the teats. Upon breaking, the pustules form red scabs which, in turn, may leave ulcerations that can take a month to heal (Tripathy *et al.*, 1981).

In man, lesions are found on the hands and sometimes on the face and arms. Most cases present fever, local edema, and lymphadenitis. Human disease is relatively severe and generally does not go unnoticed.

The outbreaks caused by viruses similar to CP virus in zoos in Moscow and Great Britain included two clinical forms: a fulminant pulmonary form without cutaneous lesions, and a dermal form with prolonged eruption. Many animals died as a consequence of the disease (Marennikova *et al.*, 1977; Baxby *et al.*, 1982). The disease in domestic cats is characterized by scabby skin lesions or erythematous papules 5 to 7 mm in diameter, distributed over the entire body. In some cases signs of respiratory difficulty are observed. Although most cats recover from the disease, some die (Hoare *et al.*, 1984).

Source of Infection and Mode of Transmission: In recent years it has been confirmed that the infection is not enzootic among bovines in Great Britain and that human cases have occurred without contact with cattle. In view of this information, it has been suggested that bovines acquire the infection from an unknown animal source, perhaps rodents, and that man becomes infected from the same animal reservoir or from sick bovines. The multiple bovine cases observed in Friesland, the Netherlands, are still unexplained; it is possible that the cows were in close contact with the unknown animal reservoir (Baxby, 1977).

In cats, the original lesion is often observed around a bite, which suggests that they could acquire the infection from an animal source while hunting.

The source of infection for zoo or circus animals in several pox outbreaks due to viruses related to CP virus has not been discovered; however, the origin of the two outbreaks in the Moscow zoo was white rats used to feed the wild cats and pumas. As for the several clinical human cases that occurred in Moscow and other outbreaks, they were presumably due to contact with sick animals. Isolation from rodents of viruses related to the CP and whitepox viruses suggests that these animals could be a reservoir for those viruses (Marennikova, 1979).

Diagnosis: The virus can be isolated in various tissue culture and chick embryo systems. Cowpox virus is distinguishable from vaccinia virus by serologic tests (see Etiology). The appearance and histology of focal lesions in the chorioallantoic membrane and on rabbit skin facilitates differential diagnosis. A combination of biological tests is required to distinguish CP virus from other similar ones (Baxby *et al.*, 1979).

Control: Current knowledge does not allow the establishment of preventive measures.

Bibliography

Andrewes, C. H., and H. G. Pereira. *Viruses of Vertebrates*, 3rd ed. Baltimore, Maryland, Williams and Wilkins, 1972.

Andrewes, C. H., and J. R. Walton. Viral and bacterial zoonoses. *In*: Brander, G. C. (Ed.), *Animal and Human Health*. London, Baillière Tindall, 1977.

Baxby, D. Poxvirus hosts and reservoirs. *Arch Viol* 55:169-179, 1977.

Baxby, D., and A. D. Osborne. Antibody studies in natural bovine cowpox. *J Hyg (Camb)* 83:425-428, 1979.

Baxby, D., W. B. Shackleton, J. Wheeler, and A. Turner. Comparison of cowpox-like viruses isolated from European zoos. *Arch Virol* 61:337-340, 1979.

Baxby, D., D. G. Ashton, D. M. Jones, and L. R. Thomsett. Outbreak of cowpox in captive cheetahs: virological and epidemiological studies. *J Hyg (Camb)* 89:365-372, 1982.

Bruner, D. W., and J. H. Gillespie. *Hagan's Infectious Diseases of Domestic Animals*, 6th ed. Ithaca, New York, Cornell University Press, 1973.

Dekking, F. Cowpox and vaccinia. *In*: Van der Hoeden, J. (Ed.), *Zoonoses*. Amsterdam, Netherlands, Elsevier, 1964.

Downie, A. W. Poxvirus group. *In*: Horsfall, F. L., and I. Tamm (Eds.), *Viral and Rickettsial Infections of Man*, 4th ed. Philadelphia, Lippincott, 1965.

Food and Agriculture Organization of the United Nations/World Health Organization/International Office of Epizootics. *Animal Health Yearbook, 1971* and *1975*. Rome, FAO, 1972 and 1976.

Hoare, C. M., M. Bennet, R. M. Gaskell, and D. Baxby. Cowpox in cats. *Vet Rec* 14:22, 1984.

Marennikova, S. A., N. N. Maltseva, V. I. Korneeva, and N. M. Garanina. Outbreak of pox disease among carnivora (Felidae) and Edentata. *J Infect Dis* 135:358-366, 1977.

Marennikova, S. S., E. M. Shelukhina, and V. A. Fimina. Pox infection in white rats. *Lab Anim* 12:33-36, 1978.

Marennikova, S. S. Field and experimental studies of poxvirus infections in rodents. *Bull WHO* 57:461-464, 1979.

Odend'hal, S. *The Geographical Distribution of Animal Viral Diseases*. New York, Academic Press, 1983.

Tripathy, D. N., L. E. Hanson, and R. A. Crandell. Poxviruses of veterinary importance: diagnosis of infections. *In*: Kurstak, E., and C. Kurstak (Eds.), *Comparative Diagnosis of Viral Diseases*, vol. 3. New York, Academic Press, 1981.

CRIMEAN-CONGO HEMORRHAGIC FEVER

(065.0)

Synonyms: Central Asian hemorrhagic fever, Congo fever.

Etiology: RNA genome virus, genus *Nairovirus*, family Bunyaviridae. Epidemiologically, this virus belongs to the group of tick-borne hemorrhagic fever viruses, together with the Omsk hemorrhagic fever and Kyasanur jungle disease viruses.

Geographic Distribution: The virus has been isolated from the southern part of the European USSR, Bulgaria, Greece, several Soviet Republics in central Asia, and Pakistan; the African countries of Zaire, Kenya, Uganda, Nigeria, Senegal, Central African Republic, and Ethiopia; and, more recently, from Iran (Sureau *et al.*, 1980), Iraq (Tantawi *et al.*, 1980), South Africa (Swanepoel *et al.*, 1983), and

Mauritania (Saluzzo *et al.*, 1985). Seroepidemiologic studies on humans and animals indicate that the geographic distribution area is much wider and that enzootic foci exist with or without the occurrence of human cases. Antibodies against the virus have been found in Hungary and Yugoslavia in Europe (in the latter country there have been clinical cases during several years); Turkey, the United Arab Emirates, Afghanistan, and India in Asia; and Tanzania, Egypt (Hoogstraal, 1979), and Zimbabwe (Blackburn *et al.*, 1982) in Africa.

Occurrence in Man: Crimean-Congo hemorrhagic fever (CCHF) usually occurs as isolated cases. The distribution and incidence of cases are scattered, in space as well as time. In four areas of Eurasia a large number of cases occurred. During World War II, 92 to 200 cases were recorded in Crimea in 1944 and some 100 cases in 1945, in both military personnel and civilians. In Astrakhan, USSR, 104 cases with 18 deaths were reported between 1953 and 1963, with a peak of 44 cases during the last year; only one case occurred annually in the majority of the villages or agricultural cooperatives. In Rostov, on the Don River, 323 cases occurred from 1963 to 1969, with a peak of 131 cases in 1968 and 16% fatality. The greatest number of cases was recorded outside the USSR: 717 cases occurred in Bulgaria between 1953 and 1965, with 0.7% morbidity and 17% fatality. From 1968 to 1972 there were 121 confirmed cases in that country. Distribution was also sporadic. In 79% of the foci, the disease appeared only once (Hoogstraal, 1979).

Epidemic situations were always related to environmental modification, be it the effects of war as in Crimea or the widening of agricultural areas due to collectivization as in the USSR and Bulgaria. The incidence of cases parallels the population density of adult ticks of the complex *Hyalomma marginatum*: it is low at the start of spring, peaks in early summer, and declines and later disappears in early autumn.

Familial and nosocomial outbreaks—sometimes with numerous cases and high fatality rates—have been recorded in several Asian and European countries, arising from direct contact with the patient during the hemorrhagic period. In African countries cases have been less numerous.

Occurrence in Animals: The main natural hosts of the CCHF virus are hares and hedgehogs (hosts for immature ticks), and bovines, ovines, goats, equines, and swine (hosts for adult ticks). According to seroepidemiologic research, the rate of reactors varies greatly within endemic areas, depending on the region, season, and animal species. There are large periodic differences in the rate of infected animals related to the population dynamics of vector ticks. In general, the rate of animals with antibodies is null or low where human cases do not occur and high where the disease is recorded.

The Disease in Man: The period of intrinsic incubation, from tick bite to appearance of symptoms, lasts from 3 to 7 days. Onset of the disease is sudden, with high fever, chills, headache, vertigo, and diffuse myalgia. The fever lasts some 8 days and can be continuous or biphasic. Abdominal pain, nausea, vomiting, diarrhea, and bradycardia are frequent. Hyperemia of the face and neck and conjunctival congestion are common signs; leukopenia and thrombocytopenia are almost always present and proteinuria is common. Hemorrhages begin on the fourth day of illness; petechiae in the mouth and on the skin vary in frequency and intensity, with a distinct hemorrhagic purpura occurring in some patients. The most common hemorrhagic manifestations are epistaxis, gingival hemorrhage, hematuria, and hemorrhage of the gastric mucosa. Death is generally due to shock as a result of blood loss or to neurologic complications, pulmonary hemorrhages, or intercurrent infections. Almost a third of the patients suffer hepatomegaly and splenomegaly.

Convalescence is characterized by asthenia, headaches, general malaise, and sometimes neuritis and temporary alopecia.

The infection in man does not always follow the severe course described; mild febrile cases without hemorrhages and even asymptomatic cases also occur.

The Disease in Animals: Although viremia has been confirmed in different animal species, the infection is asymptomatic or causes a mild illness in bovines and ovines, as was confirmed by experimental inoculation. Newborn rodents may die as a consequence of infection, as has been observed in some experiments.

Source of Infection and Mode of Transmission: The virus has been isolated or confirmed by immunofluorescence in 19 tick species and subspecies in Eurasia and nine species in Africa. Most of these ticks belong to the genera *Hyalomma*, *Dermacentor*, *Rhipicephalus*, and *Boophilus*. Several species of *Hyalomma* have a prominent role as vectors and reservoirs. Most of the cases in Bulgaria and the USSR were transmitted by *Hyalomma m. marginatum*. The larva and nymph stages of this tick feed on hares, hedgehogs, and birds, while the adult tick feeds on large animals, both domestic and wild, and is easily attracted by man. Main vectors in each enzootic region are the tick species that predominate among domestic animals. CCHF epidemic situations are closely related to the abundance of one or another species of *Hyalomma* in different ecologic areas (Hoogstraal, 1979).

The survival mechanism of the virus during the rigorous winters of the USSR is based on transstadial and transovarial transmission in ticks, as has been confirmed in *Hyalomma m. marginatum*, *Rhipicephalus rossicus*, and *Dermacentor marginatus*. Domestic animals, hares (*Lepus europaeus* and *L. capensis*), hedgehogs (*Erinaceus albiventris* and *Hemiechinus auritus*), and possibly some other animals serve as amplifers of the virus and a food source for the ticks. Upon contracting the infection from the vectors, all these animals have viremia that lasts at least a week and serve, in turn, as a source of infection for uninfected ticks. High rates of serologic reactors have been found among mammals in enzootic areas. Birds do not become infected, but play an important role as a food source for immature ticks and as a means of dispersal of these vectors to distant places (Hoogstraal, 1979).

Human disease occurs in rural areas. Persons engaged in farming and livestock raising are the most exposed. Man acquires the infection by the bite of infected ticks. He can also become infected by crushing ticks with his hands, when the virus penetrates abraded skin. Likewise, man may become infected directly from viremic animals during their sacrifice and skinning as suggested by episodes in Kazakhstan and Uzbekistan in the USSR. Numerous cases, mostly fatal, have occurred by interhuman transmission to relatives and hospital personnel exposed to hemorrhages of CCHF patients (Hoogstraal, 1979).

Diagnosis: Diagnosis can be confirmed by isolation of virus from blood of patients in the acute phase of the disease or from autopsy materials, by means of intracerebral inoculation in newborn mice. Serologic diagnosis can be carried out using the complement fixation, neutralization in newborn mice, indirect hemagglutination inhibition, radial gel diffusion, and immunofluorescence tests. Most of these tests have low sensitivity. More recently, the ELISA test has been perfected, and the authors (Donets *et al.*, 1982) consider it more sensitive and specific as well as faster and more reproducible.

Control: Measures are similar to those recommended for other tick-borne infections. In Bulgaria and the USSR, an inactivated vaccine has been tried with promising results. Isolating the patient, especially one with hemorrhages, is important to avoid interhuman transmission. Blood excretions should be treated with heat or chlorinated disinfectants. Personnel in charge of patients must be provided with protective clothing.

Bibliography

Andrewes, C., and H. G. Pereira. *Viruses of Vertebrates*, 3rd ed. Baltimore, Maryland, Williams and Wilkins, 1972.

Blackburn, N. K., L. Searle, and P. Taylor. Viral haemorrhagic fever antibodies in Zimbabwe. *Trans R Soc Trop Med Hyg* 76:803-805, 1982.

Casals, J. Antigenic similarity between the virus causing Crimean hemorrhagic fever and Congo virus. *Proc Soc Exp Biol Med* 131:233-236, 1969.

Casals, J., H. Hoogstraal, K. M. Johnson, A. Shelokov, N. H. Wiebenga, and T. H. Work. A current appraisal of hemorrhagic fevers in the USSR. *Am J Trop Med Hyg* 15:751-764, 1966.

Casals, J., B. E. Henderson, H. Hoogstraal, K. M. Johnson, and A. Shelokov. A review of Soviet viral hemorrhagic fevers, 1969. *J Infect Dis* 122:437-453, 1970.

Casals, J., and G. H. Tignor. Neutralization and hemagglutination-inhibition tests with Crimean hemorrhagic fever-Congo virus. *Proc Soc Exp Biol Med* 145:960-966, 1974.

Centers for Disease Control of the USA. *International Catalogue of Arboviruses*, 2nd ed. Berge, T. O. (Ed.). Atlanta, Georgia, 1975 (DHEW Publ. CDC 75-8301.).

Donets, M. A., G. V. Rezapkin, A. P. Ivanov, and E. A. Tkachenk. Immunosorbent assays for diagnosis of Crimean-Congo hemorrhagic fever (CCHF). *Am J Trop Med Hyg* 31:156-162, 1982.

Hoogstraal, H. The epidemiology of tick-borne Crimean-Congo hemorrhagic fever in Asia, Europe and Africa. *J Med Entomol* 15:307-417, 1979.

Saluzzo, J. F., P. Aubry, J. McCormick, and J. P. Digoutte. Haemorrhagic fever caused by Crimean-Congo haemorrhagic fever virus in Mauritania. *Trans R Soc Trop Med Hyg* 79:268, 1985.

Sureau, P., J. N. Klein, J. Casals, J. P. Digoutte, J. J. Salaun, N. Piazak, and M. A. Calvo. Isolement des virus Thogoto, Wad Madani, Wanowrie et de la fièvre hemorrhagique de Crimée-Congo en Iran à partir de tiques d'animaux domestiques. *Ann Virol* (*Inst Pasteur*) 131E:185-200, 1980.

Swanepoel, R., J. K. Struthers, A. J. Shepherd, G. M. McGillivray, M. J. Nel, and P. G. Jupp. Crimean-Congo hemorrhagic fever in South Africa. *Am J Trop Med Hyg* 32:1407-1415, 1983.

Tantawi, H. H., M. I. Al-Moslih, N. Y. Al-Janabi *et al*. Crimean-Congo haemorrhagic fever virus in Iraq: isolation, identification and electron microscopy. *Acta Virol* 24:464-467, 1980.

Yen Yu-chen, Kong Ling-Xiong, Lee Ling, Zhang Yu-Qin, Li Feng, Cai Bao-Jian, and Gao Shou-yi. Characteristics of Crimean-Congo hemorrhagic fever virus (Xinjiang strain) in China. *Am J Trop Med Hyg* 34:1179-1182, 1985.

DENGUE
(POSSIBLE WILD CYCLE)

(061)

Etiology: RNA virus of the genus *Flavivirus* (formerly group B of the arboviruses) of the family Togaviridae. Four serotypes are known (1-4). Immunity against the homologous type is complete and prolonged, but for the heterologous types it is partial and of short duration.

Geographic Distribution: Tropical Asia, eastern and western Africa, Polynesia and Micronesia, Caribbean region, Central America, and northern South America.

Occurrence in Man: The disease appears in endemic (often undiagnosed) and epidemic forms. Four epidemics occurred in the Americas in the last two decades. The first epidemic, in 1963, was caused by dengue 3 and affected some Caribbean islands and Venezuela. A second one in 1969, caused by dengue 2, also affected some Caribbean islands and spread to Colombia. The third one, caused by dengue 1, started in 1977 in Jamaica, where it affected more than 60,000 people, and expanded to other Caribbean islands, Mexico, Central America, and Venezuela (Figueroa *et al.*, 1982). The fourth epidemic occurred in 1981 and was caused by dengue 4. It started in San Bartolomé (French Antilles) and spread to other Caribbean islands and Belize (Pan American Health Organization, 1982). Puerto Rico was seriously affected during all four epidemics. After the relatively high degree of dengue activity in 1981 and 1982, when the first dengue epidemic in 50 years occurred in Brazil, most countries reported only sporadic cases in 1983. Notwithstanding, Mexico, Colombia, and El Salvador had important localized outbreaks in 1983 (Pan American Health Organization, 1984).

A serologic study carried out in Honduras determined that the 1978-1980 epidemic there involved at least 134,000 cases. Some towns in that country, including the capital, had few or no cases, probably because of the low density of the vector, *Aedes aegypti* (Figueroa *et al.*, 1982). A high rate of reactors to serologic tests is found among the population of endemic regions of Asia and Africa. In a study carried out in four ecological areas of Nigeria to determine the prevalence and distribution of immunity to the dengue (DEN) virus, 45% of 1,816 persons were found to be immune to DEN-2 using the serum neutralization test; prevalence of immunity was higher in adults than in children and in urban than in rural inhabitants (Fagbami *et al.*, 1977). Similar rates can be found in tropical Asia.

Occurrence in Animals: Dengue is essentially a human disease transmitted by mosquitoes of the genus *Aedes*. However, there are indications that, besides the human cycle, a wild cycle might exist between nonhuman primates and mosquitoes (*Aedes* spp.).

In Malaysia, of 223 serum samples taken from monkeys in areas away from towns, 62.8% were positive to the serum neutralization test (Rudnick, 1966). Research carried out in jungle areas of Nigeria also suggests the possible existence of a wild cycle, independent of man (Monath *et al.*, 1974; Fagbami *et al.*, 1977).

The Disease in Man: In its common form, dengue is an acute and benign febrile disease. The incubation period (from the mosquito bite to the onset of clinical symptoms) lasts from 5 to 8 days. Onset is sudden, with fever, chills, cephalalgia, retro-ocular pain, photophobia, and muscle and joint pains. In addition, there is often nausea, vomiting, and a sore throat. A general erythema is common at the onset of the disease, and 3 or 4 days later a maculopapular or scarlatiniform rash may appear on the trunk and spread to other parts of the body. Lymph nodes enlarge and are palpable. Fever, which is sometimes diphasic, lasts from 5 to 7 days. Convalescence may take several weeks, with signs of fatigue and depression. Case fatality is very low (American Public Health Association, 1985; Tesh, 1982).

In tropical Asia a severe and often fatal form of the disease, hemorrhagic dengue (hemorrhagic fever), is seen. This form occurs mainly in children and can be caused by any of the four serotypes. The disease may start as common dengue, but hemorrhaging, circulatory insufficiency, hypotension, and shock syndrome appear after several days of fever.

In May 1981 in Cuba, there was an explosive outbreak of dengue hemorrhagic fever with cases of severe hemorrhage, shock, and death. At the end of the epidemic (October 1981), 344,203 cases had been reported; 9,203 were considered severe, 1,109 were very severe, and 159 deaths occurred among children and adults. Serologic studies and isolation of the virus suggest that serotype DEN-2 was the cause of the epidemic (Kourí et al., 1982; Guzmán et al., 1984).

The Disease in Animals: Experimental infection of nonhuman primates with the dengue virus is clinically inapparent.

Source of Infection and Mode of Transmission: The basic cycle develops between man and a mosquito of the genus *Aedes*. The source of infection for the mosquito is man during the viremic period, which can last 5 to 6 days. Upon feeding on the blood of a febrile patient, the mosquito ingests the virus, which multiplies and infects its salivary glands. After about 10 days, the mosquito can transmit the disease to other nonimmune people. The main vector is *Aedes aegypti*, a mosquito that breeds in containers in or near houses, is highly anthropophilic, and feeds in daylight. Outside the American continent, *A. albopictus* and several species of the *A. scutellaris* complex act as vectors. Dengue is an illness of the rainy season, when *A. aegypti* is most abundant, but in hyperendemic areas or areas in the tropics where precipitation is not markedly seasonal it can occur year-round.

The Caribbean epidemics described above (see Occurrence in Man) could only have occurred by infestation or reinfestation of *A. aegypti* in the countries of the region.

In August 1985 *A. albopictus* was discovered in Harris District, Houston, Texas. This was the first report of this vector's presence and establishment in the Americas (Centers for Disease Control, 1986). Since that time, the presence of *A. albopictus* has been recorded in 10 states in the United States and three states in Brazil (Pan American Health Organization, 1987).

Even though the dengue virus has not been isolated in nonhuman primates, which would be conclusive proof, considerable serological evidence exists (high neutralizing titers for dengue 1 and 2) for a wild cycle of the infection that has monkeys as its reservoir and is independent of the man-*Aedes*-man cycle. The vector could be *A. albopictus*, which is abundant in the jungle. It is generally accepted that dengue's origin is southeastern Asia and that *A. aegypti* is of African origin. If this is so, *A. albopictus*, native to Asia, would have a very old association with the dengue virus. A review of the information about both natural and experimental transmission of the DEN virus by *A. albopictus* proves without doubt this mosquito's efficacy as a vector for epidemic dengue and its hemorrhagic complications. Moreover, transovarial transmission of all four serotypes of dengue virus has been proven in *A. albopictus*. These facts, along with its great susceptibility, its extensive habitat, and the density of its hosts (mammals and birds), are evidence that this vector plays an important role in the maintenance of the dengue virus cycle and the survival of the virus in a geographic area during interepidemic periods. The occurrence of human cases in areas free of *A. aegypti* but where *A. albopictus* is found indicates that man could be an accidental host in this cycle (Rudnick, 1966). In the total epidemiologic framework, the existence of a wild cycle between monkeys and mosquitoes would be very important. The presence of *A. albopictus* in the Americas thus merits particular study of its public health impact, especially in Brazil.

Diagnosis: Laboratory diagnosis can be done by introducing blood from the febrile patient into tissue cultures or by intrathoracic inoculation of mosquitoes. Serologic tests (hemagglutination inhibition, complement fixation, serum neutralization) can be useful to verify seroconversion, but it is often difficult to interpret the results if the patient has previously been infected by another dengue serotype or another flavivirus.

Control: The prevention of epidemics primarily depends on the control and eradication of *A. aegypti*.

Bibliography

American Public Health Association. *Control of Communicable Diseases in Man*, 14th ed. (Ed. by A. S. Benenson). Washington, D.C., APHA, 1985.

Centers for Disease Control of the USA. Summary Report, Meeting of Consultants and Local and State Health Department Personnel on *Aedes albopictus* infestation, Harris County, Texas, March 12-14, 1986, USPHS/CDC, 1986.

Fagbami, A. H., T. P. Monath, and A. Fabiyi. Dengue virus infections in Nigeria: a survey for antibodies in monkeys and humans. *Trans R Soc Trop Med Hyg* 71:60-65, 1977.

Figueroa, M., R. Pereira, H. Gutiérrez, C. de Mejía, and N. Padilla. Dengue epidemic in Honduras, 1978-1980. *Bull Pan Am Health Organ* 16:130-137, 1982.

Guzmán, M. G., G. Kourí, L. Morier, M. Soler, and A. Fernández. Casos mortales de dengue hemorrágico en Cuba, 1981. *Bol Of Sanit Panam* 97(2):111-117, 1984.

Halstead, S. B. Dengue. *In*: Warren, K. S., and A. A. F. Mahmoud (Eds.), *Tropical and Geographical Medicine*. New York, McGraw-Hill Book Company, 1984.

Kourí, G., P. Más, M. G. Guzmán, M. Soler, A. Goyenechea, and L. Morier. Dengue hemorrágico en Cuba, 1981. Diagnóstico rápido del agente etiológico. *Bol Of Sanit Panam* 93(5):414-420, 1982.

Monath, T. P., V. H. Lee, D. C. Wilson, A. Fagbami, and O. Tomori. Arbovirus studies in Nupeko forest, a possible natural focus of yellow fever virus in Nigeria. Description of the area and serological survey of humans and other vertebrate hosts. *Trans R Soc Trop Med Hyg* 68:30-38, 1974.

Pan American Health Organization. Dengue 4 in the Americas. *Epidemiol Bull* 3:7, 1982.

Pan American Health Organization. Dengue in the Americas, 1983. *Epidemiol Bull* 5:1-3, 1984.

Pan American Health Organization. *XXII Pan American Sanitary Conference, 22-27 September 1986. Verbatim Records*. Washington, D.C., PAHO, 1987. (Official Document 209.)

Rudnick, A. Studies of the ecology of dengue in Malaysia. *Bull WHO* 35:78-79, 1966.

Shroyer, D. A. *Aedes albopictus* and arboviruses: a concise review of the literature. *J Am Mosq Control Assoc* 2:224-228, 1986.

Tesh, R. B. Dengue. *In*: Wyngaarden, J. B., and L. H. Smith (Eds.), *Cecil Textbook of Medicine*, 16th ed., vol. 2. Philadelphia, Saunders, 1982.

EASTERN EQUINE ENCEPHALITIS

(062.2)

Synonyms: Eastern equine encephalomyelitis, eastern encephalitis.

Etiology: RNA virus belonging to the genus *Alphavirus* (formerly group A of the arboviruses) of the family Togaviridae. The EEE virus is part of the complex of viruses transmitted by mosquitoes. Antigenic variants of the virus occur in nature, and use of the modified hemagglutination inhibition test has determined that the strains in North America, Jamaica, and the Dominican Republic differ from those in Panama, Trinidad and Tobago, and South America.

Geographic Distribution: The virus has been isolated in Canada (eastern), the United States (Gulf and Atlantic coasts), Mexico, Guatemala, Panama, Colombia, Venezuela, Trinidad and Tobago, Jamaica, Cuba, the Dominican Republic, Haiti, Guyana, Brazil, Argentina, and Peru. There are reports that the EEE virus has also been isolated in Czechoslovakia, Poland, the Soviet Union, Thailand, and the Philippines, but some doubts exist about the validity of these isolations. At any rate, no known epidemics have occurred outside the Americas.

The South American strain of the EEE virus has also been isolated from migratory birds in the southern United States, but there is no proof that infection cycles in the local bird and vector populations were started or that enzootic foci were established (Calisher *et al.*, 1981).

Occurrence in Man: Eastern equine encephalitis (EEE) is less common than western equine or St. Louis encephalitis, but it is more serious, causing high mortality.

From 1955 to 1978 only 136 clinical cases occurred in the United States. The largest epidemic outbreak on record took place in 1938 in Massachusetts, with 38 cases. The rate of incidence is low in the United States, and in Central and South America the disease is even rarer (or the cases are not recognized). This difference is attributed to the distinct habits of the vectors that transmit the virus outside the natural foci. While *Aedes sollicitans* in North America is anthropophilic and active in daylight, *Culex taeniopus*—the indicated vector in Panama, Trinidad and Tobago, and Brazil—is predominantly a jungle mosquito, is active at twilight, and does not go into houses; thus, its only role would be as enzootic vector. During the 1973 epizootic in Panama that affected 100 horses (with 40 deaths), no reactors were found among the 1,700 samples of human serum taken from areas of activity of the virus (Dietz *et al.*, 1980).

Epidemic outbreaks occur in late summer, concurrently with epizootics in horses. These epizootics generally begin 1 or 2 weeks before the appearance of human cases. The age groups most affected are persons under 15 and over 50 years of age. Subclinical infection is less common with EEE virus than with the western equine and St. Louis encephalitis viruses. In the Dominican Republic, 2 to 3 months after the epidemic of 1948-1949, antibodies were found in 32 of 827 persons examined. In New Jersey (USA), after the outbreak of 1959, 69 of 1,600 residents examined had antibodies. During this last outbreak it was estimated that there was one recognized case of encephalitis for every 16 to 32 clinically inapparent infections. In Europe and Asia, epidemics have not been recorded in man or in horses.

Occurrence in Animals: EEE manifests itself clinically in horses and pheasants. The true incidence of EEE will only be known when a surveillance system is instituted and an attempt is made to establish specific diagnoses for cases of encephalitis among horses. During the epidemiologic surveillance begun in the United States in 1971 as a result of the large epizootic of Venezuelan equine encephalitis, the EEE virus was isolated from 67 of 1,551 sick and healthy horses living on the same properties. Even though 1971 had not been considered an epizootic year for the EEE virus, these results showed that the disease occurs every year with a similar frequency (Maness and Calisher, 1981). Epizootics with high mortality have been recorded in horses in several areas, and the epizootics were sometimes but not always accompanied by outbreaks in the human population. According to data from the U.S. Department of Agriculture, from 1956 to 1970 there were 26,468 cases of encephalitis, but only 2,620 could be specifically diagnosed; of these, 605 cases were due to the EEE virus and 2,015 cases were due to western equine encephalitis. The most serious epizootic occurred among horses in Louisiana in 1947, with an estimated 11,927 deaths (Dietz *et al.*, 1980); this epizootic was unusually large. Information from Cuba and Panama is also of interest. Cuba recorded a series of extensive epizootics and smaller outbreaks in horses during 1914-1915 and in 1972. Mortality decreased steadily and subsequently disappeared, starting from 1971 when vaccination coverage reached 86.7%. By 1973, with an immunization coverage of 94%, there was practically no susceptible equine population. In Panama, the most recent outbreak occurred in 1973, coincident with a high density of *Culex taeniopus* mosquitoes. In a 3-week period (June-July) 40 equine deaths were recorded. The latest known outbreaks in Latin America occurred in 1976 in Venezuela and in 1978 in the Dominican Republic. In this last outbreak, it was estimated that some 3,600 horses were infected and the case fatality rate was on the order of 34 per 1,000. There were no human cases (Calisher *et al.*, 1981).

Outbreaks occur frequently on pheasant-breeding farms on the Atlantic coast of the United States.

The Disease in Man: EEE is characterized by high mortality (about 65% of clinical cases) and high frequency of permanent sequelae in patients who survive. The incubation period is from 7 to 10 days. Onset is sudden, with fever, cephalalgia, conjunctivitis, vomiting, and lethargy, and the disease progresses rapidly to delirium and coma. Neurologic signs consist primarily of neck stiffness, convulsions, spasticity of the muscles of the extremities, and altered reflexes. A biphasic course is common in children, beginning with fever, vomiting, and headaches for 1 or 2 days, followed by apparent recovery, and ending with fulminant encephalitis. In children under 5 years of age who survive the disease, neurologic sequelae such as mental retardation, convulsions, and paralysis are frequently observed.

The Disease in Animals: The clinical symptomatology in horses is similar to that of western equine encephalitis (see corresponding section), but EEE has a shorter course and is highly fatal. The disease has a biphasic febrile course. Fever starts 18 to 24 hours after infection and lasts about 1 day. A second febrile period begins 4 to 6 days after infection and lasts from 1 to 4 days. It is during the second febrile period that nervous symptoms appear. The animal suffers profound depression, stands with its legs apart, keeps its head close to the ground, and has flaccid lips; also common are diarrhea or constipation and substantial weight loss. Some animals are easily excited, walk in circles, and stumble over obstacles. Finally they fall and are unable to get up. Death occurs 5 to 10 days after infection (Walton, 1981). Mortality in horses showing signs of encephalitis is approximately 75 to 90%, and brain damage is common in surviving animals.

In the eastern United States, many outbreaks of EEE have occurred among pheasants, causing a fatality rate of 5 to 75%. The symptomatology in these birds consists of fever, depression, profuse diarrhea, voice changes, ataxia, tremors, partial or complete paralysis of one or both extremities, or involuntary circular movements. Some pheasants suffer paralytic effects for several weeks. Mortality from EEE has also been observed in other domestic fowl, such as Pekin ducks. The high virulence of the EEE virus in these species contrasts with the clinically inapparent infection or benign disease course in native wild fowl.

Source of Infection and Mode of Transmission (Figure 36): The basic cycle of the infection develops between wild fowl and mosquitoes. The EEE virus has been isolated from the blood of a large number of wild bird species, both resident and migratory. During interepidemic years, the infection rate is low in wild fowl, while it is very high during epidemic periods.

In the eastern United States the virus circulates permanently between birds—especially passeriforms—and mosquitoes in many natural foci in fresh-water swamps. The vector in this geographic region is *Culiseta melanura*, an ornithophilic mosquito. This vector has sometimes been observed to feed on horses, but very rarely feeds on man. A similar role is attributed to *C. morsitans* (Morris and Zimmerman, 1981). When the virus breaks out of its endemic natural foci into adjacent areas, a new cycle begins between local birds and mosquitoes. On the Atlantic coast of the United States, *Aedes sollicitans* is thought to play an important role as vector. This mosquito is common in coastal brackish marshes and feeds on birds as well as horses and man. *A. sollicitans* is believed to be the main vector during outbreaks in human and horse populations. A study on mosquito food sources in southeastern Massachusetts suggests that *Coquilletidia perturbans, Aedes canadensis*, and *A. vexans* could be the vectors of the virus for horses and man (Nasci and Edman, 1981).

Initial infection of pheasants follows the same pattern as in man or equines, but later the disease can spread from one bird to another through pecking and cannibalism, without the intervention of vectors.

In the tropical countries of the Americas, the main vectors appear to be *Culex nigripalpus, C. taeniopus, Aedes taeniorhynchus*, and probably some other species

Figure 36. Eastern equine encephalitis. Transmission cycle of the virus in the United States.

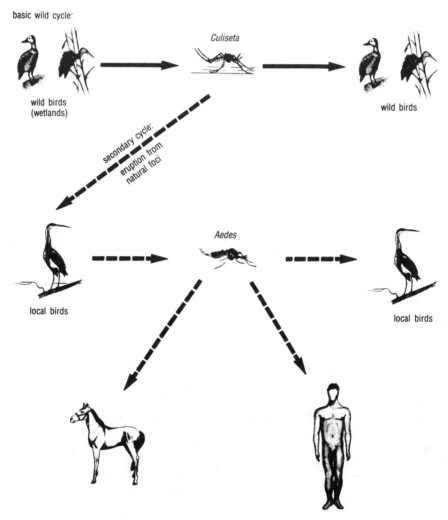

basic wild cycle:

Culiseta

wild birds
(wetlands)

wild birds

secondary cycle:
eruption from
natural foci

Aedes

local birds

local birds

of mosquitoes. Recently, during a study in the Venezuelan Guajira, multiple isolations of the virus were obtained from *C. panacossa* and *C. dunni* mosquitoes in an interepizootic period (Walder *et al.*, 1984). This fact would seem to indicate that such vectors play an important role in the maintenance of the virus in enzootic foci. These mosquitoes feed on marsupials and rodents and breed in swamps and jungles. Studies in the area around Belém in northeastern Brazil show that the EEE virus is enzootic in the rain forest, but it has not been possible to clarify the basic cycle of the virus.

Since the infection produces low-level viremia in man and horses, it is thought that these species do not play a role in maintaining the infection in nature. On one occasion the EEE virus was isolated from *C. melanura* larvae, which suggested the possibility of transovarial transmission, but later attempts to repeat such isolation were not successful. On the other hand, the virus has been isolated from rodents during the winter season, indicating that these animals might play a role in maintaining the agent during harsh weather. In the Venezuelan Guajira, hemagglutination-inhibiting antibodies were found in 7.4% of 54 opossums (*Didelphis marsupialis*) with titers of 1:20 or greater. It has been suggested that these animals could serve as natural hosts for the EEE virus (Walder *et al.*, 1984).

It has not been determined if outbreaks in the Caribbean are due to native enzootic foci or to the introduction of the virus by migratory birds from the United States. Autumn conditions in the Caribbean region, when birds migrate south from the United States, would favor circulation of the virus. However, outbreaks in Cuba, the Dominican Republic, and Jamaica, caused by the North American strain of the virus, have preceded or coincided with outbreaks of EEE in the southeastern United States (Calisher *et al.*, 1981).

Role of Animals in the Epidemiology of the Disease: Humans, horses, and pheasants are accidental hosts. The reservoir is wild fowl, among which the infection is propagated by mosquitoes.

Diagnosis: Specific diagnosis can be carried out by isolation of the virus from the brain of persons or horses who have died from the disease. In patients who survive, serologic diagnosis can be done based on an increase in the titer of serial blood samples. Since inapparent infections are not very frequent, serologic diagnosis in horses could be done using a single blood sample, especially when there is an outbreak of the disease in the area. The serologic tests available for diagnosis are hemagglutination inhibition, complement fixation, indirect immunofluorescence, and serum neutralization. Due to the rapid course of the disease, blood samples should be taken at short intervals.

Control: The only practical measure for individual prophylaxis for man lies in preventing mosquito bites through the use of protective clothing and repellents and the installation of mosquito netting and screens in dwellings. Control of specific vectors in the region may help to reduce the transmission of the disease.

To protect horses, monovalent as well as bivalent (eastern and western virus) inactivated vaccines are available, produced in chick embryos or, more recently, in tissue culture. A trivalent (EEE, WEE, and VEE) inactivated vaccine has also been developed. The study carried out during the epizootic outbreak in Panama questioned the efficacy and duration of protection that might be conferred by the North American strain of EEE against the South American strain. This aspect merits thorough study (Dietz *et al.*, 1980).

It should be taken into account that although vaccination protects horses, it does not modify the risk to which man is exposed.

Bibliography

Andrewes, C., and H. G. Pereira. *Viruses of Vertebrates*, 3rd ed. Baltimore, Maryland, Williams and Wilkins, 1972.

Barber, T. L., T. E. Walton, and K. J. Lewis. Efficacy of trivalent inactivated encephalomyelitis virus vaccine in horses. *Am J Vet Res* 39:621-625, 1978.

Calisher, C. H., E. Levy-Koenig, C. J. Mitchell, F. A. Cabrera, L. Cuevas, and J. E. Pearson. Encefalitis equina del este en la República Dominicana, 1978. *Bol Of Sanit Panam* 90:19-31, 1981.

Casals, J., and D. H. Clarke. Arboviruses; Group A. *In*: Horsfall, F. L., and I. Tamm (Eds.), *Viral and Rickettsial Infections of Man*, 4th ed. Philadelphia, Lippincott, 1965.

Centers for Disease Control of the USA. *Neurotropic Viral Diseases Surveillance. Annual Summary, 1972.* Atlanta, Georgia, 1974. (DHEW Publ. CDC 75-8252.)

Centers for Disease Control of the USA. *International Catalogue of Arboviruses*, 2nd ed. (Ed. by T. O. Berge). Atlanta, Georgia, 1975. (DHEW Publ. CDC 75-8301.)

Dietz, W. H., P. Galindo, and K. M. Johnson. Eastern equine encephalomyelitis in Panama: the epidemiology of the 1973 epizootic. *Am J Trop Med Hyg* 29:133-140, 1980.

Downs, W. G. Arboviruses. *In*: Evans, A. S. (Ed.), *Viral Infections of Humans. Epidemiology and Control*. New York, Plenum, 1976.

Faddoul, G. P., and G. W. Fellows. Clinical manifestations of eastern equine encephalomyelitis in pheasants. *Avian Dis* 9:530-535, 1965.

Maness, K. S., and C. H. Calisher. Eastern equine encephalitis in the United States, 1971; past and prologue. *Current Microbiol* 5:311-316, 1981.

McLean, R. G., G. Frier, G. L. Parham, D. B. Francy, T. P. Monath, E. G. Campos, A. Therrien, J. Kerschner, and C. H. Calisher. Investigations of the vertebrate hosts of eastern equine encephalitis during an epizootic in Michigan, 1980. *Am J Trop Med Hyg* 34:1190-1202, 1985.

Morris, C. D., and R. H. Zimmerman. Epizootiology of eastern equine encephalomyelitis virus in upstate New York. III. Population dynamics and vector potential of adult *Culiseta morsitans* (Diptera: Culicidae). *J Med Entomol* 18:313-316, 1981.

Nasci, R. S., and J. D. Edman. Blood feedings patterns of *Culiseta melanura* (Diptera: Culicidae) and associated sylvan mosquitoes in southeastern Massachusetts eastern equine encephalitis foci. *J Med Entomol* 18:493-500, 1981.

Ordóñez, J. V., W. F. Scherer, and R. W. Dickerman. Isolation of eastern encephalitis virus in Guatemala from sentinel hamsters exposed during 1968. *Bol Of Sanit Panam* 70:371-375, 1971.

Stamm, D. D. Arbovirus studies in birds in south Alabama, 1959-1960. *Am J Epidemiol* 87:127-137, 1968.

Theiler, M., and W. G. Downs. *The Arthropod-Borne Viruses of Vertebrates*. New Haven and London, Yale University Press, 1973.

Venezuelan Ministry of Health and Social Assistance. *Bol Epidemiol* No. 19, 1976.

Walder, R., O. M. Suárez, and C. H. Calisher. Arbovirus studies in the Guajira region of Venezuela: Activities of eastern equine encephalitis and Venezuelan equine encephalitis viruses during an interepizootic period. *Am J Trop Med Hyg* 33:669-707, 1984.

Walton, T. E. Venezuelan, eastern and western encephalomyelitis. *In*: Gibbs, E. P. J. (Ed.), *Virus Diseases of Food Animals*, vol. 2. New York, Academic Press, 1981.

Work, T. H. Eastern equine encephalomyelitis. *In*: Beeson, P. B., W. McDermott, and J. B. Wyngaarden (Eds.), *Cecil Textbook of Medicine*, 12th ed. Philadelphia and London, Saunders, 1967.

EBOLA DISEASE

(078.8)

Synonyms: Ebola hemorrhagic fever, African hemorrhagic fever (also includes Marburg disease).

Etiology: RNA virus (EBO), with similar morphology to the Marburg (MBG) virus but antigenically different. The taxonomy of the EBO and MBG viruses has been highly debated and different names have been proposed. A group of virologists from several countries (Kiley *et al.*, 1982) proposed incorporating both viruses into a new family, Filoviridae, genus *Filovirus*.

The EBO virus isolated in Sudan and Zaire belongs to two different biotypes, which differ in their biological, immunologic, genetic, and chemical properties (McCormick *et al.*, 1983).

Geographic Distribution and Occurrence: The virus has been isolated only in Sudan and Zaire, in central Africa. The disease first appeared in June 1976 in southwest Sudan, with 284 persons affected and a 53% fatality rate. This epidemic lasted until November of the same year. At the end of July 1976, a second epidemic began in northwest Zaire, with 318 cases and 88% fatality, also ending in November of the same year. The epidemic affected 55 out of approximately 250 villages located in the epidemic area of Zaire. The rate of attack was 10 to 14 per 1,000 inhabitants. The majority of the cases occurred in adults and very few cases were observed in children under 10 years old. Women were affected in 56% of the cases (Johnson, 1982).

Only one sporadic case occurred in Zaire in 1977; a second outbreak occurred in Sudan in August-September 1979, with 33 confirmed clinical cases and 22 deaths.

At first, the 1976 epidemics in Sudan and Zaire were believed to be epidemiologically related. However, the distance of 850 km between the two areas and the lack of communication between them indicated that the epidemics had independent origins. In addition, laboratory investigations demonstrated that two different biotypes of the virus (see Etiology) were at work in Sudan and Zaire, leaving no doubt that the two epidemics were independent of each other.

The fact that only one case of Ebola hemorrhagic fever was confirmed in 1977, in a locality situated 325 km to the west of the area where the 1976 epidemic occurred, indicates that the virus is endemic and perhaps enzootic in the Zaire River basin (Heymann *et al.*, 1980).

Several serologic studies using the indirect immunofluorescence (IIF) test have been carried out to determine the prevalence of the infection in the general population. In Sudan, 19% of the people in contact with patients had antibodies to the EBO virus, and in Zaire, 1% of persons outside the epidemic area had antibodies (International Commission, 1978). In several countries of central Africa, an average prevalence rate of 8% reactors has been found (Bouree and Bergmann, 1983). The specificity of the IIF test to titers of 1:4 to 1:64 was placed in doubt after "antibodies" at that level were found in four of 200 serum samples taken from Cuna Indians of San Blas Island, Panama, since it is unlikely that they were infected by EBO virus. In various studies in Africa, very high titers (1:512 to 1:1,024) were found in the general population (Ivanoff *et al.*, 1982; Knobloch *et al.*, 1982). This result could indicate recent infections as well as activity of the virus outside the areas where the epidemics occurred. It may likewise indicate that the virus is endemic or enzootic in several African countries and that the disease can be asymptomatic in man.

The Disease in Man: The clinical manifestations vary from a mild illness to a rapidly fatal disease. The incubation period lasts about a week and the disease has a sudden onset with fever and headache. A high proportion of patients experience thoracic pain, diarrhea, vomiting, dry and sore throat, and skin eruption and desquamation (52%). More than 90% of the patients who died and 48% of those who recovered had hemorrhages. In patients with hemorrhages, melena was the most common, but hematemesis, epistaxis, and hemorrhaging of other organs and tissues were also frequent. Convalescence was prolonged, sometimes requiring 2 months (World Health Organization, 1978).

Source of Infection and Mode of Transmission: The reservoir of the virus in nature is unknown. In Zaire and Sudan more than 1,000 animals, mostly mammals, were captured, but it was not possible to isolate the virus from them or demonstrate the presence of antibodies.

A high titer to the virus was found in 1980 in a domestic rabbit from the same region of Zaire where the 1977 sporadic case of the disease occurred (Johnson *et al.*, 1981). More recently, in Kenya, titers from 1:64 to 1:128 were found with the IIF test in three out of 184 baboons. Although experimental infection is always fatal in primates, the researchers (Johnson, B. K., *et al.*, 1982) believe the infection can occur subclinically under certain circumstances. Nevertheless, neither of these findings points to these animals as principal hosts for maintaining the virus in nature. Epidemiologic studies in Sudan and Zaire indicated that the majority of the patients acquired the infection through close contact with a previous acute case, and that the lack of sterilization of needles and syringes and other inappropriate practices caused a multiplication of cases in the hospital. It is important to note that each of the outbreaks originated from one or a few sporadic cases (whose source of infection is unknown) and then successive cases occurred by interhuman transmission. In the locality of Nzara, Sudan, where the first cases of the 1976 epidemic occurred, 14 of the 67 patients had no prior contact with a sick person. Nine of these 14 patients worked in a cotton factory, and it is possible that they may have introduced the infection to the human population of the area (World Health Organization, 1978).

The rate of 5 to 8% of the population with antibodies to the EBO virus that has been found in different countries of tropical Africa could indicate that the virus resides in the rain forest and that a mild or subclinical form of the infection is common when there is no secondary human transmission (Johnson, K. M., 1982). It is also possible that sporadic cases are not recognized due to the lack of adequate laboratories in the region.

Diagnosis: The virus can be isolated from the blood of gravely ill patients, but this procedure must be reserved exclusively for the few laboratories with P4 (biosecurity level 4) maximum security installations so that the personnel and the general population are not exposed to the infection.

The serologic test most often used is indirect immunofluorescence.

Control: Preventive measures should be principally aimed at avoiding interhuman transmission. The patient must be isolated and strict containment nursing practices must be instituted immediately; likewise, all samples for diagnosis, all patient excretions, and any other material that has been in contact with the patient should be considered infectious and be handled and decontaminated in an appropriate manner.

Personnel in charge of patient care must be properly trained, minimal in number, and provided with protective clothing (gowns, gloves, masks, glasses, caps, and overshoes) (Simpson, 1978).

Bibliography

Bouree, P., and J. F. Bergmann. Ebola virus infection in man: a serological and epidemiological survey in the Cameroons. *Am J Trop Med Hyg* 32:1465-1467, 1983.

Heymann, D. L., J. S. Weisfeld, P. A. Webb, K. M. Johnson, T. Cairns, and H. Berquist. Ebola hemorrhagic fever: Tandala, Zaire, 1977-1978. *J Infect Dis* 142:372-376, 1980.

International Commission. Ebola haemorrhagic fever in Zaire, 1976. *Bull WHO* 56:271-293, 1978.

Ivanoff, B., P. Duquesnoy, G. Languillat, J. F. Saluzzo, A. Georges, J. P. Gonzalez, and J. McCormick. Haemorrhagic fever in Gabon. I. Incidence of Lassa, Ebola and Marburg viruses in Haut-Ogooué. *Trans R Soc Trop Med Hyg* 76:719-720, 1982.

Johnson, B. K., L. G. Gitau, A. Gichogo, P. M. Tukei, J. G. Else, M. A. Suleman, R. Kimani, and P. D. Sayer. Marburg, Ebola and Rift Valley fever virus antibodies in East African primates. *Trans R Soc Trop Med Hyg* 76:307-310, 1982.

Johnson, K. M., C. L. Scribner, and J. B. McCormick. Ecology of Ebola virus: a first clue? *J Infect Dis* 143:749-751, 1981.

Johnson, K. M. African hemorrhagic fevers due to Marburg and Ebola viruses. *In*: Evans, A. S. (Ed.), *Viral Infections of Humans*, 2nd ed. New York and London, Plenum, 1982.

Kiley, M. P., E. T. W. Bowen, G. A. Eddy, M. Isaacson, K. M. Johnson, J. B. McCormick, F. A. Murphy, S. R. Pattyn, D. Peters, O. W. Prozesky, R. L. Regnery, D. I. H. Simpson, W. Slenczka, P. Sureau, G. van der Groen, P. A. Webb, and H. Wulff. Filoviridae: a taxonomic home for Marburg and Ebola viruses? *Intervirology* 18:24-32, 1982.

Knobloch, J., E. J. Albiez, and H. Schmitz. A serological survey on viral haemorrhagic fevers in Liberia. *Ann Virol (Inst Pasteur)* 133E:125-128, 1982.

McCormick, J. B., S. P. Bauer, I. H. Elliot, P. A. Webb, and K. M. Johnson. Biologic differences between strains of Ebola virus from Zaire and Sudan. *J Infect Dis* 147:264-267, 1983 (see also the three articles that follow).

Simpson, D. I. H. Infecciones por virus Marburgo y Ebola: guía para su diagnóstico, tratamiento y control. *Bol Of Sanit Panam* 85:54-72, 1978.

World Health Organization. Report of a WHO/International Study Team. Ebola haemorrhagic fever in Sudan, 1976. *Bull WHO* 56:247-270, 1978.

ENCEPHALOMYOCARDITIS

(049.9)

Synonyms: Columbia-SK disease, meningoencephalomyelitis, MM virus infection, three-day fever.

Etiology: RNA virus belonging to the genus *Cardiovirus* of the family Picornaviridae.

Geographic Distribution: The virus is ubiquitous and has been isolated in the United States, Cuba, Panama, Colombia, Brazil, Uganda, Great Britain, the Netherlands, Germany, India, Australia, and New Zealand.

Occurrence in Man: Rare. Besides sporadic cases, an epidemic outbreak was recorded in 1945-1946 among U.S. troops in the Philippines ("three-day fever").

The virus was isolated from children in Germany and the Netherlands and from a laboratory worker in Uganda. The diagnosis of "three-day fever" on a US military post in the Philippines was based on positive results to the neutralization test for EMC virus in 38.6% of 44 serum samples from convalescing soldiers.

In neutralization studies done on human serum samples from various regions of the world, antibodies to EMC virus were present in 1 to 33.9% of children and in 3.2 to 50.6% of adults. This fact indicates that infection by the virus is common and that most cases occur asymptomatically or are not recognized (Tesh, 1978).

Occurrence in Animals: The encephalomyocarditis (EMC) virus has multiple animal hosts and has been isolated from various species of rodents and monkeys, as well as from mongooses, raccoons, horses, cattle, swine, elephants, and several species of wild birds.

In the United States (Florida), Australia (New South Wales), Panama, Cuba, and New Zealand, epizootic outbreaks have occurred in swine, producing considerable mortality. Several countries have reported the disease and resultant death in non-human primates.

The Disease in Man: The symptomatology is variable. In 14 cases in children, fever and involvement of the central nervous system were observed, with lympho-cytic pleocytosis and, in some cases, paralysis. In the outbreak that occurred among the US troops in the Philippines, the disease was of sudden onset with intense cephalalgia and fever that lasted 2 to 3 days. Other symptoms frequently observed were pharyngitis, stiffness of the neck, and reflex disorders. Pleocytosis was constant. All the patients recovered without sequelae in 4 or 5 days.

In contrast to the disease in swine, myocarditis is not observed in man.

The Disease in Animals: Swine are the animals most affected. In this species the disease is characterized by sudden death without prodromal symptoms. It can also occur in a less acute form with variable clinical manifestations, such as fever, anorexia, and progressive paralysis. Most deaths in swine are seen in suckling pigs from 3 to 20 weeks of age. Anatomopathologic damage consists of myocardial lesions, hydrothorax, hydropericarditis, and ascites. The cardiac muscle is pale with small white or yellowish foci. Histopathologic examination reveals a degeneration of the myocardial fibers. Meningitis and some areas of nerve cell degeneration can also be found (Murnane, 1981). In a 1970 epizootic in Australia that affected 22 premises and caused the deaths of 277 pigs, the predominant lesion was focal or diffuse necrosis of the myocardium, especially pronounced in the right ventricle, which corresponded to the pale areas of the muscle observed in autopsy. In one of the outbreaks, 42 of 57 animals in the herd died. In outbreaks that occurred in Cuba, mortality varied from 6.6 to 47.7% in different production units (Lavicka *et al.*, cit. in Gómez *et al.*, 1982).

The disease in cattle and monkeys is likewise characterized by lesions of the myocardium, and mild encephalitis has also been observed in monkeys.

Experimentally infected mice and hamsters become ill with signs of encephalitis and die. Myocarditis is frequent.

Source of Infection and Mode of Transmission: The natural history of EMC virus has not yet been clarified. The agent has been isolated from a large number of species of mammals and wild birds. Rodents, especially the genus *Rattus*, have been considered the main reservoir of the virus, and it has been suggested that oral transmission is important in spreading the virus among them and to other vertebrates. This hypothesis is based on the high rate of seroreactors among rodents and the large number of virus isolations. However, these results may represent a statistical bias since no similar quantity of sampling has been carried out for other animal species. The findings of different researchers are also contradictory concerning intestinal transport of the virus by rodents and its transmission by contact. While the virus has been isolated from the feces of rodents, swine, and humans, transmission by contact has only been proven on a few occasions. In light of these facts, the capacity of rodents as reservoirs has been questioned, since they could be merely indicators of viral activity (Tesh and Wallace, 1978).

The virus was also isolated from several species of mosquitoes in Brazil, the United States, and Uganda, and from ticks in India. Nevertheless, there is no proof that the infection might be transmitted by arthropods.

The mode of transmission is probably oral, given the susceptibility of many species to infection via this route (Tesh and Wallace, 1978).

The quantity of virus in the tissues of rodents is much higher than in their fecal matter, and it is possible that swine become infected upon ingesting dead rodents. This theory would not explain outbreaks in which a large number of animals are affected, unless the feces of adult swine, who can become infected without becoming ill, served as a source of infection for suckling pigs. However, experiments carried out in Australia, in which suckling pigs 6 to 8 weeks old were infected, showed that the infection could be transmitted orally with high doses of the virus or with inoculated mice, but the infection was not transmitted to direct contacts, even when the feces remained in the cages (Littlejohns and Acland, 1975). Consequently, the animal reservoir that maintains the virus in nature, the sources of infection, and the circumstances producing outbreaks in swine or human cases are still not known with certainty. Because the virus is widespread in nature, it is unclear why outbreaks in swine are not more frequent or do not occur in other regions, and why more human cases do not occur.

Man contracts the infection only occasionally. Transmission possibly occurs by the oral route, but the source of infection is still unknown.

Diagnosis: The virus can be isolated by intracerebral inoculation of mice using serum or cerebrospinal fluid taken from patients at the beginning of the illness.

Serologic diagnosis can be made by neutralization and hemagglutination inhibition tests, using serum obtained during the acute and convalescent phases. Given the pantropic character of the virus, isolations can be made from a variety of organs (heart, spleen, brain, lungs, intestines, and lymph nodes) of domestic and wild animals that have died or have been destroyed. The virus has also been isolated from the excreta of swine and rats.

Control: In Florida, USA, where many outbreaks have been recognized in swine, the development of a vaccine for that species is considered a necessity.

The few human cases recorded and the knowledge gaps that exist concerning the epidemiology of the disease neither justify nor permit adoption of control measures for human protection.

Bibliography

Acland, H. M., and I. R. Littlejohns. Encephalomyocarditis virus infection of pigs. *Aust Vet J* 51:409-415, 1975.

Andrewes, C. *Viruses of Vertebrates*. Baltimore, Maryland, Williams and Wilkins, 1964.

Gainer, J. H. Encephalomyocarditis virus infections in Florida, 1960-1966. *J Am Vet Med Assoc* 151:421-425, 1967.

Gainer, J. H., J. R. Sandefur, and W. J. Bigler. High mortality in a swine herd infected with encephalomyocarditis virus; and accompanying epizootiological survey. *Cornell Vet* 58:31-47, 1968.

Gómez, L., M. Lorenzo, J. R. Ramos, M. J. Luya, D. Mayo, and T. Giral. Aislamiento del virus de la encefalomiocarditis en una cerda y su feto. *Rev Cuba Cienc Vet* 13:21-24, 1982.

Lennette, E. N., and N. J. Schmidt. *Diagnostic Procedures for Viral and Rickettsial Infections*, 4th ed. New York, American Public Health Association, 1969.

Links, I. J., R. J. Whittinston, D. J. Kennedy, A. Grewal, and A. J. Sharrock. An association between encephalomyocarditis virus infection and reproductive failure in pigs. *Aust Vet J* 63:150-152, 1986.

Littlejohns, I. R., and H. Acland. Encephalomyocarditis virus infection of pigs. 2. Experimental disease. *Aust Vet J* 51:416-422, 1975.

Murnane, T. G. Encephalomyocarditis. *In*: Beran, G. W. (Section Ed.), *CRC Handbook Series in Zoonoses*. Section B, vol. 2. Boca Raton, Florida, CRC Press, 1981.

Rhodes, A. J., and C. E. van Rooyen. *Textbook of Virology*. Baltimore, Maryland, Williams and Wilkins, 1962.

Tesh, R. B. The prevalence of encephalomyocarditis virus neutralizing antibodies among various human populations. *Am J Trop Med Hyg* 27:144-149, 1978.

Tesh, R. B., and G. D. Wallace. Observations on the natural history of encephalomyocarditis virus. *Am J Trop Med Hyg* 27:133-143, 1978.

Warren, J. Encephalomyocarditis viruses. *In*: Horsfall, F. L., and I. Tamm (Eds.), *Viral and Rickettsial Infections of Man*, 4th ed. Philadelphia, Lippincott, 1965.

EPIDEMIC POLYARTHRITIS

(066.3)

Synonym: Ross River fever.

Etiology: RNA genome River Ross (RR) virus, belonging to the genus *Alphavirus* (group A of the arboviruses), family Togaviridae. Antigenic differences have been found between the strains from northern Queensland and from the coast of New South Wales (Woodroofe *et al.*, 1977).

RR virus belongs to the Semliki complex, which also includes the Mayaro, Chikungunya, O'nyong-nyong, Bebaru, and Getah[1] viruses.

Geographic Distribution: The virus was known only in Australia, New Guinea, and the Solomon Islands until 1979, when the geographic area was extended to the South Pacific island groups of Fiji, American Samoa, New Caledonia, and Cook.

Occurrence: The disease occurs in Australia in sporadic and epidemic form. Epidemic outbreaks have been rather small and have occurred approximately every 3 years. The most extensive epidemic occurred in the Pacific islands, where the virus appeared for the first time in 1979 and the population was completely susceptible. There were an estimated 50,000 clinical cases in Fiji, and about 300,000 of 630,000 inhabitants of the islands were infected according to serologic studies (Miles and Mataika, 1981). About 13,500 of 31,000 inhabitants of American Samoa might have been affected (Tesh *et al.*, 1981). On Rarotonga, the most populous of the Cook Islands, the infection reached the majority of the inhabitants (Rosen *et al.*, 1981).

The disease occurs in summer and autumn. Epidemics usually occur after heavy rains, when the vector mosquitoes are most abundant.

In all areas where the virus is active, high rates of serologic reactors have been found in domestic and wild mammals.

The Disease in Man: The period of incubation is estimated at 3 to 7 or more days. The symptomatology can vary from a few days of fever (often no higher than 38°C) to classic polyarthritis. Arthritis does not occur in children, but it can be severe and persistent in older people. The disease preferentially attacks previously injured joints, but may affect any joint. Some patients suffer arthralgias for several months. Arthritis is the most prominent sign and the name "epidemic polyarthritis" derives from that fact. Another frequent symptom is cutaneous eruption, both in children and adults.

Polyarthritis is the clinical picture shared by this disease with diseases caused by four other alphaviruses: Mayaro, Chikungunya, O'nyong-nyong, and Sindbis (Tesh, 1982).

---

[1]Getah virus has been isolated from equines and swine. It caused an epizootic with manifestations of febrile exanthem and edema of the rear extremities in equines in Japan. The virus, mosquito-borne, is active in the USSR, Japan, Malaysia, Kampuchea, and the northern part of Australia. It has been isolated repeatedly from *Aedes vexans* and other mosquitoes.

The Disease in Animals: In Australia, the RR virus is thought to affect the central nervous system in equines and to also cause arthritis and muscular illness. Although there is certain serologic evidence in this regard, virologic confirmation is lacking (Gard *et al.*, 1977).

On the other hand, infections by RR virus occur subclinically in domestic animals, including (even if the few cases of disease in horses really were caused by this agent) most equines.

Source of Infection and Mode of Transmission: Infection is transmitted by mosquitoes. The main vectors in Australia are *Aedes vigilax* and *Culex annulirostris*, and in the Fiji, American Samoa, and Cook Islands the most probable vector is *A. polynesiensis*.

The reservoir of the virus has not yet been determined. The frequency with which antibodies are found in domestic and wild animals suggests that they serve as reservoir or amplifying host of the virus. In Australia, a probable and important role is assigned to large marsupials, and in New South Wales, to a certain local mouse species. Experimentally infected lambs showed a high-titer viremia and thus they may serve as amplifying hosts of the virus.

In Australia, the disease occurs predominantly in the rural environment. RR virus is enzootic and probably circulates among wild animals by means of vectors; man would be a casual host.

The epidemiologic differences between the disease in Australia and in the South Pacific islands are several. Epidemic polyarthritis in the latter area had an explosive character and affected urban populations. Another interesting feature is the ease of virus isolation from human patients in the islands. While in Australia the agent has been isolated only once (from a febrile child without arthritis—Doherty *et al.*, 1972), in the Cook Islands RR virus was isolated from almost half of 100 patients with arthritis who did not yet have antibodies (Rosen *et al.*, 1981). The causes of this difference have not been completely clarified, but it might be due to a biologic change in the virus, which would cause relatively high-titer viremia in man—as has been confirmed—and which could explain the intensity of the island epidemics by possible person-to-person transmission via vectors (Rosen *et al.*, 1981). The possibility that man served as an amplifying host of the virus is also suggested by the fact that in American Samoa the proportion of animals with antibodies was low compared with the proportion of the human population (Tesh *et al.*, 1981). Also of interest was evidence of transplacental transmission of the virus in the Fiji Islands, where IgM antibodies were detected in the umbilical cord blood of 11,368 babies born to mothers who were pregnant during the 1979 epidemic. Since IgM antibodies normally do not cross the placenta, this finding indicates the existence of an immune response to intrauterine infection. The babies had no signs of disease (Aaskov *et al.*, 1981).

As yet unresolved and unknown is how the virus was introduced to the Pacific islands. A viremic person or animal or infected mosquitoes could have brought the virus, but there is no evidence to this effect. It is also not known if the virus established itself in an enzootic form in these islands (Miles and Mataika, 1981).

Role of Animals in the Epidemiology of the Disease: The virus seems to circulate enzootically between wild animals and mosquitoes in Australia, while man could have been the main host during epidemics in the Pacific islands.

Diagnosis: During epidemics in the Pacific islands, the virus was isolated easily from the blood of patients in the acute phase of the disease before the appearance of antibodies. Under conditions in Australia, isolations were difficult.

Serologic confirmation of diagnosis is the most common procedure, using the hemagglutination inhibition and complement fixation tests with paired sera samples to demonstrate seroconversion.

Control: In cases of epidemics, measures should be taken against the vectors. For individual protection, repellents and other antimosquito measures can be used. No vaccines are available.

Bibliography

Aaskov, J. G., K. Nair, G. W. Lawrence, D. A. Dalglish, and M. Tucker. Evidence for transplacental transmission of Ross River virus in humans. *Med J Aust* 2:20-21, 1981.

Doherty, R. L., J. G. Carley, and J. C. Best. Isolation of Ross River virus from man. *Med J Aust* 1:1083-1084, 1972.

Gard, G. P., I. D. Marshall, K. H. Walker, H. M. Acland, and W. G. De Sarem. Association of Australian arboviruses with nervous disease in horses. *Aust Vet J* 53:61-66, 1977.

Miles, J. A. R., and J. U. Mataika. On the spread of Ross River virus through the islands of the Pacific. *In*: Fowler, M. E. (Ed.), *Wildlife Diseases of the Pacific Basin and Other Countries. Proceedings, 4th International Conference of the Wildlife Disease Association.* Sidney, Australia, August 25-28, 1981.

Rosen, L., D. J. Gubler, and P. H. Bennet. Epidemic polyarthritis (Ross River) virus infection in the Cook Islands. *Am J Trop Med Hyg* 30:1294-1302, 1981.

Tesh, R. B., R. G. McLean, D. A. Shroyer, C. H. Calisher, and L. Rosen. Ross River (Togaviridae: *Alphavirus*) infection (epidemic polyarthritis) in the American Samoa. *Trans R Soc Trop Med Hyg* 75:426-431, 1981.

Tesh, R. B. Undifferentiated Arboviral Fevers. *In*: Warren K. S., and A. A. F. Mahmoud (Eds.), *Tropical and Geographical Medicine*. New York, McGraw-Hill Book Co., 1984.

Tesh, R. B. Arthritides caused by mosquito-borne viruses. *Ann Rev Med* 33:31-40, 1982.

Woodroofe, G., I. D. Marshall, and W. P. Taylor. Antigenically distinct strains of Ross River virus from North Queensland and Coastal New South Wales. *Aust J Exp Biol Med Sci* 55:79-97, 1977.

FEVERS CAUSED BY GROUP C BUNYAVIRUSES

(066.3)

Etiology: The group is composed of RNA genome viruses of serogroup C of the genus *Bunyavirus*, family Bunyaviridae. Table 4 shows the classification of the group C viruses and their distribution.

A virus recently isolated in São Paulo, Brazil, from *Culex* (*Melanoconion*) *sacchettae* mosquitoes must be added to this group. The name Bruconha has been proposed for this virus (Calisher *et al.*, 1983).

Table 4. Classification of the group C bunyaviruses.

Complexes	Virus	Subtype	Distribution
Caraparu	Caraparu (CAR)	Ossa (OSSA)	Panama to Brazil
	Apeu (APEU)		Brazil
	Madrid (MAD)		Panama
Marituba	Marituba (MTB)	Murutucu (MUR)	
		Restan (RES)	Trinidad to Brazil
	Nepuyo (NEP)	Gumbo Limbo (GL)	Southern Florida (USA), Mexico, and Mesoamerica
Oriboca	Oriboca (ORI)		French Guiana to Brazil
	Itaqui (ITQ)		Brazil

Source: Centers for Disease Control of the USA. *International Catalogue of Arboviruses*, 2nd ed. Berge, T. O. (Ed.). Atlanta, Georgia, 1975. (DHEW Publ. CDC 75-8301). Table reproduced in Scherer *et al.*, 1983.

Geographic Distribution: The viruses of this group have been isolated only in the Americas and are native to tropical America. Most of the isolations have been made in Pará, Brazil. Human cases caused by various group C viruses have also been confirmed in Peru, French Guiana, Suriname, Trinidad, Panama, Central America, Mexico, and Florida, USA.

Occurrence: The *International Catalogue of Arboviruses* records 42 cases, mostly caused by Oriboca (14 cases) and Caraparu (10 cases) viruses. Inapparent infections are common, judging by a serologic study carried out in Belém, Brazil, where 102 out of 534 persons examined were positive to the hemagglutination inhibition test for one or more of the Oriboca, Murutucu, and Caraparu viruses.

The Disease in Man: The incubation period is estimated at less than 2 weeks. The infection produces an undifferentiated fever lasting 2 to 6 days. The symptomatology consists of pyrexia, cephalalgia, dorsalgia, and myalgia. Some patients experience chills, malaise, photophobia, vertigo, and nausea. Recuperation is complete but convalescence can take several weeks.

The Disease in Animals: The virus has been isolated from different species of rodents, marsupials, sloths, and bats. Even when there is confirmed viremia, the disease is usually asymptomatic.

Figure 37. Fevers caused by group C bunyaviruses. Transmission cycle.

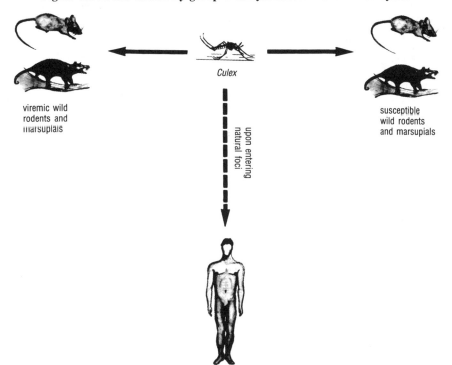

viremic wild
rodents and
marsupials

Culex

upon entering
natural foci

susceptible
wild rodents
and marsupials

Source of Infection and Mode of Transmission (Figure 37): The reservoirs are jungle rodents and marsupials. In Bush Bush, Trinidad, the main hosts are species of *Oryzomys* and *Zygodontomys*, and in Pará, Brazil, *Proechimys guyannensis* and *Oryzomys capito*. The vectors are *Culex* mosquitoes, especially *C. (Melanoconion) vomerifer* in Belém and *C. portesi* in Trinidad. The viremia reaches a high titer in rodents, and mosquitoes are easily infected upon biting them. The virus multiplies in the mosquitoes, which then transmit the infection to other susceptible rodents.

Man is an accidental host, infected by the bite of infected mosquitoes when he enters jungle areas for work.

Diagnosis: The virus can be isolated from a patient's blood by intracerebral mouse inoculation. Newborn mice die in 1 to 3 days. The tests that are used for serologic diagnosis are hemagglutination inhibition, complement fixation, and neutralization in VERO cell cultures.

Control: Preventive measures are the same as for other mosquito-borne arboviruses and are difficult to apply in the tropical jungles of the Americas.

Bibliography

Buckley, S. M., J. L. Davis, J. Madalengoitia, W. Flores, and J. Casals. Arbovirus neutralization tests with Peruvian sera in VERO cell cultures. *Bull WHO* 46:451-455, 1972.

Calisher, C. H., T. L. M. Coimbra, O. Souza Lopes, D. J. Muth, L. de Abreu Sacchetta, D. B. Francy, J. S. Lazuick, and C. B. Cropp. Identification of new Guamá and group C serogroup bunyaviruses and an ungrouped virus from southern Brazil. *Am J Trop Med Hyg* 32:424-431, 1983.

Casals, J., and D. H. Clarke. Arboviruses other than group A and B. *In*: Horsfall, F. L., and I. Tamm (Eds.), *Viral and Rickettsial Infections on Man*, 4th ed. Philadelphia, Lippincott, 1965.

Centers for Disease Control of the USA. *International Catalogue of Arboviruses*, 2nd ed. (Ed. by T. O. Berge). Atlanta, Georgia, 1975 (DHEW Publ. CDC 75–8301.).

Jonkers, A. H., L. Spence, W. G. Downs, and T. H. G. Aitken. Arbovirus studies in Bush Bush Forest, Trinidad, W. I., September 1959–December 1964. VI. Rodent-associated viruses (VEE and agents of group C and Guamá): Isolations and further studies. *Am J Trop Med Hyg* 17:285-298, 1968.

Scherer, W. F., R. W. Dickerman, and J. V. Ordoñez. Enfermedad humana causada por el virus Nepuyo, un bunyavirus de Mesoamérica transmitido por mosquitos. *Bol Of Sanit Panam* 95:111-117, 1983.

Spence, L., A. H. Jonkers, and L. S. Grant. Arbovirus in the Caribbean Islands. *Progr Med Virol* 10:415-486, 1968.

FOOT-AND-MOUTH DISEASE

(078.4)

Synonyms: Aphthosis, aftosa, hoof-and-mouth disease, aphthous fever, epizootic aphthae.

Etiology: RNA virus, genus *Aphthovirus*, family Picornaviridae. Seven different types are known: A, O, C, SAT_1, SAT_2, SAT_3, and Asia 1. The agent is endowed with a high degree of antigenic plasticity, with a tendency towards mutations that have produced many subtypes. The emergence of new subtypes in a region results in vaccine protection failures and gives rise to outbreaks of the disease.

Geographic Distribution: Areas free from foot-and-mouth disease (FMD) are North and Central America, the Caribbean islands, Chile, Scandinavia, Ireland, Poland, Hungary, Rumania, Bulgaria, Albania, Japan, Australia, and New Zealand. Types A, O, and C have the widest distribution and cause epizootics in South America, Europe, Asia, and Africa. The SAT types occur in the African continent; in 1962 SAT_1 spread to the Middle East, Turkey, and Greece, but its advance was contained and it has not been found outside of Africa since 1970. Type Asia 1 occurs on that continent; in 1973 it invaded the Middle East and reached Turkey (Pereira, 1981). In 1984, outbreaks of Asia 1 were detected in Greece and Israel (FAO/WHO/OIE, 1985).

Occurrence in Man: Rare. Man is quite resistant to the FMD virus, considering the high incidence of the disease in domestic animals in many countries and the opportunities for exposure in the field and in the laboratory. While man's susceptibility to the virus was debated for many years, today no doubt remains that FMD is a zoonosis, although of very low incidence. The virus has been isolated and typed in more than 40 human patients. Other cases have been diagnosed by reproducing the disease in animals (without typing the virus) or by serologic tests. The infection in man may be clinically apparent or asymptomatic. Massive exposure or predisposing causes that alter the susceptibility of a person are believed to be necessary for infection to occur.

Occurrence in Animals: It is common in many countries. Different epizootiological situations can be distinguished: free zones, zones where the infection occurs sporadically, and enzootic zones. Control programs have considerably reduced the number of outbreaks, the attack rates, and the severity of the disease in animals that are infected.

Extensive epizootics or panzootics involving several countries occur periodically in the world. These are caused either by an exotic type of virus that is accidentally introduced or by a "domestic" subtype that has developed in an area in which the infection was relatively inactive. The extent of epizootics depends on the density of the animal population, its susceptibility to the virus strain involved, and various environmental factors.

The number of outbreaks in Europe and South America has diminished notably in recent years. Both the rate of infected herds and general mortality have diminished in South America as a result of vaccination programs (Casas Olascoaga *et al.*, 1982), although an endemoepidemic situation still exists in many countries. Besides Chile, where the infection was eradicated, Suriname, French Guiana, and Guyana (where the last outbreak occurred in 1978) are considered free of the disease. In the majority of the continental European countries, which are not considered free from FMD, the number of known foci has been small in recent years and the intervals between reappearances of the disease are longer. Portugal and Turkey constitute an exception, since they experienced several hundred outbreaks in 1980. Great Britain, which had been free of the disease since 1968, experienced an outbreak in the Isles of Wight and Jersey in 1981 (Pereira, 1981). The situation in Asia and Africa is less well defined due to lack of surveillance in many countries.

The Disease in Man: FMD in man is benign. The incubation period is from 2 to 4 days, but can extend up to 8 days. The course of the disease is similar to that in animals. Symptoms in the initial phase are pyrexia, cephalalgia, anorexia, and tachycardia. The primary vesicle appears at the site of virus penetration (skin wound or oral mucosa); the disease then becomes generalized, with formation of secondary vesicles in the mouth and on the hands and feet. Not all lesions or symptoms described are found in all cases. When there is no secondary bacterial contamination of the aphthous ulcers, the patient recovers fully in 1 or 2 weeks.

The type of virus most frequently isolated from man is type O, followed by C and rarely A.

The disease has been found primarily in persons in close contact with infected animals or with the virus in the laboratory. Clinically, FMD may be confused with other vesicular diseases of man, especially infections caused by various serotypes of the Coxsackie A viruses, which produce lesions on the hands, feet, and in the mouth. The similarity between the symptomatology of FMD and that of other vesicular diseases invalidates any diagnosis made only on a clinical basis without laboratory confirmation.

The Disease in Animals: FMD is a disease of cloven-hoofed animals, primarily cattle, swine, sheep, and goats. It has also been found in various species of wild animals. Solipeds and carnivores are resistant.

Some FMD virus strains show a marked affinity for one animal species. Strains that have caused serious outbreaks in swine have not greatly affected cattle, and other strains isolated from cattle have presented difficulties in experimental reproduction of the disease in swine. This adaptation to host is only relative, and after being maintained for years in a given animal species, the virus can increase in virulence and attack other species.

The disease is very important economically because it spreads rapidly and causes high morbidity, losses in production, and obstacles to the marketing of livestock and animal products. The greatest impact occurs in cattle.

The incubation period ranges from less than 48 hours to 3 or 4 days.

CATTLE: After penetrating the epithelium, generally of the upper respiratory tract and the pharynx, the virus multiplies *in situ*, producing a primary vesicle that can pass clinically unnoticed. From the point of entry the virus invades the bloodstream, causing a viremia that coincides with the febrile state, which is the first observable sign. The febrile phase lasts no more than 1 or 2 days, and shortly thereafter secondary vesicles appear in the mouth, upper lip, interdigital spaces, coronary band of the foot, and, in some instances, on the teats, mammary glands, and other places with delicate skin. Other prominent signs are anorexia, delayed rumination, champing sounds, and profuse salivation. Lesions on the feet cause varying degrees of lameness. In some cases the damage to the coronary band is severe enough to cause detachment of the hooves. The animal feeds poorly and loses weight, and milk production decreases. Some cows become dry in the second half of the lactation period.

The vesicles burst after 1 to 3 days, leaving moist, painful, red erosions, which in a few days are covered with new epithelium. Some dark yellow spots remain in the mouth for a while, and scabs cover the old vesicles on the feet while new epithelial tissue is forming underneath. The pain and swelling in the feet last from 1 to 2 weeks. The most common complications are secondary bacterial infection of open vesicles in the mouth and on the feet, myiasis, and mastitis.

The case fatality rate is usually low, estimated at between 1 and 2% (4 to 5% in calves). The exception occurs when there is an epizootic of "malignant aphthosis," which causes lesions of the myocardium and can produce very high mortality, especially in calves.

SWINE: In swine, limping is the first symptom to be observed. The ungual lesion begins with red spots on the anterior part of the plantar cushion and around the heel. In other cases, vesicles appear on the coronary band, causing extensive inflammation of the surrounding skin and detachment of the hooves, especially in heavy swine that are forced to move. During the several months it usually takes for a hoof to form, the pigs remain prone and have difficulty procuring food. Vesicles can occasionally be observed on the snout of the animal and sometimes also in the mouth.

SHEEP AND GOATS: In these species, FMD is generally milder and more benign than in cattle. Nevertheless, some epizootics have been recorded in which sheep and goats were more severely affected than cattle. In small ruminants, vesicles in the mouth may be small and pass unnoticed, while vesicles on the feet and consequent lameness are clinically apparent. Secondary bacterial infections of foot lesions are frequent.

WILD ANIMALS: Natural infection has been confirmed in a large number of animal species, both free ranging and in zoos. During the FMD eradication campaign in California in 1924, lesions typical of the disease were found in 10% of 22,000 slain deer. Besides wild deer, natural infection occurs in different species of bovids, suids, and elephants. Aphthous lesions were also found in European hedgehogs (*Erinaceus europaeus*) in Great Britain, near a bovine focus of FMD. It was demonstrated that the virus can persist in these animals during hibernation. Outbreaks in zoos were described in Paris, Zurich, and Buenos Aires (Hedger, 1981).

The disease in wild animals has been studied with special attention in Africa, where free roaming ungulates share pastures with domestic animals. Of particular interest is infection of the African wild buffalo (*Syncerus caffer*), which occurs completely asymptomatically. This animal can maintain the infection independently of domestic animals (Hedger, 1981).

Source of Infection and Mode of Transmission: The natural hosts of the FMD virus are artiodactyl ungulates. An infected animal eliminates the virus in all secretions and excretions. The interval between the final phase of the prodromal state and the appearance of the vesicles (3 to 5 days after infection) is the time when the greatest amount of virus is eliminated and when the sick animal constitutes a very important source of infection. The elimination of virus then decreases and, after 8 to 10 days, the risk presented by the animal as a source of infection is minimal. The highest titers of virus are found in vesicular fluid and in the epithelium of the lesion. Large quantities of virus are eliminated in profuse salivation, which contaminates the environment and leaves small droplets containing virus suspended in the air. Lesser quantities of virus are also eliminated through the urine and feces. The virus multiplies in the mammary glands and can reach high titers in the milk, from which it has been isolated 1 to 4 days before the appearance of clinical signs. The semen of infected animals contains virus and could be a potential source of infection in artificial insemination.

There are multiple modes of transmission, both direct and indirect. Infection is transmitted mainly by aerosols, and the pharynx is perhaps the most common location for virus penetration. The virus can survive a long time in aerosols when the relative humidity is high, and can be transported to distant points. Other penetration routes of the virus are the lower respiratory tract, nasal passages, and the udder. Various inanimate objects and mechanical vectors can carry the infection from one place to another, sometimes over great distances. The copious secretions and excretions of a sick animal contaminate the environment and are probably the cause of indirect transmission of the disease, especially in endemic areas (Brooksby, 1982). The virus is resistant to environmental factors and can survive a long time outside the animal's body; viral preparations protected by organic matter can retain limited infectivity after 4 hours at 85°C (Callis, 1979).

Among the mechanical carriers of the virus is man, especially those individuals whose work involves daily visits to several livestock premises. Dogs also probably play a role by carrying contaminated material from place to place. Meat and other products of animal origin (milk, hides, wastes) can originate outbreaks in distant places. Swine frequently contribute to the start of an outbreak and serve as amplifiers of the infection because of their great susceptibility and high rate of viral excretion.

An asymptomatic carrier state has been found in cattle, sheep, and goats, but not in swine. This condition, which may last from several months to more than 2 years (Brooksby, 1982), can be demonstrated by collecting esophagopharyngeal secretions with a probang. Animals that have recovered from the disease, animals that had subclinical infection, and even vaccinated animals that come into contact with the virus can become carriers. Nevertheless, the role of carriers in the epizootiology is still uncertain, since the infection has not been successfully transmitted to susceptible animals (cattle, swine) by putting them in cohabitation with carrier animals. The amount of virus in carriers is always small. Nevertheless, epidemiologic studies suggest that carriers have been able to initiate new outbreaks. Under experimental conditions, seroconversion has been demonstrated in uninfected animals exposed to carriers. Another important consideration is that antibodies found in carriers can create selective pressure due to immunity and thus can favor the evolution of new antigenic varients of the virus (Brooksby, 1982).

Systematic vaccination in enzootic areas reduces the incidence of carriers. In a comparative study in two enzootic regions, one in which repeated vaccinations were carried out and another without any vaccination program, the carrier rates were 0.49 and 3.34%, respectively (Anderson et al., 1974).

The movement of animals is one of the most common means of diffusion of FMD. In South America cattle are commonly raised in marginal agricultural areas and are later sold at auctions or fairs (sometimes multiple times) and then sent to feedlots. In some marginal areas, intervals between vaccinations of cattle are long and coverage is poor because of the difficulty of rounding up the cattle and the cost of vaccinating them. In such regions the disease is usually endemic. The flow of animals from places where they are raised to where they are fattened creates a higher risk of disease transmission by increasing potential sources of infection (carriers) and the number of susceptible animals exposed. In this regard, a study carried out in Brazil found that 42% of the cattle raised in the Mato Grosso swamplands and destined for the west central area of the country had antibodies for the VIA[1] antigen; only 32% could be considered protected against all three types of the virus, according to serum neutralization tests (Mathias et al., 1981). This transmission mechanism is common in Brazil as well as other South American countries.

Wild animals play a role in the epizootiology of FMD only under very special conditions. One case where these tangentially infected hosts played an important part in spreading the disease was when steppe antelope (*Saiga tatarica*) contracted the infection from domestic animals in Kazakhstan, USSR, in 1967. The population of these animals had been estimated at about one million and, when they migrated, they spread the infection to cattle in distant regions. In Africa, the buffalo (*Syncerus caffer*) can be a reservoir of the virus, but transmission of the agent to cattle is very rare (Hedger, 1981).

Man is infected by contact with sick animals or infectious material through wounds or abrasions on the skin, or by drinking infected milk. Cases due to the consumption of infected meat or meat products have not been confirmed. The FMD

---

[1] VIA (Virus-infection-associated) or antigen associated with viral infection, which stimulates antibodies against VIA in infected animals for a period of 6 or more months and in repeatedly vaccinated animals for a period of several weeks to about 2 months.

virus has been isolated from human cases with vesicles up to 14 days after the onset of the disease, and also from the nasal passages of healthy persons up to 36 hours after exposure. On several occasions, sick persons are thought to have been responsible for outbreaks in animals. Although this possibility exists, it is not considered epidemiologically important and has not been proven conclusively.

Role of Animals in the Epidemiology of the Disease: FMD is an animal infection; man is an accidental host and is rarely infected. Transmission of the disease between humans has never been confirmed.

Diagnosis: Differential diagnosis to distinguish between FMD, vesicular stomatitis, and swine exanthema[2] can be done by animal inoculation. Horses inoculated intralingually are resistant to the FMD virus and are slightly susceptible to that of swine exanthema. Cattle, by contrast, are susceptible to FMD and vesicular stomatitis viruses and resistant to the exanthema virus. The animal inoculation technique is costly and is now being replaced by the complement fixation test, which not only allows differentiation of FMD virus from that of vesicular stomatitis, but also identification of the type and subtype of FMD virus. The most suitable material for the test is the epithelium of recent lingual vesicles, which is used as antigen in the cross complement fixation test together with subtype-specific sera produced in guinea pigs. The test is quantitative. The result can be confirmed by cross serum neutralization tests using suckling mice or tissue cultures. More recently, an indirect ELISA test has been perfected to detect and identify the types of FMD virus. This test is more sensitive, and anticomplementary factors do not affect it (Crowther and Abu Elzein, 1979). The ELISA test can also be used with bovine sera to quantify the antibodies against FMD.

In man, clinical diagnosis should always be confirmed by laboratory methods. The virus can be isolated by intraperitoneal inoculation of suckling mice or in tissue cultures. The complement fixation test is reliable.

Control: In the disease-free area of the Americas, the principal preventive measures are a) forbidding the introduction of animals of susceptible species, products of animal origin, and some potentially contaminated products, such as plants, from countries with FMD; b) setting up epidemiologic surveillance through inspection services in ports and quarantine stations as well as a reporting system to reveal any outbreak, with adequate laboratories for rapid diagnosis; c) providing the necessary human and economic resources to face any emergency. The FMD-free countries of the Americas have bilateral or multinational agreements to defend their borders against the disease. If an outbreak occurs, the establishments involved must be quarantined and sick and exposed animals slaughtered.

In infected areas, control programs consist primarily of systematic vaccination of cattle, until the rate of incidence of foci is reduced to a level compatible with an eradication policy. The vaccines currently in use in South America require revaccination every 4 months. Perfecting a vaccine with an oil adjuvant would allow the

---

[2] Swine exanthema, caused by a virus of serotype A of the genus *Calicivirus*, family Caliciviridae, was restricted to the Pacific coast of North America; outbreaks outside this area were only recognized in Hawaii and Ireland (Odend'hal, 1983). In 1956, the disease was officially declared eradicated. Later, the virus was isolated from marine mammals, and antibodies have been found in several species of wild land animals (Karstad, 1981).

reduction of vaccinations to twice a year (Mello *et al.*, 1975). In continental Europe ecologic and epidemiologic conditions, as well as cattle raising and handling practices, have allowed the use of a single annual vaccination, which has given excellent results in combination with the sacrifice of sick animals; eradication of the disease in the near future is a possibility.

Vaccines of proven quality should be used, and at least 80% of a susceptible population should be covered. In countries where sheep raising is important, these animals should be included in the vaccination program. A vaccine for protecting swine is not yet available, a significant drawback since many foci originate in swine. The oil emulsion vaccine would allow satisfactory vaccination of pigs, which are only partially protected with traditional aluminum hydroxide-adsorbed and saponified vaccines (Ouldridge *et al.*, 1982).

Advances in knowledge of the molecular structure and chemical composition of the FMD virus and in recombinant DNA technology have allowed the development of a vaccine with protein subunits. A vaccine produced by genetic engineering is in an experimental phase. It contains only the VP3 capsid protein of the FMD virion, which is the main immunogenic component of the virus. A synthetic peptide of 20 amino acids was also obtained, corresponding to a part of the protein surface of the virion. This peptide in conjunction with a carrier protein induced production of neutralizing antibodies in guinea pigs, and antibodies and protection in rabbits (Bittle *et al.*, 1982).

All control programs should include means for the adequate treatment of foci and perifocal areas, the control of animal movement, and the disinfection of vehicles, materials, and equipment.

Prevention of the disease in man consists mainly of controlling the disease in domestic animals. For individual prevention, wounds or abrasions of persons in contact with sick animals or with contaminated materials should be protected, and milk should be pasteurized or boiled.

Bibliography

Acha, P. N. Epidemiology of food-and-mouth disease in South America. *In:* Pollard, M. (Ed.), *Foot-and-Mouth Disease.* Notre Dame, Indiana, 1973.

Anderson, E. C., W. G. Doughty, and J. Anderson. The effect of repeated vaccination in an enzootic foot-and-mouth disease area on the incidence of virus carrier cattle. *J Hyg (Camb)* 73:229-235, 1974.

Bachrach, H. L. Foot-and-mouth disease. *Ann Rev Microbiol* 22:201-244, 1968.

Bittle, J. L., R. A. Houghten, H. Alexander, T. M. Shinninck, J. G. Suteliffe, R. A. Lerner, D. J. Rowland, and F. Brown. Protection against foot-and-mouth disease by immunization with chemically synthesized peptide predicted from the viral nucleotide sequence. *Nature* 298:30-33, 1982.

Bohm, H. O. Die Maul-und-Keluenseuche als Erkrankung des Menschen. *Fortschr Vet Med* 17:140-144, 1972.

Brooksby, J. B. Foot-and-mouth disease in man: notes on a recent case. *In: Proc Annu Meet US Livest Sanit Assoc* 71:300, 1967.

Brooksby, J. B. Wild animals and the epizootiology of foot-and-mouth disease. *In:* McDiarmid, A. (Ed.), *Diseases in Free Living Wild Animals.* New York, Academic Press, 1969.

Brooksby, J. B. Portraits of viruses: foot-and-mouth disease virus. *Intervirology* 18:1-23, 1982.

Brown, F. Vaccination against foot-and-mouth disease: past, present and future. *Ann Inst Pasteur Virol* 136E:547-552, 1985.

Cadena, J., and J. Estupiñán (Eds.). *La fiebre aftosa y otras enfermedades vesiculares en Colombia*. Bogotá, Instituto Colombiano Agropecuario, 1975. (Technical Bulletin 32.)

Callis, J. J. Foot-and-mouth disease—A world problem. *Proc Annu Meet US Anim Health Assoc* 83:261-269, 1979.

Casas Olascoaga, R., F. J. Rosenberg, and V. M. Astudillo. Situación de las enfermedades vesiculares en las Américas, 1981. *In: Actas, 3er Congreso Nacional de Veterinaria*, Montevideo, Uruguay, Sociedad de Medicina Veterinaria, 1982.

Crowter, J. R., and E. M. E. Abu Elzein. Application of the enzyme-linked immunosorbent assay to the detection and identification of foot-and-mouth disease viruses. *J Hyg (Camb)* 83:513-519, 1979.

Dawson, P. S. The involvement of milk in the spread of foot-and-mouth disease: an epidemiological study. *Vet Rec* 87:543-548, 1970.

Diego, A. I. de. La fiebre aftosa como zoonosis. *Rev Med Vet (B Aires)* 55:119-135, 1974.

DiMarchi, R., G. Brooke, C. Gale, V. Cracknell, T. Doel, and N. Mowat. Protection of cattle against foot-and-mouth disease by a synthetic peptide. *Science* 232(4750):639-641, 1986.

Donaldson, A. I. Aerobiology of foot-and-mouth disease (FMD): an outline and recent advances. *Rev Sci Technol Off Int Epizoot* 5:315-319, 1986.

Fernández, M. V. Ultimos avances en vacunas contra la fiebre aftosa. *Bol Centro Panam Fiebre Aftosa* 8:1-14, 1972.

Fletch, A. L. Foot-and-mouth disease. *In:* Davis, J. W., L. H. Karstad, and D. O. Trainer (Eds.), *Infectious Diseases of Wild Mammals*. Ames, Iowa State University Press, 1970.

Food and Agriculture Organization of the United Nations/World Health Organization/ International Office of Epizootics. *Animal Health Yearbook 1984*. Rome, FAO, 1985.

Francis, M. J., and L. Black. Response of young pigs to foot-and-mouth disease oil emulsion vaccination in the presence and absence of maternally derived neutralising antibodies. *Res Vet Sci* 41:33-39, 1986.

Gailiunas, P., and G. E. Cottral. Survival of foot-and-mouth disease virus in bovine hides. *Am J Vet Res* 28:1047-1053, 1967.

Gibson, C. F., and A. I. Donaldson. Exposure of sheep to natural aerosols of foot-and-mouth disease virus. *Res Vet Sci* 41:45-49, 1986.

Gierloff, B. C. H., and K. F. Jacobsen. On the survival of foot-and-mouth disease in frozen bovine semen. *Acta Vet Scand* 2:210-213, 1961.

Hedger, R. S. Foot-and-mouth disease. *In:* Davis, J. W., L. H. Karstad, and D. O. Trainer (Eds.), *Infectious Diseases of Wild Animals*, 2nd ed. Ames, Iowa State University Press, 1981.

Hedger, R. S., and J. B. Condy. Transmission of foot-and-mouth disease from African buffalo virus carriers to bovines. *Vet Rec* 117:205, 1985.

Hyslop, N. G. The epizootiology and epidemiology of foot-and-mouth disease. *Adv Vet Sci* 14:262-307, 1970.

Hyslop, N. S. T. G. Transmission of the virus of foot-and-mouth disease between animals and man. *Bull WHO* 49:577-585, 1973.

International Office of Epizootics. *Situación Zoosanitaria en los Países Miembros en 1984*. Paris, OIE, 1985.

Karstad, L. Miscellaneous viral infections. *In:* Davis, J. W., L. H. Karstad, and D. O. Trainer (Eds.), *Infectious Diseases of Wild Mammals*, 2nd ed. Ames, Iowa State University Press, 1981.

Manninger, R. Enfermedades infecciosas. *In:* Hutyra, F. V., J. Marek, and R. Manninger, *Patología y terapéuticas especiales de los animales domésticos*, 8th ed. Barcelona, Spain, Labor, 1948.

Mathias, L. A., E. C. Moreira, F. J. Rosenberg, and J. A. Obiaga. Estudio serológico de fiebre aftosa en bovinos procedentes del Pantanal matogrosense, Brasil. *Bol Centro Panam Fiebre Aftosa* 41-42:3-8, 1981.

Mello, P. A., V. Astudillo, I. Gomes, and T. C. García. Aplicación en el campo de vacuna antiaftosa oleosa e inactivada: vacunación y revacunación de bovinos jóvenes. *Bol Centro Panam Fiebre Aftosa* 19-20:31-38, 1975.

Odend'hal, S. *The Geographical Distribution of Animal Viral Diseases.* New York. Academic Press, 1983.

Ouldridge, E. J., M. J. Francis, and L. Black. Antibody response of pigs to foot-and-mouth disease oil emulsion vaccine: the antibody classes involved. *Res Vet Sci* 32:327-331, 1982.

Pan American Health Organization. Plan de acción a seguir en caso de un brote de fiebre aftosa. Rio de Janeiro, Pan American Foot-and-Mouth Disease Center, 1966. (Special Publication 671).

Pereira, H. G. Foot-and-mouth disease. *In:* Gibbs, E. P. J. (Ed.), *Virus Diseases of Food Animals,* vol. 2. New York, Academic Press, 1981.

Rosenberg, F. J. El conocimiento de la epidemiología de la fiebre aftosa con particular referencia a Sudamérica. Rio de Janeiro, Pan American Health Organization/Pan American Foot-and-Mouth Disease Center, 1975. (Technical Scientific Monographs 5.)

Rosenberg, F. J., and R. Goic. Programas de control y prevención de la fiebre aftosa en las Américas. *Bol Centro Panam Fiebre Aftosa* 12:1-22, 1973.

GOATPOX

(051.9)

Synonym: Variola caprina.

Etiology: DNA genome virus, genus *Capripoxvirus*, family Poxviridae. To the same genus belong the viruses of sheeppox and bovine nodular exanthema ("lumpy skin disease"). Immunologically, the ovine and caprine viruses are very closely related, and both are species-specific. However, goatpox virus attacks both species in Kenya (Tripathy *et al.*, 1981). A close antigenic relationship has been found between the virus in Kenya and bovine nodular exanthema virus: both stimulate complete cross-reactions by indirect immunofluorescence with sera prepared against one or the other virus (Davies and Otema, 1978). It has been possible to infect sheep experimentally with goatpox virus (GP) (Mohamed *et al.*, 1982).

Geographic Distribution and Occurrence in Goats: The disease is especially prevalent in African countries and in the Middle East, India, and the Far East (Tripathy *et al.*, 1981). A few outbreaks have also been recorded in several European countries.

Occurrence in Man: Rare. Several cases occurred in Sweden and India among personnel taking care of infected goats.

The Disease in Man: In the three cases diagnosed in India, an eruption was seen on various parts of the body, accompanied by a strong itching sensation. The vesicular lesions did not form pustules and dried up in 10 to 15 days. The scabs fell off without leaving scars. In the cases described in Sweden, eruption was observed only on the hands.

The Disease in Goats: The incubation period lasts approximately 1 to 2 weeks. In most outbreaks, systemic reaction is either absent or very mild. Pox lesions are seen primarily on the parts of the body not covered by hair. The disease starts with fever; lacrimation and a serous nasal discharge that may turn mucopurulent can occur also. Cutaneous eruption consists of circular papules, nodules, and plaques 0.5 to 1.5 cm in diameter which are painful to the touch. The vesicles that develop contain a serohemorrhagic exudate and hair surrounding the lesions becomes damp. The lesions are pruriginous and the animals scratch and bite themselves. Marked alopecia occurs after 8 to 10 days, and the lesions become covered by black scabs. The ulcerations left by the scabs heal in about 3 weeks. Young animals usually have more generalized lesions than adults. The picture can be aggravated by bacterial infections. Morbidity varies from 5 to 100% of animals in a flock, but mortality is low and is generally due to generalized infection (Tripathy *et al.*, 1981; Mohamed *et al.*, 1982). In northern Iraq, where GP is endemic and is considered the most important obstacle to the development of the goat-raising industry, morbidity is over 90% and case fatality, especially in young animals, is about 4% (Tantawi *et al.*, 1979). When 300 Sannen goats were introduced into the region, among the infected animals there were 62% with cutaneous lesions, 37.6% with pneumonia, 13% with keratoconjunctivitis, 10% with mastitis, and 3% with edemas of the head. Mortality was high among young goats (Karim, 1983).

Diagnosis: Laboratory confirmation can be obtained by isolation of the virus in lamb testicle cell culture, in which it produces a cytopathic effect and cytoplasmic inclusions. The virus can be cultured on the chorioallantoic membrane where it causes dark pox lesions. The immunodiffusion test with hyperimmune serum is useful for diagnosis; for that purpose, liquid from the vesicles and scabs from dermal lesions are used.

Control: In endemic areas, control is based mainly on vaccination with inactivated and modified live virus vaccines. In countries free of infection, preventive measures consist of prohibiting importation of goats from infected areas.

Bibliography

Andrewes, C. H., and H. G. Pereira. *Viruses of Vertebrates,* 3rd ed. Baltimore, Maryland, Williams and Wilkins, 1972.

Andrewes, C. H., and J. R. Walton. Viral and bacterial zoonoses. *In:* Brander, G. C. (Ed.), *Animal and Human Health*. London, Baillière Tindall, 1977.

Bruner, D. W., and J. H. Gillespie. *Hagan's Infectious Diseases of Domestic Animals,* 6th ed. Ithaca, New York, Cornell University Press, 1973.

Davies, F. G., and C. Otema. The antibody response in sheep infected with a Kenyan sheep and goat poxvirus. *J Comp Pathol* 88:205-210, 1978.

Food and Agriculture Organization of the United Nations/World Health Organization/International Office of Epizootics. *Animal Health Yearbook 1984*. Rome, FAO, 1985.

Karim, M. A. Pox among Sannen goats in Iraq. *Trop Anim Health Prod* 15:62, 1983.

Kitching, R. P., J. J. McGrane, and W. P. Taylor. Capripox in the Yemen Arab Republic and the Sultanate of Oman. *Trop Anim Health Prod* 18:115-122, 1986.

Kitching, R. P., and W. P. Taylor. Transmission of capripoxvirus. *Res Vet Sci* 39:196-199, 1985.

Kitching, R. P., and W. P. Taylor. Clinical and antigenic relationship between isolates of sheep and goat poxviruses. *Trop Anim Health Prod* 17:64-74, 1985.

Mohamed, K. A., B. E. D. Hago, W. P. Taylor, A. A. Nayil, and M. T. Abu-Samra. Goat pox in the Sudan. *Trop Anim Health Prod* 14:104-108, 1982.

Shawney, A. N., A. K. Singh, and B. S. Malik. Goatpox: an anthropozoonosis. *Ind J Med Res* 60:683-684, 1972.

Tantawi, H. H., M. O. Shony, and F. K. Hassan. Isolation and identification of the Sersenk strain of goat poxvirus in Iraq. *Trop Anim Health Prod* 11:208-210, 1979.

Tripathy, D. N., L. E. Hanson, and R. A. Crandell. Poxviruses of veterinary importance: diagnosis of infections. *In:* Kurstak, E., and C. Kurstak (Eds.), *Comparative Diagnosis of Viral Diseases.* New York, Academic Press, 1981.

HEMORRHAGIC FEVER WITH RENAL SYNDROME

(078.6)

Synonyms: Hemorrhagic nephrosonephritis (in the Soviet Far East), Korean hemorrhagic fever, epidemic nephropathy (Scandinavia).

Etiology: RNA genome virus (Hantaan), isolated for the first time in 1978 from the field mouse *Apodemus agrarius coreae* (Lee *et al.*, 1978). Definitive classification of the Hantaan virus has not yet been established, but morphologic and morphogenetic studies using electron microscopy (Hung *et al.*, 1983), as well as analysis of its biochemical and biophysical properties, indicate a relationship to members of the Bunyaviridae family (Schmaljohn *et al.*, 1983).

Based on the immune response detected by indirect immunofluorescence in patients with hemorrhagic fever with renal syndrome (HFRS) in different parts of the world, the Hantaan virus is thought to cause both the severe form of the disease, which occurs in the continental Far East, and the mild form, epidemic nephropathy, which occurs in Scandinavia and other parts of Europe. In studies of sera from cases of both forms of the disease, which have different natural reservoirs, antigenic differences have been found between strains of the virus (Cohen, 1982). Antigenic differences between virus strains from Japan and Korea have been demonstrated by the immune adherence technique (Sugiyama *et al.*, 1984). Japanese HFRS also differs from the Korean hemorrhagic fever in that it is more benign and has a different natural host.

Geographic Distribution: The disease has been clinically recognized in areas ranging from the Scandinavian peninsula and other European countries (France, Yugoslavia) to the Asian Pacific coast and Japan.

Antibodies against Hantaan virus have been detected in Alaska, Bolivia, India, Iran, Gabon, and the Central African Republic (Cohen, 1982), although not frequently and with no diagnosed HFRS human cases. Antibodies have also been found in rats captured in some cities in the United States and in inhabitants and urban rats of the Amazon region of Brazil (Pan American Health Organization, 1983). Ten of 81 *Rattus norvegicus* and one of 20 *R. rattus* captured in the port of the city of Buenos Aires had antibodies for Hantaan virus (Maiztegui *et al.*, 1983).

Occurrence: In terms of human morbidity, HFRS is the most important hemorrhagic fever in the USSR. From several hundred to several thousand cases have occurred annually in the Soviet Far East (excluding Siberia), Bashkiria, and in foci on the Upper and Lower Volga. HFRS occurs in 18 provinces in China, with an annual incidence that varies from 0.03 to 13 cases per 100,000 inhabitants in different administrative divisions (Cohen, 1982).

HFRS was an important problem, both medical and military, for United Nations troops (mainly North American) during the Korean War. From 1950 to 1953, 3,000 soldiers became ill with HFRS. The general case fatality rate was 6 to 8% and in some small outbreaks reached more than 33% (Traub and Wisseman, 1978). In rural areas of Korea, civilian hospitalized cases vary from 100 to 800 per year (American Public Health Association, 1985). Although HFRS usually occurs in rural and wild areas, 100 cases with two deaths occurred in Osaka, Japan, between 1960 and 1972. Since 1976 there have been outbreaks in laboratory personnel in Japan, with more than 100 cases and one death; the source of infection was laboratory rats (Sugiyama *et al.*, 1984). Isolated cases are also seen in rural residents in Japan (Umenai *et al.*, 1981). In 1961, 129 cases occurred among laboratory personnel at the Gamaleya Institute in Moscow after the introduction of the microtine mouse *Clethrionomys* (Traub and Wisseman, 1978).

In Scandinavia and Korea, the disease occurs as isolated cases. In Korea only 10% of multiple cases were associated with a focus, whereas in the USSR grouped infections seem to predominate (Traub and Wisseman, 1978).

The maximum incidence in Korea occurs in spring and autumn, while in the USSR it occurs in summer.

The Disease in Man: The disease starts with fever, cephalalgia, bradycardia, and conjunctival congestion; a few days later the patient experiences costovertebral and abdominal pains, nausea, vomiting, hemorrhages, and renal involvement with hematuria, oliguria, proteinuria, and output of urine with a low specific gravity (isohyposthenuria). In serious cases there is marked oliguria, acidosis, hyperkalemia, and azotemia 7 to 10 days after the onset of the disease. Death may occur during this oliguric phase. When the patient begins to improve, urine volume increases and its protein content decreases. West of the Ural Mountains, in the European part of the USSR, Scandinavia, and other European countries, hemorrhagic manifestations occur infrequently and the fatality rate is low. By contrast, in the Soviet Far East, Korea, and part of China, hemorrhagic symptoms are more frequent and mortality higher. In continental China both benign and severe forms of disease are seen. The mild form of HFRS occurs in Japan.

Blood tests show leukocytosis, lymphocytosis, thrombocytopenia, azotemia, uremia, and electrolytic imbalance; urine tests show proteinuria, hematuria, and pyuria. Convalescence is slow and generally without sequelae.

The Disease in Animals: Rodents, the natural reservoirs of the virus, do not show symptomatic infection.

Source of Infection and Mode of Transmission: The disease occurs in a variety of ecologic environments, such as agricultural fields, forests, houses, and gardens. Man contracts the infection by entering the habitat of rodents or, conversely, when rodents invade dwellings, gardens, and food supplies of man. In the USSR, major epidemics have occasionally originated during fall and winter months as a result of rodents entering dwellings and gardens. The disease primarily affects adult males when infection is contracted in woods or cultivated fields, while in urban epidemics there is no major sex or age difference in the incidence.

The reservoirs for maintenance of the virus in nature are rodents. In Korea, the main reservoir is the field mouse *Apodemus agrarius coreae*. Numerous virus isolations have been carried out from this species. Examination by immunofluorescence of tissue from 817 of these mice showed that 114 had viral antigen. On the other hand, tissue from 239 rodents of seven other species gave negative results (Lee *et al.*, 1981). In China, the virus was also isolated from *A. agrarius* in the HFRS endemic area. The mild form of the disease in China (similar to Scandinavian epidemic nephropathy), would seem, according to epidemiologic studies, to have been acquired in the patients' homes; *R. norvegicus*, from which virus was isolated, is thought to be the source of infection (Song *et al.*, 1983). In Japan, urban (Osaka) and laboratory HFRS were associated with domestic and laboratory rats, respectively. In a rural area of Japan where several human cases occurred, immunofluorescence confirmed the presence of the viral antigen in *Apodemus speciosus* and a microtine mouse, *Microtus montebelli* (Umenai *et al.*, 1981). Still undetermined is whether *R. norvegicus* is the reservoir of the virus or a temporary secondary host that serves as a bridge for transmission of the infection between field mice and man in the city (Lee *et al.*, 1981). In Europe, the main reservoir is the microtine mouse *Clethrionomys glareolus* (Brummer-Korvenkontio *et al.*, 1980). In the European USSR this microtine is also the main reservoir, but the presence of the viral antigen was also confirmed with the ELISA test in seven other species of small mammals (Gavrilovskaya *et al.*, 1983).

Viremia in rodents lasts about 7 to 10 days, but the agent persists in tissues at least 100 days (observation period of experimental infection of *A. agrarius coreae*), without clinical symptoms. The lengthy persistence of the virus in their tissues seems to indicate that these animals can contaminate the environment for a long time with their excretions and secretions (Lee *et al.*, 1981). The virus has been detected in the brown fat of *C. glareolus* and other rodents, indicating that these rodents could be an important mechanism for virus survival during winter (Gavrilovskaya *et al.*, 1983).

At the present time, no role in the transmission of the infection is attributed to arthropods, and it is thought that rodents act as both reservoirs and a source of infection for man. Man apparently becomes infected by contact with rodents and their excreta, as occurs with Bolivian and Argentine hemorrhagic fevers. Urban epidemics probably originate primarily as a result of food contaminated by excreta of rodents that invade dwellings and places where food is stored. The most likely modes of penetration of the etiologic agent are the respiratory and digestive tracts. The source of infection for laboratory as well as military and civilian personnel has probably been aerosols, through inhalation of dust during dry periods. This would explain the multiple cases at some foci.

Diagnosis: Laboratory diagnosis is accomplished mainly by indirect immunofluorescence. Viral antigen has been detected in rodents both by immunofluorescence and ELISA.

Control: Rodent control measures in villages and towns have made it possible to reduce the intensity of outbreaks.

Bibliography

American Public Health Association. *Control of Communicable Diseases in Man,* 14th ed. (Ed. by A. S. Benenson). Washington, D.C., APHA, 1985.

Brummer-Korvenkontio, M., A. Vaheri, T. Hovi, C. H. von Bensdorff, J. Vourimies, T. Manni, K. Penttinen, N. Oker-Blom, and J. Lahdevirta. Nephropathia epidemica: detection of antigen in bank voles and serologic diagnosis of human infection. *J Infect Dis* 141:131-134, 1980.

Casals, J., H. Hoogstraal, K. M. Johnson, A. Shelokov, N. H. Wiebenga, and T. H. Work. A current appraisal of hemorrhagic fevers in USSR. *Am J Trop Med Hyg* 15:751-764, 1966.

Casals, J., B. E. Henderson, H. Hoogstraal, K. M. Johnson, and A. Shelokov. A review of Soviet viral hemorrhagic fevers, 1969. *J Infect Dis* 122:437-453, 1970.

Chen, Hua-Xin, Fu-Xi Qiu, Bi-Jun Dong, Shao-Zhong Ji, Yan-Ting Li, and Yuan Wang. Epidemiological studies on hemorrhagic fever with renal syndrome in China. *J Infect Dis* 154:394-398, 1986.

Cohen, M. S. Epidemic hemorrhagic fever revisited. *Rev Infect Dis* 4:992-997, 1982.

Gavrilovskaya, I. N., N. S. Apekina, Y. A. Myasnikov, A. D. Bernshtein, E. V. Ryltseva, E. A. Gorbachkova, and M. P. Chumakov. Features of circulation of hemorrhagic fever with renal syndrome (HFRS) virus among small mammals in the European USSR. *Arch Virol* 75:313-316, 1983.

Hung, T., S. M. Xia, T. X. Zhao, J. Y. Zhou, G. Song, G. X. Liao, W. W. Ye, Y. L. Chu, and C. S. Hang. Morphological evidence for identifying the viruses of hemorrhagic fever with renal syndrome as candidate members of the Bunyaviridae family. *Arch Virol* 78:137-144, 1983.

LeDuc, J. W., G. A. Smith, J. E. Childs, F. P. Pinheiro, J. I. Maiztegui, B. Niklasson, A. Antoniades, D. M. Robinson, M. Khin, K. F. Shortridge, M. T. Wooster, M. R. Elwell, P. L. T. Ilbery, D. Koech, E. S. T. Rosa, and L. Rosen. Global survey of antibody to Hantaan-related viruses among peridomestic rodents. *Bull WHO* 64:139-144, 1986.

LeDuc, J. W., G. A. Smith, J. E. Childs, F. P. Pinheiro, J. I. Maiztegui, B. Niklasson, A. Antoniades, D. M. Robinson, M. Khin, K. F. Shortridge, M. T. Wooster, M. R. Elwell, P. L. T. Ilbery, D. Koech, E. S. T. Rosa, and L. Rosen. Global survey of antibody to Hantaan-related viruses among peridomestic rodents. *Bull WHO* 64:139-144, 1986. hemorrhagic fever. *J Infect Dis* 137:298-308, 1978.

Lee, H. W., G. R. French, P. W. Lee, L. J. Baek, K. Tsuchiya, and R. S. Foulke. Observations on natural and laboratory infection of rodents with the etiologic agent of Korean hemorrhagic fever. *Am J Trop Med Hyg* 30:477-482, 1981.

Lloyd, G., and H. Jones. Infection of laboratory workers with hantavirus acquired from immunocytomas propagated in laboratory rats. *J Infect* 12:117-125, 1986.

Maiztegui, J. I., J. L. Becker, and J. W. LeDuc. Actividad de virus de la fiebre hemorrágica de Corea o virus muroide en ratas del puerto de la Ciudad de Buenos Aires. *In: 28a Reunión Científica Anual de la Sociedad Argentina de Investigación Clínica.* Mar del Plata, 21-24 November 1983.

Pan American Health Organization. Importance of viroses transmitted by arthropods and rodents for public health in the Americas. *Epidemiol Bull* 4(3):1-4, 1983.

Schmaljohn, C. S., S. E. Hasty, S. A. Harrison, and J. M. Dalrymple. Characterization of Hantaan virions, the prototype virus of hemorrhagic fever with renal syndrome. *J Infect Dis* 148:1005-1012, 1983.

Song, G., C. S. Hang, X. Z. Qui, D. S. Ni, H. X. Liao, G. Z. Gao, Y. L. Du, J. K. Xu, Y. S. Wu, J. N. Zhao, B. X. Kong, Z. S. Wang, Z. Q. Zhang, H. K. Shen, and N. Zhou. Etiologic studies of epidemic hemorrhagic fever (hemorrhagic fever with renal syndrome). *J Infect Dis* 147:654-659, 1983.

Sugiyama, K., Y. Matsuura, C. Morita, S. Shiga, Y. Akao, T. Komatsu, and T. Kitamura. An immune adherence assay for discrimination between etiologic agents of hemorrhagic fever with renal syndrome. *J Infect Dis* 149:67-73, 1984.

Traub, R., and C. L. Wisseman, Jr. Korean hemorrhagic fever. *J Infect Dis* 138:267-272, 1978.

Umenai, T., M. Watanabe, H. Sekino, S. Yokoyama, T. Kaburagi, K. Takahashi, H. W. Lee, and N. Ishida. Korean hemorrhagic fever among rural residents in Japan. *J Infect Dis* 144:460-463, 1981.

Vasyuta Yu, S. The epidemiology of hemorrhagic fever with renal syndrome in the RSFSR. *Zh Mikrobiol Epidemiol Immunobiol* 32:49:56, 1961.

Yanagihara, R., C. T. Chin, M. B. Weiss, D. C. Gajdusek, A. R. Diwan, J. B. Poland, K. T. Kleeman, C. M. Wilfert, G. Meiklejohn, and W. P. Glezen. Serological evidence of Hantaan virus infection in the United States. *Am J Trop Med Hyg* 34:396-399, 1985.

HERPES SIMPLEX (TYPE 1)

(054)

Synonyms: Herpesvirus hominis, human herpesvirus (types 1 and 2).

Etiology: Herpes simplex virus (HSV), a DNA virus belonging to the subfamily Alphaherpesvirinae, family Herpesviridae. There are two types of herpes simplex, 1 and 2. Both have a common antigen which causes serologic cross-reactions; they can be differentiated by the neutralization and immunofluorescence tests. Epidemiologically, they differ in their transmission route: type 1 is transmitted orally and type 2 venereally.

Geographic Distribution: Worldwide.

Occurrence in Man: It is estimated that 70 to 90% of the adult population has antibodies for herpes simplex virus.

Occurrence in Animals: Two outbreaks have been recorded in owl monkeys, *Aotus trivirgatus*, shipped from South America to the United States. One group was assembled for shipment in Barranquilla, Colombia, and the other in Iquitos, Peru. Another epizootic outbreak occurred in a colony of 84 splenectomized white-handed gibbons (*Hylobates lar*). The disease affected six animals, three of which showed excoriated areas at the commissure of the lips; the other three had small vesicles which rapidly became ulcerated and necrotic. Four of the six gibbons died of encephalitis; they had signs of ataxia, convulsions, paralysis of the tongue and swallowing muscles, and a descending progressive paralysis that ended in death. Herpes simplex virus was isolated from three animals. Neutralizing antibodies for HSV were found in 16 of the 84 animals in the colony (Smith *et al.*, 1969). The virus was also isolated from naturally infected skunks and lemurs (Emmons, 1983) and tree shrews (*Tupaia glis*) from Thailand that were shipped to the United States (McClure *et al.*, 1972).

The Disease in Man: Primary infection with type 1 occurs chiefly during early infancy and is generally asymptomatic. It is estimated that only 10% of the primary infections present clinical manifestations. The disease is expressed as acute herpetic gingivostomatitis with a systemic reaction that varies in severity. Pharyngitis with vesicular lesions is more common in adolescents. Keratoconjunctivitis can also occur and, rarely, meningoencephalitis. A fatal generalized infection has been observed in newborns (congenital herpes simplex) (American Public Health Association, 1985). HSV infection is characterized by its latency. After the primary infection and the formation of antibodies, the virus seems to persist in the tissues for the lifetime of the person. The infection can reactivate and cause repeated attacks, usually in the form of herpes labialis (fever blisters) without systemic reaction.

The Disease in Animals: Infection in the two groups of owl monkeys mentioned above was characterized by a generalized and highly fatal disease that began with conjunctivitis, coryza, and lethargy; only 4 to 7 days elapsed between the appearance of symptoms and death. Autopsy revealed necrotic plaques and ulcers on the tongue (although not in all animals), necrotic foci in the liver, enlarged adrenal glands with a speckled cortical region, and petechiae on the lymph nodes.

The clinical picture in gibbons was characterized by cutaneous lesions and encephalitis (see Occurrence in Animals).

Source of Infection and Mode of Transmission: Man is the natural reservoir of the virus. The most important mode of transmission between humans is direct contact with saliva of carriers. The virus can be isolated from the saliva of asymptomatic adults.

The infection was probably transmitted to the owl monkeys by contact with human carriers.

The virus-host relationship is characterized by the benign nature of HSV infection in its usual host, man, and by the highly fatal disease it causes in an accidental host, such as the owl monkey or gibbon. An analogous situation exists with respect to infection caused by herpesvirus simiae in its natural reservoir, the rhesus monkey, in which the course of disease is mild or asymptomatic, while it is highly fatal in the accidental host, man.

Diagnosis: It may be confirmed by isolation of virus or by means of the serum neutralization test, by proving an increase in the level of specific antibodies.

Control: Practical measures are not available to prevent transmission of the infection from man to monkeys.

Bibliography

American Public Health Association. *Control of Communicable Diseases in Man,* 14th ed. (Ed. by A. S. Benenson). Washington, D.C., APHA, 1985.

Emmons, R. W. Earlier reports dealing with herpesvirus hominis. Letter. *J Am Vet Med Assoc* 182:764, 1983.

McClure, H. M., M. E. Keeling, B. Olberding, R. D. Hunt, and L. V. Meléndez. Natural herpesvirus hominis infection of tree shrews *(Tupaia glis). Lab Anim Sci* 22:517-521, 1972.

Meléndez, L. V., C. España, R. D. Hunt, M. D. Daniel, and F. G. García. Natural herpes simplex infection in the owl monkey *(Aotus trivirgatus). Lab Anim Care* 19:38-45, 1969.

Smith, P. C., T. M. Yuill, R. D. Buchanan, J. S. Stanton, and V. Chaicumpa. The gibbon *(Hylobates lar):* A new primate host for herpesvirus hominis. I. Natural epizootic in a laboratory colony. *J Infect Dis* 120:292-297, 1969.

HERPESVIRUS SIMIAE

(049.8)

Synonym: B virus infection.

Etiology: Herpesvirus simiae (herpesvirus B), closely related antigenically to herpesvirus hominis (herpes simplex virus) and SA-8 (a baboon and *Cercopithecus* sp. herpesvirus); a DNA virus, subfamily Alphaherpesvirinae, family Herpesviridae.

Geographic Distribution: The infection occurs naturally among primates of the genus *Macaca* in Asia. In India, disease incidence has been seen to increase during and after the monsoon season. An antigenically closely related herpetic virus (SA-8 virus) has been isolated from African green monkeys (*Cercopithecus aethiops*) and baboons (*Papio* spp.). Herpesvirus simiae does not occur naturally in the forests of America. Primates of other genera may possibly acquire the infection by contact when brought together with infected specimens of the genus *Macaca* in research institutes or production centers for biologicals.

Occurrence in Man: Rare. Since the first isolation of the virus in 1934, about 20 cases have been recognized. The disease occurred in persons who handled monkeys or their tissues in research centers or in vaccine production plants. The highest incidence was recorded in 1957, as a result of the increased use of rhesus monkeys for producing poliomyelitis vaccines. In recent years these monkeys have largely been replaced by African green monkeys (*Cercopithecus*).

Occurrence in Animals: In newly captured rhesus monkeys *(Macaca mulatta)* the rate of reactors to the serum neutralization test is 10 to 20%, but after captivity in closed groups the rate may reach 90 to 100% in about 2 months. Other species of *Macaca* (*M. fuscata* and *M. arctoides*), and especially the cynomolgus monkey *M. fascicularis*, are very susceptible and easily become infected.

The prevalence of herpesvirus simiae among *Macaca mulatta* varies with age. In one study the rate of animals with antibodies increased from 11.2% at 1 year of age to 33% at 3 years or more. The general rates of occurrence in animals of different origins were 4.2% in rhesus monkeys captured in India, 16.6% in those from China, and 35% in *M. irus* from the Philippines and Thailand (Rawls, 1979). Epizootiologic data are often difficult to interpret because of the different serologic methods used by laboratories (Hutt *et al.*, 1981).

The Disease in Man: Herpesvirus simiae produces a highly fatal disease in man. Only 15% of cases have survived and all had neurologic sequelae (Rawls, 1979).

Man is probably not very susceptible to the virus, judging from the large number of monkeys that are handled and the number of bites they inflict on persons who tend them. Nevertheless, given the high mortality observed in individuals with clinical manifestations, this infection merits special interest and surveillance.

The incubation period is not well known, but it is estimated to be between 1 and 5 weeks from the time of exposure. If the infection is produced by a bite or scratch, there may be vesiculation at the wound site, followed by lymphangitis and lymphadenitis. The generalized disease is characterized by fever, cephalalgia, nausea, abdominal pain, and diarrhea. Vesicular pharyngitis, urinary retention, and pneumonia can also occur (Rawls, 1979). Neurologic symptoms start with muscular pains, vertigo, diaphragmatic spasms, difficulty in swallowing, and abdominal pain. Later there is flaccid paralysis of the lower extremities which spreads to the upper extremities and thorax, ending with respiratory collapse. The manifestations of encephalitis or encephalomyelitis may last from 3 to 21 days. The histopathology is similar to that of generalized infection caused by herpesvirus hominis in children, with encephalitic lesions, myelitis, and necrotic foci in the liver, spleen, lymph nodes, and adrenal glands.

The Disease in Animals: The infection in monkeys produces a benign disease that often goes unnoticed. The disease is similar to that produced by herpesvirus hominis (herpes simplex) in man. The primary infection occurs in young animals. The most common lesion is localized in the mouth, usually on the tongue, and consists of a vesicle that leaves an ulcer when it breaks and then becomes covered with a fibrinous necrotic scab. The entire process lasts no longer than 7 to 14 days and does not leave scars or affect the general condition of the animal. Unless the animal is anesthetized and its mouth carefully examined, the lesions may pass unnoticed. The herpetiform eruption can also occur on the mucocutaneous border of the lips and sometimes on the conjunctiva and skin. Occasionally, a mucopurulent nasal secretion and conjunctivitis are seen. The primary infection is followed by a state of latency in a manner similar to human infection by herpes simplex virus, and the agent can be isolated from the trigeminal ganglia.

The disease in cynomolgus monkeys (*M. fascicularis*) seems to be more severe than in rhesus monkeys. Many of the infected monkeys become lifetime carriers of the virus, eliminating the agent intermittently in the saliva. The virus has also been isolated from primary kidney cultures of animals with no macroscopic lesions.

In a polio vaccine production laboratory in England, 2.3% of 14,400 monkeys housed in shared surroundings were found to have lingual lesions (Perkins, 1968). Histologically, the lesions consist of degeneration and necrosis of epithelial cells in which inclusion bodies can be observed within the nuclei. Necrosis of neurons and gliosis can be seen in the central nervous system, as well as a small perivascular lymphocytic infiltration.

Source of Infection and Mode of Transmission (Figure 38): The main natural reservoir is the rhesus monkey, *M. mulatta*. Other monkeys of the same genus can be a source of infection for man. One human case has also been recorded as a result of the bite of an African green monkey that lived with rhesus monkeys. The infection is transmitted within a colony of monkeys by direct contact, bites, scratches, contamination of food and water with saliva, and probably by aerosols.

Man contracts the infection through bites or skin abrasions contaminated with monkey saliva, and possibly also by aerosols that enter through the conjunctiva,

Figure 38. Herpesvirus simiae. Transmission cycle.

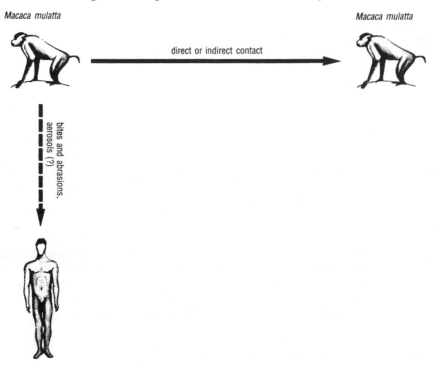

nose, or pharynx. One case of accidental laboratory infection is known to have resulted when a flask containing monkey kidney culture was broken.

Role of Animals in the Epidemiology of the Disease: Man is an accidental host. Herpesvirus simiae is not transmitted from man to man. Human infection always depends on the animal source, rhesus monkeys being the natural host of the virus.

Diagnosis: In any individual with signs of encephalitis who has been in contact with monkeys or their tissues, the possibility of herpesvirus simiae infection should be considered. Most human cases have been confirmed post-mortem by isolation of virus from the brain or medulla oblongata. When the duration of disease permits the appearance of antibodies, diagnosis can be made by means of the serum neutralization test.

Complement-fixing and neutralizing antibodies appear in monkeys after primary infection. The titers decline with time. Diagnosis can be made by serology and by isolation of the virus. Given the risk involved in handling the virus, diagnosis should be carried out only in high-security laboratories.

A correct serologic diagnosis is very important in order to establish nonhuman primate colonies free of herpesvirus simiae. Differentiation of herpesvirus simiae, herpesvirus hominis, and SA-8 is difficult because of the antigenic similarity between them. The frequency of infection of nonhuman primates by human strains must be considered in differential diagnosis. Recent studies have confirmed that it is not enough to subject simian sera to a neutralization test with herpesvirus hominis because a considerable number (about 50%) can be negative to this antigen and positive to herpesvirus simiae (Kalter *et al.*, 1978; Hutt *et al.*, 1981).

Control: All recently imported monkeys should be quarantined for 6 to 8 weeks, and any animal with herpetiform lesions should be eliminated. The animals should not be kept in large groups, and cohabitation of *M. mulatta* with other species should be avoided. It is recommended that no more than two monkeys be housed per cage. Once the carrier state has been confirmed, the best method of control is to eliminate reactors to the serum neutralization test and to repeat the test periodically.

Personnel tending the monkeys should be provided with protective clothing, and any wound or bite should be treated quickly and appropriately. Strict safety measures should be observed in laboratories where work with monkey tissues is done. Studies on rabbits—an animal very susceptible to experimental infection—have tentatively demonstrated that acyclovir might be useful in postexposure prophylaxis. Rabbits who received the treatment within 24 hours of infection did not develop disease and those treated within 5 days experienced greatly reduced mortality (Boulter *et al.*, 1980). Favorable results were also obtained when large doses of specific antiserum were administered intravenously to rabbits (Boulter *et al.*, 1981).

Bibliography

Boulter, E. A., B. Thornton, D. J. Bauer, and A. Bye. Successful treatment of experimental B virus (herpesvirus simiae) infection with acyclovir. *Br Med J* 280:681-683, 1980.

Boulter, E. A., H. T. Zwartouw, and B. Thornton. Postexposure immunoprophylaxis against B virus (herpesvirus simiae) infection. *Br Med J* 283:1495-1497, 1981.

Centers for Disease Control of the USA. B-virus infection in humans—Pensacola, Florida. *Morb Mortal Wkly Rep* 36(19):289-296, 1987.

Hunt, R. D., and L. V. Meléndez. Herpes virus infections of nonhuman primates. A review. *Lab Anim Care* 19:221-234, 1969.

Hutt, R., J. E. Guajardo, and S. S. Kalter. Detection of antibodies to herpesvirus simiae and herpesvirus hominis in nonhuman primates. *Lab Anim Sci* 31:184-189, 1981.

Kalter, S. S., R. Hutt, J. E. Guajardo, R. L. Heberling, T. L. Lester, and L. C. Pleasant. Serodiagnosis of herpesvirus infection in primates. *Dev Biol Stand* 41:235-240, 1978.

Keeble, S. A. B virus infection in man and monkey. *In:* Graham-Jones, O. (Ed.), *Some Diseases of Animals Communicable to Man in Britain*. Oxford, Pergamon Press, 1968.

Kissling, R. E. Herpes virus. *In:* Hubbert, W. T., W. F. McCulloch, and P. R. Schnurrenberger (Eds.), *Diseases Transmitted from Animals to Man,* 6th ed. Springfield, Illinois, Thomas, 1975.

Love, F. M., and W. C. Stone. Virus B infection. *In:* Davis, J. W., L. H. Karstad, and D. O. Trainer (Eds.), *Infectious Diseases of Wild Mammals*. Ames, Iowa State University Press, 1970.

Palmer, A. E. B-virus, herpesvirus simiae, historical perspective. *J Med Primatol* 16:99-130, 1987.

Perkins, F. T. Precautions against B virus in man. *In:* Graham-Jones, O. (Ed.), *Some Diseases of Animals Communicable to Man in Britain*. Oxford, Pergamon Press, 1968.

Rawls, W. E. Herpes simplex virus types 1 and 2 and herpesvirus simiae. *In:* Lennette, E. H., and N. J. Schmidt (Eds.), *Diagnostic Procedures for Viral, Rickettsial and Chlamydial Infections,* 5th ed. Washington, D.C., American Public Health Association, 1979.

ILHEUS FEVER

(066.9)

Etiology: RNA genome virus belonging to the genus *Flavivirus* (group B arboviruses), family Arenaviridae.

Geographic Distribution: The virus has been isolated in Argentina, Brazil, Colombia, Trinidad, Panama, Honduras, and Guatemala.

Occurrence: The virus has been isolated from five human cases with mild fever, from one case with encephalitis, and from two asymptomatic cases. In endemic areas the rate of seropositive reactors can be high. In a serologic study carried out at a penal colony in the forest region of Araracuara in southeastern Colombia, 76 (21%) of 368 serum samples gave positive results to the neutralization and hemagglutination inhibition tests (Prías-Landínez *et al.*, 1968). Studies done in Brazil, Trinidad, and Panama also show that inapparent clinical infections are frequent.

The Disease in Man: Most of the time, Ilheus virus infection in man is probably clinically inapparent or produces an undifferentiated and mild febrile disease. In Trinidad, a natural case with encephalitis occurred. Out of nine patients with inoperable neoplasms who were inoculated with the virus in order to induce oncolysis, three showed symptoms of encephalitis with a benign course.

The Disease in Animals: The virus has been isolated from various species of birds. Although viremia has been confirmed, the disease is generally asymptomatic.

Source of Infection and Mode of Transmission: Numerous isolations have been obtained from mosquitoes of the genera *Psorophora* and *Aedes*, which appear to be the main vectors of the virus. It has also been shown experimentally that the mosquitoes *P. ferox*, *Aedes aegypti*, and *A. serratus* can transmit the virus to suckling mice by biting them. Birds constitute the most likely reservoir. In Panama and Trinidad, the virus has been isolated from several species of birds. Antibodies have been found in mammals, but isolations have not been attained. The few studies that have been done do not allow a reservoir to be determined with certainty at the present time.

Man acquires the infection accidentally by the bite of infected mosquitoes.

Diagnosis: The virus can be isolated from patients' serum by mouse inoculation.

Control: Given the low incidence of the disease, special control measures do not appear necessary at this time.

Bibliography

Centers for Disease Control of the USA. *International Catalogue of Arboviruses,* 2nd ed. (Ed. by T. O. Berge). Atlanta, Georgia, 1975 (DHEW Publ. CDC 75-8301.).

Clarke, D. H., and J. Casals. Arboviruses; group B. *In:* Horsfall, F. L., and I. Tamm (Eds.), *Viral and Rickettsial Infections of Man,* 4th ed. Philadelphia, Lippincott, 1965.

Prías-Landínez, E., C. Bernal-Cubides, and A. Morales-Alarcón. Isolation of Ilheus virus from man in Colombia. *Am J Trop Med Hyg* 17:112-114, 1968.

Prier, J. E. *Basic Medical Virology.* Baltimore, Maryland, Williams and Wilkins, 1966.

INFLUENZA

(487)

Synonym: Grippe.

Etiology: RNA genome virus, family Orthomyxoviridae. Based on the specificity of its soluble (S) internal antigens, which are ribonucleoprotein in nature, three types are recognized: A, B, and C. Types A and B are included in the genus *Influenzavirus;* type C is in a separate genus without an approved name. The surface antigens are of special immunologic and epidemiologic interest. These antigens, which are found in different protein subunits of the viral envelope, are the hemagglutinating (H) antigen and the neuraminidase (N) antigen. Numerous subtypes of type A have been found in which these two surface antigens vary. At the present time, 12 subtypes for the hemagglutinating antigens (H1 to H12) and nine subtypes for the neuraminidase antigens (N1 to N9) are recognized (World Health Organization, 1980). According to new nomenclature, the influenza strains are identified as follows: 1) type of virus (A, B, or C); 2) host of origin, except man (equine, swine, avian, and others); 3) geographic origin; 4) strain number; 5) year of isolation; and 6) antigenic description of subtype A strains in parenthesis. For example, a duck A strain isolated in the Ukraine in 1963 would be designated A/duck/Ukraine/1/63 (H3N8). In the case of strains isolated from man, the host of origin is omitted.

The virus A genome has eight segments of single-stranded RNA, three of which code for the main H and N antigens that distinguish the subtypes and for the nucleoprotein (NP) that determines the type. This property of the virus points to the possibility of genetic recombinations between different subtypes.

There are 108 possible combinations of hemagglutinin and neuraminidase subtypes; this fact suggests the enormous potential for antigenic variation of the type A virus (Shortridge, 1982).

Variations in the main H and N antigens cause changes in the epidemiology and epizootiology of type A influenza (Kaplan, 1982). All type A viruses show variations over time, which can either be minor or signify the emergence of a new subtype. The study of these antigenic changes, as well as the possible role of animals in providing genetic material (or part of the material) for new human influenza subtypes, occupies a large part of the attention of investigators in this field who are trying to elucidate the emergence of pandemics due to new subtypes. Formerly, it was thought that types B and C were exclusively human. However, isolation of 15 strains of type C from swine has been reported in China and serologic studies indicate that this influenza virus type has been present in swine since 1979 (Laver *et al.*, 1984). Antigenic variations have been found in type B also, but they are not as marked or frequent as in type A. Type C, on the other hand, has stable antigenic characteristics.

Geographic Distribution: Worldwide.

Occurrence in Man: Influenza usually occurs in epidemic form and is characterized by high morbidity and low mortality. The largest epidemics and pandemics of this century (1918, 1957, 1968) were due to type A. Type B influenza generally causes less extensive epidemics at longer intervals than type A, while type C infection produces limited outbreaks or sporadic cases and a high incidence of subclinical cases.

During epidemics, the attack rate varies from less than 15 to 49%. During the 1957-1958 pandemic caused by Asian virus H2N2, in two months there were an estimated 70 million new cases in the USA and 5 million people were bedridden at some time during that period. In the USSR it was estimated that 30% of the total population was affected during the same epidemic. In institutions, such as schools, the attack rate frequently reached 70%. Although case fatality is generally low, mortality increases in relation to the expected nonepidemic rate. In the United States, there were approximately 62,000 excess deaths during the 1957-1958 pandemic and 27,900 from A/Hong Kong/68 (H3N2) in the 1968-1969 pandemic.

In temperate climates influenza occurs primarily in autumn and winter, extending into spring, while in the tropics it generally shows no seasonal relationship.

Occurrence in Animals: Influenza caused by type A virus occurs especially in swine, equines, and numerous species of wild and domestic birds.

SWINE: Swine influenza has been known since 1918 when it appeared in the midwestern United States. During the last 3 or 4 months of that year, millions of swine became ill and thousands died. The coincidence of this epizootic with the 1918-1919 pandemic (determined by serological methods to have been H1N1), during which 20 million persons died worldwide, and the similarity of symptoms observed in swine and man gave rise to the hypothesis that swine might have contracted the infection from man. However, some researchers support the opposite possibility, that is, that the human infection originated in swine (Kaplan, 1982). Retrospective serologic studies of elderly persons indicated that in 1918-1919 a virus similar to that of swine influenza was circulating in the human population. Since 1918-1919, outbreaks in swine due to subtype H1N1 (Hsw1N1) have occurred almost annually in the United States, and it is possible that this classic strain of swine influenza virus circulates all year in that country. Recent investigations indicate that there could be a low prevalence of this strain in several countries in the world and that the infection is probably enzootic in continental China, Hong Kong, and Singapore. A moderate antigenic variation has been observed between 1930 and 1977 in this type of swine influenza (Schild, 1981). Transmission of infection from man to swine is possible, as has been demonstrated in the last few years. During the human pandemic of 1968-1969 due to H3N2 virus, one strain was isolated from 139 pigs examined in December 1969 in Taiwan and 11 strains from 276 animals examined in January 1970. Serologic and virologic studies have confirmed the presence of this human subtype in swine in Hong Kong, the United States, and many other countries. The H3N2 viruses are very similar to the human prototype strain A/Hong Kong/68. Some studies have confirmed a high prevalence of antigenic variants of the H3N2 virus with low pathogenicity for swine. An interesting fact is that the virus could be isolated from swine in Hong Kong in 1976, several years after it had disappeared among humans. The isolation of the H3N2 virus from swine when it had ceased to circulate among the human population may indicate that it established itself in Asian swine and that this species might serve as reservoir with subsequent transmission to man (Shortridge *et al.*, 1977). Nevertheless, in other places, such as Hawaii (Wallace, 1979a) and Spain (Pérez Breña *et al.*, 1980), where infection of swine by human H3N2 virus occurred, it could not be confirmed that this subtype A strain had persisted in swine. In the human population, H3N2 virus underwent antigenic variations with respect to the prototype strain A/Hong Kong/68, but the human H3N2 strains that continued to circulate among swine were closer to the antigenic configuration of earlier strains than to human strains that emerged later. Oligonucleotide mapping confirmed that the A/swine/Hong Kong/3/76 virus was more similar to the early strains of A/Hong Kong/68 than to the H3N2 virus strains circulating in the human population in 1976. Notwithstanding, one of the strains isolated from swine (A/swine/Hong Kong/4/76) had an oligonucleotide map similar to a contemporary human strain. It was concluded that the A/swine/Hong Kong/3/76 strain represents a virus similar to the 1968 human one, which underwent genetic mutations without a pronounced change in its antigenicity while it circulated in the swine population (Nakajima *et al.*, 1982).

In 1979, during an epizootic outbreak of swine influenza in Belgium, it was possible to isolate a subtype H1N1 antigenically related to strain Hsw1N1 previously isolated from wild ducks, which would indicate that an avian virus can be transmitted to swine (Pensaert *et al.*, 1981).

Most outbreaks in the United States occur in autumn and extend through winter. The seasonal nature of the disease is attributed to stress produced by fluctuations in ambient temperature and changes in feed. In a given area, the disease appears simultaneously on many farms and affects practically all animals. These multi-centric outbreaks are generally not related to movement of pigs from one farm to another, which would indicate that the infection persists in the herd from one season to another, although the maintenance mechanism of the virus during the inter-epizootic periods is not known. In this respect, two hypotheses have been postulated: one maintains that the virus has as an intermediate host the nematode *Meta-strongylus elongatus*, a pulmonary parasite of swine; and the other holds that some recovered animals become carriers, maintaining and spreading the virus. At the present time, little importance is attributed to the role of the pulmonary parasites in the epizootiology of swine influenza, and the persistence of the virus has been confirmed in regions where the parasite does not exist (Wallace, 1979). Animals infected experimentally were able to transmit the virus to contacts up to 3 months after being inoculated. On the other hand, the classic swine influenza virus H1N1 (Hsw1N1) has been found to circulate all year, which contributes to its persistence.

HORSES: Equine influenza is caused by two different subtypes of type A. Subtype A/equine/Prague/1/56 (H7N7) or equine virus 1 was isolated in Czechoslovakia in 1956, and later in different parts of the world. The H antigen of equine virus 1 is antigenically related to the fowl plague virus (H7N7) and can protect birds against lethal doses. The second subtype, A/equine/Miami/1/63 (H3N8), was isolated for the first time in the United States during an epizootic which spread throughout that country, then to Canada, and in the same year to Uruguay and then Brazil. Two years after the beginning of the epizootic in the United States, this subtype appeared in Europe, causing large epizootics in Great Britain and France and spreading to Switzerland, and then passed to Japan.

The behavior of these viruses varies with the immunologic state and the density of the equine population, and also depends on other factors. When the virus affects a population that has had no previous experience with it, an explosive outbreak occurs, with attack rates of 60 to 90%. In populations which have suffered previous infections, the disease is observed only in young animals or in animals introduced from unaffected areas. Since its isolation in 1963, equine virus 2 has undergone a pronounced antigenic variation with respect to the prototype strain. In the 1978-1979 epizootic, horses vaccinated with antigen A/equine/Miami/63 were not protected against the acting equine virus (Van Oirschot *et al.*, 1981).

Both subtypes continue to cause outbreaks of equine influenza around the world, without A/eq-2 having displaced the previous subtype, as commonly occurs with human influenza viruses. Serologic studies have shown that between 1889 and 1895 human populations in the United States, Great Britain, and the Netherlands were affected by A/eq-2 virus or an antigenically similar virus. This subtype is also antigenically related to A/Hong Kong/1/68 (H3N2). In one study, human volunteers exposed to A/equine/Miami/1/63 fell ill, and the virus could be isolated during the first 6 days after infection; in 4 out of 15 persons virus was recovered up to the tenth day. Horses exposed to Hong Kong ("human") virus developed a mild febrile illness, and virus could be isolated up to 5 days after infection. It was not possible, however, to verify if these cross-infections occur naturally (Beveridge, 1977).

BIRDS: Numerous subtypes of virus A have been found in birds, suggesting great potential for development of antigenic recombinations. Influenza viruses have been isolated from domestic fowl (chickens, ducks, turkeys) and wild birds such as terns (*Sterna hirundo*), shearwaters (*Puffinus pacificus*), wild ducks, and other species. The etiologic agent of fowl plague is one of the influenza A viruses (H7N7). A strain similar to that of fowl plague has been isolated from a person. Outbreaks of influenza in birds generally have a focal nature. In 1983-1984, a severe influenza epizootic exploded in Pennsylvania, USA, and 11 million birds died or were sacrificed in three states. Additionally, 125,593 birds died in 10 establishments in Virginia. The appearance of this epizootic was surprising, as there had been only three cases of avian influenza in the United States since 1929 (Anon., 1984). The virus was identified as subtype H5N2 (International Office of Epizootics, 1983). The antigenic composition of avian viruses is not necessarily related to virulence, and even completely avirulent strains that are antigenically very closely related to those of fowl plague have been isolated (Schild, 1981; World Health Organization, 1981).

Since birds constitute a possible source for recombination of influenza virus because they harbor a great abundance of subtype genes, studies have been carried out in recent years on domestic and wild birds, and many strains have been isolated from numerous species in diverse parts of the world.

A characteristic feature of influenza in birds is that the virus multiplies both in the respiratory system and the intestine and is thus shed with the feces, contaminating the environment. Waterfowl, especially domestic and wild ducks, have aroused special interest. The virus can be isolated from the cloaca of these birds and from ponds where they swim. Clinical manifestations of influenza are seen in domestic ducks but have not been observed in wild ducks. In a study carried out over a 4-year period on domestic birds in southern China and Hong Kong, viruses with 46 different combinations of H and N subtypes were isolated, the majority (43) from ducks. The diversity of viruses in the duck population of this region can be explained by the large numbers of these birds that are produced for human consumption and the continuous oral-fecal transmission to young susceptible ducks in the small ponds. In addition, this zone is of great interest because it is a route for migratory birds that can introduce new antigenic combinations from different areas and because certain pandemic viruses seem to have originated there (Shortridge, 1982).

Viruses similar or identical to those of classic swine influenza (Hsw1N1) have been isolated recently from wild ducks (*Anas platyrhynchos*) in Germany and earlier in Canada, the United States, and Hong Kong. These viruses exhibit a difference in biological behavior related to their origin. The viruses isolated from wild ducks multiply both in the trachea and intestines of ducks, while those isolated from swine multiply only in the respiratory tract of these birds. It was possible to infect suckling pigs, via the nasal route and by cohabitation, with virus isolated from wild ducks in Germany and to reisolate the virus from the piglets, some of which displayed mild clinical symptomatology but no serologic conversion (Ottis and Bachman, 1980). On a property where both swine and birds were kept, serologic and epidemiologic evidence was obtained of infection of ducks with an agent related to the virus of classic swine influenza (Mohan *et al.*, 1981).

OTHER SPECIES: A virus A antigenically similar to H1N1 (Hsw1N1) of avian origin was isolated from Pacific Ocean whales (*Balaenoptera acutorostrata*) in the USSR. Antibodies for a human serotype have also been found in fur seals (*Callorhinus ursinus*). During the winter of 1979-1980 on the Cape Cod peninsula, USA, there was a die-off of harbor seals (*Phoca vitulina*); a virus similar to fowl plague virus (H7N7) was isolated from their lungs and brains. From the biologic point of view, the virus behaved more like a mammalian than an avian strain. In transmission experiments, the virus multiplied little in chicken and turkey chicks, did not cause disease, and could be isolated again only from the respiratory tract. On the other hand, it multiplied easily in ferrets, cats, and suckling pigs, but without causing clinical signs (Lang *et al.*, 1981; World Health Organization, 1981). The personnel in contact with the seals contracted conjunctivitis, and the virus was isolated from one of the members of the staff (Webster *et al.*, 1981).

The human virus A/Hong Kong/68 (H3N2) was isolated from dogs in the USSR and Taiwan. Antibodies for H3N2 and H1N1 have been found in dogs in Italy and several other countries (Buonavoglia and Sala, 1983).

The Disease in Man: The incubation period is from 1 to 2 days. The onset of the disease is sudden, with fever, chills, cephalalgia, myalgia, fatigue, and sometimes prostration. Common symptoms are conjunctival inflammation, intense lacrimation, nonproductive coughing, sneezing, and runny nose. The course of the disease is short, with recuperation in 2 to 7 days. Convalescence is generally rapid but coughing may persist for some time. In older persons, convalescence is more prolonged. The most common complications consist of secondary bacterial infections expressed as bronchitis and bronchopneumonia. These complications are more frequent in children and persons older than 50. In the periodic epidemics the pneumonic complications do not exceed 1% of the cases, but in some pandemics the rate of complications is much higher. The symptomatologies of influenza types A and B are similar. The infection caused by type C virus produces a milder disease with more pronounced coryza.

The Disease in Animals: The symptomatology is generally similar to that of human influenza.

In swine, the disease is characterized by sudden onset, loss of appetite, coughing, nasal and ocular secretions, dyspnea, fever, prostration, and rapid recuperation. Lesions in the respiratory apparatus develop and clear up rapidly, except in cases in which there are complications. Animals with antibodies may have an asymptomatic infection. The fatality rate when there are no complications is from 1 to 3%.

Equine influenza has an incubation period of 2 to 3 days. It is characterized by high fever, acute nasal catarrh with a serous discharge, coughing, dyspnea, and depression. The course is from 2 to 10 days and convalescence from 1 to 3 weeks. The disease is generally serious in young colts in which it causes viral pneumonia, often fatal. Mortality in adult horses is practically nil. Equine virus 2 (H3N8) generally produces a more severe disease than virus 1 (H7N7).

In seals the disease was characterized by pneumonia and high mortality (estimated at 20% of the affected population), but it is not known if other agents intervened in this pathology.

In birds, the effect of the infection caused by influenza viruses varies from a serious disease, such as fowl plague, to a mild or subclinical symptomatology. The recent epizootic (1983-1984) of subtype H5N2 avian influenza in the United States (see Occurrence in Animals) shows that fowl plague (H7N7) is not the only grippe subtype that can ravage domestic birds. The usual symptomatology consists of anorexia, decreased egg production, loss of egg pigment (especially in turkeys), and deformed eggs that sometimes lack a shell. Common signs are coughing, sneezing, lacrimation, sinusitis, facial edema, cyanosis, nervous disorders, and diarrhea. Mortality can be pronounced in chicks.

The infection in wild birds is usually subclinical. In South Africa, an outbreak with a high fatality rate occurred in terns *(Sterna hirundo)* in 1961.

Source of Infection and Mode of Transmission: Infection between humans occurs through direct contact by means of Flügge droplets that penetrate by way of the upper respiratory tract. The virus can also be transmitted by objects recently contaminated by secretions from an infected person. Closed or crowded locations facilitate transmission. The infection confers immunity for the specific subtype. The resistance acquired is generally lower, less strictly specific, and shorter-lasting in children than in adults. With increased age and successive exposures to antigenically related viruses, the immunologic base broadens. A community that has experienced a large outbreak almost always has a low incidence of influenza of the same subtype for some 3 or 4 years.

One of the most notable features and the one that most seriously affects the epidemiology of human influenza is the change in antigenic composition of the virus and the appearance of new subtypes or variants within subtypes. Two kinds of variations can be differentiated: a minor and gradual change (drift), which the viruses undergo with the passage of time from their first appearance, without essential changes in the subtype; and a major change (shift), which involves the substitution of one or both surface antigens (H and N). The most pronounced variation has been observed in type A, and the most widespread epidemics and pandemics occurred as a result of the emergence of new subtypes. The H1N1 virus was prevalent from the time of its identification in 1933 until 1956. In 1957, a completely new subtype arose, with composition H2N2; it replaced the former subtype and caused the pandemic of Asian influenza. This subtype was active until 1967. In 1968 another subtype, A/Hong Kong/68 (H3N2), arose which also caused a pandemic. Then, in 1977, subtype H1N1 reappeared after 20 years. These sudden changes allow influenza virus A to expand rapidly, since the human population lacks antibodies for the new subtypes. In the case of the reappearance of H1N1, the epidemic affected primarily children and adolescents, who had no prior experience with this subtype. A minor variant of Hong Kong virus (H3N2) was also active in 1977 and both subtypes could be isolated in the same community. Another minor variant of H3N2 (A/Bangkok/79) and a variant of H1N1 (A/Brazil/78) continued originating outbreaks in 1981. Until then, simultaneous activity of two subtypes had not occurred (Stuart-Harris, 1981). The minor variations (drift) can be explained by passage of virus through partially immune populations. The greater problem is posed in explaining the origin of sudden changes (shift), which involve total replacement of one or both surface antigens and the appearance of a new subtype. There are two hypotheses in that respect: one proposes that the new antigenic subtypes arise by mutation, due to pressure caused by acquired immunity in the population; the other suggests that the new pandemic strains arise by recombination of preexisting human and animal strains. The second hypothesis is receiving increasing support because it has been found experimentally that subtypes from various hosts easily recombine when cultured together in chick embryo or in animal hosts (swine or turkeys) under simulated natural conditions. The accumulated evidence points to fowl as possible primitive hosts of virus A and the principal laboratory for genetic recombinations that form variants. In this respect, the large number of virus A subtypes that have been isolated from birds and the fact that all of the antigens of the mammalian strains are present in the avian subtypes should be borne in mind. It is also thought that mammals, especially swine, can be involved in these recombinations. By contrast, the mutation hypothesis has lost popularity since the discovery that the A/Hong Kong/68 (H3N2) strain had a hemagglutinating (H) antigen completely distinct from the strains immediately preceding the 1968 pandemic; it is difficult to believe that such a radical change could have occurred in a single mutation. The advocates of the recombination hypothesis are inclined to believe that the new virus type arose as a hybrid of a human strain and an animal strain; the neuraminidase would have been contributed by an old Asian strain from man and the hemagglutinin by an animal strain; it should be remembered that each subtype is composed of a combination of one of the nine N antigens (neuraminidase) and one of the 12 H antigens (hemagglutinin). The possibility that animals contribute to the common genetic fund of the human virus A is supported by the fact that sudden changes in the surface antigens do not happen in the type B human virus, which has no counterparts in the lower animals (Stuart-Harris, 1981). One of the major objections of the hypothesis of recombination of human and animal viruses was that human viruses are infrequently transmitted to animals and transmission from animals to man rarely occurs (Kilbourne, 1978). Presently, this objection is held to be less valid owing to confirmation of Hong Kong virus (H3N2) in swine, bovines, dogs, and birds in various parts of the world after the human pandemic of 1968. It is true that transmission from animals to man occurs with low frequency and, when it does happen, originates few if any secondary cases. The species-specific barrier is not strict and, as indicated above, an avian strain caused an epidemic outbreak in marine mammals (in seals in the United States and whales in the Pacific Ocean). Many questions are still unresolved. Under the auspices of the World Health Organization, intensive studies are being carried out to elucidate this problem, which is of undoubted importance in epidemiology and prevention.

Given the role that influenza virus A from lower mammals and birds may have in the origin of pandemic human subtypes, it is important to briefly summarize the cases of transmission of animal viruses to man. In Minnesota and Wisconsin, USA, sporadic cases of influenza have been confirmed since 1974 in persons who were in contact with swine, and the viruses isolated were identified as Hsw1N1 of classic swine influenza. In all these episodes, human secondary cases were infrequent (Easterday, 1978). Human infections by a virus similar to swine influenza virus also occur in persons without known contact with swine or turkeys. A recent case occurred in 1982 in an immunosuppressed girl with acute lymphoblastic leukemia, who died of fulminating pneumonia and from whom a virus with a close antigenic relationship to A/New Jersey/8/76 (H1N1) was isolated (see below). Although five of 47 members of the hospital staff had elevated titers for this virus, this might represent an anamnestic or heterotypic response to other H1N1 viruses. At any rate, interhuman transmission of the swine virus seems to be limited and, in its current state, this agent has low potential for causing epidemic outbreaks in man (Patriarca *et al.*, 1984).

An influenza outbreak on the military base at Fort Dix, New Jersey, USA, caused alarm when a virus with characteristics of the swine influenza A/New Jersey/8/76 (Hsw1N1) was isolated from several recruits. The cause of worry was that the 1918 pandemic with numerous deaths had been attributed to a similar subtype, which many researchers related to swine. Interhuman transmission of this strain was rather limited. An epidemiologic study confirmed that 500 people out of the 12,000 on the military base had been infected with the swine strain; this is a low rate considering that the recruits, because of their age, could not have had antibodies against epidemic subtype H1N1. The virus's period of activity was also limited and lasted less than 5 weeks, while virus A/Victoria/3/75 (H3N2), a variant of the Hong Kong strain which circulated simultaneously at the base, continued active. The initial source of the swine virus infection, which caused almost 10% of the influenza cases registered at the military base, could not be confirmed. The importance of this episode lies in the confirmation for the first time that the swine virus can propagate man-to-man without the need for direct exposure to infected pigs. In the United States, antibodies for the swine influenza virus or a similar one have been found in persons older than 50 years of age, which suggests that, until 1930, antigenically similar viruses were prevalent in the human population. There are also indications that more recent infections with swine virus may have occurred among persons in frequent contact with swine.

The episode of transmission from seals to man (see Occurrence in Animals) of a virus similar to fowl plague (H7N7) likewise demonstrates that in certain circumstances the influenza agent can cross species barriers. In addition, a virus similar to that of fowl plague was isolated from the blood of a patient with hepatitis.

Influenza among animals also spreads by aerosols, through direct or indirect contact. Although epizootics are generally seasonal, it is thought that these viruses, like those of human influenza, are active throughout the year, producing sporadic cases that are usually not diagnosed. A short-term carrier state has been confirmed experimentally in swine, but more studies on animal species are necessary. Among birds the virus can be transmitted by aerosols and the fecal-oral route.

Role of Animals in the Epidemiology of the Disease: Although the role of viruses from lower mammals and birds in the genesis of human strains has not been confirmed, many researchers tend to accept this hypothesis.

Influenza fits the definition of zoonosis proposed by the World Health Organization, though the known cases of infection by "animal" viruses transmitted to man by lower mammals and birds are few. Reverse transmission, from man to animals, also occurs.

Diagnosis: During an epidemic, diagnosis is generally based on the clinical picture. Cases that may occur in interepidemic periods are rarely diagnosed. Laboratory confirmation is obtained by isolation of the virus; for this purpose chick embryos and cell cultures are inoculated with washings or swabs taken from the throat and nose during the first days of illness. Various serologic techniques are used to identify and classify the virus. Serologic diagnosis is made by showing an increase (fourfold or more) in the antibody titer between samples obtained in the acute and convalescent phases. Hemagglutination inhibition, complement fixation, and serum neutralization tests can be used.

Control: Preventive measures include protecting persons at higher risk, such as the elderly and chronic lung, heart, kidney, or metabolic deficiency patients, by vaccination. The degree of protection conferred by inactivated vaccines depends on their potency and whether their antigenic components, do or do not correspond to the viruses involved in the epidemic. Attenuated live virus vaccines are being studied for wide-scale use in the face of a pandemic in some part of the world that would allow sufficient time for the advance preparation and application of the vaccine before the arrival of the epidemic wave.

Crowds should be avoided during epidemics.

Physicians should report cases of influenza to the national authorities who, in turn, should report them to the World Health Organization.

For the protection of horses, an inactivated bivalent vaccine (A/eq-1 and A/eq-2) is available. Horses should be vaccinated with two doses, spaced 6 to 12 weeks apart, and receive a booster every year.

Vaccines against swine influenza have been used successfully in Czechoslovakia.

Bibliography

Andrewes, C., and H. G. Pereira. *Viruses of Vertebrates,* 3rd ed. Baltimore, Maryland, Williams and Wilkins, 1972.

Anon. Avian influenza outlook improving. *J Am Vet Med Assoc* 184:629-630, 1984.

American Public Health Association. *Control of Communicable Diseases in Man,* 14th ed. (Ed. by A. S. Benenson). Washington, D.C., APHA, 1985.

Arikava, J. Ecological studies of influenza virus infection among humans, ducks and swine. *Jpn J Vet Res* 33:153-158, 1985.

Beare, A. S. Live viruses for immunization against influenza. *Progr Med Virol* 20:49-83, 1975.

Beveridge, W. I. B. The origin of influenza pandemics. Geneva. *WHO Chronicle* 29:471-473, 1975.

Beveridge, W. I. B. *Influenza: The Last Great Plague.* London, Heinemann, 1977.

Bibrack, B. Vergleichende serologische Untersuchungen uber das Vorkommen von Schweine-influenza und Influenza A2/Hong Kong-Infektionen bei Schweinen in Bayern. *Zentralbl Veterinarmed* 19:397-405, 1972.

Bryans, J. T., E. R. Doll, J. C. Wilson, and W. H. McCollum. Immunization for equine influenza. *J Am Vet Med Assoc* 148:413-417, 1966.

Buonavoglia, C., and V. Sala. Indagini sierological in cani sulla presenza di anticorpi verso ceppi di virus influenzali humani tipo A. *Clin Vet (Milan)* 106:81-83, 1983.

Centers for Disease Control of the USA. Influenza—United States. *Morb Mortal Wkly Rep* 25:47-48, 1976.

Clements, M. L., M. H. Snyder, A. J. Buckler-White, E. L. Tierney, W. T. London, and B. R. Murphy. Evaluation of avian-human reassortant influenza A/Washington/897/80 x A/Pintail/119/79 virus in monkeys and adult volunteers. *J Clin Microbiol* 24:47-51, 1986.

Davenport, F. M. Influenza viruses. *In:* A. S. Evans (Ed.), *Viral Infections of Humans. Epidemiology and Control.* New York, Plenum, 1976.

Deibel, R., D. F. Emord, W. Dukelow, V. S. Hinshaw, and J. M. Wood. Influenza viruses and paramyxoviruses in ducks in the Atlantic flyway, 1977-1983, including an H5N2 isolate related to the virulent chicken virus. *Avian Dis* 29:970-985, 1985.

Easterday, B. C. Swine influenza. *In:* Dunne, H. W. (Ed.), *Diseases of Swine,* 3rd ed. Ames, Iowa State University Press, 1970.

Easterday, B. C. Influenza. *In:* Hubbert, W. T., W. F. McCulloch, and P. R. Schnurren-berger (Eds.), *Diseases Transmitted from Animals to Man,* 6th ed. Springfield, Illinois, Thomas, 1975.

Easterday, B. C. The enigma of zoonotic influenza. *Proceedings, 3rd Munich Symposium on Microbiology,* Munich, 1978.

Francis, T., and H. F. Maassab. Influenza viruses. *In:* Horsfall, F. L., and I. Tamm (Eds.), *Viral and Rickettsial Infections of Man,* 4th ed. Philadelphia, Lippincott, 1965.

Haesebrouck, F., P. Biront, M. B. Pensaert, and J. Leunen. Epizootics of respiratory tract disease in swine in Belgium due to H3N2 influenza virus and experimental reproduction of the disease. *Am J Vet Res* 46:1926-1928, 1985.

Harkness, J. W., G. C. Schild, P. H. Lamont, and C. M. Brand. Studies on relationships between human and porcine influenza. I. Serological evidence of infection in swine in Great Britain with an influenza A virus antigenically like human Hong Kong/68 virus. *Bull WHO* 46:709-719, 1972.

International Office of Epizootics. Otras enfermedades. *Bull OIE* 95:30-32, 1983.

Kaplan, M., and W. I. B. Beveridge. WHO coordinated research on the role of animals in influenza epidemiology. *Bull WHO* 47:439-443, 1972.

Kaplan, M. The epidemiology of influenza as a zoonosis. *Vet Rec* 110:395-399, 1982.

Kilbourne, E. D. Pandemic influenza: molecular and ecological determinants. *In:* Kurstak, E., and K. Marmoresch (Eds.), *Viruses and Environment.* New York, Academic Press, 1978.

Kundin, W. D. Hong Kong A2 influenza infection among swine during a human epidemic in Taiwan. *Nature* 228:857, 1970.

Lang, G., A. Gagnon, and J. R. Geraci. Isolation of an influenza A virus from seals. *Arch Virol* 68:189-195, 1981.

Laver, W. G., R. G. Webster, and C. M. Chu. Summary of a meeting on the origin of pandemic influenza viruses. *J Infect Dis* 149:108-115, 1984.

McQueen, J. L., J. H. Steele, and R. Q. Robinson. Influenza in animals. *Adv Vet Sci* 12:285-336, 1968.

Mohan, R., Y. M. Saif, G. A. Ericson, G. A. Gustafson, and B. C. Easterday. Serologic and epidemiologic evidence of infection in turkeys with an agent related to the swine influenza virus. *Avian Dis* 25:11-16, 1981.

Nakajima, K., S. Nakajima, K. F. Shortridge, and A. P. Kendal. Further genetic evidence for maintenance of early Hong Kong-like influenza A (H3N2) strains in swine until 1976. *Virology* 116:562-572, 1982.

Nascimento, J. P., M. M. Krawczuk, L. F. Marcopito, and R. G. Baruzzi. Prevalence of antibody against influenza A viruses in the Kren-Akorore, an Indian tribe of Central Brazil, first contacted in 1973. *J Hyg (Camb)* 95:159-164, 1985.

Nerome, K., Y. Yoshioka, S. Sakamoto, H. Yasuhara, and A. Dya. Characterization of a 1980-swine recombinant influenza virus possessing H1 hemagglutinin and N2 neuraminidase similar to that of the earliest Hong Kong (H3N2) virus. *Arch Virol* 86:197-211, 1985.

Ottis, K., and P. A. Bachman. Occurrence of Hsw1N1 subtype influenza A viruses in wild ducks in Europe. *Arch Virol* 63:185-190, 1980.

Patriarca, P. A., A. P. Kendal, P. C. Zakowski, N. J. Cox, M. S. Trautman, J. D. Cherry, D. M. Auerbach, J. McCusker, R. R. Belliveau, and K. D. Kappus. Lack of significant person-to-person spread of swine influenza-like virus following fatal infection in an immunocompromised child. *Am J Epidemiol* 119:152-158, 1984.

Pensaert, M. B., and F. Haesebrouck. Les virus influenza chez le pork: un problème pour l'animal et l'homme. *Ann Med Vet* 130:295-298, 1986.

Pensaert, M., K. Ottis, J. Vandeputte, M. M. Kaplan, and P. A. Bachman. Evidence for the natural transmission of influenza A from wild ducks to swine and its potential importance for man. *Bull WHO* 59:75-78, 1981.

Pérez Breña, M. P., C. López Galindez, A. Llácar, E. Nájera, E. Valle, and R. Nájera. Estudio sero-epidemiológico en la especie humana y en cerdos de la nueva cepa de influenza de tipo porcino. *Bol Of Sanit Panam* 88:146-154, 1980.

Profeta, M. L., and G. Palladino. Serological evidence of human infections with avian influenza viruses. *Arch Virol* 90:355-360, 1986.

Robinson, R. Q., and W. R. Dowdle. Influenza-A global problem: *In:* Sanders, M., and M. Schaeffer (Eds.), *Viruses Affecting Man and Animals.* St. Louis, Missouri, Green, 1971.

Schild, G. C. Influenza infections in lower mammals and birds. *In:* Kurstak, E., and C. Kurstak, *Comparative Diagnosis of Viral Diseases,* vol. 4. New York, Academic Press, 1981.

Schild, G. C., C. M. Brand, J. W. Harkness, and P. H. Lamont. Studies on relationships between human and porcine influenza. 2. Immunological comparisons of human A/Hong Kong/68 virus with influenza A viruses of porcine origin. *Bull WHO* 46:721-728, 1972.

Shortridge, K. F., R. G. Webster, W. K. Butterfield, and C. H. Campbell. Persistence of Hong Kong influenza virus variants in pigs. *Science* 196:1454-1455, 1977.

Shortridge, K. F. Avian influenza A viruses of southern China and Hong Kong: ecological aspects and implications for man. *Bull WHO* 60:129-135, 1982.

Stuart Harris, C. Virus of the 1918 influenza pandemic. *Nature* 225:850-851, 1970.

Stuart Harris, C. The epidemiology and prevention of influenza. *Am Sci* 69:166-172, 1981.

Tumova, B., and G. C. Schild. Antigenic relationships between type A influenza viruses of human, porcine, equine and avian origin. *Bull WHO* 47:453-460, 1972.

Van Oirschot, J. T., N. Masurel, A. D. N. H. J. Huffels, and W. J. J. Anker. Equine influenza in the Netherlands during winter of 1978-1979; antigenic drift of the A-equi 2 virus. *Vet Q* 3:80-84, 1981.

Wallace, G. D. Natural history of influenza in swine in Hawaii: swine influenza virus Hsw1N1 in herds not infected with lungworms. *Am J Vet Res* 40:1159-1164, 1979.

Wallace, G. D. Natural history of influenza in swine in Hawaii: prevalence of infection with A/Hong Kong/68 (H3N2) subtype virus and its variants, 1974-1977. *Am J Vet Res* 40:1165-1168, 1979.

Webster, R. G., and W. G. Laver. Antigenic variation of influenza viruses. *In:* Kilbourne, E. D. (Ed.), *The Influenza Viruses.* New York, Academic Press, 1975.

Webster, R. G., W. G. Laver, and B. Tumova. Studies on the origin of pandemic influenza viruses. V. Persistence of Asian influenza virus hemagglutinin (H2) antigen in nature. *Virology* 67:534-543, 1975.

Webster, R. G., J. R. Geraci, G. Petursson, and K. Skirnisson. Conjunctivitis in humans exposed to seals infected with an influenza A virus. *N Engl J Med* 304:911, 1981.

World Health Organization. Révision du systéme de nomenclature des virus grippaux: Memorandum. *Bull OMS* 58:877-883, 1980.

World Health Organization. The ecology of influenza viruses: a WHO memorandum. *Bull WHO* 59:869-873, 1981.

World Health Organization. Influenza in the world, 1985-86. *Wkly Epidemiol Rec* 62(5):21-23, 1987.

JAPANESE B ENCEPHALITIS

(062.0)

Synonym: Japanese encephalitis type B.

Etiology: RNA virus belonging to the genus *Flavivirus* (formerly group B of the arboviruses) of the family Togaviridae; it forms part of the complex of viruses that produce St. Louis, Murray Valley, Rocio, and West Nile encephalitides.

Geographic Distribution: The infection is widespread in large parts of Asia: the maritime provinces of the Soviet Far East, China, Taiwan, Japan, the Philippines, Vietnam, Laos, Burma, Korea, Malaysia, Okinawa, Singapore, Thailand, Indonesia, Sri Lanka, and India.

Occurrence in Man: Japanese B encephalitis (JE) occurs endemically in man in tropical areas; clinical cases are seen sporadically all year and epidemic outbreaks occur during the rainy season. In countries with temperate climates, the disease is epidemic and seasonal, occurring in late summer and early autumn. It used to recur annually in Japan with an incidence that varied from small outbreaks to more than 8,000 cases per year. During the serious epidemic of 1958, there were 5,700 clinical cases with 1,322 deaths in Korea; 1,800 cases with 519 deaths in Japan; and 142 cases with 50 deaths in Taiwan. In Japan, a substantial decrease in the incidence of human cases has been seen in the last few years and, currently, less than 100 cases occur annually. In the Republic of Korea, in spite of 80% vaccination coverage of schoolchildren, an epidemic in 1982 in the southwest part of the country produced 1,179 serologically confirmed cases. There are 10,000 cases annually in China with a 10% fatality rate, and 3,000 to 4,000 annual cases in India; there were 2,143 cases in Thailand in 1980 and 843 cases in Nepal in 1982; and in Burma less than 100 cases occur annually (World Health Organization, 1984).

The most affected age group, according to data from China (Huang, 1982), is 3 to 6 years of age. Later, the morbidity rate decreases as a consequence of immunity acquired by both apparent and inapparent infections. Most human infections are clinically inapparent. According to seroepidemiologic studies, one clinical case is recognized for every 500 to 1,000 infected individuals. In some epidemics, however, the ratio of clinical to inapparent cases has been 1:25 in adults.

Occurrence in Animals: In the periods immediately preceding epidemics, the infection in swine reaches extremely high rates. Infected pigs are the principal source for virus amplification as this species is the most abundant domestic animal in some areas of Asia, such as Japan and Taiwan. Porcine infection also constitutes a serious economic problem because of the neonatal mortality it causes in that species. High antibody levels have also been found in equines, cattle, and various species of wild and domestic fowl. In China, a proportion of more than 20% reactors has been found in ducks.

The Disease in Man: The course of the disease is generally subclinical. There are also indications that in an undetermined proportion of cases this infection may cause mild systemic disease without neurologic symptomatology. The clinical form most often seen is encephalitis, with the fatality rate ranging between 20 and 50%. The incubation period is from 4 to 14 or more days. The disease is generally of rapid onset, with hyperpyrexia, severe cephalalgia, vomiting, and cerebral and meningeal manifestations such as stiffness of the neck, convulsions (in children), confusion, disorientation, delirium, paresis, and paralysis. Convalescence is prolonged, and psychic and motor sequelae are frequent. In fatal cases, death occurs within the first 10 days of the disease.

The variability of the clinical picture could be due to differences in pathogenicity of the different strains of the JE virus (Huang, 1982).

The Disease in Animals: In several Asian countries the infection causes considerable losses because of the high rate of abortion and neonatal mortality in swine. In Japan, during the 1947-1949 epidemic, some regions recorded an abortion or neonatal mortality rate in swine of 50 to 70%. The fetuses are often mummified and hydrocephalic. Infected adult pigs either manifest no clinical symptoms or suffer a brief febrile illness. The virus can be eliminated in semen, as was proven by experimental inoculation of the virus into boars. Although signs of encephalitis have occasionally been noted in suckling pigs under 3 months of age, the most prominent disease features are abortion and neonatal death.

In equines the infection is generally inapparent, but some clinical cases occur each year. For the period from 1948 to 1967, morbidity in the endemic areas of Asia has been estimated at 44.8 per 100,000 equines; in Japan, during the great epidemic of 1948, it reached 337.1 per 100,000. Studies of some outbreaks indicate that case fatality can be as high as 25%. Clinical manifestations consist of pyrexia, depression, photophobia, muscular tremors, incoordination, and ataxia.

Morbidity in cattle, goats, and sheep is low.

Source of Infection and Mode of Transmission (Figure 39): In Japan, China, and several other countries, *Culex tritaeniorhynchus* is the most important vector in the transmission of the virus to wild birds as well as to swine and cattle. The same vector transmits the infection to man. This mosquito reproduces in rice fields and in natural bodies of fresh water. It has a predilection for the blood of domestic animals, birds, and, to a lesser extent, man. It is most active at twilight and does not enter dwellings, a fact which leads to limited morbidity in children under 3 years of age, who are generally indoors after sunset (Huang, 1982). The virus has been isolated very frequently from this mosquito. In some regions of Asia, other culicid mosquitoes play an important role as vectors.

Antibodies against the Japanese encephalitis virus have been detected in various species of wild and domestic birds. Among the wild fauna, ardeid birds appear to play an important role as hosts of the virus, since the agent has been isolated from night-herons (*Nycticorax nycticorax*) and from two species of *Egretta*.

Figure 39. Japanese B encephalitis. Transmission cycle.

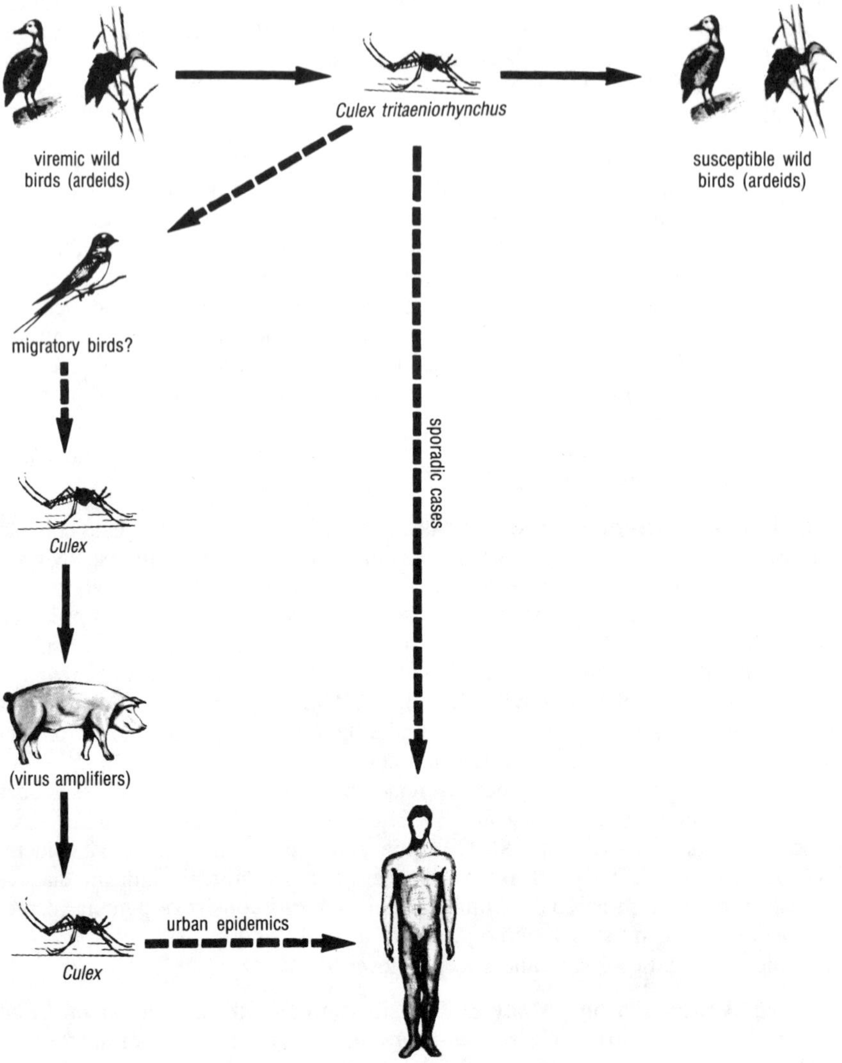

Swine play a very important role as amplifiers of the virus, since these animals are abundant in the countries affected, are prolific, have a short lifespan, and can therefore continuously provide susceptible generations. Pigs attract the vector; their viremia lasts for 2 to 4 days, which allows for infection of the mosquitoes. From the ecologic point of view, equines and cattle are not very important due to their low levels of viremia and their relatively long life spans.

The infection is probably spread from rural to urban areas by migrating viremic birds.

Epidemiologic studies carried out in Japan suggest a direct relationship between the rate of positive serologic reactors in swine and the ocurrence of epidemics in rural residents. In 1963, in one study area, antibodies were detected in only 5% of the pigs, and only three human cases were seen in a population of 1.8 million inhabitants. In 1964, by contrast, all the swine examined in the area were found to be seropositive and one of the largest epidemics of the last 10 years occurred. The infection rate of mosquitoes (*C. tritaeniorhynchus*) is higher near places where swine are raised; in epidemic years it may reach 2% or more. In addition, a positive correlation exists between vector density and epidemics (Maeda *et al.*, 1978).

Infection in swine (with an epidemiologic level sufficient to infect mosquitoes) precedes human infection by about 18 days. This period includes 4 days of viremia in the swine and 14 days incubation of the virus in the vectors.

The continuous activity of the vectors in tropical countries explains the presence of JE throughout all seasons of the year, as well as its endemicity. By contrast, the seasonal activity of the vectors in temperate areas determines the periodicity of epidemic outbreaks. The survival mechanism of the virus during winter in temperate climates is not as yet precisely understood. A study carried out from 1963 to 1965 on bats in the principal geographic regions of Japan demonstrated persistent infection in populations of these mammals throughout the year, thus providing a possible overwintering mechanism for the virus. Lizards were infected experimentally by *Culex pipiens pallens*, and the behavior of the virus was observed during a simulated hibernation. Upon coming out of hibernation, the lizards were viremic for several weeks. Lizards (*Eumeces latiscutatus*) captured in the field showed a reactivity rate of 14.3% to the hemagglutination inhibition test, but it was not possible to isolate the virus. To confirm the role of lizards in maintaining the virus during winter in temperate climates, it is necessary to demonstrate that this mechanism operates in the natural ecosystem (Doi *et al.*, 1983).

In tropical countries, the mechanism for maintenance of the agent consists of its continuous transmission between mosquitoes, swine, and birds (Monath and Trent, 1981). Transovarial transmission has been demonstrated experimentally in *C. tritaeniorhynchus*, but has not yet been confirmed in nature.

Diagnosis: The etiologic agent can be isolated from brain tissue of dead humans or animals and from swine fetuses. The virus has been on occasion isolated from blood and cerebrospinal fluid. In human patients, diagnosis is based primarily on demonstrating serologic conversion by the use of hemagglutination inhibition (HI), neutralization (N), and complement fixation (CF) tests on samples obtained during the acute and convalescent phases of the disease. The HI antibodies appear early in the disease; the increase in CF antibodies occurs during the third or fourth week, and some patients never react to the CF test. Detection of specific IgM antibodies to the JE virus with the HI test eliminates cross-reactions with St. Louis, West Nile, or Murray Valley viruses (Gatus and Rose, 1983).

A solid-phase antibody-capture radioimmunoassay has recently been described for human patients (Burke and Nisalak, 1982).

Control: Control measures are based on vaccination. For human protection, an inactivated tissue culture vaccine is used; recently, a modified live virus vaccine has been developed in China and Japan and has given satisfactory results. The use of live vaccines makes multiple vaccinations unnecessary.

Vaccination of swine has great importance from both the public health and economic standpoints. It serves to prevent viremia in swine and subsequent virus amplification as well as abortions and neonatal mortality. An inactivated vaccine and, more recently, a modified live virus vaccine have been used with satisfactory results.

Protection of horses is based on similar measures.

The reduction of human and animal morbidity rates in China and Japan is attributed to mass vaccination of humans and swine and to local use of insecticides.

Bibliography

Andrewes, C., and H. G. Pereira. *Viruses of Vertebrates*, 3rd ed. Baltimore, Maryland, Williams and Wilkins, 1972.

Burke, D. S., and A. Nisalak. Detection of Japanese encephalitis virus immunoglobulin M antibodies in serum by antibody capture radioimmunoassay. *J Clin Microbiol* 15:353-361, 1982.

Buescher, E. L., and W. F. Scherer. Ecologic studies of Japanese encephalitis virus in Japan. IX. Epidemiologic correlation and conclusions. *Am J Trop Med Hyg* 8:719-722, 1959.

Centers for Disease Control of the USA. *International Catalogue of Arboviruses*, 2nd ed. Berge, T. O. (Ed.). Atlanta, Georgia, 1975. (DHEW Publ. CDC 75-8301.)

Clarke, D. H., and J. Casals. Arboviruses: Group B. *In*: Horsfall, F. L., and I. Tamm (Eds.), *Viral and Rickettsial Infections of Man*, 4th ed. Philadelphia, Lippincott, 1965.

Doi, R., A. Oya, A. Shirasaka, S. Yabe, and M. Sasa. Studies on Japanese encephalitis virus infection in reptiles. II. Role of lizards on hibernation of Japanese encephalitis virus. *Jpn J Exp Med* 53:125-134, 1983.

Downs, W. G. Arboviruses. *In*: A. S. Evans (Ed.), *Viral Infections of Humans. Epidemiology and Control*. New York, Plenum, 1976.

Fujisaki, Y., T. Sugimori, T. Morimoto, Y. Miura, Y. Kawakami, and K. Nakano. Immunization of pigs with the attenuated S-strain of Japanese encephalitis virus. *Nat Inst Anim Health Q* 15:55-60, 1975.

Gatus, B. J., and M. R. Rose. Japanese B encephalitis: epidemiological, clinical and pathological aspects. *J Infect* 6:213-218, 1983.

Goto, H., K. Shimzu, and T. Shirahata. Studies on Japanese encephalitis of animals in Hokkaido. I. Epidemiological observation on horses. *Res Bull Obihiro Univ* 6:1-8, 1969.

Hsu, S. T., L. C. Chang, S. Y. Lin, T. Y. Chuang, C. H. Ma, K. Inoue, and T. Okuno. The effect of vaccination with a live attenuated strain of Japanese encephalitis virus on still births in swine in Taiwan. *Bull WHO* 46:465-471, 1972.

Huang, C. H. Studies of Japanese encephalitis in China. *Adv Virus Res* 27:72-101, 1982.

Inoue, Y. K. An attenuated Japanese encephalitis vaccine. *Progr Med Virol* 19:247-256, 1975.

Kodama, K., N. Sasaki, and Y. K. Inoue. Studies of live attenuated Japanese encephalitis vaccine in swine. *J Immunol* 100:194-200, 1968.

Konishi, E., and M. Yamaoka. Evaluation of enzyme-linked immunosorbent assay for quantitation of antibodies to Japanese encephalitis virus in swine sera. *J Virol Methods* 5:247-253, 1952.

Konno, J., K. Endo, H. Agatsuma, and N. Ishida. Cyclic outbreaks of Japanese encephalitis among pigs and humans. *Am J Epidemiol* 84:292-300, 1966.

Maeda, O., T. Karaki, A. Kuroda, Y. Karoji, O. Sasaki, and K. Takenokuma. Epidemiological studies of Japanese encephalitis in Kyoto city area, Japan. *Jpn J Med Sci Biol* 31:39-51, 1978.

McIntosh, B. M., and J. H. S. Gear. Mosquito-borne arboviruses primarily in the eastern hemisphere. *In*: Hubbert, W. T., W. F. McCulloch, and P. R. Schnurrenberger (Eds.),

Diseases Transmitted from Animals to Man, 6th ed. Springfield, Illinois, Thomas, 1975.

Monath, T. P., and D. W. Trent. Togaviral diseases of domestic animals. *In*: Kurstak, E., and C. Kurstak (Eds.), *Comparative Diagnosis of Viral Diseases*, vol. 2. New York, Academic Press, 1981.

Ochi, Y. L'encéphalite japonaise des porcs. *Bull Off Int Epizoot* 40:504-517, 1953.

Rosen, L. The natural history of Japanese encephalitis virus. *Annu Rev Microbiol* 40:395-414, 1986.

Sulkin, S. E., R. Allen, T. Miura, and K. Toyokawa. Studies on arthropod-borne virus infections in Chiroptera. VI. Isolation of Japanese B encephalitis virus from naturally infected bats. *Am J Trop Med Hyg* 19:77-87, 1970.

Umenai, T., R. Krzysko, T. A. Bektimirov, and F. A. Assad. Encéphalite japonaise: la situation actuelle dans le monde. *Bull WHO* 64:15-21, 1986.

World Health Organization. *Report of a Working Group on the Prevention and Control of Japanese Encephalitis*. Tokyo, 19-21 December 1983, Regional Office for the Western Pacific of the World Health Organization, Manila, 1984.

World Health Organization. Japanese encephalitis. *Wkly Epidemiol Rec* 61(11):82, 1986.

KYASANUR FOREST DISEASE

(065.2)

Etiology: RNA virus, genus *Flavivirus* (formerly group B of the arboviruses), family Togaviridae; belongs to the Russian spring-summer encephalitis and ovine encephalomyelitis complex of tick-borne viruses.

Geographic Distribution: The virus has been isolated only in Mysore, India, but some serologic studies indicate that other foci of activity of the virus exist in that country outside the Mysore area.

Occurrence in Man and Animals: The disease was first recognized in 1957 during an epidemic in Mysore, India, accompanied by mortality in two species of monkeys (*Presbytis entellus* and *Macaca radiata*). In this outbreak, 466 human cases were recorded, and the following year, 181. Not all of the cases were laboratory-confirmed, and some of them might have had a different etiology. Such was the case in the outbreak in 1959, when the virus was confirmed by isolation or by serologic methods in only 13 of 28 persons with a presumptive diagnosis of the disease.

In the Mysore endemic area human cases occur every year but the number of cases varies greatly, fluctuating from five cases in 1961 to 226 in 1975. A statistically significant correlation has been found between the intensity of infection in the main vector, *Haemaphysalis spinigera*, and the number of human cases in the different years (Banerjee and Bhat, 1977).

Clinically inapparent infection occurs in man as well as in nonhuman primates.

The Disease in Man: The incubation period is about 8 days. The disease has a sudden onset with fever, cephalalgia, myalgia, anorexia, and insomnia. Leukopenia is common. Less frequent symptoms are coughing and abdominal pain. Local hemorrhage was sometimes observed in the original outbreaks but was absent in later cases. Bradycardia and hypotension are prominent symptoms. The fever lasts from 6 to 11 days. Following an afebrile period of 9 to 21 days, a large proportion of cases displayed a second phase of pyrexia, which lasted for 2 to 12 days and generally included neurologic symptoms such as stiffness of the neck, mental confusion, tremors, and abnormal reflexes. Gastrointestinal and bronchial problems are common. Convalescence is prolonged. Case fatality is about 5%.

Source of Infection and Mode of Transmission: Kyasanur forest disease emerged as a result of increases in the human and domestic animal populations, which altered the ecosystem in places where the virus had formerly circulated only between wild animals and its vectors. Epidemic outbreaks occur primarily in the dry season when farm workers go into forest areas more frequently and ticks are more active. Cases in humans and mortality among monkeys cease with the monsoon rains.

The natural cycle of this disease is still not well known. The chief vector is most likely the tick *Haemaphysalis spinigera*, from which many isolations of the virus have been made and which has been shown to transmit the infection by biting. In addition, transovarial transmission has been confirmed in that tick. The virus was also isolated from *H. turturis,* where the agent persists all year in the nymphs, as well as from six other species of *Haemaphysalis*, from several species of *Ixodes*, and from an argasid tick, *Ornithoros chiropterphila*, a parasite of insectivorous bats (Harwood and James, 1979).

Humans are infected by the bite of *H. spinigera* nymphs. The adult stage of this tick prefers large wild or domestic animals. The introduction of cattle into the jungle allowed wider dissemination of this vector, an increase in its density, and broader circulation of the virus. Moreover, cattle brought the tick closer to the human population (Harwood and James, 1979). In a year-long study, 1,260 ticks were found on 493 out of 4,668 farmers examined, and 85% of the ticks were *H. spinigera*. In addition, the effects of deforestation, which altered the forest vegetation from perennial to deciduous, favored *H. spinigera* to the detriment of other ticks (Banerjee and Bhat, 1977).

The virus has been isolated from a large number of *Presbytis* and *Macaca* monkeys. Many infected monkeys become ill and die but others survive, as shown by serologic examinations on healthy specimens. As with jungle yellow fever, mortality in monkeys may act as a warning that the virus is active and that an epidemic is imminent. Nevertheless, monkeys are not believed to constitute the reservoir of the virus in nature. In that regard, small jungle mammals for which the infection is not fatal are being studied. In natural foci, the virus has been isolated from several species of rodents and the existence of neutralizing antibodies in them has been confirmed. The shrew *Suncus murinus* and the jungle rat *Rattus blanfordi* are indicated as natural reservoirs by their population density, their high level of experimentally induced viremia, and their susceptibility to natural infection as confirmed by virus isolation. However, other rodents may also play a role in the virus cycle.

The disease affects mainly agricultural workers whose villages are near cultivated lands adjacent to forest areas. Man is infected by the bite of *H. spinigera* nymphs.

Cattle serve as hosts for the adult stage of *H. spinigera*, which is a three-host tick: the larval and nymphal stages parasitize small mammals and the adult stage parasitizes wild or domestic ungulates. Very few larvae or nymphs are found in the rainy season, while adult ticks are abundant. This fact helps explain the seasonal nature of the disease.

Diagnosis: The virus is easily isolated from the sera of patients by means of mouse inoculation. For serologic diagnosis, the complement fixation, hemagglutination inhibition, neutralization, and ELISA tests can be used with serum samples from the acute and convalescent periods of the disease.

Control: The usual individual human protection measures against ticks, such as protective clothing and repellents, are difficult to employ in the endemic area. A formalin-inactivated cell culture vaccine tested on laboratory personnel showed 72.5% seroconversion. A field test of the vaccine in the endemic area showed only 59% seroconversion. The presence of antibodies to other flaviviruses, especially the West Nile virus, seems to interfere with the efficacy of the vaccine. Seroconversion was 1.85% in a control group (Dandawate *et al.*, 1980).

A live vaccine with an attenuated strain of the Langat[1] virus is being developed. A single administration in mice confers 70 to 100% protection against large doses of the Kyasanur forest virus for a minimum of 18 months. Previously, this attenuated strain was given to human volunteers; they experienced no secondary effects and the vaccine did not cause adverse reactions in terminal carcinoma patients (Thind, 1981).

Bibliography

Banerjee, K., and H. R. Bhat. Correlation between the number of persons suffering from Kyasanur Forest disease and the intensity of infection in the tick population. *Indian J Med Res* 66:175-179, 1977.

Centers for Disease Control of the USA. *International Catalogue of Arboviruses*, 2nd ed. (Ed. by T. O. Berge). Atlanta, Georgia, 1975. (DHEW Publ. CDC 75-8301.)

Clarke, D. H., and J. Casals. Arboviruses: Group B. *In*: Horsfall, F. L., and I. Tamm (Eds.), *Viral and Rickettsial Infections of Man*, 4th ed. Philadelphia, Lippincott, 1965.

Dandawate, C. N., S. Upadhyaya, and K. Banerjee. Serological response to formalized Kyasanur Forest disease virus vaccine in humans at Sagar and Sorab talukas of Shimoga district. *J Biol Stand* 8:1-6, 1980.

Downs, W. G. Arboviruses. *In*: A. S. Evans (Ed.), *Viral Infections of Humans. Epidemiology and Control*. New York, Plenum, 1976.

Fiennes, R. *Zoonoses of Primates*. Ithaca, New York, Cornell University Press, 1967.

Harwood, R. F., and M. T. James. *Entomology in Human and Animal Health*, 7th ed. New York, MacMillan, 1979.

Rhodes, A. J., and C. E. van Rooyen. *Textbook of Virology*, 4th ed. Baltimore, Maryland, Williams and Wilkins, 1962.

Thind, I. S. Attenuated Langat E5 virus as a live virus vaccine against Kyasanur forest disease virus. *Indian J Med Res* 73:141-149, 1981.

Webb, H. E. Kyasanur Forest disease virus in three species of rodents. *Trans R Soc Trop Med Hyg* 59:205-211, 1965.

---

[1] Langat is a flavivirus belonging to the same complex as the Kyasanur forest disease virus. The Langat virus was isolated from the ticks *Ixodes granulatus* in Malaysia and *Haemaphysalis papuana* in Thailand. The reservoir of the virus seems to be jungle rats. No human cases caused by this virus are known. In carcinoma patients inoculated with a field strain of the virus, fever and encephalitis were observed.

Webb, H. E., and R. L. Rao. Kyasanur Forest disease: A general clinical study in which some cases with neurological complications were observed. *Trans R Soc Trop Med Hyg* 55:284-298, 1961.

Work, T. H., F. R. Rodríguez, and P. N. Bhatt. Virological epidemiology of the 1958 epidemic of Kyasanur Forest disease. *Am J Public Health* 49:869-874, 1959.

LASSA FEVER

(078.8)

Etiology: RNA genome virus belonging to the genus *Arenavirus*, family Arenaviridae. The virus is antigenically related to the lymphocytic choriomeningitis (LCM) virus. A very similar virus has been isolated from a variety or subspecies of *Mastomys natalensis* in Mozambique (Mozambique virus), and antibodies for this virus have been found in man in Zimbabwe, but it is not known if it is pathogenic. Another virus antigenically related to Lassa virus has been isolated from the rodent *Praomys* in the Central African Republic (Odend'hal, 1983).

Geographic Distribution and Occurrence in Man: Lassa fever (LF) was recognized for the first time in 1969, in a missionary nurse in Lassa, Nigeria. Another two nurses contracted the disease while taking care of the index case in a hospital in Jos, Nigeria. Two of the three died and the third suffered a severe and prolonged illness. From 1969 to 1975 six more outbreaks occurred in three West African countries: Nigeria (1970, 1974, 1975), Liberia (1972), and Sierra Leone (1970-1972, 1973-1975); an isolated case also occurred in Nigeria in 1975. With the exception of the Sierra Leone outbreak in 1970-1972, the other outbreaks were nosocomial, spreading within hospitals where the index case was confined. Secondary and tertiary cases have occurred among hospitalized patients, hospital personnel, and some family members. In contrast to the nosocomial outbreaks, in Sierra Leone most human cases originated within the affected communities. The fatality rate of hospitalized cases was from 20 to 66% in the different outbreaks, with an average of 36% (Casals, 1976; Monath, 1975).

Recent observations indicate that benign cases of the disease as well as clinically inapparent infections occur. Seroepidemiologic studies suggest that LF virus is probably distributed multifocally in western Africa. Out of 458 serum samples collected from human patients in 1965-1966 at 48 different localities in northern Nigeria, neutralizing antibodies were found in 10 samples from inhabitants of five regions. Of another 281 serum samples collected over 5 years from nomadic herders in Nigeria, 23 showed positive results. In Sierra Leone, 11% of inhabitants in one locality and 3.5% in another had complement-fixing antibodies (Monath, 1975).

Infection in Sierra Leone is endemic and cases occur all year long in several rural areas, while the nosocomial outbreaks in Nigeria and Liberia coincided with the dry season.

Serologic studies indicate that the infection exists in Guinea, the Central African Republic, Mali, Senegal, Cameroon, and Benin (Casals, 1982).

Two LF cases, one fatal, occurred in personnel of a research institute in the USA.

Occurrence in Animals: Because of the relationship that exists between the LF virus and other arenaviruses, it was thought from the beginning that the reservoir of the agent might be rodents.

In 1972, during the outbreak of LF in Sierra Leone, 641 small vertebrates were captured, including specimens of 15 species of rodents, 6 bats species, 1 insectivore, 1 primate, and 2 species of reptiles. The LF virus was isolated from only one murine species, *Mastomys natalensis*; 17% of the 82 specimens processed were found to be infected. A high prevalence of infected *Mastomys* was observed in homes of LF patients. *M. natalensis* is widely distributed south of the Sahara; its habitat is both domestic and peridomestic. In a more recent study in Sierra Leone, distribution of the infection in *Mastomys* in houses in an endemic area was found to be rather focal. In homes where there had been cases of disease in the family, 39% of these rodents had viremia, compared with 3.7% in control (no LF cases) homes. In one village near a diamond mine, 79% of all rodents captured in houses were *M. natalensis* (Keenlyside *et al.*, 1983).

The Disease in Man: The incubation period is generally about 7 days, but it can be as long as 3 weeks. Onset of the disease is gradual, with fever, asthenia, muscular pains, and cephalalgia; it affects many organ systems. The intestinal tract is frequently affected, with vomiting, diarrhea, and abdominal pain. Also common are pharyngitis, tonsillitis, coughing, stertorous breathing, and thoracic pain. Ulcerative pharyngitis occurs in about 80% of the cases. Many patients manifest albuminuria, a low level of serum albumin, and an increase in urea nitrogen in the blood. Cervical adenopathies, tumefaction, edema of the face and neck, and a tendency toward hemorrhages are frequently observed. When the disease course is severe, high fever persists, the toxic state increases, and the patient becomes apathetic. In addition, vomiting, diarrhea, capillary hemorrhages, complications of the central nervous system, respiratory failure, oliguria, and shock are present, and circulatory collapse often occurs. Death is generally due to cardiac failure. The fatality rate among hospitalized patients—usually those who are suffering serious illness—varies from 30 to 50%. It has been estimated that 10 to 20 infections occur in the population for each patient hospitalized, and therefore the proportion of infected people who die from LF would be 1 to 2% (Johnson *et al.*, 1982).

In contrast to Argentine and Bolivian hemorrhagic fevers, viremia in LF patients can last 10 to 16 days and the severity of the disease is directly related to the level of viremia (Johnson *et al.*, 1982).

The disease is often milder in children than in adults. Following an outbreak in a village of Sierra Leone, a serologic study was conducted in 20 family homes; antibodies for the virus were found in 20.4% of children (age group 0 to 14 years) without recorded cases of disease (Sharp, 1982).

Patients who recover have a long convalescence; the most frequent sequelae are partial deafness and alopecia.

The Disease in Animals: Natural infection caused by LF virus has been found so far in *M. natalensis* rodents captured in Sierra Leone during the epidemic and, more recently, in northern Nigeria during an interepidemic period. Experimental studies with a race of *M. natalensis* in Zimbabwe demonstrated that the animals acquire a chronic infection with viremia and viruria when they are inoculated during the first 4 days of life. Carrier females give birth to the same number of offspring as normal females (in contrast to female *Calomys callosus* with Machupo virus, in which fetal mortality is almost total) and all offspring become infected within 2 weeks (Johnson, 1981).

No clinical signs of the disease have been described in *M. natalensis*. A comparative study between virus carrier and noncarrier *M. natalensis* captured in a house in a Sierra Leone village revealed that infected rodents are smaller and weigh less than uninfected ones and that inflammatory lesions (spleen follicular hyperplasia, myocarditis, and myositis among others) are more frequent in them (Demartini *et al.*, 1975).

Source of Infection and Mode of Transmission: The facts indicate that the reservoir of virus is the domestic and peridomestic rodent *M. natalensis*. This species is the most common rodent in houses in certain villages of western Africa, and its rate of infection is high where there have been human cases (see Occurrence in Animals). Experiments have demonstrated that the virus is transmitted horizontally among these rats and perhaps also vertically. Transmission is continuous in house colonies because susceptible animals are contaminated by excreta of those with persistent infection.

In general, nosocomial outbreaks have originated from an index patient who acquired the disease at home or some other place in the community and then infected hospital personnel. Currently, it is thought that secondary cases are due mainly to contact with blood (viremia is often high-titer and prolonged) and excreta from the index patient, but airborne transmission cannot be ruled out (see below).

It is not known how the LF virus is transmitted from rodent to man, but it is suspected that the mechanism is similar to that of other agents of the arenavirus group, that is, by means of close contact between the rodent and man, permitting contamination of the human environment with infected urine and other rodent excretions and secretions. The mode of transmission could be direct contact with the reservoir animals or their urine and saliva, consumption of raw rodent meat, or contamination of food and water by rodent urine (Casals, 1982).

The virus is easily transmitted from person to person, as shown by the outbreaks that occurred in hospitals where LF patients were treated. Infection by LF virus represents a great risk for hospital and laboratory personnel. For example, 14 nurses and a physician who took care of patients contracted the disease. The possibility of airborne transmission is also being considered, since virus is found in pharyngeal washings in the acute phase of the disease. The portals of entry would be the upper respiratory or digestive tract; early manifestations of the disease are pharyngitis and tonsillitis. During the 1970 epidemic in Jos, Nigeria, a nurse with pulmonary involvement was the source of infection for 16 other cases. Cases of the infection contracted through skin wounds are also known.

The fact that more than one-third of recognized LF cases are nosocomial in origin raises the possibility that secondary cases might occur in other parts of the world as a result of hospitalizing a patient who had acquired the infection in Africa.

Diagnosis: Specific diagnosis is obtained by virus isolation or by serologic tests. Virus has been isolated from 82% of blood samples and 50% of pharyngeal washings or swabs taken from patients within 14 days after the appearance of the disease. Viruria is less common, but it has been observed up to 32 days after onset of disease. The virus is easily isolated in VERO cells from serum obtained from the patient between the third and fourteenth day of illness. The virus's cytopathic effect can be observed beginning on the fourth day after culture. Diagnosis can be accelerated by daily examination of the culture by direct immunofluorescence.

Serologic diagnosis consists in confirming the development of complement-fixing or neutralizing antibodies in blood samples obtained at the beginning of the illness and during convalescence. The complement fixation test is not satisfactory for early diagnosis. Indirect immunofluorescence allows antibody detection from the seventh to the tenth day after appearance of the disease; it is currently the most used test because of the enormous importance of early diagnosis for preventing secondary cases. The technique of virus isolation by tissue culture and immunofluorescence is the most appropriate for an early diagnosis, but few labs in the world have the biosecurity installations required for this work.

Control: The control measures consist of treating suspected patients in rigorously isolated units and providing masks, gloves, and protective clothing to service and nursing personnel attending patients. Diagnostic material should be handled exclusively in a laboratory that provides maximum safety measures for personnel.

Control of the *M. natalensis* population could be a very important means of preventing infection. However, a recent attempt to that effect in family houses in a Sierra Leone village yielded inconclusive results (Keenlyside *et al.*, 1983).

Bibliography

Buckley, S. M., and J. Casals. Lassa fever, a new virus disease of man from West Africa. III. Isolation and characterization of the virus. *Am J Trop Med Hyg* 19:680-691, 1970.

Carey, D. E., G. E. Kemp, H. A. White, L. Pinneo, R. F. Addy, A. L. M. D. Fuom, G. Stroh, J. Casals, and B. E. Henderson. Lassa fever. Epidemiological aspects of the 1970 epidemic, Jos, Nigeria. *Trans R Soc Trop Med Hyg* 66:402-408, 1972.

Casals, J. Arenaviruses. *In*: A. S. Evans (Ed.), *Viral Infections of Humans. Epidemiology and Control*. New York, Plenum, 1976.

Casals, J. Arenaviruses. *In*: Evans, A. S. (Ed.), *Viral Infections of Humans*, 2nd ed. New York, Plenum, 1982.

Casals, J., and S. Buckley. Lassa fever. *Progr Med Virol* 18:111-126, 1974.

Demartini, J. C., D. E. Green, and T. P. Monath. Lassa fever infection in *Mastomys natalensis* in Sierra Leone. Gross and microscopic findings in infected and uninfected animals. *Bull WHO* 52:651-663, 1975.

Frame, J. D., J. M. Baldwin, D. J. Gocke, and J. M. Troup. Lassa fever, a new virus disease of man from West Africa. I. Clinical description and pathological findings. *Am J Trop Med Hyg* 19:670-675, 1970.

Henderson, B. E., G. W. Gary, R. E. Kissling, J. D. Frame, and D. E. Carey. Lassa fever. Virological and serological studies. *Trans R Soc Trop Med Hyg* 66:409-416, 1972.

Johnson, K. M. Arenaviruses: diagnosis of infection in wild rodents. *In*: Kurstak, E., and C. Kurstak (Eds.), *Comparative Diagnosis of Viral Diseases*. New York, Academic Press, 1981.

Johnson, K. M., J. B. McCormick, P. A. Webb, and J. W. Krebs. The comparative biology of Old World (Lassa) and New World (Junin-Machupo) arenaviruses. *In*: Pinheiro, F. P. (Ed.), Simposio Internacional de Arbovirus dos Trópicos e Febres Hemorrágicas. Belém, Pará, 14-18 April 1980. Brazilian Academy of Sciences, 1982.

Keenlyside, R. A., J. B. McCormick, P. A. Webb, E. Smith, L. Elliot, and K. M. Johnson. Case-control study of *Mastomys natalensis* and humans in Lassa virus-infected households in Sierra Leone. *Am J Trop Med Hyg* 32:829-837, 1983.

Monath, T. P. Biological hazards associated with *Mastomys*. *WHO Chronicle* 29:241, 1975.

Monath, T. P. Lassa fever: review of epidemiology and epizootiology. *Bull WHO* 52:577-592, 1975.

Monath, T. P., V. F. Newhouse, G. E. Kemp, H. W. Setzer, and A. Cacciopuoti. Lassa virus isolation from *Mastomys natalensis* rodents during an epidemic in Sierra Leone. *Science* 185:263-265, 1974.

Odend'hal, S. *The Geographical Distribution of Animal Viral Diseases.* New York, Academic Press, 1983.

Sharp, P. C. Lassa fever in children. *J Infect* 4:73-77, 1982.

Troup, J. M., H. A. White, A. L. M. D. Fuom, and D. E. Carey. An outbreak of Lassa fever on the Jos Plateau, Nigeria, in January-February 1970. A preliminary report. *Am J Trop Med Hyg* 19:695-696, 1970.

White, H. A. Lassa fever. A study of 23 hospital cases. *Trans R Soc Trop Med Hyg* 66:390-398, 1972.

LOUPING-ILL

(063.1)

Synonym: Infectious ovine encephalomyelitis.

Etiology: RNA genome virus of the genus *Flavivirus* (formerly group B of the arboviruses) in the family Togaviridae; it belongs to the complex of tick-borne viruses (Russian spring-summer encephalitis complex).

Geographic Distribution: Ireland, Scotland, northern England, and Wales. The distribution is not uniform. An antigenically similar virus has been isolated from sheep in Turkey (Martin, 1981).

Occurrence in Man and Animals: Louping-ill is rare in man. About 35 cases are known, 26 acquired in the laboratory and 9 contracted naturally (Smith and Varma, 1981). Serologic studies indicate that sheepherders are less exposed to the infection than laboratory or slaughterhouse workers. The infection is enzootic in several areas of Great Britain. The animal species most affected is sheep, but the disease also occurs naturally in cattle, equines, deer, small mammals (*Apodemus sylvaticus* and *Sorex araneus*), and some birds (*Lagopus lagopus scoticus*). Recently, the disease was described in suckling pigs (Bannatyne *et al.*, 1980). The regional incidence in sheep is about 5%, but it can be higher in some flocks. The greatest losses are experienced when sheep free of the infection are introduced into enzootic areas.

The Disease in Man: The incubation period is from 2 to 8 days. The disease is biphasic. The first phase, which lasts 2 to 12 days, is characterized by fever, retro-ocular pain, cephalalgia, and malaise. After an asymptomatic interval of about 5 days, the second phase begins, characterized by nervous symptomatology. The symptoms are quite variable in this phase, and the disease may take the form of meningoencephalitis or resemble paralytic poliomyelitis. Convalescence may be prolonged but mortality is nil (Smith and Varma, 1981). In laboratory and slaughterhouse workers the disease may be limited to the first phase and can thus be confused with influenza. Subclinical infections probably occur in laboratory personnel.

The Disease In Animals: The incubation period may last a few days or extend to several weeks. The disease also takes the form of biphasic pyrexia in sheep. Many animals recover after the first febrile and viremic phase, while in others the virus invades the central nervous system causing encephalomyelitis. The most prominent symptoms are fever, motor incoordination, tremors, salivation, and apathy. The sick animal's characteristic hopping gait is produced by its advancing the hind legs simultaneously and then the front legs. After 1 or 2 days of illness, the affected animals fall to the ground and remain prostrate, with violent movements of the extremities. Only about 50% of the animals with symptoms of encephalomyelitis recuperate. The disease occurs mainly in spring and autumn when the vector *Ixodes ricinus* is most abundant. In enzootic areas sporadic cases also occur in cattle.

Similarly, the louping-ill virus causes disease and death in the red grouse, *Lagopus lagopus scoticus*. In areas heavily infested with *I. ricinus*, a very high proportion of these gallinaceous birds have antibodies against the virus; many of their young are infected during the first 2 months of life and only a small number of those infected survive. By the end of July in areas lightly infested with ticks, an average brood was found to consist of 5.5 chicks, while in highly infested areas the average was barely 0.6 (Reid *et al.*, 1978).

Source of Infection and Mode of Transmission (Figure 40): Epizootics among sheep usually occur in spring, early summer, and autumn, when the vector *I. ricinus* is active. The factors that determine whether an animal will pass on to the second phase of the disease and develop signs of encephalomyelitis, or will recuperate after the first febrile phase have not been well established. It is thought that a concomitant infection with *Ehrlichia phagocytophilia*, as well as such factors as shipping, cold weather, and deficient nutrition, may favor virus invasion of the central nervous system.

Sheep appear to constitute the main reservoir and the sheep-tick-sheep cycle can perpetuate the circulation of the virus in nature. There are many species of small mammals in which antibodies have been found or from which the virus has been isolated. In some species the viremia level is too low to infect the vector; in others it has not been investigated. These animals play an important role as a source of food for the larvae and nymphs of *I. ricinus*. When the population density of some small mammals increases, the tick population also increases (Smith and Varma, 1981). In this manner, a greater tick infestation on sheep is produced and, consequently, the occurrence of epizootics in this species is favored. The red grouse (*Lagopus l. scoticus*), in spite of having a sufficiently high level of viremia to infect the ticks, serves only as a temporary virus amplifier, since its population decreases rapidly in the active foci of louping-ill. The high mortality this bird experiences indicates that it is not a primary host and that its contact with the virus is rather recent; its first large-scale contact was possibly when sheep-breeding was introduced into Scotland in the 19th century, which increased the tick population and the circulation of the virus (Reid *et al.*, 1978).

Figure 40. Louping-ill. Transmission cycle.

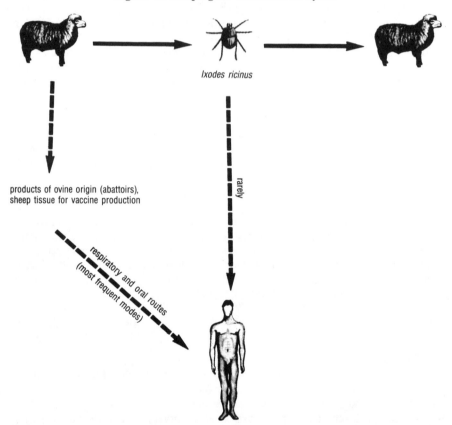

Ixodes ricinus

products of ovine origin (abattoirs),
sheep tissue for vaccine production

rarely

respiratory and oral routes
(most frequent modes)

The larvae or nymphs become infected with the virus when feeding on viremic sheep. The virus survives the winter in the tick, which then transmits it to sheep the following spring (Martin, 1981). In this vector, transstadial (but not transovarial) transmission has been verified; a larva that becomes infected when feeding on a viremic animal can transmit the virus to the nymph stage and hence to the adult tick.

The fact that clinical and subclinical infections in man are rare in rural environments and are more frequent among laboratory and slaughterhouse workers indicates that inhalation and needle prick accidents may be more important than tick bites in the transmission of the disease. The reason that man rarely becomes infected in nature may be that the vector rarely attaches itself to man.

Diagnosis: In man, the virus can be isolated from the blood during the first phase of the disease by inoculation into mice, embryonated eggs, and sheep kidney cell cultures. During the second phase of the disease, cerebrospinal liquid must be used. The virus can also be isolated from brain tissue and the medulla oblongata of animals with symptoms of encephalomyelitis, which either died or were sacrificed. Diagnosis is accomplished by the neutralization, complement fixation, and hemagglutination inhibition tests as well as by histopathology.

Control: For prevention in man, no measures are called for other than laboratory safety.

For the immunization of sheep, an inactivated vaccine with oil adjuvant, produced in cell culture, is available.

Bibliography

Bannatyne, C. C., R. L. Wilson, H. W. Reid, D. Buxton, and I. Pow. Louping-ill virus infection of pigs. *Vet Rec* 106:13, 1980.

Centers for Disease Control of the USA. *International Catalogue of Arboviruses*, 2nd ed. (Ed. by T. O. Berge). Atlanta, Georgia, 1975. (DHEW Publ. CDC 75-8301.)

Goldblum, M. Group B arthropod-borne viral diseases. *In*: Van der Hoeden, J. (Ed.), *Zoonoses*. Amsterdam, Netherlands, Elsevier, 1964.

Gordon, W. S. Louping-ill in animals and in man. *In*: Gordon-Jones, O. (Ed.), *Some Diseases of Animals Communicable to Man in Britain*. Oxford, Pergamon Press, 1968.

Gordon Smith, C. E., M. G. R. Varma, and D. McMahon. Isolation of louping-ill virus from small mammals in Ayrshire. *Nature* 203:992-993, 1964.

Jensen, R. *Diseases of Sheep*. Philadelphia, Lea and Febiger, 1974.

Martin, W. B. Virus diseases of sheep and goats. *In*: Gibbs, E. P. J. (Ed.), *Virus Diseases of Food Animals*, vol. 1. New York, Academic Press, 1981.

Reid, H. W., J. S. Duncan, J. D. P. Phillips, R. Moss, and A. Watson. Studies on louping-ill virus (Flavivirus group) in wild red grouse (*Lagopus lagopus scoticus*). *J Hyg (Camb)* 81:321-329, 1978.

Reid, H. W., and I. Pow. Excretion of louping-ill virus in ewes' milk. *Vet Rec* 117:470, 1985.

Ross, C. A. C. Louping-ill in man. *In*: Graham-Jones, O. (Ed.), *Some Diseases of Animals Communicable to Man in Britain*. Oxford, Pergamon Press, 1968.

Smith, C. E. G., and M. G. R. Varma. Louping-ill. *In*: Beran, G. W. (Section Ed.), *CRC Handbook Series in Zoonoses*. Section B, vol. 1. Boca Raton, Florida, CRC Press, 1981.

Stamp, J. T. Some viral diseases of sheep. *In*: Food and Agriculture Organization of the United Nations/International Office of Epizootics, *International Conference on Sheep Diseases*. Rome, 1966.

Timoney, P. J. Recovery of louping-ill virus from the red grouse in Ireland. *Br Vet J* 128:19-23, 1972.

LYMPHOCYTIC CHORIOMENINGITIS

(049.0)

Synonym: Armstrong's disease.

Etiology: RNA virus of the genus *Arenavirus*, family Arenaviridae.

Geographic Distribution: In contrast to other arenaviruses, which have limited geographic distributions, the lymphocytic choriomeningitis (LCM) virus has been found in the Americas, Europe, and Asia. Human cases of LCM have occurred in Japan, several European countries, the United States, El Salvador, Brazil, and Argentina. Doubts exist, however, about whether the infection was identified correctly in some cases. The agent has not been found in Africa or Australia.

Occurrence in Man: The disease is sporadic and not very common, but outbreaks occasionally occur. The human infection related to house mice—which are the main reservoir of the agent—is distributed in accordance with the presence of the virus in animal colonies. Sporadic cases can occur for several years in the same block of a city or town. In the Federal Republic of Germany, clinical cases associated with mice were recorded only in the north and northwest, where the rate of serologic reactors in the rural population reached 10% in some studies. By contrast, in the south of the country, where clinical cases have not been observed, the rate of reactors varied from 0.18 to 1.6%. The incidence of clinical cases per year is very low; it is estimated that there are about 1,000 infections by the virus annually in West Germany (Ackermann, 1982). In a study of nearly 1,600 cases of central nervous system illnesses among military personnel in the United States over an 18-year period, only 8% were found to have been caused by the LCM virus, with only about seven cases occurring per year (Casals, 1982).

Because of the widespread custom in recent years of keeping hamsters as pets, cases related to these animals have turned up in the Federal Republic of Germany (47 cases from November 1968 to May 1971, distributed throughout the country) and in the United States (181 cases from December 1973 to April 1974 in 12 states, with 57 cases each in New York and California). All the hamsters that gave rise to the United States outbreak came from a single commercial breeder, although the animals were acquired from different retail suppliers.

Cases of the disease have also occurred among laboratory personnel who worked with the virus or with infected animal colonies. In the United States, three outbreaks with 65 cases were recorded in 1973-1975 in laboratory staff who handled hamsters with tumor grafts containing lymphocytic choriomeningitis virus (Gregg, 1975). An epidemiologic study carried out by two institutes showed that the outbreaks were due to lines of tumoral tissue (of hamster origin) acquired from a single biological products company.

Occurrence in Animals: Many animal species are susceptible to choriomeningitis virus, and various naturally infected species have been found. Nevertheless, there is no doubt that the host and natural reservoir is the house mouse (*Mus musculus*). In the Federal Republic of Germany, where various species of mice have been studied, a high incidence of choriomeningitis has been found in house mice and in the field mouse, *Apodemus sylvaticus*. In the buildings of research institutes where human cases have been recorded, the infection was found in approximately 40% of the mouse colonies; about 50% of the rodents were carriers of the virus.

The Disease in Man: The course of the infection varies from clinically inapparent to fatal in some (rare) cases. In general, it is a benign disease. Most cases have a symptomatology similar to that of influenza. The incubation period is from 1 to 2 weeks. The clinical form similar to influenza can clear up in a few days, or the patient may suffer a relapse with meningeal symptoms. Meningitis may also develop initially without prior symptoms, but in this case the incubation period is longer (2 to 3 weeks). The symptoms are stiffness of the neck, fever, cephalalgia, malaise, and muscular pains. Cerebrospinal fluid contains from under 100 to over 3,000 cells per ml, 80 to 95% of which are lymphocytes. On rare occasions, there may be meningoencephalitis with alteration of the deep reflexes, paralysis, cutaneous anesthesia, and somnolence. Chronic sequelae are not very common, and death occurs in very few cases.

The infection can interfere with gestation as well as cause prenatal damage to the child (encephalitis, hydrocephaly, chorioretinitis) (Ackermann, 1982).

The Disease in Animals: Naturally infected animals, including the house mouse, generally do not show clinical symptoms.

The course of the infection in a naturally infected mouse colony was observed in a laboratory. Although 50% of the animals were infected, morbidity was less than 20%. Many of the young mice were stunted in growth, but about 40% recovered completely. Those which were infected *in utero* maintained the virus throughout their lives. The proportion of mice with persistent tolerant infection (PTI) increased with time, and after 4 years high titers of virus could be found in all animals without illness. Infection in this colony was transmitted only congenitally, in contrast to what had been observed previously, when some animals born without the virus became infected shortly after birth by contact.

It is believed that in nature the infection is maintained in mice by transovarial transmission and that congenital infection is the rule.

Experimental infection in adult mice produces acute disease after an incubation period of 5 to 6 days. The disease may end in death or complete recuperation with a normal immune response and elimination of the virus. During the course of the disease the animal experiences a characteristic and frequently fatal convulsive attack if grasped by the tail and twirled. Acute lymphocytic choriomeningitis is associated with general immunosuppression, which appears during the second week of infection and persists for several weeks. The immunosuppression mechanism consists of viral interference with the maturation of T-cells (Thomsen *et al.*, 1982). A completely different picture is seen in mice infected in the perinatal period, during the first 5 days of life. Although normal development is retarded several weeks in these animals and a certain number of them may die, survivors recover completely even though the virus continues to replicate and high titers are found in all organs during the entire life of the mouse. This immunologic tolerance for the choriomeningitis virus has been the subject of numerous studies. These animals display a marked suppression of cellular immunity and neutralizing antibodies, although the latter can be detected by the immunofluorescence and complement fixation tests. Mice with PTI (especially those that acquire the infection shortly after birth) generally suffer from glomerulonephritis, which will reduce their life expectancy by a few months. The lesion is due to the deposit of the virus-antibody complex in the kidneys.

The reaction of laboratory mice to infection is conditioned by their age, the strain of the virus, and the mode of administration.

The patterns of both natural and experimental infection lead to the conclusion that horizontal infection is of little epidemiologic importance; in contrast, vertical infection becomes chronic and persists in mice so that they become a continuous source of environmental contamination through their excreta (Johnson, 1981).

Source of Infection and Mode of Transmission (Figure 41): The primary and probably sole reservoir is the mouse. All other species of animals, including man, contract the infection from mice. The infection in mice is persistent, while in man and other animals it is of limited duration. Mice eliminate the virus through nasal secretions, urine, semen, and milk, as well as through the feces. Congenital and neonatal infection is very important in this species. Transmission of the virus is both vertical and horizontal.

The mode of transmission of the infection from mouse to man is not well understood, but some observations indicate that the routes of entry may be varied. Human cases have resulted from mouse bites (and bites of other rodents) and from handling dead mice. The infection can probably be introduced through the upper digestive tract when foods contaminated by rat feces or urine are eaten. Laboratory

Figure 41. Lymphocytic choriomeningitis. Transmission cycle.

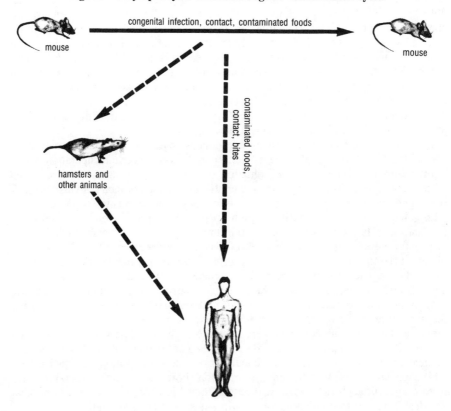

infections are probably due to virus penetration via the respiratory tract or conjunctiva. The respiratory route is also thought to be important in other circumstances, even though the agent is not very hardy in the environment.

The virus can be transmitted experimentally by arthropod vectors (ticks, lice, bedbugs, and mosquitoes), but it is not known if this mode of transmission occurs in nature. The virus has been isolated from fleas, wild rodents, *Culicoides*, various species of *Aedes*, ticks, and cockroaches. The prevalent opinion among researchers is that arthropods play a limited role, if any, in transmission.

Mice can transmit the infection to other species of animals and through these to man. Infections at some hamster and guinea pig farms have probably been contracted from mice and have given rise to many human cases.

Role of Animals in the Epidemiology of the Disease: Lymphocytic choriomeningitis is a zoonosis. Cases of human-to-human transmission are exceptional; one case is known in which the infection was acquired while performing an autopsy and another in which it was probably acquired *in utero*. Mice are essential to the maintenance of the infection.

Diagnosis: Laboratory confirmation is based on serologic tests and isolation of the virus. The complement-fixing antibodies appear during the first or second week of the disease and disappear in less than 6 months. Neutralizing antibodies appear later and last for years. A high titer in the complement fixation (CF) test is good diagnostic evidence. The serum neutralization test must always be based on an increase in titers between the period of disease and convalescence. The indirect immunofluorescence test will probably replace the CF test because it allows earlier detection of the disease. The virus is isolated by intracerebral inoculation of mice with blood from febrile patients or with cerebrospinal fluid from patients with meningitis. For obvious reasons, the test mice must originate from colonies that are choriomeningitis-free.

Infection of laboratory animals with the choriomeningitis virus, in addition to being a risk for laboratory staff, presents a problem for research and may invalidate experimental results. Many strains of virus maintained or passaged in laboratory mice have been contaminated with lymphocytic choriomeningitis. A serologic diagnosis is possible in an infected colony using the CF test (the serum neutralization test does not work because of immunologic tolerance) or the immunofluorescence test, using livers from suspect mice. Diagnosis can also be confirmed by experimental inoculation. Intracerebral inoculation with neurotropic strains of LCM will cause the characteristic disease and death of normal mice, but not of carriers of the virus. Another method is inoculation of guinea pigs with a suspension of organs from suspect mice.

Control: Consists mainly of controlling the mouse population in houses by means of environmental hygiene and the use of rodenticides. Mice captured or killed should under no conditions be handled with bare hands.

When the disease was transmitted by other animals, for example hamsters, the origin of these animals should be investigated and their sale to the public should be avoided until the breeding colony is free of the infection.

Periodic surveillance of colonies of laboratory mice by means of serologic tests should be practiced. Breeding units and installations should be rodent-proof.

Pregnant women should not keep hamsters or other rodents in their homes.

Bibliography

Ackermann, R. Infektionen mit dem Virus der Lymphozytaeren Choriomeningitis. *Bundesgesundhbl* 25:240-243, 1982.

Ackermann, R., W. Stille, W. Blumenthal, E. B. Helm, K. Keller, and O. Baldus. Syrische Goldhamster als Ubertrager von lymphozytaren Choriomeningitis. *Dtsch Med Wochensch* 97:1725-1731, 1972.

Casals, J. Arenaviruses. *In*: Evans, A. S. (Ed.), *Viral Infections of Humans. Epidemiology and Control*. New York, Plenum, 1976.

Casals, J. Arenaviruses. *In*: Evans, A. S. (Ed.), *Viral Infections of Humans*, 2nd ed. New York and London, Plenum, 1982.

Centers for Disease Control of the USA. Follow-up on hamster-associated LCM infection. *Morb Mortal Wkly Rep* 23:131-132, 1974.

Gregg, M. B. Recent outbreaks of lymphocytic choriomeningitis in the United States of America. *Bull WHO* 52:549-554, 1975.

Hotchin, J. The biology of lymphocytic choriomeningitis infection: virus-induced immune disease. *Cold Spring Harbor Symposia on Quantitative Biology* 27:479-499, 1962.

Hotchin, J. Persistent and Slow Virus Infections. *Monograph in Virology*, vol. 3. Basel, Switzerland, Karger, 1971.

Hotchin, J. E., and L. M. Benson. Lymphocytic choriomeningitis. *In*: Davis, J. W., L. H. Karstad, and D. O. Trainer (Eds.), *Infectious Diseases of Wild Mammals*. Ames, Iowa State University Press, 1970.

Hotchin, J., and E. Sikora. Laboratory diagnosis of lymphocytic choriomeningitis. *Bull WHO* 52:555-560, 1975.

Hotchin, J., W. Kinneh, and E. Sikora. Some observations on hamster-derived human infection with lymphocytic choriomeningitis virus. *Bull WHO* 52:561-566, 1975.

Johnson, K. M. Arenaviruses: diagnosis of infection in wild rodents. *In*: Kurstak, E., and C. Kurstak (Eds.), *Comparative Diagnosis of Viral Diseases*, vol. 4. New York, Academic Press, 1981.

Maurer, F. D. Lymphocytic choriomeningitis. *Lab Anim Care* 14:415-419, 1964.

Swango, L. J. Lymphocytic choriomeningitis. *In*: Hubbert, W. T., W. F. McCulloch, and P. R. Schnurrenberger (Eds.), *Diseases Transmitted from Animals to Man*, 6th ed. Springfield, Illinois, Thomas, 1975.

Thomsen, A. R., K. Bro-Jorgensen, and B. L. Jensen. Lymphocytic choriomeningitis virus-induced immunosuppression; evidence for viral interference with T-cell maturation. *Infect Immun* 37:981-986, 1982.

Wilsnack, R. E. Lymphocytic choriomeningitis. *In*: *Symposium on Viruses of Laboratory Rodents*. Bethesda, Maryland, National Cancer Institute, 1966. (Monograph 20.)

MARBURG DISEASE

(078.8)

Synonyms: African hemorrhagic fever (also includes Ebola disease); green monkey disease.

Etiology: RNA virus (MBG), for which creation of the genus *Filovirus*, family Filoviridae, was proposed. Besides the MBG virus, this proposed family would include the Ebola disease virus; for now, these would be the only two members of the taxon (Kiley *et al.*, 1982).

Geographic Distribution and Occurrence: Marburg disease was recognized for the first time in 1967 in Marburg and Frankfurt, West Germany, and in Belgrade, Yugoslavia. Its name derives from the city where the pathogenic agent was first isolated and identified. The disease occurred in laboratory personnel who had handled viscera, body fluids, or tissue cultures (kidney) obtained from African green monkeys (*Cercopithecus aethiops*). There were 25 primary cases, of which seven died. Five secondary cases also occurred as a result of contact with the blood and tissues of the primary patients, and in a sixth case the infection was apparently contracted through sexual contact. The monkeys that gave rise to the outbreak came from the Kyoga Lake region of Uganda and were shipped to Europe, in two lots of 100 animals each, from Entebbe, Uganda.

Three human cases occurred in 1975 in South Africa, one of whom died. The first case, an Australian tourist, had traveled for 2 weeks in Zimbabwe before becoming ill. The other two cases, one of them a nurse, were infected by contact. In 1980 there were two cases, one of them fatal, in the western part of Kenya.

In a study in Liberia using the indirect immunofluorescence test, seven reactive people with titers from 1:16 to 1:128, were found out of 481 tested (Knobloch *et al.*, 1982). In the Central African Republic, 499 sera were examined with the same technique, and two sera with titers of 1:64 or more were found (Saluzzo *et al.*, 1982).

The Disease in Man: The incubation period varies from 4 to 9 days. In primary cases a fatality rate of 29% has been observed. The onset of the disease is sudden, with fever, cephalalgia, prostration, arthralgia, myalgia, vomiting, diarrhea, and occasionally conjunctivitis. These symptoms are followed by a maculopapular eruption, gastrointestinal hemorrhages, epistaxis, other hemorrhagic signs, and also lymphadenopathy and hepatitis. In some cases there are central nervous system alterations, myocarditis, and other complications. Leukopenia is present and transaminase values are high. Convalescence is prolonged.

The Disease in Animals: No clinical symptomatology was observed in the green monkeys that gave rise to the human infection in Germany and Yugoslavia during the 1967 outbreak. Infection produced by experimental inoculation in other species of monkeys is generally fatal, although the symptoms consist only of a febrile reaction, with lethargy, anorexia, and sometimes petechial eruptions occurring in the terminal phase of the disease. The pathologic picture is the same as in man; death occurs on the seventh or eighth day after inoculation. The virus is not pathogenic for mice; in guinea pigs, however, after three to five passages of the virus mortality is 100%.

Source of Infection and Mode of Transmission: The human cases occurring in South Africa and Kenya would indicate that the virus is active in areas very remote from each other, perhaps in a focal and enzootic form. Neither the reservoir of the virus nor the mode of transmission is known. On the basis of serologic studies using the complement fixation test, green monkeys were thought to be the main reservoirs; however, later studies have shown that the antigen used, obtained from the organs of infected guinea pigs, was not sufficiently specific. More recently, antibodies to the indirect immunofluorescence test were found in 4 of 136 captive green monkeys in Kenya (Johnson *et al.*, 1982), but this species is no longer considered to play the role of primary reservoir. New studies are needed in order to discover the natural reservoir of this infection.

During the 1967 episode, most of the human primary cases contracted the infection during the course of bleeding or eviscerating green monkeys; some contracted the disease while preparing kidney cultures or by cleaning test tubes used for tissue cultures. The disease was transmitted by direct contact with the viscera or body fluids. Personnel exposed only to live animals did not become ill. Five of the six secondary cases contracted the infection by accidentally pricking themselves with hypodermic needles used for taking blood samples or for injecting the primary patients, by contact with blood taken from patients, or by contact with viscera and body fluids during autopsy. The sixth secondary case involved sexual transmission of the infection to a woman from her husband, who had recovered from the disease and from whose semen the virus was later isolated. The disease has never been confirmed in the United States, in spite of the large number of green monkeys imported there from Africa. Though it remains unproven, the possibility of transmission by vectors was considered in the South African cases, since the first case was not directly exposed to animals but was bitten by arthropods while sleeping outdoors in Zimbabwe. Artificially infected monkeys spread the infection both by direct contact and indirectly by cohabitation in the same environment in separate cages. Monkeys have been infected experimentally by aerosols, and the infected animals can excrete the virus through the urine and saliva.

Diagnosis: Specific diagnosis can be made by isolating the virus in tissue culture, by inoculating guinea pigs and monkeys, by electron microscopy, and by serologic tests using antigens obtained from tissue cultures.

Control: In view of the present lack of knowledge, it is impossible to set up efficient control measures. Patients should be kept in isolation wards and personnel attending them should be provided with protective clothing. Bodies of dead animals, their viscera, body fluids, and any other contaminated materials should be destroyed. Instruments used should be rigorously accounted for and sterilized.

Bibliography

American Public Health Association. *Control of Communicable Diseases in Man*, 14th ed. (Ed. by A. S. Benenson). Washington, D.C., APHA, 1985.

Borwen, E. T. W., G. S. Platt, G. Lloyd, *et al*. Viral hemorrhagic fever in southern Sudan and northern Zaire. *Lancet* 1:571-573, 1977.

Centers for Disease Control of the USA. *International Catalogue of Arboviruses*, 2nd ed. (Ed. by T. O. Berge). Atlanta, Georgia, 1975. (DHEW Publ. CDC 75-8301.)

Centers for Disease Control of the USA. Update on viral hemorrhagic fever—Africa. *Morb Mortal Wkly Rep* 25:339, 1976.

Gear, J. S. S., G. A. Cassel, A. J. Gear, *et al*. Outbreak of Marburg virus disease in Johannesburg. *Br Med J* 4:489-493, 1975.

Johnson, K. M., P. A. Webb, J. V. Lange, *et al*. Isolation and partial characterization of a new virus causing acute hemorrhagic fever in Zaire. *Lancet* 1:569-571, 1977.

Johnson, B. K., L. G. Gitan, A. Gichogo, P M. Tukei, J. G. Else, M. A. Suleman, R. Kimani, and P. D. Sayer. Marburg, Ebola and Rift Valley fever virus antibodies in East African primates. *Trans R Soc Trop Med Hyg* 76:307-310, 1982.

Kiley, M. P., E. T. W. Bowen, G. A. Eddy, M. Isaacson, K. M. Johnson, J. B. McCormick, F. A. Murphy, S. R. Pattyn, D. Peters, O. W. Prozesky, R. L. Regnery, D. I. H. Simpson, W. Slenczka, P. Sureau, G. van der Groen, P. A. Webb, and H. Wulff. Filoviridae: a taxonomic home for Marburg and Ebola viruses? *Intervirology* 18:24-32, 1982.

Kissling, R. E. Epidemiology of Marburg disease. *In*: Sanders, M., and M. Schaeffer (Eds.), *Viruses Affecting Man and Animals*. St. Louis, Missouri, Green, 1971.

Kissling, R. E. Marburg virus. *In*: Hubbert, W. T., W. F. McCulloch, and P. R. Schnurrenberger (Eds.), *Diseases Transmitted from Animals to Man*, 6th ed. Springfield, Illinois, Thomas, 1975.

Kissling, R. E., F. A. Murphy, and B. E. Henderson. Marburg virus. *Ann NY Acad Sci* 174:932-945, 1970.

Knobloch, J., E. J. Albiez, and H. Schmitz. A serological survey on viral haemorrhagic fevers in Liberia. *Ann Virol (Inst Pasteur)* 133E:125-128, 1982.

Saluzzo, J. F., J. P. González, and A. J. Georges. Mise en evidence d'anticorps anti-virus Marburg dans les populations humaines du sud-est de la Republique Centrafricaine. *Ann Virol (Inst Pasteur)* 133E:129-131, 1982.

Slenczka, W., G. Wolff, and R. Siegert. A critical study of monkey sera for the presence of antibody against the Marburg virus. *Am J Epidemiol* 93:496-505, 1971.

World Health Organization. Viral haemorrhagic fever surveillance. Marburg and Ebola diseases. *Wkly Epidemiol Rec* 39:300-301, 1984.

MAYARO FEVER

(066.3)

Etiology: RNA genome virus (MAY), belonging to the genus *Alphavirus* (group A of the arboviruses), family Togaviridae; it is closely related to the virus of Semliki forest fever (see footnote 2 in Chikungunya Fever). Presently, the Bolivian Uruma virus is considered a strain of the Mayaro virus.

Geographic Distribution: The Mayaro virus has been isolated in Bolivia, Brazil, Suriname, Colombia, Trinidad, and Panama, as well as from a migratory bird in Louisiana, USA. According to seroepidemiologic studies, the virus also appears to circulate in Guyana, Peru, and Costa Rica.

Occurrence: The infection is endemic in several tropical regions of South America. Studies carried out in Bolivia, Brazil, Guyana, and Trinidad using the neutralization test show that 10 to 50% of the stable resident population in endemic areas has antibodies to the Mayaro virus.

In 1955, an outbreak of 50 cases occurred in Pará, Brazil. In 1954-1955, in Uruma, Santa Cruz Department, Bolivia, an epidemic of "forest fever" occurred among 400 settlers from Okinawa, Japan. Approximately half of them fell ill, and 10 to 15% of the cases were attributed to Uruma (Mayaro) virus. In 1977-1978, another epidemic occurred in Belterra, Pará State, Brazil. Nearly 20% of the 4,000 residents were infected and a large proportion of them became ill. The epidemic started at the beginning of the rainy season and ended with the start of the dry season (LeDuc *et al.*, 1981).

The Disease in Man: The symptomatology is similar to that of other "jungle fevers," without any special characteristics. It is a febrile, benign, and brief illness, accompanied by pyrexia, frontal cephalalgia, conjunctival congestion and photophobia, myalgia, and occasionally arthralgia. The duration of fever is usually 3 days, but in some cases it lasts a few days longer.

In the epidemic of 1977-1978 in Belterra, Brazil, 55 clinical cases confirmed by laboratory tests were studied. It is of interest to note that in all patients arthralgias were a prominent sign. The wrists, fingers, ankles, and toes were the most frequently affected, and some 20% of patients manifested joint edema. Arthralgias appeared at the onset of disease and were the cause of temporary disability. A macropapular or micropapular cutaneous eruption was observed in two-thirds of the patients towards the fifth day of the illness. Leukopenia was constant (Pinheiro *et al.*, 1981).

Other mosquito-borne alphaviruses, such as the viruses of Chikungunya, O'nyong-nyong, Ross River, and Sindbis fevers, also affect the joints (Tesh, 1982). No deaths attributable to Mayaro fever have been recorded.

Source of Infection and Mode of Transmission: Mayaro fever (MF) occurs in jungle areas of the American tropics. The epidemic of Mayaro fever in Belterra coincided with an outbreak of yellow fever, and it was theorized that the same vector could transmit both diseases. Nine thousand insects of two species were processed, but MF virus was isolated only from *Haemagogus janthinomys*. Out of 62 pools which contained 736 of these mosquitoes, captured during the peak of the epidemic, nine strains of MAY virus and two of yellow fever were isolated. The minimum infection rate of *H. janthinomys* in the field was 1:82 for Mayaro virus and 1:368 for yellow fever. There is no doubt that *H. janthinomys* was the main and perhaps only vector of MAY virus in the Belterra epidemic. In other places, the virus has been isolated from *Culex, Mansonia, Aedes, Psorophora,* and *Sabethes* mosquitoes, but more frequently from *Haemagogus* spp. than from other species (Hoch *et al.*, 1981).

During the same epidemic in Belterra, attempts were made to identify the most probable animal host of the virus using the hemagglutination inhibition test. Out of 1,200 birds examined, 1.3% were positive, and out of 585 mammals, 5.6% had antibodies. The only reactive mammals were marmosets (*Callithrix argentata*), 32 (27%) out of 119 of which had antibodies, and the one howler monkey examined. The virus was isolated from one of the marmosets, and experimental inoculation of these animals produced a level of viremia which, although of short duration, was perhaps sufficiently high to infect the vector. Even though in this epidemic episode marmosets were very probably the amplifying hosts of the virus, there is evidence indicating that birds or rodents, or both, are reservoirs for maintenance of the virus in enzootic cycles. Other studies have found 29% positive reactors among *Columbigallina* spp. doves in the jungle near Belém, Brazil, and the virus has been isolated from a migratory bird (*Icterus spurius*) in Louisiana, USA. Among the rodents *Oryzomys*, *Proechimys*, and *Nectomys* a high rate of reactors to MAY virus has been found (Hoch *et al.*, 1981).

In conclusion, studies of the epidemic in Belterra have advanced knowledge about the immediate mechanism responsible for that episode, and primates would seem to have been the reservoir of the virus; however, much information is still needed to completely elucidate the natural history of the MAY virus.

Man is an accidental host who is infected upon entering jungle areas, where the virus circulates among wild vertebrates by means of mosquitoes.

Diagnosis: Virus can be easily isolated from the blood of febrile patients at the beginning of disease. The most suitable procedure for isolation is intracerebral inoculation of newborn mice.

Serologic diagnosis is carried out by means of the hemagglutination inhibition and complement fixation tests by confirming an increase of antibody titers with samples from the acute and convalescent periods.

Control: Individual preventive measures are the same as for other mosquito-borne diseases: protective clothing, repellents, mosquito netting, and window and door screens to keep mosquitoes out of houses. In practice, these measures are difficult to carry out in tropical regions of the Americas. On the other hand, as this disease is usually benign, no special control measures are justified in tropical America.

Bibliography

Andrewes, C., and H. G. Pereira. *Viruses of Vertebrates*, 3rd ed. Baltimore, Maryland, Williams and Wilkins, 1972.

Casals, J., and D. H. Clarke. Arboviruses: Group A. *In*: Horsfall, F. L., and I. Tamm (Eds.), *Viral and Rickettsial Infections of Man,* 4th ed. Philadelphia, Lippincott, 1965.

Centers for Disease Control of the USA. *International Catalogue of Arboviruses,* 2nd ed. (Ed. by T. O. Berge). Atlanta, Georgia, 1975 (DHEW Publ. CDC 75-8301.).

Groot, H., A. Morales, and H. Vidales. Virus isolations from forest mosquitoes in San Vicente de Chucuri, Colombia. *Am J Trop Med Hyg* 10:397-402, 1961.

Hoch, A. L., N. E. Peterson, J. W. LeDuc, and F. P. Pinheiro. An outbreak of Mayaro virus disease in Belterra, Brazil. III. Entomological and ecological studies. *Am J Trop Med Hyg* 30:689-698, 1981.

LeDuc, J. W., F. P. Pinheiro, and A. P. A. Travassos da Rosa. An outbreak of Mayaro virus disease in Belterra, Brazil. II. Epidemiology. *Am J Trop Med Hyg* 30:682-688, 1981.

Metselaar, D. Isolation of arboviruses of group A and group C in Surinam. *Trop Geogr Med* 18:137-142, 1966.

Pinheiro, F. P., R. B. Freitas, J. F. Travassos da Rosa, Y. B. Gabbay, W. A. Mello, and J. W. LeDuc. An outbreak of Mayaro virus disease in Belterra, Brazil. I. Clinical and virological findings. *Am J Trop Med Hyg* 30:674-681, 1981.

Schaeffer, M., D. C. Gajdusek, A. Brown, and H. Eichenwald. Epidemic jungle fevers among Okinawan colonists in the Bolivian rain forest. *Am J Trop Med Hyg* 8:372-396, 1959.

Tesh, R. B. Arthritides caused by mosquito-borne viruses. *Annu Rev Med* 33:31-40, 1982.

Work, T. H. Semliki Forest-Mayaro virus disease. *In*: Beeson, P. B., W. McDermott, and J. B. Wyngaarden (Eds.), *Cecil Textbook of Medicine,* 15th ed. Philadelphia, Saunders, 1979.

MEASLES

(055)

Synonym: Morbilli.

Etiology: RNA genome virus, genus *Morbillivirus*, family Paramyxoviridae. The same genus includes the antigenically related viruses of distemper (Carré's disease) and bovine plague ("rinderpest").

Geographic Distribution: The virus has a worldwide distribution.

Occurrence in Man: Prior to the use of vaccines, the disease was very common in childhood, with more than 90% of children having had measles by 10 years of age. The disease was endemic in cities and epidemics occurred approximately every 2 years. In areas where effective infant vaccination programs have been carried out, the disease is more common among adolescents and adults. In temperate climates, measles occurs more frequently in late winter and early spring (American Public Health Association, 1985).

Occurrence in Animals: Besides man, the disease is observed only in captive nonhuman primates. Measles epizootics have been described in several nonhuman primate species, among them rhesus monkeys (*Macaca mulatta*), cynomolgous monkeys (*M. fascicularis*), colobus monkeys (*Colobus guereza*), langurs (*Presbytis cristatus*), and marmosets (*Saguinus oedipus, Callithrix jacchus*). Antibodies have also been found in chimpanzees, orangutans, and gibbons (Montrey *et al.*, 1980). Infection occurs only in captive animals in primate centers, research institutes, and zoos. The rate of serologic reactors to measles virus can reach 100% of animals in some institutes (Soave, 1981). Negative results have been obtained from serologic studies on free-ranging monkeys in their jungle habitat. A study of 170 *Macaca radiata* and 195 *Presbytis entellus* captured in the jungle around Mysore, India, found no antibodies to measles virus in any of them (Bhatt *et al.*, 1966). Likewise, baboons (*Papio* spp.) in their natural habitat or those that have had limited contact with people rarely have antibodies (Kalter *et al.*, 1967).

The Disease in Man: The incubation period, from exposure to appearance of fever, lasts 8 to 13 days. Prodromal signs consist of fever, conjunctivitis, coryza, cough, and Koplik's spots on the oral mucosa above the first and second upper molars. Inflammation of the pharynx and upper respiratory tract is common. Between the third and seventh day after onset of disease, a reddish brown maculopapular eruption appears on the face and later becomes generalized. The eruption lasts 4 to 7 days, ending in scaly desquamation. Possible complications are otitis media, pneumonia, and encephalitis. Measles is more severe in malnourished children, in whom it can cause a 5 to 10% fatality rate (American Public Health Association, 1985).

The Disease in Nonhuman Primates: Many infections occur subclinically. Since most clinical measles outbreaks have appeared in recently imported animals, it is thought that stress caused by capture, confinement, and transport is an important factor in the appearance of clinical infection (Karstad, 1981). Symptomatology is variable from one outbreak to another and may or may not include cutaneous eruption or some of the other signs. In the outbreak that occurred among *P. cristatus*, 24 of 31 monkeys had a maculopapular eruption, especially on the ventral surface of the body, which lasted 6 to 9 days and ended in desquamation over a period of 2 weeks. Some animals had mucopurulent coryza and conjunctivitis (Montrey *et al.*, 1980). In the outbreak among colobus monkeys (*C. guereza*), the predominant signs consisted of rhinitis, conjunctivitis, pneumonia, dry cough, and periorbital and facial edema, but no cutaneous eruption (Hime and Keymer, 1975). Deaths occurred in some of the outbreaks, but it could not be established with certainty that they were due to measles virus.

Source of Infection and Mode of Transmission (Figure 42): Man is the only known reservoir. The virus has been isolated from nasopharyngeal secretions of man both in the prodromal period and during the first days of eruption. This fact indicates

Figure 42. Measles. Transmission cycle.

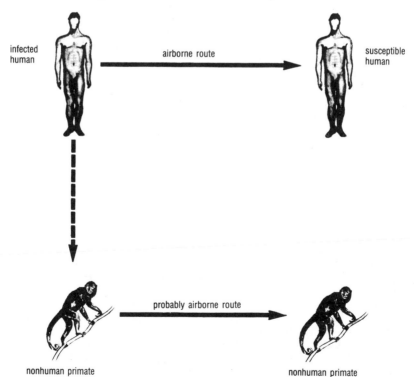

infected human

airborne route

susceptible human

probably airborne route

nonhuman primate

nonhuman primate

that infection is transmitted from person to person mainly via the airborne route. The transmission period starts shortly before the onset of the prodromal symptomatology and lasts up to 4 days after appearance of the eruption; it is minimal after the second day of eruption.

All evidence indicates that nonhuman primates acquire infection by exposure to man, although the source could not be identified in all cases. It is probable that infection propagates among monkeys in the same manner as in humans (Yamanouchi *et al.*, 1969). Retransmission of infection from monkey to man has not been observed up to now.

Diagnosis: Specific diagnosis can be made by isolation of the virus or by serology. Virus can be isolated in tissue culture during the prodromal period or from pharyngeal washings, blood, or urine during the first days of eruption. Serologic examination to confirm seroconversion is done by complement fixation and hemagglutination inhibition tests.

Control: Potent attenuated live virus vaccines are now available. With the introduction in 1963 of immunization in the USA, the annual incidence of approximately 500,000 cases was reduced to 14,000 by 1980 (Katz, 1982). Although these vaccines have been very effective in preventing the disease in developed countries, their use on children in tropical regions has not had the same success. This is due to the fact that infection with wild virus can occur in the short period, which varies with age, between the loss of maternal antibodies and the time the vaccine takes effect (Black, 1984).

To prevent contagion of nonhuman primates from a human source and to permit their use in measles research, their strict isolation is recommended from the time of capture to their incorporation into colonies, always keeping them in individual cages and providing personnel with masks and protective clothing (Yamanouchi *et al.*, 1969). If the monkeys are not to be used for measles research they can be vaccinated, but the susceptibility of different species to attenuated (vaccine) viruses must be kept in mind. A very attenuated Edmonston virus strain vaccine has been used successfully on rhesus monkeys, but it causes clinical measles and death in marmosets and owl monkeys. For highly susceptible species, the use of an inactivated vaccine is suggested, followed by vaccination with a modified live virus vaccine 1 month later (Karstad, 1981).

Bibliography

American Public Health Association. *Control of Communicable Diseases in Man*, 14th ed. (Ed. by A. S. Benenson). Washington, D.C., APHA, 1985.

Bhatt, P. N., C. D. Brandt, R. A. Weiss, J. P. Fox, and M. F. Shaffer. Viral infections of monkeys in their natural habitat in southern India. *Am J Trop Med Hyg* 15:561-566, 1966.

Black, F. L. Measles. *In*: Warren, K. S., and A. A. F. Mahmoud (Eds.), *Tropical and Geographical Medicine*, New York, McGraw-Hill Book Co., 1984.

Hime, J. M., and I. F. Keymer. Measles in recently imported colobus monkeys (*Colobus guereza*). *Vet Rec* 97:392-394, 1975.

Kalter, S. S., J. Ratner, G. V. Kalter, A. R. Rodríguez, and C. S. Kim. A survey of primate sera for antibodies to viruses of human and simian origin. *Am J Epidemiol* 86:552-568, 1967.

Karstad, L. Miscellaneous viral infections. *In*: Davis, J. W., L. H. Karstad, and D. O.

Trainer (Eds.), *Infectious Diseases of Wild Mammals*, 2nd ed. Ames, Iowa State University Press, 1981.

Katz, S. L. Measles. *In*: Wyngaarden, J. B., and L. H. Smith, Jr. (Eds.), *Cecil Textbook of Medicine*, 16th ed., vol. 2. Philadelphia, Saunders, 1982.

Montrey, R. D., D. L. Huxsoll, P. K. Hildebrandt, B. W. Booth, and S. Arimbalam. An epizootic of measles in captive silver leaf-monkeys (*Presbytis cristatus*) in Malaysia. *Lab Anim Sci* 30:694-697, 1980.

Soave, O. Viral infections common to human and non-human primates. *J Am Vet Med Assoc* 179:1385-1388, 1981.

Yamanouchi, K., A. Fakuda, F. Kobune, M. Hikita, and A. Shishido. Serologic survey with the sera of monkeys in regard to their natural infection with measles virus. *Jpn J Med Sci Biol* 22:117-121, 1969.

MURRAY VALLEY ENCEPHALITIS

(062.4)

Synonym: Australian X disease.

Etiology: RNA virus belonging to the genus *Flavivirus* (formerly group B of the arboviruses) of the family Togaviridae; it is a member of the complex of viruses that produce Japanese B, St. Louis, West Nile, and Rocio encephalitides.

Geographic Distribution: Australia and New Guinea.

Occurrence in Man: Since 1917-1918, when an unknown human disease (X disease) responsible for 134 cases of encephalitis was recognized in southern Australia, several epidemics have occurred at irregular intervals in the same area of that country, most recently in 1971 and 1974. The virus was isolated in 1951 and was named Murray Valley encephalitis (MVE) virus for the place where it was isolated. Although cases of the infection have been confirmed in all of the Australian states and in New Guinea, epidemics have occurred only in the most populous part of southern Australia. According to serologic studies, only one clinical case of encephalitis occurs per 500 to 1,000 inapparent infections. Other parts of Australia report sporadic cases or small outbreaks, but not epidemics.

Seroepidemiologic studies carried out in the Northern Territory of Australia indicate that endemic foci of the virus exist. In 11 areas studied, neutralizing antibodies were found in 7 to 89% of the aborigines; in three of these areas the prevalence of seropositives varied between 86 and 89%. There are also endemic areas in New Guinea.

Occurrence in Animals: High rates of seroreactors have been found in equines, cattle, dogs, foxes, marsupials, and wild and domestic birds.

The Disease in Man: The symptomatology of MVE is similar to that of Japanese B encephalitis. The rate of attack is highest in children under 10 years of age. The symptoms consist of fever, cephalalgia, myalgia, vomiting, and encephalitis. Case fatality rates (over 40%) and rates of nervous sequelae are high. Epidemics have occurred during the second half of summer.

The Disease in Animals: Domestic mammals become infected, but do not manifest clinical symptoms. A few years ago, on the basis of serologic tests, an association was suggested between infection with MVE virus and a disease of the central nervous system in equines. Nevertheless, such a cause and effect relationship has not been verified because the virus has not been isolated in these cases (Gard *et al.*, 1977).

Source of Infection and Mode of Transmission: The natural history of the disease is not yet clear. In endemic areas of northern Australia and New Guinea, the virus might circulate between aquatic birds and mosquitoes. The virus has been isolated from *Culex annulirostris*, considered the main vector, and from two other mosquito species. The only virus isolation from a bird was obtained from the heron *Ardea novaehollandiae* during the 1974 epidemic. The role of domestic and wild mammals as amplifiers of the virus is also undefined. According to experimental data, many species of birds and mammals could play that role (Kay *et al.*, 1981).

The origin of the important epidemic outbreaks that have occurred in southern Australia (Murray Valley), sometimes at 15-year intervals, remains in doubt. One hypothesis was that the virus disappeared during interepidemic periods and then broke out again from endemic areas in the North, carried by young birds. Once the virus was introduced, domestic and aquatic birds would play an important role as a source of infection for the arthropod vector. Amplification of the infection through birds and mosquitoes, along with the presence of a dense and susceptible human population, would favor epidemics.

However, serum samples from wild pigs from several localities in New South Wales, studied in the years preceding the 1974 epidemic, showed that the MVE virus was active in this interepidemic period. A high rate of reactors to the hemagglutination inhibition test was found in wild pigs in swampy areas of the region. Some of the positive sera were examined by the neutralization test for the MVE as well as the Kunjin[1] virus; much higher titers were obtained for MVE than for Kunjin, except in a few samples (Gard *et al.*, 1976). In that region, when rivers flood and more food becomes available, populations of pigs, aquatic birds, and mosquitoes increase greatly. Studies on the habits of *C. annulirostris* found that the vector feeds principally on mammals (Kay *et al.*, 1981). The sometimes contradictory results of the research to date have identified the vector, but the hosts and amplifiers of the virus and factors leading to epidemic situations have not been defined.

Diagnosis: The virus has only been isolated from the central nervous system of fatal cases, by means of inoculation of mice and chick embryos. Serologic diagnosis is done with hemagglutination inhibition, complement fixation, and neutralization tests. This last test is important to distinguish MVE antibodies from those resulting from other flaviviruses, especially the Kunjin virus.

---

[1] The Kunjin virus is another Australian flavivirus, antigenically related to MVE, transmitted by the same vector (*C. annulirostris*), and probably maintained by a wild bird-mosquito cycle or a mammal-mosquito cycle (Liehne *et al.*, 1976); a few cases of mild febrile illness in man have been recorded (Doherty, 1981).

Control: Vaccines are not available. In an epidemic, control should be directed against the vector.

Bibliography

Andrewes, C., and H. G. Pereira. *Viruses of Vertebrates*, 3rd ed. Baltimore, Maryland, Williams and Wilkins, 1972.

Centers for Disease Control of the USA. *International Catalogue of Arboviruses*, 2nd ed. (Ed. by T. O. Berge). Atlanta, Georgia, 1975. (DHEW Publ. CDC 75-8301.)

Clarke, D. H., and J. Casals. Arboviruses: Group B. *In*: Horsfall, F. L., and I. Tamm (Eds.), *Viral and Rickettsial Infection of Man*, 4th ed. Philadelphia, Lippincott, 1965.

Doherty, R. L. Arboviral zoonoses in Australasia. *In*: Beran, G. W. (Section Ed.), *CRC Handbook Series in Zoonoses*. Section B, vol. 1. Boca Raton, Florida, CRC Press, 1981.

Downs, W. G. Arboviruses. *In*: Evans, A. S. (Ed.), *Viral Infections of Humans. Epidemiology and Control*. New York, Plenum, 1976.

Gard, G. P., J. P. Giles, R. J. Dwyer-Gray, and G. M. Woodroofe. Serological evidence of interepidemic infection of feral pigs in New South Wales with Murray Valley encephalitis virus. *Aust J Exp Biol Med Sci* 54:297-302, 1976.

Gard, G. P., I. D. Marshall, K. H. Walker, H. M. Acland, and W. G. De Sarem. Association of Australian arboviruses with nervous disease in horses. *Aust Vet J* 53:61-66, 1977.

Kay, B. H., P. L. Young, I. D. Fanning, and R. A. Hall. Which vertebrates amplify Murray Valley encephalitis virus in Southern Australia? *In*: Fowler, M. E. (Ed.), *Wildlife Diseases of the Pacific Basin and Other Countries. Proceedings, 4th International Conference of the Wildlife Diseases Association* (Sydney, Australia, August 1981). Davis, University of California, 1981.

Liehne, C. G., N. F. Stanley, M. P. Alpers, S. Paul, P. F. S. Liehne, and K. H. Chan. Ord River arboviruses—serological epidemiology. *Aust J Exp Biol Med Sci* 54:505-512, 1976.

Miles, J. A. R. Epidemiology of the arthropod-borne encephalitides. *Bull WHO* 22:339-371, 1960.

NEWCASTLE DISEASE

(077.8)
(372.0)

Synonyms: Pneumoencephalitis, pseudoplague of fowl, pseudo–fowl pest, paramyxovirus 1, Ranikhet disease.

Etiology: RNA virus belonging to the genus *Paramyxovirus* of the family Paramyxoviridae. At least six other paramyxoviruses of birds form part of the same taxonomic group, along with the parainfluenza viruses and the infectious parotitis (mumps, urlian fever) virus. In nature, several genetically distinct types of the virus exist, which differ in their virulence and the pathology they produce in birds.

According to how quickly they cause the death of inoculated chick embryos (among other parameters), they have been classified as follows: a) lentogenic viruses of attenuated virulence, b) velogenic viruses of high virulence, and c) mesogenic viruses of intermediate virulence. To these three types must be added the viscerotropic viruses. Thus, Newcastle disease (ND) viruses are classified into four pathogenic types, or pathotypes. There are no indications that the neurotropic lentogenic, mesogenic, or velogenic viruses can change into the viscerotropic pathotype, also called the Asian or exotic type.

Formerly, it was thought that the strains of the ND virus were antigenically uniform, according to results of the hemagglutination inhibition test. But the crossed plaque reduction serum neutralization test has demonstrated antigenic variation among the strains from different countries; however, this finding lacks importance in protection efforts. In a recent project that utilized monoclonal antibodies to study 40 strains of the virus, eight antigenic groups were differentiated. The viruses of each group seemed to have biological and epizootiological properties in common (Russell and Alexander, 1983).

Geographic Distribution: The disease in fowl is distributed worldwide.

Occurrence in Man and Animals: Newcastle virus infection is seen in domestic, semidomestic, and wild fowl. It is one of the most important diseases of domestic fowl and occurs enzootically and epizootically, producing large economic losses. An especially important panzootic caused by the velogenic-viscerotropic virus appeared in 1966-1968 in the Middle East, in 1970 in parts of South America and Europe, and in 1970-1971 in the United States and Canada. This form of the disease is characterized by a superacute course, high mortality, and an affinity for the viscera, especially the digestive tract, where it produces hemorrhages and necrotic areas. The viscerotropic type of the virus is probably responsible for the disease that was recognized in 1926 in Indonesia and in 1927 in Newcastle, England, for which the illness was named. In India, Southeast Asia, and parts of Africa, outbreaks of a highly fatal disease have been recorded, probably due to the same pathotype of the virus.

On the other hand, enzootics with a variable clinical picture and caused by a less virulent virus occur continually in many countries of the world.

The disease occurs infrequently in humans, primarily among poultry slaughterhouse workers, laboratory personnel, and vaccinators applying live virus vaccines. In a poultry slaughterhouse in Minnesota, USA, which employed 90 workers, an outbreak with 40 clinical cases was described. In an agricultural school in Israel, 17 cases occurred among kitchen staff, but none were seen among persons who worked with poultry on the school farm. It is possible that many sporadic cases of conjunctivitis caused by the Newcastle disease virus occur in which either medical attention is not sought due to the benign course of the disease, or laboratory diagnosis is not provided. The infection may also be subclinical, as indicated by a serologic study carried out at a poultry slaughterhouse. Here, using the serum neutralization test, high titers were found in 64% of exposed personnel who had not demonstrated any clinical symptoms. In other studies the prevalence of reactors was low, especially in professional groups that did not have contact with birds.

The Disease in Man: The incubation period is usually from 1 to 2 days, but may extend up to 4 days. The clinical picture consists primarily of conjunctivitis, with congestion, lacrimation, pain, and swelling of the subconjunctival tissues. The preauricular lymph glands are often affected. The conjunctivitis is generally unilateral, and systemic reactions are rare. The patient recovers in 1 week without sequelae. Some cases have involved a generalized infection lasting 3 or 4 days with a symptomatology similar to that of influenza, including a slightly elevated temperature, chills, and pharyngitis. This form of the infection has occurred after exposure to aerosols of the virus.

Man is susceptible to all pathotypes of the virus, including the lentogenic vaccine viruses.

The Disease in Animals: The virus has been isolated from numerous species of birds. The natural disease occurs in domestic fowl, especially chickens, turkeys, and pigeons; ducks and geese are more resistant. Several forms of the disease have been observed, depending on the pathotype of the infecting virus and the host's resistance. The incubation period averages 5 to 6 days, but varies between 2 and 15 or more days. The most commonly observed clinical forms worldwide are the following:

a) Pneumoencephalitic or neurotropic form, characterized by neurologic symptoms that appear a few days after the onset of a respiratory syndrome. Tremors, torticollis, and opisthotonos are common. Mortality can vary between 10 and 90% from one poultry farm to another. This form attacks birds of all ages and does not cause hemorrhagic lesions in the digestive tract. It is produced by velogenic strains.

b) Respiratory syndrome, which affects adult fowl and manifests itself in chicks as respiratory and neurologic symptoms. Mortality in chicks is 10 to 50%, but is insignificant in adult fowl. This form is caused by some mesogenic strains.

c) Inapparent infection in adult fowl and mild respiratory symptoms in chicks, with an insignificant mortality rate. This form is caused by lentogenic viruses.

In Australia a special situation exists. The last outbreaks of the infection with clinical manifestations occurred in 1930 and 1932. A serologic study done in 1964 found no reactors. A few years later a strain of the virus was isolated in Queensland and subsequent serologic studies found that the infection was widespread in the country. The isolated strains had very low pathogenicity for embryos and chicks and produced no symptomatic infection. These avirulent strains of unknown origin demonstrated good immunogenic capacity (Westbury, 1981).

In the Americas the first outbreak of the velogenic-viscerotropic type was recognized in Paraguay in 1970. It caused great losses, estimated at 1 million birds, to the incipient poultry industry of that country. In the same year the illness also appeared in Europe and the United States. This form of the disease is considered to be similar or identical to that originally described in 1927 in Newcastle, which later disappeared. It has been estimated that the viscerotropic form of the disease has caused losses in Europe of about £100 million. This superacute or exotic form is characterized by a short incubation period of 2 to 4 days, sudden onset, diarrhea, and frequent tracheal discharge. The tremors and torticollis of the neurotropic form are rare, but paralysis sometimes occurs. This form is highly fatal, with death occurring 1 to 3 days after the onset of symptoms. Some cases exhibit edema of the wattles, eyelids, and face; this was formerly considered to be a characteristic sign of fowl plague.

The "domestic" forms of the disease, caused by less virulent viruses, produce macroscopic lesions that are usually located in the trachea; splenomegaly is sometimes found. By contrast, the exotic form mainly produces hemorrhagic lesions of the intestinal tract, especially in the proventriculus and sometimes in the gizzard and small intestine. Hemorrhages can also be found in the trachea, and edema in the underlying tissues.

The disease causes losses not only from the deaths and stunted growth of fowl, but also from a large reduction in egg laying. Affected hens stop laying for at least a week. At the start of an outbreak, hens lay eggs with abnormal shells, an irregularity that may persist temporarily or permanently.

Source of Infection and Mode of Transmission (Figure 43): Fowl constitute the reservoir of the virus. The original reservoir may possibly have been some species of wild bird from Southeast Asia, as evidenced by the explosive and highly fatal nature of the outbreaks in domestic birds recognized in 1926 in Indonesia. Outbreaks of this nature would indicate that the virus was poorly adapted to domestic fowl and that these animals would have difficulty acting as the reservoir. At the present time the agent-host relationship has changed, so that domestic fowl, especially poultry,

Figure 43. Newcastle disease. Transmission cycle.

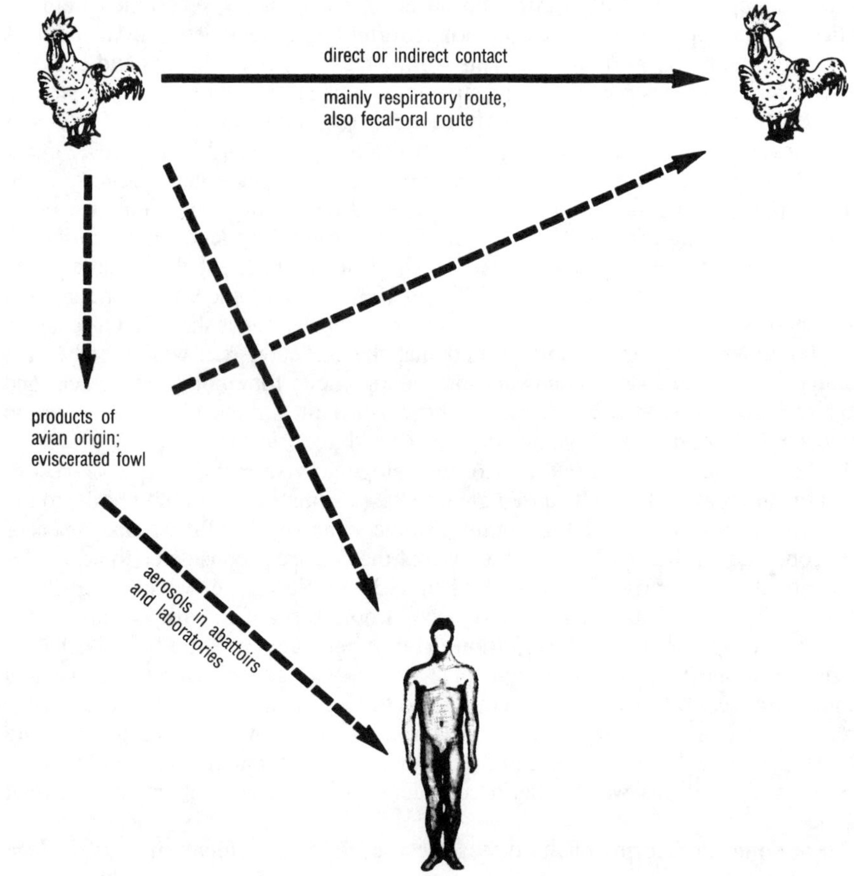

are the main hosts of the virus, at least for pathotypes less virulent than the viscerotropic virus.

On a poultry farm the virus is spread from bird to bird by direct or indirect contact, generally by the respiratory route and, less frequently, by the digestive route. The changes introduced in the last 50 years in poultry operations played an essential role in the persistence of the virus. Transmission of this disease, as with any other disease transmitted by aerosols, depends on population density, and on modern poultry farms the concentration of birds is enormous (Hanson, 1978). The infection is introduced onto a farm by infected birds and contaminated objects, as well as by people's clothing, shoes, and hands. Fowl vaccinated with mesogenic strains eliminate the virus in their droppings for 15 to 19 days, and this may constitute another source of infection. The lentogenic vaccinal strain B1 can be propagated from vaccinated to susceptible fowl only by direct contact.

A permanent carrier state is rare in chickens. It has been shown experimentally that after 34 days chickens cease to transmit the infection by contact. Shedding of the virus seems to be more prolonged in turkeys.

Infected live fowl are the most important source of virus transmission from one country to another and within the same country. Fowl killed for consumption and wastes from poultry slaughterhouses are also very important sources of infection both in international and national trade. The disease was thought to have been introduced into several countries by importation of frozen eviscerated chickens. It has been shown experimentally that the virus can survive 300 days or more in bone marrow, and up to 190 days in lungs and skin. Survival of the virus, of course, depends on the storage temperature. Contaminated truck beds, cages, and cartons constitute other vehicles of virus dissemination. On several occasions biologicals such as avian pox and laryngotracheitis vaccines that were contaminated with the Newcastle disease virus have produced infection foci. The infection can also be spread to neighboring establishments by wind, the movement of personnel, and, less frequently, by free-ranging birds. In some instances the virus has been introduced from one country to another by the importation of pheasants and partridges.

The panzootic of the viscerotropic form of the disease in the late 1960s and early 1970s drew the attention of researchers to the role played by various wild or captive undomesticated fowl and by recreational domestic fowl. Velogenic-viscerotropic virus has been repeatedly isolated in Europe and the United States from imported parrots and related birds. Another important source of the virus has been illegally introduced fighting cocks. So far, there is no reliable evidence that migratory birds transmit the virus from one country to another. The hypothesis has been formulated that two reservoirs of the virus exist in nature: migratory waterfowl of the Neartic for the mild respiratory type virus, and tropical jungle birds for the viscerotropic virus (Hanson, 1976).

In an area of the United States where the viscerotropic form of the disease was epizootic in domestic fowl, a study was carried out (Pearson and McCann, 1975) to determine the role of wild, semidomestic, and exotic birds in the epizootiology of the disease. Out of 9,446 wild noncaptive birds, the virus was isolated from only three house sparrows (*Passer domesticus*) and one crow (*Corvus brachyrhynchos*), which had all been in contact with infected chickens. Out of 4,367 semidomestic fowl the virus was isolated from 33 (0.76%), mainly ducks, pheasants, and pigeons; out of 3,780 exotic birds kept in captivity, the agent was found in 38 (1.01%), mostly psittacines, pittas, and toucans. These results suggest that the disease is primarily linked to confinement.

During studies on the role of migratory waterfowl, strains of virus classified as lentogenic and heat stable were isolated from ducks and geese. The latter characteristic differentiates these strains from those isolated from chickens. The scant contact between waterfowl and domestic poultry, together with the thermostability of these waterfowl strains, would indicate that infection of wild geese and ducks occurs independently in nature (Spalatin and Hanson, 1975).

The main source of the virus for man is poultry and poultry products, as well as virus cultures in the laboratory. The disease is transmitted by aerosols in poultry slaughterhouses and in laboratories, or by contact when rubbing the eyes with hands contaminated by handling infected fowl or the virus. On farms the infection can be acquired during the administration of powdered or aerosol vaccines.

Diagnosis: In the event that Newcastle disease is suspected in a human patient, an attempt should always be made to isolate the virus, since serologic response is absent in a large proportion of infected persons. The virus may be isolated from conjunctival or nasopharyngeal secretions, saliva, or urine, after inoculation into chick embryos, susceptible chickens, or tissue culture. Serologic diagnosis is performed using blood samples obtained during the acute phase of the disease and 2 or 3 weeks later, by means of the neutralization, hemagglutination inhibition, and gel precipitation tests.

The same procedures are used for poultry. Samples for the isolation tests should be obtained from birds in the first phase of the disease and should consist of tracheal exudate, spleen, or lung tissue for inoculations or culture. Besides the currently used hemagglutination inhibition and neutralization tests, the ELISA test for one serum dilution has recently been perfected and will prove useful once standardization is achieved among laboratories (Snyder *et al.*, 1983).

Control: The chief control measures for domestic fowl consist of good hygiene practices and routine vaccination. The vaccines most widely used are those containing live lentogenic virus type B1. Inactivated vaccines have also been used and, according to data from Great Britain, considerably reduced the incidence of the disease. Although they confer shorter duration immunity, inactivated vaccines have the advantage of not producing the secondary effects induced by live vaccines in laying hens. On the other hand, live vaccines permit mass vaccination, a great advantage in the modern poultry industry with large concentrations of birds since individual vaccination is practically impossible owing to costs. The aerosolization technique is used for mass vaccination. The vaccine can also be administered in drinking water, but this method is less efficient. On smaller establishments (poultry breeding farms), individual application of the vaccine by instilling one drop into the conjunctival sac can be done. By preventing the disease, vaccines have allowed poultry production to continue under the present concentrated and confined conditions, but the infection has not been eradicated yet and it is widely distributed (Hanson, 1978).

In the laboratory, precautions should be taken to avoid the formation of aerosols and contamination of eyes by the hands. The risk of infection to vaccinators can be reduced by the use of masks to protect them against ocular or respiratory exposure.

Bibliography

Allan, W. H. The problem of Newcastle disease. *Nature* 234:129-131, 1971.

Andrewes, C., and H. G. Pereira. *Viruses of Vertebrates*, 3rd ed. Baltimore, Maryland, Williams and Wilkins, 1972.

Benson, H. N., D. R. Wenger, and P. D. Beard. Efficacy of a commercial Newcastle vaccine against velogenic viscerotropic Newcastle disease virus. *Avian Dis* 19:566-572, 1975.

Brandly, C. A. The occupational hazard of Newcastle disease to man. *Lab Anim Care* 14:433-440, 1964.

Francis, D. W., and E. Rivelli. Case report—Newcastle disease in Paraguay. *Avian Dis* 16:336-342, 1972.

Hanson, R. P. Newcastle disease. *In*: Hofstad, N. S. (Ed.), *Diseases of Poultry*. Ames, Iowa State University Press, 1971.

Hanson, R. P. Paramyxovirus infections. *In*: Hubbert, W. T., W. F. McCulloch, and P. R. Schnurrenberger (Eds.), *Diseases Transmitted from Animals to Man*, 6th ed., Springfield, Illinois, Thomas, 1975.

Hanson, R. P. Avian reservoirs of Newcastle disease. *In*: Page, L. A. (Ed.), *Wildlife Diseases*. New York, Plenum, 1976.

Hanson, R. P. Newcastle disease. *In*: Hofstad, N. S., B. W. Calnek, C. F. Hemboldt, W. M. Reid, and H. W. Yoder, Jr. (Eds.), *Diseases of Poultry*. Ames, Iowa State University Press, 1978.

Hanson, R. P., J. Spalarin, and G. S. Jacobson. The viscerotropic pathotype of Newcastle disease virus. *Avian Dis* 17:354-361, 1973.

Lancaster, J. E. Newcastle disease—modes of spread. *Vet Bull* 33:221-226 and 279-285, 1963.

Pearson, G. L., and M. K. McCann. The role of indigenous wild, semidomestic, and exotic birds in the epizootiology of velogenic viscerotropic Newcastle disease in Southern California, 1972-1973. *J Amer Vet Med Assoc* 167:610-614, 1975.

Russell, P. H., and D. J. Alexander. Antigenic variation of Newcastle disease virus strains detected by monoclonal antibodies. *Arch Virol* 75:243-253, 1983.

Snyder, D. B., W. W. Marquardt, E. T. Mallinson, and E. Russek. Rapid serological profiling by enzyme-linked immunosorbent assay. I. Measurement of antibody activity titer against Newcastle disease virus in a single serum dilution. *Avian Dis* 27:161-170, 1983.

Spalatin, J., and R. P. Hanson. Epizootiology of Newcastle disease in waterfowl. *Avian Dis* 19:573-582, 1975.

Walker, J. W., B. R. Heron, and M. A. Mixson. Exotic Newcastle disease eradication programs in the United States. *Avian Dis* 17:486-503, 1973.

Westbury, H. A. Newcastle disease virus in Australia. *Aust Vet J* 57:292-298, 1981.

OMSK HEMORRHAGIC FEVER

(065.1)

Etiology: RNA genome virus of the genus *Flavivirus* (arbovirus complex B), family Togaviridae; antigenically, it belongs to the complex that includes tick-borne Russian spring-summer encephalitis and ovine encephalomyelitis. Two antigenic varieties of the virus have been described.

Geographic Distribution: The virus has only been isolated in western Siberia, USSR.

Occurrence: Formerly it occurred among rural workers and children in the steppes of the Omsk region; more recently it has been observed in the Novosibirsk, Kurgan, and Tyumen regions.

The Disease in Man: The incubation period is from 3 to 7 days. It is an acute febrile disease of sudden onset, with or without hemorrhagic manifestations. Bronchopneumonia is frequent; leukopenia is common. Generally, the central nervous system is not affected. In 25 to 40% of the cases the fever is biphasic, with an intermediate afebrile interval. Alopecia during convalescence is frequent. The fatality rate is 1 to 2%.

The Disease in Animals: The virus has been isolated from various species of rodents and other small mammals. The muskrat, *Ondatra zibethicus,* is very susceptible and many die as a consequence of the infection. In this species, experimental inoculation often produces a hemorrhagic disease with high viremia that can last more than 3 weeks. In some other small mammals, experimental infection causes only a mild and transitory illness with asthenia and lethargy, and in other species it is asymptomatic (Seymour and Yuill, 1981).

Source of Infection and Mode of Transmission: The main vector is *Dermacentor pictus*, a tick which requires three hosts for its development: the larvae and nymphs feed on small mammals and the adults on large domestic and wild animals. The tick also acts as a reservoir, since it can transmit the virus transovarially.

The virus has been isolated frequently from the muskrat, *O. zibethicus,* which was introduced from the Americas. Epizootics with high mortality occur among muskrats. It is probable that the real reservoirs for maintenance of the virus in nature are not muskrats but small rodents and insectivores, such as *Arvicola terrestris*, *Microtus oeconomus*, and *Sorex araneus*, from which the virus has been isolated. The first of these mammals maintains close contact with muskrats, sharing their burrows in winter. Urine is probably the source of infection for the rodents. The virus has been isolated from the urine of naturally infected muskrats and *A. terrestris* mice and from experimentally inoculated *M. oeconomus* and *Citellus erythrogenus*. It was also possible to confirm infection via the oral route in some of these animals (Seymour and Yuill, 1981).

Man can become infected by tick bites and by direct transmission from muskrats. Most cases now occur among persons whose work involves muskrats (hunters, trappers, skinners). Human cases have occurred in winter, when ticks are inactive. Laboratory infections are common and are probably contracted from aerosols.

Diagnosis: The virus can be isolated from the blood of febrile patients. Serologic diagnosis can be made by using the neutralization, complement fixation, and hemagglutination inhibition tests.

Control: An inactivated vaccine of mouse brain origin is available and has given satisfactory results.

Bibliography

Andrewes, C., and H. G. Pereira. *Viruses of Vertebrates*, 3rd ed. Baltimore, Maryland, Williams and Wilkins, 1972.

American Public Health Association. *Control of Communicable Diseases in Man*, 14th ed. (Ed. by A. S. Benenson). Washington, D.C., APHA, 1985.

Casals, J., B. E. Henderson, H. Hoogstraal, K. M. Johnson, and A. Shelokov. A review of Soviet viral hemorrhagic fevers, 1969. *J Infect Dis* 122:437-453, 1970.

Centers for Disease Control of the USA. *International Catalogue of Arboviruses*, 2nd ed. (Ed. by T. O. Berge). Atlanta, Georgia, 1975 (DHEW Publ. CDC 75-8301).

Clarke, D. H., and J. Casals. Arboviruses, group B. *In*: Horsfall, F. L., and I. Tamm (Eds.), *Viral and Rickettsial Infections of Man*, 4th ed. Philadelphia, Lippincott, 1965.

Downs, W. G. Arboviruses. *In*: A. S. Evans (Ed.), *Viral Infections of Humans. Epidemiology and Control*. New York, Plenum, 1976.

Kharitonova, N. N., and Y. A. Leonor (M. P. Chumakov, Ed.-in-chief). *Omsk Hemorrhagic Fever: Ecology of the Agent and Epizootiology*. New Delhi, India, National Library of Medicine, Amerinol Publishing Co., Pvt. Ltd., 1985.

Prier, J. E. *Basic Medical Virology*. Baltimore, Maryland, Williams and Wilkins, 1966.

Seymour, C., and T. M. Yuill. Arboviruses. *In*: Davis, J. W., L. H. Karstad, and D. O. Trainer, *Infectious Diseases of Wild Mammals*, 2nd ed. Ames, Iowa State University Press, 1981.

OROPOUCHE FEVER

(066.3)

Etiology: RNA genome virus (ORO), genus *Bunyavirus*, family Bunyaviridae. Serologically, ORO is classified in the Simbu group.

Geographic Distribution and Occurrence in Man: The virus was isolated for the first time in 1955 from a forest worker with fever who came from the locality Vega de Oropouche in Trinidad, giving the disease its name. The serum neutralization test on 46 forest workers from the island found antibodies present in only three of them (Anderson *et al.*, 1961).

From 1961 to 1978 seven epidemics of Oropouche fever (OF) occurred in Pará State, Brazil, all in the most populous part, south of the Amazon River. In two of these epidemics, in Belém in 1961 and in Santarém in 1975, the number of persons affected was estimated at 11,000 and 14,000, respectively (Pinheiro *et al.*, 1981). It has been estimated that at least 165,000 persons were infected during these epidemics. In 1978, another outbreak started in the small town of Quatro Bocas (Pará) and later spread in a northerly direction to other rural communities until it reached epidemic proportions in Belém (capital of the state) in 1979-1980 (LeDuc *et al.*, 1981).

In the neighboring state of Amazonas the disease appeared for the first time in two epidemics, one in the city of Barcelos from May to July 1980 and the other in Manaus from October 1980 to February 1981. The prevalence of hemagglutination-inhibiting antibodies in 496 randomly selected persons in six Manaus neighborhoods was 4.2% at the beginning of the outbreak and 16.7% at the end of the epidemic. According to one estimate, 97,000 persons among the 650,000 inhabitants of Manaus were infected during the outbreak (Borborema *et al.*, 1982).

Up to now, epidemics have occurred only in the Brazilian Amazon region, but lately they have become more frequent and have affected a growing number of persons (LeDuc *et al.*, 1981).

Epidemics occur during the rainy season. It is probable that unrecognized sporadic cases also occur, as happened in Trinidad when the virus was first isolated in man. Subclinical infections have been confirmed by serologic studies carried out during postepidemic periods and in portions of the Brazilian Amazon outside the epidemic areas (Pinheiro *et al.*, 1981).

Besides northern Brazil and Trinidad, it is possible that the virus exists in Colombia, where neutralizing antibodies have been found in nonhuman primates in the Magdalena valley (Centers for Disease Control, 1975).

Occurrence in Animals: The ORO virus has been isolated only from the three-toed sloth, *Bradypus tridactylus,* in Brazil (Pinheiro *et al.*, 1981). Neutralizing antibodies have been found in 9 of 26 howler monkeys (*Alouatta saniculus insularis*) and in 8 of 26 *Cebus* spp. in Trinidad (Anderson *et al.*, 1961). Out of a large number of vertebrates (mostly birds) captured in the Brazilian Amazon region, hemagglutination-inhibiting antibodies were found in 1% of rodents, 11.9% of primates, 4.1% of sloths, and 2.8% of birds (Pinheiro *et al.*, 1981).

The Disease in Man: The incubation period lasts 4 to 8 days. The disease is of sudden onset. The main symptomatology consists of pyrexia, which can reach 40°C, intense cephalalgia, chills, myalgia, arthralgia, asthenia, and photophobia. Some patients also manifest nausea, vomiting, diarrhea, and conjunctival congestion. In less than 5% of the cases a maculopapular exanthematic eruption is observed on the trunk, arms, and sometimes the lower extremities. The acute phase lasts 2 to 5 days. Nearly 60% of patients experience one or more recurring crises 1 or 2 weeks after disappearance of the initial manifestations. During the 1980 epidemic wave, some patients displayed symptoms of meningitis (Pinheiro *et al.*, 1982a). No deaths attributable to this disease have been confirmed.

The Disease in Animals: The disease occurs asymptomatically in lower animals. Sloths and primates inoculated subcutaneously with the ORO virus develop viremia that lasts several days (Pinheiro *et al.*, 1981).

Source of Infection and Mode of Transmission (Figure 44): The natural history of the ORO virus has not yet been completely elucidated. Research points to the existence of two different cycles, one wild and another urban (Pinheiro *et al.*, 1981).

Figure 44. Oropouche fever. Possible circulation of the virus.
(Adapted from Pinheiro *et al.*, 1981.)

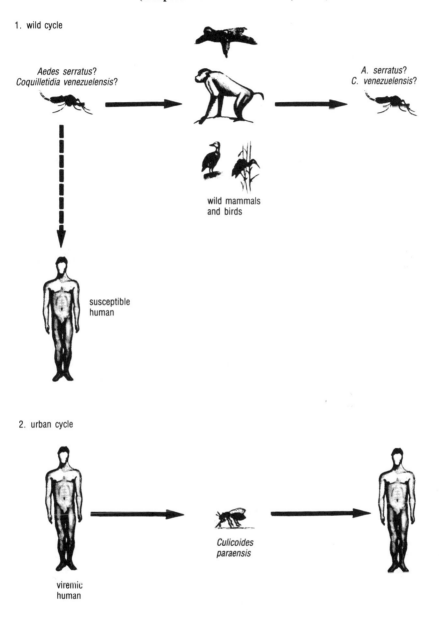

1. wild cycle

Aedes serratus?
Coquilletidia venezuelensis?

A. serratus?
C. venezuelensis?

wild mammals
and birds

susceptible
human

2. urban cycle

Culicoides
paraensis

viremic
human

Neither the main reservoir of the virus in nature nor the vector of the wild cycle is known precisely. The virus has been isolated only from sloths (*Bradypus tridactylus*), and antibodies have been found in primates, rodents, and birds (especially of the family Formicariidae). When the primates *Cebus*, *Saimiri*, and *Saguinus* are experimentally infected, a viremia is produced that can last up to one week. Accordingly, it is possible that sloths, primates, and birds constitute the ORO virus reservoir. Information regarding what vector transmits the virus in the jungle is limited. The virus was isolated once from the jungle mosquito *Coquilletidia venezuelensis* in Trinidad and once also from *Aedes serratus* in Brazil, in spite of the fact that more than one million hematophagous insects have been examined in that country (up to now with the exclusion of wild *Culicoides*). As for the urban cycle, the most notable epidemiologic facts are the following: a) the disease occurs where there is a high density of the midge *Culicoides paraensis*; b) this insect was an efficient vector in experimental transmission to hamsters; c) man develops viremia of a sufficient level to infect these midges and they can, in turn, retransmit the virus to hamsters (Pinheiro *et al.*, 1982b).

In urban situations the disease incidence is not uniform. In Manaus, the rate of reactors to the hemagglutination inhibition test in samples taken at the end of the epidemic varies between 0 and 40.6%, depending on the neighborhood in the city. Such a variation in the rate of infection might depend on whether or not ecological conditions in each neighborhood favor breeding of the vector (Borborema *et al.*, 1982).

Investigators have noted the very low rate of virus isolations (compared to other infections transmitted by insects) from *C. paraensis*, calculated at 1:12,500. Nevertheless, it seems that the low proportion of infected vectors is compensated by their diffusion of the virus resulting from their great abundance. This would explain the high rate of human infection during epidemics (LeDuc *et al.*, 1981).

The nexus between the wild and urban cycles is man when he penetrates the natural foci of infection in the jungle, acquires infection, and infects *C. paraensis* upon returning to the urban population in a viremic state; in this way the urban cycle might be initiated between the vector and the human population (Pinheiro *et al.*, 1981). Thus, man would be a virus amplifier under urban conditions.

Diagnosis: The ORO virus can be isolated from the blood of febrile patients by intracerebral inoculation in suckling mice or adult hamsters. Serologic diagnosis consists of confirming seroconversion by the hemagglutination inhibition test.

Control: Measures must be directed towards the urban vector to prevent epidemics or shorten them when they begin.

Bibliography

Anderson, C. R., L. Spence, W. G. Downs, and T. H. G. Aitken. Oropouche virus: a new human disease agent from Trinidad, West Indies. *Am J Trop Med Hyg* 10:574-578, 1961.

Borborema, C. A. T., F. P. Pinheiro, B. C. Albuquerque, A. P. A. Travassos da Rosa, F. S. Travassos da Rosa, and H. V. Dourado. Primeiro registro de epidemias causadas pelo virus Oropouche no estado do Amazonas. *Rev Inst Med Trop S Paulo* 24:132-139, 1982.

Centers for Disease Control of the USA. *International Catalogue of Arboviruses*, 2nd ed. (Ed. by T. O. Berge). Atlanta, Georgia, 1975 (DHEW Publ. CDC 75-8301.).

LeDuc, J. W., A. L. Hoch, F. P. Pinheiro, and A. P. A. Travassos da Rosa. Epidemic Oropouche virus disease in northern Brazil. *Bull Pan Am Health Organ* 15:97-103, 1981.

Pinheiro, F. P., A. P. A. Travassos da Rosa, J. F. S. Travassos da Rosa, R. Ishak, R. B. Freitas, M. L. C. Gomes, J. W. LeDuc, and O. F. P. Oliva. Oropouche virus. I. A review of clinical, epidemiological and ecological findings. *Am J Trop Med Hyg* 30:149-160, 1981.

Pinheiro, F. P., A. G. Rocha, R. B. Freitas, B. A. Ohana, A. P. A. Travassos da Rosa, J. S. Rogerio, and A. C. Linhares. Meningite associada as infecçoes por virus Oropouche. *Rev Inst Med Trop S Paulo* 24:246-251, 1982a.

Pinheiro, F. P., A. P. A. Travassos da Rosa, M. L. Gomes, J. W. LeDuc, and A. L. Hoch. Transmission of Oropouche virus from man to hamster by the midge *Culicoides paraensis*. *Science* 215:1251-1253, 1982b.

ORUNGO FEVER

(066.3)

Etiology: RNA genome virus belonging to the genus *Orbivirus*, family Reoviridae.

Geographic Distribution: The virus has been isolated in Uganda, Nigeria, Central African Republic, and Senegal. There is serologic evidence that the virus is also active in Sierra Leone (Tomori, 1978).

Occurrence in Man and Animals: In Africa some 60 human cases have been recorded. In 1972 near Jos, Nigeria, three outbreaks of the disease occurred (Fabiyi *et al.*, 1975).

A serologic study carried out in different ecologic areas of Nigeria using the neutralization test confirmed that infection was very widespread. Of 1,197 human sera examined, 23% were positive, with the highest prevalence in the savannah to the north of the country and the lowest in the rain forest areas. The prevalence of seropositives increased with age (Tomori and Fabiyi, 1976). In the same study, antibodies were found in 52% of 44 sheep, 14% of 99 cattle, and 24% of specimens of three species of *Cercopithecus* monkeys.

The Disease in Man: The disease is characterized by fever which lasts 3 to 7 days, cephalalgia, nausea, vomiting, myalgia, and cutaneous eruption. Diarrhea was an additional symptom in one of the outbreaks. A case of progressive paralysis was described in a girl who recovered without sequelae. Autopsy of two fatal cases found edema and congestion of the spleen, meningeal congestion, and ecchymosis of the cerebellum (Fabiyi *et al.*, 1975).

The Disease in Animals: No clinical symptoms have been described in animals. Antibodies were found in experimentally inoculated lambs, but no signs of disease or viremia were observed (Tomori and Fabiyi, 1977).

Source of Infection and Mode of Transmission: The virus was isolated for the first time in 1962, from a pool of *Anopheles funestus* mosquitoes in Orungo, Uganda. In Nigeria it has been isolated from *Aedes dentatus* and in the Central African Republic from *Culex perfuscus* and *Anopheles gambiae* (Tomori, 1978). The virus is transmitted by *Anopheles* and *Aedes* vectors to man and his domestic animals in urban areas, and between wild animals (primates) in enzootic rural areas (Tomori and Fabiyi, 1976). Ovines, in which a high rate of reactors has been found, do not play a role as reservoirs or virus amplifiers, since they do not experience viremia. The virus has not yet been isolated from nonhuman primates nor have they been examined experimentally to determine if they develop viremia and to what degree; consequently, whether they play a role as reservoir in a probable enzootic cycle is unknown.

Diagnosis: The virus can be isolated from the blood of febrile patients by inoculation into suckling mice. The serologic methods utilized are complement fixation and neutralization tests using paired samples (from acute and convalescent phases) to confirm seroconversion.

Control: No control methods against the disease have been tried.

Bibliography

Fabiyi, A., O. Tomori, and M. S. M. El-Bayoum. Epidemic of a febrile illness associated with UgMP 359 virus in Nigeria. *W Afr Med J* 23:9-11, 1975.

Tomori, O. Orungo (ORU). Strain UgMP 359. *In*: Karabastos, N. (Ed.), Supplement to International Catalogue of Arboviruses Including Certain Other Viruses of Vertebrates. *Am J Trop Med Hyg* 27(2, part 2):406-408, 1978.

Tomori, O., and A. Fabiyi. Neutralizing antibodies to Orungo virus in man and animals in Nigeria. *Trop Geogr Med* 28:233-238, 1976.

Tomori, O., and A. Fabiyi. Susceptibility of laboratory and domestic animals to experimental infection with Orungo virus. *Acta Virol* 21:133-138, 1977.

POWASSAN ENCEPHALITIS

(063.8)

Etiology: RNA virus (POW) of the genus *Flavivirus* (formerly group B of the arboviruses) of the family Togaviridae; it belongs to the tick-borne arbovirus complex (Russian spring-summer encephalitis complex). The virus takes its name from the locality in Canada where it was first isolated.

Geographic Distribution: The virus has been isolated in Canada (Ontario and Quebec) and in the United States (New York, New England, South Dakota, Colorado, and California). Antibodies for the Powassan virus have also been found in Sonora, Mexico. Based on serology, the virus is present throughout North America. Outside this continent, the virus is also found in the USSR (central Asia, southern Far East) (Lvov, 1978).

Occurrence in Man: In spite of its widespread distribution in nature, human cases are rare. This fact could be explained by the infrequency with which the tick vectors of the virus bite man. Some 17 cases of encephalitis or meningoencephalitis are known from Canada and the United States (Odend'hal, 1983). There were no known human cases from the USSR. Less than 1% of the population in enzootic areas has antibodies for the virus (Monath, 1979).

Occurrence in Animals: The Powassan encephalitis virus circulates between wild animals and ticks in several enzootic areas. High rates of reactors to the neutralization test have been found in several animal species. The virus has been isolated from several species of Rodentia, especially squirrels, as well as from weasels and a fox.

The Disease in Man: The few cases observed were characterized by fever, cephalalgia, prostration, meningitis, spastic paresis, and pleocytosis.

The Disease in Animals: The infection is probably subclinical. Parenteral inoculation of the virus in marmots produces viremia during the first week but without clinical symptomatology. One case of encephalitis and death possibly caused by the POW virus has been described in a grey fox (*Urocyon cinereoargenteus*).

Source of Infection and Mode of Transmission (Figure 45): Wild animals such as marmots, squirrels, mice, rabbits, and mustelids constitute the natural reservoir. The infection is transmitted among them by ticks of the genera *Ixodes* and *Dermacentor*. The ticks *Ixodes cookei* and *I. marxi* in Canada and *I. spinipalpis*, *I. cookei*,

Figure 45. Powassan encephalitis. Transmission cycle.

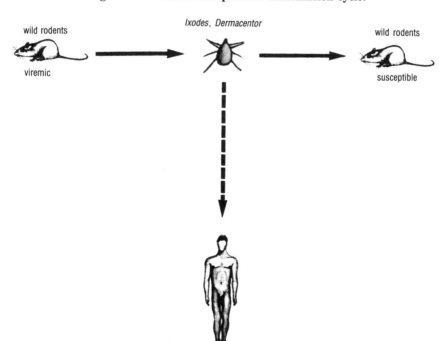

and *Dermacentor andersoni* in the United States have been indicated as vectors. In the USSR, the virus was isolated from *Haemaphysalis longicornis*. It has been shown experimentally that *D. andersoni* transmits the virus after feeding on viremic rabbits. Man is occasionally infected by the bite of ixodids.

Diagnosis: The virus has been isolated from the brain of deceased patients by intracerebral inoculation of mice. Serologic diagnosis can be made by using the complement fixation, hemagglutination inhibition, or neutralization test.

Control: The few cases observed do not justify control measures. Individual prophylaxis consists of protection against ticks.

Bibliography

Andrewes, C., and H. G. Pereira. *Viruses of Vertebrates*, 3rd ed. Baltimore, Maryland, Williams and Wilkins, 1972.

Centers for Disease Control of the USA. *International Catalogue of Arboviruses*, 2nd ed. (Ed. by T. O. Berge). Atlanta, Georgia, 1975. (DHEW Publ., CDC 75-8301.)

Centers for Disease Control of the USA. Powassan virus—New York. *Morb Mortal Wkly Rep* 24:379, 1975.

Johnson, H. N. Isolation of Powassan virus from a spotted skunk in California. *J Wildl Dis* 23:152-153, 1987.

Lvov, D. K. Epizootiology and ecology of viral zoonoses transmitted by ticks. *In: Proceedings, Third Munich Symposium on Microbiology*. Munich, WHO Collaborating Center for Collection and Evaluation of Data on Comparative Virology, 1978.

Monath, T. P. Arthropod-borne encephalitis in the Americas. *Bull WHO* 57:513-533, 1979.

Odend'hal, S. *The Geographical Distribution of Animal Viral Diseases*. New York, Academic Press, 1983.

Whitney, E. Serologic evidence of group A and B arthropod-borne virus activity in New York State. *Am J Trop Med Hyg* 12:417-424, 1963.

PSEUDOCOWPOX

(051.1)

Synonyms: Milkers' nodules, pseudovaccinia, paravaccinia.

Etiology: DNA genome virus, belonging to the genus *Parapoxvirus*, family Poxviridae. Pseudocowpox virus is antigenically closely related to the papular bovine stomatitis and contagious ecthyma viruses. Some researchers maintain that viruses of pseudocowpox and papular bovine stomatitis may be identical (Nagington *et al.*, 1967). Parapoxvirus is antigenically different from cowpox and vaccinia viruses.

Geographic Distribution and Occurrence: Since the time of Jenner, the disease has been recorded sporadically in cattle and man. Distribution is worldwide, as proven by confirmation of the disease in several countries on all continents (Tripathy *et al.*, 1981; Hernández-Pérez and Serpas de López, 1981). The frequency of disease in animals and man is still not well known. A study carried out in a slaughterhouse in Great Britain found 46 of 358 milch cows (13%) clinically affected. Serologic studies in the USA have confirmed that the disease is widespread and probably clinically inapparent for the most part. In countries where milking is done by hand, human disease (milkers' nodules) is relatively frequent but seldom diagnosed. In El Salvador, Central America, 46 cases have been diagnosed on a single dairy farm (Hernández-Pérez and Serpas de López, 1981; Tripathy *et al.*, 1981).

The Disease in Man: The disease is known as "milkers' nodules." The incubation period is from 5 to 7 days. It is a benign disease, without systemic reaction, which begins with an erythematous and pruriginous papule, generally located on the fingers or hand but sometimes found on other parts of the body. The development of the lesion may take 4 to 6 weeks, eventually becoming a firm nodule ranging in color from gray to reddish blue or brown and in size from 0.5 to 2 cm in diameter. The lesion heals without leaving a scar.

The Disease in Animals: The disease occurs in milch cows. The lesions, which are located mainly on the udder and teats, start with a small focal area of erythema, which turns into a papule with a small central vesicle. There is also umbilication of the lesion and a pustular phase, although these sometimes go unnoticed. The pustules break in 2 or 3 days and form dark red scabs. The scabs drop off in about 2 weeks. Individual lesions heal in 7 to 10 days, but in some animals lesions can persist for months. One of the characteristics of pseudocowpox is periodic recurrence of the lesions. In nursing calves, buccal lesions can be found (Nagington *et al.*, 1967).

Source of Infection and Mode of Transmission (Figure 46): Milch cows are the natural host of the virus. The infection is spread between cows by the hands of milkers or the cups of mechanical milking machines. The virus has been isolated from lesions up to 6 months after their appearance; this fact could explain the persistence of the agent in a herd (Tripathy *et al.*, 1981). Man contracts the infection while milking by contact with lesions on the udders and teats of cows, or by contact with lesions in calves' mouths. Skin abrasions facilitate infection.

Diagnosis: The clinical disease can be confused with cowpox, vaccinia virus infection, and mamillitis produced by bovine herpesvirus, type 2. Pseudocowpox virus can be isolated from the lesions in primary bovine kidney cell cultures, in which it causes a cytopathic effect. By contrast, the agent does not replicate in the chorioallantoic membrane of the chick embryo or on rabbit skin, both of which are good substrates for the multiplication of vaccinia and cowpox viruses. Electron microscopy is very useful in diagnosis of pseudocowpox, as the virus has the cylindrical morphology typical of parapoxviruses. Calves vaccinated against cowpox vaccine are not resistant to the pseudocowpox virus.

Control: No vaccines are available. Natural immunity is of short duration. Prevention consists primarily of hygienic measures during milking.

Figure 46. Pseudocowpox. Mode of transmission.

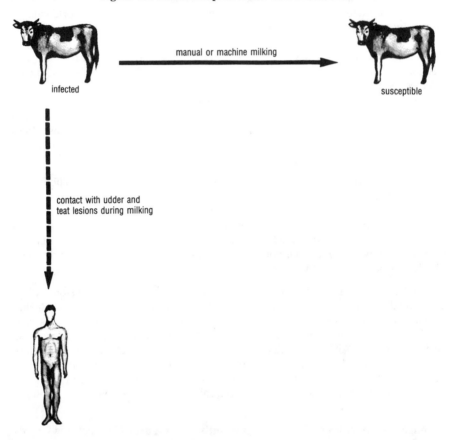

Bibliography

Andrewes, C. H., and H. G. Pereira. *Viruses of Vertebrates*, 3rd ed. Baltimore, Maryland, Williams and Wilkins, 1972.

Andrewes, C. H., and J. R. Walton. Viral and bacterial zoonoses. *In*: Brander, G. C. (Ed.), *Animal and Human Health*. London, Baillière Tindall, 1977.

Bruner, D. W., and J. H. Gillespie. *Hagan's Infectious Diseases of Domestic Animals*, 6th ed. Ithaca, New York, Cornell University Press, 1973.

Cheville, N. F., and D. L. Shey. Pseudopox in dairy cattle. *J Am Vet Med Assoc* 150:855-861, 1967.

Dekking, F. Milker's nodules. *In*: Van der Hoeden, J. (Ed.), *Zoonoses*. Amsterdam, Netherlands, Elsevier, 1964.

Hernández-Pérez, E., and M. E. Serpas de López. Nódulo de los ordeñadores. *Dermatología (México)* 25:142-149, 1981.

Mitra, K., and A. Chatterjee. Milker's nodule contracted from pox in water buffaloes. *Int J Zoonoses* 13:141-142, 1986.

Nagington, J., L. M. Lander, and J. S. Smith. Bovine papular stomatitis, pseudocowpox and milker's nodules. *Vet Rec* 81:306-313, 1967.

Tripathy, D. N., L. E. Hanson, and R. A. Crandell. Poxviruses of veterinary importance: Diagnosis of infections. *In*: Kurstak, E., and C. Kurstak (Eds.), *Comparative Diagnosis of Viral Diseases*, vol. 3. New York, Academic Press, 1981.

RABIES

(071)

Synonyms: Hydrophobia, lyssa.

Etiology: The rabies virus is a bullet-shaped RNA virus belonging to the genus *Lyssavirus*, family Rhabdoviridae. It has two main antigens: an internal group-specific nucleoprotein, and a glycoprotein surface antigen that induces neutralizing antibodies. The "classic" rabies virus and morphologically similar viruses recently isolated in Africa (see Viruses Related to Rabies Virus) have the group-specific antigen in common, that is, the internal nucleoprotein antigen. On this basis, designation of the genus *Lyssavirus* within the rhabdoviruses has been proposed. The viruses related to rabies virus are differentiated by their surface antigens or glycoproteins by means of the neutralization and cross-protection tests; monoclonal antibodies directed against the nucleocapsid are also used (Wiktor *et al.*, 1980).

The classic rabies viruses are divided into the "street viruses" and the "fixed viruses." Street virus refers to virus that has been recently isolated from animals and has not undergone modifications in the laboratory. These strains are characterized by a highly variable incubation period, which is sometimes quite prolonged, and by their capacity to invade the salivary glands. Fixed virus, by contrast, refers to strains adapted to laboratory animals by serial intracerebral passages; they have a short incubation period of only 4 to 6 days and do not invade the salivary glands. The WHO Expert Committee on Rabies has pointed out that, under certain conditions, the fixed virus can be pathogenic for man and animals (World Health Organization, 1984a). Cases of rabies are known to have occurred in persons who received poorly inactivated antirabic vaccine, and one case occurred by inhalation of the virus during the preparation of a concentrated vaccine.

It has long been suspected that rabies viruses differ in their antigenic composition, and cross-protection assays, neutralization tests, kinetic neutralization studies, and counterimmunoelectrophoresis have provided evidence for this idea (Díaz and Varela-Díaz, 1980). The advent of monoclonal antibody techniques has proved the existence of great antigenic variation among rabies viruses. Analysis of several fixed and street viruses using a monoclonal antibody panel directed against glycoprotein antigens revealed great diversity in reactivity (Wiktor *et al.*, 1980). This new knowledge and these new techniques allowed the recent confirmation of rabies of vaccine origin, due to modified live virus vaccines, in dogs, cats, and a fox. The existence of a reactive pattern identical to that of the vaccine virus was confirmed when a panel of eight monoclonal antibodies was used to analyze viruses isolated from 14 animals that had been vaccinated with modified virus and dead rabies virus

(Whetstone *et al.*, 1984). Intensive research work is being carried out in several countries to correlate the antigenic differences between vaccine viruses and the virus present in the animal population in an attempt to explain why protection failure sometimes occurs in persons vaccinated on time with the complete indicated course for postexposure prophylaxis.

A recent study which tested 204 strains of street rabies virus from Europe, Asia, and Africa by directing a panel of 20 monoclonal antibodies against the nucleocapsid found that the strains from Madagascar, Thailand, and Iran differed markedly from the others (Sureau *et al.*, 1983).

Viruses Related to Rabies Virus: Five of these viruses have been discovered since 1975, isolated in sub-Saharan Africa:

a) Lagos bat virus (LBV), isolated from three species of frugivorous bats in Nigeria, Central African Republic, and South Africa.

b) Mokola virus (MOK), isolated from African shrews (*Crocidura* spp.), from two human cases, and recently from cats and one dog (Foggin, 1983) in Nigeria, Cameroon, and Zimbabwe.

c) Duvenhage virus (DUV), isolated from man in South Africa.

d) Kotonkan virus (KOT), isolated from *Culicoides* in Nigeria.

e) Obodhiang virus (OBOD), isolated from mosquitoes (*Mansonia uniformis*) in Sudan.

None of these viruses similar to rabies virus are presently thought to have much epidemiologic importance, although MOK and DUV have caused some cases of human disease and death. The isolation of MOK virus from cats and a dog in Zimbabwe (Foggin, 1983) indicates that the possibility of its transmission to man must be borne in mind.

A virus apparently identical to DUV was isolated from three bats in the Hamburg-Bremen region, West Germany. It is suspected that the agent was introduced by ships from South Africa, but it also might be native to the bat population in Europe (World Health Organization, 1983).

The KOT virus apparently causes a disease in bovines similar to ephemeral bovine fever (Crick, 1981).

These viruses can present a certain degree of cross-reaction with the rabies virus in immunofluorescence and complement fixation tests; therefore, some confusion in rabies diagnosis is possible. The introduction of these African viruses in other countries would complicate diagnosis of the disease and would mandate preparation of specific immunoreagents for these agents. Likewise, it must be taken into account that rabies vaccine does not confer protection against related viruses.

Comparative studies of pathogenesis in hamsters caused by strains of classic rabies, Lagos, and MOK viruses have confirmed that the three are similar in their tropism and the course of infection. Experimentation has also demonstrated that mice, hamsters, dogs, and monkeys are susceptible to intracerebral inoculation of the African viruses (Lagos and MOK) and that the agents can then be isolated from the brain and salivary glands; on the other hand, inoculation of those serotypes by other routes rarely results in death of the animals. Strains isolated from mosquitoes (OBOD) are pathogenic only to suckling mice inoculated intracerebrally. Neutralizing antibodies for KOT virus, isolated from *Culicoides,* are frequently found in bovines, ovines, and equines, as well as rodents and insectivores in northern Nigeria.

Geographic Distribution: Rabies occurs on all continents, but not in most of Oceania. Several countries are currently free of the infection, among them Uruguay, Barbados, Jamaica, and several other Caribbean islands in the Americas; Japan in Asia; and several Scandinavian countries, Ireland, Great Britain, the Netherlands, Bulgaria, Spain, and Portugal in Europe (World Health Organization, 1984b). Rabies is not uniformly distributed in the infected countries, where there may exist areas free of disease, low and high endemicity areas, and other areas with epizoodemic outbreaks.

Occurrence: Two rabies cycles are distinguished: urban and wild. Most human cases by far are recorded in cities and are due to bites of rabid dogs. In countries in which canine rabies has been controlled or eradicated and where wild rabies exists, the number of human cases has been reduced to a very low level. This is the situation in the United States, where there were 47 human cases in 1938, while in recent years the number has fluctuated between zero and two per year.

Partial data obtained by the World Health Organization in 1984 reported 1,135 human cases in the world: 90 in Africa, 213 in America, 831 in Asia, and one in Europe, contracted in Sudan. Epidemiologic surveillance is deficient in many developing countries and case notification is incomplete. According to an estimate for the year 1981, in the tropical areas of the world there were 20,482 human cases, of which 272 (1.3%) occurred in America, 133 (0.6%) in Africa and the Middle East, 20,070 (98%) in Asia, 3 (0.01%) in Oceania, and 3 (0.01%) in Europe. Maps 3 and 4 contain information by geographical region about notified animal cases of rabies and human deaths from rabies in 1981 (Acha and Arambulo III, 1985). The public health importance of rabies is not based on the number of cases, which is low as evidenced by these data, but on the high fatality rate, which is practically 100% of the patients. No less important is the mental and emotional impact, the suffering and

Map 3. Notified cases of rabies in animals, by geographic region, 1981.

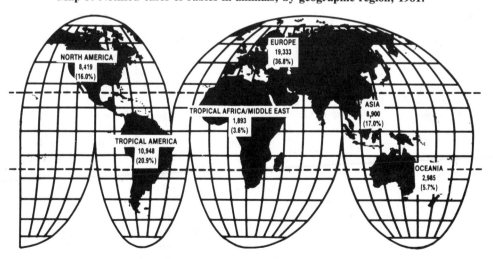

Source: Acha, P. N., and P. V. Arambulo III. Rabies in the Tropics—History and Current Status. *In: Rabies in the Tropics,* ed. by E. Kuwert *et al.* Heidelberg, Springer-Verlag, 1985.

Map 4. Human deaths from rabies, by geographic region, 1981.

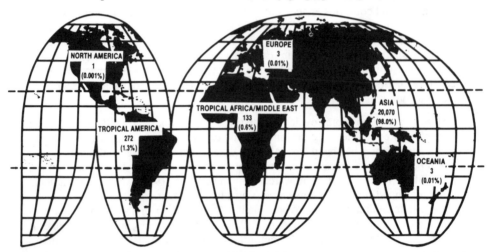

Source: Acha, P. N., and P. V. Arambulo III. Rabies in the Tropics—History and Current Status. *In: Rabies in the Tropics,* ed. by E. Kuwert *et al.* Heidelberg, Springer-Verlag, 1985.

the anxiety of bitten persons faced with fear of contracting the disease. Another consideration is the economic impact of man-hours lost in antirabic treatment. According to the World Survey of Rabies (World Health Organization, 1984b), 390,661 persons received the postexposure antirabic treatment in 1981 and 77% of these treatments were done in America.

In the decade 1970-1979, 2,796 human cases occurred in the Americas, or an average of 280 cases per year. Sixty-five per cent of the total was recorded in two countries, Brazil and Mexico; the majority of cases occurred in about 12 large cities. The following countries had more than 100 human cases during 1970-1979: Brazil, Peru, Ecuador, Colombia, and Mexico (Honigman, 1981). Figure 47 shows cases of rabies in man, dogs, cats, and wild animals in the Americas from 1970 to 1982.

Natural infection occurs in almost all domestic and wild mammals, although different animal species show distinct degrees of susceptibility. Dogs are the main source of infection for man in cities, followed by cats. Between 1970 and 1979, on average some 18,640 dogs and 1,174 cats were diagnosed with rabies annually in the Americas. During that decade, only 1.2% of dogs and 15.8% of cats with a positive rabies diagnosis were found in the United States and Canada. This fact explains the difference in the incidence of human hydrophobia to the north and south of the Rio Grande. In Latin America during the period 1970-1983, there were 3,662 human rabies cases and 224,684 cases of rabies in dogs in large urban areas (Fernandes and Arambulo III, 1985).

With respect to rabies in wild animals (including bats) in the Americas, 89% of cases from 1970 to 1979 were diagnosed in the United States and Canada, mainly in skunks (*Mephitis mephitis*), foxes (*Vulpes fulva* and *Urocyon cinereoargenteus*), bats, and raccoons (*Procyon lotor*). This great preponderance of cases in North America compared with the rest of the hemisphere probably does not reflect reality, since wildlife rabies has received little attention outside the United States and

**Figure 47. Cases of rabies in humans, dogs, cats, and wild animals in
the Americas, 1970-1982.**

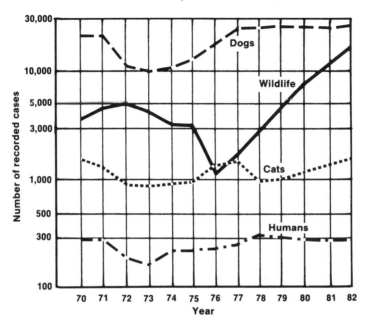

Source: Acha, P. N., and P. V. Arambulo III. Rabies in the Tropics—History and Current
Status. In: Rabies in the Tropics, ed. by E. Kuwert et al. Heidelberg, Springer-Verlag,
1985.

Canada, and surveillance has been deficient. Wild rabies is important in Europe,
where around 1940 an epizootic in red foxes (*Vulpes vulpes*) started in Poland. It
subsequently spread to a large part of the continent and is still active. In northern
regions rabies is maintained in arctic foxes (*Alopex lagopus*); in the Middle East, the
Indian subcontinent, and Africa, jackals are important hosts of the rabies virus, as
are wolves in eastern Europe and a large part of Asia. Rabies in wild carnivores is
also present in other parts of the world. When it occurs enzootically it generally goes
unnoticed, but when it reaches epizootic proportions the wild cycle affects man and
domestic animals.

Mongooses are rabies vectors in South Africa, Zimbabwe, Nigeria, India, and Sri
Lanka, where they contribute to human infection. In the 19th century the Indian
mongoose (*Herpestes auropunctatus*) was introduced to several Caribbean islands to
control rats. Mongooses currently are hosts for rabies in Grenada, Puerto Rico,
Cuba, and the Dominican Republic and are responsible for infections in humans and
other mammals.

Rabies virus has been isolated from rats and other rodents in various parts of the
world, but the potential for its transmission to man is thought to be low. Up to 1975,
63 cases of rabies in rats were diagnosed in the Americas, most of them (32 cases) in
Colombia. Three human cases were attributed to rat bites. A special situation has
been found in wild rats in several European countries; a rabies virus of very low
virulence has been isolated from these animals, without the rodents presenting any
clinical symptoms. These viruses are apparently adapted to wild mice, and 10 or

more passes in laboratory mice are required to detect them. On the other hand, intrauterine transmission of the virus has been confirmed. In an area of Czechoslovakia, some 25% of *Microtus arvalis* had neutralizing antibodies for rabies virus (Beran, 1981). Likewise, a virus of very low virulence has been found in the multimammate African mouse (*Mastomys natalensis*), in which the virus can persist asymptomatically and be transmitted vertically (Schoop, 1977).

Rabies in bats is a problem independent of the infection cycles in other mammals and is of interest only in the Americas. The significance of the infection is different in hematophagous compared with nonhematophagous bats. Rabies in nonhematophagous bats occurs in both North and South America and has been confirmed in numerous species of insectivorous as well as several frugivorous, omnivorous, and piscivorous bats. There have been several human cases of rabies transmitted by the bite of these bats, mainly in the United States, since the first case was recognized in 1953 in Florida. Rabies in bats has been diagnosed in all states in that country except Hawaii. The number of cases varies from about 150 to 500 per year and is lower than in skunks and foxes (2,095 and 645 cases, respectively, in 1972) (Centers for Disease Control of the USA, 1975). Outside the American continent, thousands of bats have been examined in parts of Asia and Africa with negative results, while in Europe and Thailand some infected specimens have been found.

Rabies in hematophagous or vampire bats is a problem limited to Latin America and Trinidad and Tobago. Infection has been confirmed in the three species of hematophagous bats, *Desmodus rotundus*, *Diphylla ecaudata*, and *Diaemus youngi*, but only the first species is of epidemiologic importance. The distribution of vampire bats (*D. rotundus*) comprises an area that extends from Mexico to central Argentina. *Desmodus* is responsible for significant losses in the livestock industry in Latin America, especially from bovine rabies, which has prevented the development of new regions of the American tropics. It is very difficult to establish the true magnitude of losses due to bovine rabies, since in many countries this disease occurs in marginal cattle-raising areas where the limited number of veterinarians and the lack of diagnostic laboratories prevent confirmation and accurate reporting of the outbreaks. A recent study estimated that losses due to rabies transmitted by vampire bats, in terms of cattle mortality, loss of meat and milk, and devaluation of hides exceeds US$40 million per year in the enzootic areas of Latin America (Acha and Málaga Alba, 1987). In South America, only Chile and Uruguay have no reported cases of rabies transmitted by vampire bats. Also free from desmodine rabies are the Caribbean islands except Trinidad. Since 1929, when human rabies attributed to a vampire bat bite was observed for the first time, more than 180 human cases have been recorded in Latin America.

Urban rabies has been eradicated in several European countries, North America, and Japan. In Latin America, Uruguay has remained free of rabies for several years, and the successful campaigns in Argentina, Chile, and in several cities of the continent are noteworthy. In 1945, 8,505 cases of canine rabies were diagnosed in the United States, while in 1982 only 153 cases were diagnosed; since 1963 no human cases of rabies transmitted by dogs or cats have been confirmed in that country (some cases were of unknown origin). The cases of rabies in dogs which still occur are transmitted by wild animals and not from one dog to another. In Canada, where wildlife rabies still persists but canine rabies has been controlled, no human cases have been recorded since 1971.

The Disease in Man: The incubation period is from 2 to 8 weeks, but it may vary from 10 days to 8 months or more. Of 500 cases studied, 4 to 10% had incubation periods of 6 months or more. Longer or shorter incubation may depend on the dose of virus injected by the bite, the site of the bite, and the severity of the wound. The incubation period is longer when the wound is farther away from the central nervous system.

The disease begins with a feeling of anxiety, cephalalgia, a small increase in body temperature, malaise, and indefinite sensory changes, frequently around the site of the bite. The patient usually feels pain and irritation in the region of the wound. The excitation phase that follows includes hyperesthesia and extreme sensitivity to light and sound, dilation of the pupils, and an increase in salivation. As the disease progresses, there are spasms of the deglutitory muscles, and liquids are violently rejected by muscular contraction. This swallowing dysfunction is seen in most patients, many of whom experience spasmodic laryngopharyngeal contractions simply when looking at a liquid and stop swallowing their own saliva ("hydrophobia"). There may also be spasms of the respiratory muscles and generalized convulsions. The excitation phase may persist until death, or it may be replaced by a generalized paralysis. In some cases the excitation phase is very short, with the paralytic symptomatology predominating throughout most of the disease course. The disease lasts from 2 to 6 days, although sometimes longer, and almost invariably ends in death.

The Disease in Animals: Two forms are distinguished, furious rabies and paralytic or dumb rabies, according to the predominant nervous symptomatology.

DOGS: The incubation period lasts from 10 days to 2 or more months. In the prodromal phase, dogs exhibit a change in behavior, hide in dark corners, or show unusual agitation and walk around restlessly. Reflex excitability is enhanced, the animal being startled by the least stimulus. There is anorexia, irritation in the region of the bite, stimulation of the genitourinary tract, and a slight increase in body temperature. After 1 to 3 days, symptoms of excitation and agitation increase notably. The dog becomes dangerously aggressive, with a tendency to bite objects, animals, and man, including its owner; often it will bite itself and inflict serious wounds. Salivation is profuse since the animal does not swallow its saliva because of paralysis of the deglutitory muscles, and its bark changes to a prolonged and hoarse howl because of partial paralysis of the vocal cords. Rabid dogs often wander from their homes and travel long distances, furiously attacking other dogs and animals along the way. In the terminal phase of the disease, generalized convulsions are frequently observed, followed by muscular incoordination and paralysis of the muscles of the trunk and extremities.

The dumb form is characterized by predominantly paralytic symptoms, the excitation phase being very short or sometimes absent. Paralysis begins with the muscles of the head and neck region and the animal has difficulty swallowing. Its owner may suspect that it swallowed a bone and may become exposed to the infection by trying to help the dog. The disease progresses to paralysis of the extremities, general paralysis, and death. The course of the disease lasts from 1 to 11 days.

In western Africa a special form of rabies, called "oulou fato," occurs in dogs. It is characterized by dumb rabies without the furious phase, inclusion bodies that differ from Negri bodies, a short incubation period, diarrhea, and progressive paralysis. The "oulou fato" is thought to be produced by an attenuated rabies virus (Beran, 1981).

CATS: Generally, the disease is the furious type, with symptomatology similar to that in dogs. Paralysis of the posterior third of the body follows 2 to 4 days after the excitation symptoms appear.

CATTLE: Rabies transmitted by vampire bats tends to have a long incubation period, from 25 to 150 or more days. The predominant symptoms are paralytic, and thus the disease is called paretic or paralytic bovine rabies. Affected animals move away from the herd; some show dilated pupils and raised hair, others somnolence and depression. Abnormal movements of the posterior extremities can be observed, as well as lacrimation and nasal catarrh. Fits of fury are rare, but there may be muscular tremors, restlessness, priapism, and hypersensitivity at the site of the bite which causes the animal to scratch the area to the point of causing ulcerations. As the disease progresses, muscular incoordination and tonic-clonic contractions of the muscle groups of the neck, trunk, and extremities occur. The animals have difficulty swallowing and cease to ruminate. Finally, they fall, cannot rise again, and die. Prominent symptoms are emaciation, foamy yellowish spittle covering the snout, and constipation. The paralytic signs usually occur the second or third day after the appearance of symptoms. The disease lasts 2 to 5 days but occasionally extends to 8 to 10 days. On the basis of symptomatology, it is not possible to differentiate bovine rabies caused by vampire bat bites from that caused by the bites of dogs or other animals, especially if the occurrence is sporadic. Epizootiologic data such as the presence of hematophagous bats, discovery of bites caused by these bats, the occurrence of multiple cases, the preponderance of paralytic manifestations, and, above all, the absence of canine rabies in the region lead to the suspicion of vampire-transmitted rabies. It is hoped that the monoclonal antibody technique will detect antigenic differences that will allow viruses transmitted by bats to be distinguished from those transmitted by dogs.

OTHER DOMESTIC ANIMALS: The symptomatology of rabies in equines, ovines, and goats is not very different from bovine rabies. After an excitation period of variable length and intensity, paralytic symptoms occur which cause difficulty in swallowing, followed by incoordination of the extremities. Taste is altered and many animals ingest indigestible objects. In all cases there is a change in behavior. In swine, the disease begins with very violent excitation, and the symptomatology is generally similar to that in dogs. Rabies in ovines, goats, and swine is not frequent.

BIRDS: Naturally acquired rabies is exceptional in this class.

WILD ANIMALS: Rabies occurs naturally in many species of Canidae and other mammals. Based on experimental and some epidemiologic data, foxes, coyotes, jackals, and wolves are considered to be the most susceptible. Skunks, raccoons, bats, and mongooses manifest a lesser degree of susceptibility. Opossums are more resistant. Experiments have shown that the dose of virus necessary to infect skunks is 100 times greater than the quantity needed to infect foxes. The incubation period is variable, but rarely less than 10 days or greater than 6 months. Clinical symptomatology in experimentally infected foxes, skunks, and raccoons is similar to that in dogs; most animals manifest furious rabies, but some exhibit dumb rabies. The disease lasts from 2 to 4 days in foxes and 4 to 9 days in skunks. In bats, both hematophagous and nonhematophagous, furious and sometimes dumb rabies are observed.

Pathogenesis: The rabies virus inoculated subcutaneously or intramuscularly, as happens naturally through a bite, spreads from the point of inoculation to the central nervous system through the axoplasm of peripheral nerves. Neurectomy of the regional nerves prior to inoculation with a fixed virus prevents the development of the disease in laboratory animals. Of great importance is the experimental finding that the virus remains at the site of inoculation for a variable period of time without propagating. In the great majority of mice inoculated in the plantar cushion with street virus it was possible to prevent rabies by amputation of the inoculated foot up to 18 days after the experimental exposure. In the period prior to neural invasion the virus was found to multiply in myocytes at the site of inoculation. The time that elapses between inoculation of the virus and neural invasion is possibly the only period in which prophylactic vaccinal postexposure "treatment" can give satisfactory results.

Once infection of the central nervous system occurs, the virus spreads centrifugally to salivary glands and other organs and tissues by means of peripheral nerves, in the same manner as centripetal progression occurs.

Higher viral titers have been found in the salivary glands than in the brain, and high titers have also been found in the lungs, indicating that the agent may replicate outside the central nervous system. Virus has been isolated or detected in different organs and tissues, such as the adrenal glands, brown fat (interscapular gland) of bats, kidneys, bladder, ovaries, testicles, sebaceous glands, germinal cells of hair follicles, cornea, tongue papillae, intestinal wall, and others. Nevertheless, distribution of the virus is not uniform and the frequency of infection of different organs is variable. It is important to point out that whenever the virus is isolated from the salivary glands it will also be found in the central nervous system.

The appearance of rabies virus in saliva is of special interest in the epidemiology, since biting is the main mode of transmission of infection. In most cases, elimination in saliva begins with the start of disease, but appearance of the agent in saliva has been confirmed in animals of many species before clinical symptoms were observed. In dogs the virus was detectable 1 to 3 days and in some cases 14 days before the disease was manifested. A recent study on dogs experimentally exposed to street virus revealed that four of nine dogs that contracted rabies after exposure to a virus of Ethiopian origin excreted it up to 13 days before showing clinical manifestations, and 8 of 16 rabid dogs inoculated with a virus of Mexican origin shed virus up to 7 days before. It was concluded that the time of appearance of virus in saliva depends not only on the dose but also on the virus strain. Given that the virus can be excreted for more than 10 days and that this is the length of time recommended for observation of biting dogs, that period should be extended (Fekadu *et al.*, 1982). Shedding of virus in saliva has been confirmed 1 to 3 days before clinical symptoms in cats, 1 to 2 days in bovines, up to 14 days in skunks, and for an undetermined period in clinically healthy arctic foxes as well as in vampire bats and nonhematophagous bats (Beran, 1981).

On several occasions, an early, brief, low-titer viremia has been demonstrated, but it has not been possible to show convincingly that hematogenous dissemination of the virus occurs or that it plays some role in the pathogenesis of rabies.

Source of Infection and Mode of Transmission: Animal hosts that maintain rabies virus in nature are carnivores and bats. Herbivores and other nonbiting animals, rodents, and lagomorphs do not play any role in the epidemiology of the disease.

URBAN RABIES **(Figure 48):** Dogs are the main vector of urban rabies. The infection is transmitted from dog to dog and from dog to man and to domestic animals by bites. In spite of the fatal outcome of the disease, rabies in cities and towns is maintained by a significant proportion of susceptible dogs. The high density and high rate of annual reproduction of canines are important factors in canine rabies epizootics in Latin America and other geographic areas. Another important factor in the maintenance of the virus is the long incubation period in some dogs. On several occasions, the virus has been found in the saliva a few days (from 2 or 3 up to 13 days) before onset of the disease, and virus elimination by this route can continue until the animal dies. Nevertheless, not all rabid dogs eliminate virus in saliva and, consequently, some bites are not infectious. It is estimated that 60 to 75% of rabid dogs eliminate the virus in saliva, and this may vary from scarcely a trace to very high titers. Obviously, the risk of the virus being transmitted to man by a bite or abrasion is greater when the dose of virus is higher. Likewise, the risk of contracting the infection is greater when the bite is on the face, neck, or

Figure 48. Urban rabies. Transmission cycle.

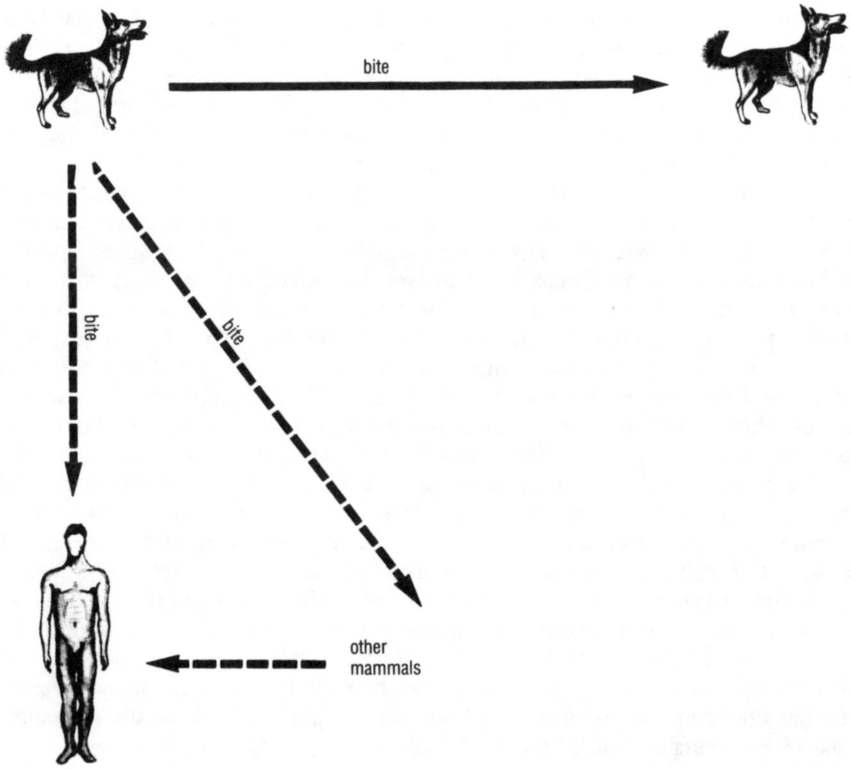

bite

bite

bite

other
mammals

hands and less when it is on the trunk or lower extremities. Many minor bites or scratches do not introduce enough virus to cause disease, especially if the lesion is inflicted through clothing. Before the establishment of postexposure prophylaxis schedules, it was estimated that only 20% of persons bitten by rabid dogs became infected.

According to current estimates, in Latin America and the Caribbean more than 370,000 persons are bitten every year and 260,000 seek treatment. A study in an industrialized suburb of Buenos Aires, Argentina, found that 3,295 persons (854 per 100,000 inhabitants) had attended the rabies center for treatment of dog bites. The group most at risk was children under 15 years of age, especially males. Because of their short stature, a fourth of them had been bitten on the face and neck. Some 43.8% of the total number of persons bitten had been attacked by loose dogs near their owners' home; 47.9% of the wounds were puncture or punctiform and a significant number required medical and/or surgical treatment. Most bites occur in the summer months (Szyfres *et al.*, 1982).

Cats are second to dogs in the number of confirmed rabies cases in urban areas. It is thought that cats are accidental hosts of the virus and perhaps do not play an important role in the natural disease cycle, but they can serve as an important source of human infection and therefore their vaccination coverage should be increased (Diesch *et al.*, 1982). Cats may acquire rabies from infected dogs or wild animals with which they come in contact.

It is appropriate to discuss here "abortive" rabies in dogs and the carrier state. Some mice inoculated with rabies virus in the laboratory become ill and then recover. Numerous facts suggest that rabies is not always fatal. Cases of abortive rabies, although few in number, have been described in several animal species, including man. In an enzootic area of Buenos Aires, Argentina, the cerebro-neutralization test was used to examine the brains of 1,015 dogs and 114 cats that had given negative results to isolation procedures and immunofluorescence tests for rabies diagnosis. The brain specimens of two dogs and one cat out of all those examined showed significant titers to the cerebro-neutralization test (in the absence of the virus), which is accepted as proof that the animals had recovered from the disease, since in vaccinated animals or those that have died of rabies this test is negative (Díaz *et al.*, 1975). Judging from this study, the incidence of "abortive" rabies is very low.

One aspect that has given rise to long-term controversy is the possible existence of carriers, that is, clinically normal animals that eliminate virus in their saliva. Until recently, there was no convincing proof that such a rabies virus carrier state existed. In Ethiopia and India, however, the virus has been isolated during very prolonged periods from the saliva of several asymptomatic dogs. Out of 1,083 apparently healthy dogs examined in Ethiopia, five were intermittent salivary excretors of virus. The carrier state was confirmed more recently in an experimentally infected bitch that contracted rabies and then recuperated. This dog was inoculated intramuscularly with virus isolated from saliva of an apparently healthy dog from Ethiopia; 42, 169, and 305 days after she recovered, virus was isolated from her saliva. Sixteen months after her recovery this dog died giving birth to two stillborn pups; the presence of viable rabies virus was confirmed in her tonsils but not in the brain or other organs (Fekadu *et al.*, 1981; Fekadu *et al.*, 1983).

Interhuman rabies transmission is exceptional. In this category are included the two known rabies cases transmitted by corneal transplant, one in the United States and the other in France. These cases occurred because rabies had not been suspected in the donors. The presence of rabies virus in the cornea of animals and man has been confirmed by the impression technique and direct immunofluorescence (see discussion of airborne transmission, below).

RABIES IN WILDLIFE: Rabies in wildlife is maintained in a form similar to urban rabies. In a given ecosystem, one or two species of mammals, especially carnivores and bats, are responsible for perpetuating rabies. In different parts of the world several wild species maintain the rabies virus cycle in their different ecosystems (see Occurrence). In the United States, different animal species maintain more or less independent epizootics in various areas. In the eastern part of that country, from New England to the southern Atlantic states, foxes (*Vulpes fulva* and *Urocyon cinereoargenteus*) are the main hosts and vectors of rabies, while skunks (*Mephitis mephitis*) are the main hosts and vectors in the midwestern states, and raccoons (*Procyon lotor*) in Florida and Georgia and the mid-Atlantic region. None of these species is a true reservoir, since all of the animals from whose saliva the virus has been isolated die a few days after falling ill. No known healthy carriers of the virus exist among other species of wild animals. Rabies virus has been isolated occasionally from apparently healthy arctic foxes (*Alopex lagopus*). However, it is unknown whether some or all of the isolations were done during the incubation period of rabies (Beran, 1981). Epizootics and enzootics among these animals depend mainly on population dynamics. When the population density is high, rabies takes on epizootic proportions and a large number of animals die. It is estimated that up to 60% of a population of foxes may die during an epizootic. When the density is low, rabies may occur enzootically or disappear entirely with time. New epizootic outbreaks occur when there is a new and susceptible generation. The annual renewal rate for fox populations is very high (up to 70% of the total population), and repeated outbreaks may result if the increase in population density is uncontrolled. It is not known, however, what population density has to be reached by an animal species in order to create epizootic conditions. The variable incubation period, which in some animals may be very long, facilitates continuous propagation of the virus.

Antibodies against rabies virus have been found in several wild species, such as foxes, raccoons, mongooses, and insectivorous bats, indicating that rabies infection does not always lead to disease and death. In less susceptible animals, such as raccoons, the rate of reactors may be high in the postepizootic period. Low virus titers have been found in salivary glands of rabid mongooses; this fact suggests that they could transmit sublethal doses by bite. Even in highly susceptible species, such as foxes, some specimens are found with a very low virus titer in the salivary glands. In a 4-year-long study carried out in Grenada, 498 out of 1,675 mongooses examined (30%) were found to have neutralizing antibodies for rabies virus (Everard *et al.*, 1981). It is believed that naturally acquired immunity in a population of wild animals is an important factor in determining whether or not an epizootic outbreak will occur in a given species and area. That is, a high proportion of animals with antibodies may permit sporadic transmission of the virus but would make it difficult for transmission to reach epizootic proportions (Bigler *et al.*, 1983).

The epizootiology of rabies in bats follows the same lines as in other mammals. A carrier state in bats has long been believed to exist but has not yet been proven. Bats die when they contract rabies, and the virus has never been isolated from the salivary gland without virus also being found in the brain. Some bats can eliminate virus in their saliva for 10 days or more before death, but this phenomenon has also been seen in other animal species; the agent has been isolated from the saliva of skunks for at least 18 days and from foxes for 17 days. Likewise, some bats probably recover from the disease and, as in other wild mammals, neutralizing antibodies are found in vampire bats in areas where outbreaks of bovine rabies occur. In such an area in Argentina, antibodies were found in the serum of 24 of 99 vampire bats examined; however, no virus was found in the brain or other tissues, nor were neutralizing antibodies found in the central nervous system, which would indicate that the animals had not been sick with rabies (Lord *et al.*, 1975). The serum antibodies may have been due to repeated sublethal infections, but experimental evidence is lacking in that regard.

Wild rabies is a permanent danger for man and domestic animals. When wild animals are rabid, they approach towns and may attack man and his animals. It should also be borne in mind that a larger proportion of wild carnivores than dogs eliminate the virus in their saliva. The main victims are generally bovines, in Europe as well as in Canada and the United States. In areas where canine rabies has been eradicated, the disease may be reintroduced by wild carnivores if the population of dogs is not adequately immunized.

The transmission of both wild and urban rabies occurs mainly when an animal that is shedding virus in its saliva bites another susceptible animal, including man. The disease can also be transmitted by other means, and human cases of rabies acquired by airborne transmission have been identified. Two cases occurred in scientists who stayed for a few hours without being bitten in a cave in Texas (Frio Cave) where millions of free-tailed bats (*Tadarida brasiliensis*) live during the summer (Constantine, 1971). In the same cave, airborne transmission of the disease was also demonstrated in coyotes and foxes kept in bat- or arthropod-proof cages. The aerosols were probably produced by the saliva (and urine) of the insectivorous bats. The virus was also collected from the cave air with special devices and inoculated into foxes, which became sick and died of rabies. Another case occurred in a laboratory; the victim was a microbiologist who was preparing a concentrated vaccine. An epizootic outbreak was described in an experimental station in Las Cruces, New Mexico, USA, where different species of wild animals (including foxes, coyotes, and opossums) were kept in individual cages, without any possibility of direct contact and transmission by biting (Winkler, 1972). Transmission was attributed to airborne dissemination of the virus, which was probably of bat origin and would have been especially adapted to aerosol transmission. Laboratory animals have been infected experimentally through the digestive tract, and infection through cannibalism has been confirmed in dams of suckling mice inoculated with rabies virus. This mode of transmission is believed to play some role in rabies propagation among wild animals. Human cases of rabies acquired by ingestion are not known, even when the virus has been detected in the milk of some rabid cows.

Diagnosis: The preferred test is the direct immunofluorescence test, which is rapid, highly sensitive, and specific. The effectiveness of the test depends on the competence of the technician and the quality of the reagents, especially the conjugate. The WHO Expert Committee on Rabies recommends that when this test is introduced into a laboratory, it should be used simultaneously with inoculation into suckling mice for at least a year (World Health Organization, 1984a). It is also recommended that inoculation of mice with cerebral material from the suspected animal be carried out if the immunofluorescence test is negative. Another advantage of the immunofluorescence technique over other tests is that it can be done while the patient or rabid animal is still alive, using corneal impressions, scrapings of the lingual mucosa, bulbar tissue of the hair follicles, and frozen skin sections. The sensitivity of the test under these conditions is limited; a positive result confirms diagnosis, but a negative result does not exclude the possibility of infection. Use of these tests on biting animals is very helpful for instituting early prophylactic treatment of exposed persons.

Intracerebral inoculation of mice for isolation of the virus continues to be one of the most useful tests for the diagnosis of rabies. In this case, use of suckling mice up to 3 days old is recommended, since they are more sensitive than older animals. This test gives best results if it is combined with an immunofluorescence test. In order to obtain a rapid diagnosis, so important for making a decision regarding prophylactic treatment of exposed persons, a larger group of mice can be inoculated with the material from the biting animal and then sacrificed daily from the fourth day after inoculation and their brains examined with the immunofluorescence test.

In developing countries, microscopic examination for Negri bodies, a simple, rapid, and economical procedure, continues to be useful for diagnosis. Although it is a less sensitive method, experienced personnel can obtain a correct diagnosis in 80 to 90% of the cases, especially in dogs dead of furious rabies. Detection of Negri bodies using Seller's, May-Grünwald, and Mann stains or other techniques confirms the diagnosis of rabies, but their absence does not exclude the possibility of infection.

Examinations should not be limited to nervous tissue, but should also include a search for the virus in the salivary glands, especially the submaxillary glands.

It is very important that samples arrive at the laboratory properly preserved. A recent study carried out with tissue in gradual deterioration showed that the first test that gives negative results is examination for Negri bodies, then the mice inoculation test, and finally the immunofluorescence test.

Serologic tests are usually used to find out the immunogenic capacity of vaccines and the immune response of persons subjected to pre- or postexposure treatment. In addition to the plaque reduction neutralization test in mice or the fluorescent focus inhibition test, other quick tests that have been perfected include the modified counterimmunoelectrophoresis test (Díaz, 1983), the immunoadherence hemagglutination test (Budzko et al., 1983) and ELISA[1] (Nicholson and Prestage, 1982). All tests that measure neutralizing antibodies are useful to determine the degree of resistance against the infection.

Control: The following should be considered: 1) control and eradication programs for urban rabies; 2) control measures for wildlife rabies; 3) regulations regarding international transport of animals; and 4) procedures for both pre- and postexposure vaccination of individuals against human rabies.

1. Control and eradication of urban rabies: The most rational approach for preventing human rabies consists of control and eradication of the infection in domestic animals, especially dogs.

The procedures used in control and eradication programs for urban rabies aim at rapidly reducing the population of susceptible animals by immunizing domestic

---

[1] A simplified ELISA-type kit is being tested by the Pasteur Institute, France, and promises to be applicable to field conditions in developing countries.

dogs and cats and eliminating street dogs. To stop urban epizootics, it is recommended that, in as short a time as possible, at least 80% of the entire canine population of the city and adjacent areas be vaccinated. Once the epizootic is interrupted, vaccination should continue, both in old generation animals not previously vaccinated and in those entering the canine population by birth or introduction from other areas. Vaccination campaigns can be carried out by house-to-house visits, in fixed stations, or in mobile clinics that go where dogs are concentrated in each district; the first procedure is preferable when resources permit.

At the present time, a large number of safe and highly effective vaccines are available for use in dogs, both the inactivated and the modified live virus (MLV) types. The first type includes vaccines prepared with fixed virus in nervous tissue and those of cell culture origin. Among the live virus vaccines are those prepared in chick embryo after a few passages ("low egg passage," LEP) or after many passages ("high egg passage," HEP) and vaccine made in swine kidney cells (ERA strain). Although rabies cases brought on by MLV vaccines in dogs and cats are few, inactivated virus vaccines give the best guarantee of safety.

The most widely used vaccines in Latin America are inactivated suckling mouse brain (SMB) vaccines followed at present in numerical importance by several vaccines prepared in tissue culture (Pan American Zoonoses Center, 1980). Comparative studies of different types of animal vaccines have shown that MLV cell culture vaccine and Flury LEP chick embryo vaccine confer immunity for 3 years after a single injection, and that the inactivated SMB vaccine protects all dogs for 1 year and 80% for 3 years (Sikes, 1975). Consequently, the two types of vaccine most widely used in Latin America are of proven effectiveness. Each lot of vaccine of any type should be submitted to official tests for safety and activity. A vaccine produced in BHK cells and inactivated with ethylenamine (PV-BHK-EI) that was developed at the Pan American Zoonoses Center protected 100% of dogs exposed to street virus 12 and 25 months after vaccination, and 89% after 3 years (Larghi et al., 1979).

In mass vaccination campaigns, the WHO Expert Committee on Rabies recommends that primary immunization be practiced annually on all dogs between the ages of 3 months and 1 year. Dogs should be revaccinated in accordance with the duration of immunity conferred by the type of vaccine used. Pups less than 3 months old may be vaccinated with an inactivated vaccine, but they should be revaccinated as soon as possible after they reach that age.

Cats can be vaccinated with an inactivated vaccine or a modified live virus vaccine, with the exception of Flury LEP vaccine, which can be pathogenic for these animals. The recommended vaccination age is the same as for dogs. Cats should be revaccinated annually until more information becomes available on the duration of immunity in these animals.

Dogs or cats bitten by a rabid animal should be destroyed. An exception may be made when it is certain that the bitten animal was vaccinated with an active vaccine and that it is still within the anticipated period of immunity conferred by that vaccine. If the bitten animal is not destroyed, it should be kept confined and under observation for at least 3 months.

The control of stray dogs can be carried out by means of selective poisoning programs or capture by animal pounds. In the latter case, the dog can be returned to its owner upon payment of a fine and vaccination against rabies.

2. Control of wildlife rabies: The following types should be considered: a) bat-transmitted rabies and b) rabies transmitted by carnivores.

a) Control of rabies transmitted by hematophagous bats is of special interest for Latin America. The main control procedures consist of vaccination of cattle in exposed areas and reduction of the vampire bat population. Excellent vaccines are currently available, among which the ERA vaccine stands out, providing adequate protection for more than 3 years. Other useful vaccines are the Flury HEP chick embryo vaccine and the SMB and PV-BHK-EI vaccines with an aluminum hydroxide adjuvant, which protect for more than 1 year. In Mexico, the Acatlán strain vaccine, prepared in a tissue culture of vampire bat cells, is used.

The epizootiology of bovine rabies is still not well known, but observations from several countries indicate that this infection has a focal nature; thus it would be possible to protect cattle by means of focal and perifocal vaccination, without having to resort to costly mass vaccinations. For this purpose epizootiologic studies and an adequate surveillance system are needed.

The other method developed in recent years is the use of anticoagulants, such as diphenadione, to reduce vampire bat populations in places where bovine rabies occurs. Vampire bats are captured with nylon nets ("mist nets") set up around corrals or pastures, their backs are smeared with a mixture of vaseline and diphenadione, and they are released. When they return to their roosts the treated vampires are licked during grooming by other colony members, which then die as a result of internal hemorrhages caused by the ingestion of diphenadione. Pilot studies show that this procedure is effective in achieving a significant reduction in the number of vampire bats in colonies and in preventing bovine and human rabies caused by these animals. However, the possibility exists that the vampire bat bodies constitute a danger for animals of other species. Accordingly, the residues of anticoagulant in dead vampire bats were examined by means of gas chromatography; only 1.17% of the diphenadione used to treat them was found. Although this study indicated that the risk for other species was low, the authors (Burns and Bullard, 1980) recommend caution in anticoagulant use because the susceptibility of different species to the compound is unknown. Another technique consists of intramuscular inoculation of bovines with warfarin, which kills bats when they feed on the cow's blood (Flores Crespo et al., 1979).

To prevent human cases caused by nonhematophagous bats, the public and especially children should be instructed to refrain from touching or picking up bats that are on the ground or from capturing those seen flying during the day. Likewise, the entry of bats into buildings should be prevented by sealing entry and exit ways. On the other hand, insectivorous bats are beneficial to agriculture and they should not be destroyed indiscriminately.

b) The control of rabies transmitted by wild, ground-dwelling carnivores consists primarily of reducing the populations of the main vector species responsible for maintaining the virus transmission cycle, such as the fox in Europe and the fox, skunk, and raccoon in the United States. By significantly reducing the density of the main host of wildlife rabies in a given area, a large reduction in the number of cases of infection can be achieved and the infection will cease to propagate. For this purpose, baits poisoned with sodium fluoroacetate or thallium sulphate for mongooses and strychnine for skunks are used, as well as fumigation of fox dens with poison gases (cyanide or hydrogen phosphate compounds) during the parturition period. An auxiliary but less efficient measure is to hunt the animals with firearms and traps. In some areas of Europe where the density of the fox population has been reduced to 0.2 foxes per km^2, rabies has disappeared and has not been reintroduced. The following parameters are used to evaluate the destruction of foxes in areas of wildlife rabies: a) the critical population density level, below which transmission of infection ceases; b) annual renewal of the population not affected by rabies or control measures; and c) the growth rate of a reduced population to reach its original level (Bogel *et al.*, 1981). Several researchers have expressed opposition to the procedure of reducing the animal population, as it involves the indiscriminate sacrifice of both immune and susceptible animals, and the latter could increase upon repopulation of the area. This argument seems worthwhile particularly when animal species relatively resistant to rabies virus are involved, such as raccoons and mongooses (Everard *et al.*, 1978; Carey *et al.*, 1978). Experiments have shown that foxes can be immunized orally by means of baits containing modified live virus vaccines, especially ERA or WIRAB (derived from the former and cultured in BHK). This procedure is still in the experimental phase and its possible impact on other components of the fauna, especially rodents, is being studied.

3. Control of international transport of animals: Countries that are free of rabies should prohibit the importation of dogs and cats from infected areas, as is done in Australia, or establish a prolonged quarantine of 6 months and simultaneously immunize the animals introduced into the country with an inactivated vaccine. In countries where rabies exists and a prolonged quarantine is not possible, only dogs and cats with a valid official vaccination certificate should be permitted entry and they should be confined in the owner's home, under veterinary supervision, until a reduced quarantine is completed.

Wild animals should be submitted to the same measures. As far as possible, introduction of animals from enzootic areas should be prohibited. The use of inactivated vaccines is recommended as MLV may be pathogenic for some wild species.

4. Prevention of human rabies (Table 5): Prophylaxis prior to exposure is limited to groups exposed to high risk, such as laboratory workers, personnel of city animal pounds and of rabies control programs, veterinarians, and naturalists. Mass vaccination is not currently recommended, even in epizootic areas, since no vaccine is completely safe. In Latin America, SMB vaccine is used for pre-exposure immunization. With this vaccine, which is highly immunogenic and relatively free of encephalitogenic effects, high neutralizing titers are obtained by administering three 2 ml doses every other day, thus completing the vaccination program in just 5 days. Three to four weeks after the final dose, a blood sample should be taken to determine the antibody titer, and if it is found to be low, one or more additional doses should be administered. A booster should be given at 1- to 3-year intervals. Vaccinated persons who have a satisfactory antibody response should receive one or more boosters when they are exposed to the infection. In developed countries, the human diploid cell vaccine (HDCV) is used in prophylaxis prior to exposure; it is highly immunogenic, but its cost makes it inaccessible to developing countries. The vaccine can be administered intramuscularly with 1 ml or intradermally with 0.1 ml. Serologic conversion is achieved in more than 99% of those treated and lasts 2 years in 100% of persons vaccinated if three doses are administered on days 0, 7, and 28. Intradermal inoculation is much less costly and is as effective as intramuscular administration. Undesirable side effects are observed in less than 1% of those immunized and consist of muscular pain, cephalalgia, and pain at the site of injection (Turner *et al.*, 1982; Dreesen *et al.*, 1982). According to recent data from

Table 5. Specific systemic treatment of rabies.

| Nature of exposure | Status of biting animal irrespective of previous vaccination | | Recommended treatment |
	At time of exposure	During 10-day[a] observation period	
I. Contact, but no lesions; indirect contact; no contact	Rabid	—	None
II. Licks of the skin; scratches or abrasions; minor bites (covered areas of arms, trunk, and legs)	a) Suspected as rabid[b]	Healthy	Start vaccine. Stop treatment if animal remains healthy for 5 days[a,c]
		Rabid	Start vaccine; administer serum upon positive diagnosis and complete the course of vaccine
	b) Rabid: wild animal,[d] or animal unavailable for observation		Administer serum + vaccine
III. Licks of mucosa; major bites (multiple or on face, head, finger, or neck)	Suspect[b] or rabid domestic or wild[d] animal, or animal unavailable for observation		Administer serum + vaccine. Stop treatment if animal remains healthy for 5 days[a,c]

[a] Observation period applies only to dogs and cats.

[b] All unprovoked bites in endemic areas should be considered suspect unless proved negative by laboratory examination (brain fluorescent antibody (FA) test).

[c] Or if its brain is found negative by FA examination.

[d] In general, exposure to rodents and rabbits seldom, if ever, requires specific antirabic treatment.

the United States, over a period of 46 months there were 108 (11 per 10,000 persons vaccinated with HDCV) cases of generalized allergic reactions, from urticaria to anaphylaxis. A few cases required hospitalization, but none died as a consequence of these reactions. Of the 108 cases, 9 were immediate hypersensitivity, presumably type I; 87 were of late onset (2 to 21 days after one or more doses were administered), presumably type III (deposit of the antigen-antibody complex in tissues, activation of the complement, and inflammation); and 12 were cases of undetermined type (World Health Organization, 1984c).

The prevention of rabies after exposure consists basically of local treatment of the wound and passive and active immunization of the individual.

a) Local treatment of the wound is extremely important and on its own can prevent many cases of rabies by eliminating or inactivating the inoculated virus. The wound should be washed as soon as possible under a strong jet of water and cleaned with soap or detergent and water, followed by application of 40-70% alcohol, tincture of iodine, iodized alcohol, or 0.1% quaternary ammonium compounds. The wound should not be sutured immediately. Tests carried out on laboratory animals show that infiltration of the wound with antirabic serum is a very effective means of preventing infection; therefore, infusion of serum in and around the wound is recommended.

b) Because of the long incubation period typical of most cases of human rabies, postexposure prophylactic immunization is possible. Vaccination must be started as soon as possible to ensure that the individual will be immunized before the rabies virus reaches the central nervous system. An estimated 500,000 to 1,500,000 persons worldwide, possibly more, are subjected to antirabic treatment each year. Treatment consists of daily administration of a vaccine dose for 14 to 21 days in some countries and 7 to 10 days in others. When the shortened schedule is used, it is recommended that booster doses be administered at 10, 20, and 90 days.

Combined administration of serum and vaccine is the most effective method of antirabic prophylaxis. It may be used in all cases, but is especially indicated when severe exposures are involved. The sera used may be heterologous, obtained by hyperimmunization of various animal species (horses, rabbits, and others) or homologous rabies immunoglobulin (of human origin). The serum is administered just once, intramuscularly, at a rate of 40 international units (IU) per kg body weight for heterologous serum, or 20 IU per kg for homologous serum. At the same time, the first dose of vaccine is administered at another body site and treatment is continued until completion of the 14 doses, followed by booster doses at 10, 20, and 90 days after the end of the initial series. The serum should be administered as soon as possible, no matter how much time has elapsed since exposure, in an attempt to neutralize the virus inoculated by the bite.

For human prophylaxis, only the use of inactivated vaccines is indicated. The WHO Expert Committee on Rabies recommends that the use of vaccines such as the Fermi type (produced in nerve tissue and inactivated with phenol at 22°C), containing residual live virus, be suspended. Inactivated vaccine can be produced with fixed virus in nerve tissue of adult animals (Semple type), in brain tissue of suckling animals (rabbits, rats, and mice), and in cell culture. Formerly, a duck embryo vaccine was used in the United States, but its production was discontinued at the end of 1981 mainly because it was not very active. A significant advance was development of the human diploid cell culture vaccine (HDCV), which has replaced all other vaccines for human use in Europe, the United States, and Canada. This is a very active vaccine and has much less frequent secondary local or systemic effects than other vaccines (Wiktor et al., 1977; Plotkin, 1980; Meyer, 1980). The high immunogenicity of the vaccine allowed reduction of the postexposure immunization schedule; on day 0, immunoglobulin and the first dose of vaccine are administered, and then vaccine doses are applied on days 3, 7, 14, and 28. WHO recommends a booster on day 90. The recommended dose of human immunoglobulin is being revised (Mertz et al., 1982).

In Latin America, the Fuenzalida (SMB) vaccine has practically replaced all other types. It has the advantage of being much more potent and safer than the Semple vaccine, causing much less frequent neurologic postvaccinal accidents. Because of the high immunogenic value of the vaccine, it is currently being used in a reduced schedule in Argentina, Colombia, Chile, and Venezuela, with daily application for 7 days and three boosters on days 10, 20, and 60 after the last dose of the initial series (Held et al., 1972; Díaz et al., 1979).

When prescribing prophylactic treatment in man, it should be borne in mind that both the serum and vaccine may cause complications. The heterologous serum may cause an anaphylactic reaction; before its administration, an intradermal or ophthalmic sensitivity test should be done. It is estimated that 15 to 25% of those treated with equine serum suffer from anaphylactic reactions with characteristics of so-called serum sickness. Complications with homologous serum are rare, but unfortunately this serum is costly to produce and not readily available.

With respect to vaccines in general use, none is completely innocuous. The incidence of neuroparalytic complications with nerve tissue vaccines varies from country to country between 1.2 and 34 per 10,000 persons vaccinated. The number of postvaccinal accidents in Latin America dropped significantly as the use of SMB vaccine spread, but even so, in the period from 1970 to 1980, there were 141 cases of neurologic complications with an annual average of 13 accidents, out of more than three million postexposure treatments in the 11 years (Acha, 1981). Although HDCV is considered the safest vaccine, one case of Guillain-Barré syndrome reported in Norway (Boe and Nyland, 1980) and one case of transitory neuroparalytic disease in the United States (Bernard *et al.*, 1982) were associated in their timing with postexposure treatment.

For the reasons discussed, every effort should be made to avoid unnecessary treatment. In enzootic or epizootic areas the treatment of a bitten person should begin immediately, but subsequent doses should not be administered if the dog or cat that inflicted the bite is found to be healthy after its capture and observation for 10 days. If the bite is caused by a wild animal, it is recommended that the animal be killed immediately and its brain tissue tested by immunofluorescence. At the present time, technological advances in genetic engineering raise the possibility of developing a vaccine containing only the rabies virion subunits that induce immunity. Recently, biosynthesis of virus glycoprotein (GP) has been achieved by transfer of rabies virus genes to *Escherichia coli* (Yelverton *et al.*, 1983). If a vaccine could be developed on the basis of this fraction, it probably would not have side effects and would be less costly, to the point of allowing its use on man and animals. Using recombinant DNA techniques, protection against rabies infection has been obtained experimentally in mice with a recombinant vaccinia-rabies virus vaccine (Lecocg *et al.*, 1985).

Studies with monoclonal antibodies, of much interest in rabies immunization, are currently being done to correlate antigenically the vaccine viruses with the viruses active in the animal population of a given region. Although it is premature to attribute some of the failures of postexposure immunization to antigenic variation— since several experiments have demonstrated that an active vaccine can confer protection against different antigenic strains—it is certain that more studies are needed in different areas of the world to clarify this problem.

Bibliography

Acha, P. N. Epidemiología de la rabia bovina paralítica y de la rabia del murciélago. *In*: *Primer Seminario Internacional sobre Rabia en las Américas*. Washington, D.C., Pan American Health Organization, 1968. (Scientific Publication 169).

Acha, P. N. A review of rabies prevention and control in the Americas, 1970-1980. Overall status of rabies. *Bull Off Int Epizoot* 93:9-52, 1981.

Acha, P. N., and P. V. Arambulo III. Rabies in the Tropics—History and Current Status. *In*: Kuwert, E., C. Merieux, H. Koprowski, and K. Bögel, *Rabies in the Tropics*. Heidelberg, Springer-Verlag, 1985.

Acha, P. N., and A. A. Málaga Alba. Economic losses due to *Desmodus rotundus*. Chap. 14 *in*: Greenhall, A., and U. Schmidt (Eds.), *Natural History of Vampire Bats*. Boca Raton, Florida, CRC Press, in press.

Anderson, R. M. Rabies control. Vaccination of wildlife reservoirs. *Nature* 322:304-305, 1986.

Andrewes, C. H., and J. R. Walton. Viral and bacterial zoonoses. *In*: Brander, G. C. (Ed.), *Animal and Human Health*. London, Baillière Tindall, 1977.

Atanasiu, P. Étude sur les voies d'élimination du virus rabique. *In*: *International Symposium on Rabies (II), Lyon, 1972*. Basel, Switzerland, Karger, 1974.

Baer, G. M. Rabies: mode of infection and pathogenesis. *In*: *International Symposium on Rabies (II), Lyon, 1972*. Basel, Switzerland, Karger, 1974

Baer, G. M. (Ed.). *The Natural History of Rabies*, vols. 1 and 2. New York, Academic Press, 1975.

Baer, G. M., M. K. Abelseth, and J. G. Debie. Oral vaccination of foxes against rabies. *Am J Epidemiol* 93:487-490, 1971.

Bell, J. F., G. J. Moore, and G. H. Raymond. Protracted survival of rabies infected insectivorous bat after infective bite. *Am J Trop Med Hyg* 18:61-68, 1969.

Beran, G. W. Rabies and infections by rabies-related viruses. *In*: Beran, G. W. (Section Ed.), *CRC Handbook Series in Zoonoses*. Section B, vol. 2. Boca Raton, Florida, CRC Press, 1981.

Bernard, K. W., P. W. Smith, F. J. Kader, and M. J. Merand. Neuroparalytic illness and human diploid cell rabies vaccine. *JAMA* 248:3136, 1982.

Bernard, K. W., D. B. Fishbein, K. D. Miller, R. A. Parker, S. Waterman, J. W. Sumner, F. L. Reid, B. K. Johnson, A. J. Rollins, C. M. Oster, L. B. Schonberger, G. M. Baer, and W. G. Winkler. Pre-exposure rabies immunization with human diploid cell vaccine: decreased antibody responses in persons immunized in developing countries. *Am J Trop Med Hyg* 34:633-647, 1985.

Bigler, W. J., G. L. Hoff, J. S. Smith, R. G. McLean, H. A. Trevino, and J. Ingwersen. Persistence of rabies antibody in free-ranging raccoons. *J Infect Dis* 148:610, 1983.

Blancou, J. Les vaccins et la vaccination antirabique des animaux domestiques et sauvages en Europe. *Rev Sci Tech Off Int Epizoot* 4:235-241, 1985.

Blancou, J., M. P. Kieny, R. Lathe, J. P. Lecocq, P. P. Pastoret, J. P. Soulebot, and P. Desmettre. Oral vaccination of the fox against rabies using a live recombinant vaccinia virus. *Nature* 322:373, 1986.

Blenden, D. C., W. Creech, and M. J. Torres-Anjel. Use of immunofluorescence examination to detect rabies virus antigen in the skin of humans with clinical encephalitis. *J Infect Dis* 154:698-701, 1986.

Boe, E., and H. Nyland. Guillain-Barré Syndrome after vaccination with human diploid cell rabies vaccine. *Scand J Infect Dis* 12:231-232, 1980.

Bogel, K., H. Moegle, F. Steck, W. Krocza, and L. Andral. Assessment of fox control in areas of wildlife rabies. *Bull WHO* 59:269-279, 1981.

Bruner, D. W., and J. H. Gillespie. *Hagan's Infectious Diseases of Domestic Animals*, 6th ed. Ithaca, New York, Cornell University Press, 1973.

Budzko, D. B., L. J. Charamella, D. Jelinek, and G. R. Anderson. Rapid test for detection of rabies antibodies in human serum. *J Clin Microbiol* 17:481-484, 1983.

Burns, R. J., and R. W. Bullard. Diphacinone residue from whole bodies of vampire bats: a laboratory study. *Bull Pan Am Health Organ* 13:365-369, 1979.

Carey, A. B., R. H. Giles, and R. G. McLean. The landscape epidemiology of rabies in Virginia. *Am J Trop Med Hyg* 27:573-580, 1978.

Centers for Disease Control of the USA. Changes in rabies control. *CDC Vet Public Health Notes*, February 1975.

Centers for Disease Control of the USA. Rabies surveillance. Annual Summary 1985. Atlanta, CDC, December 1986.

Constantine, D. G. Bat rabies: current knowledge and future research. *In*: Nagano, Y., and F. M. Davenport (Eds.), *Rabies*. Baltimore, Maryland, University Park Press, 1971.

Constantine, D. G. Absence of prenatal infection of bats with rabies virus. *J Wildl Dis* 22:249-250, 1986.

Crane, L. S., and G. M. Baer. Reported canine and feline rabies in the United States between 1980 and 1983. *Rabies Information Exchange, CDC/USPHS* 15:38-43, December 1986.

Crick, J. Rabies. *In*: Gibbs, E. P. J. (Ed.), *Virus Diseases of Food Animals*, vol. 2. New York, Academic Press, 1981.

Dean, D. J., and M. K. Abelseth. The fluorescent antibody test. *In*: Kaplan, M. M., and H. Koprowski (Eds.), *Laboratory Techniques in Rabies*, 3rd ed. Geneva, World Health Organization, 1973. (Monograph Series 23).

Debbie, J. C. Rabies. *Progr Med Virol* 18:241-256, 1974.

Delpietro, H., A. M. C. de Díaz, E. Fuenzalida, and J. F. Bell. Determinación de la tasa de ataque de rabia en murciélagos. *Bol Of Sanit Panam* 73:222-230, 1972.

Díaz, A. M. Rabies neutralizing antibodies determination by the modified counterimmunoelectrophoresis test and the rapid fluorescent focus inhibition test. *Zentralbl Bakteriol Mikrobiol Hyg* [A]256:1-6, 1983.

Díaz, A. M., E. Fuenzalida, and J. F. Bell. Non-fatal rabies in dogs and cats. *Ann Microbiol (Inst Pasteur)* 126B:503-509, 1975.

Díaz, A. M., G. González Resigno, A. Fernández Munilla, O. P. Larghi, N. Marchevsky, and J. C. Arrossi. Vacuna antirrábica de cerebro de ratón lactante. Esquemas reducidos de inmunización posexposición. *Rev Argent Microbiol* 11:42-44, 1979.

Díaz, A. M., and V. M. Varela-Díaz. Persistence and variation of mangosta street rabies virus antigens during adaptation into mice. *Zentralbl Bakteriol Mikrobiol Hyg* [B]171:73-78, 1980.

Diesch, S. L., S. L. Hendricks, and R. W. Currier. The role of cats in human rabies exposure. *J Am Vet Med Assoc* 181:1510-1512, 1982.

Dreesen, D. W., J. W. Sumner, J. Brown, and D. T. Kemp. Intradermal use of human diploid cell vaccine for preexposure rabies immunization. *J Am Vet Med Assoc* 181:1519-1523, 1982.

Everard, C. O. R., D. Murray, and P. K. Gilbert. Rabies in Grenada. *Trans R Soc Trop Med Hyg* 66:878-888, 1972.

Everard, C. O. R., G. M. Baer, M. E. Alls, and S. A. Moore. Rabies serum neutralizing antibody in mongooses from Grenada. *Trans R Soc Trop Med Hyg* 75:654-666, 1981.

Fekadu, M. Asymptomatic non-fatal canine rabies. *Lancet* 1:569, 1975.

Fekadu, M., J. H. Shaddock, and G. M. Baer. Intermittent excretion of rabies virus in the saliva of a dog two and six months after it had recovered from experimental rabies. *Am J Trop Med Hyg* 30:1113-1115, 1981.

Fekadu, M., J. H. Shaddock, and G. M. Baer. Excretion of rabies virus in the saliva of dogs. *J Infect Dis* 145:715-719, 1982.

Fekadu, M., J. H. Shaddock, F. W. Chandler, and G. M. Baer. Rabies virus in the tonsils of a carrier dog. *Arch Virol* 78:37-47, 1983.

Fernandes, M. V., and P. V. Arambulo III. Rabies as an International Problem. *In*: Koprowski, H., and S. A. Plotkin (Eds.), *World's Debt to Pasteur*. The Wistar Symposium Series, vol. 3. New York, Alan R. Liss, Inc., 1985.

Fishbein, D. B., A. J. Belotto, R. E. Pacer, J. S. Smith, W. G. Winkler, S. R. Jenkins, and K. M. Porter. Rabies in rodents and lagomorphs in the United States, 1971-1984: increased cases in the woodchuck (*Marmota monax*) in Mid-Atlantic States. *J Wildl Dis* 22:151-155, 1986.

Flores Crespo, R., S. Said Fernández, D. Anda López, F. Ibarra Velarde, and R. M. Anaya. Intramuscular inoculation of cattle with warfarin: a new technique for control of vampire bats. *Bull Pan Am Health Organ* 13:147-161, 1979.

Foggin, C. M. Mokola virus infection in cats and a dog in Zimbabwe. *Vet Rec* 113:115, 1983.

Fuenzalida, E. Human pre-exposure rabies immunization with suckling mouse brain vaccine. *Bull WHO* 46:561-563, 1972.

Fuenzalida, E., P. N. Acha, P. Atanasiu, O. Larghi, and B. Szyfres. Rabies immunity in vaccinated cattle. *Proc Annu Meet US Anim Health Assoc* 73:307-322, 1969.

Held, J. R., E. Fuenzalida, H. López Adaros, J. C. Arrossi, N. O. R. Poles, and A. Scivetti. Inmunización humana con vacuna antirrábica de cerebro de ratón lactante. *Bol Of Sanit Panam* 72:565-575, 1972.

Honigman, M. N. *La rabia en las Américas, 1970-1979. Análisis y comentarios.* Buenos Aires, Pan American Zoonoses Center, 1981. (Special Publication 3).

Johnson, R. T. The pathogenesis of experimental rabies. *In*: Nagano, Y., and F. M. Davenport (Eds.), *Rabies*. Baltimore, Maryland, University Park Press, 1971.

Koprowski, H. The mouse inoculation test. *In*: Kaplan, M. M., and H. Koprowski (Eds.), *Laboratory Techniques in Rabies*, 3rd ed. Geneva, World Health Organization, 1973. (Monograph Series 23).

Koprowski, H. Rabies. *In*: Beeson, P. B., W. McDermott, and J. B. Wyngaarden (Eds.), *Cecil Textbook of Medicine*, 15th ed. Philadelphia, Saunders, 1979.

Larghi, O. P., E. González, and J. R. Held. Evaluation of the corneal test as a laboratory method for rabies diagnosis. *Appl Microbiol* 25:187-189, 1973.

Larghi, O. P., and E. Jiménez. Methods for accelerating the fluorescent antibody test for rabies diagnosis. *Appl Microbiol* 21:611-613, 1971.

Larghi, O. P., V. L. Savy, A. E. Nebel, and A. Rodríguez. Vacuna antirrábica inactivada con etilenimina. Duración de inmunidad en perros. *Rev Argent Microbiol* 11:102-107, 1979.

Lecocg, J. P., M. P. Kieny, Y. Lemoine, R. Drillien, T. Wiktor, H. Koprowski, and R. Lathe. New Rabies Vaccines; Recombinant DNA Approaches. *In*: Koprowski, H., and S. A. Plotkin (Eds.), *World's Debt to Pasteur*, The Wistar Symposium Series, vol. 3. New York, Alan R. Liss, Inc., 1985.

Lewis, V. J., and W. L. Thacker. Limitations of deteriorated tissue for rabies diagnosis. *Health Lab Sci* 11:8-12, 1974.

Lord, R. D., E. Fuenzalida, H. Delpietro, O. P. Larghi, and A. M. O. de Díaz. Observations on the epizootiology of vampire bat rabies. *Bull Pan Am Health Organ* 9:189-195, 1975.

Málaga Alba, A. Rabia bovina transmitida por vampiros. *In*: *Memorias del Primer Seminario Internacional y Tercer Seminario Nacional de Rabia*. Cali, Colombia, Ministry of Public Health, 1974.

Mayr, A., H. Kraft, O. Jaeger, and H. Haacke. Orale Immunisierung von Füchsen gegen Tollwut. *Zentralbl Veterinarmed* 19:615-625, 1972.

Mertz, G. J., K. E. Nelson, V. Vithayasai, S. Makornkakeyoon, E. I. Rosanoff, H. Tint, and T. J. Wiktor. Antibody responses to human diploid cell vaccine for rabies with and without human rabies immunoglobulin. *J Infect Dis* 145:720-727, 1982.

Meyer, H. M. Rabies vaccine. *J Infect Dis* 142:287-289, 1980.

Nagano, Y., and F. M. Davenport (Eds.). *Rabies: Proceedings of a Working Conference on Rabies, Japan–United States Cooperative Medical Science Program*. Baltimore, Maryland, University Park Press, 1971.

Nicholson, K. G., P. R. Farrow, U. Bijok, and R. Barth. Pre-exposure studies with purified chick embryo cell culture rabies vaccine and human diploid-cell vaccine: serological and clinical responses in man. *Vaccine* 5:208-210, 1987.

Nicholson, K. G., and H. Prestage. Enzyme-linked immunosorbent assay: a rapid reproducible test for the measurement of rabies antibodies. *J Med Virol* 9:43-49, 1982.

Ogunkoya, A. B., and F. Macconi. Emergence of antirabies vaccine of unknown origin for human treatment in Nigeria. *Vaccine* 4:77-78, 1986.

Okoh, A. E. Investigation of possible rabies reservoirs in rodents in Nigeria. *Int J Zoonoses* 13:1-5, 1986.

Pan American Zoonoses Center. *Encuesta sobre laboratorios productores de vacunas antirrábicas en América Latina y el Caribe. Año 1980.* Buenos Aires, CEPANZO, 1980.

Perrin, P., P. E. Rollin, and P. Sureau. A rapid rabies enzyme immunodiagnosis (RREID): a useful and simple technique for the routine diagnosis of rabies. *J Biol Stand* 14:217-222, 1986.

Plotkin, S. A. Rabies vaccine prepared in human cell cultures: progress and perspectives. *Rev Infect Dis* 2:433-448, 1980.

Pybus, M. J. Rabies in insectivorous bats of western Canada. *J Wildl Dis* 22:307-313, 1986.

Rausch, R. Observations on some natural-focal zoonoses in Alaska. *Arch Environ Health* 25:246-252, 1972.

Rosatte, R. C., M. J. Pybus, and J. R. Gunson. Population reduction as a factor in the control of skunk rabies in Alberta. *J Wildl Dis* 22:459-467, 1986.

Schneider, L. G. Oral immunization of wildlife against rabies. *Ann Inst Pasteur Virol* 136E:469-474, 1985.

Schneider, L. G., and U. Schoop. Rabies-like viruses. *In: International Symposium on Rabies (II), Lyon, 1972*. Basel, Switzerland, Karger, 1974.

Schoop, U. *Praomys (Mastomys) natalensis*: an African mouse capable of sustaining persistent asymptomatic rabies infection. *Ann Microbiol (Inst Pasteur)* 128B:289-296, 1977.

Shope, R. E. Rabies. *In*: Evans, A. S. (Ed.), *Viral Infections of Humans. Epidemiology and Control*. New York, Plenum, 1976.

Sikes, R. K. Rabies. *In*: Davis, J. W., L. H. Karstad, and D. O. Trainer (Eds.), *Infectious Diseases of Wild Mammals*. Ames, Iowa State University Press, 1970.

Sikes, R. K. Rabies. *In*: Hubbert. W. T., W. F. McCulloch, and P. R. Schnurrenberger (Eds.), *Diseases Transmitted from Animals to Man*, 6th ed. Springfield, Illinois, Thomas, 1975.

Steck, F. Epizootiology of rabies. *In: International Symposium on Rabies (II), Lyon, 1972*. Basel, Switzerland, Karger, 1974.

Sureau, P., P. Rollin, and T. J. Wiktor. Epidemiologic analysis of antigenic variations of street rabies virus: detection by monoclonal antibodies. *Am J Epidemiol* 117:605-609, 1983.

Szyfres, L., J. C. Arrossi, and N. Marchevsky. Rabia urbana: el problema de las lesiones por mordeduras de perro. *Bol Of Sanit Panam* 92:310-327, 1982.

Tierkel, E. S. Rapid microscopic examination for Negri bodies and preparation of specimens for biological test. *In*: Kaplan, M. M., and H. Koprowski (Eds.), *Laboratory Techniques in Rabies*, 3rd ed. Geneva, World Health Organization, 1973. (Monograph Series 23.)

Thompson, R. D., C. G. Mitchell, and R. J. Burns. Vampire bat control by systemic treatment of livestock with an anticoagulant. *Science* 177:806-808, 1972.

Turner, G. S., K. G. Nicholson, D. A. J. Tyrrell, and F. Y. Aoki. Evaluation of a human diploid cell strain rabies vaccine: final report of a three year study of pre-exposure immunization. *J Hyg (Camb)* 89:101-110, 1982.

Whetstone, C. A., T. O. Bunn, R. W. Emmons, and T. J. Wiktor. Use of monoclonal antibodies to confirm vaccine-induced rabies in ten dogs, two cats and one fox. *J Am Vet Med Assoc* 185:285-288, 1984.

Wiktor, T. J., S. A. Plotkin, and H. Koprowski. Development and clinical trials of the new human rabies vaccine of tissue culture (human diploid cell) origin. *Dev Biol Stand* 40:3-9, 1977.

Wiktor, T. J., A. Flamand, and H. Koprowski. Use of monoclonal antibodies in diagnosis of rabies virus infection and differentiation of rabies and rabies related viruses. *J Virol Meth* 1:33-46, 1980.

Winkler, W. G., E. F. Baker, and C. C. Hopkins. An outbreak of nonbite transmitted rabies in a laboratory animal colony. *Am J Epidemiol* 95:267-277, 1972.

Winkler, W. G., J. H. Shaddock, and L. W. Williams. Oral rabies vaccine: evaluation of its infectivity in three species of rodents. *Am J Epidemiol* 104:294-298, 1976.

World Health Organization. Report of an International Conference: Rabies in the Tropics. Tunis, 3-6 October 1983.

World Health Organization. *WHO Expert Committee on Rabies, Seventh Report*. Geneva, WHO, 1984a. (Technical Report Series 709.)

World Health Organization. World survey of rabies XXI (for years 1982/1983). (WHO/Rabies/84.195, 1984b.)

World Health Organization. Rabies surveillance. Systemic allergic reactions following immunization with human diploid cell rabies vaccine. *Wkly Epidemiol Rec* 46:354-356, 1984c.

World Health Organization. Bat rabies. *Wkly Epidemiol Rec* 61:109-110, 1986.

World Health Organization. Bat rabies cases in the Federal Republic of Germany. *Rabies Bull Eur* 10:8, 1986.

World Health Organization. Bat rabies in Europe. *Wkly Epidemiol Rec* 61(34):257, 1986.

Yelverton, E., S. Norton, J. F. Obijeski, and D. V. Goeddel. Rabies virus glycoprotein analogs: biosynthesis in *Escherichia coli*. *Science* 219:614-620, 1983.

RIFT VALLEY FEVER

(066.3)

Synonym: Enzootic hepatitis.

Etiology: RNA genome virus, belonging to the genus *Phlebovirus*, family Bunyaviridae; forms part of the complex of mosquito-borne viruses.

Geographic Distribution: Occurs in a large part of the African continent. Virus activity has been confirmed in at least 24 African countries if it is taken into account that the Zinga virus[1] is identical to the Rift Valley fever (RVF) virus (Meegan *et al.*, 1983).

Occurrence: Since 1931, when the virus was isolated from a sheep on a ranch in the Rift Valley, Kenya, several epizootics of the disease have occurred at irregular intervals. The most serious was recorded in South Africa during the summer of 1950-1951, during which about 100,000 sheep and cattle died and some 20,000 human cases occurred. In the same region of the South African high plateau, new outbreaks appeared in the animal and human population in 1953, 1956, and 1969. Another extensive epizootic among domestic animals and numerous human cases with at least four deaths occurred in 1974-1976. This characteristic of enzootic periods followed at variable intervals by epizootics has been observed in other countries. Extensive epizootics among domestic ruminants, accompanied by human cases, were recorded in eight countries in southern and eastern Africa (Shimshony and Barzilai, 1983).

Up to 1977 the disease was confined to the countries south of the Sahara. That year an alarming outbreak occurred in Egypt, causing from 20,000 to 200,000 human cases with about 600 deaths from October to December; during 1978 there were at least 400 other cases. The fatality rate in the civilian population was estimated at 3%. The prevalence of antibodies ranged from less than 1 to 25% in the

---

[1] The Zinga virus has been isolated from mosquitoes and human beings in the Central African Republic and Senegal, where it caused a febrile disease ("Zinga fever"). Antibodies against this virus have also been found in the inhabitants of Congo-Brazzaville.

different provinces and the number of infected persons has been estimated at one million (Brés, 1981).

The disease had a devastating impact on livestock production because of abortions and mortality in sheep, cattle, and buffaloes. The disease in animals preceded human cases by several months. A serologic study carried out in the Nile Valley using the hemagglutination inhibition test found a high rate of reactors in sheep (35.7%), cattle (56.6%), buffaloes (19.3%), and camels (31.4%), and lower rates in goats and burros (Hoogstraal et al., 1979). The average rates of abortions and stillbirths on government ranches during 1978 were 28% in sheep, 18.8% in cattle, and 12.1% in buffaloes; mortality on the same ranches was 20% in sheep, 17.5% in cattle, and 20.4% in buffaloes (Malik, 1981).

The unexpected and dramatic appearance of RVF in Egypt caused worry for several reasons: the presence of the disease in an ecologic region completely different from those where it was known until then, the severity of some previously unknown clinical pictures, and the high morbidity and mortality that were without antecedents in the history of the disease.

Numerous cases have also occurred among laboratory personnel and veterinarians who performed necropsies. Cases of the disease have been recorded not only in Africa but also in laboratories in the United States, Great Britain, and Japan.

The extensive epizootics have generally occurred after heavy rains, when the population of the vector mosquito increases. In Egypt RVF occurred in the Nile Delta, an irrigated area without much precipitation and with high population densities of humans and animals—favorable conditions for mosquito breeding.

The Disease in Man: The disease as described in the sub-Saharan countries was generally mild, with few complications. The incubation period is from 4 to 6 days. The patients suffer from fever, intense cephalalgia, myalgia, arthralgia, and photophobia. Sometimes there is also vertigo, prostration, nausea, vomiting, and vision changes. The disease lasts only a few days, but the fever can reappear around the sixth day. Recuperation of the patient is generally complete, except in some cases with lesions of the retina which can last for months or years. In the 1974-1976 epidemic in South Africa, 12 patients had encephalitis and four died from a hemorrhagic form of the disease.

A study of patients during the epidemic in Egypt established the following clinical forms (Meegan et al., 1981): RVF without complications, which is the most common form; hemorrhagic RVF with meningoencephalitis; and RVF with ocular complications.

The hemorrhagic syndrome is the major cause of mortality. The patients suffer from fever for 2 to 4 days and then have jaundice and hemorrhages such as hematemesis, melena, hemorrhagic gingivitis, and petechiae and purpura on the skin. Hepatic necrosis was one of the lesions found in corpses. The meningoencephalitic syndrome occurred in some patients 5 to 15 days after the febrile period, with disorientation, hallucination, and vertigo. Meningitis and pleocytosis were common. The 80 patients studied with ocular complications had loss of visual acuity 5 to 15 days after the febrile period and had retinal lesions that were frequently bilateral. Nearly half of the patients with more severe macular lesions of the retina suffered permanent loss of central vision (Meegan et al., 1981).

Patients have high-titer viremia that can persist more than a week, suggesting that man can participate in amplification of the virus during epidemics such as the one in Egypt.

The Disease in Animals: RVF occurs naturally in sheep, goats, cattle, and buffaloes. In some outbreaks the disease is seen only in lambs, while in others it also occurs in adult sheep and cattle.

The incubation period is very short, and in experimental infections the first symptoms can be seen from 20 to 72 hours after inoculation. In newborn lambs the disease has a rapid course, without a definite symptomatology, and is highly fatal. Mortality among newborns can sometimes reach 95%. In pregnant ewes, abortion is common during the illness or convalescence, and approximately 20% of those that abort die. In nonpregnant adult sheep, vomiting is sometimes the only observable symptom. Cattle may exhibit abortions, a short-lasting fever, loss of appetite, profuse salivation, abdominal pains, and diarrhea. Mortality in this species is generally low. In necropsy of sheep, the most commonly found lesion is a focal necrosis of the liver which in lambs can affect the whole organ, giving it a greasy appearance and a bright yellow color. Acidophilic cytoplasmic degeneration of hepatocytes progresses to form hyaline bodies, accompanied by changes in the nuclei. Abortions and deaths can also occur among dogs and cats.

Source of Infection and Mode of Transmission: The virus has been isolated from 20 species of mosquitoes of six different genera, as well as from *Culicoides* and *Simulium* spp. Seventeen species of mosquitoes have been studied to evaluate their capacity to transmit the virus to laboratory and domestic animals; 14 of them were capable of doing so (Shimshony and Barzilai, 1983). In South Africa and Zimbabwe, the most important epizootics have occurred in the high plains of areas that do not appear to be the usual habitat of the virus, and it is assumed that the agent was introduced there from an as yet unidentified enzootic area. Three species of naturally infected mosquitoes (*Aedes caballus*, *A. lineatopennis*, and *Culex theileri*) have been found capable of transmitting the infection experimentally (Davies, 1975). The two species of *Aedes* mosquitoes are very numerous after heavy rains, but they disappear rapidly in the dry season. These vectors transmit infection among domestic animals by biting. Sheep and cattle, and perhaps also goats, have very high-titer viremia for 1 to 7 days and are efficient amplifiers of infection for mosquitoes.

Little is known of the basic circulation cycle of the virus in nature. It has been suggested that rodents could be the natural reservoirs, but this suspicion has not been confirmed. The role of wild ruminants in the cycle has not been defined, and thus the primary host of the virus is still unknown. It is likely that the cycle involving domestic animals and mosquitoes is only tangential to a still undetermined wildlife cycle.

On the other hand, the conclusion reached in Zimbabwe is that RVF is enzootic in areas where livestock epizootics occur; consequently, these outbreaks would be due more to an intensification of virus activity than to introduction of the agent from an unknown enzootic area. Heavy rains may be one of the factors that precipitate epizootics, by increasing the density of the vector population. The interepizootic intervals could be periods of increase in the number of susceptible animals (Swanepoel, 1981).

Based on field observations and experimentation, the main vector in Egypt is thought to be *Culex pipiens*, a very abundant mosquito in the Nile Delta which feeds on domestic animals and also man. The low rate of virus isolation from this vector is compensated by its abundant population. The importance of other arthropods in circulation of the virus is still undetermined.

The maintenance mechanism of the virus in nature is still unknown. Research has not confirmed transstadial or transovarial transmission in mosquitoes. However, the virus was recently isolated from larvae of *A. lineatopennis* in Kabete, Kenya; therefore, the agent could persist in the mosquito's eggs during interepizootic periods (International Office of Epizootics, 1983).

In summary, the principal mode of virus transmission among animals is mosquitoes. In contrast, man contracts the infection by contact with infected animals during their slaughter or necropsy, or during food preparation or laboratory work. The source of infection could be apparently healthy animals, as demonstrated by isolation of virus from the spleen of lambs that had recovered from an experimental infection 11 to 21 days after inoculation (Yedloutschnig *et al.*, 1981). Transmission by vectors has not been reliably demonstrated, but it could have played a role during the epidemic in Egypt. Virus probably penetrates through the skin and mucosae, but other routes are also indicated. Experiments have demonstrated that aerosols of the virus are highly infectious for mice; consequently, the airborne route could be important in infection of slaughterhouse workers, veterinarians, and laboratory personnel (Brown *et al.*, 1981). Several investigators who were present when a sheep was slaughtered but had no direct contact with the animal became ill 3 days later, and it is probable that aerosol originating from the blood was the source of infection (Hoogstraal *et al.*, 1979). Although virus has been isolated from milk of an experimentally infected cow, there are no indications that the digestive tract can serve as a portal of entry for the virus. Man is not only susceptible to field viruses but also to modified viruses, as demonstrated by cases observed among laboratory personnel who handled strains attenuated by multiple passages (up to 300) in mice.

It is not known with certainty how the virus was introduced into Egypt. It may have come from Sudan, which borders Egypt to the south and where an epizootic occurred in 1976, by means of viremic camels or humans, or also by arthropods carried on the wind from the Intertropical Convergence Zone to the Aswan area, where it could have been amplified in domestic animals (Shimshony and Barzilai, 1983).

Diagnosis: Diagnosis in man is confirmed by isolation of virus from blood from the acute phase of disease by mouse inoculation (in addition, the virus replicates in most tissue culture systems). Serologic tests, especially the neutralization, complement fixation, hemagglutination inhibition, gel diffusion, indirect immunofluorescence, and ELISA tests, can be used for comparison of titers in sera from the acute and convalescent phases.

One of the fastest methods currently in use to confirm diagnosis is a combination of seeding blood or autopsy material in cell cultures and employing the immunofluorescence test, which can be done the day after seeding.

Diagnosis of the disease in animals is possible by examining histopathologic liver preparations and finding lesions considered to be pathognomonic (necrosis and presence of intranuclear acidophilic inclusions). Virus can be isolated from blood and various organs. Special attention should be given to differential diagnosis with Wesselsbron disease, which has similar symptomatology and epidemiology.

Special precautions should be taken in autopsies and the handling and sending of materials to the laboratory, as well as in the processing of samples.

Control: The unforeseen manner in which outbreaks in animals occur makes it difficult to apply systematic prophylaxis against RVF. In animals, the best way to prevent disease is vaccination. Inactivated vaccines have been used in South Africa for years. It is also thought that immunization of domestic animals, which are the main amplifying hosts of the virus, might prevent epizootics and epidemics that may originate by invasion of the virus from a neighboring country. For this reason, faced with the potential risk that the RVF virus might be introduced from Egypt, in 1978 Israel carried out a national campaign of sheep and cattle vaccination. A modified live virus vaccine for animals is also available, which can be used in females prior to breeding. Vaccination of pregnant females can cause abortion. This vaccine should also not be used in newborn animals, nor is it recommended for use in areas free of RVF because of the possibility that the virus could turn virulent. In South Africa and Kenya this vaccine has been very useful in limiting epizootics, as it is easy to prepare and low in cost (Shope *et al.*, 1982).

In the case of an epizootic, precautions should be taken in handling sick or dead animals and protective clothing should be provided to personnel. Likewise, strict precautionary measures should be taken in laboratories. A formalin-inactivated vaccine has been developed which can be used to protect persons exposed to high risk, such as laboratory personnel and veterinarians.

Bibliography

Allam, I. H., F. M. Feinsod, R. McN. Scott, C. J. Peters, A. J. Saah, S. A. Ghaffar, S. El-Said, and M. A. Darwish. Rift Valley fever surveillance in mobile sheep flocks in the Nile Delta. *Am J Trop Med Hyg* 35:1055-1060, 1986.

Andrewes, C., and H. G. Pereira. *Viruses of Vertebrates*, 3rd ed. Baltimore, Maryland, Williams and Wilkins, 1972.

Brès, P. Prevention of the spread of Rift Valley fever from the African Continent. *Contrib Epidemiol Biostat* 3:178-190, 1981.

Brown, J. L., J. W. Dominik, and R. L. Morrissey. Respiratory infectivity of a recently isolated Egyptian strain of Rift Valley fever virus. *Infect Immun* 33:848-853, 1981.

Centers for Disease Control of the USA. *International Catalogue of Arbovirus*, 2nd ed. (Ed. by T. O. Berge). Atlanta, Georgia, 1975. (DHEW Publ. CDC 75-8301.)

Davies, F. G. Observations on the epidemiology of Rift Valley fever in Kenya. *J Hyg (Camb)* 75:219-230, 1975.

Davies, F. G., J. Koros, and H. Mbugua. Rift Valley fever in Kenya: the presence of antibody to the virus in camels (*Camelus dromedarius*). *J Hyg (Camb)* 94:241-244, 1985.

Davies, F. G., K. J. Linthicum, and A. D. James. Rainfall and epizootic Rift Valley fever. *Bull WHO* 63:941-943, 1985.

Easterday, B. C. Rift Valley Fever. *Adv Vet Sci* 10:65-127, 1965.

Henning, M. W. *Animal Diseases in South Africa*, 3rd ed. Pretoria, Central News Agency, 1956.

Hoogstraal, H., J. M. Meegan, G. M. Khalil, and F. K. Adham. The Rift Valley fever epizootic in Egypt 1977-78. 2. Ecological and entomological studies. *Trans R Soc Trop Med Hyg* 73:624-629, 1979.

International Office of Epizootics. Aislamiento del virus de la fiebre del Valle de Rift en unas larvas de *Aedes lineatopennis. Bull OIE* 95:47, 1983.

Malik, S. K. A. Epidemiology of Rift Valley fever in domestic animals in Egypt. *In: Rift Valley Fever*. Paris, International Office of Epizootics, 1981. (Tech. Ser. 1.)

McIntosh, B. M., and J. H. S. Gear. Mosquito-borne arboviruses, primarily in the eastern hemisphere. *In*: Hubbert, W. T., W. F. McCulloch, and P. R. Schnurrenberger (Eds.), *Diseases Transmitted from Animals to Man*, 6th ed. Springfield, Illinois, Thomas, 1975.

Meegan, J. M., R. H. Watten, and L. W. Laughlin. Clinical experience with Rift Valley fever in humans during the 1977 Egyptian epizootic. *Contrib Epidemiol Biostat* 3:114-123, 1981.

Meegan, J. M., J. P. Digoutte, C. J. Peters, and R. E. Shope. Monoclonal antibodies to identify zinga virus as Rift Valley fever virus. *Lancet* 1:641, 1983.

Shimshony, A., and R. Barzilai. Rift Valley fever. *Adv Vet Sci* 27:347-425, 1983.

Shope, R. E., C. J. Peters, and F. G. Davies. The spread of Rift Valley fever and approaches to its control. *Bull WHO* 60:299-304, 1982.

Swanepoel, R. Observation on Rift Valley fever in Zimbabwe. *Contrib Epidemiol Biostat* 3:83-91, 1981.

Yedloutschnig, R. J., A. H. Dardiri, and J. S. Walker. Persistence of Rift Valley fever virus in the spleen, liver, and brain of sheep after experimental infection. *Contrib Epidemiol Biostat* 3:72-76, 1981.

ROCIO ENCEPHALITIS

(062.9)

Etiology: RNA virus belonging to the genus *Flavivirus* (group B of the arboviruses) of the family Togaviridae.

Geographic Distribution: Rocio encephalitis is an emerging zoonosis that was first recognized in March 1975 on the southern coast of the state of São Paulo, Brazil. Between March 1975 and July 1978, 821 human cases occurred with 10% fatality. No cases have been reported since that date. The epidemic spread to 20 municipalities (districts) in Vale do Ribeira and Baixada Santista. The region is low-lying, very humid and hot, covered with residual forests, and thus favorable to the accumulation of standing water and the breeding of mosquitoes (Iversson, 1980).

Of 153 wild birds examined by the hemagglutination inhibition test, 34 (22.2%) had antibodies for the Rocio virus. The agent was isolated from the blood of one rufous-collared sparrow (*Zonotrichia capensis*) out of 1,007 specimens examined. High rates of reactors were also found in rodents and marsupials (Lopes, 1978a).

The Disease in Man: The incubation period lasts an average of 12 days. Clinical manifestations are variable. The disease has a sudden onset with fever and cephalalgia; slightly more than 50% of the patients experience vomiting and some 20% have abdominal pains. The neurologic symptoms consist of stiffness of the neck, mental confusion, and motor and equilibrium disturbances. About 20% of patients who survive experience a significant decrease in mental functions. Histologic lesions of the brain are the same as produced by other acute viral encephalitides, but characteristically affect mostly the thalamus, the dentate nucleus, and the hypothalamic nuclei (Rosemberg, 1977).

Source of Infection and Mode of Transmission: Epidemiologic investigations indicated that in 75% of the cases the disease affected only one family member, leading to the supposition that interhuman transmission was not important. Nor were there cases among hospital personnel who cared for patients. These facts and the antigenic relationship of the Rocio virus with other flaviviruses transmitted by mosquitoes support the theory that the infection is transmitted by an arthropod (Lopes *et al.*, 1978b). It is also noteworthy that the epidemic occurred in a highly agricultural area and that most of the cases were in males in close contact with the rural environment, especially farmers and fishermen (Iversson, 1980).

Entomologic studies carried out in the area's residual forest, where the epidemic occurred, showed that *Aedes scapularis* and *A. serratus* were the mosquitoes most frequently attracted by human bait. Both species are diurnal with moderate nocturnal activity. *A. scapularis* is active both inside and outside the forest and is more likely to come in contact with the human population (Forattini *et al.*, 1981). In an attempt to isolate the virus from mosquitoes, 2,230 pools containing 38,896 mosquito specimens of several species (including *A. scapularis* and *A. serratus*) were examined; the virus was isolated from only one of the 47 pools of the species *Psorophora ferox* (Lopes *et al.*, 1981). This is the only isolation of the virus from mosquitoes in nature. Nevertheless, this mosquito is probably not a competent vector of the virus. Only a few female *P. ferox* were successfully infected experimentally by oral inoculation. Since the most abundant species in the epidemic area was *A. scapularis*, its competence as a vector was investigated experimentally; it was found to be susceptible to oral infection and highly capable of transmitting the virus by bite to 2-day-old chicks (Mitchell and Forattini, 1984). Although *A. scapularis* is strongly presumed to be the main vector, its infection in nature has not been proven.

The high rate of wild birds with antibodies for the Rocio virus makes them suspect as the natural reservoir of the infection. Mammals have been discounted due to their small numbers in the region.

In summary, the natural history of the disease is still poorly known, although little doubt exists that the infection is transmitted to man by mosquito bites. Likewise, it is not known how this epidemic emerged and why it disappeared. The highest incidence of the disease was in April 1975, with about 55 cases per 100,000 inhabitants, and at about the same time of year in 1976, with 90 per 100,000. Few cases were reported in 1977 and 1978 (Iversson, 1980). According to seroepidemiologic studies carried out on the population in the area, the rate of inapparent infection was low, leading to an assumption that the epidemic's disappearance was not due to lack of a susceptible human population but was perhaps related to the population dynamics of the vector or the reservoirs (Iversson *et al.*, 1982). As for the origin of the epidemic, it was suggested that the virus might have circulated in a sylvatic cycle between nonanthropophilic vectors and primary hosts, and could have broken out into the human population when anthropophilic vectors acquired the infection (Iversson, 1980).

Diagnosis: The virus was isolated from the brains of patients who died of the disease, by means of intracerebral inoculation of the material in 2-day-old mice. Serologic diagnosis is done by hemagglutination inhibition, complement fixation, and neutralization tests using paired serum samples to evaluate seroconversion.

Control: No vaccines are available. In case of epidemics, the same general prevention procedures as for other arboviruses should be followed.

Bibliography

Forattini, O. P., A. C. Gomes, J. L. F. Santos, E. A. B. Galati, E. X. Rabello, and D. Natal. Observaçoes sobre atividade de mosquitos Culicidae em mata residual no Vale do Ribeira, S. Paulo, Brasil. *Rev Saúde Pública* 15:557-586, 1981.

Iversson, L. B. Aspectos da epidemia de encefalite por arbovirus na Região do Vale do Ribeira, S. Paulo, Brasil, no periodo de 1975 a 1978. *Rev Saúde Pública* 14:9-35, 1980.

Iversson, L. B., A. P. A. T. Rosa, J. T. Rosa, and C. S. Costa. Estudos serologicos para pesquisa de anticorpos de arbovirus em populaçao humana da região do Vale do Ribeira. *Rev Saúde Pública* 16:160-170, 1982.

Lopes, O. S. Rocio (ROC) strain: SPH 34675. *Am J Trop Med Hyg* 27:418-419, 1978a.

Lopes, O. S., L. A. Sacchetta, T. L. M. Coimbra, G. H. Pinto, and C. M. Glasser. Emergence of a new arbovirus disease in Brazil. II. Epidemiologic studies on 1975 epidemic. *Am J Epidemiol* 108:394-401, 1978b.

Lopes, O. S., L. A. Sacchetta, D. B. Francy, W. L. Jakob, and C. H. Calisher. Emergence of a new arbovirus disease in Brazil. III. Isolation of Rocio virus from *Psorophora ferox* (Humboldt, 1819). *Am J Epidemiol* 113:122-124, 1981.

Mitchell, C. J., and O. P. Forattini. Experimental transmission of Rocio encephalitis virus by *Aedes scapularis* (Diptera: Culicidae) from the epidemic zone in Brazil. *J Med Entomol* 21:34-37, 1984.

Rosemberg, S. Neuropathological study of a new viral encephalitis: the encephalitis of São Paulo south coast (preliminary report). *Rev Inst Med Trop S Paulo* 19:280-282, 1977.

ROTAVIRAL GASTROENTERITIS

(008.6)

Synonyms: Infantile gastroenteritis; acute gastroenteritis of children, calves, suckling pigs, foals, and lambs; neonatal calf diarrhea; Nebraska calf diarrhea; suckling mouse diarrhea.

Etiology: In recent years, several RNA viruses that are morphologically similar and antigenically related have been isolated from children, calves, piglets, foals, lambs, dogs, cats, nonhuman primates, deer, antelopes, rabbits, birds, and suckling mice. It has been suggested that these viruses be grouped together and called rotaviruses (proposed genus *Rotavirus*) in the family Reoviridae. Rotaviruses differ from both the reoviruses and orbiviruses of this family in morphologic and serologic characteristics as well as in polypeptide composition. The diameter of the viral particle of rotaviruses is 60 to 70 nm. According to recent studies, rotaviruses could constitute the most important cause of gastroenteritis in children.

Under electron microscopy, human and animal rotaviruses are morphologically identical. The virion capsid has two layers (for that reason rotaviruses were previously called "duoviruses"). All rotaviruses have a common group-specific antigen, which is found in the inner layer and can be revealed by the complement fixation, immunofluorescence, and ELISA tests. The serotype-specific antigens, related to specificity to an animal species, are found on the outer layer of the capsid. Recent evidence has confirmed that at least some serotypes (see below) are not strictly species-specific. In this regard, strains isolated from dogs, monkeys, swine, and equines have been found not to differ from human strains assigned to the tentative human serotype 3 (Hoshino *et al.*, 1983a).

Rotaviruses of human origin can be transmitted to suckling pigs, calves, lambs, dogs, and newly born rhesus monkeys, causing either diarrheal disease or only infection, as in dogs. In experiments, it was possible to transmit bovine rotavirus through a series of five passes in gnotobiotic suckling pigs, and each pass caused diarrhea. Also, suckling pigs were infected with rotaviruses of equine and simian origin (Holmes, 1979). Cats experimentally infected with bovine rotaviruses eliminated the agent in the feces for 2 weeks; cats and dogs exposed to these cats by cohabitation became infected and also eliminated virus, but without becoming ill (Schwers *et al.*, 1982). These findings indicate that the animal species barrier is not strict; nevertheless, it is not known to what degree such interchange of viruses among different species occurs naturally. The identification of serotype strains common to man and some animals also suggests that the viruses can cross animal species barriers.

Of interest epidemiologically and from the viewpoint of protection is the existence of different serotypes, which has been established by several immunobiologic methods. The recurrence of disease in some children long after the first diarrheic episode is indicative of this finding (Rodríguez *et al.*, 1978). The number of virus serotypes in humans is still a subject of controversy, both because of the antigenic affinity of the different strains and the lack of sensitivity or specificity of different techniques used. However, three to five serotypes with uniform geographic distribution and stability over time are generally accepted (Lambert *et al.*, 1983).

Two serotypes have been found in bovines, using the cross neutralization test. When calves deprived of colostrum were inoculated with type 1 or 2 of bovine rotavirus, they produced neutralizing antibodies only against the homologous type. In naturally infected herds, calves that react to one type only can be found, but the majority have neutralizing antibodies for both types, perhaps due to successive infections (Murakami *et al.*, 1983). As happens in children, the disease usually recurs in calves (Woode and Bridger, 1975). Two serotypes, H1 and H2, have been found in equines, using the plaque reduction neutralization test. Type H1 was similar or identical to swine rotavirus; type H2 was similar or identical to simian rotavirus, which in turn is antigenically related to strains of human serotype 3 (this serotype includes the canine and feline rotaviruses in addition to the simian) (Hoshino *et al.*, 1983b). Likewise, a serotypic diversity has been confirmed in birds (McNulty *et al.*, 1980) and swine (Bohl, 1980).

The rotavirus genome consists of 11 segments of double-stranded RNA. Genes 4 and 5 have some degree of species specificity, but this is not absolute. The common morphology and antigens of the rotaviruses and their potential for crossing the species barrier seem to indicate a common evolutionary origin (Schroeder *et al.*, 1982).

Recently, atypical rotaviruses (pararotaviruses) have been found in man and other vertebrates (chicks, piglets, calves). They lack the common rotavirus group antigen, but are morphologically indistinguishable from typical rotaviruses under the electron microscope. Infections by these atypical rotaviruses cannot be diagnosed by the

ELISA test, which today largely replaces examination by electron microscopy. Their relative frequency is very poorly known but seems to be low (Chasey and Davies, 1984).

Geographic Distribution: Worldwide.

Occurrence in Man: Gastroenteritis is the most common disease of infants and children throughout the world and constitutes one of the main causes of infant morbidity and mortality. Since 1973, when rotavirus was detected for the first time in Australia in stools of children with diarrhea, morphologically identical viruses have been described in several European, Asian, African, and American countries. In a 1-year study (Davidson *et al.*, 1975) of children with enteritis in a hospital in Melbourne, Australia, rotavirus was found in more than half of the patients. The disease primarily affects children up to 5 years of age, and the highest incidence is observed in the 6 months to 1 year age group. However, in a 2-year-long study of hospitalized children in Buenos Aires, Argentina, the highest frequency was found in children under 6 months old, with the highest rate among those who were not breast-fed (Plaza *et al.*, 1982).

The infection also occurs in newborns, but is usually mild or asymptomatic. In the Baltimore area, USA, sudden infant death syndrome (SIDS) was described in five children between 8 days to 5 months old in the course of 3 weeks. The syndrome was attributed to rotavirus, which was the only agent isolated from feces of the five children and was also found in the trachea of two of them (Yolken and Murphy, 1982). The disease also occurs among school-age children and among adults, but is rarer in these groups.

In developed countries rotaviruses are the most important etiologic agents of acute gastroenteritis requiring hospitalization of children. In developing countries in Asia, Africa, and Latin America, where hundreds of millions of cases of diarrhea occur every year with 5 to 10 million associated deaths, the relative role of rotaviruses in morbidity and mortality is not yet well known, but it is known to be an important agent (Kapikian *et al.*, 1980). According to other sources, 20 to 40% of diarrhea in hospitalized children up to 5 years old in tropical countries is due to rotaviruses, while in temperate countries the rate is 40 to 60%. Studies of communities in Guatemala and El Salvador have demonstrated that 7 to 14% of all episodes of diarrhea before age 3 were due to rotavirus and that almost all the children suffered at least one episode of diarrhea by rotavirus during the first 3 years of life (Pan American Health Organization, 1982). In a study over several years in Costa Rica that considered nonhospitalized diarrheic children, rotaviruses were found to be the most common agent, with a rate of 45.3%, and enterotoxigenic *Escherichia coli* placed second, with a rate of 13.4% (Mata *et al.*, 1983).

The greatest incidence of the disease is observed in the cold winter months in temperate climates and the dry, cool season of tropical climates.

A study carried out in Washington, D.C., using the immunofluorescence and complement fixation tests, indicated that by the time children were 1 year old, 60% of them had been infected by rotavirus, and by the time they were 4 years old, few had escaped the infection (Pan American Health Organization, 1982).

Occurrence in Animals: From the economic point of view, neonatal diarrhea in domestic animals is important because of the high morbidity and mortality it occasions. The large number of bacterial and viral agents that cause diarrhea, and the frequency of mixed infections, make it difficult to establish the rate of incidence of a single etiologic agent. Bacterial infections often occur concurrently with viral infections and aggravate the clinical picture.

Viral and serologic studies indicate that 90 to 100% of suckling pigs and calves and 38% of lambs acquire infection by rotavirus at a very early age. In suckling pigs and calves, infection by rotavirus is usually responsible for lower mortality than infection due to *E. coli* or coronavirus, although some epizootics causing up to 90% mortality have been recognized (World Health Organization, 1980). Subclinical infections are probably frequent, which could be because of passive immunity conferred by the mother's colostrum or strains of the virus with low pathogenicity (Woode, 1978).

A study of rotavirus-associated diarrheas in dairy herds and beef cattle in the United Kingdom found a history of enzootic or sporadic gastroenteritis and epizootic outbreaks in all herds. In units where calves were fed milk from pails, the outbreaks were almost always explosive in 3- to 14-day-old calves that were in contact. On the other hand, in pasturing beef cattle, outbreaks occurred among calves 4 to 6 weeks old; the infection then spread to the majority of calves, especially newborns, in the course of a week (Woode, 1978).

A high rate of reactors (more than 70%) was found in various localities of Japan in horses, sheep, swine, calves, rabbits, and rats by a serologic study using the complement fixation test. The highest titers were found in sera from sheep, rabbits, and calves (Takahashi *et al.*, 1979).

The Disease in Man: The incubation period is usually less than 2 days, but can last up to 7 days. Vomiting precedes the onset of watery diarrhea in the majority of cases. The feces contain mucus in about 25% of the cases, but rarely blood. Low-level pyrexia occurs in 30 to 50% of patients. The disease lasts about 1 week; elimination of virus in the feces can last up to 10 days. The more severe cases can include dehydration and electrolyte imbalance. The fatality rate is low. In a study carried out in Australia, four of 396 children who had virus in the feces died.

A syndrome of hemolytic uremia or diffuse intravascular coagulation has been observed in several infected children. More recently, disease of the respiratory tract and SIDS have been described in nursing babies and small children. Rotavirus was identified in the trachea and feces of two of five children who died of SIDS and in the feces of the other three (Yolken and Murphy, 1982).

The rotaviruses infect the absorbent epithelial cells of the villi of the small intestine and cause a shortening of villi, proliferation of crypt cells, and lymphocytic infiltration of the lamina propria. These changes indicate that the diarrhea could be related to a diminished capacity for absorption within the small intestine.

The Disease in Animals: The disease occurs primarily in newborns and young animals, but it can occur at any age. In experimentally infected gnotobiotic animals the incubation period was 18 hours. The symptomatology consists of depression, anorexia, and diarrhea. Vomiting has been observed only in suckling pigs. The disease is usually afebrile if other microorganisms are not involved. Prolonged diarrhea can result in dehydration and death.

Gnotobiotic calves experimentally inoculated with rotavirus had diarrhea for 6 to 8 hours only and then recovered. When an invasive strain of *E. coli* was introduced prior to virus inoculation, the clinical picture became much more serious and frequently proved fatal. It is probable that the epithelial lesion of the small intestine caused by rotavirus allows proliferation of other microorganisms which complicate the clinical picture.

Source of Infection and Mode of Transmission: The epidemiology of the disease has not yet been completely clarified. The virus is resistant and can survive for months in feces at environmental temperatures; consequently, contamination of the environment can be a source of infection for animals, since animals such as suckling pigs and calves can eliminate 10^7 to 10^{11} infective doses per gram of fecal material for 5 to 9 days (Woode, 1978). In obstetric hospitals, neonatal infection by rotavirus is very common and causes epidemic or endemic diarrhea; sometimes, however, 70 to 90% of the infections are asymptomatic. In day nurseries, children 5 to 10 days old who were eliminating the virus have been found (Holmes, 1979). Given the high incidence of disease and the occurrence of reinfections, it is possible that the virus perpetuates itself by this mechanism (Gillespie and Timoney, 1981). Transmission is by direct or indirect contact. As in other intestinal infections, the mode of transmission is evidently fecal-oral both in man and animals. Oral administration of the virus resulted in infection both in animals and human volunteers. There are several indications that outbreaks of gastroenteritis in human populations were due to contamination of tap water with rotavirus (Hopkins *et al.*, 1984). Samples of drinking water from Mexico and Egypt have been found to contain viable rotavirus particles (Pan American Health Organization, 1982).

Diarrhea by rotavirus in suckling mice was prevented by covering their cages with filters; consequently, it would seem that at least in these animals airborne transmission is important.

Rotaviruses are not strictly species-specific, and experimental cross-infections with human or animal rotaviruses in several animal species have been confirmed. The finding of serotypes common to man and various animal species might indicate that some serotypes can infect both (see Etiology). In England, a rotavirus isolated from a child was found to have a close serologic relationship to a bovine strain, and a strain isolated from a suckling pig was more closely related to a bovine rotavirus than to a porcine strain (World Health Organization, 1980). However, the natural occurrence of cross-infections between species and the possible role of animals in the epidemiology of the disease in humans are still unknown.

Diagnosis: In enteritis in children, the most abundant virus elimination in fecal matter occurs between the third and fifth day after onset of disease, and the agent is rarely detectable after the eighth day. The presence of virus can be confirmed in extracts of fecal matter by electron microscopy. In the last few years other methods to detect virus in the feces have been perfected which do not require such costly equipment, such as immunoelectrophoresis, a modified complement fixation test, ELISA (with blocking reagents), immunoassays using red blood cells as carriers (passive hemagglutination, etc.), and radioimmunoassay. Latex agglutination is a recently perfected, simple test that can be used in clinical practice (Haikala *et al.*, 1983). It is as sensitive as electron microscopy but less specific, and therefore is indicated as a screening test. Also, the difficulties in isolating human rotavirus in cell cultures have recently been surmounted, constituting a great advance. It was possible to culture these viruses in a stable cell line (MA 104) derived from embryonic rhesus monkey kidneys in the presence of trypsin (Sato *et al.*, 1981).

The presence of antibodies can be confirmed using immune electron microscopy (now almost obsolete), complement fixation, radial immunodiffusion, indirect immunofluorescence, radioimmunoassay, agar gel electrophoresis of the viral RNA, and ELISA. The radioimmunoassay, ELISA, and immunofluorescence tests can also be used to measure the different types of immunoglobulins (IgM, IgG, and IgA). Currently, the ELISA test is the most widely used. Although electrophoresis of the viral RNA (Espejo *et al.*, 1978) is less sensitive than the indirect ELISA, it could be of great use in developing countries because of its high specificity, ease of application, and low cost (Avendaño *et al.*, 1984).

Diagnosis of rotaviral diarrhea in animals can be made with the same methods. It has been possible to isolate the rotaviruses involved in animal disease in cell cultures for a long time.

Control: Given the fecal-oral route as the main mode of transmission, the prevention of disease in children must be based on education and observation of basic rules of personal hygiene. Several studies have shown that breast-fed babies have a lower incidence of disease than bottle-fed babies. In hospitals and nurseries good hygiene practices are essential. The rotaviruses have a relatively high resistance to chlorine and other common chemical disinfectants. Treatment with 5 mM of tetracetic ethylenediaminic acid or ethyleneglycolic acid has been found effective in destroying the virus. In the developing world, a problem underlying mortality from all types of diarrhea is malnutrition.

Since rotaviral diarrhea in animals occurs primarily in the first days of life and thus there is no time to actively immunize young animals, the attention of investigators has centered on passive protection. Ingestion of the maternal colostrum is not always sufficient to prevent disease. To be effective, the colostrum has to possess a high antibody titer, as was demonstrated in a recent attempt to vaccinate mothers using a modified virus vaccine with Freund's incomplete adjuvant (Saif *et al.*, 1983). It has been proposed to supply colostrum as a milk supplement during the whole period in which animals are at risk.

In humans, on the other hand, the greatest incidence of disease occurs after the age of 5 or 6 months, allowing time for active immunization. It is still not known whether one human serotype protects against a heterologous human serotype and whether an animal rotavirus can confer immunity against human rotaviruses. The results of studies are contradictory; some tests suggest that some rotaviruses of different serotypes give cross-protection, while other experiments have demonstrated the opposite (Gaul *et al.*, 1982). The current ability to propagate human rotaviruses in cell cultures might lead to the availability of polyvalent vaccines in the future.

Bibliography

Anderson, E. L., R. B. Belshe, J. Bartram, F. Crookshanks-Newman, R. M. Chanock, and A. Z. Kapikian. Evaluation of rhesus rotavirus vaccine (MMW18006) in infants and young children. *J Infect Dis* 153:823-831, 1986.

Avendaño, L. F., S. Dubinovasky, and H. D. James, Jr. Comparison of viral RNA electrophoresis and indirect ELISA methods in the diagnosis of human rotavirus infections. *Bull Pan Am Health Organ* 18:245-249, 1984.

Bohl, E. H. Enteric viral infections as related to diarrhea in swine. *In*: Acres, S. D. (Ed.), *Proceedings of the Third International Symposium on Neonatal Diarrhea*. Saskatoon, Saskatchewan, Canada, 1980. Cit. Hoshino *et al.*, 1983.

Chasey D., J. C. Bridger, and M. A. McCrae. A new type of atypical rotavirus in pigs. *Arch Virol* 89:235-243, 1986.

Chasey, D., and P. Davies. Atypical rotaviruses in pigs and cattle. *Vet Rec* 114:16-17, 1984.

Clark, H. F., P. A. Offit, K. T. Dolan, A. Tezza, K. Gogalin, E. M. Twist, and S. A. Plotkin. Response of adult human volunteers to oral administration of bovine and bovine/ human reassortant rotaviruses. *Vaccine* 4:25-31, 1986.

Davidson, G. P., R. F. Bishop, R. R. W. Townley, I. H. Holmes, and B. J. Ruck. Importance of a new virus in acute sporadic enteritis in children. *Lancet* 1:242-246, 1975.

Espejo, R., P. Romero, E. Calderón, and N. González. Diagnóstico de rotavirus por electroforesis del RNA viral. *Bol Med Hosp Infant Mex* 35:323, 1978.

Flewett, T. H., A. S. Bryden, H. Davies, G. N. Woode, J. C. Bridger, and J. M. Derrick. Relation between viruses from acute gastroenteritis of children and newborn calves. *Lancet* 2:61-63, 1974.

Flores, J., I. Pérez-Schael, M. González, D. García, M. Pérez, N. Daoud, W. Cunto, R. M. Chanock, and A. Z. Kapikian. Protection against severe rotavirus diarrhoea by rhesus rotavirus vaccine in Venezuelan infants. *Lancet* 882-884, April 1987.

Fragoso, M., A. Kumar, and D. L. Murray. Rotavirus in nasopharyngeal secretions of children with upper respiratory tract infection. *Diagn Microbiol Infect Dis* 4:87-88, 1986.

Gaul, S. K., T. F. Simpson, G. N. Woode, and R. W. Fulton. Antigenic relationships among some animal rotaviruses virus neutralization in vitro and cross-protection in piglets. *J Clin Microbiol* 16:495-503, 1982.

Gerna G., N. Passarani, A. Sarasini, and M. Battaglia. Characterization of serotypes of human rotavirus strains by solid-phase immune electron microscopy. *J Infect Dis* 152:1143-1151, 1985.

Gillespie, J. H., and J. F. Timoney. *Hagan and Bruner's Infectious Diseases of Domestic Animals*, 7th ed. Ithaca, Cornell University Press, 1981.

Haikala, O. J., J. O. Kokkonen, M. K. Leinoen, T. Nurmi, R. Mantyjarvi, and H. K. Sarkkinen. Rapid detection of rotavirus in stool by latex agglutination. *J Med Virol* 11:91-97, 1983.

Hoblet, K. H., L. J. Saif, E. M. Kholer, K. W. Theil, S. Bech-Nielsen, and G. A. Stitzlein. Efficacy of an orally administered modified-live porcine-origin rotavirus vaccine against post weaning diarrhea in pigs. *Am J Vet Res* 47:1697, 1986.

Holmes, I. H. Viral gastroenteritis. *Progr Med Virol* 25:1-36, 1979.

Hopkins, R. S., B. Gaspard, F. P. Williams, R. J. Karlin, G. Cukor, and N. R. Blacklow. A community waterborne gastroenteritis outbreak: evidence for rotavirus as the agent. *Am J Public Health* 74:263-265, 1984.

Hoshino, Y., R. G. Wyatt, H. B. Greenberg, A. R. Kalica, J. Flores, and A. Z. Kapikian. Serological comparison of canine rotavirus with various simian and human rotaviruses by plaque reduction neutralization and haemagglutination inhibition tests. *Infect Immun* 41:169-173, 1983a.

Hoshino, Y., R. G. Wyatt, H. B. Greenberg, A. R. Kalica, J. Flores, and A. Z. Kapikian. Isolation, propagation and characterization of a second equine rotavirus serotype. *Infect Immun* 41:1031-1037, 1983b.

Kapikian, A. Z., J. Flores, Y. Hoshino, R. I. Glass, K. Miothun, M. Gorziglia, and R. M. Chanock. Rotavirus: the major etiologic agent of severe infantile diarrhea may be controllable by a "Jennerian" approach to vaccination. *J Infect Dis* 153:815-822, 1986.

Kapikian, A. Z., Hyun Wha Kim, R. G. Wyatt, W. J. Rodríguez, W. L. Cline, R. H. Parrott, and R. M. Chanock. Reovirus-like agent in stools: association with infantile diarrhea and development of serologic tests. *Science* 185:1049-1053, 1974.

Kapikian, A. Z., R. G. Wyatt, H. B. Greenberg, A. R. Kalica, H. W. Kim, C. D. Brandt, W. J. Rodríguez, R. H. Parrott, and R. M. Chanock. Approaches to immunization of infants and young children against gastroenteritis due to rotaviruses. *Rev Infect Dis* 2:459-469, 1980.

Lambert, J. P., D. Marissens, P. Marbehant, and G. Zissis. Prevalence of subgroups 1, 2, and 3 rotaviruses in Belgian children suffering from acute diarrhea (1978-1981). *J Med Virol* 11:31-38, 1983.

Mata, L., A. Simhon, R. Padilla, M. del Mar Gamboa, G. Vargas, F. Hernández, E. Mohs, and C. Lizano. Diarrhea associated with rotaviruses, enterotoxigenic *Escherichia coli, Campylobacter* and other agents in Costa Rican children, 1976-1981. *Am J Trop Med Hyg* 32:146-153, 1983.

McNulty, M. S., G. M. Allan, D. Todd, J. B. McFerran, E. R. McKillop, D. S. Collins, and M. McCracken. Isolation of rotaviruses from turkeys and chickens: demonstration of distinct serotypes and RNA electrophoretypes. *Avian Pathol* 9:363-375, 1980.

Mebus, C. A., R. G. Wyatt, R. L. Sharpee, M. M. Sereno, A. R. Kalica, A. Z. Kapikian, and M. J. Twiehaus. Diarrhea in gnotobiotic calves caused by the reovirus-like agent of human infantile gastroenteritis. *Infect Immun* 14:471-474, 1976.

Middleton, P. J., M. Petric, and M. T. Szymanski. Propagation of infantile gastroenteritis virus (Orbi-group) in conventional and germfree piglets. *Infect Immun* 12:1276-1280, 1975.

Mochizuki, M., and M. Yamakawa. Detection of rotaviruses in cat feces. *Jpn J Vet Sci* 49:159-160, 1987.

Much, D. H., and I. Zajac. Purification and characterization of epizootic diarrhea of infant mice virus. *Infect Immun* 6:1019-1024, 1972.

Murakami, Y., N. Nishioka, Y. Hashiguchi, and C. Kuniyasu. Serotypes of bovine rotaviruses distinguished by serum neutralization. *Infect Immun* 40:851-855, 1983.

Newman, J. F. E., F. Porown, J. C. Bridger, and G. N. Woode. Characterization of a rotavirus. *Nature* 258:631-633, 1975.

Pan American Health Organization. The rotaviruses. *Epidemiol Bull* 3(5):12-15, 1982.

Plaza, A., S. Grinstein, G. Muchinik, M. Valvano, and J. Gómez. Estudio clínico y epidemiológico de la diarrea por rotavirus en la infancia. *Arch Argent Pediatr* 80:289-308, 1982.

Rodríguez, W. J., H. W. Kim, C. D. Brandt, R. H. Yolken, J. O. Arrobio, A. Z. Kapikian, R. M. Chanock, and R. H. Parrott. Sequential enteric illnesses associated with different rotavirus serotypes. *Lancet* 2:37, 1978.

Rotaviruses of man and animals. (Editorial) *Lancet* 1:257-262, 1975.

Saif, L. J., D. R. Redman, K. L. Smith, and K. W. Theil. Passive immunity to bovine rotavirus in newborn calves fed colostrum supplements from immunized or nonimmunized cows. *Infect Immun* 41:1118-1131, 1983.

Sato, K., Y. Inaba, T. Shinozaki, R. Fujii, and M. Matsumoto. Isolation of human rotavirus in cell cultures. *Arch Virol* 69:155-160, 1981.

Schroeder, B. A., J. E. Street, J. Kalmakoff, and R. Bellamy. Sequence relationships between the genome segments of human and animal rotavirus strains. *J Virol* 43:379-385, 1982.

Schwers, A., P. Hoyois, G. Chappuis, L. Dagenais, and P. P. Pastoret. Propagation of bovine rotavirus by cats and dogs. *Ann Rech Vet* 13:303-308, 1982.

Simhon, A. Virología de los rotavirus y epidemiología de la diarrea por rotavirus. *Bol Of Sanit Panam* 98:295-310, 1985.

Spence, L. Rotavirus. *In*: Warren, K. S., and A. A. F. Mahmoud (Eds.), *Tropical and Geographical Medicine*. New York, McGraw-Hill Book Company, 1984.

Stair, E. L., M. B. Rhodes, R. G. White, and C. A. Mebus. Neonatal calf diarrhea; purification and electron microscopy of a coronavirus-like agent. *Am J Vet Res* 33:1147-1156, 1972.

Takahashi, E., Y. Inaba, K. Sato, H. Kurogi, H. Akashi, K. Satoda, and T. Omori. Antibody to rotavirus in various animal species. *Nat Inst Anim Health Q* 19:72-73, 1979.

Theil, K. W., L. J. Saif, P. D. Moorhead, and R. E. Whitmoyer. Porcine rotavirus-like (group B Rotavirus): characterization and pathogenicity for gnotobiotic pigs. *J Clin Microbiol* 21:340-345, 1985.

Torres-Medina, A., R. G. Wyatt, C. A. Mebus, N. R. Underdahl, and A. Z. Kapikian. Diarrhea caused in gnotobiotic piglets by the reovirus-like agent of human infantile gastroenteritis. *J Infect Dis* 133:22-27, 1976.

Vesikari, T., A. Z. Kapikian, A. Delem, and G. Zissis. A comparative trial of rhesus monkey (RRV-1) and bovine (RIT 4237) oral rotavirus vaccine in young children. *J Infect Dis* 153:832-839, 1986.

White, R. G., C. A. Mebus, and M. J. Twiehaus. Incidence of herds infected with a neonatal calf diarrhea virus (NCDV). *Vet Med* 65:487-490, 1970.

Woode, G. N. Transmissible gastroenteritis of swine. *Vet Bull* 39:239-248, 1969.

Woode, G. N. Epizootiology of bovine rotavirus infection. *Vet Rec* 103:44-46, 1978.

Woode, G. N., J. C. Bridger, G. Hall, and M. J. Dennis. The isolation of reovirus-like agent associated with diarrhea in colostrum-deprived calves in Great Britain. *Res Vet Sci* 16:102-105, 1974.

Woode, G. N., and J. C. Bridger. Viral enteritis of calves. *Vet Rec* 96:85-88, 1975.

World Health Organization, Working Group. Rotavirus and other viral diarrheas. *Bull WHO* 58:183-198, 1980.

Yolken, R., and M. Murphy. Sudden infant death syndrome associated with rotavirus infection. *J Med Virol* 10:291-296, 1982.

Yolken, R. H., G. A. Losonsky, S. Vonderfecht, F. Leister, and S. B. Wee. Antibody to human rotavirus in cow's milk. *New Engl J Med* 312, 1985.

RUSSIAN AND CENTRAL EUROPEAN SPRING-SUMMER ENCEPHALITIS

(063.0)

Synonyms: Tick-borne group B virus encephalitis, Far East spring-summer encephalitis, biphasic meningoencephalitis.

Etiology: RNA virus belonging to the genus *Flavivirus* (group B of Casals arboviruses) of the family Togaviridae. The virus is part of a complex that includes the Powassan encephalitis, louping-ill, Kyasanur Forest disease, Omsk hemorrhagic fever, and Langat viruses. Two antigenic variants are recognized: the Far East (oriental virus) and the Central Europe (occidental virus).

Geographic Distribution: The virus has been isolated in the European and Asiatic regions of the USSR, Finland, Sweden, Norway, Denmark, the German Democratic Republic, Poland, Czechoslovakia, Hungary, Austria, Switzerland, and Bulgaria. The occidental variant of the virus is present in European countries, the oriental variant is found in Asia, and both variants have been isolated in the western Soviet Union.

Occurrence in Man: The disease caused by tick bites is sporadic and mainly affects adults. Infection due to consumption of goat's milk contaminated by the occidental virus shows up as outbreaks involving the whole family, with children as well as adults affected. In 1951 there was an epidemic with 660 cases in Czechoslovakia. Every year several hundred to 2,000 cases occur, with a morbidity rate of up to 20 per 100,000 inhabitants (Monath, 1982).

Inapparent clinical infections are frequent in man in endemic areas, as shown by seroepidemiologic studies. The disease occurs in summer, when ticks are abundant.

Occurrence in Animals: The virus has been isolated from small mammals, mainly rodents, and from goats and cattle.

The Disease in Man: The disease caused by the oriental variant is generally more severe than that caused by the European or occidental type. In the Soviet Far East, the infection is of sudden onset, with intense cephalalgia, rapidly rising pyrexia, vomiting, hyperesthesia, and photophobia. Symptomatology characteristic of encephalomyelitis is common in that region, with temporary or permanent flaccid paralysis, nystagmus, visual disorders, deafness, vertigo, somnolence, epileptiform convulsions, delirium, and coma. Convalescence is extended and sequelae are common, consisting primarily of paralysis of the upper extremities and back muscles. Sometimes, motor disorders and paralysis may appear months or even years after the acute phase of the disease. There is evidence, as yet unproven, that these late syndromes may be due to the persistence of the virus in the nervous system (Asher, 1979). Case fatality is approximately 20%.

In Europe and in part of Siberia, the disease is more benign and generally follows a biphasic course. The first phase corresponds to the viremic period and is characterized by a mild febrile illness resembling influenza and lasting about 1 week. The patient improves but relapses after a few days, with fever, cephalalgia, stiffness of the neck, and vomiting. The disease frequently takes the course of aseptic meningitis or mild meningoencephalitis. Serious cases with paralysis or death are rarer than with the oriental variant of the virus. Convalescence is lengthy, and the fatality rate is usually 1 to 2%.

The tick-borne infection has an incubation period of 8 to 20 days, while that of the infection caused by consumption of contaminated milk is only 4 to 7 days.

The Disease in Animals: The infection is usually asymptomatic and only occasionally causes disease in dogs and lambs. Experimental inoculation of the virus in adult sheep results in a viremia that may last up to 5 days, and elimination of the virus from the second to the seventh day. In lambs it causes viremia, encephalitis, and death in 5 to 6 days (Gresíková and Beran, 1981).

Source of Infection and Mode of Transmission (Figure 49): The infection is nidal in character and occurs in woods or pastures within forest areas. The virus circulates between small mammals, especially rodents, and ticks. The main vectors are *Ixodes persulcatus* for the oriental variant of the virus and *I. ricinus* for the occidental variant, but other tick species, such as *Haemaphysalis concinna*, *H. japonica douglasi*, and several species of *Dermacentor*, can also act as vectors. Both transstadial and transovarial transmission of the virus have been proven in the two principal vectors (*I. persulcatus* and *I. ricinus*). Transovarial transmission occurs irregularly, in about 6% of the infected vectors.

The tick larvae feed on and infect small mammals. These animals serve as amplifiers of the virus in spring and summer. At least 10 species of wild rodents have been found to have high viremia titers that persist for a long time (Gresíková and Beran, 1981). Larvae transmit the infection to nymphs, and they, in turn, to

**Figure 49. Russian and central European spring-summer encephalitis.
Transmission cycle.**

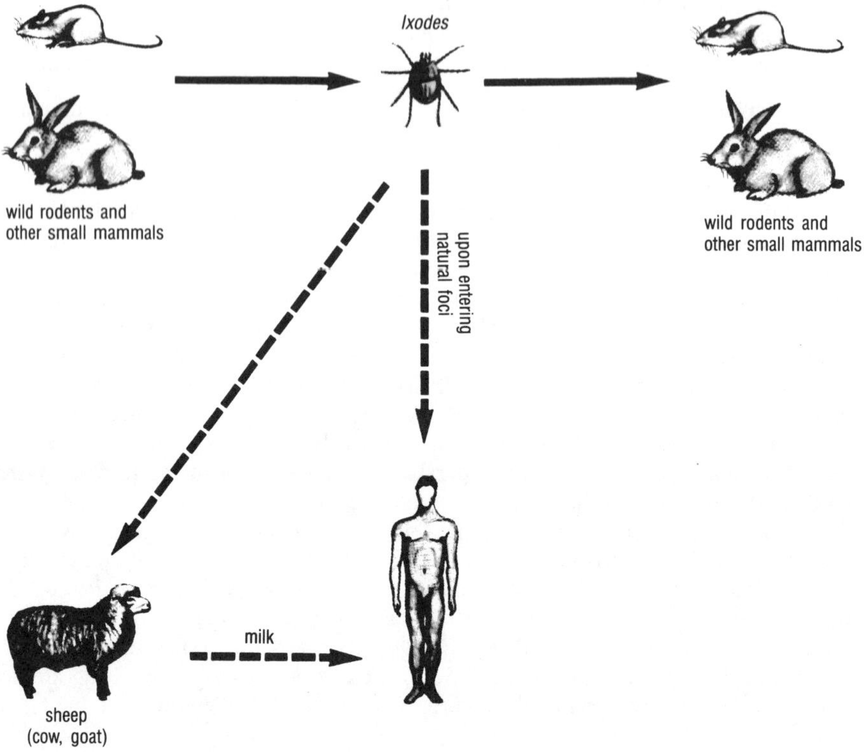

wild rodents and
other small mammals

Ixodes

upon entering
natural foci

wild rodents and
other small mammals

sheep
(cow, goat)

milk

adult ticks. Nymphs and adult ticks feed on large animals including sheep, goats, and cattle.

It has been shown experimentally that several species of small mammals and wild birds, after peripheral inoculation or tick bite, develop prolonged viremia, the infection remaining clinically inapparent in most cases. In some animals, such as the hedgehog, dormouse, and bats, the virus persists in the blood for a long time during hibernation.

Man and domestic animals, such as goats and cattle, contract the infection through tick bites upon entering the natural foci of the virus. Man can also contract the infection by ingesting contaminated goat's or sheep's milk or cottage cheese. Goats and sheep are infected by ticks when they graze in enzootic areas, and they eliminate the virus in their milk. The bite of infected ticks has been shown experimentally to produce viremia and excretion of the virus in the milk of cattle and sheep. However, no human cases are known to have resulted from drinking cow's milk.

The disease in man is seasonal and is related to the time of tick activity. In the Soviet Far East this period occurs in spring and early summer, while in Europe activity can extend until autumn.

Role of Animals in the Epidemiology of the Disease: In addition to being vectors, ticks are also reservoirs of the virus because of their transstadial and transovarial transmission. Wild rodents serve as amplifiers. Likewise, the virus can hibernate in wild rodents. In Europe and a part of the Far East, infected goats and sheep that eliminate the virus through milk serve as a source of infection for man.

Man is an accidental host who becomes infected by means of tick bites or consumption of goat's milk or cottage cheese. In the USSR, the incidence of the disease increased as man penetrated the natural foci when developing forested areas of Siberia and the Far East.

Diagnosis: The virus can be isolated from the blood of patients, especially during the first phase of the disease, by means of intracerebral inoculation in mice and hamsters or by cellular culture. Serologic diagnosis consists of proving seroconversion (at least a four-fold increase in the titer) by means of the complement fixation, hemagglutination inhibition, neutralization, and, more recently, ELISA tests (Roggendorf *et al.*, 1981; Hofmann *et al.*, 1983).

Control: In eastern Europe and the USSR, an inactivated vaccine is used to protect groups exposed to high risk (forestry workers, military personnel, farmers). An attenuated vaccine is still experimental. To avoid epidemic outbreaks, it is important to pasteurize or boil milk. Use of protective clothing and tick repellents for individual protection is recommended in endemic areas.

Bibliography

Andrewes, C., and H. G. Pereira. *Viruses of Vertebrates*, 3rd ed. Baltimore, Maryland, Williams and Wilkins, 1972.

Asher, D. M. Persistent tick-borne encephalitis infection in man and monkeys: relation to chronic neurologic disease. *In*: Kurstak, E. (Ed.), *Arctic and Tropical Arboviruses*. New York, Academic Press, 1979.

Centers for Disease Control of the USA. *International Catalogue of Arboviruses*, 2nd ed. (Ed. by T. O. Berge). Atlanta, Georgia, 1975. (DHEW Publ. CDC 75-8301.)

Clarke, D. H., and J. Casals. Arboviruses: Group B. *In*: Horsfall, F. L., and I. Tamm (Eds.), *Viral and Rickettsial Infections of Man*, 4th ed. Philadelphia, Lippincott, 1965.

Fox, J. P. Russian spring-summer encephalitis and louping-ill. *In*: Beeson, P. B., W. McDermott, and J. B. Wyngaarden (Eds.), *Cecil Textbook of Medicine*, 12th ed. Philadelphia, Saunders, 1967.

Goldblum, N. Group B arthropod-borne viral disease. *In*: Van der Hoeden, J. (Ed.), *Zoonoses*. Amsterdam, Netherlands, Elsevier, 1964.

Gresíková, M., and G. W. Beran. Tick-borne encephalitis (TBE). *In*: Beran, G. W. (Section Ed.), *CRC Handbook Series in Zoonoses*. Section B, vol. 1. Boca Raton, Florida, CRC Press, 1981.

Hofmann, H., F. X. Heinz, and H. Dippe. ELISA for IgM and IgG antibodies against tick-borne encephalitis virus: quantification and standardization of results. *Zentralbl Bakteriol Mikrobiol Hyg* [A] 255:448-455, 1983.

Hubalek, Z., J. Mitterpak, J. Prokopic, Z. Juricova, and J. Kilik. A serologic survey for Bhanja and tick-borne encephalitis viruses in sheep of eastern Slovakia. *Folia Parasitol (Praha)* 32:279-283, 1985.

McNeill, J. G., W. M. Lednar, S. K. Stansfield, R. E. Prier, and R. N. Miller. Central European tick-borne encephalitis: assessment of risk for persons in armed services and vacationers. *J Infect Dis* 152:650-651, 1985.

Monath, T. P. Arthropod-borne viral encephalitides. *In*: Wyngaarden, J. B., and L. H. Smith, Jr. (Eds.), *Cecil Textbook of Medicine*, 16th ed., vol. 2. Philadelphia, Saunders, 1982.

Rhodes, A. J., and C. E. van Rooyen. *Textbook of Virology*, 4th ed. Baltimore, Maryland, Williams and Wilkins, 1962.

Roggendorf, M., F. Heinz, F. Deinhardt, and C. Kunz. Serological diagnosis of acute tick-borne encephalitis by demonstration of antibodies of the IgM class. *J Med Virol* 7:41-50, 1981.

ST. LOUIS ENCEPHALITIS

(062.3)

Synonyms: Type C lethargic encephalitis.

Etiology: RNA virus belonging to the genus *Flavivirus* (formerly group B of the arboviruses) of the family Togaviridae; forms part of the virus complex including Murray Valley, West Nile, and Japanese B encephalitides.

There are indications that strains of the virus isolated in different zones differ in their capacity to produce viremia in birds (Bowen, 1980), virulence in 3-week-old mice, and neurovirulence in rhesus monkeys (Monath, 1979). By the technique of nucleotide mapping, considerable genetic variation among the strains of the virus was demonstrated, and it was proposed to name these geographic variants as topotypes (Trent *et al.*, 1981).

Geographic Distribution: The agent is distributed from Argentina to Canada. The disease is unknown outside the Americas.

Occurrence in Man: The disease is seen in endemic and sporadic form and only occasionally in epidemic form in the western United States; on the other hand, east of the Mississippi River periodic epidemic outbreaks occur. Epidemics have also occurred in Canada and Mexico (Monath, 1979). In other parts of the Americas a few isolated cases occur. Sporadic cases have been reported in Jamaica, Trinidad, French Guyana, Argentina, and possibly Curaçao (Spence, 1980). Less than 25 clinical cases have been observed since 1953 outside the United States, Canada, and Mexico, the majority of them without neural symptomatology (Monath, 1979).

St. Louis encephalitis (SLE) occupies first or second place—according to the year—among the arboviral encephalitides in the United States. The great majority of the cases (about 75%) occur in the eastern section of the country. Since 1933, several outbreaks of variable magnitude have occurred at irregular intervals in a large area of the United States; in some outbreaks, up to 500 clinical cases were confirmed and, in others, more than 1,000. In 1975 there was an epidemic in 28 states and the District of Columbia, with 1,367 confirmed cases, 574 presumptive cases, and 95 deaths. In 1976, 379 cases were reported in 15 states (Centers for Disease Control of the USA, 1976), and in 1977 and 1978, 132 and 26 cases, respectively, were reported.

In 1974, an epidemic outbreak took place in the city of Hermosillo, Mexico, with an incidence of 19 per 100,000 inhabitants, 51 patients hospitalized, and 20% fatality. The first outbreak in Ontario, Canada, occurred in 1975, with 22 cases.

As with other arboviruses, the number of inapparent infections with the SLE virus is much greater than the number of recognized clinical cases. After an epidemic in the Tampa Bay area of Florida in 1962, a serologic study showed a rate of inapparent infections among the population of Clearwater of 4,291 per 100,000 inhabitants, while the rate of clinical cases was 109.6 per 100,000. Following an epidemic in 1964 in Houston, Texas, a random sample study carried out among the inhabitants of that city revealed 8% inapparent infections; in the primary epidemic area, which corresponded to the poorest socioeconomic sector, the rate was 34%. The relation between clinical cases and inapparent infections is 1:800 in children up to 9 years old and 1:85 in persons older than 60 years (Monath, 1982).

Inapparent human infections are also common in Central America, the Caribbean, and South America, as indicated by serologic studies (Monath, 1979).

St. Louis encephalitis occurs in the second half of summer and in early autumn.

Occurrence in Animals: The virus has been isolated from many species of wild birds and mammals in the United States and elsewhere in the hemisphere. Serologic studies have found the infection in many other animal species, including equines.

The infection is subclinical in animals.

The Disease in Man: The clinical infection presents a wide spectrum, from an undifferentiated febrile disease similar to influenza to severe encephalitis. Three syndromes can be distinguished: febrile disease, aseptic meningitis, and encephalitis. The febrile syndrome usually has a benign course, with fever and intense cephalalgia lasting several days, followed by complete recovery. The aseptic meningitis has a sudden onset, with fever, stiffness of the neck, and positive Kernig and Brudzinski signs, but without neurologic dysfunction. Pleocytosis is common. The disease characterized by encephalitis also begins suddenly, with fever and one or more signs of brain inflammation, such as personality changes, confusion, delirium, lethargy, paresis, convulsions, and others (Brinker and Monath, 1980). The encephalitis syndrome is more frequent in elderly persons; its frequency increases from 56% in patients up to 20 years old to 87% in those over 60. Convalescence in these cases lasts several weeks.

The incubation period is estimated at 4 to 21 days.

In the United States, the case fatality rate in 2,261 confirmed clinical cases between 1955 and 1968 was 5 to 10%. The majority of deaths were in persons over 50 years old, among whom the fatality rate can be as high as 30% or more (Luby *et al.*, 1969). During the 1962 epidemic in Tampa Bay, Florida, the highest fatality rate (36.3%) was recorded in patients 65 years of age and older in Pinellas County, where a large number of retired persons live. In that county the general mortality rate was 22.2%, while the rate was 9.8% in the remaining three counties in that area (Bond *et al.*, 1965).

In Central and South America, most of the small number of recorded patients did not exhibit impairment of the central nervous system.

The Disease in Animals: The infection is subclinical in animals. Experimental peripheral inoculation of the virus produces viremia without clinical symptoms in domestic and wild fowl and in various species of insectivorous bats.

When the disease occurs in man, antibodies for SLE are generally found in horses and in some other mammals. In contrast to western, eastern, and Venezuelan equine encephalitides, St. Louis encephalitis does not cause clinical illness in equines. Some equines inoculated experimentally develop viremia.

Source of Infection and Mode of Transmission (Figure 50): The basic cycle of the infection involves wild birds and ornithophilic mosquitoes. *Culex salinarius*, from which the SLE virus has been isolated, could be the vector in the wild enzootic cycle. In the United States, two different epidemiologic situations are known, depending on the habits of the primary vector and other ecologic conditions. West of the Rocky Mountains the disease is rural and sporadic because the vector, *C. tarsalis*, is sparse and the widely scattered human population has a high rate of subclinical infection, protecting it against reinfection. Though the vector and birds reach high concentrations in areas flooded by irrigation water, human cases are not numerous for the reasons given. In the south-central and north-central states of the country, by contrast, the disease is urban-suburban in character, primarily because the vectors are the peridomestic and domestic mosquitoes *C. quinquefasciatus* and *C. pipiens*. These vectors proliferate where water contaminated with organic wastes collects, that is, in poorer urban and suburban areas deficient in environmental sanitation. The same conditions favor the proliferation of sparrows, pigeons, and other birds that feed among household wastes. Peridomestic birds and domestic fowl serve as amplifiers of the virus; that fact, together with the increased density of the human population, creates the conditions necessary for epidemics. During the 1964 epidemic in Houston, the virus was isolated from geese, domestic pigeons, and various other species of birds. In addition, antibodies were found in 20% of the birds, especially house sparrows (*Passer domesticus*), and in almost all poultry examined. How the virus gets into urban areas is not yet established, but it is suspected that migratory wild birds may introduce it.

In the epidemic in Hermosillo, Mexico, the vector was *C. tarsalis*. The incidence was higher in children than in adults, perhaps because older age groups had been previously exposed to the virus and were immune.

In the 1962 epidemic in Florida, the vector was *C. nigripalpus*, a mosquito of tropical and subtropical regions that breeds in a wide variety of habitats and feeds on human and avian blood.

In Jamaica, SLE virus has been isolated from this same mosquito species. In South and Central America the virus has been isolated from numerous species of mosquitoes. The relative importance of the different species as vectors (vectorial competence) has not yet been evaluated. *C. pipiens quinquefasciatus*, which is an efficient vector of the SLE virus east of the Mississippi River in the United States, is also found in the Caribbean and South America. Recently, the virus has been isolated from this species of mosquito in the province of Santa Fe, Argentina. Argentine mosquitoes that were bred in the laboratory in the United States and infected orally with the Argentine virus demonstrated the same ability to acquire the infection and transmit it to chicks as was found in *C. pipiens quinquefasciatus* of United States origin. On the other hand, no differences were observed between the Argentine and United States strains of the virus in their capacities to infect these mosquitoes and be transmitted by them (Mitchell *et al.*, 1980).

Several hypotheses have been formulated to explain why epidemics of SLE do not occur in the Caribbean and Central and South America, but none of them are totally satisfactory. Several strains isolated in Central and South America were classified as

Figure 50. St. Louis encephalitis. Probable cycle of the virus.

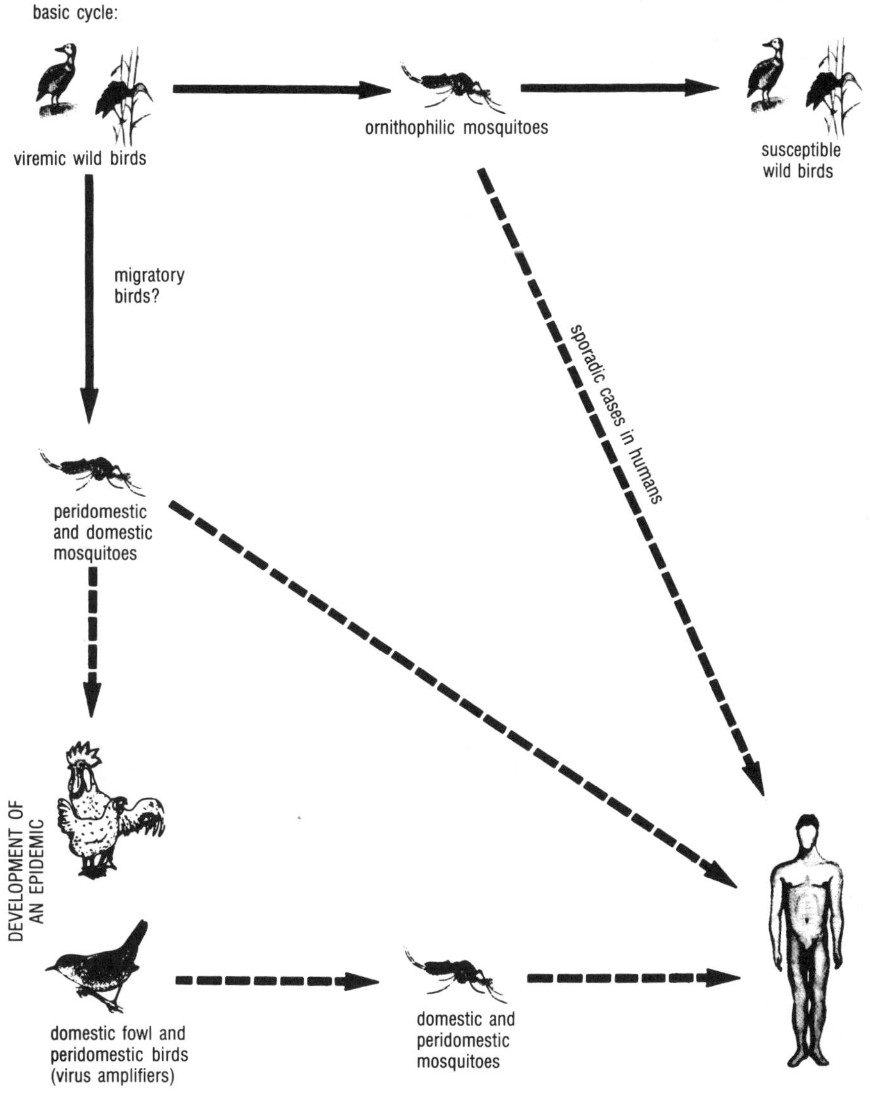

very virulent (Monath *et al.*, 1980). This region also has efficient vectors that are prone to attack man (Mitchell *et al.*, 1980). Thus, neither lack of virulence of the agent nor vector inefficiency could explain the absence of epidemics. A hypothesis supported by several researchers is that people in South America, Central America, and the Caribbean acquire immunity very early in life, and continue to accumulate it with age. The prevalence of antibodies in the population is high, and immunity in persons in the older age groups, for whom the infection tends to have clinical manifestations, could be a factor in preventing epidemic outbreaks (Mitchell *et al.*, 1980).

As is true for many other arboviruses, the mechanism that allows the virus to overwinter in temperate climates is not fully known. The virus has been isolated from hibernating adult female *C. pipiens,* which indicates that the virus can persist in the vector during the winter in temperate climates (Bailey *et al.*, 1978). It also has been proven experimentally that low-level transovarial transmission occurs in *C. pipiens* (Francy *et al.*, 1981).

Role of Animals in the Epidemiology of the Disease: Man is an accidental host of the virus and does not play any role in the natural maintenance cycle. The basic reservoir is wild birds and perhaps the vector mosquitoes; poultry and peridomestic and domestic birds act as amplifiers of the virus, which circulates from one host to another by means of mosquitoes. Wild and domestic mammals are not thought to play a role in the virus cycle because their viremia is low-level and transitory and virus strains isolated from them possess low virulence (Monath *et al.*, 1980). In Panama, sloths inoculated with the SLE virus developed prolonged high-titer viremia, but the role of these animals under natural conditions has not been determined. Likewise, bats may be involved in the virus's overwintering within enzootic foci in temperate climates, as well as in its dissemination to epizootic foci, a subject that requires further study (Herbold *et al.*, 1983).

Diagnosis: SLE may be confused clinically with other febrile diseases or with encephalitides and aseptic meningitis caused by different agents. Laboratory confirmation is essential. Laboratory diagnosis is based primarily on serology; only on a few occasions has it been possible to isolate the etiologic agent from the blood of viremic patients. Most successful isolations have been made from the brain of patients who died a short time after contracting the disease.

Diagnosis is based on demonstrating serologic conversion in the patient by comparing titers of serum samples taken during the acute phase with those taken during convalescence. The most widely used tests are complement fixation, neutralization (which is the most specific), and hemagglutination inhibition. Antibodies can be detected during the first week of the disease by the hemagglutination inhibition and neutralization tests, while the complement fixation antibodies appear during the second or third week. In Latin American and Caribbean countries, where infections due to several flaviviruses occur, tests must include all of the other viruses of the group known to be present in the area.

Control: The only preventive measure available is control of the vector. Programs of epidemiologic surveillance and vector control have given satisfactory results in California against *C. tarsalis,* in Florida against *C. nigripalpus,* and in Texas against *C. quinquefasciatus.* An effective vaccine is not yet available.

Bibliography

Allen, R., S. K. Taylor, and S. E. Sulkin. Studies of arthropod-borne virus infections in Chiroptera. VIII. Evidence of natural St. Louis encephalitis virus infection in bats. *Am J Trop Med Hyg* 19:851-859, 1970.

Andrewes, C., and H. G. Pereira. *Viruses of Vertebrates*, 3rd ed. Baltimore, Maryland, Williams and Wilkins, 1972.

Bailey, C. L., B. F. Eldridge, D. E. Hayes, D. M. Watts, R. F. Tammariello, and J. M.

Dalrymple. Isolation of St. Louis encephalitis virus from overwintering *Culex pipiens* mosquitoes. *Science* 199:1346-1349, 1978.

Bond, J. O., D. T. Quick, J. J. Witte, and H. C. Oard. The 1962 epidemic of St. Louis encephalitis in Florida. I. Epidemiologic observations. *Am J Epidemiol* 81:392-404, 1965.

Bowen, G. S., T. P. Monath, G. E. Kemp, J. H. Kerschner, and L. J. Kirk. Geographic variation among St. Louis encephalitis virus strains in the viremic responses of avian hosts. *Am J Trop Med Hyg* 29:1411-1419, 1980.

Brinker, K. R., and T. P. Monath. The acute disease. *In*: Monath, T. P. (Ed.), *St. Louis Encephalitis*. Washington, D.C., American Public Health Association, 1980.

Centers for Disease Control of the USA. *International Catalogue of Arboviruses*, 2nd ed. (Ed. by T. O. Berge). Atlanta, Georgia, 1975. (DHEW Publ. CDC 75 8301.)

Centers for Disease Control of the USA. Arboviral infections in the United States—1975. *Morb Mortal Wkly Rep* 25:116, 1976.

Centers for Disease Control of the USA. St. Louis Encephalitis—United States. *Morb Mortal Wkly Rep* 25:294, 1976.

Centers for Disease Control of the USA. Arboviral infections of the central nervous systems—United States, 1986. *Morb Mortal Wkly Rep* 36(27):450-455, 1987.

Clarke, D. H., and J. Casals. Arboviruses: Group B. *In*: Horsfall, F. L., and I. Tamm (Eds.), *Viral and Rickettsial Infections of Man*, 4th ed. Philadelphia, Lippincott, 1965.

Chamberlain, R. W. Arbovirus infections of North America. *In*: Sanders, M., and M. Schaeffer (Eds.), *Viruses Affecting Man and Animals*. St. Louis, Missouri, Green, 1971.

Downs, W. G. Arboviruses. *In*: A. S. Evans (Ed.), *Viral Infections of Humans. Epidemiology and Control*. New York, Plenum, 1976.

Fox, J. P. St. Louis encephalitis. *In*: Beeson, O. B., W. McDermott, and J. B. Wyngaarden (Eds.), *Cecil Textbook of Medicine*, 15th ed. Philadelphia and London, Saunders, 1979.

Francy, D. B., W. A. Rush, M. Montoya, D. S. Inglish, and R. A. Bolin. Transovarial transmission of St. Louis encephalitis virus by *Culex pipiens* complex mosquitoes. *Am J Trop Med Hyg* 30:699-705, 1981.

Herbold, J. R., W. P. Heuschele, and R. L. Berry. Reservoir of St. Louis encephalitis virus in Ohio bats. *Am J Vet Res* 44:1889-1893, 1983.

Luby, J. P., S. E. Sulkin, and J. P. Sanford. The epidemiology of St. Louis encephalitis: a review. *Annu Rev Med* 20:329-350, 1969.

Mitchell, C. J., T. P. Monath, and M. S. Sabattini. Transmission of St. Louis encephalitis virus from Argentina by mosquitoes of the *Culex pipiens* (Diptera: Culicidae) complex. *J Med Entomol* 17:282-285, 1980.

Monath, T. P. Arthropod-borne encephalitides in the Americas. *Bull WHO* 57:513-533, 1979.

Monath, T. P., C. B. Cropp, G. S. Bowen, G. E. Kemp, C. J. Mitchell, and J. J. Gardner. Variation in virulence for mice and rhesus monkeys among St. Louis encephalitis virus strains of different origin. *Am J Trop Med Hyg* 29:948-962, 1980.

Monath, T. P. Arthropod-borne viral encephalitides. *In*: Wyngaarden, J. B., and L. H. Smith, Jr. (Eds.), *Cecil Textbook of Medicine*, vol. 2., 16th ed. Philadelphia, Saunders, 1982.

Philips, C. A., and J. L. Melnick. Urban epidemic encephalitis in Houston caused by a group B arbovirus (SLE). *Progr Med Virol* 9:159-175, 1967.

Quick, D. T., R. E. Serfling, I. L. Sherman, and H. L. Casey. The 1962 epidemic of St. Louis encephalitis in Florida. III. A survey for inapparent infections in an epidemic area. *Am J Epidemiol* 81:415-427, 1965.

Spence, L. P. St. Louis encephalitis in tropical America. *In*: Monath, T. P. (Ed.), *St. Louis Encephalitis*. Washington, D.C., American Public Health Association, 1980.

Trent, D. W., J. A. Grant, A. V. Vorndam, and T. P. Monath. Genetic heterogenicity among St. Louis encephalitis virus isolates of different geographic origin. *Virology* 114:319-332, 1981.

SINDBIS FEVER

(066.3)

Etiology: RNA genome virus, genus *Alphavirus* (group A of arboviruses), family Togaviridae; it is antigenically related to the virus of western equine encephalitis.

Geographic Distribution: The Sindbis virus (SIN) has been isolated in several countries in Africa (Egypt, Nigeria, Central African Republic, Senegal, Cameroon, Uganda, Mozambique, and South Africa), in Asia (Israel, India, the Philippines, Malaysia, Borneo), and in Australia, Czechoslovakia, and the USSR.

Occurrence: The infection manifests itself clinically only in man. Just over 30 clinical cases are known. Seroepidemiologic studies done in the Nile Delta region of Egypt and in Sudan show that the rate of clinically inapparent infections is high in endemic areas. Human cases occur in summer, when the vector mosquitoes are abundant. Antibodies have been found in wild birds, bovines, ovines, and equines.

The Disease in Man: In 1961, the first human cases were recognized in Uganda. The symptomatology consisted of fever, cephalalgia, and articular pain; in two out of five patients mild jaundice was observed. In South Africa, where manifestations of the disease have been more severe, a maculopapular eruption on the trunk and extremities, with a tendency to form vesicles especially on the feet and palms of the hands, has also been observed. Some patients experience periocular pain, nausea and vomiting, sore throat, asthenia, and lymphadenopathies. The acute disease disappears rapidly, but arthralgia may persist for several weeks. A case described in Australia included hemorrhagic manifestations, had several recrudescences, and lasted 4 months (Guard *et al.*, 1982).
  The SIN virus is one of the alphaviruses that cause arthritis. The others are Mayaro, Chikungunya, O'nyong-nyong, and Ross River (epidemic polyarthritis) (Tesh, 1982).

The Disease in Animals: The infection is subclinical in domestic animals, and viremia has not been confirmed. Infection in wild birds, the natural reservoir of the virus, may be asymptomatic. Experimentally inoculated chicks have high-titer viremia, and some die.

Source of Infection and Mode of Transmission: The SIN virus has been isolated from several species of wild birds and in some countries antibodies have been found within the populations of those birds. The facts indicate that the basic cycle of infection occurs between birds and ornithophilic mosquitoes. The most probable vectors, and those mosquitoes from which the virus has been isolated repeatedly, are *Culex univittatus* in Africa and *C. annulirostris* in Australia. SIN virus has also been isolated from other mosquitoes, especially culicines, such as *C. pseudovishnui* in Borneo.
  Man is only an accidental host.

Diagnosis: The virus is isolated with some difficulty from viremic patients during the first 3 days of disease by inoculation into suckling mice. Another diagnostic method consists of confirming serologic conversion in patients by using the hemagglutination inhibition test.

Control: Measures are based on individual protection against mosquito bites.

Bibliography

Casals, J., and D. H. Clarke. Arboviruses: group B. *In*: Horsfall, F. L., and I. Tamm (Eds.), *Viral and Rickettsial Infections of Man*, 4th ed. Philadelphia, Lippincott, 1965.

Centers for Disease Control of the USA. *International Catalogue of Arboviruses,* 2nd ed. (Ed. by T. O. Berge). Atlanta, Georgia, 1975 (DHEW Publ. CDC 75-8301.).

Guard, R. W., M. J. McAuliffe, N. D. Stallman, and B. A. Bramston. Haemorrhagic manifestations with Sindbis infection. Case report. *Pathology* 14:89-90, 1982.

McIntosh, B. M., and J. H. S. Gear. Mosquito-borne arboviruses, primarily in the eastern hemisphere. *In*: Hubbert, W. T., W. F. McCulloch, and P. R. Schnurrenberger (Eds.), *Diseases Transmitted from Animals to Man*, 6th ed. Springfield, Illinois, Thomas, 1975.

Tesh, R. B. Arthritides caused by mosquito-borne viruses. *Annu Rev Med* 33:31-40, 1982.

SLOW VIRUSES (DEGENERATIVE ENCEPHALOPATHIES) AND RETROVIRUSES OF MAN AND ANIMALS

(046)   Slow virus infection
(279.8) Retrovirus infection

From the points of view of comparative pathology, etiology, and epidemiology, the study of subacute spongiform encephalopathies caused by "slow viruses" is of great interest. This group of diseases of man and animals is characterized by the absence of inflammatory lesions, similar histopathology of the central nervous system, similar etiologic agents (not yet well characterized), and an unusually prolonged incubation period. The first disease recognized, the best studied, and the model for the other diseases in the group is lumbar prurigo of sheep and goats, better known as "scrapie." The study of scrapie has served as a basis for better knowledge of two similar human diseases, kuru and Creutzfeldt-Jakob disease (CJD), as well as transmissible mink encephalopathy and chronic wasting disease of mule deer, Odocoileus hemionus.

Both natural and experimental disease in animals can serve as models for human disease, but it has also been suggested that the closely related agents of all these diseases are really strains of the same virus modified by adaptation to different hosts (Gajdusek, 1977). This thesis is based on the fact that when the agent of scrapie is passaged through nonhuman primates, its host spectrum alters and it no longer causes disease in the original hosts, sheep and goats.

Etiology: The agents of this group of diseases have been called slow or unconventional viruses. They are distinguished from the conventional viruses in that 1) they have long incubation periods, extending for months or years both in natural and experimental hosts; 2) they cause degeneration in the nerve cells of the central nervous system without producing inflammation or specific antibodies; 3) they are impossible to detect by electron microscopy; and 4) they can only be detected by inoculation into animals in which they cause the degenerative nerve disease (Marsh, 1983). The agents are characterized by their resistance to heat, formalin, ultraviolet rays, ionizing radiation, and pH changes (Eklund and Hadlow, 1981). These peculiarities and indirect measurements led to the theory that these agents had a nonviral structure such as viroids (infectious agents of some plants) or prions (infective proteinaceous particles). However, more recent studies have indicated that resistance to inactivators is limited to a small subpopulation, while most of these agents are very sensitive to them. The researcher (Rohwer, 1984) maintains that the scrapie agent is similar to a small virus and that its unusual resistance to inactivators is due to the protection provided by cerebral tissue. The recent purification of the infective proteinaceous particle (prion) allowed identification of a protease-resistant protein (Pr P 27-30) as a major component of the prion and the production of an antiserum that reacts with that protein, which has structural and histochemical characteristics of an amyloid. The antiserum produced in rabbits not only reacts with this scrapie protein but also with the Creutzfeldt-Jakob disease protein, demonstrating that prions of the two diseases share antigenic determinants (Bendheim et al., 1984).

SLOW VIRUS DISEASES OF ANIMALS

1. Scrapie

Synonyms: Lumbar prurigo, enzootic ovine paraplegia.

Geographic Distribution: The disease has been diagnosed in Iceland, Great Britain (England, Scotland), Germany, France, Canada, and the USA. With the importation of British sheep, it was also introduced into Kenya, South Africa, and Australia, but prompt diagnosis and the sacrifice of affected animals eradicated the infection (Eklund and Hadlow, 1981). The disease was also diagnosed in a sheep in Rio Grande do Sul, Brazil (Fernándes et al., 1978). Overall distribution of the disease is not yet completely known.

In the United States, the infection occurs primarily in Suffolk sheep, due perhaps to a genetic predisposition of the breed, to the viral strain (biotype introduced from Great Britain), or to control measures which have prevented the extension of infection to other breeds. In certain Suffolk lines, up to 50% of sheep can be affected.

Observations in the United States show that death due to scrapie occurs in sheep 30 to 50 months old (Eklund and Hadlow, 1981). In other affected countries, most flocks are either free from infection or the incidence is insignificant; however, on some premises the disease constitutes an important economic problem since it kills 10 to 15% of the infected sheep (Stamp, 1980).

The Disease in Sheep and Goats: Scrapie is mainly a disease of sheep, but on occasion it can affect goats who share a common pasture. The incubation period is very long, estimated at 1 to 4 years for natural infection. The disease is of insidious onset. The affected individuals are more excitable and present slight tremors of the head and neck, which gave rise to the French name "maladie tremblante." The most obvious symptom and usually the first to be observed is the intense pruritus that attacks affected animals. Pruritis starts in the lumbar region ("lumbar prurigo") and can extend to other parts. The intense itching forces the animal to rub against wire fences or other objects and to bite its sides and extremities. The loss of wool can extend to large areas. In advanced stages the animal becomes emaciated. Motor disorders and incoordination are frequent. The disease can last from several weeks to several months and generally ends in death.

Necropsy uncovers no macroscopic lesions other than skin abrasions caused by the intense pruritus. Histopathology reveals a spongiform encephalopathy, hypertrophy of astrocytes, and degeneration and vacuolation of neurons. The most pronounced lesions are found in the cerebellar cortex, medulla oblongata, bridge of Varolius, mesencephalon, diencephalon, and corpus striatum, while the cerebral cortex is rarely affected (Eklund and Hadlow, 1981).

Source of Infection and Mode of Transmission: There is clear genetic predisposition in sheep which, to some degree, controls their susceptibility to disease. Experimental genetic selection has produced lines of high and low susceptibility to the scrapie agent and has demonstrated that response to the infection is controlled by one gene, with the allele that confers susceptibility being dominant (Kimberlin, 1981). Additionally, the scrapie agent was found not to be uniform, and differences in virulence and pathogenicity among different strains or subpopulations could determine the disease course and perhaps even the potential for its establishment in certain breeds or genetic lines.

Of special interest is confirmation that the scrapie agent multiplies slowly in lymphoreticular tissue during the long incubation period before invading the central nervous system. Moreover, the agent is first detectable in the intestinal tract before progressing to regional lymph nodes, spleen, and the central nervous system (Hadlow *et al.*, 1982), indicating that sheep could be infected orally. Animals in cohabitation with infected sheep or living in an infected environment have contracted the disease. Experimentally, sheep can be infected orally, by scarification, and by the conjunctival route. The agent is found in many tissues and in large numbers in the fetal membranes. Consequently, it is very probable that sheep can contract infection in contaminated pastures, since the agent, or part of its population, is highly resistant to environmental factors. On infected farms in Iceland that were kept without animals for 1 to 3 years and then repopulated with sheep from farms free of disease, the sheep acquired the infection in following years, which indicates that the agent can survive for a long time in the environment (Kimberlin, 1981). Transmission from mother to offspring also takes place, but it is not known whether it occurs pre- or postnatally.

Diagnosis: Diagnosis is based mainly on histopathology of the central nervous system and, if necessary, animal inoculation. The infection can be reproduced in mice (with a minimum incubation period of 100 days) or hamsters (with an incubation period of 50 days). Up to now, antibodies cannot be detected against the agent and, therefore, no serologic tests are available for diagnosis (Stamp, 1980; Marsh, 1983). More recent work (Bendheim *et al.*, 1984) suggests that some immunoassay techniques will be available in the future, both for scrapie and other diseases in the group.

Control: Areas free of infection should prohibit importation from endemic areas. Australia was able to free itself of scrapie by early diagnosis and sacrifice of imported animals, their progeny, and contacts. In endemic areas, the infection and its propagation can be reduced by sacrifice of animals on affected farms. Eradication is difficult to achieve due to the resistance of the agent to environmental factors.

2. Transmissible Mink Encephalopathy

This is a rare disease that occurs in establishments that feed sheep organs and tissues to mink. Only 14 outbreaks of the disease are known, some causing a high mortality rate among adults. Mink can be infected experimentally (via the oral route), but the incubation period is much longer than that estimated for natural infection. The infection can also be transmitted, as has been demonstrated experimentally, by one mink biting another, especially when being fed (Kimberlin, 1981).

This disease is of interest because it demonstrates that infection by the scrapie agent or a similar one can occur in carnivores and that the species-specificity barrier is not strict. It is probable that, on crossing that barrier, natural selection creates a subpopulation of the agent which can multiply in the new host.

It has also been suggested, but not confirmed, that man acquires Creutzfeldt-Jakob disease by ingestion of ovine tissue infected with the scrapie agent.

The agent of mink encephalopathy can be transmitted to hamsters and nonhuman primates (Marsh, 1983).

3. Chronic Wasting Disease of Deer

In recent years a communicable spongiform encephalopathy has been confirmed among 53 *Odocoileus hemionus hemionus* and one *O. hemionus colombianus* mule deer kept in captivity in Colorado and Wyoming, USA (Williams and Young, 1980). Clinical signs observed in adult deer consisted of behavioral changes, progressive weight loss, and death in 2 weeks to 8 months. Histopathologic lesions of the central nervous system were identical to scrapie. The infection can be transmitted experimentally to ferrets and spider monkeys. Natural disease has also been recognized in the wapiti, *Cervus canadensis* (Marsh, 1983).

HUMAN SLOW VIRUS DISEASES

1. Kuru

Geographic Distribution and Occurrence: The disease is limited to Papua New Guinea; 80% of the cases occurred in the Fore linguistic group in the eastern highlands of the island. From 1957 (when the disease was first confirmed) to 1975, more than 2,500 deaths attributable to kuru occurred. The incidence of disease began to decline when the traditional ritual of honoring dead relatives by consuming their bodies was prohibited. Currently, kuru is disappearing (Gajdusek, 1977). Kuru affected all age groups, and was more common among women than adult males. The disease disappeared first in children and adolescents.

Clinical Manifestations: Kuru begins insidiously. The disease is characterized by cerebellar ataxia and tremors, progressing to complete motor incapacity and death within a year. Speech difficulty is very common and progressive. No fever or convulsions are observed.

The incubation period is very long, a minimum of 4 to a maximum of 30 years (American Public Health Association, 1985).

Histopathologic lesions of kuru are similar to those of other diseases in the group, consisting of spongiform alterations of the gray matter, loss of neurons, and astrocytosis (Eklund and Hadlow, 1981).

Source of Infection and Mode of Transmission: The source of infection was tissue from corpses, especially the central nervous system tissues, which were consumed during mourning rituals. Proof of this mode of transmission is that since cannibalism ceased, the disease has declined and practically disappeared. The much higher incidence among women and children is explained by the fact that the women officiated during the ritual and distributed the brain, containing a million infective doses of the agent per gram, to the children. Men and initiated young males rarely participated in the burial rituals and even less in the preparation and cooking of meat from the dead. The portal of entry was possibly the skin, conjunctiva, or oral mucosa (Gajdusek, 1977).

The epidemiology of kuru is similar to that of transmissible mink encephalopathy in that the infection is transmitted by ingestion of or contact with infected tissue.

Kuru may have originated from a case of Creutzfeldt-Jakob disease (which has a worldwide distribution) and then spread in a chain of transmission produced by the special cultural habits of the Fore group in Papua.

Diagnosis: Diagnosis is based on discovery of the typical clinical symptomatology in the affected population and on histopathologic examination of central nervous system tissue.

The agent is transmissible to many primate species and also to mice.

2. Creutzfeldt-Jakob Disease

Geographic Distribution and Occurrence: A rare disease of worldwide distribution. Creutzfeldt-Jakob disease (CJD) is always fatal; the mean annual mortality rate is under 1 per million, with a variation of 0.1 to 30 cases per million annually in different populations (American Public Health Association, 1985). In the USA, the estimated incidence is 200 cases per year. In a study carried out in Israel among inhabitants of various origins, a much higher incidence (31.3 per million) was confirmed among Jews from Libya, followed by those from Iraq, than in those from other countries. Among the different Jewish communities in the United States a similar pattern of incidence has been observed (Kahana *et al.*, 1974).

A family history of the disease is present in 10 to 15% of the cases, but whether this is due to transmission from the mother or horizontally from others in the family, or to genetic factors, is not known (Kimberlin, 1981).

Clinical Manifestations: The disease generally appears in patients between 40 and 65 years old. The incubation period is unknown in the majority of cases. In a case linked to corneal transplantation, the disease started 18 months later, and in another case it appeared 27 to 30 months after the application of intracerebral electrodes. The disease is of insidious onset and is characterized by rapidly progressing dementia. Early myoclonic spasms appear, and extrapyramidal signs, cerebellar ataxia, and visual and behavioral disorders are also frequent. The electroencephalogram is abnormal soon after onset of the disease. On the average, CJD lasts about 7 months, but it can continue up to 4 years; it is invariably fatal (American Public Health Association, 1985; Johnson, 1982). Histopathology of the central nervous system is similar to other diseases in the group.

Source of Infection and Mode of Transmission: Except in some cases of iatrogenic transmission, as by transplant of a cornea from a person dead of CJD or the application of insufficiently sterilized intracerebral electrodes, the mode of transmission has not been determined.

It has been suggested that consumption of brains and other tissue from sheep or goats infected with scrapie could give rise to human CJD cases, much as mink acquire infection from these animals. In this regard, the greater incidence of the disease among Libyan and North African Jews who customarily consume the brains and eyes of sheep and goats is cited (Gajdusek, 1977). However, data about the occurrence of scrapie in small ruminants in Libya or other North African countries are not available. Another argument against this hypothesis is that the incidences of CJD are similar in Great Britain (where scrapie is enzootic), Australia (where scrapie does not occur), and Japan (where sheep are scarce and infection is nonexistent in these animals). It is more probable that man is a reservoir for the agent of CJD; although transmission of the agent or agents from another animal species is possible, as demonstrated in the case of mink, experimental adaptation of the agent to a new species is a slow process which requires several passages. Consequently, man is probably more easily infected by an agent adapted to humans than one adapted to other animals (Marsh, 1983). Notwithstanding, concern persists that man could occasionally acquire CJD by consumption of organs or tissue infected by the agent of scrapie, as inferred from experimental oral transmission to squirrel monkeys (*Saimiri sciureus*) by means of infected brain, kidney, and spleen (Gibbs *et al.*, 1980).

Diagnosis: It is based on clinical signs and histopathologic examination of the central nervous system.

RETROVIRUSES

Retroviruses are RNA viruses characterized by the presence and peculiar action of the enzyme reverse-transcriptase (RTC). Through the action of RTC, retroviruses utilize viral RNA as a template for making DNA, which then integrates itself into the chromosomes of the host cell and there serves as the basis for viral replication through the production of further viral RNA (Gallo, 1986); they owe their name to this process.

The retroviruses should be discussed, even if briefly, in a treatise on the zoonoses for a number of reasons. For example, there are suggestions that the feline leukemia virus (FeLV) may infect human cells under experimental conditions (Olsen, 1981), although there is no evidence of natural pathogenicity to humans. Definitive proof exists that the human immunodeficiency virus (HIV)[1] may be experimentally transmitted to the chimpanzee (Saltzman, 1986), and the same virus may have originated from the green monkeys in Africa (Gallo, 1986; Gallo, 1987). The latter two conclusions would make acquired immunodeficiency syndrome (AIDS) of humans (HAIDS) an authentic zoonoses, even by the most orthodox definitions.

---

[1]The virus associated with human acquired immunodeficiency syndrome (HAIDS) has been recently renamed, in a necessary but fiat action, as HIV. Chronologically, however, it had been named in a pathologically descriptive manner as lymphadenopathy virus (LAV); in a biologically descriptive way as human T-lymphocyte virus type three (HTLV-III); and in a clinically descriptive way as AIDS-related virus (ARV). See Table 6.

The most important aspects of the retroviruses *vis-à-vis* the zoonoses have arisen from the widespread concern with this emergent human disease. The inclusion of a discussion of the retroviruses in this book on the zoonoses relates more to a philosophical expansion of the definition of zoonoses (Schwabe, 1984) to include the diseases *shared* by man and animals. Such a definition is the basis of comparative medicine, and no better justification for this approach exists than the subject of HAIDS, since the manifestion of AIDS in several species presents us with the best possible approach for the study of the human disease. The presently recognized animal models for HAIDS are the simian AIDS model (SAIDS) (Arthur *et al.*, 1986; Saltzman, 1986), and the feline AIDS model (FAIDS) (Hardy and Essex, 1986; Saltzman, 1986). (See Table 6.)

Table 6. Different animal retrovirus models of acquired immunodeficiency syndrome.

Species	Acronym	Retroviruses
Human	HAIDS	HIV
		LAV
		HTLV-III
		ARV
Primate (Simian)	SAIDS	SIV
		SAIDS-D
Cat (Feline)	FAIDS	FeLV
		FTLV

The first model (SAIDS) has been intensively studied from the outset of the interest in HAIDS for obvious reasons. But even the second (FAIDS) has also been a highly regarded model, not only because of the historical similarities between the viruses which, through extrapolation from the more studied FeLV, contributed to the recent discovery of HIV (Gallo, 1986), but because of the outstanding similarities between the diseases. These two aspects were recognized in the call for grant proposals on the biology of FeLV by the National Institute of Allergy and Infectious Diseases (NIAID), National Institutes of Health (NIH), in 1986.

The utilization of animal models of HAIDS based on the retroviruses of animal origin has been recently recognized in a meeting and publication, again sponsored by NIH (Saltzman, 1986). This publication expanded the concept from the SAIDS and FAIDS models, which were also thoroughly reviewed, to other retroviruses, particularly the "slow" disease-producing viruses (lentiviruses). Such an expanded concept has also been recently endorsed by the call for research proposals on the pathogenicity and immunology of animal lentivirus, again by NIAID, NIH, in 1987. The lentiviruses studied from this point of view are the caprine arthritis-encephalitis virus, the Visna/Maedi viruses of sheep, and the virus of equine infectious anemia (EIA).

The comparison of the animal retroviruses with HAIDS provides an interesting illustration of the reciprocal flow of knowledge in research. For example, in the study of FAIDS with respect to HAIDS, advances in knowledge about the latter stimulated questions with respect to the former; it has been recently documented that in the case of HAIDS there is a definitive involvement of the brain, particularly in infants and children (Gallo, 1987). In FAIDS, however, there was a conspicuous hiatus in this respect, since even the most comprehensive treatises (Olsen, 1981) did not consider the brain as a possible target organ. The difference was important since the involvement of the central nervous system could have dramatic importance in explaining AIDS in both species. It was also an interesting difference in that the brain is known to share antigenic determinants with the T-lymphocytes (thy). Inoculation of FeLV into the brain of kittens gave rise to an accelerated early fatal disease syndrome (EFDS) indistinguishable from FeLV-FAIDS and with the appearance of FeLV immunoreactivity in the brain (Torres-Anjel, 1987). This finding could become even more important with the recent discovery of a non-FeLV T-lymphotropic FAIDS-producing lentivirus (FLTV) in felines (Pedersen, 1987), bringing HAIDS and the FAIDS model even closer together, and the topic of the retroviruses even more in line with the concept of the zoonoses.

In summary, the subject of the human immunodeficiencies associated with retroviruses, like many other study areas, has benefited enormously from and will continue to depend heavily on animal studies, in order to reach the goals of full treatment, understanding, prevention, management, and successful immunization.

Bibliography

American Public Health Association. *Control of Communicable Diseases in Man*, 14th ed. (Ed. by A. S. Benenson). Washington, D.C., APHA, 1985.

Arthur, L. O., R. V. Gilden, P. A. Marx, and M. B. Gardner. Simian acquired immunodeficiency syndrome. *In*: E. Klein (Ed.), *Acquired Immunodeficiency Syndrome, Progress in Allergy*, vol. 37, pp. 332-352. Basel-New York, Karger, 1986.

Bendheim, P. E., R. A. Barry, S. J. De Armond, D. P. Stites, and S. B. Prusiner. Antibodies to a scrapie prion protein. *Nature* 310:418-421, 1984.

Carp, R. I., P. A. Merz, R. J. Kascsak, G. S. Merz, and H. M. Wisniewski. Nature of scrapie agent: current status of tests and hypotheses. *J Gen Virol* 66:1357, 1985.

Davanipour, Z., M. Alter, E. Sobel, D. M. Asher, and D. C. Gajdusek. A case-control study of Creutzfeldt-Jakob disease: dietary risk factors. *Am J Epidemiol* 122:443-451, 1985.

Dawson, M. Pathogenesis of maedi-visna. *Vet Rec* 120:451-454, 1987.

Eklund, C. M., and W. J. Hadlow. Characteristics of the slow viral diseases. *In*: Beran, G. W. (Section Ed.), *CRC Handbook Series in Zoonoses*, Section B, vol. 2. Boca Raton, Florida, CRC Press, 1981.

Fernándes, R. E., C. M. Real, and J. C. T. Fernándes. "Scrapie" em ovinos no Rio Grande do Sul (Relato de um caso). *Arq Fac UFRGS (Porto Alegre)* 6:139-143, 1978.

Gajdusek, D. C. Unconventional viruses and the origin and disappearance of kuru. *Science* 197:943-960, 1977.

Gallo, R. C. The first human retrovirus. *Scientific American* 255(6):88-98, 1986.

Gallo, R. C. The AIDS virus. *Scientific American* 256(1):46-56, 1987.

Gibbs, Jr., C. J., H. L. Amyx, A. Bacote, C. L. Masters, and D. C. Gajdusek. Oral transmission of kuru, Creutzfeldt-Jakob disease, and scrapie to nonhuman primates. *J Infect Dis* 142:205-208, 1980.

Hadlow, W. J., R. C. Kennedy, and R. E. Race. Natural infection of Suffolk sheep with scrapie virus. *J Infect Dis* 146:657-664, 1982.

Hardy, W. D., Jr., and M. Essex. FeLV-induced feline acquired immune deficiency syndrome. A model for human AIDS. *In*: E. Klein (Ed.), *Acquired Immunodeficiency Syndrome, Progress in Allergy*, vol. 37, pp. 353-376. Basel-New York, Karger, 1986.

Johnson, R. T. Slow infections of the nervous system. *In*: Wyngaarden, J. B., and L. H. Smith (Eds.), *Cecil Textbook of Medicine*, 16th ed., vol. 2. Philadelphia, Saunders, 1982.

Kahana, E., M. Alter, J. Braham, and D. Sofer. Creutzfeldt-Jakob disease: focus among Libyan Jews in Israel. *Science* 183:90-91, 1974.

Kimberlin, R. H. Scrapie as a model slow virus disease: problems, progress and diagnosis. *In*: Kurstak, E., and C. Kurstak (Eds.), *Comparative Diagnosis of Viral Diseases*, vol. 3. New York, Academic Press, 1981.

Manuelidis, L., and E. E. Manuelidis. Recent developments in scrapie and Creutzfeldt-Jakob disease. *Prog Med Virol* 33:78-81, 1986.

Marsh, R. F. Animal models of unconventional slow virus infections. *ILAR News* 26:19-22, 1983.

Olsen, R. *Feline Leukemia*. Boca Raton, Florida, CRC Press, 1981.

Pedersen, N. C., M. W. Ho, M. L. Brown, and J. K. Yamamoto. Isolation of a T-lymphotropic virus from domestic cats with an immunodeficiency-like syndrome. *Science* 235:790-793, 1987.

Prusiner, S. B., and M. P. McKinley (Eds.). *Prions: Novel Infectious Pathogens Causing Scrapie and Creutzfeldt-Jakob Disease*. Orlando, Florida, Academic Press, 1987.

Rohwer, R. G. Scrapie infectious agent is virus-like in size and susceptibility to inactivation. *Nature* 308:658-662, 1984.

Saltzman, L. A. *Animal Models of Retrovirus Infection and Their Relationship to AIDS*. New York, Academic Press, 1986.

Schwabe, C. W. *Veterinary Medicine and Human Health*, 3rd ed. Baltimore, Williams and Wilkins, 1984.

Seale, J. R. Pathogenesis and transmission of AIDS. *Vet Rec* 120:454-459, 1987.

Stamp, J. T. Slow virus infections of the nervous system of sheep. *Vet Rec* 107:529-530, 1980.

Torres-Anjel, M. J. Accelerated wasting syndrome induced by intracerebral inoculation of feline leukemia virus (FLV) in infant felines. *American Society of Microbiology, Annual Meeting, Abstracts* 87:(T27), 1987.

Williams, E. S., and S. Young. Chronic wasting disease of captive mule deer: a spongiform encephalopathy. *J Wildl Dis* 16:89-98, 1980.

SMALLPOX OF NONHUMAN PRIMATES

(051.9)

In 1980, the 33rd World Health Assembly declared human smallpox to be eradicated worldwide. The eradication campaign, through massive vaccination and epidemiological surveillance, was started by the World Health Organization in 1958 and intensified in 1967. The result was unprecedented success, with no human smallpox cases having occurred since October 1977 (except two cases due to accidental exposure in a British laboratory in 1978).

The Global Commission for Certification of Smallpox Eradication, whose work preceded the declaration of the World Health Assembly, formulated several recom-

mendations for the posteradication period, among them, permanent surveillance of presumed smallpox cases, especially those contracted from nonhuman primates in western and central Africa. The possible existence of an animal reservoir of human smallpox virus has been a constant concern for the World Health Organization and researchers in this field, since it obviously would have been an insurmountable obstacle in the eradication campaign. However, up to now such a reservoir has not been found; instead, animal poxviruses that can be transmitted to man are known. These viruses, with a low potential for interhuman transmission, require continued surveillance and research.

Nonhuman primate viruses, which are occasionally transmitted to man, are considered here. Infection of monkeys in their natural habitat by these viruses has been confirmed in the African jungles only.

Prior to 1958, when monkeypox virus was identified, a disease similar to human smallpox had been described in seven outbreaks in monkeys which had occurred both in the natural habitat (India, Brazil, Trinidad, Panama) and zoos. In four of these outbreaks the disease was attributed to human smallpox, but the virus was isolated in only one outbreak, and in that case its exact identification was not possible due to the loss of the strain.

Although monkeys can be infected experimentally with human smallpox and can transmit the virus, the infection has not been demonstrated to exist naturally in these animals. Moreover, countries with large monkey populations have remained free of variola with the eradication measures they had taken.

1. Monkeypox

Etiology: Monkeypox virus forms part of the genus *Orthopoxvirus* with human smallpox (variola), vaccinia, and cowpox viruses, among others. There is a close antigenic relationship between this virus and the variola and vaccinia viruses, and the neutralization and hemagglutination inhibition tests produce cross-reactions. Each virus has type-specific antigens that can be detected by several techniques. Antibodies for these viruses can be differentiated by cross adsorption with heterologous antigens; specific antibodies are detected by the immunodiffusion and immunofluorescence techniques. For that purpose, radioimmunoassay is a simpler process; after only one adsorption with crude antigenic preparations it allows direct measurement of the relative concentration of residual antibodies for each virus (Hutchinson *et al.*, 1977). More recently, the ELISA test has been perfected (Marennikova *et al.*, 1981). Monkeypox virus causes hemorrhagic lesions on rabbit skin, while variola virus does not infect it (Tripathy *et al.*, 1981). Differentiation between monkeypox and variola infection is essential in posteradication epidemiologic surveillance, as the diseases are clinically identical.

Geographic Distribution (Map 5): The virus occurs naturally only in western and central Africa.

Occurrence in Man: Between 1970 (when the first human case of monkeypox was discovered in Zaire) and 1984, 165 cases were recorded in seven African countries, of which 148 occurred in Zaire (Table 7). Observations in this region showed that the majority of patients were children and only seven were older than 15. Of 179 persons who had not been vaccinated with smallpox vaccine and who were in close contact with the primary cases, only six became sick; this means a secondary attack rate of less than 4%, much lower than is produced by variola (25 to

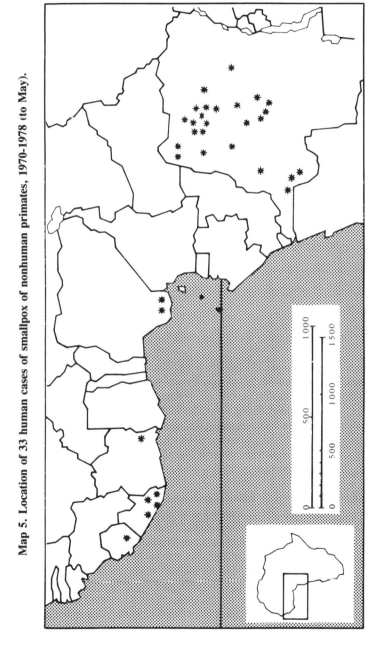

Map 5. Location of 33 human cases of smallpox of nonhuman primates, 1970-1978 (to May).

Source: Breeman and Arita (WHO). *Third Symposium on Microbiology.* Munich, 1978.

40%). Eight of 63 hospitalized patients died, signifying a fatality rate close to 13%, comparable to that from human smallpox in the same region. Only five of the patients had been vaccinated (Arita and Gromyko, 1982).

Table 7. Number of human cases of orthopoxviroses (smallpox of nonhuman primates) reported in western and central Africa, by country and year, 1970-1984.

Country	Number of cases															
	1970	71	72	73	74	75	76	77	78	79	80	81	82	83	84[a]	Total
Cameroon										2						2
Central African Republic															5	5
Ivory Coast		1										1				2
Liberia	4															4
Nigeria		2							1							3
Sierra Leone	1															1
Zaire	1		5	3	1	3	5	6	12	7	3	6	37	56	3	148
Total	6	3	5	3	1	3	5	6	13	9	3	7	37	56	8	165

[a] January and February only.

Source: Bull WHO 63(2):256, 1985.

Occurrence in Monkeys: Since the virus was recognized in 1958, only 10 outbreaks have been reported in captive monkeys in research centers or zoos in Europe and the USA. It should be noted that there were no cases among personnel who had been in contact with these animals. In a serologic study carried out using 2,242 serum samples from African and Asian monkeys, no reactors with significant titers were found. From this study it has been inferred that the infection is not very widespread in the natural environment and perhaps is localized in small areas (Arita *et al.*, 1972). Serologic investigations in western and central Africa confirmed the presence of neutralizing antibodies in seven nonhuman primates and three other mammals out of 372 specimens examined (Foster *et al.*, 1972). Following a case that occurred in a 5-year-old child in Ivory Coast, a serologic study was done on 115 specimens from 10 rodent and six other mammalian species. Neutralizing antibodies were found in seven of the 10 rodent species and in two groups of birds examined (Breman *et al.*, 1977). Later, in the area of western Africa where human cases had occurred, 195 primate specimens were examined; 8% were positive with high titers to the hemagglutination inhibition test (sera had been pretreated to reduce non-specific reactions), and 21% to the neutralization test (Breman *et al.*, 1977). These results indicated that nonhuman primates and other animals such as the African giant squirrel, porcupines, and pangolins had been infected by a virus of the genus *Orthopoxvirus,* but not necessarily the monkeypox virus. In Asia, where no human cases of monkeypox have occurred, no neutralizing antibodies were found in nonhuman primates.

The Disease in Man: The signs and symptoms are similar to human smallpox. The incubation period lasts 7 to 15 days. In the 2-to-3-day prodromal period, the patient suffers extreme fatigue, fever, and muscular and back pains. The eruption appears at approximately the same time on the face and body. Evolution of maculas to papules, vesicles, pustules, and scabs takes about 10 days, and desquamation can last about 3 weeks. Lesions are more abundant on the extremities.

The Disease in Monkeys: In captive monkeys, lesions have been observed to consist of multiple and discrete papules that vary from 1 to 4 mm in diameter. Lesions are abundant on the palms of the hands, but also can be found on the whole trunk and tail. The content of the papules is very thick and similar to pus. Lesions are frequently umbilicated. Sometimes ulcerative circular lesions appear in the mouth. Histopathologically, the lesions consist of epidermal proliferation followed by necrosis. Likewise, foci of acanthosis are found.

Source of Infection and Mode of Transmission: Human cases caused by the monkeypox virus have occurred only in Africa. It is believed that the reservoir is a species of monkey of that continent, but the possibility remains that other animal species maintain the virus in nature. In the zoo in Rotterdam, Netherlands, an outbreak started following the introduction of two giant anteaters that became ill and transmitted the infection to primates. In the few human cases that have occurred in Africa, the infection was possibly acquired through close contact with monkeys hunted for food. The outbreaks in Asian monkeys in research centers could have originated from cohabitation with African monkeys.

The potential for infection by monkeypox virus is low for man; secondary cases have been scarce. Smallpox vaccination protects against monkeypox virus infection. It is possible that the number of human monkeypox cases will increase with the cessation of smallpox vaccination, but the world will remain smallpox-free (American Public Health Association, 1985).

Diagnosis: Virus can be isolated from skin lesions, including the scabs. The isolated strain should be sent to a reference laboratory for correct identification. Confirmation of an increase in titers with sera taken from the acute and convalescent periods can aid in diagnosis, but special tests (see Etiology) should be used to confirm the existence of specific antibodies against monkeypox virus.

Control: Patients should be isolated and, preferably, persons taking care of them should have been vaccinated. The small number of human cases does not justify any other measures. Preventive measures in animal colonies are the same as for tanapox (see below).

2. Tanapox

Etiology: Unclassified DNA virus, family Poxviridae; the virus has some antigenic relationship to Yabapox.

Occurrence in Man: In 1957 and 1962, two outbreaks were recorded in a tribe living along the Tana River in Kenya, which affected several hundred people in that isolated area. A study carried out in Zaire during 1978-1981 detected more than 163 cases of tanapox (Arita and Gromyko, 1982). In 1966 in the United States, 23 human cases occurred among personnel who worked with monkeys affected by pox at three primate centers.

Occurrence in Monkeys: Outbreaks by this virus occurred in several primate centers in the United States; the attack rate reached 30% in the breeding colony of one institute and affected several species of *Macaca*. Nothing is known of the disease's occurrence in the jungle. A serologic study carried out on 263 monkeys of Asian origin (*Macaca*) revealed a 15% rate of reactors to the neutralization test; in 55 green monkeys (*Cercopithecus aethiops*) of African origin the rate was 76%. The neutralizing titer among green monkeys was high (Hall and McNulty, 1967).

The Disease in Man: The incubation period could not be determined during the epidemic in Kenya. The illness began with a febrile period of 3 or 4 days, sometimes accompanied by pronounced cephalalgia and prostration. The lesions were at first similar to smallpox lesions, but did not evolve into pustules. Papules and umbilicated vesicles formed on the arms, face, neck, and trunk, but not on the hands, legs, or feet; a notable characteristic is that patients had no more than one or two lesions. Histopathologic study of the lesions revealed pronounced hyperplasia of the epithelium of the skin with little damage to underlying dermis. No destructive alterations of epithelium were observed, as in lesions caused by vaccinia or variola viruses. The disease in personnel working with sick monkeys in the United States was similar to that described in the cases in Kenya.

The Disease in Monkeys: The disease observed in monkeys of the genus *Macaca* in United States research centers was characterized by single lesions in some animals and multiple lesions in others (*M. fuscata*). The lesions were located primarily on the face, mainly around the lips and nostrils, but they were also found on other parts of the body. The lesions consisted of an enlarged circle of skin, with umbilication and an adherent scab in the center. There was no vesiculation, pustulation, or hemorrhaging. Vaccination with vaccinia virus did not confer resistance to infection caused by tanapox virus. Morbidity was high, but there were no deaths. Regression of the more severe lesions occurred in 6 to 8 weeks.

Source of Infection and Mode of Transmission: The high prevalence of serologic reactors among African green monkeys without clinical symptomatology seems to indicate that this species is the natural host of the virus. Also, epidemics in man have occurred in jungle areas of Africa. Asian monkeys (*Macaca* spp.) contract the infection by direct or indirect contact with green monkeys in primate centers. Transmission may also occur through aerosols or vectors. Human cases in the laboratory have resulted from contamination of abrasions and skin scratches. In the Kenya epidemics transmission might have occurred mechanically by means of arthropods, since *Mansonia* spp. mosquitoes were very abundant.

Diagnosis: Laboratory confirmation can be obtained by isolation of the virus. The isolated strain should be sent to a reference laboratory for correct identification.

Control: Prevention of pox in research center primates depends on employing proper handling practices. Asian and African monkey species should not be kept in common environments. Likewise, special care should be taken in the use of potentially contaminated gloves and equipment.

If a tanapox virus outbreak occurs in a colony of monkeys, they can be vaccinated with that virus. The vaccinia virus does not protect against tanapox.

Medical attention should be given to wounds and skin abrasions in personnel in charge of the animals.

3. Yabapox

Unclassified virus of the family Poxviridae, antigenically related to tanapox but not to viruses of the genus *Orthopoxvirus*.

Nonhuman primate infection by this virus produces subcutaneous tumors on the extremities and, less frequently, on the face. The disease starts with one tumor which then propagates via the lymphatic system and produces multiple similar lesions. Yabapox affects only mesodermal cells, while tanapox infects epidermal tissue. Spontaneous regression of the lesions is observed (Tripathy *et al.*, 1981). The first outbreak was recognized in 1958 in a colony of *M. mulatta* located in Yaba, Nigeria; it affected 20 of 35 rhesus monkeys and a baboon. In 1969, an outbreak occurred in a colony in the United States. An accidental human case resulted from puncture with a contaminated needle in a laboratory. Four months after the accident a nodule appeared at the puncture site (Bruestle *et al.*, 1981).

4. "Whitepox"

Six strains of "whitepox" virus have been isolated, two from monkey kidney tissue culture in a laboratory in the Netherlands and four from monkey and rodent renal tissue during a study in Zaire. These "whitepox" strains cannot be distinguished from some strains of variola by biologic tests or DNA restriction analysis. The first two strains isolated were found to be the result of contamination by a variola virus from India. Although the remaining four strains are still being studied, there was no epidemiologic evidence of transmission of such viruses to man (Arita and Gromyko, 1982). Because contamination accidents can occur in laboratories where poxviruses are studied, the origin of these four strains, as well as the "monkeypox" mutants obtained by monkeypox cloning, is in doubt, but it is hoped that their true identity will be clarified in the future.

Bibliography

Andrewes, C. H., and J. R. Walton. Viral and bacterial zoonoses. *In*: Brander, G. C. (Ed.), *Animal and Human Health*. London, Baillière Tindall, 1977.

Arita, I., R. Grispen, S. S. Kalter, *et al.* Outbreaks of monkeypox and serological surveys in non-human primates. *Bull WHO* 46:625-631, 1972.

Arita, J., and D. A. Henderson. Smallpox and monkeypox in non-human primates. *Bull WHO* 39:277-283, 1968.

Arita, I., and A. Gromyko. Surveillance of orthopoxvirus infections, and associated research, in the period after smallpox eradication. *Bull WHO* 60:367-375, 1982.

Arita, I., Z. Jezek, L. Khodakevich, and K. Ruti. Human monkeypox: a newly emerged orthopoxvirus zoonosis in the tropical rain forests of Africa. *Am J Trop Med Hyg* 34:781-789, 1985.

American Public Health Association. *Control of Communicable Diseases in Man*, 14th ed. (Ed. by A. S. Benenson). Washington, D.C., APHA, 1985.

Breman, J. G., J. Bernadou, and J. H. Nakano. Poxvirus in West African nonhuman primates: serological survey results. *Bull WHO* 55:605-612, 1977.

Breman, J. G., J. H. Nakano, E. Coffi, H. Godfrey, and G. Gauton. Human poxvirus disease after smallpox eradication. *Am J Trop Med Hyg* 26:273-281, 1977.

Bruestle, M. E., J. G. Golden, A. Hall III, and A. R. Banknieder. Naturally occurring Yaba tumor in a baboon. *Lab Anim Sci* 31:286-294, 1981.

Committee on Orthopoxvirus Infections. The current status of human monkeypox: Memorandum from a WHO Meeting. *Bull WHO* 62:703-713, 1984.

Downie, A. W., and C. España. Comparison of Tanapox virus and Yabalike viruses causing epidemic disease in monkeys. *J Hyg (Camb)* 70:23-32, 1972.

Downie, A. W., C. H. Taylor-Robinson, A. E. Caunt, *et al.* Tanapox: a new disease caused by a poxvirus. *Br Med J* 1:363-368, 1971.

Foster, S. O., E. W. Brink, D. L. Hutchins, J. M. Pifer, B. Lourie, C. R. Moser, E. C. Cummings, O. E. K. Kuteyi, R. E. A. Eke, J. B. Titus, E. A. Smith, J. W. Hicks, and W. H. Foege. Human monkeypox. *Bull WHO* 46:569-576, 1972.

Hall, A. S., and W. P. McNulty. A contagious pox disease in monkeys. *J Am Vet Med Assoc* 151:833-838, 1967.

Hutchinson, H. D., D. W. Ziegler, D. E. Wells, and J. H. Nakano. Differentiation of variola, monkeypox, and vaccinia antisera by radioimmunoassay. *Bull WHO* 55:613-623, 1977.

Jezek, Z., S. S. Marennikova, M. Mutumbo, J. H. Nakano, K. M. Paluko, and M. Szczeniowski. Human monkeypox: a study of 2,510 contacts of 214 patients. *J Infect Dis* 154:551-555, 1986.

Jezek, Z., I. Arita, M. Szczeniowski, K. M. Paluku, K. Ruti, and J. H. Nakano. Human tanapox in Zaire: clinical and epidemiological observations on cases confirmed by laboratory studies. *Bull WHO* 63:1027-1035, 1985.

Marennikova, S. S., E. M. Seluhina, N. N. Malceva *et al.* Isolation and properties of the causal agent of a new variola-like disease. *Bull WHO* 46:599-611, 1972.

Marennikova, S. S., N. N. Malceva, and N. A. Habahpaseva. ELISA—a simple test for detecting and differentiating antibodies to closely related orthopoxviruses. *Bull WHO* 59:365-369, 1981.

Munz, E. Afrikanische virusbedingte Zoonosen. *Munch Med Wochenschr* 115:1-9, 1973.

Tripathy, D. N., L. E. Hanson, and R. A. Crandell. Poxviruses of veterinary importance: diagnosis of infections. *In*: Kurstak, E., and C. Kurstak (Eds.), *Comparative Diagnosis of Viral Diseases*. New York, Academic Press, 1981.

Tsuchiya, Y., and J. Tagaya. Sero-epidemiological survey on Yaba and 1,211 virus infections among several species of monkeys. *J Hyg (Camb)* 69:445-451, 1971.

World Health Organization. Smallpox: post-eradication surveillance. First isolation of monkeypox virus from a wild animal infected in nature. *Wkly Epidemiol Rec* 60:393-394, 1985.

SWINE VESICULAR DISEASE

(079.2)

Etiology: RNA virus, genus *Enterovirus,* family Picornaviridae.

It has been suggested that this virus be classified as serotype 9 of the porcine enterovirus. More recent investigations indicate that, considering its serologic and biochemical properties, classification as a porcine strain of Coxsackie B5 virus[1] would be more appropriate (Knowles *et al.*, 1979).

---

[1] Coxsackie B is a biological subgroup of the genus *Enterovirus* that comprises six immunotypes of human enteroviruses.

The extraordinary resistance of the SVD virus to environmental factors is very important from the epidemiological point of view. In slaughterhouse drains the agent persists for 4 to 6 weeks at 18 to 22°C; in the presence of organic matter it resists desiccation, as well as fermentation and smoking of pork products. In dry sausage the virus can survive 400 days, and in treated tripe up to 780 days (Loxam and Hedger, 1983).

Geographic Distribution and Occurrence: Swine vesicular disease (SVD) was recognized for the first time in 1966 in Lombardy, Italy, where outbreaks occurred on two farms. A second episode was recorded in Hong Kong 5 years later, in 1971. From the second half of 1972 onwards, outbreaks of the disease were confirmed in the following 13 countries, which are important in international commerce: Great Britain, Belgium, the Netherlands, the Federal Republic of Germany, Poland, Austria, Switzerland, France, Italy, Malta, Greece, Hong Kong, and Japan. Only three of these countries reported disease foci in 1980 and 1981 (Great Britain, with 60 and 12 outbreaks, respectively; Italy, 29 and 5; and Germany, 1 and 1) (Loxam and Hedger, 1983).

In the winter of 1972-1973 the disease occurred among staff working with the SVD virus at the Animal Virus Research Institute in Pirbright, England. Immunodiffusion tests on serum from a patient convalescing from aseptic meningitis provided indirect evidence that the causal agent was the SVD virus. So far, no human cases contracted in the field are known.

This disease aroused much interest because of its clinical similarity to foot-and-mouth disease in swine and its spread throughout several European and Asian countries.

The Disease in Man: The disease in the laboratory staff was similar to that caused by Coxsackie B5 virus. There were no cases with vesicular eruption. In view of the fact that Coxsackie B5 antiserum neutralizes SVD virus and that SVD antiserum has the same effect on Coxsackie B5 virus, it had to be determined which virus caused the cases. It was found by means of immunodiffusion that, in addition to common antigens, each virus has a specific antigen. Using serum from a member of the laboratory staff convalescing from aseptic meningitis, the presence of antibodies for the specific antigen of SVD was demonstrated by immunodiffusion. Later, the two viruses were differentiated by means of the neutralization test. Inoculation of swine with the human Coxsackie virus did not cause SVD.

The Disease in Animals: SVD is primarily a disease of swine. No clinical symptomatology has been observed in any other species of domestic animal in contact with sick pigs. The incubation period in swine lasts some 3 to 7 days. The symptomatology of the disease is very similar to that of other vesicular diseases of swine, among them foot-and-mouth disease. In some herds the infection spreads rapidly and the morbidity is very high, while in other herds the disease spreads slowly and is accompanied by low morbidity. The first clinical manifestation is fever, which can reach 41°C and disappears in 2 or 3 days. The vesicles are seen primarily on the lateral part of the coronet and, upon rupturing, leave an eroded area with granulation tissue and loose epithelium at the edges. Vesicles are not commonly found in the interdigital space, but one or more supernumerary digits may be affected a few hours before lesions are observed on the main hoofs. A prominent symptom of SVD is limping, which is seen primarily when the animal has to move over hard ground. The limping ceases when the vesicles rupture. Separation of the hoof from adjacent tissue frequently occurs and always starts along the coronet; however, the hoofs rarely fall off completely as happens with foot-and-mouth disease. Between 5 and 10% of the pigs develop vesicles on the snout, in the mouth, and sometimes on the nipples. Nervous symptomatology has also been noted in some outbreaks in Europe.

The clinical picture varies greatly. The most serious symptomatology appears in suckling pigs, but even they recover rather quickly and suffer insignificant mortality (Loxam and Hedger, 1983).

During an outbreak, some animals in a herd will not exhibit clinical symptoms but will have antibodies for the SVD virus. Subclinical infection is attributed to exposure of the animals to small doses of the agent.

Source of Infection and Mode of Transmission: Swine are the only natural hosts of the virus. Other domestic species do not become infected under natural conditions. Replication of the virus has been observed in sheep living in prolonged proximity to sick swine, and the agent has been isolated from their pharynx; it is very doubtful, however, that this species can contract the infection under natural conditions or play any role in transmission of the virus.

The major source of the virus is the vesicles which, because they are located primarily on the feet, contaminate the soil when they rupture.

Most primary foci have originated as a result of ingestion of or contact with raw wastes; secondary foci have resulted from movement of animals, contact with infected animals at auctions, use of contaminated vehicles, and consumption of uncooked kitchen wastes. The SVD virus can enter the body of swine by several routes. Experimental studies have shown that abraded skin is the tissue most susceptible to infection. A smaller amount of the virus was required to infect an animal by this route than via the mouth, nose, or conjunctiva. The dermal route is probably the most frequent when a focus begins. In such a case, one or two pigs might become infected by exposure to relatively small amounts of the virus contained in raw wastes or contaminated objects. Infection probably occurs through the most sensitive route, that is, damaged skin, especially the commonly injured coronet area of the foot (Mann and Hutchings, 1980). The virus is eliminated in large quantities in the secretions and excretions of the infected pig. The first 2 weeks constitute the most infective period, and other swine can easily become infected by contact. This cycle would end quickly when there were no longer susceptible animals, were the virus not able to survive for a long time outside an animal (see Etiology), survive in pork and its by-products, and resist pH changes caused by rigor mortis (Mann, 1981). Raw wastes and the movement of animals are the most frequent means for the spread of the disease from one establishment or one country to another.

The few known human cases have resulted from handling the virus or from contact with sick animals during laboratory studies. The risk for man is apparently insignificant, since veterinarians who work in the control of the disease have so far shown neither clinical signs nor antibodies.

Because of its similarity to the Coxsackie B5 "human" virus, it has been speculated the SVD virus could have originated by a mutation of that virus in an infection transmitted from man to swine.

Diagnosis: Differential diagnosis is important between swine vesicular disease and the other vesicular diseases, such as foot-and-mouth disease, vesicular stomatitis, and swine vesicular exanthema. The differential diagnosis can only be done by means of laboratory tests. The virus can be isolated in tissue culture or by inoculation into laboratory animals. In monolayers of primary swine kidney cells or in the 1B-RS-2 continuous line of swine kidney cells, a cytopathic effect is obtained in 1 to 3 days. This cytopathic effect is not seen in BHK 21 cultures or in calf kidney cultures, in contrast to the activity of foot-and-mouth disease and vesicular stomatitis viruses. The SVD virus can also be isolated in suckling mice. A rapid diagnosis can be made by means of the complement fixation test, using vesicle epithelium as an antigen and a hyperimmune serum obtained from guinea pigs with purified virus in an oil adjuvant. The recommended serologic tests for diagnosis and seroepidemiologic studies are counterimmunoelectrophoresis, ELISA, and double gel immunodiffusion. The neutralization test is used mainly to corroborate the results of the previous tests.

Control: Swine vesicular disease has not been verified in the Americas, Africa, Australia, and a large part of Asia, and it should be treated as an exotic disease to prevent its introduction. In case of accidental introduction, all sick and exposed animals should be destroyed immediately.

Bibliography

Brown, F., P. Talbot, and R. Burrows. Antigenic difference between isolates of swine vesicular disease virus and their relationship to Coxsackie B5 virus. *Nature* 245:315-316, 1973.

Brown, F., D. Goodridge, and R. Burrows. Infection of man by swine vesicular virus. *J Comp Pathol* 86:409-414, 1976.

De Simone, F., G. F. Panina, and E. Lodetti. Diagnosi sierologica della malattia vescicolare dei suini da enterovirus. *Vet Ital* 25:218-228, 1974.

Dhennine, L., and L. Dhennine. La maladie vesiculeuse du porc. *Bull Acad Vet Fr* 46:47-51, 1973. Summary *Vet Bull* 43(10):4470, 1973.

Graves, J. H. Serological relationship of swine vesicular disease virus and Coxsackie B5 virus. *Nature* 245:314-315, 1973.

Knowles, N. J., L. S. Buckley, and H. G. Pereira. The classification of porcine enteroviruses by antigenic analysis and cytopathic effects in tissue culture: description of three new serotypes. *Arch Virol* 62:201-208, 1979.

Loxam, J. G., and R. S. Hedger. Enfermedad vesicular del cerdo: síntomas, diagnóstico, epidemiología y control. *Rev Sci Tech Off Int Epizoot* 2:41-55, 1983.

Mann, J. A. Swine vesicular disease. *In*: Gibbs, E. P. J. (Ed.), *Virus Diseases of Food Animals*, vol. 2. New York, Academic Press, 1981.

Mann, J. A., and G. H. Hutchings. Swine vesicular disease: pathways of infection. *J Hyg (Camb)* 84:355-363, 1980.

Mowat, G. M., J. H. Darbyshire, and J. F. Huntley. Differentiation of a vesicular disease of pigs in Hong Kong from foot-and-mouth disease. *Vet Rec* 90:618-621, 1972.

Nardelli, L. Malattia vescicolare dei suini (da enterovirus). *Sel Vet* 14:105-113, 1973.

Nobuto, K. The first case of swine vesicular disease in Japan. *Bull Off Int Epizoot* 82:561-566, 1974.

Pohlenz, J., D. M. Williams, and H. Keller. Die Vesikularkranheit des Schweines bei ihrem Auftreten in der Schweiz. *Schweiz Arch Tierheilkd* 116:413-422, 1974. Summary *Vet Bull* 45(2):670, 1975.

Saurat, P., and J. P. Ganiere. La maladie vesiculeuse des suides. *Rev Med Vet* 126:1487-1506, 1975.

S.V.D. Fewer outbreaks. *Vet Rec* 97:42, 1975.

Swine vesicular disease. *Vet Rec* 92:234-235, 1973.

Swine vesicular disease and Coxsackie infection. *Nature* 245:285, 1973.

VACCINIA VIRUS INFECTION

(—)

This is an infection of the past, since smallpox has been officially eradicated throughout the world and smallpox vaccine is no longer administered.

Synonyms: Vaccinia, poxvirus officinalis.

Etiology: Vaccinia virus is a DNA virus belonging to the genus *Orthopoxvirus*, family Poxviridae. This genus includes, among others, the smallpox, cowpox, monkeypox, whitepox, and ectromelia viruses. The history and origin of laboratory strains of the vaccinia virus are not well known. The properties and characteristics of most of the strains seem to indicate that this virus is derived from cowpox virus.

The strains of vaccinia virus that are used to produce smallpox vaccine in different laboratories vary in their virulence for animals and man.

The vaccinia virus is being used as the principal recombinant vector for experiments in immunization against rabies (Blancou *et al.*, 1986), hepatitis B, vesicular stomatitis, and other viruses. It shows great promise for new utilizations and effectiveness in widespread and innovative immunization programs (Quinnan, 1985).

Geographic Distribution: Smallpox vaccine was used universally in the control and the later eradication of smallpox. The potential of transmission of vaccinia virus to cattle and from them to man existed everywhere.

Occurrence in Man and Cattle: It is very difficult to determine the frequency with which outbreaks occurred because data for the viruses of vaccinia, cowpox, and even milker's nodule (pseudocowpox) are not well differentiated. The confusion was due primarily to the similarity in the clinical symptomatology of the infection caused by the vaccinia and cowpox viruses in both man and cows.

The human vaccinia virus infection contracted from cows was almost exclusively a disease of milkers. Outbreaks of the disease have been described in several Latin American countries.

The Disease in Man: The disease occurred only in milkers who had not been vaccinated against smallpox. The incubation period was from 2 to 7 days. The lesion or lesions appeared mainly on the fingers and hands, although sometimes they were found on other parts of the body. The lesion started as a papule that turned into a vesicle and then a pustule, with characteristic umbilication. The patient experienced itching and sometimes pain. After a few days, the lesion dried and was covered by a scab that fell off after 10 to 14 days. In general, the lesions were not very numerous, but if the patient suffered from eczema the disease could involve large areas of skin. Some cases included fever and malaise, which required the patient to stop working for a or more day.

The Disease in Cattle: The lesions were similar to those found in man and were localized on the teats and the skin of the udder. Milking ulcerated the skin and retarded the healing process. The most common complication was mastitis.

Source of Infection and Mode of Transmission: The source of infection for cattle was persons who had been recently vaccinated against smallpox. By scratching the vaccination lesion and then milking an animal, the milker inoculated the virus into the animal with his fingers and fingernails. The infection was passed from one cow to another during the milking process, and other milkers could contract the disease from cows with lesions.

Diagnosis: The vaccinia virus can be isolated, and then identified, in various primary cell cultures and in continuous tissue culture lines, as well as in the chorioallantoic membrane of embryonated eggs. In addition to cattle, guinea pigs and hamsters are very susceptible to the virus. Smallpox virus cannot be propagated in series in cattle or rabbits, and, besides man, only monkeys are susceptible. The appearance and histology of the focal lesions in the chorioallantoic membrane and on rabbit skin help distinguish infections caused by the vaccinia virus from those caused by cowpox virus (see also "Cowpox").

Control: With the cessation of smallpox vaccination, the possibility of infection by vaccinia virus disappeared.

Bibliography

Bruner, D. W., and J. H. Gillespie. *Hagan's Infectious Diseases of Domestic Animals*, 6th ed. Ithaca, New York, Cornell University Press, 1973.

Dekking, F. Cowpox and vaccinia. *In*: Van der Hoeden, J. (Ed.), *Zoonoses*. Amsterdam, Elsevier, 1964.

Downie, A. W. Poxvirus group. *In*: Horsfall, F. L., and I. Tamm (Eds.), *Viral and Rickettsial Infections of Man*, 4th ed. Philadelphia, Lippincott, 1965.

Lum, G. S., F. Soriano, A. Trejos, and J. Llerena. Vaccinia epidemic and epizootic in El Salvador. *Am J Trop Med Hyg* 16:332-338, 1967.

Quinnan, G. V. (Ed.). *Vaccinia Viruses as Vectors for Vaccine Antigens*. New York, Elsevier, 1985.

VENEZUELAN EQUINE ENCEPHALITIS

(066.2)

Synonyms: Venezuelan equine encephalomyelitis, Venezuelan encephalitis.

Etiology: RNA virus, belonging to the genus *Alphavirus* (formerly group A of the arboviruses) of the family Togaviridae. Recognition of the existence of different antigenic variants is very important epidemiologically. A study (Young and Johnson, 1969) using the kinetic hemagglutination inhibition test on a large number of strains from different regions made it possible to classify the viruses that make up this complex into four subtypes (I to IV), subtype I having five antigenic variants (including the new variant I-F).

The most important distinction from the epidemiologic standpoint is between epizootic (or epidemic) and enzootic variants. The AB and C variants of subtype I (I-AB and I-C) are highly virulent for equines and are responsible for epizoodemics (epizootics-epidemics). The D, E, and F variants of subtype I (I-D, I-E, I-F) and the subtypes II (Everglades), III (Mucambo), and IV (Pixuna) are enzootic strains, not pathogenic to equines. In subtype III, two variants (III-A Mucambo and III-B Tonate virus) have been recently recognized. More variants and subtypes possibly exist (Walton, 1981), as was demonstrated recently in southern Brazil when an enzootic variant of subtype I was isolated from a *Culex* spp. mosquito and from a bat; classification of this variant as I-F has been proposed (Calisher *et al.*, 1982).

Geographic Distribution (Table 8): Venezuelan equine encephalitis (VEE) virus is native to the Americas, and its presence has not been confirmed outside this hemisphere. In tropical and subtropical America several natural foci of VEE are known, where enzootic antigenic variants of the virus circulate between lower vertebrates and mosquitoes. The recognized enzootic foci are located in Belém, Brazil (Mucambo and Pixuna viruses); Paramaribo, Suriname; Magangué, Colombia; Almirante, Panama; Veracruz, Mexico; Bush Bush, Trinidad and Tobago; southern Florida, USA; and also in Guatemala, Honduras, and Belize. Recently, circulation of the virus (I-D) in the Peruvian Amazon as well as in the western United States (Tonate virus, Bijou Bridge strain) has been confirmed, and it is likely that other as yet unrecognized natural foci exist in different tropical and subtropical regions of the Americas. Numerous isolations of the VEE complex virus have been obtained from *Culex delpontei* in the provinces of Chaco and Corrientes, Argentina, pointing to the existence of enzootic foci in that country (Sirivanakarn and Jakob, 1981). Other recently discovered enzootic foci exist in the south of Brazil with I-F virus (Calisher *et al.*, 1982) and the Venezuelan Guajira with I-D virus (Walder *et al.*, 1984).

Epizoodemics have occurred from the area south of Ica, Peru, to Texas, USA (see Occurrence).

Occurrence in Man and Animals: Since the VEE virus was isolated in 1938, many outbreaks and epizoodemics have occurred in the Americas. Twelve countries have been affected by VEE epizoodemics (from south to north): Peru, Ecuador, Colombia, Venezuela, Trinidad and Tobago, Costa Rica, Nicaragua, Honduras, El Salvador, Guatemala, Mexico, and the United States. Between 1935 and 1961 the

Table 8. Geographic distribution of eastern equine encephalitis (EEE), western equine encephalitis (WEE), and Venezuelan equine encephalitis (VEE) and the dates of the most recent known outbreaks in the countries of the Americas, 1969-1978.

Country	EEE Countries with epidemic outbreaks in the last 10 years	EEE Year of last known outbreak	WEE Countries with epidemic outbreaks in the last 10 years	WEE Year of last known outbreak	VEE Countries with epidemic outbreaks in the last 10 years	VEE Year of last known outbreak
Argentina	X	1972	X	1972		—
Barbados	—			—		—
Bolivia	X	1975		—		—
Brazil	(X)	—		—		—
Canada	X	1972	X	1977		—
Chile		—		—		—
Colombia		—		—	X	1973
Costa Rica	(X)	—		—	X	1971
Cuba	X	1972		—		—
Ecuador		—		—	X	1972
El Salvador		—		—	X	1969
Guatemala		—		—	X	1969
Guyana	X	1977	X	1977	X	1977
Haiti		—	X	1974		—
Honduras		—		—	X	1978
Jamaica	(X)	(1962)		—		—
Mexico		—		—	X	1972
Nicaragua		—		—	X	1970
Panama	X	1973		—	(X)	—
Paraguay		—		—		—
Peru		—		—		—
Suriname		—		—		—
United States of America	X	1978	X	1978	X	1971
Uruguay		—	X	1973/1974		—
Venezuela	X	1976		—	X	1973

Note: (X) refers to outbreaks in the 1960s.
Source: Bull Pan Am Health Organ 14(4):361, 1980

outbreaks were limited to Colombia, Venezuela, Trinidad and Tobago, and Peru (especially the first two countries). From 1962 to 1972 outbreaks of VEE occurred every year, and they spread to Central America, Mexico, and the United States. The greatest epizoodemic wave began in 1969 and was caused by subtype I-AB. It extended from Ecuador to Guatemala and then to the other Central American countries and Mexico, finally reaching Texas, USA, in June 1971. In just two years, the epizoodemic covered 4,000 km and caused tens of thousands of human cases of the disease as well as considerable morbidity and mortality in equines.

VEE epidemics are very often explosive, as was the outbreak of 1962, which began in the Colombian portion of La Guajira. Between October and December of that year this outbreak resulted in 3,000 human cases with 20 deaths in Colombia, and 6,762 cases with 43 deaths occurred in just 2 months in Venezuela. The 1969 epizoodemic, which seems to have started in Ecuador, caused about 31,000 human cases with 310 deaths in that country. In general, the epidemics are characterized by a high attack rate that may exceed 10% of the human population in the affected region. There was a lack of epidemic activity from 1972 until 1977, when small outbreaks, possibly due to the VEE virus, occurred in horses in Guyana, northern Peru, and the peninsula of La Guajira in Venezuela (Monath, 1979).

Epizootics in equines begin before epidemics, and the epidemics usually end when animal cases cease. The economic impact is very serious. Equine mortality in affected areas can be 20 to 40%. The proportion of sick horses that die varies from 38 to 83%. It has been estimated that in the epizoodemic that began in 1969, between 38,000 and 50,000 horses died. During that epizootic, Ecuador lost about 20,000 horses, valued at US$1,200,000. In addition, equine mortality affects the rural economy, since many rural people use these animals for farming and for transporting produce.

The Disease in Man: The incubation period is from 2 to 5 days. The symptomatology may vary from undifferentiated fever similar to that of influenza to serious encephalitis. In most cases, it is characterized by a rapid onset of fever accompanied by malaise, chills, myalgia, cephalalgia, and, frequently, nausea, vomiting, and diarrhea. Pronounced leukopenia is often observed in samples taken soon after the fever begins. The disease course lasts 1 to 4 days or more, and convalescence takes a greater or lesser period of time depending on the duration of the fever. Patients with fever of short duration recuperate fully and rapidly. Those with prolonged illness experience marked asthenia, and convalescence lasts several weeks.

The symptoms of encephalitis are more common in children than in adults. In one outbreak in Colombia, the incidence of encephalitis was estimated at 4% of the infections in children and 0.4% of the adult cases. The various peripheral neurologic symptoms of flaccid or spastic paralysis and alterations in reflexes are similar to the neurologic symptoms of other arboviral encephalitides. Meningitis rarely occurs. The fatality rate is low, estimated at 0.2 to 1% of the clinical cases. The rate of subclinical infections is high, based on postepidemic serologic studies.

The enzootic subtypes and variants of the virus sometimes cause sporadic cases of undifferentiated fever and meningitis.

The Disease in Animals: The VEE virus of the epizootic type (variants AB and C of subtype I) has been isolated from 21 different species of domestic and wild vertebrates, and serologic studies demonstrate that many other species contract the infection naturally. Nevertheless, the infection is clinically apparent and economically important only in equines, and not in other animal species. The incubation period is from 1 to 3 days. The symptomatology of the disease in the Equidae (horses, mules, asses) varies with the degree of severity. In some animals the infection manifests itself as a benign febrile disease, with pyrexia for 1 or 2 days, anorexia, and depression. These symptoms are accompanied by mild leukopenia and low-titer viremia or none at all. Neutralizing antibodies appear in 4 to 6 days. The animals recuperate without further sequelae. Other animals develop the characteristic course of the disease, which is encephalomyelitis. The disease begins suddenly with high fever, deep depression, pronounced anorexia and weight loss, grinding of the teeth, diarrhea, or constipation. There is a high-titer viremia and commonly leukopenia. The encephalitic symptoms are similar to those of western and eastern equine encephalitis (WEE and EEE). Some sick horses experience profound stupor, have difficulty maintaining balance and must support the head on some object, are unwilling to move, and often fall and are unable to get up. Other animals manifest signs of excitation and are hypersensitive to touch and sound; they may also be aggressive, walk in circles, bump into obstacles, and experience increasingly frequent convulsions. The fatality rate among equines that develop encephalitic symptoms is very high, sometimes reaching 80% of the cases.

Source of Infection and Mode of Transmission (Figures 51 and 52): The natural foci of the enzootic infection are found in the rain forests of tropical America, usually in swampy areas. The infection cycle develops between rodents and mosquitoes. The main reservoirs are rodents of the genera *Sigmodon*, *Proechimys*, *Peromyscus*, and *Oryzomys* and also marsupials. Several species of *Culex* (*Melanoconion*) mosquitoes, especially *C. aikenii*, *C. opisthopus*, and *C. portesi,* serve as vectors to transmit the infection from viremic to susceptible animals. The infection in rodents is asymptomatic, but the viremia is sufficiently high to infect the

Figure 51. Venezuelan equine encephalitis. Epizoodemic cycle.

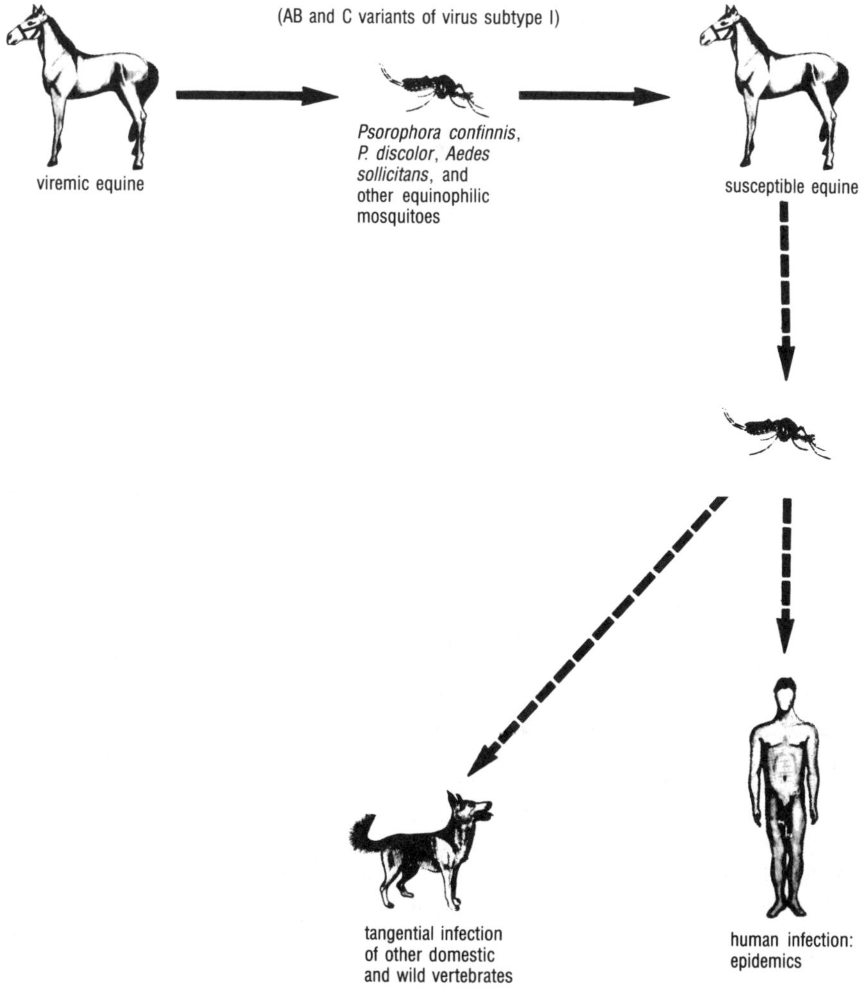

(AB and C variants of virus subtype I)

viremic equine

Psorophora confinnis, P. discolor, Aedes sollicitans, and other equinophilic mosquitoes

susceptible equine

tangential infection of other domestic and wild vertebrates

human infection: epidemics

Figure 52. Venezuelan equine encephalitis. Enzootic wildlife cycle.

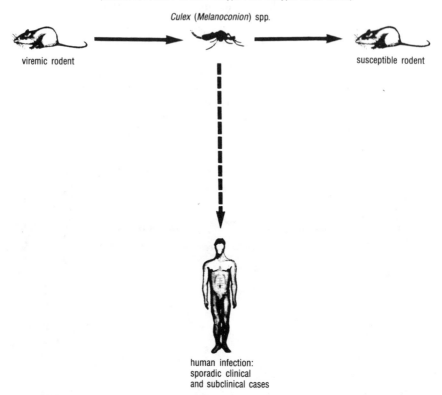

(variants D, E, and F of virus subtype I and subtypes II, III, and IV)

Culex (*Melanoconion*) spp.

viremic rodent

susceptible rodent

human infection:
sporadic clinical
and subclinical cases

vectors. Birds are the reservoir for the cycle of the Tonate variant (III-B). Seasonal variations exist in viral activity, which is more pronounced in the rainy season. Nevertheless, activity is continuous; in the dry season there is still a low level of transmission between rodents and mosquitoes, especially more slowly developing *Culex* (*Melanoconion*) species *C. portesi* and *C. cedecei*, thus allowing the cycle to be maintained. Man is infected by the enzootic viruses upon entering their natural foci. Cases are sporadic and the enzootic viruses (variants D and E of subtype I and subtypes II, III, and IV) have never given rise to large epidemics or epizootics; only occasionally have they broken out from their natural foci and invaded adjacent areas to produce small outbreaks in susceptible human populations. Communities in the endemic areas have high rates of seropositivity and immunity to these viruses, as shown by studies on Indian reservations in southern Florida, USA. The main reason for the nonepidemic behavior of these virus strains is their lack of pathogenicity for equines. Experimental inoculation of horses with nonepidemic viruses (enzootic viruses) produces fever and mild leukopenia, moderate antibody titers, and low-titer viremia insufficient to infect the vector mosquitoes. In contrast, horses inoculated with epizootic strains develop high-level viremia accompanied by disease symptoms and high antibody titers. The high-level viremia in a horse infected with an epidemic strain (variants AB and C of subtype I) is sufficient for a single animal to infect several thousand mosquitoes in 1 day. These titers sometimes persist for 4 or 5 days in the infected horse. Thus, equines play an essential role in the propagation of epizootics and epidemics, for without them as amplifiers of the virus, epizoodemics could not occur.

The epidemic virus has been isolated numerous times from 34 species of mosquitoes belonging to eight different genera. One or more species of mosquitoes can predominate as transmitters of the infection in an area. A high rate of infection has been found in some species of mosquitoes, which could explain the explosive character of VEE. Laboratory and field tests have proven certain mosquito species, such as *Psorophora confinnis*, *Aedes aegypti*, *A. sollicitans*, *Mansonia tittilans*, *M. indubitans*, *Culex tarsalis*, and *A. taeniorhynchus*, to be very efficient vectors (Monath and Trent, 1981). The relationship between the mosquito and the host is of indisputable importance, especially given the mosquito's habit of feeding on epizootic hosts, the Equidae. The viremia in horses is of such magnitude that it also permits mechanical transmission of the virus by biting flies such as *Culicoides* and *Simulium*. The virus has been isolated from these insects, and they played an important role in the epidemic of 1967 in Colombia (Sanmartín *et al.*, 1973).

In summary, the epizootic viruses depend on equines as primary hosts, and circulation of the virus is accomplished by means of equinophilic mosquitoes that transmit the infection from a viremic to another susceptible equine, as well as to man and other vertebrates.

The origin of the epidemic virus and its maintenance during interepizootic periods are not known. One possibility is low-level transmission of the virus from one equine to another. The virus would propagate slowly until a large susceptible equine population existed and conditions for an epizootic were created. In contrast to epizootics of western and eastern equine encephalitis, which begin and end suddenly within a few months, VEE epizootics progress more slowly and may continue to spread for several years, as occurred in the most recent epizoodemic. In Venezuela during the period 1953-1961, between 7 and 60 sporadic equine cases of VEE occurred annually. These facts suggest that the virus can perpetuate itself in interepizootic periods by passing from one equine to another by means of vectors. The possibility that the epidemic virus originates by mutation from the enzootic virus in the jungle foci of VEE is being investigated, but so far has not been proven. Recently, very sensitive techniques have been introduced (absorption chromatography) to detect minuscule amounts of epidemic virions within isolated strains in enzootic foci. Sentinel guinea pigs are also being used for that purpose, as they are very sensitive to the epizootic virus (Monath, 1979). According to findings so far, there does not seem to be a relationship between the enzootic viruses found in the natural foci of the Americas and the epizootic viruses that cause epizoodemics. On that continent, there are areas with jungle enzootic foci where outbreaks of VEE in equines have never been observed. The two cycles would seem to be independent of each other, and the cycle involving epizootic viruses could be maintained continuously by low-level transmission during the dry season between equines and either surviving epizootic vectors or drought-resistant species of mosquitoes that feed on equines. Nevertheless, other mechanisms for the origin and maintenance of the epidemic virus during the interepizootic periods are possible, and it is hoped that research now in progress will resolve this much-debated topic.

Epizootics occur more frequently in arid or semiarid regions or in areas with moderate seasonal rainfall. Epizoodemics always begin with an initial outbreak in equines followed in a few weeks by epidemics. Transmission of the disease to man occurs by means of mosquitoes, but many cases resulting from fly bites or acquired in the laboratory by inhalation of the virus are also known.

Role of Animals in the Epidemiology of the Disease: The main reservoirs for the enzootic viruses responsible for the wildlife cycle are rodents and, for some strains such as the III-B subtype, birds. The virus circulates between these animals and vector mosquitoes (*Culex* spp.), with infection generally limited to the natural focus. Human cases with clinical symptomatology occur sporadically or in small outbreaks and only when man enters natural niches. The cycle for epizootic viruses is maintained between equines and various species of equinophilic mosquitoes. Infection of other vertebrates, including man, plays a secondary role in the life cycle of the virus.

Diagnosis: In man, specific diagnosis is based on isolation of the virus and on serologic tests. The virus can be easily isolated from the blood and from the nasopharyngeal exudate of patients during the initial phase of the infection. Serologic diagnosis is based on the use of the complement fixation (CF), hemagglutination inhibition, or neutralization test, by establishing the difference between titers in serum samples obtained during the acute phase of the disease and convalescence. The neutralizing and hemagglutination-inhibiting antibodies appear during the first week of the disease and complement-fixing antibodies during the second week.

Diagnosis in equines is based on the same procedures, but it must be borne in mind that in animals with clinical symptoms the viremia may already have disappeared. Similar difficulty may be experienced in attempting to isolate the virus from the brain of animals that die following a lengthy illness. For this reason, blood samples for virus isolation or serology should be taken from asymptomatic animals in contact with sick animals or from animals in the early febrile period.

Control: In geographic areas exposed to the risk of epizoodemics, the most practical and effective control method on a national level is the systematic vaccination of equines. This measure makes it possible to eliminate from the epizoodemic cycle the main source (susceptible equines) of the virus for mosquitoes. Epizootics, with accompanying economic losses and subsequent epidemics with high human morbidity, are thus prevented.

At the present time an attenuated live vaccine is available (TC-83), and it has given very satisfactory results in equine immunization. The vaccine is prepared from an epizootic strain of VEE isolated in Trinidad in 1943 from the brain of a burro. It is attenuated by passages in guinea pig fetal heart cells, with passage 83 being utilized in the product. The vaccine was originally developed for human immunization. Over 6,000 persons received the vaccine, 90% of whom developed antibodies after 2 weeks and maintained them for prolonged periods. In a high proportion (about 25%) of individuals, however, severe systemic reactions, such as fever, myalgia, and leukopenia, were observed.

During recent years, over 15 million equines have been vaccinated with TC-83 vaccine. Experience has shown that when vaccinations are carried out during the course of an epizootic, equine mortality from the disease ceases 8 to 10 days after vaccinations begin. Since death rarely occurs before the fifth or sixth day after infection in equines, it is thought that the vaccine confers immunity in only 3 to 4 days. In all cases in which the vaccine was administered correctly, the seroconversion rate approached 100%, with antibodies persisting for at least 2 years. Systemic reactions were rare, with the exception of transitory fever.

A few immunization failures have been recorded, due to exposure of the vaccine to high tropical temperatures or to interference phenomena from preexisting antibodies for WEE or EEE produced either by earlier vaccinations against these diseases or by previous natural infection. Preexisting antibodies for WEE and EEE interfere with the replication of the attenuated virus of the TC-83 vaccine and, consequently, interfere with immune response. TC-83 vaccine should not be used in areas where the disease does not occur. The viremia produced by the vaccine is of a low level, and generally insufficient to infect mosquitoes. Nevertheless, in Louisiana, USA, a VEE virus with biological characteristics of the TC-83 strain was isolated from one of 928 pools of *P. confinnis* mosquitoes captured 12 days after vaccination of the horses in the area. The establishment of a horse-mosquito-horse cycle is a remote possibility because mosquitoes rarely become infected with the vaccinal strain. However, caution is recommended, mostly because the TC-83 virus could conceivably revert to a more virulent state. Passage of the TC-83 virus in suckling mouse brain results in increased virulence of the strain. It is assumed that such a phenomenon could occur in nature under suitable ecologic conditions if a mosquito-rodent-mosquito cycle developed, and that the progressively increasing virus virulence in such a cycle could give rise to epizootics.

Because of the limitations of the present attenuated vaccine and the severe systemic reactions that it often causes in man, an inactivated vaccine has been developed using the same TC-83 strain (Cole *et al.*, 1974). A vaccine made with the attenuated strain in chick embryo cell culture and inactivated by formalin gave very satisfactory results in mice, and a trivalent vaccine (EEE, WEE, and VEE) has been tried on equines with satisfactory results (Barber *et al.*, 1978). This vaccine presents no risk, and previous vaccinations with EEE and WEE vaccines do not interfere with the immune response; however, the duration of the immunity it confers is shorter and annual vaccinations are required. It is recommended that, confronted with a definite epizoodemic, the modified live virus vaccine should be used, as experience has shown it to be extremely valuable in such circumstances. An illustrative example of the effectiveness of this vaccine was the mass vaccination of equines in Texas, which in 1971 held back the advance of the epizoodemic to other regions of the United States.

Of special interest for Latin America, because of the high risk which it implies, is the use of inactivated chick embryo vaccines prepared from virulent strains of VEE. This type of vaccine is very difficult to inactivate and frequently contains residual live virus not detected by usual laboratory methods. The residual virus may multiply in the vaccinated horse and thus be responsible for outbreaks of VEE. Several outbreaks are suspected to have started in this way following the use of such "inactivated" vaccines, and the surprising leap of the infection from Ecuador to Guatemala during the great epizoodemic of 1969 could have had this origin. In addition, the handling of virulent strains of VEE poses a risk for staff in industrial laboratories.

A formalin-activated vaccine made with the attenuated strain TC-83 has been evaluated in 28 human volunteers. Only occasional minor local and systemic reactions have been observed. The vaccine was administered subcutaneously in two doses at a 28-day interval, followed by a third dose 6 months later. In volunteers without previous vaccinations against equine encephalitides, the vaccine produced high neutralizing titers that lasted at least 14 months (Edelman *et al.*, 1979).

In addition to vaccination, another very valuable measure for controlling epizoodemics is prohibition of the transport of horses, thus preventing spread of the infection to other areas. In emergency situations, the vectors can be controlled by aerial ultralow-volume application of insecticides such as malathion. The optimum period for insecticide application is during the peak of adult mosquito emergence, before they have time to feed on horses and before the virus completes its extrinsic incubation period in the vectors. The operation is always costly, and opportune application can prove difficult.

For personal prevention, protective clothing, repellents, and mosquito screens on windows and doors can be used.

Bibliography

Andrewes, C., and H. G. Pereira. *Viruses of Vertebrates*, 3rd ed. Baltimore, Maryland, Williams and Wilkins, 1972.

Barber, T. L., T. E. Walton, and K. J. Lewis. Efficacy of trivalent inactivated encephalomyelitis vaccine in horses. *Am J Vet Res* 39:621-625, 1978.

Bigler, W. J., A. K. Ventura, A. L. Lewis, F. M. Welling, and N. J. Ehrenkrantz. Venezuelan equine encephalomyelitis in Florida: Endemic virus circulation in native rodent population of Everglades hammocks. *Am J Trop Med Hyg* 23:513-521, 1974.

Calisher, C. H., R. M. Kinney, O. de Souza Lopes, D. W. Trent, T. P. Monath, and D. B. Francy. Identification of a new Venezuelan equine encephalitis virus from Brazil. *Am J Trop Med Hyg* 31:1260-1272, 1982.

Calisher, C. H., T. P. Monath, C. J. Mitchell, M. S. Sabattini, C. B. Cropp, J. Kerschner, A. R. Hunt, and J. S. Lazvick. Arbovirus investigations in Argentina, 1977-1980. III. Identification and characterization of virus isolated, including new subtypes of western and Venezuelan equine encephalitis viruses and four new bunyaviruses (Las Mayolas, Resistencia, Barranqueras and Antequera), *Am J Trop Med Hyg* 34:956-965, 1985.

Cole, F. E., Jr., S. W. May, and G. A. Eddy. Inactivated Venezuelan equine encephalomyelitis vaccine prepared from attenuated (TC-83 strain) virus. *Appl Microbiol* 27:150-153, 1974.

Chamberlain, R. W. Arbovirus infections of North America. *In*: Sanders, M., and M. Schaeffer (Eds.), *Viruses Affecting Man and Animals*. St. Louis, Missouri, Green, 1971.

De Diego, A. I., M. E. Grela, and J. G. Barrera-Oro. Anticuerpos contra encefalomielitis equina venezolana en infecciones accidentales humanas en la República Argentina. *Gac Vet (B Aires)* 37:404-418, 1975.

Downs, W. G. Arboviruses. *In*: A. S. Evans (Ed.), *Viral Infections of Humans. Epidemiology and Control*. New York, Plenum, 1976.

Eddy, G. A., F. E. Cole, Jr., C. E. Pedersen, Jr., and R. O. Spretzel. Vacunas atenuadas de arbovirus del grupo A: ventajas e inconvenientes de su uso en equinos. *Conferencia Internacional sobre Vacunas contra las Encefalitis Equinas (Maracay, Venezuela, August 1974)*. Buenos Aires, Pan American Health Organization/Pan American Zoonoses Center, 1974.

Edelman, R., M. S. Ascher, C. N. Oster, H. H. Ramsburg, F. E. Cole, and G. A. Eddy. Evaluation in humans of a new, inactivated vaccine for Venezuelan equine encephalitis virus (C-84). *J Infect Dis* 140:708-715, 1979.

Groot, H. The health and economic impact of Venezuelan equine encephalitis. *In*: *Venezue-*

lan Encephalitis. Washington, D.C., Pan American Health Organization, 1972. (Scientific Publication 243.)

Jahrling, R. W. T. O., and W. F. Scherer. Homogeneity of Venezuelan encephalitis virion populations of hamster-virulent and benign strains, including the attenuated TC-83 vaccine. *Infect Immun* 7:905-910, 1973.

Johnson, K. M. Vacunas vivas para encefalitis equina venezolana (VEE). *In: Conferencia Internacional sobre Vacunas contra las Encefalitis Equinas (Maracay, Venezuela, August 1974).* Buenos Aires, Pan American Health Organization/Pan American Zoonoses Center, 1974.

Kissling, R. E. Epidemic behavior of Venezuelan encephalitis infection. Diseased hosts: Equines. *In: Venezuelan Encephalitis*. Washington, D.C., Pan American Health Organization, 1972. (Scientific Publication 243.)

La Monte, S. de, F. Castro, N. J. Bonilla, A. G. de Urdaneta, and G. M. Hutchins. The systemic pathology of Venezuelan equine encephalitis virus infection in humans. *Am J Trop Med Hyg* 34:194-202, 1985.

Lord, R. D., C. H. Calisher, W. D. Sudia, and T. H. Work. Ecological investigations of vertebrate hosts of Venezuelan equine encephalomyelitis virus in South Florida. *Am J Trop Med Hyg* 22:116-123, 1973.

McKinney, R. W. Inactivated and live VEE vaccine—A review. *In: Venezuelan Encephalitis*. Washington, D. C., Pan American Health Organization, 1972. (Scientific Publication 243.)

Monath, T. P. Arthropod-borne encephalitides in the Americas. *Bull WHO* 57:513-533, 1979.

Monath, T. P., and D. W. Trent. Togaviral diseases of domestic animals. *In*: Kurstak, E., and C. Kurstak (Eds.), *Comparative Diagnosis of Viral Diseases*, vol. 4. New York, Academic Press, 1981.

Pan American Health Organization. *Vigilancia de las encefalitis en las Américas*. Semiannual Report, vol. 1, July-December 1972. Buenos Aires, Pan American Zoonoses Center, 1973.

Pedersen, C. E., Jr., D. M. Robinson, and F. E. Cole, Jr. Isolation of the vaccine strain of Venezuelan equine encephalomyelitis virus from mosquitoes in Louisiana. *Am J Epidemiol* 95:490-496, 1972.

Sanmartín, C. Epidemic behavior of Venezuelan encephalitis infection. Diseased hosts: Man. *In: Venezuelan Encephalitis*. Washington, D.C., Pan American Health Organization, 1972. (Scientific Publication 243.)

Sanmartín, C., R. B. Mackenzie, H. Trapido, P. Barreto, C. H. Mullenax, E. Gutiérrez, and C. Lesmes. Encefalitis equina venezolana en Colombia. *Bol Of Sanit Panam* 74:108-137, 1973.

Scherer, W. F., J. Madalengoitia, W. Flores, and M. Acosta. Ecologic studies of Venezuelan encephalitis virus in Peru during 1970-1971. *Am J Epidemiol* 101:347-355, 1975.

Scherer, W. F., and K. Anderson. Antigenic and biologic characteristics of Venezuelan encephalitis virus strains including a possible new subtype isolated from the Amazon region of Peru in 1971. *Am J Epidemiol* 101:356-361, 1975.

Sirivanakarn, S., and W. L. Jakob. Notes on the distribution of *Culex (Melanoconion)* mosquitoes in northeastern Argentina (Diptera: Culicidae). *Mosquito Systematics* 13: 195-200, 1981.

Spretzel, R. O., and R. W. McKinney. Venezuelan equine encephalomyelitis in Central America and Mexico. *Milit Med* 137:441-445, 1972.

Stanick, D. R., M. E. Wiebe, and W. F. Sherer. Markers of Venezuelan encephalitis virus which distinguish enzootic strains of subtype I-D from those of I-E. *Am J Epidemiol* 122:234-244, 1985.

Sudia, W. D., L. Fernández, V. F. Newhouse, R. Sanz, and C. H. Calisher. Arbovirus vector ecology studies in Mexico during the 1972 Venezuelan equine encephalitis outbreak. *Am J Epidemiol* 101:51-58, 1975.

Sudia, W. D., and V. F. Newhouse. Epidemic Venezuelan equine encephalitis in North America. A summary of virus-vector-host relationships. *Am J Epidemiol* 101:1-13, 1975.

Sudia, W. D., V. F. Newhouse, L. D. Beadle, D. L. Miller, J. G. Johnston, Jr., R. Young, C. H. Calisher, and K. Maness. Epidemic Venezuelan equine encephalitis in North America in 1971. Vector studies. *Am J Epidemiol* 101:17-35, 1975.

Trapido, H. Geographic distribution and ecologic setting. *In: Venezuelan Encephalitis.* Washington, D. C., Pan American Health Organization, 1972. (Scientific Publication 243.)

Walder, R., O. M. Suárez, and C. H. Calisher. Arbovirus studies in the Guajira region of Venezuela: Activities of eastern equine encephalitis and Venezuelan equine encephalitis viruses during an interepizootic period. *Am J Trop Med Hyg* 33:699-707, 1984.

Walton, T. E. Venezuelan, eastern and western encephalomyelitis. *In*: Gibbs, E. P. J. (Ed.), *Virus Diseases of Food Animals*, vol. 2. New York, Academic Press, 1981.

Walton, T. E., and K. M. Johnson. Epizootiology of Venezuelan equine encephalomyelitis in the Americas. *J Am Vet Med Assoc* 161:1509-1525, 1972.

Walton, T. E., O. Alvarez, M. Ross, R. M. Buckwalter, and K. M. Johnson. Experimental infection of horses with enzootic and epizootic strains of Venezuelan equine encephalomyelitis virus. *J Infect Dis* 128:271-282, 1973.

Work, T. H. Venezuelan equine encephalomyelitis. *In*: Beeson, P. B., W. McDermott, and J. B. Wyngaarden (Eds.), *Cecil Textbook of Medicine*, 15th ed. Philadelphia and London, Saunders, 1979.

Young, N. Origin of epidemics of Venezuelan equine encephalitis. *J Infect Dis* 125:565-567, 1972.

Young, N. A., and K. M. Johnson. Antigenic variants of Venezuelan equine encephalitis virus: Their geographic distribution and epidemiologic significance. *Am J Epidemiol* 89:286-307, 1969.

VESICULAR STOMATITIS

(079.8)

Synonym: Sore mouth of cattle and horses.

Etiology: RNA virus belonging to the genus *Vesiculovirus* of the family Rhabdoviridae.

Vesicular stomatitis (VS) in domestic animals, which is found only in the Americas, is caused by two serotypes, New Jersey and Indiana. The latter includes three immunologic subtypes: subtype 1 (Indiana), subtype 2 (Cocal-Argentina), and subtype 3 (Alagoas).[1]

---

[1] Other recognized types of vesiculovirus—which are not agents of vesicular stomatitis in domestic animals—are Piry, endemic in some areas of Brazil; Chandipura in India and Nigeria, antigenically related to Piry; and Isfahan, endemic in certain areas of Iran. Natural and laboratory infections with the Piry and Chandipura viruses indicate that they can produce the disease in man and therefore should be considered zoonotic agents.

Geographic Distribution: Vesicular stomatitis is limited to the Western Hemisphere. In the United States, Mexico, Central America and Panama, Venezuela, Colombia, Ecuador, and Peru there are enzootic areas of the New Jersey type and Indiana subtype 1. Indiana subtype 2 (Cocal-Argentina) was isolated in the Bush-Bush jungle in Trinidad and in Belém, Brazil, from mites from a rodent of the genus *Oryzomys*; no association with clinical vesicular stomatitis was shown, even though antibodies were found in equines in Trinidad. Although the disease was clinically diagnosed in horses in Argentina in 1939, infection was not confirmed by isolation of the virus until 1963 when an outbreak in horses occurred in Salta Province and, later, in Buenos Aires Province. The virus, which apparently affected only equines, was identified as Indiana subtype 2 (Cocal Argentina), that is, the same as in Trinidad. In Brazil, the disease was confirmed for the first time in 1964 during an outbreak in Alagoas state that affected primarily mules and horses, although cases were also seen in cattle and humans. The virus was identified as a new Indiana subtype (subtype 3 or Alagoas). Currently, the subtypes recognized in Brazil are Indiana 3 in Alagoas and Minas Gerais and Indiana 2 in São Paulo and Rio Grande do Sul. In this last state, an outbreak in the summer of 1978-1979 affected horses at 15 establishments; the diagnosis was confirmed serologically (Prado *et al.*, 1979).

Occurrence in Man: The frequency of the clinical disease is not yet known precisely. The disease is often not recognized due to its benign course, its similarity to influenza, and the difficulty in isolating the virus from man. Most human cases have been diagnosed in laboratory personnel. Out of 74 persons who were exposed to virulent material or who were in charge of infected animals in a laboratory, 54 had antibodies for vesicular stomatitis, and of these, 31 (57.4%) manifested clinical symptoms (Johnson *et al.*, 1966). Clinical cases are also observed in the field, although most of these may not be correctly identified. Man is susceptible to both types of the virus, and the prevalence of the infection in some populations in enzootic areas may be very high (more than 90% of adults in a rural locality in Panama), judging from serologic studies. As in other endemic situations, the rate of reactors increases with age. In four selected rural communities in Panama, the rates of positive reaction to the serum neutralization test were 21 and 9% in the 0-to-5-years age group and 80 and 63% in the 16-to-20-years age group for the New Jersey and Indiana types, respectively (Tesh *et al.*, 1961).

Occurrence in Animals: The infection occurs in cattle, equines, swine, and wild animals. Cases in sheep have been recorded in Colombia. In a study carried out in Panama, antibodies were found for the Indiana type (subtype 1) in arboreal and semiarboreal species, and for the New Jersey type in bats, carnivores, and some rodents (Shrihongse, 1969).

VS is endemic in the forested plains of tropical and subtropical areas of the Americas, where the virus persists in a wild host or hosts, as yet unidentified, and the disease reappears in domestic animals practically every year. In temperate areas, on the other hand, VS appears irregularly and epidemically, and there is no evidence that the virus persists during interepidemic periods (Hanson, 1981).

In enzootic areas the disease is propagated slowly, and the number of animals with clinical symptoms is relatively low. Serologic studies in cattle have demonstrated the presence of antibodies in animals of all ages, with an increase in the reactor rate in older animals. Explosive outbreaks, principally in swine, have been recorded in several Central American countries and have resulted in great losses.

Epizootics occur at irregular intervals both to the north and south of the endemic tropical area. Extensive outbreaks have been recorded in the United States approximately every 10 years, in the upper Mississippi Valley, in the Appalachians, and in the Rocky Mountains. The infection's spread is commonly irregular rather than contiguous, with adjacent farms often unaffected. VS is generally propagated more slowly than foot-and-mouth disease and usually affects fewer animals, with an attack rate varying between 10 and 100%.

The latest epizootic in the United States, caused by the New Jersey (NJ) virus, began in May 1982 in Arizona and extended to 14 states; to the north it reached Oregon, Washington, and Wyoming. This epizootic is thought to have originated in Central America, passed through Mexico, and extended to Arizona. It affected 829 livestock premises (American Veterinary Medical Association, 1983).

Inapparent infection is always more frequent than apparent infection. Epidemiologic studies carried out during this last epizootic in the United States found that the rate of sick animals in 16 livestock establishments was 7% in cattle and 42% in horses, while the incidence of serologic reactors was 74% and 67% in cattle and equines, respectively (Reif *et al.*, 1983).

Outbreaks of the disease also occur in endemic areas, such as Central America and northern South America. In some countries the importance of VS among vesicular diseases can be significant, as shown by data from Colombia, where 283 samples were positive for foot-and-mouth disease and 145 positive for vesicular stomatitis (109 New Jersey and 36 Indiana types) out of a total of 477 samples received for diagnosis in 1972 (Cadena and Estupiñán, 1975).

The disease is seasonal in character, occurring in summer in temperate climates and immediately after the rainy season in tropical climates.

The Disease in Man: Man is susceptible to both types of the virus. The incubation period is from 1 to 2 days. The symptomatology is acute and resembles influenza, with pyrexia lasting 1 to 2 days, cephalalgia, retro-ocular pain, and myalgia. Other signs and symptoms are occasionally present, such as vesicles in the mouth or pharynx or on the hands, nausea, vomiting, and diarrhea.

The patient recovers in a few days. Although the disease course is short and mild, some cases may require hospitalization.

The Disease in Animals: The incubation period is from 2 to 4 days. Symptomatology is similar to that of foot-and-mouth disease, with which SV can easily be confused. The disease is characterized by a short febrile period and the appearance of papules and vesicles in the mouth, on the udder, in interdigital areas, and on the coronary band. Profuse salivation is often a prominent sign. In cattle the papules do not always become vesiculated. Experiments show that only 30% of the animals develop evident vesiculation. The site of the lesions can vary in different outbreaks; in some, oral vesicles predominate, and in others, mammary vesicles. Pedal lesions are not present in every outbreak and are more frequent in swine. Generally, animals recover in a week. The disease caused by the New Jersey type virus is usually more severe than that produced by the Indiana type (Mason, 1978). The most common complications are secondary bacterial infections, myiasis, and mastitis. Case fatality is low. The disease can cause appreciable economic losses, primarily when it affects dairy cattle and swine.

Source of Infection and Mode of Transmission: The ecology of the VS virus is still not well understood, and there continue to be many gaps in knowledge of the basic cycle of infection. Many questions still exist as to where and how the virus is maintained in nature, how it is transmitted from one animal to another, and how it is introduced into herds free from infection. It is possible that the Indiana and New Jersey viruses have different cycles. Infection with the Indiana virus in enzootic areas is common in wild arboreal or semiarboreal animals, and the agent has been isolated from sandflies and *Aedes* mosquitoes. In addition, the sandfly *Lutzomyia trapidoi* has been found to transmit the infection transovarially to its progeny and, in experiments, to mice by biting them. Similarly, serologic conversion has been observed in sentinel monkeys placed in individual cages in the forest of Panama (endemic area). These observations, along with the fact that the disease occurs when arthropods are most abundant, suggest that, at least for the Indiana virus, there may be a cycle between wild animals and arthropods. Nevertheless, several objections to this hypothesis have been raised, for example, that the viremia in various experimentally exposed animals is insufficient to infect biting arthropods and that the rate of infection in arthropods is low. Moreover, transmission by arthropods could not account for the presence of oral lesions (vesiculation in the oral cavity is only produced experimentally by inoculation); the disease's irregular distribution during outbreaks, when it sometimes does not affect contiguous farms; and epizootics during which attempts to isolate the virus from arthropods have failed. Other hypotheses suggest that the virus is in the soil or pasture and that the animals become infected by inoculation, either through the skin or oral mucosa, or that the reservoir of the virus is a plant or insect and that vertebrates are only accidental hosts. It has also been suggested that in enzootic situations arthropods could play an important role in transmission, while in epizootic situations several mechanisms could be involved at the same time.

Replication of the New Jersey virus in arthropods that fed on a natural host has not yet been confirmed. During the epizootic of 1982 in the United States, this virus was isolated from several dipterans: *Culicoides variipennis,* which in the United States is the vector for blue tongue disease; several species of Simuliidae, Chloropidae, and Anthomyiidae; and *Musca domestica* and *M. autumnalis.* It is still unknown whether any of these insects can act as a biological or mechanical vector (Walton *et al.*, 1983).

In endemic tropical areas a large number of wild animal species react to serologic tests, which may indicate a relationship to the ecology of the VS virus. However, so far it is not known whether they are reservoirs for the maintenance of the agent in nature or simply accidental hosts. In an ecologic study carried out in Antioquia, Colombia, a very high rate (between 30 and 40%) of wild animals with antibodies was found for the New Jersey and Indiana viruses, both near the mountains and in the coastal plain. The presence of high rates of reactors among wild animals in wooded areas near the mountains, where the domestic animal population is small, would indicate that the VS viruses might circulate in the wild, independent of equines, cattle, or swine (Zuluaga and Yuill, 1979).

Although the ecology and epidemiology of VS are not yet clear, it has been confirmed that milking allows the infection to be transmitted directly from a cow with infected teats to another healthy cow. The infection can also be transmitted by ingestion when there are preexisting wounds or abrasions in the epithelium. This latter mode of transmission has been demonstrated experimentally by feeding swine embryonated acarids together with the virus; this practice produced vesicles on snouts that were already injured. The presence of virus in saliva and the frequency of preexisting lesions in animals (skin and oral mucosa) indicate that direct contact could play a considerable role, at least in transmission of the disease caused by New Jersey virus, although several researchers downplay its importance. During the New Jersey virus epizootic of 1982 in the United States, the disease was shown to have started in four states with the arrival of infected cattle from another state. Another salient finding was that animals recovering from the disease developed new lesions after being transported to other areas, signaling the possibility of latent infections that turn into apparent infections when triggered by stress.

None of the hypotheses about persistence and transmission of the virus are satisfactory. In the hypotheses of vector transmission and of transmission through plants or direct contact, gaps and unanswered questions remain (Mason, 1978). Data from the 1982 epizootic in the United States suggest the possibility that the virus is transmitted by direct contact and that it persists inapparently in the animal. New research is required to clarify the ecology and epidemiology of VS.

Man contracts the infection by contact with domestic animals, either through the nasopharyngeal route, through abrasions in the skin, or by aerosols. The direct sources of infection may be saliva, the exudate or epithelium of open vesicles, or the virus itself when it is handled in laboratories. The virus is not eliminated in milk, and infections contracted through the digestive tract are not known.

Diagnosis: The diagnosis of VS in man is based primarily on the complement fixation and serum neutralization tests. Two blood samples should be obtained, one at the beginning of the disease and the other 2 weeks later, to determine the increase in the antibody titer. Viremia in man lasts a very short time, and it is difficult to isolate the virus from the blood. When there are vesicles, an attempt should be made to isolate the agent.

Rapid laboratory diagnosis is very important in domestic animals to distinguish VS from foot-and-mouth disease. The most useful test is complement fixation, using the epithelium of vesicles as antigen. The virus can easily be isolated from vesicles (epithelium or fluid) of the animal.

Control: To prevent disease in man, safety rules should be observed in laboratories, particularly to avoid the production of aerosols. Personnel who work with sick animals in the field (veterinarians, dairymen, and others) should be provided with protective clothing and gloves. Wounds should be cared for properly.

Because of gaps in our knowledge of the epidemiology of VS, it is not possible to set up programs for controlling the infection in animals, but the immobilization of sick and exposed animals can help decrease the spread of the disease. Natural immunity is of short duration. Not only do cattle that have recovered from the disease caused by one type of the virus continue to be susceptible to the other type, but some herds have become reinfected by the same type of virus three times in the course of a year. Swine appear to be more resistant to reinfection.

Vaccines are in the experimental stage. Some have proven useful during epizootics and under enzootic conditions. Inactivated live vaccines with different adjuvants have been studied (Arbaláez *et al.*, 1982).

Bibliography

American Veterinary Medical Association. Vesicular stomatitis hits two more states. News. *J Am Vet Med Assoc* 182:450, 1983.

Arbaláez, G., J. R. Rocha, U. Cardona, and W. Ríos. Ensayos de vacunas contra la estomatitis vesicular. II. Observación experimental de campo. *Rev Asoc Col Med Vet Zoot* 6:27-34, 1982.

Bruner, D. W., and J. H. Gillespie. *Hagan's Infectious Diseases of Domestic Animals*, 6th ed. Ithaca, Cornell University Press, 1973.

Cadena, J., and J. Estupiñán (Eds.). *La fiebre aftosa y otras enfermedades vesiculares en Colombia*. Bogotá, Instituto Colombiano Agropecuario, 1975. (Technical Bulletin 32.)

Federer, K. E., R. Burrows, and J. B. Brooksby. Vesicular stomatitis virus: the relationship between some strains of the Indiana serotype. *Res Vet Sci* 8:103-113, 1967.

Food and Agriculture Organization of the United Nations/World Health Organization/ International Office of Epizootics. *Animal Health Yearbook 1984*. Rome, FAO, 1985.

Hansen, D. E., M. C. Thurmond, and M. Thorburn. Factors associated with the spread of clinical vesicular stomatitis in California dairy cattle. *Am J Vet Res* 46:789-795, 1985.

Hanson, R. P. Discussion of the natural history of vesicular stomatitis. *Am J Epidemiol* 87:264-266, 1968.

Hanson, R. P. Vesicular stomatitis. *In*: Gibbs, E. P. J. (Ed.), *Virus Diseases of Food Animals*. New York, Academic Press, 1981.

Hanson, R. P., J. Estupiñán, and J. Castañeda. Estomatitis vesicular en las Américas. *In*: *Primera Reunión Interamericana sobre el Control de la Fiebre Aftosa y Otras Zoonosis*. Washington, D.C., Pan American Health Organization, 1968. (Scientific Publication 172.)

Jenney, E. W. Vesicular stomatitis in the United States during the last five years (1963-1967). *Proc Annu Meet US Livest Sanit Assoc* 71:371-385, 1967.

Johnson, K. M., J. E. Vogel, and P. H. Peralta. Clinical and serological response to laboratory-acquired human infection by Indiana type vesicular stomatitis virus. *Am J Trop Med Hyg* 15:244-246, 1966.

Jonkers, A. H. The epizootiology of vesicular stomatitis viruses; a reappraisal. *Am J Epidemiol* 86:286-291, 1967.

Mason, J. La epidemiología de la estomatitis vesicular. *Bol Centro Panam Fiebre Aftosa* 29-30:13-33, 1978.

Patterson, W. C., L. O. Mott, and E. W. Jenney. A study of vesicular stomatitis in man. *J Am Vet Med Assoc* 133:57-62, 1958.

Pérez, E. P. La estomatitis vesicular como zoonosis. *Bol Of Sanit Panam* 68:223-229, 1970.

Prado, J. A. P., S. A. Petzhold, P. E. Reckziegel, and E. N. Jorgens. Estomatite vesicular no estado Rio Grande do Sul (Brasil). *Bol Inst Pesq Vet D Finamor* 6:73-77, 1979.

Reif, J. S., P. A. Webb, T. P. Monath, T. E. Walton, J. K. Emerson, D. W. MacVean, D. B. Francy, J. D. Poland, G. E. Kemp, and G. Cholas. Vesicular stomatitis: epidemiologic and zoonotic aspects of the 1982 outbreak (Abstract). *J Am Vet Med Assoc* 183:350, 1983.

Srihongse, S. Vesicular stomatitis virus infections in Panamanian primates and other vertebrates. *Am J Epidemiol* 90:69-76, 1969.

Stallknecht, D. E., V. F. Nettles, G. A. Erickson, and D. A. Jessup. Antibodies to vesicular stomatitis virus in populations of feral swine in the United States. *J Wildl Dis* 22:320-325, 1986.

Tesh, R. B., and K. M. Johnson. Vesicular stomatitis. *In*: Hubbert, W. T., W. F. McCulloch, and P. R. Schnurrenberger (Eds.), *Diseases Transmitted from Animals to Man*, 6th ed. Springfield, Illinois, Thomas, 1975.

Tesh, R. B., P. H. Peralta, and K. M. Johnson. Ecologic studies of vesicular stomatitis. I. Prevalence of infection among animals and humans living in an area of endemic V.S.V. activity. *Am J Epidemiol* 90:255-261, 1961.

Walton, T. E., P. A. Webb, and D. B. Francy. Vesicular stomatitis virus in wild caught insects. *Foreign Anim Dis Rep* (USDA) 11:2, 1983. Reproduced in *Bull OIE* 95:48, 1983.

Webb, P. A., R. G. McLean, G. S. Smith, J. H. Ellenberger, D. B. Francy, T. E. Walton, and T. P. Monath. Epizootic vesicular stomatitis in Colorado, 1982: some observations on the possible role of wildlife populations in an enzootic maintenance cycle. *J Wildl Dis* 23:192-198, 1987.

Zuluaga, F. N., and T. M. Yuill. Estudios ecológicos de los virus de estomatitis vesicular en Antioquia, Colombia. *Bol Of Sanit Panam* 87:389-404, 1979.

VIRAL HEPATITIS OF MAN AND NONHUMAN PRIMATES

(070)

Currently, at least three etiologically different forms of the disease are distinguished, designated hepatitis A (HA), hepatitis B (HB), and non-A non-B hepatitis (NANBH); to these should be added hepatitis associated with the delta antigen. Viral hepatitides constitute an important public health problem, but only the zoonotic aspects—their intercommunicability between man and other primates—are discussed here. Deinhardt and Gust (1983) have done an up-to-date revision on the most important aspects of viral hepatitides for the participants in a meeting of specialists called by the World Health Organization.

Synonyms: Viral hepatitis A: epidemic hepatitis, epidemic jaundice, infectious hepatitis.
Viral hepatitis B: Serum hepatitis, Australian antigen hepatitis.

Etiology: Hepatitis A virus has recently been characterized and classified as an RNA virus, a picornavirus that is very similar to members of the genus *Enterovirus*, family Picornaviridae (Gust *et al.*, 1983). The virus of hepatitis B is a DNA virus and as yet has no official taxonomic placement. Its inclusion in the new family Hepadnaviridae, together with similar viruses found in marmosets, California ground squirrels, and Pekin ducks, has been proposed (Melnick, 1982). The agents (it is not clear if they are two different viruses or two serotypes) of non-A non-B hepatitis have not been characterized; their name is derived from the fact that they are serologically different from HA and HB viruses. There are recent indications that the NANBH agents are retroviruses. The delta antigen seems to be a defective RNA virus that requires HB virus synthesis for its replication. This agent can be found in acute coinfection with the HB virus (HBV) or in superinfection in HBV carriers.

Geographic Distribution: The hepatitis viruses are distributed worldwide.

Occurrence: Since the first outbreak, which occurred in 1958-1960 on an Air Force base in the USA, there have been more than 200 human cases in which the infection was related to nonhuman primates. Only two secondary cases have been observed in two separate outbreaks (Deinhardt, 1976). All the cases were probably due to HA virus. Chimpanzees are the main species that has been implicated, but others have also been involved.

In recent years, several studies have been carried out to determine the prevalence of HA and HB viruses in nonhuman primates. In captive chimpanzees, the prevalence of HB antibodies (anti-HB$_s$) has been noted to increase with age; in animals older than 10 years, it is sometimes higher than 80%. Up to 25% of chimpanzees captured in the jungle had these antibodies when examined weeks or months after their arrival at their final destination. Ten out of 26 chimpanzees kept by a distributor in Africa were found to be already positive to HB$_s$Ag.[1] These findings indicate that the infection could have occurred via human transmission shortly after capture, but HB virus might also occur naturally among these primates (Deinhardt, 1976). In a US primate center, tests on sera from seven species of nonhuman primates and from human personnel revealed that 2.4% of 82 chimpanzees and 1.6% of 62 humans were positive for HB$_s$Ag; 29.9% of chimpanzees, 36.2% of baboons (*Papio cynocephalus*), 5% of squirrel monkeys (*Saimiri sciureus*), and 11.3% of humans had antibodies for HB surface antigen (Eichberg and Kalter, 1980). In a London zoo five of nine chimpanzees were HB virus carriers and the other four had antibodies. Three of the carriers were born in the zoo to a carrier mother or father so perinatal transmission could have occurred, as happens in man (Zucherman *et al.*, 1978). With respect to HA virus antibodies in the primate center mentioned above, the prevalence rate was even higher and the number of reactive species increased. In Panama, only two out of 145 owl monkeys (*Aotus trivirgatus*) had antibodies soon after capture, while almost all had a serologic reaction after being kept 100 days in the colony of a scientific institute there (Lemon *et al.*, 1982).

The Disease in Man: The disease associated with nonhuman primates is generally mild, of short duration, and clinically indistinguishable from HA, which is usually acquired by contact with infected persons or by consuming contaminated food or water. The incubation period lasts 3 to 6 weeks, that is, shorter than that of hepatitis B (serum hepatitis), which on the average lasts 60 to 90 days. The disease is of sudden onset with fever, nausea, and anorexia. The patient may or may not have jaundice. In some individuals the disease was identified only by means of hepatic function tests. No deaths have been recorded.

The Disease in Animals: As far as is known, the only animals that become infected naturally are nonhuman primates, especially chimpanzees. Generally, the infection is clinically inapparent. It has been suggested that the hepatic affection and other clinical symptoms associated with some cases might have been caused by an intercurrent disease.

The chimpanzee serum that caused a recent outbreak in Pennsylvania, USA, with five human cases, had 85 IU (normal: 0 to 15 IU) glutamic oxaloacetic transaminase and 2 mg% of bilirubin (normal: 0.1 to 0.5 mg%).

After the natural transmission of the infection from nonhuman primates to humans was recognized and this infection was confirmed to be biochemically and histologically similar to the one which occurs in man, efforts to utilize these animals as models were renewed. As a consequence, there has been a great advance in

---

[1] HB surface antigen, which can be detected in human serum several weeks before the appearance of symptoms and from days to months afterward, and which persists in chronic infections.

knowledge of viral hepatitis A and B in man. Currently, the animals most often used in these studies are marmosets, *Saguinus mystax* being the most susceptible. The infection in marmosets can be transmitted regularly in series, both parenterally and orally. Some specimens of experimentally infected *S. mystax* develop clinical disease and even die of acute hepatic insufficiency, but in general they recover; no chronic hepatitis or cirrhosis has been found in these animals (Deinhardt, 1976).

Source of Infection and Mode of Transmission (Figure 53): It is probable that all human infections have been due to HA virus, acquired through close contact with nonhuman primates. Out of 173 human cases that had contact with only one species of these animals, 151 contracted the disease from chimpanzees and the other 22 from other simians. Almost all cases occurred through contact with recently imported young animals, which usually require more intensive care; no human infection was caused by animals in captivity longer than 6 months. Cases have occurred among personnel of research institutes, primate centers, and zoos; persons employed in the importation of simians; and, sometimes, members of families who kept monkeys in their homes.

Figure 53. Hepatitis A transmitted by nonhuman primates.
Probable transmission cycle.

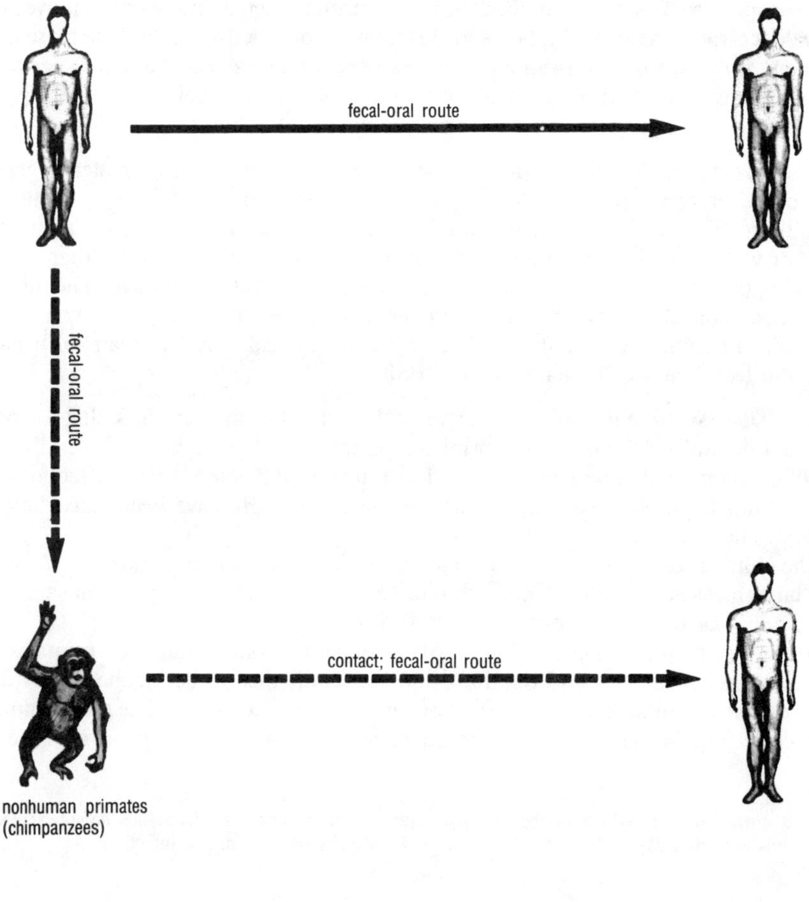

The most probable route of infection is the fecal-oral route. Since chimpanzees customarily handle their feces and even ingest them, man has ample opportunity to become infected by contact with the hands, mouth, and skin of these primates. It is believed that chimpanzees acquire hepatitis from infected persons and can transmit it to man only for a short period, about 1 month. In Africa it is common practice to capture a young chimpanzee and keep him in the home in close contact with people. On the other hand, many chimpanzees approach human dwellings in search of food in cultivated plots and thus may also become infected by contaminated wastes. Also, collectors inoculate some of these animals with human serum in order to protect them against human diseases, possibly explaining their infection by HB virus.

In the study carried out on the colony of *Aotus trivirgatus* in Panama (Lemon *et al.*, 1982), the HA virus was present in the feces of the majority of infected monkeys before the appearance of antibodies. These viruses could not be distinguished from the human HA virus. Thus, the virus evidently spreads from one nonhuman primate to another, and on occasion the infection can be transmitted to man.

That chimpanzees are the primary nonhuman primate implicated in transmitting the HA virus to humans could be explained by the fact that these animals, especially young ones, are in much closer contact with man than are other primates. However, the infection can be transmitted to man by other primates, as has been seen on several occasions.

In spite of the high prevalence of the HB virus in nonhuman primates, there are no confirmed cases of its transmission to man. In the London zoo, even though some chimpanzees had a high level of infection caused by HB virus, no human cases occurred. This could be explained by lack of prolonged contact between personnel and chimpanzees, which appears necessary for nonparenteral transmission of hepatitis B to man (Kessler *et al.*, 1982). In this respect, it should be remembered that the HB virus usually is transmitted by transfusions, contaminated syringes (multiple use), and exposure to contaminated blood. Transfer of infection from a carrier mother to a newborn infant is an important mode of transmission and possibly occurs in nonhuman primates. The virus is not transmitted by the fecal-oral route as happens with HA virus.

Most probably, the original source of infection of nonhuman primates is man; the virus then propagates among these animals and occasionally is retransmitted to man.

Role of Animals in the Epidemiology of the Disease: The participation of nonhuman primates in the epidemiology of human hepatitis is minimal. Man is the main reservoir of the viruses and nonhuman primates are only secondary hosts.

The real importance of having confirmed natural infection in these animals and its transmission to man was their later use as models for the human disease, which led to a great advance in the knowledge of hepatitis.

Diagnosis: Human cases of hepatitis contracted from nonhuman primates have been classified as hepatitis A and differentiated from hepatitis B on the basis of the shorter incubation period and the invariably negative results of tests for the surface antigen of hepatitis B ("Australian antigen"). The specific diagnosis of hepatitis A can be done by confirming the presence of particles of the virus or specific antigens (HAAg) in the feces, or by confirming the rise in titer and detecting IgM anti-HA virus antibodies (anti-HAV IgM); this last test constitutes the method of choice (Deinhardt and Gust, 1983). Different associations of serological markers have been established for HB virus to indicate the degree of infectivity of blood or the degree of acquired immunity (Deinhardt and Gust, 1983). Recently, an ELISA test for a non-A non-B hepatitis antigen has been developed, and it was possible to infect a chimpanzee with a patient's serum containing that antigen (Durmeyer *et al.*, 1983).

Control: The following measures are recommended to prevent transmission of hepatitis A from nonhuman primates to man: a) good personal hygiene and use of protective clothing when handling primates or their excreta; b) prophylactic doses of immunoglobulin administered to persons who are in continual or frequent contact with young, recently imported simians, especially chimpanzees; and c) a limit to the number of persons assigned to look after recently imported nonhuman primates.

Bibliography

American Public Health Association. *Control of Communicable Diseases in Man*, 14th ed. (Ed. by A. S. Benenson). Washington, D.C., APHA, 1985.

Centers for Disease Control of the USA. *Hepatitis Surveillance Reports*. Atlanta, Georgia, Nos. 34 and 36, September 1972 and September 1973.

Centers for Disease Control of the USA. Nonhuman primate-associated hepatitis—Pennsylvania. *Morb Mortal Wkly Rep* 24:115, 1975.

Deinhardt, F. Hepatitis in primates. *Adv Virus Res* 20:113-157, 1976.

Deinhardt, F., and J. B. Deinhardt. Association of nonhuman primates with human hepatitis. *In*: Geraty, R. J. (Ed.), *Hepatitis A*. Orlando, Florida, Academic Press, 1984.

Deinhardt, F., and I. D. Gust. L'hépatite virale. *Bull WHO* 61:199-232, 1983.

Durmeyer, W., R. Stute, and J. A. Hellings. An enzyme-linked immunosorbent assay for an antigen related to non-A, non-B hepatitis and its antibody. *J Med Virol* 11:11-21, 1983.

Eichberg, J. W., and S. S. Kalter. Hepatitis A and B: serologic survey of human and nonhuman primate sera. *Lab Anim Sci* 30:541-543, 1980.

Feinstone, S. M., A. Z. Kapikian, and R. H. Purcell. Hepatitis A: Detection by immune electron microscopy of a virus-like antigen associated with acute illness. *Science* 182:1026-1028, 1973.

Gust, I. D., C. J. Burrell, A. G. Coulepis, W. S. Robinson, and A. J. Zuckerman. Taxonomic classification of human hepatitis B virus. *Intervirology* 25:14-29, 1986.

Gust, I. D., A. G. Coulepis, S. M. Feinstone, S. A. Locarnini, Y. Maritsugu, R. Najera, and G. Siegl. Taxonomic classification of hepatitis A virus. *Intervirology* 20:1-7, 1983.

Held, J. The public health implications of nonhuman primates in the transmission of hepatitis to man. *Proc Annu Meet Am Vet Med Assoc* 100:183-185, 1963.

Hollinger, F. B., D. W. Bradley, J. E. Maynard, G. R. Dreesman, and J. L. Melnick. Detection of hepatitis A viral antigen by radioimmunoassay. *J Immunol* 115:1464-1466, 1975.

Kessler, H., K. N. Tsiquaye, H. Smith, D. M. Jones, and A. J. Zuckerman. Hepatitis A and B at the London Zoo. *J Infect* 4:63-67, 1982.

Kissling, R. E. Simian hepatitis. *In*: Hubbert, W. T., W. F. McCulloch, and P. R. Schnurrenberger (Eds.), *Diseases Transmitted from Animals to Man*, 6th ed. Springfield, Illinois, Thomas, 1975.

Lemon, S. M., J. W. LeDuc, L. N. Binn, A. Escajadillo, and K. G. Ishak. Transmission of hepatitis A virus among recently captured Panamanian owl monkeys. *J Med Virol* 10:25-36, 1982.

Melnick, J. L. Classification of hepatitis A virus as enterovirus type 72 and of hepatitis B virus as Hepadnavirus type 1. *Intervirology* 18:105-106, 1986.

Neefe, J. R., and E. N. Willey. Hepatitis viral. *In*: Top, F. H., and P. H. Wehrle (Eds.), *Communicable and Infectious Diseases*. St. Louis, Missouri, Mosby, 1972.

Pattison, C. P., and J. E. Maynard. Subhuman primate-associated hepatitis. *J Infect Dis* 132:478-479, 1975.

World Health Organization. *Viral Hepatitis. Report of a WHO Scientific Group.* Geneva, WHO, 1973. (Technical Report Series 512.)

Zuckerman, A. J., A. Thornton, C. R. Howard, K. N. Tsiquaye, D. M. Jones, and M. R. Brambell. Hepatitis B outbreak among chimpanzees at the London Zoo. *Lancet* 2:652-654, 1978.

WESSELSBRON DISEASE

(066.3)

Synonym: Wesselsbron fever.

Etiology: RNA virus, genus *Flavivirus* (formerly group B of the arboviruses), family Togaviridae; forms part of the complex of the mosquito-borne viruses.

Geographic Distribution: The Wesselsbron (WSL) virus has been isolated from animals or mosquitoes in South Africa, Zimbabwe, Cameroon, Nigeria, Uganda, the Central African Republic, Senegal, and Thailand (in this last country only from mosquitoes). According to serologic surveys, it may also exist in Mozambique, Angola, Madagascar, Botswana, and possibly Ethiopia. Serologic studies have shown that the infection occurs throughout a wide area of Africa.

Occurrence in Man and Animals: The virus has a large number of hosts among mammals and possibly among birds. In the low-lying areas of Natal, South Africa, the prevalence of neutralizing antibodies in cattle, sheep, and goats reaches 50%. Several serious epizootic outbreaks have occurred in sheep in southern Africa. Subclinical infection is also common among the human population of enzootic areas. In studies using the serum neutralization test, positive reactions were obtained in 36 out of 83 individuals examined among the populations of northern Kenya, 17 out of 54 in Angola, and 48 out of 141 in Uganda (Henderson *et al.*, 1970). In this last country prevalence varied between regions, from zero in mountainous areas to high in the Nile basin. Clinical infection occurred on at least nine occasions in laboratory staff or field workers who had worked with the virus or had handled contaminated material. In spite of the wide diffusion of the virus and the number of infected persons, few cases of the clinical disease have been recorded, and even fewer cases due to mosquito bites.

The Disease in Man: The incubation period is from 2 to 4 days. The symptomatology consists of fever, cephalalgia, arthralgia, myalgia, and sometimes cutaneous hyperesthesia and a mild skin eruption. The fever lasts 2 to 3 days, but muscular pains may persist much longer. The high prevalence of reactors to the serum neutralization test in endemic areas indicates that the infection is generally subclinical, or if mild clinical symptoms occur, such as slight fever, they are attributed to other causes.

The Disease in Animals: The distribution, epizootiology, and clinical symptomatology of the disease are similar to those of Rift Valley fever. The most susceptible animal species is sheep. The incubation period is from 1 to 4 days, as deduced from experimental infection. Sheep of all ages are susceptible to natural or experimental infection, and neonatal mortality may reach high proportions. Pregnant ewes frequently abort and also suffer high mortality rates due to complications. Nonpregnant females display only a febrile reaction, without other clinical manifestations. Nevertheless, during an outbreak in 1957 in South Africa, jaundice, nasal secretion, diarrhea, swelling in various parts of the head, and a high fatality rate were noted. It is not known whether that outbreak included some other concurrent disease. However, it is believed that the WSL virus, which is hepatotropic, might trigger "enzootic jaundice," caused in that region by chronic copper intoxication. This would explain the high mortality as well as the atypical symptomatology and pathology. Experimental inoculation of adult sheep and goats with the WSL virus resulted in a moderate to severe febrile reaction, but not in other clinical symptoms or death. Histopathologic studies have demonstrated that the liver was affected and that the damage consisted of small necrotic foci (Coetzer and Theodoridis, 1982).

Experimental inoculation of cattle, equines, and swine evokes a febrile reaction without any other symptomatology. Notwithstanding, infection by the WSL virus is suspected to cause some abortions in cattle. In Zimbabwe, where the WSL virus is the predominant flavivirus and about 50% of the cattle have antibodies against it, fetal pathologic abnormalities or abortions only occasionally can be attributed to it. Cattle inoculated experimentally show a febrile reaction and viremia. One heifer gave birth to a weak calf that died shortly after birth; the calf had antibodies that may have indicated intrauterine infection (Blackburn and Swanepoel, 1980).

Source of Infection and Mode of Transmission: Wesselsbron virus infection occurs primarily in low-lying, humid areas where mosquitoes are abundant. The disease is seasonal, occurring in late summer and in autumn. The virus has been repeatedly isolated from *Aedes circumluteolus* and *A. caballus*, species that have been shown experimentally to be capable of transmitting the infection. *A. lineatopennis* may also be an important vector. The infection is transmitted from animal to animal and from animal to man by mosquito bites. The clinical disease in man has occurred primarily in laboratory staff or field workers handling the virus or material containing it; they acquired the infection by contact or from aerosols.

The mechanism by which the virus is maintained in nature is not yet completely clear. Sheep and cattle have a high-titer viremia for 3 or 4 days and can serve as a source of infection for mosquitoes. The virus has been isolated from a wild rodent, *Desmodillus*, which has been shown to develop viremia lasting 1 week. Antibodies against the virus have been found in several species of wild birds, and viremia has been confirmed in experimentally infected birds.

Diagnosis: The disease can be diagnosed with certainty only by laboratory methods: isolation of the virus and serology. Virus isolation can be done by inoculating serum from a febrile patient into suckling mice. On one occasion, the virus was successfully isolated from a pharyngeal wash. The virus can be isolated from the blood (or serum), liver, and brain of aborted sheep fetuses, or from the spleen and liver of dead lambs, by inoculating the materials either into suckling mice or into a lamb kidney cell culture. Serologic diagnosis consists of confirming a significant increase in antibody titers between acute and convalescent sera.

Control: An attenuated live virus vaccine is available for sheep and is used simultaneously with Rift Valley fever vaccine. The vaccine can cause abortion in pregnant ewes, and for this reason it should be administered about 3 weeks before breeding. Lambs of immune ewes acquire passive immunity through the colostrum, and it is recommended that such lambs be vaccinated after 6 months of age.

Precautions should be taken in laboratories so as not to expose staff to the virus or contaminated materials. Gloves, protective clothing, and control measures against the production of aerosols are required. The same precautions should be taken in performing autopsies and field work.

Bibliography

Blackburn, N. K., and R. Swanepoel. An investigation of flavivirus infections of cattle in Zimbabwe Rhodesia with particular reference to Wesselsbron virus. *J Hyg (Camb)* 85:1-33, 1980.

Centers for Disease Control of the USA. *International Catalogue of Arboviruses*, 2nd ed. (Ed. by T. O. Berge). Atlanta, Georgia, 1975. (DHEW Publ. CDC 75-8301.)

Coetzer, J. A. W., and A. Theodoridis. Clinical and pathological studies in adult sheep and goats experimentally infected with Wesselsbron disease virus. *Onderstepoort J Vet Res* 49:19-22, 1982.

Henderson, B. E., G. B. Kirya, and L. E. Hewitt. Serological survey for arboviruses in Uganda, 1967-69. *Bull WHO* 42:797-805, 1970.

Henderson, B. E., D. Metselaar, G. B. Kirya, and G. L. Timms. Investigations into yellow fever virus and other arboviruses in the northern regions of Kenya. *Bull WHO* 42:787-795, 1970.

Henning, M. W. *Animal Diseases in South Africa*, 3rd ed. Pretoria, Central News Agency, 1956.

Jensen, R. *Diseases of Sheep*. Philadelphia, Lea and Febiger, 1974.

Justines, G. H., and R. E. Shope. Wesselsbron virus infection in a laboratory worker, with virus recovery from throat washing. *Health Lab Sci* 6:46-49, 1969.

Kokernot, R. H., V. M. R. Casaca, M. P. Weinsbren, and B. M. McIntosh. Survey for antibodies against arthropod-borne viruses in the sera of indigenous residents of Angola. *Trans R Soc Trop Med Hyg* 59:563-570, 1965.

McIntosh, B. M., and H. J. S. Gear. Mosquito-borne arboviruses, primarily in the eastern hemisphere. *In*: Hubbert, W. T., W. F. McCulloch, and P. R. Schnurrenberger (Eds.), *Diseases Transmitted from Animals to Man*, 6th ed. Springfield, Illinois, Thomas, 1975.

Salaün, J. J., A. Rickenbach, P. Brès, H. Brottes, M. Germain, J. P. Eouzan, and L. Ferrara. Les arbovirus isolés à partir de moustiques au Cameroun. *Bull WHO* 41:233-241, 1969.

Weiss, K. E. Wesselsbron virus disease. *In*: Dalling, T., and A. Robertson (Eds.), *International Encyclopedia of Veterinary Medicine*. Edinburgh, Green, 1966.

WESTERN EQUINE ENCEPHALITIS

(062.1)

Synonyms: Western equine encephalomyelitis, western encephalitis.

Etiology: RNA virus belonging to the genus *Alphavirus* (formerly group A of the arboviruses) of the family Togaviridae; it is part of the group of arboviruses transmitted by mosquitoes.

Geographic Distribution: The virus has been isolated in Canada, the United States, Mexico, Guyana, Brazil, Argentina, and Uruguay.

Occurrence in Man: From 1955 to 1978, 941 human cases of western equine encephalitis (WEE) were recorded in the United States. The annual incidence is quite variable. In 1975 there were 133 cases with four deaths in the United States, while only one case was recorded in 1976 and none in 1982 (Centers for Disease Control of the USA, 1981 and 1982). In that country, WEE ranks third overall among the arboviral encephalitides, after St. Louis encephalitis and California encephalitis. Both human and equine cases have occurred west of the Mississippi River. The most extensive epidemic took place in 1941 in the North Central states of the United States and neighboring provinces of Canada, affecting more than 3,000 people and several hundred thousand horses. Clinical cases of WEE have also been seen in Brazil.

As in other diseases caused by arboviruses, there are many more cases of inapparent than of clinical infection. It has been estimated that in persons older than 15 years of age, one case of clinical encephalitis occurs for every 1,150 subclinical infections. In children under 5 years of age the ratio is estimated at 1 to 58. Serologic studies carried out using the hemagglutination inhibition and neutralization tests have shown that the prevalence of reactors varies and that it can reach very high rates in hyperendemic areas.

Occurrence in Animals: In the western United States, epizootics or sporadic cases of the disease occur every year. Nearly 174,000 horses in 1937 and another 184,000 in 1938 were affected by equine encephalitides (eastern and western types). From 1966 to 1970, 7,683 cases of encephalitis occurred in horses, with 1,773 deaths. Most of these cases were due to WEE. Serologic studies (neutralization test) have shown that the rate of reactors is very high in hyperendemic areas. A virus of the same complex, Highlands J (HJ), is active in the eastern part of the United States, but illness caused by this virus is rare in horses and unknown in humans. The WEE virus has also been isolated from horses in Brazil and Argentina. An epizootic in Argentina in late 1982 and early 1983 affected about 300 horses, and the disease was found in provinces where it had not been known before (Pan American Zoonoses Center, 1983). Human cases were not seen, or perhaps were not recognized.

The Disease in Man: The disease occurs during the summer months, the highest attack rate being observed in young adults and children under 1 year of age. The incubation period is from 5 to 10 or more days. In adults, disease onset is sudden, with fever, cephalalgia, stiffness of the neck, and lethargy; mental confusion is common. In children, fever, cephalalgia, and malaise precede the neurologic symptoms by a few days; convulsions are common, as are vomiting, stiffness of the neck, and headaches. Flaccid and spastic paralyses and abnormal reflexes are seen more frequently in children than in adults. The febrile state lasts from 7 to 10 days. In general, adult patients recover completely. Permanent sequelae are rare in adults, but frequent in children, who may undergo personality changes, and suffer from mental retardation, spastic paralysis, and recurrent convulsions. The case fatality rate varies between 3 and 14%.

The Disease in Animals: The WEE virus has multiple hosts, but only manifests itself clinically in horses. The disease is usually sporadic at the beginning of summer; it can later reach epizootic proportions, and then ceases in winter with the disappearance of mosquitoes. The incubation period is 1 to 3 weeks. Fever is the only clinical manifestation before the appearance of neurologic symptoms. As in man, only some horses develop encephalitis. By the time neurologic symptoms appear, the viremia and fever have disappeared. The principal neurologic symptoms are restlessness, unsteady gait, lack of coordination, and somnolence. The sick animal attacks any obstacle, walks in circles, and loses all sense of orientation. During the lethargic phase, it is common to see the animal immobile and supporting its head on a fence or other object. In the final paralytic phase, the animal is incapable of getting up after falling, has a dangling lower lip, and experiences difficulty swallowing. Death may occur 1 or 2 days after the neurologic symptoms appear. Animals who recover frequently show nervous sequelae, especially abnormal reflexes. The fatality rate in horses affected by encephalomyelitic symptomatology varies between 20 and 30%, but can reach 50%.

Source of Infection and Mode of Transmission (Figure 54): The natural reservoirs of the WEE virus are domestic fowl and wild birds. The virus has been isolated from many species of birds, especially passerine birds such as sparrows. In endemic areas of the western United States, antibodies have been found in at least 15 different bird species. When infected, birds develop viremia with a sufficiently high titer to infect vector mosquitoes. In experimentally infected wild birds, the virus can be isolated up to 10 months after inoculation.

The main vector in the western United States is *Culex tarsalis*, which is also responsible in this same area for transmission of the St. Louis encephalitis virus. *Aedes dorsalis* is probably involved in the transmission in areas where it predominates. The basic cycle of infection is maintained by transmission from a viremic to a susceptible bird, by means of one or more vectors. Viral activity reaches its peak in early and midsummer. Wild birds, especially young ones (because of their susceptibility), constitute the enzootic and amplifying link in the circulation of the virus. The vector, *C. tarsalis*, is very widespread, living in irrigated farming areas, flooded pasture land, and at lake edges. In spring and early summer, the vector is mainly ornithophilic, but by midsummer it feeds more and more often on mammals (Monath and Trent, 1981). Different populations of *C. tarsalis* have been shown to vary significantly in their competence as vectors of the virus (Hardy *et al.*, 1979). *C. tarsalis* infects man and horses when it feeds on them but may or may not produce clinical disease. Nevertheless, both man and horses are accidental hosts in which the virus provokes a low-titer viremia and, for this reason, neither species is involved in the basic cycle. The role of the horse in the epidemiology of this disease thus differs notably from its role in Venezuelan equine encephalitis, in which it serves as an important amplifier of the virus.

Figure 54. Western equine encephalitis. Transmission cycle of the virus.

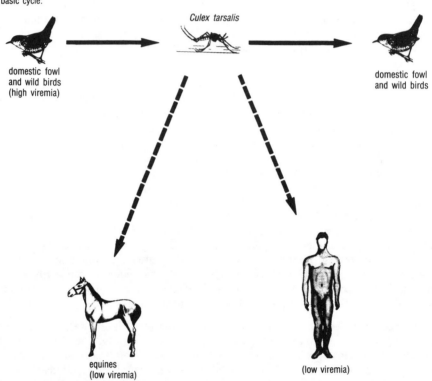

The name "equine" encephalitis (western or eastern) derives only from the fact that the virus was isolated for the first time in this animal species, and it should not be construed that horses are a reservoir of the etiologic agent.

The maintenance mechanism of the virus during the winter months is not yet fully known, but there are indications that reptiles could play a role. In Utah (USA) the virus has been isolated from the blood of 37 out of 84 snakes of three genera (*Thamnophis*, *Coluber*, and *Pituophis*) captured and examined at the beginning of spring. Viremia in these animals is cyclic, appearing and disappearing with changes in ambient temperature. During hibernation the viremia disappears, but the virus reappears when the ambient temperature increases. The titer of the viremia is sufficiently high to infect a large percentage of *C. tarsalis*. Viremia has also been found in the progeny of infected snakes. In Canada, the virus has been isolated from snakes of the genus *Thamnophis* and from frogs (*Rana pipiens*); neutralizing antibodies were found in 50 of 179 frogs examined. Even so, great doubts exist that infection of reptiles and amphibians is the mechanism by which the virus is maintained in winter.

In western Canada epizootics in horses have occurred in areas where *C. tarsalis* is scarce, and it is suspected that the vector in these cases might be *Culiseta inornata*, a mosquito adapted to colder climates (Monath, 1979).

In the eastern United States the main vector is *Culiseta melanura*, which transmits the infection between wild birds but rarely infects horses. The strains of virus that have been isolated from birds, mosquitoes, or sentinel mice in this region and along the Gulf of Mexico all correspond to a prototype (Highlands J), and they can be distinguished antigenically from strains of the virus from the western United States and Canada. Although the eastern strains are closely related to the WEE virus, they are considered to be a different virus of the same complex. The absence of the disease in man and its rarity in horses in the eastern United States might be explained by the habitat (freshwater swamps) of *C. melanura*, its decidedly ornithophilic habits, or the limited virulence of the Highlands J strain for mammals (Hayes and Wallis, 1977).

Recently, several isolations of the WEE virus have been obtained from *Culex ocossa* in Chaco and Corrientes provinces of Argentina (Sirivanakarn and Jakob, 1981). As a result of the most recent epizootic in Argentina, systematic studies were begun to clarify the ecology of the disease, which has been studied little in Latin America.

Diagnosis: Specific diagnosis can be made by virus isolation or by serology. It is difficult to isolate the virus from ill persons or horses. Most isolations have been obtained from brain tissue of people or animals who have died from the infection. In the case of horses, samples are best obtained by destroying the seriously ill animal. Serologic diagnosis consists of demonstrating a four-fold or more increase in the titer of antibodies by the complement fixation, hemagglutination inhibition, serum neutralization, or immunofluorescence test with sera obtained during the acute and convalescent phases of the disease.

It is often difficult to obtain more than one serum sample from horses. If the serum neutralization test (which, alone, detects 80% of infections) is used along with the complement fixation test (which detects 56.3%) and the hemagglutination inhibition test (which detects 43.8%), a presumptive diagnosis can be reached with only one sample in more than 90% of the cases (Calisher *et al.*, 1983).

Control: Preventive measures are directed toward control of the vector. Results have been satisfactory in areas where control programs have been established against *C. tarsalis*. For individual protection, the use of protective clothing, repellents, mosquito netting, and screens in dwellings is recommended.

For the protection of horses, a formalin-inactivated chick embryo vaccine is available. The vaccine may be monovalent (WEE virus only), bivalent, or trivalent, including eastern and Venezuelan equine encephalitides (see "Eastern Equine Encephalitis"). Vaccination is carried out annually during the spring, using two intradermal doses 7 to 10 days apart. Immunity is established approximately 2 weeks after the first dose. Recently, an inactivated tissue culture vaccine and an attenuated live virus vaccine (clone 15B 628) have given satisfactory results in laboratory and field tests, but their use is not yet authorized.

An epizootic outbreak in horses, which usually precedes human cases by a week or more, should be a warning to public health authorities to institute control measures.

An epidemiological surveillance program should take into account the density of the vector population, its rate of infection, seroconversion in sentinel birds, and the rate of infection in birds born that year.

Bibliography

Andrewes, C., and H. G. Pereira. *Viruses of Vertebrates*, 3rd ed. Baltimore, Maryland, Williams and Wilkins, 1972.

Bruner, D. W., and J. N. Gillespie. *Hagan's Infectious Diseases of Domestic Animals*, 6th ed. Ithaca and London, Cornell University Press, 1973.

Calisher, C. H., J. K. Emerson, D. J. Muth, J. S. Lazuick, and T. P. Monath. Serodiagnosis of western equine encephalitis virus infections: relationship of antibody titer and test to observed onset of clinical illness. *J Am Vet Med Assoc* 183:438-440, 1983.

Calisher, C. H., M. I. Mahmud, A. D. el-Kafrawi, J. K. Emerson, and D. J. Muth. Rapid and specific serodiagnosis of western equine encephalitis virus infection in horses. *Am J Vet Res* 47:1296-1299, 1986.

Calisher, C. H., T. P. Monath, C. J. Mitchell, M. S. Sabattini, C. B. Cropp, J. Kerschner, A. R. Hunt, and J. S. Lazvick. Arbovirus investigations in Argentina, 1977-1980. III. Identification and characterization of virus isolated, including new subtypes of western and Venezuelan equine encephalitis viruses and four new bunyaviruses (Las Mayolas, Resistencia, Barranqueras and Antequera). *Am J Trop Med Hyg* 34:956-965, 1985.

Casals, J., and D. H. Clarke. Arboviruses: Group A. *In*: Horsfall, F. L., and I. Tamm (Eds.), *Viral and Rickettsial Infections of Man*, 4th ed. Philadelphia, Lippincott, 1975.

Centers for Disease Control of the USA. *Neurotropic Viral Diseases Surveillance. Annual Summary, 1972*. Atlanta, Georgia, 1974. (DHEW Publ. CDC 75-8252.)

Centers for Disease Control of the USA. Current trends in arboviral diseases. United States, August 1974. *Morb Mortal Wkly Rep* 23:293-294, 1974.

Centers for Disease Control of the USA. *International Catalogue of Arboviruses*, 2nd ed. (Ed. by T. O. Berge). Atlanta, Georgia, 1975. (DHEW Publ. CDC 75-8301.)

Centers for Disease Control of the USA. Arboviral infections in the United States. *Morb Mortal Wkly Rep* 25:116, 1976.

Centers for Disease Control of the USA. *Encephalitis Surveillance. Annual Summary 1978*. Atlanta, Georgia, CDC, 1981.

Centers for Disease Control of the USA. Arboviral encephalitis—United States, 1982. *Morb Mortal Wkly Rep* 31:433-435, 1982.

Pan American Zoonoses Center. Informe encefalomielitis (Argentina). *Comunicaciones Epidemiológicas* 3, May 1983.

Chamberlain, R. W. Arbovirus infections of North America. *In*: Sanders, M., and M. Schaeffer (Eds.), *Virus Affecting Man and Animals*. St. Louis, Missouri, Green, 1971.

Downs, W. G. Arboviruses. *In*: A. S. Evans (Ed.), *Viral Infections of Humans. Epidemiology and Control*. New York, Plenum, 1976.

Gebhardt, L. P., S. C. St. Yeor, G. J. Stanton, and D. A. Stringfellow. Ecology of western encephalitis virus. *Proc Soc Exp Biol Med* 142:731-733, 1973.

Gebhardt, L. P., G. J. Stanton, D. W. Hill, and C. Collett. Natural overwintering hosts of the virus of western equine encephalitis. *N Engl J Med* 271:172-177, 1964.

Gutekunst, D. E., M. J. Martin, and P. H. Langer. Immunization against equine encephalomyelitis with a new tissue culture origin vaccine. *Vet Med* 61:348-351, 1966.

Hardy, J. L., W. C. Reeves, W. A. Rush, and Y. D. Nir. Experimental infection with western encephalomyelitis virus in wild rodents indigenous to Kern County, California. *Infect Immun* 10:553-564, 1974.

Hardy, J. L., W. C. Reeves, J. P. Bruen, and S. B. Presser. Vector competence of *Culex tarsalis* and other mosquito species for western equine encephalomyelitis virus. *In*: Kurstak, E. (Ed.), *Arctic and Tropical Arboviruses*. New York, Academic Press, 1979.

Hayes, R. O., L. C. Lamotte, and P. Holden. Ecology of arboviruses in Hale County, Texas, during 1965. *Am J Trop Med Hyg* 16:675-687, 1967.

Hayes, C. G., and R. C. Wallis. Ecology of western equine encephalomyelitis in the eastern United States. *Adv Virus Res* 21:37-83, 1977.

Holden, P., R. O. Hayes, C. J. Mitchell, D. B. Francy, J. S. Laznick, and T. B. Hughes. House sparrows, *Passer domesticus* (L.), as hosts of arboviruses in Hale County, Texas. I. Field studies, 1965-1969. *Am J Trop Med Hyg* 22:244-253, 1973.

Hughes, J. P., and H. N. Johnson. A field trial of a live-virus western encephalitis vaccine. *J Am Vet Med Assoc* 150:167-171, 1967.

Monath, T. P. Arthropod-borne encephalitides in the Americas. *Bull WHO* 57:513-533, 1979.

Monath, T. P., M. S. Sabattini, R. Pauli, J. F. Daffner, C. J. Mitchell, G. S. Bowen, and C. B. Cropp. Arbovirus investigations in Argentina, 1977-1980. IV. Serologic surveys and sentinel equine program. *Am J Trop Med Hyg* 34:966-975, 1985.

Monath, T. P., and D. W. Trent. Togaviral diseases of domestic animals. *In*: Kurstak, F., and C. Kurstak (Eds.), *Comparative Diagnosis of Viral Diseases*. New York, Academic Press, 1981.

Sirivanakarn, S., and W. L Jakob. Notes on the distribution of *Culex* (*Melanoconion*) mosquitoes in northeastern Argentina (Diptera: Culicidae). *Mosquito Syst* 13:195-200, 1981.

Theiler, M., and W. G. Downs. *The Arthropod-Borne Viruses of Vertebrates*. New Haven and London, Yale University Press, 1973.

Work, T. H. Western equine encephalomyelitis. *In*: Beeson, P. B., W. McDermott, and J. B. Wyngaarden (Eds.), *Cecil Textbook of Medicine*, 15th ed. Philadelphia and London, Saunders, 1967.

WEST NILE FEVER

(066.3)

Etiology: RNA genome virus, genus *Flavivirus*, family Togaviridae; forms part of the complex of the St. Louis, Murray Valley, Japanese B, and Rocio encephalitides viruses.

Geographic Distribution: The virus has been isolated from man, other mammals, birds, and arthropods in Africa (Egypt, Uganda, Zaire, Mozambique, Central African Republic, Nigeria, and South Africa), in Asia (Israel, India, Pakistan, Borneo, and the USSR), and in Europe (France and Cyprus). Moreover, serologic evidence (serum neutralization) suggests that the infection is present in practically all of the African continent and in Thailand, the Philippines, Malaysia, Turkey, and Albania.

Occurrence: West Nile fever (WNF) is endemic and epidemic. In hyperendemic areas, infection occurs at an early age and the majority of the adult population is immune. In regions where the virus is less active, occasional epidemics occur among persons of all ages (Tesh, 1982). The disease is endemic in the Nile Delta where it primarily affects children. In Israel, it occurs in epidemic form and clinical disease is observed in a large number of persons. In South Africa, the disease is sporadic, with some small epidemic outbreaks occurring regularly during the summer. In 1974, in the Karroo region and the northern part of Cape of Good Hope Province, South Africa, the largest ever epidemic of WNF occurred concurrently with Sindbis fever. The serologic study carried out after the epidemic revealed that 55% of the population of the area had been infected by WNF virus and 16% by Sindbis (McIntosh *et al.*, 1976). In serologic studies using the serum agglutination test, high reactor rates have been found among human populations of some endemic areas. Of 1,168 human serum samples obtained in an endemic region of the Nile Delta in Egypt, 61% contained neutralizing antibodies for the disease virus (Taylor *et al.*, 1956). The virus has been isolated from several species of birds, horses, camels, and a bat. High reactor rates to the neutralization test have been found in horses (183 out of 375 examined in Egypt), nonhuman primates, and bovines.

The Disease in Man: Infection in man can be subclinical or the symptomatology can vary in severity from temporary fever to serious encephalitis. The disease is generally mild in children and more severe in the elderly. The incubation period is from 3 to 6 days. Onset of disease is sudden, with fever, cephalalgia, lymphadenopathy, and a cutaneous maculopapular eruption mainly on the trunk. Other symptoms that sometimes occur are ocular, muscular, and articular pains and gastrointestinal upset. Less frequently there is myocarditis, meningitis, and encephalitis. Mortality is insignificant. Viremia in humans is low-level and lasts about 6 days. The disease occurs during summer when mosquitoes are abundant.

The Disease in Animals: Among domestic animals, clinical manifestations have been observed only in horses, but even in this species most infections are asymptomatic. The characteristic picture is that of meningoencephalitis. A WNF outbreak in 1962-1964 in La Camargue, France, caused 10% morbidity and a fatality rate of 25%.

Little is known about the course of infection in birds. The mortality rate was high in crows (*Corvus corone sardonius*) infected experimentally by mosquito bites. In nature, many of these birds have neutralizing antibodies, indicating that a large number survive infection. Other species of birds probably fall ill because of this virus, as evidenced by a domestic pigeon captured in Egypt which had clinical symptoms and from which the etiologic agent was isolated (Taylor *et al.*, 1965).

Source of Infection and Mode of Transmission (Figure 55): Virus of this disease infects a large number of vertebrate hosts, among them man, domestic animals, and several species of fowl. Only birds meet the criteria for a reservoir, since they have a high-titer and prolonged viremia that would enable them to serve as a source of infection for the arthropod vector. Moreover, in areas where the virus is found, many birds reproduce at a sufficient rate to provide enough susceptible young to maintain an infection cycle. The virus has been isolated from pigeons (*Columba livia*), from a species of crow (*Corvus corone sardonius*) in Egypt, from *Sylvietta rufescens* in South Africa, and from turtledoves (*Streptopelia turtur*) in Israel. The virus has also been isolated from wild birds in Borneo, Cyprus, and Nigeria. The presence of neutralizing antibodies has been demonstrated in various other countries.

Ornithophilic mosquitoes of the genus *Culex* act as the vector, becoming infected by feeding on blood from a viremic bird and transmitting the infection by biting a susceptible host, either bird or mammal. Virus has been isolated from several species of *Culex*, but *C. univittatus* undoubtedly plays a primary role in the transmission of infection and in maintaining the circulation of the virus in nature in

Figure 55. West Nile fever. Transmission cycle.

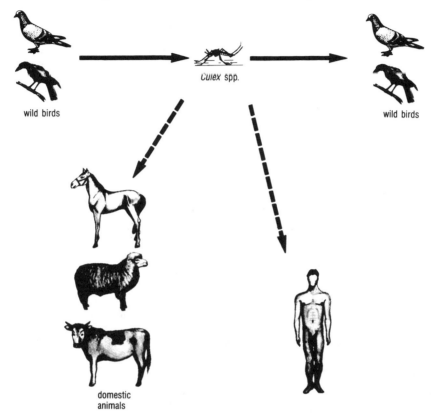

wild birds   *Culex* spp.   wild birds

domestic
animals

Egypt, Israel, and South Africa. In other areas, the main vector has not yet been positively identified. The *vishnui* complex seems to be important in India. In La Camargue, France, the role of vector is attributed to *C. modestus*.

As yet, the manner in which the virus is maintained during winter is not fully understood. It is thought that the mechanism consists of delayed transmission by mosquitoes that remain active during the cold months. Some female *C. univittatus* have been found feeding in winter on occasional warm days, and virus has been isolated from sentinel pigeons during the same season.

Role of Animals in the Epidemiology of the Disease: WNF is a zoonosis transmitted from birds to man and other mammals by means of mosquitoes of the genus *Culex*. Man, horses, sheep, and cattle are only accidental hosts of the virus and are not involved in the basic cycle of the agent. Viremia in horses, sheep, and cattle is low-level (it may even be absent in cattle) and is incapable of infecting a vector.

Diagnosis: Laboratory confirmation is through isolation of virus by inoculating mice with blood obtained from patients during the acute phase of disease, or through demonstrating serologic conversion, primarily by means of the neutralization test.

Control: A mixed vaccine to prevent human infection with the WNF virus and other group B arboviruses is in an experimental stage.

At present, control of the vector is difficult, since the species of mosquitoes that transmit the infection to man in different countries are not well known and *Culex* mosquitoes are ornithophilic, but not always anthropophilic. In some countries it is likely that there is a vector that serves as a link between the wild cycle and infection in man. In that case, controlling the population of this connecting vector would be the most logical measure.

Bibliography

Andrewes, C., and H. G. Pereira. *Viruses of Vertebrates*, 3rd ed. Baltimore, Maryland, Williams and Wilkins, 1972.

Centers for Disease Control of the USA. *International Catalogue of Arboviruses*, 2nd ed. (Ed. by T. O. Berge). Atlanta, Georgia, 1975. (DHEW Publ. CDC 75-8301.)

Clarke, D. H., and J. Casals. Arboviruses: Group B. *In*: Horsfall, F. L., and I. Tamm (Eds.), *Viral and Rickettsial Infections of Man*, 4th ed. Philadelphia, Lippincott, 1965.

Goldblum, N. Group B. Arthropod-borne viral diseases. *In*: Van der Hoeden, J. (Ed.), *Zoonoses*. Amsterdam, Elsevier, 1964.

Jouber, L., and J. Oudart. La meningoencefalitis equina por el virus del Nilo occidental en la zona mediterránea de Francia. *Bull Soc Sci Vet Med Comp* 76:255, 1974. Summary *Sel Vet* 16:675, 1975.

McIntosh, B. M., and J. H. S. Gear. Mosquito-borne arboviruses, primarily in the eastern hemisphere. *In*: Hubbert, W. T., W. F. McCulloch, and P. R. Schnurrenberger (Eds.), *Diseases Transmitted from Animals to Man*, 6th ed. Springfield, Illinois, Thomas, 1975.

McIntosh, B. M., P. G. Jupp, I. Dos Santos, and G. M. Meenehan. Epidemics of West Nile and Sindbis viruses in South Africa with *Culex univittatus* Theobald as vector. *S Afr J Sci* 72:295-300, 1976.

Nir, Y., R. Golwasser, Y. Lasowski, and A. Avivi. Isolation of arboviruses from wild birds in Israel. *Am J Epidemiol* 86:372-378, 1967.

Taylor, R. M., T. H. Work, H. S. Hurblut, and F. Rizk. A study of the ecology of West Nile virus in Egypt. *Am J Trop Med Hyg* 5:579-620, 1956.

Tesh, R. B. West Nile fever. *In*: Wyngaarden, J. B., and L. H. Smith (Eds.), *Cecil Textbook of Medicine*, vol. 2, 16th ed. Philadelphia, Saunders, 1982.

YELLOW FEVER

(060)

Synonym: Black vomit.

Etiology: RNA genome virus, genus *Flavivirus* (formerly group B of the arboviruses), family Togaviridae; forms part of the complex of mosquito-borne viruses. There is an antigenic difference between the African and American strains.

Geographic Distribution: Yellow fever has never been found outside Africa and America. In the past, urban yellow fever (UYF), transmitted between humans by *Aedes aegypti*, afflicted the American population from the eastern United States to Argentina. Currently, infection in the Americas is limited to an exclusively jungle cycle, while in Africa it also occurs in urban areas. The infection exists enzootically in jungles, circulating between monkeys (and probably other mammals) and mosquitoes. In Latin America, the areas of greatest activity of the jungle virus are the basins of the Amazon, Orinoco, and Magdalena rivers, and also the Brazilian areas of Ilhéus (in the northeast) and Mato Grosso. The endemic zone in Africa lies between latitudes 16°N and 10°S. The annual incidence of cases is characterized by larger outbreaks than in the Americas with no predictable periodicity or localization. Urban-type yellow fever outbreaks transmitted by *A. aegypti* have been notified in rural areas on several occasions, but no large center has been hit since 1946 (World Health Organization, 1986).

Jungle yellow fever (JYF) is in continuous movement within its enzootic areas or ecologic niches. Under favorable conditions the infection spreads from permanent foci to adjacent areas by means of nonhuman primates and mosquitoes. An epizootic wave that began in 1950 spread from the Isthmus of Panama to the border between Guatemala and Mexico—the northern limit of the nonhuman primate hosts of the virus. Cases have also occurred at various times in northern Argentina. In the Americas, no outbreaks of UYF transmitted by *A. aegypti* have occurred since 1942, with the exception of a few cases recorded in 1954 in Trinidad. Nevertheless, almost every year human cases of JYF are recorded in different South American countries.

The only countries in which cases of JYF have not been observed since this epidemiologic variety was confirmed are Chile, El Salvador, and Uruguay.

Occurrence in Man and Animals (Maps 6, 7, and 8; Figure 56): In the Americas, 710 cases were reported in the period between 1975 and 1980. In 1981-1982, Bolivia, Brazil, Colombia, Ecuador, and Peru reported a total of 368 cases with 183 deaths. With the exception of an epidemic in 1981 in Rincón del Tigre, Santa Cruz, Bolivia, all other cases in the biennium occurred in the known endemic zones.

JYF is mainly an occupational disease of males (farmers, rubber plantation workers, hunters, forestry workers, and public road workers) whose work brings them into jungles or neighboring areas. In the 1972-1973 epidemic in the state of Goiás, Brazil, with 71 confirmed cases and 44 deaths, the ratio of men to women affected was 9 to 1 (Pinheiro *et al.*, 1978). In general, the population indigenous to an enzootic region is less affected than workers who come from regions free of the

Map 6. Epidemiologic patterns of yellow fever in ecologic zones of the Americas and Africa.

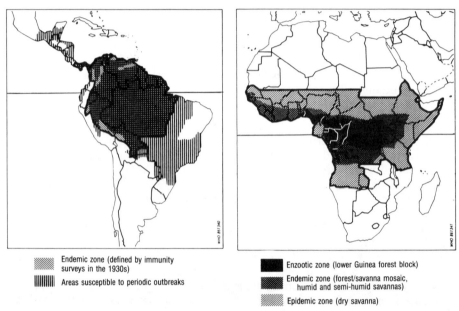

Endemic zone (defined by immunity surveys in the 1930s)

Areas susceptible to periodic outbreaks

Enzootic zone (lower Guinea forest block)

Endemic zone (forest/savanna mosaic, humid and semi-humid savannas)

Epidemic zone (dry savanna)

Source: Brès, P. L. J. *Bull WHO* 64(6):779, 1986.

disease. The 20-to-39-year-old age group is the most affected. Most cases occur during the rainy season, when the population density of the mosquito *Haemagogus*, the main vector of JYF in the Americas, is highest.

Serologic studies carried out among residents of jungle regions reveal a high reactor rate for group B arboviruses, which includes the yellow fever virus. Colonization programs in the jungle areas of Latin America will expose new human populations to the infection.

Urban yellow fever has disappeared from the Americas, but the danger of epidemics of this type will persist as long as its vector, *A. aegypti*, has not been completely eradicated. This mosquito's habitat in that hemisphere is domestic and peridomestic. The campaign against *A. aegypti* began in 1947, and by 1960 the mosquito was successfully eradicated from 80% of the infested area, or nearly 12 million km². Lamentably, implementation of the campaign has suffered a setback and several areas have become reinfested. Epidemics of dengue, also transmitted by *A. aegypti*, occurred in 1963, 1969, 1977, and 1981 (see Dengue). Studies have revealed high densities of the mosquito in several areas, which signals the danger of possible UYF epidemics if the virus of this disease were transported from the jungle to the urban habitat.

In the Americas, the UYF cycle develops between *A. aegypti*-man-*A. aegypti*. Four factors are thought to determine the risk of extension of the jungle cycle to cities: a) the titer and duration of viremia in man; b) the population density of *A. aegypti* and its competence as a vector; c) the frequency of exposure of the vector to viremic patients in urban areas; and d) the immunity level of the urban population

(Woodall, 1981). It has been suggested that patients are brought to a city for hospitalization when the viremic period has already passed or the viremia has lowered to a level insufficient to infect the vector and originate an urban cycle. It is also suspected that the high prevalence of antibodies for other flaviviruses, especially for dengue, could be a factor that prevents urban diffusion of yellow fever. In reality, the conditions governing the urbanization of JYF are still not well known (Groot, 1980) and, faced with such lack of knowledge, precautionary measures are advisable. As a result of an outbreak in jungle areas of Trinidad in 1978-1979, with 10 cases and 5 deaths, extensive vaccination was begun and 96.4% of the population of the island older than 1 year of age was immunized (Centers for Disease Control of the USA, 1980; Pan American Health Organization, 1983).

The pattern of jungle yellow fever outbreaks is different in East and West Africa. East Africa was included in the endemic zone after serologic surveys in the 1930s, but is usually a "silent zone" owing to the absence of notified cases, except on two occasions when very severe epidemics occurred. The first one caused 40,000 infections, more than 15,000 clinical cases, and 1,500 deaths in the Nuba mountains of Sudan in 1940; the second, in southwest Ethiopia in 1960-1962, is the most severe outbreak ever known, with 30,000 deaths among 100,000 cases in a rural population of one million. Outbreaks of jungle yellow fever are more frequent in West Africa than in East Africa. Severe outbreaks occurred recently in Ghana and Burkina Faso in 1983. Two unvaccinated French tourists, who together visited the endemic zone of Senegal in 1979, died in different intensive care units in Paris. The etiology was clinically unsuspected and remained unknown until the virus was

Map 7. Cases of jungle yellow fever in the Americas, 1981-1982.

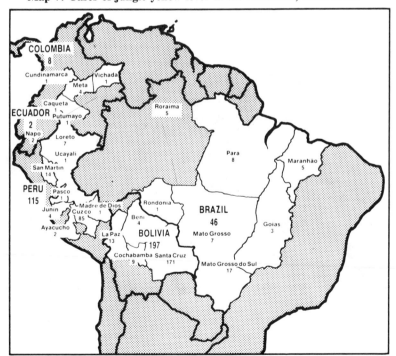

Map 8. Endemic areas of yellow fever in the Americas, 1981 and 1982.

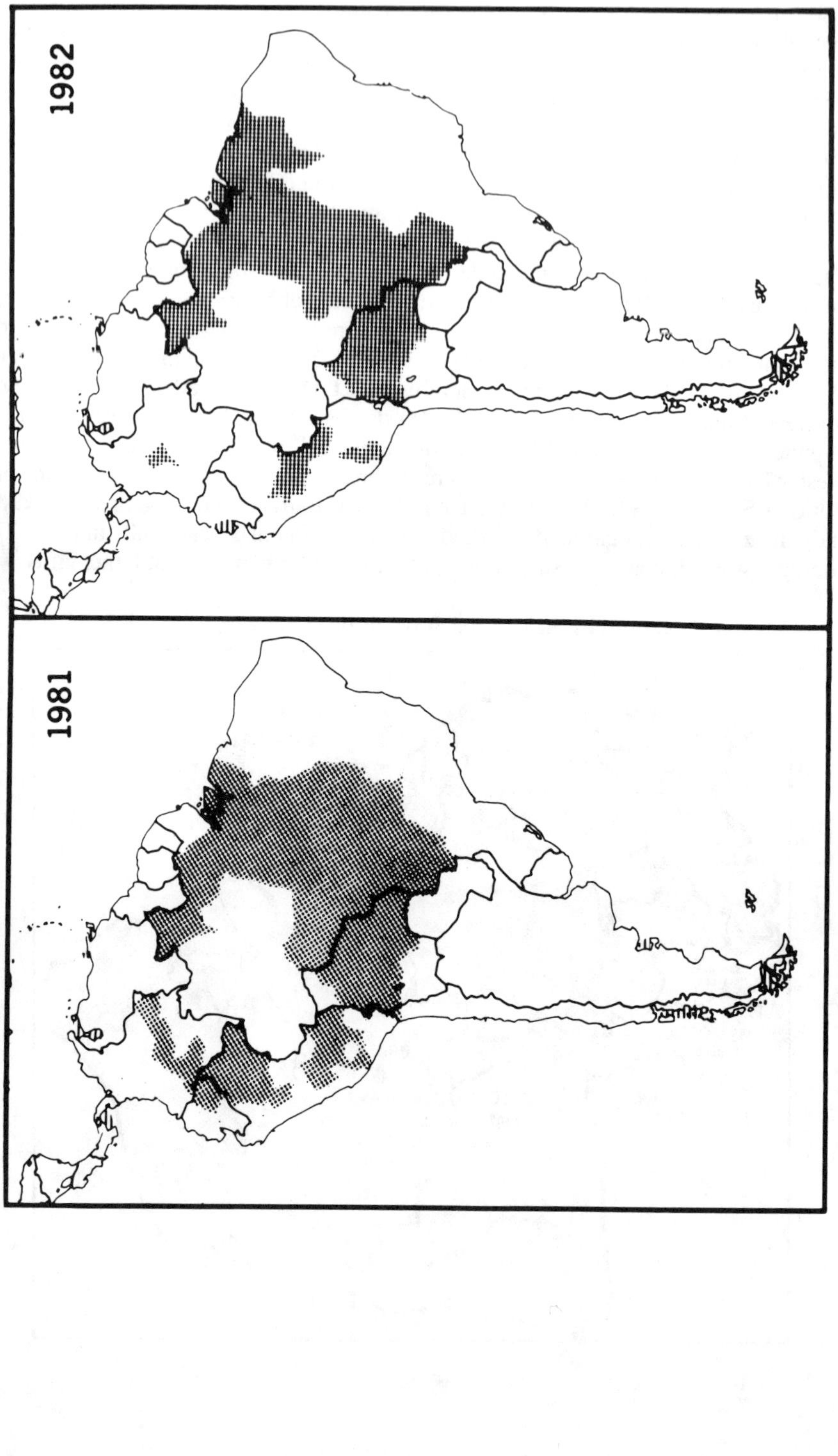

Source: PAHO Epidemiol Bull 4(1):3, 1983.

Figure 56. Monthly average of yellow fever cases in the Americas, 1981-1982.

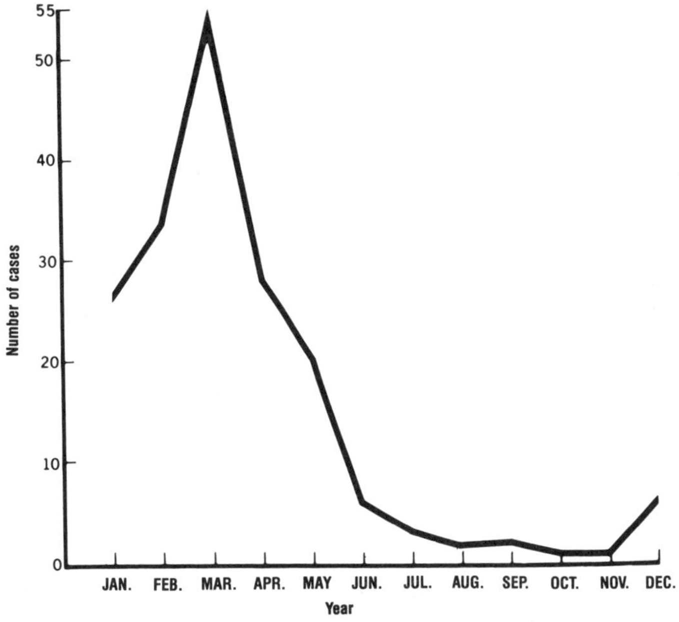

Source: PAHO Epidemiol Bull 4(1):3, 1983.

isolated after the patients died. Sporadic cases of jungle yellow fever are usually missed, either because they are generally mild or because of inadequate surveillance (Brès, 1986).

The frequency of the disease in monkeys is difficult to determine. Virus activity in Latin American forests often results in a high mortality rate in howler monkeys (*Alouatta*). Serologic studies carried out in certain enzootic areas in Africa have shown a high serologic reactor rate in different species of nonhuman primates.

The Disease in Man: The infection in man varies from clinically inapparent to a serious and potentially fatal disease. Serologic studies in Latin America have revealed reactor rates to the serum neutralization test as high as 90% of the population in enzootic areas. The incubation period is from 3 to 6 days following the bite of an infected mosquito. Mild cases present an indefinite clinical picture, difficult to distinguish from other common febrile conditions; serious cases, on the other hand, show a distinctive clinical picture. The onset of the disease is sudden, with high fever, cephalalgia, dorsalgia, chills, prostration, nausea, and vomiting. The fever is often diphasic: the first phase lasts some 3 to 4 days; the fever then subsides temporarily but returns in the second phase. This latter phase is characterized by hepatic and renal insufficiency and by a tendency toward hemorrhages. As the disease advances, the pulse rate decreases in relation to the temperature, and the patient becomes hypotensive. The patient develops epistaxis and oral and gastrointestinal hemorrhages with hematemesis ("black vomit") and melena. In addition to hemorrhages that perhaps are due to the liver's inability to synthesize sufficient quantities of coagulating factors, the hepatic disorder is manifested in varying degrees of jaundice—hence the name of the disease. Nevertheless, jaundice is not a constant symptom of yellow fever. Renal decompensation is marked by albuminuria and, sometimes, by serious renal insufficiency with concomitant oliguria and azotemia. In fulminating cases the patient dies between the third and seventh day. If the illness lasts beyond 10 days, the chance of recovery improves. In autochthonous populations within endemic areas, the fatality rate is less than 5%.

Viremia occurs during the first 4 days of the disease.

Anatomopathologic signs of yellow fever are not particularly characteristic. Jaundice, sometimes slight, may be seen, as well as hemorrhagic lesions in various organs. Histopathology reveals the most characteristic alterations. The hepatic lesions consist of splotchy necrosis of the central zones, acidophilic degeneration, and fatty metamorphosis. The lesions produced by acidophilic or eosinophilic degeneration of the infected hepatocytes, which are typical but not pathognomonic of yellow fever, are called Councilman bodies.

The Disease in Animals: Jungle yellow fever is a zoonotic infection that circulates in the rain forests of the Americas and Africa between nonhuman primates and mosquitoes.

Knowledge of the symptomatology and pathology of the disease in nonhuman primates is based on experimental exposure. Different species of primates show different degrees of susceptibility. A notable difference is observed between the susceptibility of African and American monkeys: while African primates (*Cercopithecus, Colobus, Erythrocebus, Papio*) are infected but rarely die as a result of experimental inoculation, the monkeys of various American species die a few days after contracting the disease. It is believed that this difference is due to long-term adaptation of the virus to African monkeys. In the Americas the infection is of much more recent origin and seems to have been introduced by *A. aegypti* from Africa. Experimental studies indicate that there are six genera of neotropical monkeys susceptible to the yellow fever virus: *Aotus* (owl or night monkey), *Alouatta* (howler monkey), *Cebus* (capuchin or white monkey), *Ateles* (spider monkey), *Callithrix* (marmoset), and *Saimiri* (squirrel monkey). These monkeys play different roles in the jungle cycle of yellow fever. The course of the infection in the howler and spider monkeys is almost always fatal. The *Macaca* monkeys of Asian origin are susceptible, but they are not natural hosts since there is no yellow fever in Asia.

The symptomatology and pathology of yellow fever are similar in monkeys and man.

Source of Infection and Mode of Transmission (Figure 57): Yellow fever occurs in two epidemiologic varieties, urban and jungle. It is very likely that urban yellow fever originated from the jungle cycle. The only known host of the urban variety is man, and the disease is transmitted by a biological vector, *A. aegypti*. The mosquito acquires the infection by biting the human host during the viremic phase and transmits the infection to another susceptible person after 10 to 12 days of extrinsic[1] incubation.

---

[1] In the majority of the diseases transmitted by arthropods, there are two periods of incubation: extrinsic and intrinsic. The extrinsic incubation period occurs in the biologic vector; during this time, the etiologic agent multiplies and/or transforms until it becomes infective and transmissible to the host. The intrinsic incubation period refers to the time interval between penetration of the host organism by the agent and the appearance of disease symptoms.

Figure 57. Jungle yellow fever in the Americas. Transmission cycle.

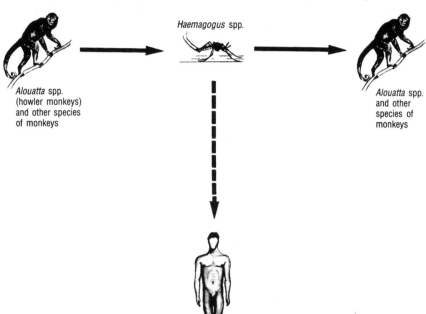

JYF, by contrast, is a zoonotic disease whose main hosts are monkeys, man being only an accidental host. The virus circulates in tropical rain forests and is transmitted from one host to another by the bite of infected mosquitoes. The urban and jungle cycles are independent and self-sufficient, but the infection can be transferred from one cycle to another when conditions are favorable.

The disease differs in several epidemiologic and ecologic aspects between Latin America and Africa. In Latin America, the primary vectors of the virus are mosquitoes of the genus *Haemagogus* (especially *H. janthinomys* and *H. spegazzini*), which live in jungle treetops. Several species of this genus are diurnal and descend to ground level in forest areas that have been cleared of trees. Tree felling is an activity that especially encourages contact between these mosquitoes and man. The range of *H. spegazzini* extends from northern Honduras to southern Ecuador. The mosquitoes *Aedes leucocelaenus* and *Sabethes chloropterus* have also been found to be naturally infected, but they are thought to play only a secondary role. *S. chloropterus* is resistant to drought and could provide the biological mechanism for the virus's survival during the dry season.

Knowledge of the animal reservoir of the virus is still incomplete. A primary role in maintaining the virus in the jungle environment is attributed to the howler monkey. These monkeys are very susceptible to the virus and die in large numbers during epizootics. The absence of their characteristic howling is a warning sign of virus activity in the jungle. One infected monkey may serve as a source of infection for many mosquitoes in a tree. The infection can be transmitted from one group of monkeys to another group in a contiguous territory, or it can be carried a greater distance by infected mosquitoes transported on air currents. However, because of the great susceptibility and mortality of howler monkeys, partially resistant monkeys, such as capuchins (*Cebus*), probably play an important role as reservoirs. Apparently, other susceptible monkeys are less important because of their distribution and habits.

In some regions where sporadic human cases occur but where the monkey population is insufficient to maintain the jungle cycle, some small arboreal mammals, among them marsupials, kinkajous, and olingos, might be involved in the epizootiology of the disease (Strano *et al.*, 1975). The high rate of serologic reactors that has been found among marsupials suggests that they may participate in the circulation of the virus, but their role has not been established (Woodall, 1981).

Man contracts the infection accidentally, from the bite of infected *Haemagogus*, when he goes into an area where the monkey-mosquito-monkey cycle exists.

In eastern and central Africa the main vector of the jungle cycle is *Aedes africanus*, a mosquito which lives in treetops and spreads the virus in the monkey population. Infected monkeys carry the virus to cultivated areas adjoining the forest, such as banana plantations. There it is transmitted from primates to man by *Aedes simpsoni*, which inhabits the vegetation around houses. The epidemic which occurred in southwest Ethiopia in 1960-1962, with 100,000 cases and 30,000 deaths among the million inhabitants of the region, was preceded by an epizootic in the jungle that developed between monkeys and *A. africanus*. Baboons (*Papio* spp.) carried the infection to banana plantations and infected *A. simpsoni*, which in turn transmitted the infection to man; there was also possibly a secondary mosquito-man-mosquito cycle. If *A. aegypti* is present in the locality, a man-*A. aegypti*-man cycle can be created.

In other regions of Africa, *A. simpsoni* is usually not anthropophilic, and it is suspected that *A. africanus* can transmit the virus directly from monkey to man.

The epidemics that have occurred in recent years in Africa have stimulated investigation of the survival mechanism of the virus during interepidemic periods. Numerous virus strains have been isolated from *A. africanus*, *A. opok*, *A. furcifer*, *A. taylori*, and *A. luteocephalus*, during interepidemic periods. Transovarial transmission in *A. aegypti*, *A. furcifer*, and *A. taylori* has been confirmed, and the virus has been isolated from eggs and adults of the cattle tick *Amblyomma variegatum*. Although these findings may explain the survival of the virus during the dry season, their real significance is still unknown. Transovarial transmission is infrequent and, when it does occur, is exhausted by the fourth ovarial cycle; this would indicate the necessity for virus amplification in vertebrate animals.

The main yellow fever hosts in Africa are green monkeys (*Cercopithecus* spp.), red monkeys (*Erythrocebus patas*), baboons (*Papio* spp.), leaf-eating monkeys (*Colobus* spp.), and *Galago* spp. (Seymour and Yuill, 1981).

Role of Animals in the Epidemiology of the Disease (Table 9): Jungle yellow fever is an infection of wild animals, chiefly nonhuman primates. Man is an accidental host. When conditions are favorable, the jungle cycle can give rise to an urban cycle in which man is the main host and *A. aegypti* the vector.

Diagnosis: Laboratory confirmation is obtained by isolation of the virus or by serologic tests. Virus isolation is the quickest and most reliable process. This method uses blood samples taken from the patient during the first 3 or 4 days of the

Table 9. Nonhuman primates and mosquitoes involved in regional transmission cycles of yellow fever.

Region and cycle	Nonhuman primates	Mosquitoes
Americas		
Enzootic forest cycle	*Alouatta* *Aotus* *Cebus* *Ateles* *Callithrix* *Saimiri*	*Haemagogus janthinomys* *H. spegazzini*
Jungle yellow fever	As above	*H. janthinomys* *Aedes leucocaelenus* *Sabethes chloropterus*
Urban yellow fever (before 1942)	Nil	*A. aegypti*
Africa		
Enzootic forest cycle	*Cercopithecus* *Colobus* (East Afr.)	*A. africanus*
Jungle yellow fever in forest-savanna mosaic and humid savanna	*Cercopithecus*	*A. africanus* *A. simpsoni* (East Afr.) *A. opok* (West Afr.)
Jungle yellow fever in a semi-humid and dry savanna	*Cercopithecus* *Erythrocebus* *Papio* *Galago*	*A. furcifer* *A. taylori* *A. luteocephalus* *A. vittatus* *A. metallicus*
Urban yellow fever	Nil	*A. aegypti*

Source: Adapted from P. L. J. Brès, *Bull WHO*, 64(6):779, 1986.

disease. The virus can be isolated in cell culture, in mice, or in rhesus monkeys. An enzymatic immunoassay (ELISA) test has been perfected to detect the virus in serum samples, using type-specific monoclonal antibodies or human serum with high titers of IgM antibodies against yellow fever virus. The process was evaluated in viremic monkeys with satisfactory results (Monath and Nystrom, 1984). Serologic examination can be done by means of the hemagglutination inhibition (HI), neutralization (N), complement fixation (CF), indirect immunofluorescence (IIF), and, recently, ELISA tests. This last test gives results comparable to the neutralization test and is more sensitive and specific than the hemagglutination inhibition and complement fixation tests (Deubel *et al.*, 1983). Antibodies for HI and N appear about 5 days after the beginning of the disease and reach maximum titers 3 to 4 weeks later. Diagnosis is based on confirmation of a significant increase between acute and convalescent serum titers.

Histopathologic examination of material from deceased persons is important for epidemiologic surveillance.

Control: The principal measure for preventing JYF is vaccination of persons who enter or live in enzootic areas. The 17D chick embryo vaccine is preferred. It is a lyophilized attenuated live virus vaccine and confers very long-lasting protection. Revaccination is recommended every 10 years. Of special importance in the Americas is the eradication of *A. aegypti* from areas still infested and the maintenance of ongoing surveillance in regions from which this vector has been eradicated.

Bibliography

American Public Health Association. *Control of Communicable Diseases in Man*, 14th ed. (Ed. by A. S. Benenson). Washington, D.C., APHA, 1985.

Brès, P. L. J. A century of progress in combating yellow fever. *Bull WHO* 64(6):775-786, 1986.

Centers for Disease Control of the USA. *Morb Mortal Wkly Rep* 22:326, 1973.

Centers for Disease Control of the USA. Follow-up on yellow fever—Trinidad. *Morb Mortal Wkly Rep* 29:52, 1980.

Clark, D. H., and J. Casals. Arboviruses: Group B. *In*: Horsfall, F. L., and I. Tamm (Eds.), *Viral and Rickettsial Infections of Man*, 4th ed. Philadelphia, Lippincott, 1965.

Deubel, V., V. Mouly, J. J. Salaun, C. Adam, M. M. Diop, and J. P. Digoutte. Comparison of the enzyme-linked immunosorbent assay (ELISA) with standard tests used to detect yellow fever virus antibodies. *Am J Trop Med Hyg* 32:565-568, 1983.

Groot, H. The reinvasion of Colombia by *Aedes aegypti:* aspects to remember. *Am J Trop Med Hyg* 29:330-338, 1980.

Johnson, K. M. Yellow fever. *In*: Hubbert, W. T., W. F. McCulloch, and P. R. Schnurrenberger (Eds.), *Diseases Transmitted from Animals to Man*, 6th ed. Springfield, Illinois, Thomas, 1975.

Kerr, J. A. (Revised by Downs, W. S.). Yellow fever. *In: Practice of Medicine*. Hagerstown, Maryland, Harper and Row, 1975.

Monath, T. P., and R. R. Nystrom. Detection of yellow fever virus in serum by enzyme immunoassay. *Am J Trop Med Hyg* 33:151-157, 1984.

Monath, T. P. Yellow Fever. *In*: Warren, K. S., and A. A. F. Mahmoud (Eds.), *Tropical and Geographical Medicine*. New York, McGraw-Hill Book Company, 1984.

Munz, E. Afrikanisch virusbedingte Zoonosen. *Munch Med Wochenschr* 115:1-9, 1973.

Pan American Health Organization. *Quadrennial Report of the Director, 1978-1981*. Washington, D.C., 1982. (Official Document 131.)

Pan American Health Organization. Primera Reunión del Comité Científico Asesor de la OPS sobre Dengue, Fiebre Amarilla y *Aedes aegypti*, Panamá, marzo de 1976. Document presented at the XXIV Meeting of the PAHO Directing Council, Mexico, D. F., September-October 1976.

Pan American Health Organization. Fiebre amarilla selvática. *Inf Epidemiol Sem* 48: 140-141, 1976.

Pan American Health Organization. Yellow fever in the Americas, 1981-1982. *Epidemiol Bull* 4(1):1-5, 1983.

Pan American Health Organization. Vaccination against yellow fever in the Americas. *Epidemiol Bull* 4(6):7-11, 1983.

Pinheiro, F. P., A. P. A. Travassos da Rosa, M. A. P. Moraes, J. C. Almeida Neto, S. Carmargo, and J. P. Figueiras. An epidemic of yellow fever in central Brazil, 1972-1973. *Am J Trop Med Hyg* 27:125-132, 1978.

Prías-Landínez, E., C. Bernal-Cúbides, S. V. de Torres, and M. Romero-León. Encuesta serológica de virus transmitidos por antrópodos. *Bol Of Sanit Panam* 68:134-141, 1970.

Ruch, T. C. *Diseases of Laboratory Primates*. Saunders, Philadelphia and London, 1959.

Seymour, C., and T. M. Yuill. Arboviruses. *In*: Davis, J. W., L. H. Karstad, and D. O. Trainer (Eds.), *Infectious Diseases of Wild Mammals*, 2nd ed. Ames, Iowa State University Press, 1981.

Strano, A. J., J. R. Dooley, and K. G. Ishak. *Syllabus—Yellow Fever and Its Histopathologic Differential Diagnosis*. Washington, D.C., American Registry of Pathology, Armed Forces Institute of Pathology, 1974.

Trapido, H., and P. Galindo. Parasitological reviews: the epidemiology of yellow fever in Middle America. *Exp Parasitol* 5:285-323, 1956.

Woodall, J. P. Summary of a symposium on yellow fever. *J Infect Dis* 144:87-91, 1981.

World Health Organization. Yellow fever in Africa. *WHO Chronicle* 21:460-463, 1967.

World Health Organization. *WHO Expert Committee on Yellow Fever. Third Report*. Geneva, WHO, 1971. (Technical Report Series 479.)

World Health Organization. *Prevention and Control of Yellow Fever in Africa*. Geneva, WHA/WHO, 1986.

World Health Organization. Yellow fever. *Wkly Epidemiol Rec* 61(8):59-60, 1986.

SUMMARY OF VIRAL ZOONOSES[1, 2]

Poxvirus group

This group includes members of *Parapoxvirus* and *Orthopoxvirus* and the unclassified tanapox virus. These zoonotic poxviruses cause only sporadic, usually benign, and localized skin infections in man, with no tendency to spread among human beings. In addition to the poxviruses from cattle, sheep, and goats (listed in the table), camelpox and buffalopox are of regional importance and may be transmitted to man. Vaccinia virus protects against cowpox and monkeypox, not against tanapox virus and members of *Parapoxvirus*.

Diagnosis: By clinical history and signs, histopathology, electron microscopy, virus isolation by inoculation of embryonated eggs. Differentiation of viruses by biological properties, serology, and restriction endonuclease analysis of virus genomes by specialized laboratories. Particularly important at present is the differentiation between monkeypox and variola, which share a similar clinical appearance in man. Members of *Parapoxvirus* have a characteristic external coat with thick filaments arranged in regular spiral coils.

Control: In view of the sporadic and benign nature of the poxviruses transmitted from cattle or sheep and goats to man, control is limited to hygienic measures, as well as vaccination of lambs and ewes. Cases of poxvirus infections transmitted from nonhuman primates to man necessitate refined etiological clarifications and epidemiological surveillance.

R	=	Reservoir	
E	=	Epizootiology/epidemiology	
PA	=	Principal animals	
PR	=	Persons at risk	
O	=	Occurrence	
CA	=	Clinical form: animals	
CM	=	Clinical form: man	

Causative agent	Disease		
Parapoxvirus group:			
Bovine pustular stomatitis virus	Bovine pustular stomatitis	R/PA.	Cattle
		E.	Common in young cattle; man rarely infected through skin abrasions.
		O.	Canada, USA, Europe, Kenya, Nigeria, Australia.
		CA.	Papulopustular lesions on skin of muzzle and buccal mucosa in cattle.

[1] See introduction to Summary of Bacterial Zoonoses.
[2] Taken from *Bacterial and Viral Zoonoses. Report of the WHO Expert Committee, with the participation of FAO.* Geneva, WHO, Tech. Rep. Ser. 682, 1982.

		R	=	Reservoir	O	=	Occurrence
		E	=	Epizootiology/epidemiology	CA	=	Clinical form: animals
		PA	=	Principal animals	CM	=	Clinical form: man
		PR	=	Persons at risk			
Causative agent	Disease						

Causative agent	Disease		Epizootiology / animals		Occurrence / clinical form
Parapoxvirus group (cont.)		PR.	Groups I and II.	CM.	Papule progressing to pustule on finger or hand; recovery protracted.
Orf virus	Contagious ecthyma (contagious pustular dermatitis, orf)	R/PA.	Sheep, goats.	O.	Worldwide, wherever sheep are raised.
		E.	Disease of sheep and goats, rarely spreading to man by direct contact.	CA.	Papular, becoming pustular, lesions on lips, mouth, nostrils, eyelids, ears, teats, and udders.
		PR.	Groups I and II.	CM.	Papule progressing to pustule on finger or hand; recovery protracted.
Milkers' nodule virus	Milkers' nodules (pseudocowpox)	R/PA.	Cattle	O.	Sporadic in cattle and man in Europe and USA.
		E.	Lesions on udder in cattle; contact-spread by milkers' hands and milking machines.	CA.	Papular, becoming pustular, lesions on teats; characteristically recur.
		PR.	Groups I and II.	CM.	Papule progressing to pustule on finger or hand; recovery protracted.
Orthopoxvirus group:					
Cowpox virus	Cowpox	R/PA.	Cattle.	O.	Worldwide.
		E.	Infection transmitted during milking; rapid spread from cow to cow and occasionally to man by direct contact.	CA/CM.	Similar to milkers' nodules (see above).
		PR.	Groups I and II.		

Causative agent	Disease	R = Reservoir E = Epizootiology/epidemiology PA = Principal animals PR = Persons at risk	O = Occurrence CA = Clinical form: animals CM = Clinical form: man
Orthopoxvirus group (cont.)			
Monkeypox virus	Monkeypox	R/PA. Unknown, but monkeys and rodents suspected.	O. West and Central Africa.
		E. Cycles of infection among wild animals, occasional transmission to man.	CA. No data on clinical symptoms in nature. In captive colonies and experimentally infected monkeys, there are fever and eruptions (in sequence—papules, vesicles, pustules, scabs).
		PR. Groups III and V.	CM. Similar to symptoms in monkeys.
Vaccinia virus	Vaccinia	R. Cattle, rabbits, and man.	O. Until recently, vaccinia virus was used worldwide as smallpox vaccine.
		E. Cycles of infection between cows and dairymen, especially when unvaccinated. By contrast, newly vaccinated persons can infect animals.	CA. In cattle, as for milkers' nodules (see above); in rabbits, generalized infections.
		PA. Cattle and man.	CM. Localized papulopustular lesions which may become generalized.
		PR. Groups I, II, and V.	
Unclassified group:			
Tanapox virus	Tanapox	R. Unknown.	O. East and Central Africa.
		PA. Wild or domestic animals suspected.	CM. Fever and one or two pustular lesions, lasting up to 6 weeks.
		E. Epidemic and sporadic (endemic) form. Transmission by mosquitoes (?) (*Mansonia* spp.).	
		PR. Groups III and V.	

Herpesvirus group

Human herpesviruses 1 and 2 (herpes simplex viruses) in man and cercopithecid herpesvirus 1 (herpesvirus simiae) in primates cause similar infections in their respective hosts. Latent infections, where the virus persists in cervical nerve ganglia, with periodic recrudescence of lesions, particularly under stress, are common.

The transmission of cercopithecid herpesvirus 1 to man, often by bites, may lead to fatal encephalitis. Human herpesvirus may cause severe generalized infections, involving in particular the respiratory tract in young primates.

Diagnosis: Demonstration by electron microscopy of characteristic virus particles in vesicular lesions. Virus isolation in tissue culture. Serological tests: serum neutralization and complement fixation tests.

Control: Avoid mutual contact, in particular monkey bites. Quarantine monkeys; avoid overcrowding, eliminate monkeys with herpes lesions. Apply strict safety measures in laboratories.

R	=	Reservoir
E	=	Epizootiology/epidemiology
PA	=	Principal animals
PR	=	Persons at risk
O	=	Occurrence
CA	=	Clinical form: animals
CM	=	Clinical form: man

Causative agent	Disease
Herpesvirus group:	
Human herpesvirus	Herpes simplex

R. Man

E. Man-to-man transmission; man infects monkeys by contact.

PA. Transmitted to nonhuman primates.

PR. Not applicable; human exposures predominantly from man.

O. Worldwide.

CA. Severe, highly fatal disease with conjunctivitis, coryza, necrotic plaques and ulcers on the tongue, necrotic hepatitis, pneumonia in young primates.

CM. Lesions anywhere on the skin including genitalia, around or in the oral cavity (gingivostomatitis), the eye (keratitis) and the fingers (whitlow). Severe, highly fatal, sporadic encephalitis. Latent infection is frequent. Recurrent lesions in some individuals.

Causative agent	Disease				
		R = Reservoir		O = Occurrence	
		E = Epizootiology/epidemiology		CA = Clinical form: animals	
		PA = Principal animals		CM = Clinical form: man	
		PR = Persons at risk			
Herpesvirus group (cont.)					
Cercopithecid herpesvirus 1	● Herpesvirus simiae	R/PA.	Rhesus monkey (*Macaca mulatta*) and other Asian *Macaca* species.	O.	Asia
		E.	Rare infection in man, from bites or laboratory contamination with saliva and aerosols.	CA.	Varies from inapparent to mild stomatitis, gingivitis, or conjunctivitis. Infected animals become lifetime latent carriers with recrudescent shedding.
		PR.	Groups IV and V.	CM.	Severe ascending myelitis and encephalitis; mortality about 85%.

Arthropod-borne virus (arbovirus) group

The zoonotic diseases include a large number of arthropod-borne infections where man is often an accidental victim. The *basic cycle* involves arthropods and birds or small mammals (rarely reptiles or amphibians). *Virus amplification* in larger birds or mammals may lead to epidemic outbreaks involving domestic animals and man. The following subgroups are recognized which often cause severe diseases in man or diseases of economic importance in domestic animals.

1. *Togaviruses* (arthropod-borne). These are divided (on the basis of antigenic structure) into:
   (a) *Alphaviruses* (formerly known as group A arboviruses): western equine encephalitis (WEE), eastern equine encephalitis (EEE), Venezuelan equine encephalitis (VEE), and Sindbis, Mayaro, Chikungunya, and Ross River fevers.
   (b) *Flaviviruses*: mosquito-borne—yellow fever, and close antigenic relationship between Japanese encephalitis, Murray Valley encephalitis, St. Louis encephalitis, West Nile fever; tick-borne—tick-borne encephalitis (TBE = Russian spring-summer encephalitis (RSSE) and its European forms), louping-ill, Omsk hemorrhagic fever, Kyasanur Forest disease, Powassan encephalitis.

2. *Bunyaviruses*: California encephalitis, Rift Valley fever, Crimean-Congo hemorrhagic fever, and hemorrhagic fever with renal syndrome.

3. *Orbivirus*: Colorado tick fever.

The basic cycle of infection is adapted to certain vectors and particular ecological conditions, which result in more or less characteristic geographical distribution patterns.

Clinical symptoms in man are those of generalized viremic infections: often biphasic fever, hemorrhages, and meningoencephalomyelitis.

Diagnosis: Mild or subclinical infections in man are often undiagnosed.

Virus isolation has to be performed under conditions which prevent infection of laboratory personnel (by the use of glove boxes or negative pressure laminar flow cabinets). Virus isolation can be performed in suckling mice, embryonated eggs, or cell cultures from blood collected during the acute viremic phase, or from postmortem specimens.

Virus differentiation should be reserved for specialized regional laboratories.

Serological diagnosis can be performed with safety and precision in any well-equipped laboratory by trained technical personnel, depending on the availability of reagents for the viruses of regional importance. It is striking (but not surprising) to note that most information about arboviruses is derived from certain specialized laboratories.

Control: Effective vaccines for man are available against yellow fever, Japanese encephalitis, tick-borne encephalitis, Rift Valley fever, WEE, EEE, VEE, and Murray Valley encephalitis.

Vaccination of domestic animal hosts has been successfully in immunizing horses and mules against WEE, EEE, and VEE. The vaccination of pigs, the amplifying host of Japanese encephalitis, has been hampered by interference due to passive immunity in young pigs and by their fast population turnover.

Attenuated live virus vaccine is available for Wesselsbron fever and louping-ill in sheep. An attenuated neurotropic vaccine against Rift Valley fever may cause abortion in cattle; newer reports describe an inactivated vaccine.

Vector control has been successful mainly in urban areas, especially control of *Aedes aegypti*, the mosquito vector of yellow fever, by the use of insecticides; however, the control of multiple vectors encounters considerable difficulties.

A reduction of the number of ticks (*Ixodes ricinus, Ixodes persulcatus*) can be attempted by alternate land use. Repellent-impregnated clothes have been successfully used to protect persons from occupational hazards.

In the case of hemorrhagic fever with renal syndrome, rodent control is indicated.

In addition to these often severe diseases mentioned above, *serological surveys indicate extensive or rare human infections* with a large number of additional arboviruses which are mostly limited to certain ecogeographical regions. Clinical symptoms are mostly absent; only a few cases of febrile illness are known. Control is limited to the avoidance of exposure to arthropods. The following list of strains is certainly incomplete and subject to periodic revision:

1. *Togaviruses*
   (a) *Alphaviruses* (mosquito-borne): extensive—O'Nyong-nyong, Semliki Forest, Sagiyama, and Whataroa; rare—Middleburg, Mucambo, Pixuna.
   (b) *Flaviviruses*. Mosquito-borne: extensive—Banzi, Bussuqara, Kokobera, Ilheus, Spondweni, Wesselsbron; rare—Kunjin, Uganda S, Zika. Dengue types 1 and 2 may have a reservoir in wild monkeys in southeast Asia and Malaysia.

Tick-borne: rare—Langat, Powassan. Unknown vectors: extensive—Rocio (outbreaks with clinical disease); rare—Dakar, Rio Bravo.

2. *Bunyaviruses:* extensive—Apeu, Bujaru, Bunyamwera, Bwamba, Cache Valley, Calovo, Caraparu, Germiston, Kairi, Murutucu, Nairobi sheep disease, Oriboca, Oropouche, Pongola, Restan, Tacaiuma, Tahyna, Tensaw, Tlacotalpan, Trivittatus; frequency of human infections un-known or rare—Bhanja, Candiru, Catu, Guama, Itaqui, Madrid, Manzanilla, Marituba, Nepuyo, Ossa, Wyeomia.

3. *Orbiviruses*. Tick-borne: rare—Kemerovo, Tribec. Phlebotomine-borne: rare—Changuinola.

4. *Rhabdovirus:* rare—Mossuril.

5. *Unclassified:* rare—"Quaranfil."

R	=	Reservoir
E	=	Epizootiology/epidemiology
PA	=	Principal animals
PR	=	Persons at risk

O	=	Occurrence
CA	=	Clinical form: animals
CM	=	Clinical form: man

Causative agent	Disease		Epizootiology/epidemiology
Alphavirus group:			
Eastern equine encephalitis virus	● Eastern equine encephalitis (EEE)	R/PA.	Wild fowl and pheasants, rodents, also horses.
		E.	Transmission by mosquito bites (*Culiseta melanura, Aedes sollicitans, Aedes vexans*). Cycle of infection in wild fowl leads to outbreaks in pheasants which amplify infection for horses and man.
		PR.	Groups III, V, VI and general public.
		O.	Eastern USA, Canada, Mexico, South America; possibly Czechoslovakia, Poland, USSR, Thailand, and the Philippines.
		CA/CM.	High mortality in horses and man. Fever, vomiting, delirium; leads to coma and death. Apparent recovery may be followed by fatal encephalitis. Excessive salivation may cause confusion with rabies.
Western equine encephalitis virus	● Western equine encephalitis (WEE)	R/PA.	Many species of birds, also snakes and amphibians; spread to horses and man.
		O.	North and South America.
		CA.	Inapparent in most hosts. Encephalitis in horses.

546

Causative agent	Disease				
		R = Reservoir		O = Occurrence	
		E = Epizootiology/epidemiology		CA = Clinical form: animals	
		PA = Principal animals		CM = Clinical form: man	
		PR = Persons at risk			
Alphavirus group (cont.)		E.	Cycles of infection between reptiles, birds, amphibians; small mammals, and mosquitoes, especially *Culex tarsalis, Culiseta melanura*. Horses and man are accidental hosts. *Note*: The horse does not amplify the virus.	CM.	Fever, leading to nervous symptoms and paralysis, especially in children who may not completely recover.
		PR.	Possibly overwintering in reptiles, amphibians, and small rodents. Groups III, V, VI and general public.		
Venezuelan equine encephalitis virus	● Venezuelan equine encephalitis (VEE)	R/PA.	Various species of rodents; may extend to horses and man.	O.	Tropical America.
		E.	Cycles of infection in rodents may extend to horses, initiating epidemics in man. Transmission by mosquitoes (*Aedes* spp. and *Mansonia* spp.). Non-immunized sentinel horses are used to detect spread.	CA.	High mortality in horses due to encephalitis.
				CM.	Low mortality in man. Acute influenza-like syndrome leading to encephalitis, especially in children.
		PR.	Groups III, V, VI and general public.		
Chikungunya virus	Chikungunya fever	R/PA.	Primates; domestic and wild animals, and birds.	O.	South and Southeast Asia, Africa.
		E.	Widespread infection in endemic areas by mosquito bites (*Culex, Aedes, Mansonia* spp.).	CM.	Biphasic fever with rash; in convalescence, swelling of joints.
		PR.	General population in endemic foci.		

Causative agent	Disease		
		R = Reservoir	O = Occurrence
		E = Epizootiology/epidemiology	CA = Clinical form: animals
		PA = Principal animals	CM = Clinical form: man
		PR = Persons at risk	

Alphavirus group (cont.)

Mayaro virus	Mayaro fever		
		R. Wild animals (?).	O. Trinidad and various South American countries.
		E. Widespread infection of population in endemic areas, transmitted by several mosquito species. Man is an accidental host.	CM. Fever, but benign and transient.
		PA. Wild animals (?) and man.	
		PR. Groups III, V, VI and general public.	

Sindbis virus	Sindbis fever		
		R. Wild birds.	O. Africa, Asia, Australia, Philippines (possibly Czechoslovakia, USSR).
		E. Cycles of infection in wild birds. Man is accidental host after mosquito bites (*Culex pseudovishnui, univittatus, annulirostris,* and other spp.).	CM. Fever, pain in joints, sometimes mild jaundice and skin vesicles; recovery usual.
		PR. Groups III, V, VI and general public.	

Ross River virus	Epidemic polyarthritis (Ross River fever)		
		R. Wild mammals and birds.	O. Northern and eastern Australia.
		E. Transmitted by vector mosquitoes (*Culex* and *Aedes* spp.) from infected hosts.	CA. Considered inapparent in nature.
		PA. Horses, cattle, kangaroos, wallabies, goats, sheep, bandicoots, dogs, rats, bats, and pigs.	CM. Polyarthritis with maculopapular or vesicular rash.
		PR. General population in endemic foci.	

Causative agent	Disease			
		R = Reservoir		O = Occurrence
		E = Epizootiology/epidemiology		CA = Clinical form: animals
		PA = Principal animals		CM = Clinical form: man
		PR = Persons at risk		

Flavivirus group (mosquito-borne):

Causative agent	Disease			
Yellow fever virus	● Yellow fever	R/PA.	Man and other primates.	O. South America and Africa.
		E.	*Jungle or forest cycle* of infection involves wild animals, particularly monkeys, with accidental transmission to man, mainly by *Haemagogus* spp. in Americas and *Aedes africanus* and *simpsoni* in Africa. Spread to man can initiate an *urban cycle* with man-to-man transmission by *Aedes aegypti*.	CM. Mild cases with fever of sudden onset. Severe cases develop hemorrhage (black vomit and melena) with liver and kidney failure (albuminuria or anuria and jaundice); high mortality.
		PR.	Groups III, V, and VI.	
Japanese encephalitis virus	● Japanese encephalitis (JE)	R.	Wild birds, mainly herons and egrets.	O. Widespread in Asia.
		E.	Virus amplification in by pigs, followed by epidemics in man in rural areas. Transmission by mosquitoes, especially *Culex tritaeniorhynchus* and *C. vishnui* complex.	CA. Asymptomatic except in pregnant sows; causes abortion and neonatal deaths in pigs.
		PA.	Birds, pigs, horses.	CM. Infection commonly inapparent in man, but occasionally encephalitis with high mortality.
		PR.	Groups I, III, V, and VI.	
Murray Valley virus	Murray Valley encephalitis (Australian encephalitis)	R.	Wild birds.	O. Australia and New Guinea.
		E.	Cycles of infection, fostered by heavy rains and irrigation schemes, between birds and mosquitoes (especially *Culex annulirostris*). Adjacent, dense human populations support the epidemics.	CM. Children especially susceptible. Fever, vomiting, and encephalitis. High mortality. Many subclinical cases.
		PR.	Group I and general public.	

Causative agent	Disease	R = Reservoir E = Epizootiology/epidemiology PA = Principal animals PR = Persons at risk		O = Occurrence CA = Clinical form: animals CM = Clinical form: man	

Flavivirus group (mosquito-borne) (cont.)

Causative agent	Disease		Epizootiology/epidemiology		Occurrence
St. Louis virus	St. Louis encephalitis	R/PA.	Wild birds, bats, horses.	O.	North and South America.
		E.	Cycles of infection rural, with transmission by *Culex tarsalis* and *C. nigripalpis*; involve man accidentally. Subclinical infection protects. Spread to urban areas may cause epidemics. Urban vectors involve many other mosquito species, especially *C. quinquefasciatus*.	CM.	Usually benign; fever can lead to encephalitis and death, particularly in the elderly.
		PR.	Group I and general public.		
West Nile virus	West Nile fever	R.	Birds.	O.	Africa and Asia, occasionally Europe.
		E.	Cycles of infection between birds and mosquitoes, especially *C. univittatus*. Man and other animals are accidental hosts.	CA.	Can be subclinical, otherwise fever and encephalitis with 25% mortality in horses and donkeys.
		PA.	Birds; also man, horses, donkeys, sheep, cattle, and camels.	CM.	Can be subclinical in man. Transient fever or even encephalitis, especially in the elderly. Mortality low.
		PR.	General public.		
Flavivirus group (tick-borne):					
Far East (RSSE) virus and European subtypes	● Tick-borne encephalitis (TBE)	R.	Wild rodents.	O.	An emerging zoonosis spreading in Asiatic USSR and Europe.
		E.	Infection in deciduous forests with cycles in wild animals. Man and domestic animals infected via ticks, es-	CA.	Little known.

Causative agent	Disease	R = E = PA = PR =	Reservoir Epizootiology/epidemiology Principal animals Persons at risk	O = CA = CM =	Occurrence Clinical form: animals Clinical form: man
Flavivirus group (tick-borne) (cont.)					
			...pecially *Ixodes persulcatus* and *I. ricinus*, giving seasonal infectivity. Transmission also through milk from infected goats and cattle.	CM.	Diphasic fever, vomiting, and meningoencephalitis that can be lethal (5–20%). RSSE more virulent than the central European form of the disease.
		PA.	Wild rodents, goats, cattle, and man.		
		PR.	Groups I, III, V and general public.		
Louping-ill virus	Louping-ill	R/PA.	Sheep, red grouse.	O.	Scotland, Northern England, Ireland.
		E.	Cycles of infection occur in sheep, spread by ticks (*Ixodes ricinus*). Infection of slaughtermen and laboratory workers by inhalation or ingestion.	CA/CM.	Fever, followed sometimes by meningoencephalitis and death. Usually much milder than RSSE and TBE.
		PR.	Groups I and II.		
Omsk hemorrhagic fever virus	● Omsk hemorrhagic fever	R/PA.	Ticks, muskrats, and other rodents.	O.	Localized in Western Siberia.
		E.	Man infected by tick bites (*Dermocentor pictus*) and, especially trappers and skinners, directly from muskrats. Laboratory infection by aerosols common.	CM.	Biphasic fever in man, gastrointestinal symptoms, hemorrhages and bronchopneumonia, lymphadenopathy; loss of hair during convalescence is frequent.
		PR.	Groups III and V.		
Kyasanur forest disease virus	● Kyasanur forest disease	R.	Monkeys and rodents.	O.	Mysore, India.
		E.	Monkeys may initiate the epidemic. High mortality gives early warning.	CM.	Fever, bradycardia and hypertension, hemorrhages; later a second fever rise

		R = Reservoir	O = Occurrence
		E = Epizootiology/epidemiology	CA = Clinical form: animals
		PA = Principal animals	CM = Clinical form: man
		PR = Persons at risk	

Causative agent	Disease	Epizootiology/epidemiology	Occurrence
Flavivirus group (tick-borne): (cont.)		Rural workers infected by tick bites, especially *Haemophysalis spinigera*, *H. turturis*, and others.	CM. with neurological signs, leukopenia; subclinical infections common.
		PR. Group I.	
Bunyavirus group:			
California encephalitis virus	California encephalitis	R/PA. Wild rodents and lagomorphs.	O. USA.
		E. Seasonal incidence linked to mosquito prevalence (*Culex tarsalis* and various *Aedes* spp.).	CM. In children, fever, vomiting, and convulsions with meningoencephalitis.
		PR. Groups I, III and general rural populations.	
Rift Valley fever virus	● Rift Valley fever (enzootic hepatitis)	R. Mainly sheep, cattle, buffaloes, sometimes goats and camels.	O. South, Central, and West Africa and Egypt. Spreading.
		PA. Sheep, cattle and goats, buffaloes, camels.	CA. Febrile disease in young lambs with high mortality. Abortion in ewes and cattle.
		E. Irregular epidemics in man during and after epizootics in animals. Mosquito transmission among animals by *Culex pipiens*, *C. theileri*, *Aedes caballus*, and others. Contact infection by droplets.	CM. Biphasic fever, vomiting with recovery. Severe cases present hemorrhages, jaundice, and neurological signs (encephalitis and characteristic retinitis) and death.
		PR. Groups I, II, V and general public.	

Causative agent	Disease			
		R = Reservoir E = Epizootiology/epidemiology PA = Principal animals PR = Persons at risk	O = Occurrence CA = Clinical form: animals CM = Clinical form: man	
Bunyavirus group (cont.)				
Crimean hemorrhagic fever virus and Congo virus	● Crimean-Congo hemorrhagic fever (Congo fever) (CHF)	R.	O.	Southern part of European USSR, Bulgaria, Central Asia, Pakistan, and several African countries.
		E.		Transmitted by ticks (especially *Boophilus decoloratus* and *Hyalomma* spp.) after amplification in animals. Migrating birds may carry ticks. Laboratory and hospital infections.
			CA.	Asymptomatic.
			CM.	Fever and leukopenia. Hemorrhages with death from blood loss.
		PR.		Group III and rural population in general.
Hemorrhagic fever with renal syndrome virus	● Hemorrhagic fever with renal syndrome (Korean hemorrhagic fever)	R.	O.	Europe and Asia.
			CA.	Not observed.
		E.	CM.	Seasonal, coinciding with rodent migration. Man infected by contact with mouse excreta. Epidemics follow contamination of food.
				Fever, vomiting, hemorrhages, and renal involvement. Some mortality.
		PA.		Wild rodents (?). In certain circumstances, laboratory mice.
		PR.		Groups I, III, VII and soldiers.
Orbivirus group:				
Colorado tick fever virus	Colorado tick fever (mountain fever)	R.	O.	Northwestern USA and Canada.

Rodents, especially ground squirrels.

Rodents (*Apodemus agrarius*, *Microtus* spp., and *Clethrionomys* spp.) have been implicated or suspected.

553

Causative agent	Disease		
		R = Reservoir	O = Occurrence
		E = Epizootiology/epidemiology	CA = Clinical form: animals
		PA = Principal animals	CM = Clinical form: man
		PR = Persons at risk	
Orbivirus group (cont.)	E. High infection rate in ticks in enzootic regions. Transmission to man by adult tick vectors, especially *Dermacentor andersoni*.	CM. Characteristically a mild febrile infection, but can be severe in children with occasional encephalitis or tendency to bleed. Deaths are uncommon.	
	PR. Groups I and III.		

Arenavirus group

This virus group includes four zoonoses with quite diverse epidemiologic and pathogenetic features:

Lymphocytic choriomeningitis (LCM) has a worldwide distribution among house mice (*Mus musculus*); it recently gained additional importance by the fact that certain breeding colonies of Syrian golden hamsters turned out to be the source of human infections.

Lassa fever, limited to the African continent, has proved to be highly contagious by direct contact, necessitating particular precautions in caring for or transporting patients and handling diagnostic specimens.

Argentine and *Bolivian hemorrhagic fevers* are limited to certain geographic areas of South America.

Transmission in all four diseases is mainly through contact with infectious excretions of reservoir rodents.

Diagnosis: *Virus isolation.* The identification of Lassa virus should be carried out in laboratories with adequate high-security facilities. Junin and Machupo virus can be isolated by intracerebral inoculation of suckling mice; LCM virus by intracerebral inoculation of weaned mice.

Serological tests are available for these infections; they may be carried out by specialized laboratories only.

Control: In *Lassa fever*: isolation of suspected patients; administration of convalescent sera to them, plus symptomatic treatment. Rodent control is directed especially at *Mastomys natalensis*.

In *LCM*: control of wild mouse populations and surveillance of laboratory animals. Establishment of LCM-free breeding colonies (in particular of Syrian golden hamsters, used as pets).

In *Argentine* and *Bolivian hemorrhagic fever*: rodent control by shrub clearance.

Causative agent	Disease	R = Reservoir E = Epizootiology/epidemiology PA = Principal animals PR = Persons at risk		O = Occurrence CA = Clinical form: animals CM = Clinical form: man	

Arenavirus group:

Causative agent	Disease	Code	Epizootiology/epidemiology	Code	Occurrence
Lymphocytic choriomeningitis virus	● Lymphocytic choriomeningitis (LCM)	R/PA.	House mouse (*Mus musculus*); focal also in laboratory animals and pets, e.g. hamsters (particularly young Syrian hamsters from certain colonies).	O.	Worldwide.
		E.	In mice, infection is by contact and vertically via the placenta. In man, infections are caused by urine and feces contamination and by respiratory transmission. Man-to-man transmission is rare.	CA.	Lymphocytic choriomeningitis in weaned and adult mice. Immune tolerance with late glomerulonephritis follows in *in utero* infections.
		PR.	Groups I, IV, V and general population.	CM.	Generally benign fever in man, sometimes mild meningitis. Death is rare.
Lassa virus	● Lassa fever	R/PA.	*Mastomys natalensis* (multimammate rat).	O.	Western and Central Africa.
		E.	Presumed spread from rat to man by excretions, followed by man-to-man transmission by contact. Laboratory specimens are a special hazard.	CM.	Long-lasting fever with insidious onset, vomiting, and diarrhea. Ulcerative pharyngitis, pneumonia, proteinuria, leukopenia, circulatory collapse, and death. Extreme caution has to be applied when caring for patients or handling diagnostic specimens.
		PR.	General population, hospital personnel, and group V.		

Causative agent	Disease				
		R =	Reservoir	O =	Occurrence
		E =	Epizootiology/epidemiology	CA =	Clinical form: animals
		PA =	Principal animals	CM =	Clinical form: man
		PR =	Persons at risk		
Arenavirus group (cont.)					
Junin virus (anti-genically closely re-lated to Machupo virus)	● Argentine hemorrhagic fever	R/PA.	Wild rodents.	O.	Argentina.
		E.	Epidemics, especially in rural popula-tions. Seasonal incidence depending on rodent contact. No man-to-man transmission (?). Frequent laboratory infections.	CM.	Fever leading to mucosal hemor-rhages and neurologic signs with 5–20% mortality.
		PR.	Groups I, III, and V.		
Machupo virus	● Bolivian hemorrhagic fever	R/PA.	Wild rodents, especially *Calomys callosus*.	O.	Bolivia.
		E.	Epidemics occur in association with rodent populations through infected urine. *C. callosus* lives in houses in close contact with man.	CM.	Fever, mucosal hemorrhages, hemo-concentration, and neurologic signs with 15–20% mortality.
		PR.	Groups I, III, and V.		

Orthomyxovirus group

Commonly known as influenza viruses, they are responsible for worldwide epidemics in man. The viruses, belonging to antigenic group A, according to their nucleoprotein antigen A, also cause infections of epidemic proportions in horses, pigs, and birds. (Fowl plague is also due to an influenza A virus.) These viruses are more or less species-specific and vary, in particular, in their hemagglutnin (HA) and neuraminidase (NA) antigens and in some of their intravirion enzymes. There are, however, a great deal of antigenic cross-reactions between strains affecting different animal species. In the laboratory, *in vitro* and *in vivo* genetic recombination experiments have shown that new viruses (e.g., viruses capable of causing epidemics in man or animals) may originate in nature by such means. Certain strains (e.g., swine influenza, A equi 2) may infect man in close contact, generally without further transmission.

Diagnosis: Virus isolation in embryonated eggs and characterization by their nucleoprotein, HA and NA antigens. Serological tests with paired serum samples by hemagglutination inhibition and complement fixation.

Control: Effective, short-lasting protection against clinical disease can be obtained by inactivated or subunit vaccines containing the essential HA and NA antigens.

Paramyxovirus group

This group has similar properties to the influenza viruses. Newcastle disease virus is, however, found only in one antigenic type. The disease is of great importance in the poultry industry. It may be introduced by wild and pet birds. Disease in man is sporadic and benign.

Diagnosis: As with orthomyxoviruses.

Control: Vaccination with live attenuated vaccines or testing and eradication of infected fowl

R = Reservoir
E = Epizootiology/epidemiology
PA = Principal animals
PR = Persons at risk
O = Occurrence
CA = Clinical form: animals
CM = Clinical form: man

Causative agent	Disease		
Paramyxovirus group:			
Newcastle disease virus (1 serotype)	Newcastle disease (pseudo–fowl pest)	R/PA.	Fowl; domestic, pet, and wild birds.
		E.	Main source of infection for man is poultry, poultry products, and pet birds. Contact infection. Aerosols in slaughterhouses and laboratories. Infection also from live vaccines.
		PR.	Groups I, II, IV, and V.
		O.	Worldwide.
		CA.	Generalized viremia with respiratory, intestinal, and neurologic signs; often with high mortality.
		CM.	Conjunctivitis with local inflammation of lymph nodes. Fever is influenza-like.

Rhabdovirus group

Among the rhabdovirus diseases, vesicular stomatitis is of economic importance in cattle, horses, and pigs; human infections are relatively rare. Several antigenically related strains of vesicular stomatitis virus exist. The strains associated with disease in man are: Indiana, New Jersey, Piry, and Chandipura. Differential diagnosis from foot-and-mouth disease is important. Precautions should be taken in laboratories against aerosols.

Rabies (Lyssa virus type 1), through its worldwide distribution and the fatal course of disease in man, is considered to be one of the most important zoonoses. Minor variants of Lyssa virus type 1, differing in antigenicity (detected by monoclonal antibody) and pathogenicity, are known to exist. The strains appear to be reservoir-adapted. Lyssaviruses of different types are related by their nucleocapsid antigen.

This same subgroup contains two antigenically related zoonotic viruses, with a similar pathogenic potential, namely Duvenhage and Mokola virus. These two viruses have been isolated only from the African continent where they have been associated with encephalitis in man. Mokola virus was originally isolated from shrews. Several other antigenically or morphologically related viruses of this group are under study.

Diagnosis of rabies: Clinical signs, immunofluorescence test, mouse inoculation, identification of Negri bodies.

Control of rabies: Control and eradication in domestic animals (and wildlife) by vaccination, reduction of population density and movements. International regulations. Human pre- and postexposure treatment.

R =	Reservoir
E =	Epizootiology/epidemiology
PA =	Principal animals
PR =	Persons at risk

O =	Occurrence
CA =	Clinical form: animals
CM =	Clinical form: man

Causative agent	Disease		
Vesicular stomatitis virus	Vesicular stomatitis (not to be confused with vesicular stomatitis caused by Coxsackie virus)	R/PA.	Wild arboreal animals, horses, cattle, sheep, and pigs.
		E.	Insect vectors (*Phlebotomus* spp.) transmit some strains.
			Slow propagation with occasional outbreaks, especially in pigs. Contact and aerosol inhalation infect man.
		PR.	Groups I and V.
		O.	North and South America.
		CA.	Papules and vesicles on mouth, udder, and hoofs.
		CM.	Disease resembles influenza, occasionally with oral or digital vesicles and diarrhea.

Rhabdovirus group:

558

Causative agent	Disease		
		R = Reservoir	O = Occurrence
		E = Epizootiology/epidemiology	CA = Clinical form: animals
		PA = Principal animals	CM = Clinical form: man
		PR = Persons at risk	

Rhabdovirus group (cont.)

Causative agent	Disease		Occurrence / Clinical
Rabies virus (Lyssavirus type 1)	● Rabies (hydrophobia)	R. Dog, fox, skunk, raccoon, mongoose, bats, and jackals.	O. Worldwide except Australia, New Zealand, most islands of Oceania and Caribbean, and where eradicated.
		E. Reservoir depending on density or mobility of host population. Virus transmitted by bites or saliva contacting open wounds or mucous membranes. Incubation periods of 14 days to > 1 year. Transmission to man is particularly through dog bites. Aerosol transmission only in certain bat caves and the laboratory.	CA. Encephalitis, paralysis, and death. Usually an initial period of altered behavior, which may be aggressive.
			CM. Encephalitis, muscular spasms of throat causing hydrophobia, paralysis, and death.
		PA. All reservoir animals plus cats, wolves, raccoon dogs, cattle, horses, deer. Occasionally all other mammals.	
		PR. Groups III, VI and general public.	

Picornavirus group

1. Foot-and-mouth disease and swine vesicular disease

The picornaviruses include viruses which are very resistant to environmental conditions. Indirect transmission, particularly with meat and bone products from infected animals but also through other fomites, regularly causes widespread epidemics.

Much international effort is being devoted to the control and containment of foot-and-mouth disease (FMD) and swine vesicular disease (SVD), which are both responsible for great economic losses in cattle and/or pigs. FMD has been proven to cause very rarely vesicular skin lesions in man; after close contact with animals at the height of infection, man may be a transient carrier of FMD virus in the nasopharyngeal area. SVD may cause a febrile disease with myalgia in laboratory workers.

Diagnosis: Direct determination of virus antigens in vesicular lesions by complement fixation test or animal inoculation. Serological tests are only in the second place.

Control: National and international eradication programs based on slaughter and/or vaccination with multivalent vaccines have eliminated foot-and-mouth disease from North America, including Mexico, and have greatly reduced the occurrence of the disease in Europe. Swine vesicular disease, with its similarities to FMD, is also subject to eradication.

In other continents, the diversity of FMD-virus strains involved and the difficulties encountered in containment of infected herds have hampered control.

Reovirus group

Rotavirus enteritis

Rotaviruses have been associated in recent years with enteritis in calves, piglets, foals, and the young of many other species including man. There appear to be numerous serotypes with a high degree of cross-reaction. Experimental cross-infection between species has been shown, but it is unclear at present if this observation is of epidemiologic importance.

Diagnosis: Owing to difficulties in culturing these viruses in cell cultures, they can best be demonstrated by direct examina-

2. *Encephalomyocarditis*

The reservoir of encephalomyocarditis virus is most likely rodents, but it has sporadically caused meningoencephalitis in man. In subtropical countries, several outbreaks in pigs have been associated with liver degeneration and myocarditis. Knowledge about its epidemiology is scanty.

3. *Viral hepatitis A*

The widely occurring hepatitis A virus has recently been identified as an enterovirus. Infection commonly occurs through fecal contamination of food or water; transmission is also possible by blood transfusion. The original reservoir was probably man who transmitted the disease to nonhuman primates. These, in turn, have transmitted the disease back to man in a number of clinical episodes.

tion of fecal matter (or intestinal contents) by electron microscopy, immunofluorescence, or the enzyme-linked immunosorbent assay (ELISA) method.

Control: Active immunization of cows or sows and peroral administration of colostrum daily during the first two weeks of life have proven to be protective, whereas humoral antibodies have no direct influence.

Active immunization with attenuated strains is used in calves.

Unclassified or suspected virus infections

Marburg disease

Limited but dramatic outbreaks of human disease associated with high mortality rates have focused attention on certain viruses of African origin. Owing to the great hazards involved in handling these virulent viruses, only specialized, high-security laboratories must be used in their study. The status of the Marburg/Ebola agent as a zoonotic agent is not yet defined.

Diagnosis: Clinically, a presumptive diagnosis is made in certain geographical areas in patients with a severe, toxic progressive illness.

In some specialized laboratories, diagnosis is made by virus isolation and serologic tests on early and late serum samples.

Control: Isolate patients suspected of being affected by Marburg disease (or Ebola fever). Avoid contact with their blood or excreta. Incinerate the corpses or use special precautions for the burial of persons dead of these diseases.

Causative agent	Disease			
		R	=	Reservoir
		E	=	Epizootiology/epidemiology
		PA	=	Principal animals
		PR	=	Persons at risk
		O	=	Occurrence
		CA	=	Clinical form: animals
		CM	=	Clinical form: man
Marburg/Ebola agent (virus unrelated to other known viruses) (long, tubular enveloped virus)	● Marburg disease (green monkey disease)	R/PA.		Green monkey (*Cercopithecus aethiops*).
		E.		Human cases by direct contact with monkeys or monkey tissues, especially under laboratory conditions. Secondary cases by man-to-man contact.
		PA.		Green monkey (*Cercopithecus aethiops*).
		PR.		Group V.
		O.		In monkeys from East Africa.
		CA.		Not clear; experimental infection in monkeys fatal.
		CM.		Acute sudden onset. Fever, vomiting, diarrhea, hemorrhages, lymphadenopathy, and hepatitis. High mortality.

561

Part V

PARASITIC ZOONOSES

SECTION A
PROTOZOOSES

AFRICAN TRYPANOSOMIASIS

(086.5)

Synonyms: Sleeping sickness, Gambian trypanosomiasis (caused by *T. brucei gambiense*), Rhodesian trypanosomiasis (caused by *T. brucei rhodesiense*).

Etiology: Two subspecies of *Trypanosoma* (*Trypanozoon*) *brucei*: *T. brucei gambiense* and *T. brucei rhodesiense*, flagellate protozoans with an undulating membrane; they are transmitted by flies of the genus *Glossina* (tsetse).

The two "human" subspecies (*T. b. gambiense* and *T. b. rhodesiense*) cannot be distinguished morphologically from one another, nor from *T. b. brucei*, a pathogen of domestic animals in Africa (dogs, horses, camels) that does not infect man. The morphologic similarity between these agents has made epidemiologic studies very difficult. Until a few years ago, differentiation between the three *T. brucei* subspecies was based on their infectivity and pathogenicity for rats, their sensitivity to the drug tryparsamide, and their pathogenicity for man. To distinguish between *T. b. brucei* and "human" trypanosomes, human volunteers were used, with the consequent risk. New techniques for identifying the parasites are now available. One method consists of incubating them in human serum or plasma and then inoculating them into rats. *T. b. brucei* loses its infectivity for rats while the human subspecies maintain it. Nevertheless, more recent studies have revealed wide variation in susceptibility to the effects of human serum, and some evidence exists that *T. b. brucei* can become resistant to serum action. This latter finding could point to a mechanism by which an animal parasite (*T. b. brucei*) becomes infective for man when transmitted to humans by flies infected by animals (Minter, 1982). Another important and increasingly used method is characterization of trypanosomes by the electrophoretic movement of isozymes, allowing distinction of different zymodemes (see definition in "American Trypanosomiasis"). On the basis of this procedure, Gibson *et al.* (1980) proposed grouping trypanosomes of the sub-genus *Trypanozoon* into a single species (*T. brucei*) comprising six main groups: two not infective to man and four human pathogens, of which two occur in western and central Africa and two in eastern Africa.

These trypanosomes occur in two main morphologic forms in vertebrates, one long and thin and about 30 microns in length, and the other short and thick and measuring about 20 microns; the latter form is considered more infective to the vector. Other forms intermediate in size are also found.

Two life cycles are distinguished for *T. brucei* trypanosomes, one in the vertebrate host and the other in the invertebrate vector. In contrast to *T. cruzi* (the agent of Chagas' disease), the trypanosomes of sleeping sickness multiply not only in the blood, but also in lymph, cerebrospinal fluid, and intercellular spaces in humans. In the insect vector, trypanosomes reproduce in the lumen of the midgut and hindgut, then migrate to the proventriculus and from there to the salivary glands, where they assume the epimastigote form (crithidia); in 2 to 5 days they transform into metacyclic trypomastigotes, which is the infective form. The entire cycle in *Glossina* is completed in approximately 3 weeks. Unlike the triatomine vector of *T. cruzi*, which infects the vertebrate host by means of its feces (called transmission from the "posterior station"), the tsetse fly inoculates trypanosomes into the host with its saliva ("anterior station").

Geographic Distribution: *T. b. rhodesiense* is distributed in eastern Africa from Botswana to Ethiopia, and *T. b. gambiense* in central and western Africa from Senegal in the northwest and Sudan in the northeast southward to Zaire and Angola.

Occurrence in Man (Map 9): The greatest number of patients with sleeping sickness has been recorded in Zaire, where there were 4,126 cases in 1972; in the rest of Africa the total of new cases during that year was 3,000 (de Raadt, 1976). Gambian trypanosomiasis is a chronic disease that tends to produce epidemics, while Rhodesian trypanosomiasis has a more acute course and occurs sporadically. In the past, devastating epidemics of Gambian trypanosomiasis ensued as a result of the migration of populations during colonization. In the Congo basin alone, approximately 500,000 persons died in one decade, and about 200,000 (two-thirds of the population) died in Busoga Province, Uganda (Goodwin, 1970). Thanks to control measures, especially chemotherapy and chemoprophylaxis, in some areas the incidence of the disease has been reduced to a very low level. Gambian trypanosomiasis is endemic in 23 African countries, placing 45 million inhabitants at risk. It is estimated that 10,000 new infections occur every year (UNDP/World Bank/WHO Consultation, 1982).

Epidemics due to *T. rhodesiense* are much less common. The infection is endemic among cattle-raising tribes of eastern Africa. It frequently affects hunters, fishermen, and travelers. The general incidence is rather low, since the people avoid living in areas infested by the vector fly.

The Disease in Man: Three phases can be distinguished: primary lesion, parasitemic phase, and invasion of the central nervous system. Two or three days after the bite of an infected fly, a chancre appears at the inoculation site; it disappears in 2 to 3 weeks. This primary lesion is more frequently observed in infection by *T. b. rhodesiense* than by *T. b. gambiense*. From the chancre site, the trypanosomes invade the bloodstream, and the patient suffers irregular and intermittent fever in synchrony with waves of parasitemia. Other signs during this acute period are lymphadenopathies, particularly of the posterior cervical lymph nodes, as well as edema of the eyelids and joints. The most common symptoms of the acute phase consist of cephalalgia, insomnia, arthralgia, weight loss, and generalized pruritus, especially in the sternal region. In the more advanced stage of the disease, the symptomatology is related to the organ affected. Invasion of the central nervous system is common and produces a great variety of psychic, motor, and sensory perturbations. The lesions produced by this invasion cause irritability, paresthesia, insomnia, and eventually can cause cerebral edema with severe headaches and edema of the optic papillae; likewise, neurologic manifestations can be produced, such as epileptic attacks, chorea, psychotic phenomena, euphoria, somnolence, mental lethargy, and coma.

Gambian trypanosomiasis generally has a slow and chronic course. Between the first and second phase, weeks or months can elapse, and between the second and third, months or years. Rhodesian trypanosomiasis follows a more acute course and the phases are less marked. It also may cause death in a few months, while a patient with Gambian trypanosomiasis can survive many years. Cardiac complications are more frequent in Rhodesian trypanosomiasis, and a certain number of patients die before reaching the neurologic phase (Greenwood and Whittle, 1980; World Health Organization, 1979).

Map 9. Principal foci of African trypanosomiasis in western Africa.

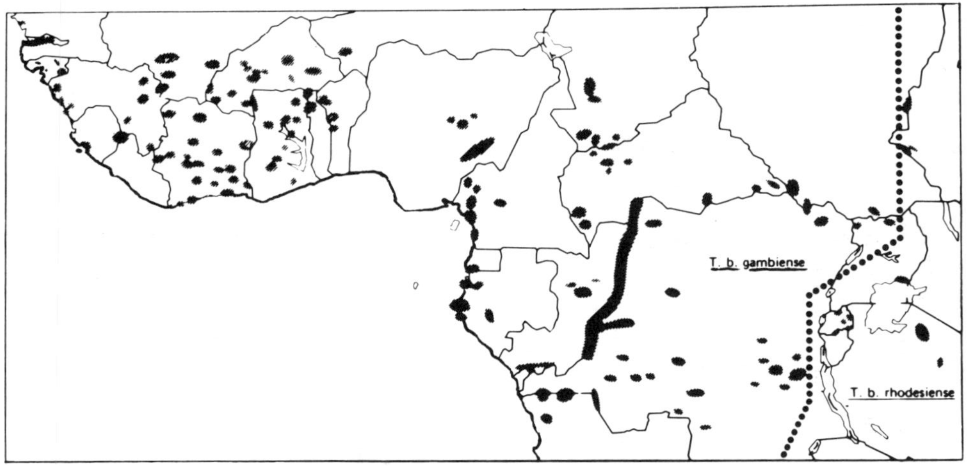

Source: Bull WHO 60(6):821, 1982

The pathogenesis of sleeping sickness is still not well known. Most of the tissue damage is probably due to an immunopathologic reaction (Greenwood and Whittle, 1980).

The Disease in Animals: Infections by *T. b. gambiense* and *T. b. rhodesiense* are generally subclinical in domestic and wild animals.

The important species causing disease in bovines in Africa are *T. congolense* and *T. vivax*, which do not infect man. Left untreated, infected animals either die in 3 or 4 weeks or, more frequently, develop a chronic illness with lymphadenopathy, intermittent fever, anemia, and progressive emaciation (Urquart, 1980). *T. b. brucei* causes an acute disease with anemia, edemas, and emaciation in equines, dogs, and camels. Another trypanosomiasis that occurs in Africa and also outside that continent is caused by *T. evansi*, which is transmitted by tabanid flies. It is especially pathogenic for camels, equines, and dogs.

Source of Infection and Mode of Transmission (Figures 58 and 59): In trypanosomiasis of western and central Africa (*T. b. gambiense*), man is the main reservoir and source of infection for the vector. Since the infection is prolonged and includes intervals between the febrile attacks during which the patient feels relatively well, the victim may move about and thus spread infection to new areas where vectors exist. Pigs, dogs, and perhaps other species can harbor the parasite, but their role in the epidemiology is secondary. Using the new methods of incubation in

Figure 58. African trypansomiasis. Cycle of *Trypanosoma brucei gambiense*.

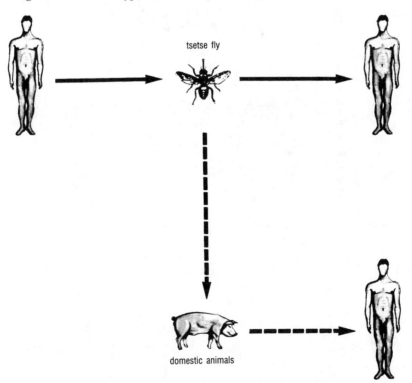

tsetse fly

domestic animals

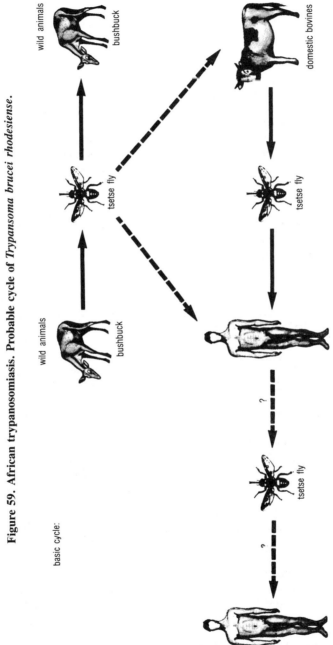

Figure 59. African trypanosomiasis. Probable cycle of *Trypansoma brucei rhodesiense*.

human serum (sensitivity or resistance to serum) and isozyme electrophoresis (see Etiology), Mehlitz *et al.* (1982) have found identical enzymatic profiles for "strains" of trypanosomes from man in Ivory Coast and from domestic pigs as well as several wild animals and a bovine in Upper Volta. Likewise, these researchers have confirmed their previous findings in Liberia that animals are reservoirs for *T. b. gambiense* and that their parasites can be infective for man. In Congo, a sheep "strain" had the same enzymatic characteristics and sensitivity to human serum as three strains from human patients (Scott *et al.*, 1983). Wild and domestic animals have been experimentally infected with *T. b. gambiense* of human origin; these infections were of long duration and were transmissible by the vector fly from one animal to another, and sometimes retransmissible to man (Molyneux, 1983). In areas where control programs have been carried out but active foci of infection have persisted, it is suspected that domestic animals, especially pigs, may constitute reservoirs. Likewise, the presence of animal reservoirs could explain how the infection is maintained in areas where isolated human cases occur at great intervals. The main vectors of the Gambian infection are the tsetse flies *Glossina palpalis*, *G. tachinoides*, and *G. fuscipes*, along with some other species of this group that live on the banks of rivers and lakes. Thus, infection most often propagates from man to *Glossina*, and from these flies back to man. Human infection almost always occurs in the vicinity of water courses or standing water near the victim's home. The tsetse fly is a biological vector, but during epidemics, when there are many parasitemic patients, it may transmit the infection mechanically. In general, the infection rate of vectors is low.

By contrast, in the case of *T. b. rhodesiense*, the agent of trypanosomiasis in eastern Africa, it has become clear that animals play an important role as reservoirs. The parasite has been isolated from a bushbuck (*Tragelaphus scriptus*), the spotted hyena (*Crocuta crocuta*), the lion (*Panthera leo*), and the red hartebeest (*Alcelaphus buselaphus cokei*), and the reservoir probably includes other wild animals of the East African savannah. The agent has also been isolated from a domestic zebu. Domestic animals are considered an accidental reservoir, while wild animals are more important in this regard because they occupy the same habitat as the tsetse fly. Strains from wild animals were proved to be identical to *T. b. rhodesiense* by inoculation into human volunteers, the only reliable method available at the time to differentiate "human" trypanosomes within the species *T. brucei*. Infection persists for a long time in several wild animal species (World Health Organization, 1979). Infected tsetse flies have been found in areas that have not been inhabited by man for several years. The main vectors in eastern Africa are *Glossina morsitans*, *G. swynnertoni*, and *G. pallipedes*. Use of the precipitation test has shown that these species of tsetse flies feed preferentially on wild animals. The zoophilic habits of the vectors are another indication that wild animals constitute the main reservoir of *T. b. rhodesiense*. Man can serve as a source of the parasite for the vector, but it is wild animals that perpetuate the infection. The human disease occurs sporadically because man comes into very little contact with the habitat of flies of the *morsitans* group, which in addition are not homophilic. The main victims of the disease are hunters, tourists, and other persons who enter the habitat of wild animals in which the infection is enzootic. These habitats seem to be circumscribed; they are especially associated with the range of the bushbuck (*T. scriptus*). In Uganda, however, an epidemic occurring between 1942 and 1944 caused 2,500 cases; the vector was *G. pallipedes* (*morsitans* group), a zoophilic fly that lives in the savannah scrub.

The possibility of controlling Rhodesian trypanosomiasis in the future has been complicated by the discovery of the parasite in domestic bovines.

Diagnosis: The main diagnostic method consists of microscopic examination for the parasite in blood, lymph, or bone marrow during the acute phase, or in the cerebrospinal fluid during the chronic phase. In patients with acute Rhodesian trypanosomiasis, which induces high-level parasitemias, the parasite's presence can be confirmed by examining thick blood films. In the Gambian disease, confirmation of the agent's presence is more difficult, because the parasitemia is low-level. Best results are obtained by puncture of affected lymph nodes and microscopic observation of the exudate obtained. Examination of the chronic phase cerebrospinal fluid should be done immediately after it is collected. A great advance in parasitologic diagnosis was the introduction of the diethylaminoethyl (DEAE) filtration technique, which requires very low cost equipment (Lumsden *et al.*, 1981), allowing its application in the field. Serologic tests have serious limitations, primarily because the antigens in the host vary with each parasitemic crisis. The indirect immunofluorescence test has given the best results. It is performed using stable antigens common to different trypanosome species; the homologous response generally produces the highest titer. More recently, an ELISA test and passive hemagglutination in capillary tubes have been introduced (World Health Organization, 1979).

Confirmation of a fourfold or greater increase in the level of IgM immunoglobulins in the cerebrospinal fluid of the patient, compared to noninfected persons, is very useful in diagnosis and is considered a pathognomonic sign that the central nervous system is affected (World Health Organization, 1979).

Control: Vaccines are not available. Control measures for Gambian trypanosomiasis consist primarily of a) detecting patients and treating them (with suramin or pentamidine), thus reducing the source of infection for the vectors; b) administering chemoprophylaxis with pentamidine to the exposed population at 6-month intervals (however, it should be borne in mind that strains resistant to the drug have arisen; in addition, this procedure of treating large masses of people can mask the infection in some individuals and prevent them from receiving treatment, and thus, at the present time, it is recommended only for high-risk groups); c) modifying the environment by clearing away the underbrush along the banks of rivers and lakes that constitutes the tsetse fly's habitat; and d) reducing the vector population by applying insecticides (DDT or dieldrin).

Control of Rhodesian trypanosomiasis is much more difficult. These patients should be treated with the same drugs as victims of the Gambian infection, but chemoprophylaxis is not justified because of the low incidence of the Rhodesian infection. The most rational long-range method is considered to be ecologic modification, which could be achieved by devoting areas infested by the tsetse fly to agriculture. Such projects would clear away the underbrush and establish conditions that do not permit reinfestation by the vectors. Exclusion of wild animals from infested areas is a problem that still lacks a satisfactory solution. The establishment of parks and reserves in which human settlements would not be permitted has been proposed. Application of insecticides to such vast areas would be very costly and impractical. Biological methods for controlling *Glossina* are being studied. More detailed information on control can be found in a recent work by Molyneux (1983), as well as in WHO publications (World Health Organization, 1979; UNDP/World Bank/WHO, 1982).

Bibliography

Abaru, D. E. Sleeping sickness in Busoga, Uganda, 1976-1983. *Trop Med Parasitol* 36: 72-76, 1985.

Belding, D. L. *Textbook of Parasitology*, 3rd ed. New York, Appleton-Century-Crofts, 1965.

Gibson, W. C., T. F. de C. Marshall, and D. G. Godfrey. Numerical analysis of enzyme polymorphism: a new approach to the epidemiology and taxonomy of trypanosomes of the subgenus *Trypanozoon*. *Adv Parasitol* 18:175-246, 1980.

Goodwin, L. G. The pathology of African trypanosomiases. *Trans R Soc Trop Med Hyg* 64:797-812, 1970.

Greenwood, B. M., and H. C. Whittle. The pathogenesis of sleeping sickness. *Trans R Soc Trop Med Hyg* 74:716-723, 1980.

Hajduk, S. L., P. T. Englund, A. A. F. Mahmoud, and K. S. Warren. African Trypanosomiasis. *In*: Warren, K. S., and A. A. F. Mahmoud (Eds.), *Tropical and Geographical Medicine*. New York, McGraw-Hill Book Company, 1984.

Leach, T. M. African trypanosomiases. *Adv Vet Sci* 17:119-162, 1973.

Lumsden, W. H. R., C. D. Kimber, P. Dukes, L. Haller, A. Stanghellini, and G. Duvallet. Field diagnosis of sleeping sickness in the Ivory Coast. I. Comparison of the miniature anion exchange/centrifugation technique with other protozoological methods. *Trans R Soc Trop Med Hyg* 75:242-250, 1981.

Mehlitz, D., U. Zillmann, C. M. Scott, and D. G. Godfrey. Epidemiological studies on the animal reservoir of Gambiense sleeping sickness. Part III. Characterization of Trypanozoon stocks by isoenzymes and sensitivity to human serum. *Tropenmed Parasitol* 33:113-118, 1982.

Minter, D. M. Trypanosomes. *In*: Manson-Bahr, P. E. C., and F. I. C. Apted (Eds.), *Manson's Tropical Diseases*, 18th ed. London, Baillière Tindall, 1982.

Molyneux, D. H. Animal reservoirs and Gambian trypanosomiasis. *Ann Soc Belge Med Trop* 53:605-618, 1973. Cit. Gibson *et al.*, 1980.

Molyneux, D. M. Selective primary health care: strategies for control of disease in developing world. VIII. African trypanosomiasis. *Rev Infect Dis* 5:945-956, 1983.

Okoth, J. O., and R. Kapaata. Trypanosome infection rates in *Glossina fuscipes fuscipes* Newst in the Busoga sleeping sickness focus, Uganda. *Ann Trop Med Parasitol* 80:459-461, 1986.

Onyango, R. J., K. van Hoeve, and P. de Raadt. The epidemiology of T. *rhodesiense* sleeping sickness in Algo Location, Central Nyanza, Kenya. I. Evidence that cattle may act as reservoir hosts of trypanosomes infective to man. *Trans R Soc Trop Med Hyg* 60:175-182, 1966.

Raadt, P. de. African sleeping sickness today. *Trans R Soc Trop Med Hyg* 70:114-116, 1976.

Scott, C. M., J. L. Frézil, A. Toudic, and D. G. Godfrey. The sheep as a potential reservoir of human trypanosomiasis in the Republic of the Congo. *Trans R Soc Trop Med Hyg* 77:397-401, 1983.

United Nations Development Program/World Bank/World Health Organization Consultation. Control of sleeping sickness due to *Trypanosoma brucei gambiense*. *Bull WHO* 60:821-825, 1982.

Urquart, G. M. The pathogenesis and immunology of African trypanosomiasis in domestic animals. *Trans R Soc Trop Med Hyg* 74:726-729, 1980.

World Health Organization. *African Trypanosomiasis*. Report of a Joint FAO/WHO Expert Committee. Geneva, WHO, 1969. (Technical Report Series 434.)

World Health Organization, *The African Trypanosomiases*. Report of a Joint WHO Expert Committee and FAO Expert Consultation. Geneva, WHO, 1979. (Technical Report Series 635.)

World Health Organization. *Parasitic Zoonoses*. Report of a WHO Expert Committee with the Participation of FAO. Geneva, WHO, 1979. (Technical Report Series 637.)

AMEBIASIS

(006 and 007.8)

Synonyms: Amebic dysentery, amebiosis.

Etiology: Of the numerous species of the genus *Entamoeba* found among animals, two hold some interest as agents of zoonoses: *E. histolytica* and *E. polecki*. The first is essentially a human parasite that can be transmitted to lower animals, and the second parasitizes mainly swine and can be transmitted to man.

Amebae are protozoans with two developmental phases, one trophic (vegetative) and the other cystic. In the trophic phase, the trophozoites multiply by binary fission in the large intestine of the host. They move by means of pseudopods. Before passing to the cystic phase, the amebae divide to form smaller cells and stop feeding. The cystic forms of *E. histolytica* are first uninucleate; the nuclei then subdivide by two consecutive mitoses and give rise to two and, when mature, four nuclei (the metacyst). The cysts are eliminated with the feces of the host to the environment. When these cysts are ingested with contaminated food or water by another host, the digestive juices of the small intestine cause them to excyst, and the multinucleate ameba (metacyst) divides into four amebae. These pass with the contents of the small intestine to the large intestine, where they start to feed and multiply; finally, they colonize the mucosa and complete the cycle (Faust *et al.*, 1974). *E. polecki* cysts, in contrast to those of *E. histolytica*, are uninucleate or, in a small proportion, binucleate (for other differential characteristics, see Diagnosis).

Although trophozoites can be eliminated with liquid feces, their resistance to environmental factors and gastric juices is minimal. Cysts, on the other hand, are more resistant. They can remain viable at least 2 weeks in feces and up to 5 weeks in water at ambient temperatures, but desiccation destroys them rapidly (Soulsby, 1982). Consequently, cysts have greater epidemiologic significance and constitute the infective element.

Geographic Distribution: Both *E. histolytica* and *E. polecki* have worldwide distribution.

Occurrence in Man: Infection by *E. histolytica* is more prevalent in developing countries than in industrialized ones. Prevalence is particularly high in Asia and Africa, where it sometimes reaches more than 30% of the population. In Latin America, this infection represents a grave public health problem, especially in Mexico and some other countries. In Canada, the USA, and Europe, the estimated prevalence is between 2 and 5%; the infection is usually asymptomatic or benign (World Health Organization, 1981).

Infection of man by *E. polecki* is rare. The number of known infections is just over 300, and the vast majority of cases have been diagnosed in Papua New Guinea. In some villages of that country, the prevalence rate varies from 20 to 25.6%, and several parasitologic surveys have recorded a total of 227 persons positive to *E. polecki* (McMillan and Kelly, 1970). In refugees arriving in the United States from Southeast Asia (Kampuchea, Laos, and Vietnam), 4.6% (68 of 1,478) were found to have this parasite, a proportion similar to those harboring *E. histolytica* (De Girolami and Kimber, 1983). Of 435 refugees from Kampuchea and Vietnam arriving in France, 14 (3.2%) were infected (Chaker *et al.*, 1982). It is believed that the true prevalence of *E. polecki* is higher than that recorded, since this species might be mistaken for *E. histolytica* in general laboratories.

Occurrence in Animals: Natural infection of dogs by *E. histolytica* has been diagnosed in many parts of the world, but is more frequent in the Far East. In the USA, the prevalence was 8.4% in Tennessee, and 1% out of 835 dogs examined in New Jersey. Natural infection is also common in nonhuman primates, especially those from Asia and Africa. *E. histolytica* has been associated with dysenteric symptoms in a cow in Africa and pulmonary amebiasis in a zebu. Rats can harbor *E. histolytica* that is indistinguishable from the human parasite (Soulsby, 1982).

E. polecki was originally identified in swine, but it can also be found in nonhuman primates. Its prevalence in animal species is not yet very well known.

The Disease in Man: Infection by *E. histolytica* can occur asymptomatically. Minute, saprophytic forms of the protozoan in the colon can remain at a subclinical level for many years, but there is always the potential danger that they will transform into large forms of *E. histolytica,* causing a progressive and invasive disease. Consequently, all infections must be considered as potentially pathogenic (World Health Organization, 1981). Intestinal disease varies from acute, fulminant dysentery, with fever, chills, and bloody or mucous diarrhea (amebic dysentery), to mild abdominal discomfort, with episodes of diarrhea containing blood or mucus alternating with periods of constipation (American Public Health Association, 1985). Fulminant intestinal amebiasis especially affects women during pregnancy or soon after childbirth; they account for 5 to 10% of cases hospitalized with intestinal amebiasis. The colon develops multiple ulcers and many perforate. Patients with prolonged intestinal amebiasis or chronic amebiasis may recuperate or may relapse with colitis; 10 to 20% of these patients need hospitalization. The most frequent extraintestinal complication is hepatic abscesses, which can be the primary ailment or a symptom associated with a progressive infection of the colon. Hepatomegaly, pain, fever, and biologic, radiographic, and echotomographic changes are present in 65 to 80% of cases (World Health Organization, 1981). Amebic necrosis and liver abscesses are particularly frequent in Southeast Asia, India, North Africa, and Mexico. In developed countries, on the other hand, amebiasis is usually benign.

Infection of man by *E. polecki* almost always occurs subclinically, but some patients manifest clinical symptoms, with diarrhea and abdominal pain. Extraintestinal invasions do not occur.

The Disease in Animals: In dogs, infection by *E. histolytica* is generally asymptomatic and frequently localized in the cecum. Occasionally, it can invade tissues and cause acute or chronic amebiasis. A generalized infection that affected the lungs, liver, kidney, and spleen has been described in a puppy (Soulsby, 1982).

Infection by *E. histolytica* has been confirmed in many species of nonhuman primates. Rhesus monkeys are generally resistant and usually experience asymptomatic infection, but chronic, mild colitis can occur. In chimpanzees, the infection can persist for a long time, in most cases subclinically, but sometimes it invades the tissues causing ulcerative colitis and hepatic abscesses. Fatal cases have been confirmed on several occasions (Miller and Bray, 1966). New World monkeys are considered more susceptible to the disease than Asian or African monkeys. A devastating outbreak occurred in a colony of 90 spider monkeys in the United States. At least half of these monkeys suffered diarrhea, and severe cases included abdominal pain and hemorrhagic evacuations. During the month-long outbreak, there were two to six deaths per week; necropsies revealed hepatic abscesses in almost 30% of the dead animals (Amyx *et al.*, 1978). Cases of clinical amebiasis in cattle have been described in Africa, although the disease seems rare in this species. Wild rats can also harbor *E. histolytica* indistinguishable from the human parasite; as in other species, the protozoan can be found in the large intestine as a commensal or it can invade the mucosa and cause amebic dysentery (Soulsby, 1982).

It is rare for *E. polecki* or other amebae to cause clinical symptomatology or lesions in swine (Dunlap, 1975).

Source of Infection and Mode of Transmission: The reservoir of *E. histolytica* is man; infection is transmitted via the fecal-oral route. The infective element is the cyst. Food and water contaminated by feces that contain cysts are the main sources of infection. The principal contributors to environmental contamination are asymptomatic carriers or individuals who suffer bouts of diarrhea intermittent with well-formed or pasty feces. These carriers eliminate cysts with the feces, while diarrheic patients eliminate trophozoites that can be destroyed by gastric juices (Faust *et al.*, 1974). Deficient sanitation, lack of personal as well as food hygiene, and crowding are all very important factors in the epidemiology of amebiasis.

Animals contract *E. histolytica* infection from a human source. Transmission from dog to dog or from dog to man does not occur or is exceptional, since only trophozoites and not cysts are found in dogs' intestines (World Health Organization, 1979). On the other hand, the infection can propagate between nonhuman primates, who can in turn retransmit it to man. When one group of 29 chimpanzees was obtained, only two had *E. histolytica*, perhaps by exposure to human carriers; 4 years later, 10 of the 29 were infected (Miller and Bray, 1966). It is probable that the infection of spider monkeys mentioned above (see The Disease in Animals) was produced by exposure of the animals to Old World nonhuman primates in the same colony (Amyx *et al.*, 1978).

The main reservoir of *E. polecki* is swine; human infection occurs by ingestion of protozoan cysts from contaminated hands or in water or food. Close contact and cohabitation with swine are important factors in transmission. Explanations of the high prevalence of *E. polecki* infections in Papua New Guinea (see Occurrence) and the higher rate of infection in women than in men are that swine often live in human dwellings and that women are in charge of raising them and may even breast-feed suckling pigs (McMillan and Kelly, 1970). Another probable source of infection is nonhuman primates. Interhuman transmission is also suspected; of three cases diagnosed in Venezuela, two had had no contact with animals (Chacin-Bonilla, 1983).

Diagnosis: Laboratory diagnosis is based on parasitologic examination and serologic tests. Direct examination of diarrheic feces almost always reveals trophozoites, whereas cysts are found in formed feces. Samples of diarrheic and pasty fecal matter should be examined as soon after collection as possible, since trophozoites are easily destroyed. In general, one preparation should be observed in saline solution and another in iodized solution. If protozoans are not seen by this method, concentration by zinc sulfate and centrifugation can be used; fresh specimens can be stained with iron hematoxylin. Since it is difficult to distinguish between the trophozoites of *E. histolytica* and *E. polecki,* attention should be directed toward the cysts. *E. polecki* cysts have only one nucleus, which occupies one-quarter to one-third of the cyst, and a large karyosome, while those of *E. histolytica* have four nuclei that occupy one-third to one-half of the cyst (immature intermediate phases with one or two nuclei can be observed) and smaller karyosomes. Chromatin is uniformly distributed in the nuclear periphery in *E. histolytica* but not in *E. polecki.* Glycogen vacuoles are commonly observed in the cytoplasm of *E. histolytica* while they are rare in *E. polecki,* where an opaque mass (inclusion mass) several times larger than the nucleus is found. Another distinctive characteristic is the number of chromatoidal bars, which is less than 10 in *E. histolytica* and can reach 30 in *E. polecki* (Levin and Armstrong, 1970).

The most used serologic tests for diagnosis of amebiasis by *E. histolytica* are indirect hemagglutination, immunodiffusion in gel, indirect immunofluorescence, counterimmunoelectrophoresis, immunoelectrophoresis, latex agglutination, complement fixation, and ELISA. Serologic tests only give positive results when the tissue is invaded, because *E. histolytica* in the commensal state does not induce antibody production. Consequently, serology can be used to distinguish disease from commensal infection. Positive reactions occur in 60 to 70% of patients with intestinal amebiasis and 90 to 95% of patients with extraintestinal forms (Parrochia, 1982). The few patients with *E. polecki* amebiasis tested with *E. histolytica* antigens gave negative results.

Control: Prophylactic measures consist mainly of environmental sanitation, provision of potable water, sanitary elimination of feces, personal hygiene, and food hygiene. Treatment with metronidazole is recommended for carriers, especially those involved in the preparation of food.

Bibliography

Amyx, H. L., D. M. Asher, T. E. Nash, C. J. Gibbs, Jr., and D. C. Gajdusek. Hepatic amebiasis in spider monkeys. *Am J Trop Med Hyg* 27:888-891, 1978.

American Public Health Association. *Control of Communicable Diseases in Man,* 14th ed. (Ed. by A. S. Benenson). Washington, D.C., APHA, 1985.

Chacin-Bonilla, L. *Entamoeba polecki* infection in Venezuela. Report of a new case. *Trans R Soc Trop Med Hyg* 77:137, 1983.

Chaker, E., M. Kremer, and T. T. Kien. Quatorze cas d'*Entamoeba polecki* chez refugies du sud-est asiatique: remarques sur l'aspect morphologique du parasite. *Bull Soc Pathol Exot* 75:484-490, 1982.

De Girolami, P. A., and J. Kimber. Intestinal parasites among Southeast Asian refugees in Massachusetts. *Am J Clin Pathol* 79:502-504, 1983.

Desowitz, R. S., and G. Barnish. *Entamoeba polecki* and other intestinal protozoa in Papua New Guinea highland children. *Ann Trop Med Parasitol* 80:399-402, 1986.

Dunlap, J. S. Protozoa. *In*: Dunne, H. W., and A. D. Leman (Eds.), *Diseases of Swine*, 4th ed. Ames, Iowa State University Press, 1975.

Faust, E. C., P. F. Russell, and R. C. Jung. *Craig and Faust's Clinical Parasitology*, 8th ed. Philadelphia, Lea and Febiger, 1970.

Levin, R. L., and D. E. Armstrong. Human infection with *Entamoeba polecki*. *Am J Clin Pathol* 56:611-614, 1970.

McMillan, B., and A. Kelly. *Entamoeba polecki* von Prowazek, 1912 in New Guinea. *Trans R Soc Med Hyg* 64:792-793, 1970.

Miller, M. J., and R. S. Bray. *Entamoeba histolytica* infections in the chimpanzee (*Pan satyrus*). *J Parasitol* 52:386-388.

Parrochia, E. Diagnóstico diferencial de la enfermedad amebiana. *Bol Hosp San Juan de Dios* (*Chile*) 29:276-282, 1982.

Soulsby, E. J. L. *Helminths, Arthropods and Protozoa of Domesticated Animals*, 7th ed. Philadelphia, Lea and Febiger, 1982.

World Health Organization. *Parasitic Zoonoses*. Report of a WHO Expert Committee with the Participation of FAO. Geneva, WHO, 1979. (Technical Report Series 637.)

World Health Organization. *Intestinal Protozoan and Helminthic Infections*. Report of a WHO Scientific Group. Geneva, WHO, 1981. (Technical Report Series 666.)

AMERICAN TRYPANOSOMIASIS

(086.2)

Synonyms: Chagas' disease, Chagas-Mazza disease.

Etiology: *Trypanosoma* (*Schizotrypanum*) *cruzi*, a flagellate protozoan with an undulating membrane; it has a complex developmental cycle, undergoing several transformations in both the vertebrate host and the triatomine vector.

Infection of man occurs when metacyclic trypomastigotes (the last phase of the parasite's development in the vector insect) enter the macrophages of the dermal connective tissue or subcutaneous tissue, where they become amastigotes (leishmanial form). This intracellular form, which lacks the flagellum and membrane, multiplies by binary fission for 4 or 5 days; the host cell then ruptures and other macrophages become infected. Some parasites from the primary focus are liberated into the bloodstream, where they again become trypomastigotes (flagellate forms with a membrane) that are carried throughout the body and invade the cells of various organs. In the cell protoplasm, they again take on the leishmanial, or amastigote, form and multiply.

The second developmental cycle occurs in the triatomine vector. These hematophagous insects ingest the trypomastigotes (free forms of trypanosomes) that abound in the bloodstream of infected lower mammals and, during febrile periods, of man. The triatomine may also ingest intracellular leishmanial forms, which undergo a new series of transformations and multiply in the insect's midgut. The parasites are in the epimastigote (crithidial) form when they multiply; after 15 to 30 days, they change into metacyclic trypomastigotes (metacyclic trypanosomes) in the insect's rectum. These forms of the parasite are eliminated with the feces of the triatomine as it feeds on man or another vertebrate host. Metacyclic trypanosomes in the vector's feces invade the host's body by way of the insect bite wound or through abrasions in the skin or mucous membranes, thus reinitiating the cycle. This sequence of events is referred to as transmission from the "posterior station," or by contamination; by contrast, in African trypanosomiasis (see corresponding section), transmission is from the "anterior station," or by inoculation. Lower vertebrates can also become infected by ingesting triatomines or their feces.

Study of different strains of *T. cruzi* has revealed great variation in the morphology of the bloodstream forms, and in the parasite's antigenic constituents, virulence, susceptibility to drugs, and infectivity for host cells (Brener, 1982). One unresolved problem is whether geographical differences in the clinicopathologic pictures and responses of patients to treatment are due to differences in the strains of *T. cruzi* prevailing in each region. For this reason, various methods have been employed to identify genetic markers in order to distinguish different strains of the agent. An interesting advance has been obtained with electrophoresis of isozymes,[1] which has allowed identification and grouping of strains of the agent according to their isozymic profiles. The name zymodeme has been given to a population of parasites with identical isozymic profiles. Miles (1983), who introduced this technique in the study of *T. cruzi*, identified three zymodemes in Brazil. Zymodeme 1 (Z1) exists in the wild, zymodeme 2 (Z2) has a domestic cycle, and zymodeme 3 (Z3) also has a wild cycle. Z2 is found in central and eastern Brazil where triatomines live in houses, and it has been isolated from chronically ill patients as well as from domestic animals. Z1 circulates mainly among arboreal wild animals and wild triatomines; it is also infective for man. Z3 has been isolated from armadillos and from some acute human cases in the Brazilian Amazon jungle. In this region, where there are no domiciliary triatomines, only sporadic cases caused by Z1 and Z3 occur. Z1 and Z3 have also been found in Venezuela, where the former predominates. Since the megacolon and megaloesophagus forms of the disease rarely occur in Venezuela, but are more frequent in endemic areas of Brazil where Z2 predominates, the possibility has been suggested that these pathologies may be related to the zymodeme (Miles *et al.*, 1980). Two principal zymodemes have been found in Bolivia, one very closely related to Brazilian Z1, and the other related to Z2 in some differential characteristics (Tibayrenc and Miles, 1983).

Geographic Distribution (Map 10): Infection by *T. cruzi* occurs from the southern United States south to Argentina and Chile. Infected wild reservoirs and/or wild triatomine vectors have been found throughout most of the Caribbean region, formerly considered to be free from the infection (Pan American Health Organization, 1984). Chagas' disease has not been confirmed outside the Americas.

Occurrence in Man: Chagas' disease is essentially a problem affecting southern Mexico and Central and South America. In the Caribbean region, where the infection cycle is sylvatic, some sporadic human cases have been described in Trinidad and Tobago, Belize, and Guyana, but the prevalence of the human disease on the Caribbean islands has not been recorded. In the southern United States,

---

[1] Isozyme: One of the multiple forms in which an enzyme may exist in a single species, the various forms differing chemically, physically, and/or immunologically but catalyzing the same reaction (*Dorland's Illustrated Medical Dictionary*, 26th ed. Philadelphia, Saunders, 1985).

Map 10. Distribution of American trypanosomiasis.

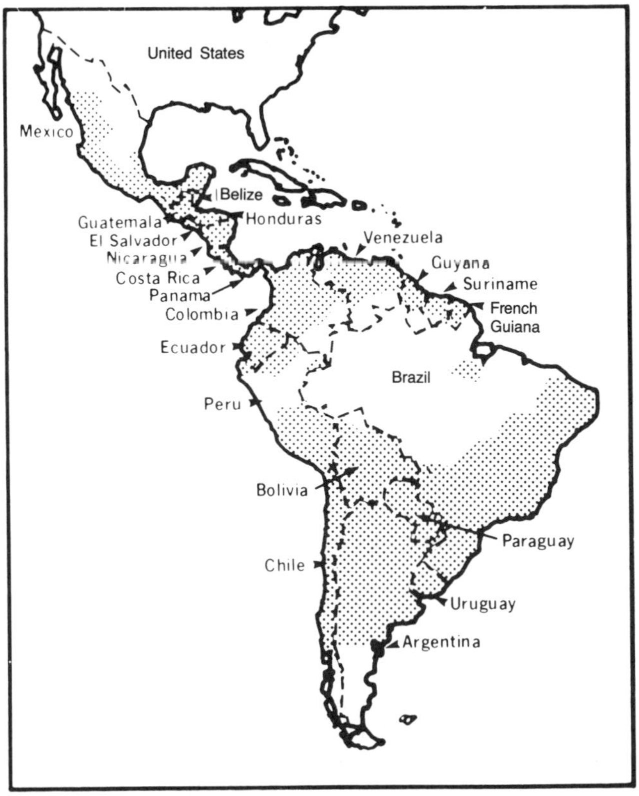

Source: PAHO Epidemiol Bull 5(2):5, 1984

where infected vectors and sylvatic reservoirs exist, only three cases of human infection have been described; in the area of Texas where the first two cases were diagnosed, antibodies against *T. cruzi* were found in nine of 500 individuals. According to estimates based on seroepidemiologic studies, 10 to 20 million persons in Latin America are infected and 65 million are exposed to risk. It is calculated that nearly 10% of those infected in South America will develop clinical signs and symptoms of chronic Chagas' disease (Pan American Health Organization, 1984). The highest prevalence of disease is found in rural and periurban areas, but the distribution is uneven and depends on the habits of the triatomine vector, that is, whether it lives in and around houses. Thus, in the Brazilian Amazon, where the infection cycle is sylvatic, only nine autochthonous human cases have been recognized, eight of them in Pará (Dorea, 1981). On the other hand, in some regions of high endemicity where the vector is domiciliary, such as Minas Gerais, Rio Grande do Sul, and Goiás, the prevalence of reactors in the general population, as determined by the indirect immunofluorescence test, was 7 to 9% (Camargo *et al.*, 1984). Some serologic surveys conducted in endemic localities have found a high rate of reactors, sometimes reaching 40% or more of the population examined. One of the most extensive studies was carried out in Brazil from 1975 to 1980, and encompassed the rural areas of the entire country except São Paulo and the Federal District; 4.2% of the more than 1,300,000 samples examined gave positive results to the immunofluorescence test (Camargo et al., 1984). The well-documented importance of Chagas' disease in public health lies mainly in the frequency with which it causes cardiopathies in chronic patients. In some areas, this disease is the most frequent cause of myocardiopathies and even of death.

Chagas' disease is a rural affliction, but its sequelae can also be seen in chronically ill patients in cities owing to the increasing migration of rural inhabitants to urban areas. A study on mortality in 10 Latin American cities (Puffer and Griffith, 1967) revealed that deaths caused by chagasic cardiopathy occurred in seven of them. The mortality rate was exceptionally high in Ribeirão Preto, Brazil, a city with a population of over 100,000. Chagas' disease caused 13% of all deaths in the age group 15 to 74 years, and 29% in males between 25 and 44 years of age; in women of the same age group the rate was somewhat less (22%). The cause of death of the Chagas' disease patients was almost always heart disease.

In Belén (Carabobo State), a rural town in Venezuela with 1,656 inhabitants, a longitudinal study carried out on 1,210 persons over 5 years of age showed a 47.3% prevalence of infection, and found cardiopathies in 17.3%. Of those who suffered from chronic myocarditis, 84.8% were serologically positive for *T. cruzi*. During the 4-year study, serologic conversion occurred in 16.3% and cardiopathies in 2.2% of 812 persons studied. The incidence of heart disease was five times higher in the seropositive group than in the seronegative group (Puigbó et al., 1968).

The accumulated data clearly demonstrate that Chagas' disease must be considered one of the most serious public health problems in Latin America.

Occurrence in Animals: Natural infection has been found in more than 100 species of domestic and wild mammals. Nevertheless, difficulties in identification make it uncertain that all of the isolated strains correspond to *T. cruzi*. Several animal species serve as reservoirs in different ecologic situations. Among domestic animals, dogs and cats are frequent and important hosts of the parasite. On several occasions the prevalence in these species in endemic areas has been found to be greater than that in man. In a number of localities in Brazil and Argentina, xenodiagnosis has revealed infection rates of more than 20% in dogs and cats. In Yaracuy Valley, Venezuela, 70 out of 140 dogs examined were positive to xenodiagnosis. Out of 3,321 dogs and 1,805 cats examined in Chile, 9.1 and 11.9%, respectively, gave positive xenodiagnostic results, while 8.4% of the humans tested by the same method were positive. The high rate in cats may be attributable to the large population of infected house mice, which could be a source of infection for the cats that hunt and feed on them. In addition, cats, mice, and many other mammals frequently ingest triatomines. Other domestic animals can also act as reservoirs (Miles, 1983). A hemagglutination serologic study in 34 rural localities in Region IV of Chile found antibodies for *T. cruzi* in 7.8% of 232 goats examined, 11.7% of 145 rabbits, and 4.8% of 42 sheep; high reactor rates were also confirmed in dogs and cats (Correa et al., 1982).

The guinea pig *Cavia porcellus*, a domestic animal of the Andean high plateau, is of great importance in the epidemiology of Chagas' disease in that region. Infection rates ranging from 10.5% to 61% have been found in these animals in different Bolivian localities.

Natural infection has been confirmed in a large number of wild animal species.

Although practically any mammal that comes in contact with infected vectors can acquire the infection, not all animal species are equally important in maintaining enzootic wild Chagas' disease. Generally, one or two species are the primary hosts in an ecologic region. Studies carried out in Brazil and Venezuela implicate opossums of the genus *Didelphis* (*D. marsupialis, D. albiventris*). Xenodiagnostic studies on 750 mammals of 31 species in the dry tropical forests of the Venezuelan high plains yielded positive results in 10 species and revealed 143 infections; 83% of the animals infected were *D. marsupialis*, which represented only 30% of the total number of mammals sampled. The infection rate increased at the end of the rainy season, when more than 80% of the opossum population was found to be infected (Telford *et al.*, 1981). Several studies carried out in Brazil by different authors have also found high rates of infection in *D. marsupialis* and *D. albiventris*. These marsupials are notable for their prolonged parasitemia, which can persist for more than 12 months (Mello, 1981; Mello, 1982). Since opossums often approach human dwellings, they serve as an important link between the wild and domestic cycle of infection by *T. cruzi*. In several countries, armadillos, which are common in Latin America, are also frequently parasitized.

The Disease in Man: The incubation period is usually from 7 to 14 days, but can last from 30 to 40 days when the infection is transmitted by blood transfusion from an infected donor.

Three phases are distinguished: acute, indeterminate, and chronic. The acute phase of infection varies from asymptomatic to a severe and fatal disease. It affects primarily children and is characterized by intermittent or continual high pyrexia. About 50% of children manifest unilateral swelling of the eyelids (Romaña's sign), related to the inoculation site. The palpebral edema is accompanied by conjunctivitis and regional adenopathy; keratitis is frequent. On other areas of the face or body, cutaneous lesions (chagomas) that resemble furuncles occur near the agent's site of entry and are always accompanied by regional adenopathy. Approximately 25% of patients show no lesions that indicate the point of entry. In some cases there may be generalized edema of the entire body. Hepatosplenomegaly is common in children but not frequent in adults. Symptoms and signs of the disease vary with the different organs affected. The febrile syndrome can be accompanied by myocarditis, with cardiac dilation, hypotension, and tachycardia. Involvement of the central nervous system can be manifested by encephalomyelitis or meningoencephalitis. Cases in which the digestive tract is affected are also seen, and include vomiting and diarrhea. The course of the acute form is from 3 to 4 weeks. Lesions are almost always of the inflammatory type. Although the parasite can be found in any part of the body, it has a certain preference for the reticuloendothelial system, the cardiac muscle or skeletal musculature, and the central nervous system; thus, the most important clinical manifestations are myocarditis and meningoencephalitis (González Cappa and Segura, 1982). The fatality rate of the acute form is around 8%; mortality occurs mostly in children with cardiac or central nervous system complications.

Primary infection can often pass unnoticed, as confirmed by the fact that many serologically positive adults have no history of the acute form.

After the acute phase, a period of latent infection follows (indeterminate phase), with low parasitemia and without clinical symptomatology. It can persist indefinitely or lead to the chronic disease form. The indeterminate phase is characterized by positive serology and/or positive xenodiagnosis, but not by clinical manifestations (cardiac, digestive, or neural) or electrocardiographic and radiologic alterations. In endemic areas, this form is found mainly in persons under 30 years of age (Dorea, 1981). Autopsies of some persons in this phase who died in accidents found foci of myocarditis and a decrease in neurons of the parasympathetic plexus. In heart biopsies, lymphocytes were found to have penetrated the cells, indicating the possibility that a sensitized population of lymphocytes might participate directly in the production of lesions (González Cappa and Segura, 1982).

The chronic form appears in 10 to 30% of affected individuals, generally 10 to 15 years after the acute phase and with chagasic cardiopathy as the most common and important effect. After the first manifestations, which almost always consist of extrasystoles and precordialgia, an electrocardiogram shows complete or incomplete blockage of the right branch of the bundle of His. In this stage, signs of cardiac insufficiency are found, and autopsies reveal thinned or aneurysmal ventricular walls. Often, the chronic phase is only apparent by abnormalities in the electrocardiogram, and not by clinical symptomatology. Histopathologic examination reveals areas of fibrosis and infiltration of mononuclears but not the presence of parasites, which are not usually found in the chronic disease. Heart lesions consist of diffuse, fibrous microfocal myocarditis. Likewise, there is a great reduction in the number of parasympathetic nerve ganglia (González Cappa and Segura, 1982). In Argentina, an estimated 20% of Chagas' patients suffer from myocarditis. Patients with the chronic disease often deny having experienced the acute form, possibly because it passed asymptomatically or because it occurred in childhood and was forgotten.

In several endemic areas of Latin America, a digestive form of Chagas' disease that produces visceromegalies, especially megaloesophagus and megacolon, is seen. Neurologic, myxedematous, and glandular forms occur less frequently.

The Disease in Animals: Infection in wild animals is clinically inapparent. Dogs, by contrast, sometimes develop symptoms similar to those in man, and acute and chronic disease forms are seen. The acute phase, which starts after an incubation period of 5 to 42 days, is manifested by moderate fever and may include palpebral edema, pronounced hepatomegaly, various adenopathies, cardiac disorders, and neurologic alterations. The acute form lasts from 10 to 30 or more days, and then progresses to the indeterminate form, which may last years without clinical manifestations. The chronic form is characterized, in dogs as in man, by myocarditis. Canine trypanosomiasis caused by *T. cruzi* is often fatal. Cardiopathies, visceromegalies, and alterations of the central nervous system have been reproduced experimentally in dogs. Dogs sacrificed during the indeterminate phase showed mild, focal, chronic myocarditis with a few microscopic foci of fibrosis. In several parts of the conduction system, especially the atrioventricular node and the distal portion of the bundle of His, focal or diffuse fibrous lesions and sclerosis were found. It is thought that these lesions are sequelae of the inflammation and necrosis produced during the acute phase (Andrade *et al.*, 1981). Puppies inoculated with high infective doses die in 2 to 3 weeks with an acute form of the disease that characteristically involves cardiac insufficiency.

Source of Infection and Mode of Transmission (Figure 60): Parasitosis caused by *T. cruzi* was originally an infection that circulated among wild mammals, as it still is in many scattered sylvatic foci in the Americas. Chagas' disease is now a significant public health problem in Latin America because some species of triatomine vectors have adapted to living in human dwellings. This has allowed the parasite to circulate among domestic animals (especially dogs, cats, and guinea

Figure 60. American trypanosomiasis. Domiciliary cycle of *Trypanosoma cruzi*.

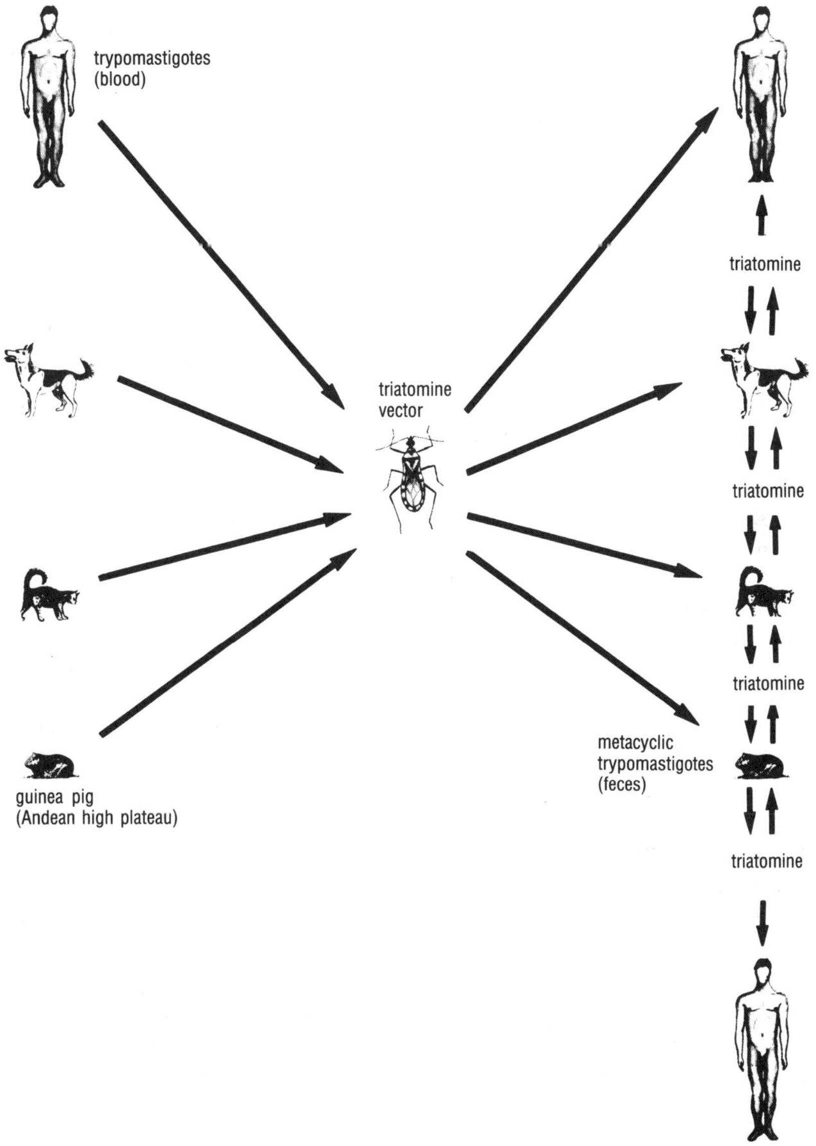

pigs), between these animals and man, and also among human, so that the cycle is now, for the most part, independent of animals. Human infection persists for life. In the acute phase of the disease, parasitemia is high-level, while during the indeterminate and chronic phases, the number of parasites circulating in the blood is low.

In areas where only the sylvatic cycle exists, infection in humans is occasional and of little public health importance; however, where there are domiciliary triatomines, Chagas' disease occurs endemically or hyperendemically.

Animal reservoirs (see The Disease in Animals) provide a significant source of infection for the vectors because of their prolonged parasitemia and the high number of trypanosomes (trypomastigotes) in their blood.

Infection is transmitted by hemipterans of the family Reduviidae, subfamily Triatominae. There are 53 known species of naturally infected triatomines, 36 of which live around and in human dwellings; of these, approximately 12 are epidemiologically important because they are highly adapted to the domestic or peridomestic ecotope.

One of the species best adapted to the human environment is *Triatoma infestans*, which is widely distributed in Peru, Bolivia, Chile, Argentina, Uruguay, Paraguay, and Brazil. Its preference for the blood of man and several species of domestic animals has been shown by the precipitation test. *Rhodnius prolixus* is an important species in Colombia, Ecuador, Venezuela, much of Central America, and also in Mexico. This triatomine can reach high densities in human dwellings; in Venezuela, it is also found on palm trees, its natural environment.

Several triatomines are in the process of adapting to human dwellings. These include *Triatoma sordida*, whose habitat in Bolivia, Argentina, and Brazil is usually peridomiciliary; *Panstrongylus magistus* in eastern Brazil, which is found in both dwellings and natural ecotopes; *T. brasiliensis* in northeastern Brazil; and *T. maculata* in Venezuela, which is the predominant triatomine in areas around houses and is associated with poultry.

Other triatomines only occasionally invade human dwellings, where they are unable to establish themselves or reproduce. Another group of these insects is found exclusively in natural niches in the wild.

A triatomine such as *T. infestans* lays about 300 eggs during its lifetime. Under laboratory conditions (25°C, 80% relative humidity, and one feeding per week) development from egg to adult, passing through five molts, takes 193 to 241 days (Schenone *et al.*, 1980). Duration of the life cycle varies in different triatomine species.

The ecology of Chagas' disease is closely connected to underdevelopment and poverty in rural and marginal urban areas of Latin America. Precarious dwellings made of adobe, mud, and cane, and roofs made of palm leaves or straw offer ideal conditions for triatomine colonization. The bugs readily infest small crevices that abound in this type of construction, and will also take up residence in furniture and various other household objects. Triatomines are also found in chicken houses, rabbit hutches, corrals, pigsties, aviaries, sheds, and wood piles around dwellings. In general, deficient socioeconomic conditions maintain endemic Chagas' disease.

The triatomine becomes infected by ingesting the blood of a vertebrate with parasitemia. The parasite multiplies in the vector's intestine; after about 20 days, the bug begins to eliminate trypanosomes with its feces, and it can continue to do so throughout its lifetime. Infection of some domiciliary species of triatomines is very common; in some endemic areas, more than 80% of *T. infestans* have been found to be parasitized.

The infection is most commonly transmitted to man by means of the triatomine vector. While feeding on human blood, the bug defecates and, with its feces, deposits metacyclic trypanosomes on the skin. If the person scratches or rubs the area, the feces can contaminate the insect bite wound or another pre-existing wound, and in this way the parasites enter the body. Likewise, the parasite can penetrate the body via contamination of the conjunctiva by vector feces. The vector attacks at night when the person is sleeping. The time a triatomine species takes between the acts of ingesting the blood and defecating is important in determining its efficiency as a vector of the parasite. The most efficient vectors are those that defecate while feeding or shortly thereafter, such as *T. infestans*. By contrast, *T. protracta*, a North American species, defecates long enough after feeding that it may already have left the host.

In addition to its domiciliary nature, defecation habits, and receptivity to *T. cruzi*, other important epidemiologic characteristics of the vector are its population density and rate of infection.

The risk of Chagas' disease transmission via blood transfusions is serious when proper precautions are not taken. In a nonendemic area of metropolitan Buenos Aires, Argentina, 5.4% of blood donors were found to be reactors to the complement fixation test (Carcavallo and Rubin de Celis, 1972); in endemic areas the rates are much higher. This mode of transmission has been confirmed on several occasions in Brazil, Argentina, Chile, and Venezuela. Blood transfusion constitutes the second most important way the infection is transmitted and, in areas free of vector insects, it can provide a source of infection, owing to the increasing migration of the rural population from endemic areas to nonendemic areas and to cities.

Chagasic placentitis can cause abortions and congenital infection. Studies in two hospitals in Salvador, Bahia, Brazil, found an incidence of chagasic infection of 2.7% in 296 fetuses examined, and 1.3% in 232 newborn infants.

Per os infection is also possible by means of foods contaminated by triatomine feces. A fatal infection via the oral route was contracted accidentally in an Argentine laboratory.

The mechanisms of transmission between animals are the same as those that operate for man. Infection via the digestive tract possibly plays a more important role among lower animals.

Diagnosis: Specific diagnostic methods consist of the following: a) demonstration of the parasite's presence directly by microscopic examination or indirectly by xenodiagnosis, inoculation of laboratory animals, or hemoculture; and b) serologic tests.

When the number of parasites in the blood is high, as it is during the acute phase of disease, the presence of the parasite can be confirmed by microscopic observation of fresh blood between slide and coverslip, and of thick films stained by Giemsa or Wright's method. A practical and very efficient method is Strout's procedure of concentrating hemoflagellates by blood centrifugation and examining wet mounts of the sediment that forms between the serum and clot layers (Flores *et al.*, 1966).

In chronic or long-term cases, the number of trypanosomes in peripheral blood decreases and the parasite's presence can only be demonstrated by indirect methods.

One very useful indirect method is xenodiagnosis. It consists of letting 40 triatomines in the third nymphal stage (if *T. infestans* is used) bite the patient and then examining the insects' feces 45 to 60 days later for the presence of parasites. For child patients, 20 nymphs can be used. The triatomines should be bred from eggs in the laboratory and fed on laboratory fowl to ensure that they are free of the infection. The procedure is effective in 100% of acute cases and 50% of chronic cases (González Cappa and Segura, 1982). Another, less sensitive method for diagnosing the chronic phase of the disease is hemoculture. Use of both xenodiagnosis and hemoculture increases the likelihood of isolation.

The most commonly used serologic tests are complement fixation (Guerreiro-Machado test), indirect hemagglutination (IH), direct agglutination (DA), and indirect immunofluorescence (IIF). All these tests give positive results in chagasic patients after 5 months of infection, the immunofluorescence test giving the earliest results. An ELISA test has recently been developed. The complement fixation (CF) test gives negative results in 30 to 50% of acute phase patients; on the other hand, in chronic patients its sensitivity is over 90%. The IIF and ELISA tests are very sensitive and specific; IIF can give cross-reactions in patients with leishmaniasis. The sensitivity of IH is comparable to CF and IIF. The latex test is less sensitive than the others; direct agglutination, for which stabilized antigens are currently available, is especially indicated for patients in the acute phase of the disease (Brener, 1982). The standardization of serologic tests is essential to ensure that results are reliable and repeatable in different laboratories, and toward that end, reference laboratories are needed in the Region of the Americas. To minimize the possibility of false positive or negative results, at least two tests should be used. Diagnosis of chagasic infection in lower animals is based on the same methods as diagnosis in man.

Cross-reactions have been observed in many cases of North American blastomycosis and in some cases of toxoplasmosis.

Control: Chagas' disease is in large measure a socioeconomic problem, and the long-term control strategy should be improvement of rural and periurban dwellings, since poor housing is the fundamental factor maintaining the endemic disease.

Control programs in the affected countries are mostly directed against the vectors. Treatment of dwellings with residual insecticides produces a marked reduction in triatomine infestation. The insecticide of choice is benzene hexachloride (gamexane), which is inexpensive and not very toxic to man or other vertebrates. However, its residual effect is short (about 1 month) and it does not affect triatomine eggs. The addition of pyrethrins to the insecticide improves its effectiveness by driving the vector from its hiding places. The spraying program should be carried out over geographic areas that are sufficiently extensive to prevent reinfestations. In each home the spray should be applied to the internal and external walls, ceilings, eaves, furniture, bed frames, mattresses, and any possible refuge of the vector. Similarly, all nearby structures and annexes, such as chicken houses, pigsties, and wood piles, should be sprayed. At the beginning of the program, tests should be conducted to determine the most appropriate interval between sprayings, which currently varies between 1 and 5 months or even a year, depending on the country. As the program advances, treatment can be limited to localized areas and then focused on infested dwellings.

Traditional vector control by chemical insecticides has been the most utilized measure because of its applicability and favorable cost-benefit ratio. However, application by the community of combined or integrated control measures should be explored in order to achieve more permanent results. A combination of residual-action insecticides, health education, improvement of rural dwellings, and promotion of rural development projects through multisectoral cooperation must constitute the basis of a new control strategy for Chagas' disease.

Currently, research is being done on juvenile hormone analogs, which inhibit the production of fertile adult triatomines. These synthetic substances act at very low doses and their effect is prolonged.

To prevent transmission of the infection via blood transfusions, donors should be subjected to serologic tests. In places where diagnosis is not possible, gentian violet

(1:4,000) should be added to the blood, which should then be kept refrigerated for 24 hours before use.

No vaccines against Chagas' disease are available at present.

Bibliography

Alonso, J. M., S. Pividori, and C. Guilleron. Antígenos circulantes de *Trypanosoma cruzi* en chagásicos de área endémica. *Medicina (B Aires)* 46:69-72, 1986.

Andrade, Z. A., S. G. Andrade, M. Sadigusky, and J. H. Maguire. Experimental Chagas' disease in dogs. *Arch Pathol Lab Med* 105:460-464, 1981.

Barreto, M. P. Reservatórios do *Trypanosoma cruzi*. *In*: Cançado, J. R. (Ed.), *Doença de Chagas*. Belo Horizonte, Imprensa Oficial do Estado de Minas Gerais, 1968.

Bittencourt, A. L., and E. Mota. Isoenzyme characterization of *Trypanosoma cruzi* from congenital cases of Chagas disease. *Ann Trop Med Parasitol* 79:393-396, 1985.

Brener, Z. Life cycle of *Trypanosoma cruzi*. *Rev Inst Med Trop S Paulo* 13:171-178, 1971.

Brener, Z. Recent developments in the field of Chagas' disease. *Bull WHO* 60:463-473, 1982.

Camargo, M. E., G. R. Silva, E. A. Castilho, and A. C. Silveira. Inquérito serológico da prevalência de infecção chagásica no Brasil, 1975/1980. *Rev Inst Med Trop S Paulo* 26:192-204, 1984.

Carcavallo, R. V., and M. Rubin de Celis. *La enfermedad de Chagas en la Provincia de Buenos Aires*. La Plata, Ministry of Social Welfare of the Province of Buenos Aires, 1972.

Cerisola, J. A., M. Alvarez, H. Lugones, and J. B. Rebosolan. Sensibilidad de las reacciones serológicas para el diagnóstico de la enfermedad de Chagas. *Bol Chile Parasitol* 24:2-8, 1969.

Correa, V., J. Briceño, J. Zuñiga, J. C. Aranda, J. Valdés, M. C. Contreras, H. Schenone, F. Villaroel, and A. Rojas. Infección por *Trypanosoma cruzi* en animales domésticos de sectores rurales de la IV Región, Chile. *Bol Chile Parasitol* 37:27-78, 1982.

Deane, L. M. Animal reservoirs of *Trypanosoma cruzi* in Brazil. *Rev Bras Malar* 16:27-48, 1964.

Dorea, R. C. C. Doença de Chagas na Amazônia: aspectos epidemiológicos regionais e considerações a propósito de um caso pediátrico. *Hileia Med (Belem)* 3:81-109, 1981.

Faust, E. C., P. C. Beaver, and R. C. Jung. *Animal Agents and Vectors of Human Disease*, 4th ed. Philadelphia, Lea and Febiger, 1975.

Flores, M. A., A. Trejos, A. R. Paredes, and A. Y. Ramos. El método de concentración de Strout en el diagnóstico de la fase aguda de la enfermedad de Chagas. *Bol Chile Parasitol* 21:38-39, 1966.

Garnham, P. C. C. The significance of inapparent infections in Chagas' disease and other forms of trypanosomiasis. *Mem Inst Oswaldo Cruz* 75:181-188, 1980.

González Cappa, S. M., and E. L. Segura. Enfermedad de Chagas. *Adel Microbiol Enferm Infecc (B Aires)* 1:51-102, 1982.

Gürtler, R. E., M. Lauricella, N. D. Solarz, M. A. Bujas, and C. Wisnivesky-Colli. Dynamics of transmission of *Trypanosoma cruzi* in a rural area of Argentina. I. The dog reservoir: an epidemiological profile. *Rev Inst Med Trop S Paulo* 28:28-35, 1986.

Gürtler, R. E., C. Wisnivesky-Colli, N. D. Solarz, M. Lauricella, and M. A. Bujas. Dynamics of transmission of *Trypanosoma cruzi* in a rural area of Argentina. II. Household infection patterns among children and dogs relative to the density of infected *Triatoma infestans*. *Bull Pan Am Health Organ* 21:280-292, 1987.

Higuchi, M. L., E. A. Lopes, L. B. Saldanha, A. C. P. Barretto, N. A. G. Stolf, G. Bellotti, and F. Pileggi. Immunopathologic studies in myocardial biopsies of patients with Chagas' disease and idiopathic cardiomyopathy. *Rev Inst Med Trop Sao Paulo* 28:87-90, 1986.

Hipólito, O., M. G. Freitas, and J. B. Figuereido. *Doenças Infeto-Contagiosas dos Animais Domésticos*, 4th ed. São Paulo, Melhoramentos, 1965.

Hosino-Shimizu, S., M. E. Camargo, and E. S. Umezawa. A rapid slide flocculation test for the diagnosis of American trypanosomiasis using *Trypanosoma cruzi* fragments preserved by lyophilization. Comparison with hemagglutination, immunofluorescence, and complement fixation tests. *Am J Trop Med Hyg* 24:586-589, 1975.

Korberle, F. Chagas' disease and Chagas' syndromes: the pathology of American trypanosomiasis. *Adv Parasitol* 6:63-116, 1968.

Luquetti, A. O., M. A. Miles, A. Rassi, J. M. de Rezende, A. A. de Souza, M. M. Povoa, and I. Rodrigues. *Trypanosoma cruzi* zymodemes associated with acute and chronic Chagas' disease in central Brazil. *Trans R Soc Trop Med Hyg* 80:462-470, 1986.

Marsden, P. D., and J. W. C. Hagstrom. Experimental *Trypanosoma cruzi* infection in beagle puppies. The effect of variations in the dose and source of infecting trypanosomes and the route of inoculation on the course of infection. *Trans R Soc Trop Med Hyg* 62:816-824, 1968.

Martínez, A., and J. A. Cichero. *Los vectores de la enfermedad de Chagas*. Buenos Aires, Ministry of Social Welfare, Subsecretariat of Public Health, 1972.

Mello, D. A. Aspectos do ciclo silvestre do *Trypanosoma cruzi* em regiões de cerrado (Municipio de Formosa, Estado de Goiás). *Mem Inst Oswaldo Cruz* 76:227-246, 1981.

Mello, D. A. Roedores, marsupiais e triatomíneos silvestres capturados no Município de Mambai-Goiás. Infecção natural pelo *Trypanosoma cruzi*. *Rev Saúde Publica (S Paulo)* 16:282-291, 1982.

Miles, M. A., S. M. Lanham, A. A. de Souza, and M. Póvoa. Further enzymic characters of *Trypanosoma cruzi* and their evaluation for strain identification. *Trans R Soc Trop Med Hyg* 74:221-237, 1980.

Miles, M. A. The epidemiology of South American trypanosomiasis—Biochemical and immunological approaches and their relevance to control. *Trans R Soc Trop Med Hyg* 77:5-23, 1983.

Morato, M. J. F., Z. Brenner, J. R. Cangado, R. M. B. Nunes, E. Chiari, and G. Gazzinelli. Cellular immune responses of chagasic patients to antigens derived from different *Trypanosoma cruzi* strains and clones. *Am J Trop Med Hyg* 35:505-511, 1986.

Mott, K. E., E. A. Mota, I. Sherlock, R. Hoff, T. M. Muniz, T. S. Oliveira, and C. C. Draper. *Trypanosoma cruzi* infections in dogs and cats and household seroreactivity to *T. cruzi* in a rural community in northeast Brazil. *Am J Trop Med Hyg* 27:1123-1127, 1978.

Otero, M. A. *et al.* El uso de pequeños gallineros como método de estudio de triatomíneos selváticos. *Bol Div Malar San Amb* 16:46-49, 1976.

Pan American Health Organization. *Informe de un grupo de estudio sobre la enfermedad de Chagas*. Washington, D.C., PAHO, 1970. (Scientific Publication 195.)

Pan American Health Organization. *New Approaches in American Trypanosomiasis Research: Proceedings of an International Symposium*. Washington, D.C., PAHO, 1975. (Scientific Publication 318.)

Pan American Health Organization. Status of Chagas' disease in the Americas. *Epidemiol Bull* 5(2):5-9, 1984.

Pereira da Silva, L. H., and E. Plessman Camargo. Ciclo evolutivo do *Trypanosoma cruzi*. *In*: Cançado, J. R. (Ed.), *Doença de Chagas*. Belo Horizonte, Imprensa Oficial do Estado de Minas Gerais, 1968.

Puffer, R. R., and G. W. Griffith. *Patterns of Urban Mortality*. Washington, D.C., Pan American Health Organization, 1967. (Scientific Publication 151.)

Puigbó, J. J., J. R. Nava, and G. C. García. A 4-year follow-up study of the rural community with endemic Chagas' disease. *Bull WHO* 39:341-348, 1968.

Rabinovich, A. El control de la enfermedad de Chagas. *In*: Sonis, A. (Ed.), *Medicina Sanitaria y Administración de Salud*. Buenos Aires, Ateneo, 1971.

Ruiz, A. M., C. Wisnivesky-Colli, R. E. Gürtler, J. Lazzari, M. A. Bujas, and E. L. Segura. Infección por *Trypanosoma cruzi* en humanos, perros y cabras en áreas rurales de la provincia de Córdoba. *Medicina (B Aires)* 45:539-546, 1985.

Schenone, H., H. A. Christensen, A. M. de Vásquez, C. Gonzales, E. Méndez, A. Rojas, and F. Villaroel. Fuentes de alimentación de triatomas domésticos y su implicancia epidemiológica en relación a la enfermedad de Chagas en áreas rurales de siete regiones de Chile. *Bol Chil Parasitol* 40:34-38, 1985.

Schenone, H., F. Villaroel, A. Rojas, and E. Alfaro. Factores biológicos y ecológicos en la epidemiología de la enfermedad de Chagas en Chile. *Bol Chile Parasitol* 35:42-54, 1980.

Siquieira, A. F. de. Diagnóstico parasitológico de molestia de Chagas. *In*: Cançado, J. R. (Ed.), *Doença de Chagas*. Belo Horizonte, Imprensa Oficial do Estado de Minas Gerais, 1968.

Telford, S. R., R. J. Tonn, J. J. González, and P. Betancourt. Dinámica de las infecciones tripanosómicas entre la comunidad de los bosques tropicales secos en los llanos altos de Venezuela. *Bol Div Malar San Amb* 21:196-209, 1981.

Tibayrenc, M., and M. A. Miles. A genetic comparison between Brazilian and Bolivian zymodemes of *Trypanosoma cruzi*. *Trans R Soc Trop Med Hyg* 77:76-83, 1983.

Turovetzky, A. *Las enfermedades infecciosas y parasitarias*. Buenos Aires, Edición de Autor, 1975.

Walton, D. Research needs in Chagas disease. *In*: *XVI Meeting of the PAHO Advisory Committee on Medical Research*. Washington, D. C., Pan American Health Organization, July 1977.

Widmer, G., C. J. Marinkelle, F. Guhl, and M. A. Miles. Isozyme profiles of *Trypanosoma cruzi* stocks from Colombia and Ecuador. *Ann Trop Med Parasitol* 79:253-257, 1985.

Wisnivesky-Colli, C., R. E. Gürtler, N. D. Solarz, M. D. Lauricella, and E. L. Segura. Epidemiological role of humans, dogs and cats in the transmission of *Trypanosoma cruzi* in a central area of Argentina. *Rev Inst Med Trop S Paulo* 27:346-352, 1985.

Wisnivesky-Colli, C., I. Pavlone, A. Perez, R. Chuit, J. Gualtieri, N. Solarz, A. Smith, and E. L. Segura. A new tool for continuous detection of the presence of triatomine bugs, vectors of Chagas disease, in rural households. *Medicina (B Aires)* 47:45-50, 1987.

World Health Organization, Working Group. Immunology of Chagas' disease. *Bull WHO* 50:459-472, 1974.

Zeledón, R. Epidemiology, modes of transmission and reservoir hosts of Chagas' disease. *In*: *Trypanosomiasis and Leishmaniasis with Special Reference to Chagas' Disease. CIBA Foundation Symposium 20*. Amsterdam, Elsevier, 1974.

Zeledón, R. Vectores de la enfermedad de Chagas y sus características ecofisiológicas. *Interciencias* 8:384-395, 1983.

BABESIOSIS

(088.8)

Synonyms: Piroplasmosis, babesiasis; the latter is a more general term for all aspects of the parasitism, while babesiosis refers specifically to clinical disease (Mahoney, 1977).

Etiology: *Babesia* spp. Within the family Babesiidae, 40 species that parasitize different domestic and wild vertebrates have been catalogued, but the taxonomy and nomenclature of many of them have not yet been precisely determined. The round, pyriform, or ameboid protozoan multiplies in the erythrocytes of vertebrate hosts by schizogenesis to form two, four, or more trophozoites. Upon being set free, these invade other erythrocytes. Under natural conditions, babesias are transmitted by various tick species. The parasite is ingested by the female tick with the host's blood and multiplies asexually in the intestine of the arthropod; it later migrates to the salivary glands where it divides by multiple fission into small forms. Sexual reproduction of babesias in tick vectors has not been confirmed up to the present time. In one-host ticks, transmission of the protozoan is transovarial, while in ticks with several hosts, transstadial transmission has been confirmed. The tick inoculates the protozoan into the vertebrate host when sucking its blood. Electron microscopy studies have confirmed that these protozoans are similar in structure to sporozoa.

The species of animal babesias of special interest as agents of human infection are *Babesia microti*, *B. bovis* (*B. argentina*), *B. divergens*, and possibly some of the equine babesias. It has been suggested that *B. divergens* may be identical to *B. bovis* (Hoare, 1980), but most researchers consider these babesias to be different species.

In the United States the main *B. microti* reservoirs are the wild mice *Peromyscus leucopus* and *Microtus pennsylvanicus*. The vector is *Ixodes dammini*, which in the larval and nymph stages feeds mainly on rodents, but is also found on man and domestic animals. The adult form of this tick parasitizes the white-tailed deer, *Odocoileus virginianus*. Bovines and deer are the reservoirs of *B. bovis*; its vectors are *Ixodes ricinus*, *I. persulcatus*, *Boophilus microplus*, *B. calcaratus*, and *Rhipicephalus bursa*. Bovines are also the hosts of *Babesia divergens*, which occurs mainly in northern Europe, and the principal vector is *I. ricinus* (Soulsby, 1982).

Geographic Distribution: Babesiasis occurs almost everywhere in the world where ticks exist. Clinical cases in man have been diagnosed only in the United States and Europe.

Occurrence in Man: Clinical disease is infrequent. The first case was confirmed in 1957, and to date more than 100 cases have been reported from the islands on the Atlantic coast of the United States (Dammin *et al.*, 1981; cit. Marcus *et al.*, 1984). Two different clinical and epidemiologic situations can be distinguished. In Europe, the disease is caused by *B. bovis* and *B. divergens* of bovine origin and occurs in splenectomized patients; in the United States, the disease is caused mainly by *B. microti* of murine origin and is seen in patients with an intact spleen. Cases in splenectomized persons have also occurred in the United States: two in California caused by babesias of supposed equine origin, and one in New York produced by an unspecified babesia. The cases caused by *B. microti* occurred on four islands off the coast of Massachusetts and New York. All the patients were 49 years of age or older (Ruebush II, 1980). In Europe a total of seven cases were diagnosed in Yugoslavia, France, Great Britain, and the USSR (Georgia). All cases occurred in splenectomized adults (Garnham, 1980). The infection can also occur asymptomatically, as was demonstrated in a rural area of Mexico, where 101 people were examined serologically and 38 were found to have antibodies. Blood of the reactors was inoculated into splenectomized hamsters, and *Babesia* spp. was isolated from three of them (Osborne *et al.*, 1976). Likewise, the parasite was observed in smears of blood from an asymptomatic blood donor in Georgia, USA. In the endemic area of Shelter Island, New York, indirect evidence of clinically inapparent infection was obtained by examining paired serum samples by indirect immunofluorescence. Of 102 persons examined, six registered a four-fold increase in their antibody titer during the summer season, while 300 other people from New York City did not produce significant titers for *B. microti* (Filstein *et al.*, 1980). In conclusion, subclinical infections are perhaps more frequent than clinically apparent ones. In malarial areas, infection by *Babesia* spp. can be confused with *Plasmodium* spp. infection.

Occurrence in Animals: Animal babesiasis is widespread throughout the world, with highest prevalence in the tropics, it is one of the most important cattle diseases in Africa, the Middle East, and parts of Asia. Bovine infection causes large economic losses in South and Central America. In the United States and Puerto Rico, bovine babesiasis was eliminated with the eradication of the tick *Boophilus annulatus*. In Europe, foci of *B. bovis* and *B. divergens* infection are found in cattle, and the vector is *Ixodes ricinus*.

B. microti occurs in wild rodents in both the United States and Europe, and possibly in other parts of the world. In an area near Munich, Federal Republic of Germany, 38% of 255 microtine mice (*Microtus agrestis*) were positive for this parasite, with a peak of 71% of those sampled at the beginning of summer (Krampitz, 1979). Nevertheless, apart from the cases on the eastern coast of the United States, no human infections are known. A study carried out on the island of Nantucket, Massachusetts, where most of the human cases have occurred, found that the white-footed mouse (*Peromyscus leucopus*) was the animal species most parasitized by *B. microti*, with an infection rate of 35.4% based on blood smears and 67% by hamster inoculation (Spielman *et al.*, 1981).

The Disease in Man: The cases of *B. bovis* or *B. divergens* infection in splenectomized persons in Europe were characterized by severe illness, often with pyrexia, anemia, prostration, hemoglobinuria, and jaundice. With the exception of two patients diagnosed in France who recovered from the disease, all died of kidney failure (Garnham, 1980). The spleen plays a very important role in the host's resistance against the parasite, and splenectomy was undoubtedly a predisposing factor in these patients. In American patients infected by *B. microti* and not splenectomized, onset of disease was gradual, with anorexia, fatigue, fever, sweating, and generalized myalgia. Some patients may develop slight splenomegaly and hepatomegaly. Mild to severe hemolytic anemia is common. Parasitemia can affect less than 1% to 10% or more of the erythrocytes. The form of *B. microti* that predominates in the blood smears closely resembles the small ring form of *Plasmodium*. Recovery is slow; malaise and fatigue persist for several months (Ruebush II, 1980). No deaths were recorded among nonsplenectomized patients infected by *B. microti*. The incubation period from tick (nymph) bite to appearance of symptoms lasts 7 to 28 days, based on observations in some patients (Ruebush II, 1980).

The Disease in Animals: The symptomatology of babesiosis is similar among different domestic species. Bovine babesiosis, which is the most important from an economic standpoint, can have a benign course with spontaneous recovery, or a severe course ending in death. The disease is manifested by fever, anorexia, anemia as a result of erythrocyte destruction, hemoglobinuria, jaundice, diarrhea or constipation, yellowish feces, and emaciation. Autopsy reveals an enlarged spleen with dark-red, soft pulp; an enlarged, yellowish brown liver; slightly edematous lungs; and hemorrhagic serous fluid in the pericardial cavity.

Young animals (calves, colts, piglets) are much more resistant to babesiosis than are adults. Infection results in a state of premunition, with the parasite persisting in the animal for several years or for life and conferring resistance to subsequent infections. Animals raised in enzootic areas acquire the infection, and thus premunition, at a very early age, which explains why animals brought in from babesiosis-free areas become ill and often die, while the local livestock is resistant. Stress factors can reactivate a latent infection and premunized animals can become ill.

Infection by *B. microti* in rodents occurs asymptomatically.

Source of Infection and Mode of Transmission (Figure 61): The reservoirs are domestic and wild animals. The infection is transmitted by ticks from one animal to another and, accidentally, to man. Transovarial and transstadial transmission have been confirmed in many tick species.

Figure 61. Babesiosis. Transmission cycle.

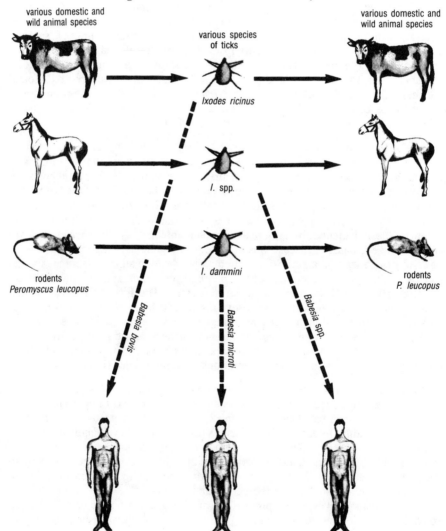

Man can be infected by different species of *Babesia*. The known cases probably represent infection due to three or four different species. Splenectomized animals are much less resistant to the initial infection, and splenectomy activates the latent infection in premunized animals.

On the coastal islands of the eastern United States, transmission of *B. microti* to man is effected by nymphs of *I. dammini*. According to studies carried out on Nantucket Island, the main reservoir is the mouse *P. leucopus*, which is the most abundant rodent and the animal most parasitized by the protozoan as well as by its vector. Parasitemia in this host is usually low-level, and few ticks (larvae and nymphs of *I. dammini*) can become infected, as indicated by the fact that only 5% of the nymphs on this island harbor the parasite. Areas with enzootic babesiasis in rodents are characterized by a large population of deer, which are hosts for adult ticks (Spielman *et al.*, 1981). The *I. dammini* nymph, which transmits the infection to man, is small; many times, the person does not notice its bite. Most human cases have occurred in the months of July and August, soon after the *I. dammini* nymph population reaches its maximum (Ruebush II, 1981). Splenectomy is not a prerequisite for human infection by *B. microti* as it is for infections by *B. bovis* and *B. divergens*, although it can be a predisposing factor.

Latent babesiosis is very common in animals. Still unknown is whether the same situation occurs in man in enzootic tropical and subtropical regions, where humans are frequently exposed to ticks infected with babesias.

Role of Animals in the Epidemiology of the Disease: Babesiosis is an animal disease transmitted by ticks. As in the majority of zoonoses, man is an accidental host. Interhuman transmission does not occur naturally, but can take place via blood transfusion, as has happened in two cases.

Diagnosis: The diagnosis of animal babesiosis can be confirmed during febrile periods by blood smears stained with Giemsa stain. Confirmation of the parasite's presence in chronic cases is difficult and is based primarily on inoculation of blood into susceptible animals.

Diagnosis in man is based on the same procedures. Babesias in human blood have been mistaken for *Plasmodium falciparum*, but these protozoans can be differentiated by the absence of pigments (hemozoin) in *Babesia*. The indirect immunofluorescence test is useful in diagnosis of infection by *B. microti*. Although cross-reactions occur among *B. bovis* (*argentina*), *B. bigamina*, *B. equi*, *Plasmodium vivax*, *P. falciparum*, and *P. brasilianum*, the highest titers are obtained with the homologous antigen (Chisholm *et al.*, 1978).

Control: Some protection against human infection can be obtained by the use of tick repellents. Blood donors, especially those from endemic areas, should be examined for the presence of the parasite.

Tick control and, where economically feasible, eradication are the most important preventive measures against the disease in bovines and other domestic animals.

Animals destined for enzootic areas can be protected with artificial premunition. This procedure is preferably applied to young animals, in which it is less likely to cause severe disease. Now that *in vitro* culture of *B. bovis* has been achieved, possibilities exist of obtaining vaccines made with antigenic fractions of the parasite or with modified live strains (Smith and Ristic, 1981).

Bibliography

Centers for Disease Control of the USA. Babesiosis—Massachusetts. *Morb Mortal Wkly Rep* 24:314, 1975.

Chisholm, E. S., T. K. Ruebush II, A. J. Sulzer, and G. R. Healy. *Babesia microti* infection in man: evaluation of an indirect immunofluorescent antibody test. *Am J Trop Med Hyg* 27:14-19, 1978.

Chisholm, E. S., A. J. Sulzer, and T. K. Ruebush II. Indirect immunofluorescence test for human *Babesia microti* infection: antigenic specificity. *Am J Trop Med Hyg* 35:921-925, 1986.

Coan, M. E., and D. Stiller. *Ixodes dammini* (Acari: Ixodidae) in Maryland, U.S.A., and a preliminary survey for *Babesia microti. J Med Entomol* 23:446-453, 1986.

Filstein, M. R., J. L. Benach, D. J. White, B. A. Brody, W. D. Goldman, C. W. Bakal, and R. S. Schwartz. Serosurvey for human babesiosis in New York. *J Infect Dis* 141:518-521, 1980.

Garnham, P. C. Human babesiosis: European aspects. *Trans R Soc Trop Med Hyg* 74:153-155, 1980.

Healy, G. R., P. D. Walzer, and A. J. Sulzer. A case of asymptomatic babesiosis in Georgia. *Am J Trop Med Hyg* 25:376-378, 1976.

Hoare, C. A. Comparative aspects of human babesiosis. *Trans R Soc Trop Med Hyg* 74:143-148, 1980.

Krampitz, H. E. *Babesia microti:* morphology, distribution and host relationship in Germany. *Zentralbl Bakteriol [Orig A]* 244:411-415, 1979.

Levine, N. D. *Protozoan Parasites of Domestic Animals and of Man*, 2nd ed. Minneapolis, Minnesota, Burgess, 1973.

Mahoney, D. F. Babesia of domestic animals. *In*: Kreier, J. P. (Ed.), *Parasitic Protozoa*, vol. 4. New York, Academic Press, 1977.

Marcus, L. C., C. J. Mabray, and G. H. Sturgis. *Babesia microti* infection in the hamster: failure of quinine and pyrimethamine in chemotherapeutic trials. *Am J Trop Med Hyg* 33:21-23, 1984.

Osorno, M., C. Vega, M. Ristic, C. Robles, and S. Ibarra. Isolation of *Babesia* spp. from asymptomatic human beings. *Vet Parasitol* 2:111-120, 1976.

Ristic, M., and R. D. Smith. Zoonoses caused by hemoprotozoa. *In*: Soulsby, E. J. L. (Ed.), *Parasitic Zoonoses*. New York, Academic Press, 1974.

Ruebush II, T. K. Human babesiosis in North America. *Trans R Soc Trop Med Hyg* 74:149-152, 1980.

Ruebush II, T. K., D. D. Juranek, A. Spielman, J. Piesman, and G. R. Healy. Epidemiology of human babesiosis on Nantucket Island. *Am J Trop Med Hyg* 30:937-941, 1981.

Ruebush II, T. K. Babesiosis. *In*: Warren, K. S., and A. A. F. Mahmoud (Eds.), *Tropical and Geographical Medicine*, New York, McGraw-Hill Book Company, 1984.

Scholtens, R. G., E. H. Braff, G. R. Healy, and N. Gleason. A case of babesiosis in man in the United States. *Am J Trop Med Hyg* 17:810-813, 1968.

Smith, R. D., and M. Ristic. Immunization against bovine babesiosis with culture-derived antigens. *In*: Ristic, M., and J. P. Kreiyer (Eds.), *Babesiosis*. New York, Academic Press, 1981.

Soulsby, E. J. L. *Helminths, Arthropods and Protozoa of Domesticated Animals*, 7th ed. Philadelphia, Lea and Febiger, 1982.

Spielman, A., P. Etkind, J. Piesman, T. K. Ruebush II, D. D. Juranek, and M. S. Jacobs. Reservoir hosts of human babesiosis on Nantucket Island. *Am J Trop Med Hyg* 30:560-565, 1981.

Western, K. A., G. D. Benson, and N. Gleason. Babesiosis in a Massachusetts resident. *N Engl J Med* 283:854-856, 1970.

CRYPTOSPORIDIOSIS

(007.8)

Etiology: *Cryptosporidium* is a protozoan genus in the family Cryptosporidiidae, suborder Eimeriina, subclass Coccidia. It was formerly subdivided into numerous species that were differentiated according to the animal species they parasitized and their anatomic localization, but research has demonstrated that the parasite is not species-specific and that it can be transmitted from one animal species to another. Consequently, *Cryptosporidium* is currently considered a monotypic genus (Tzipori *et al.*, 1980). Its life cycle is similar to that of the coccidia, with both an asexual stage of multiplication by schizogony or segmentation, and a sexual stage in which it multiplies by means of fertilization of the female cell (macrogametocyte) by the male cell (microgametocyte). Both developmental stages occur in the same host and generally on the epithelial surface of the intestine. In contrast to other coccidia, which develop and multiply inside the cell cytoplasm, *Cryptosporidium* lives outside the enterocyte, in or on the intestinal microvilli. Fertilized macrogametocytes develop into oocysts that form four sporozoites without cyst membranes, that is, without first forming sporocysts. Sporozoites develop inside the intestine and are already infective when eliminated with the feces (Tzipori, 1983). The length of time oocysts can survive outside the animal organism is not yet known, but they are highly resistant to disinfectants; in experiments they could be destroyed only with 10% formalin or 5% ammonia after 18 hours of treatment (Campbell *et al.*, 1982).

Geographic Distribution: The agent has been identified in animals or man in countries on all continents, indicating worldwide distribution.

Occurrence in Man: It is an emerging disease, unknown in man until 1976 when the first two cases in immunocompromised patients were reported. Until recently, cryptosporidiosis was considered a rare disease occurring only in immunodeficient or immunosuppressed persons. However, it is increasingly evident that *Cryptosporidium* also affects immunocompetent persons and must be considered one of the pathogens that cause diarrhea in the general population, especially among children.

In two hospitals in Melbourne, Australia, *Cryptosporidium* oocysts were found in the feces of 36 (4.1%) of 884 gastroenteritis patients (only five of them had other enteropathogens), while no oocysts were found in 320 patients without gastroenteritis. The incidence was higher in children (4.8%) than in adults (1.6%). The disease is more frequent in summer (Tzipori *et al.,* 1983).

Recently, reports of this disease have multiplied as the medical profession has become alert to it. Oocysts of the protozoan were found in 1.25% of 800 gastroenteritis patients in Denmark, and in at least 1% of those in Finland (Current, 1983). A 4.3% rate of infection by *Cryptosporidium* was found in rural and urban Costa Rican children suffering from diarrhea, while in nondiarrheic controls of the same age, the agent's presence was not confirmed. The authors (Mata *et al.*, 1984) consider that in that country *Cryptosporidium* ranks immediately behind rotavirus, enterotoxigenic *Escherichia coli, Campylobacter,* and *Shigella* in order of importance of intestinal pathogens.

In 1984, the Centers for Disease Control of the USA received reports of multiple cryptosporidiosis cases among children in day-care centers in five states (Centers for Disease Control of the USA, 1984).

Occurrence in Animals: Cryptosporidiosis has been described in 16 different species of domestic and wild mammals, birds, and reptiles. In at least 10 species there is direct or indirect evidence that infection causes disease (Tzipori, 1983). A serologic study of 10 animal species, including man, found reactors to the indirect immunofluorescence test in over 80% of individuals tested (Tzipori and Campbell, 1981). However, the criteria for positiveness to this test have been disputed (Campbell and Current, 1983).

The most frequently affected species is cattle.

The Disease in Man: Cryptosporidiosis in immunodeficient persons or those undergoing immunosuppressant therapy is a severe disease, with chronic and persistent diarrhea and malabsorption that can result in death. More than 30 cases of cryptosporidiosis have occurred among patients with acquired immunodeficiency syndrome (AIDS) during the current epidemic in the United States (Guarda *et al.*, 1983; Blagburn and Current, 1983). The number of evacuations can vary between six and 25 per day, and the volume between one and 17 liters. This protozoosis can be an important contributing factor in AIDS mortality (Schultz, 1983). In immunodeficient patients, the parasite can invade other organs besides the intestine; the protozoan has been found in the gall bladder of AIDS patients in addition to the intestine and stomach (Guarda *et al.*, 1983).

Cryptosporidiosis in immunologically normal patients is a self-limiting disease characterized by watery diarrhea lasting 3 to 14 days. Abdominal pain, nausea, and malaise are frequent. Some patients also have a slight fever.

The Disease in Animals:

CATTLE: The disease is common in Canada, the USA, Europe, and Australia. In newborn calves with diarrhea, *Cryptosporidium* often occurs in association with other enteropathogens, making it difficult to evaluate the true role of the protozoan. More recently, infection by *Cryptosporidium* has been recognized in many cases of neonatal diarrhea. Concurrent infections by other enteropathogens have been found in six out of 55 cases. In cases of diarrhea in 51 calves 1 to 15 days old from 47 herds, 17 were found to have cryptosporidiosis (Anderson, 1982). In Victoria, Australia, cryptosporidia were recognized in five out of nine recent diarrhea outbreaks (Jarret and Snodgrass, 1981). In summary, cryptosporidia can be found as the sole pathogen or in mixed infections with other agents, such as rotavirus and *E. coli* K99, in bovine neonatal diarrheas. The clinical picture varies from mild to severe. Morbidity is high, but the fatality rate is low.

OTHER DOMESTIC MAMMALS: The disease has been described in 5- to 12-day-old lambs raised artificially or naturally. The most prominent sign, as in other species, is diarrhea, from which the lambs may recover or die. Relapses can occur after recovery. The clinical picture is similar in young goats. A generalized infection has been described in immunodeficient Arabian colts; the parasite was found in the stomach, along the entire length of the intestine, in the gall bladder, and in the bile and pancreatic ducts.

BIRDS: Cryptosporidiosis associated with a disease of the upper respiratory tract has been observed in turkey poults and chicks destined for market. The respiratory disease in turkey poults was present on five of six poultry farms surveyed, causing 1 to 30% morbidity and 0.7 to 20% mortality. The affected poults were 2 to 11 weeks old. Symptoms consisted of dyspnea, cough, and stunted growth. The protozoan was observed by electron microscopy in different development stages on the surface of the tracheal mucosa, mucous glands, and in some cases in the bronchial and nasal passages (Hoerr *et al.*, 1978). A similar syndrome was described in 7-week-old, market-bound chicks, among which severe losses resulted in a week's time. In addition, an adenovirus isolated from the trachea of these birds is believed to have possibly had a synergistic effect on the course of the disease (Dhillon *et al.*, 1981). The respiratory form of cryptosporidiosis has only been confirmed in birds. Turkey poults have also been observed to suffer from the intestinal disease, with diarrhea and low mortality.

Source of Infection and Mode of Transmission: Investigations carried out in recent years have confirmed that *Cryptosporidium* is not species-specific and that strains from one animal species can infect a wide spectrum of other species. Accordingly, strains isolated from man, calves, lambs, goats, and deer have been transmitted orally to lambs, calves, and suckling pigs, in which they caused diarrhea, and to colts, chicks, and laboratory animals, in which they produced infection but not disease (Tzipori, 1983). These experiments indicated that multiple hosts and reservoirs exist in nature and that one animal species can contract infection from another. In fact, episodes of the disease in humans following contact with calves sick with cryptosporidiosis suggest that transmission from animals to man is possible. One such case involved a veterinary student who treated two infected calves and contracted cryptosporidiosis after 5 days of contact (Anderson *et al.*, 1982). In another episode, 12 of 18 persons who had direct contact over time periods ranging from 10 minutes to 6 days with the feces of calves ill with cryptosporidiosis contracted the infection; nine of them had diarrhea and abdominal pain lasting from 1 to 10 days. Protozoans isolated from these persons and calves were experimentally transmitted to calves, mice, kittens, pups, and goats, demonstrating the possibility of natural interchange of the agent between different species, man among them (Current *et al.*, 1983).

Human disease also occurs in the absence of any contact with animals, and evidence exists for interhuman transmission. In Australia, a father contracted the infection from his sick daughter. Direct transmission via anal contact was confirmed in a male homosexual. Indirect transmission can occur by ingestion of food and water contaminated by human or animal feces (Current, 1983). A laboratory accident in which a researcher became infected suggests that a small number of oocysts is sufficient to infect man (Blagburn and Current, 1983).

A study carried out in Costa Rica confirmed that infection was more frequent in bottle-fed babies than in breast-fed babies (Mata *et al.*, 1984).

As in other intestinal infections, the main transmission route is fecal-oral, in both animals and man.

Diagnosis: Diagnosis is based on confirmation of the presence of oocysts (about 4 to 5 microns in diameter) in the feces by examining films stained with the Giemsa method, modified Ziehl-Neelsen, or by flotation techniques such as Sheater. Intestinal biopsy or histology can confirm the different developmental stages of the protozoan on the epithelial microvilli.

The indirect immunofluorescence test confirmed the persistence of antibodies for at least 1 year in a recent study of a group of immunocompetent persons who had recovered from the disease. Antibodies were also found in some but not all of a group of AIDS patients. Cross-reactions with other coccidia, such as *Toxoplasma*, *Sarcocystis*, and *Isospora*, were absent or very low-level (Campbell and Current, 1983).

Control: As with other intestinal infections, personal and food hygiene are recommended. Immunodeficient or immunosuppressed patients should avoid contact with diarrheic persons or animals, since for people with compromised immune systems, cryptosporidiosis is a severe disease for which there is no adequate therapy.

Bibliography

Anderson, B. C., T. Donndelinger, R. M. Wilkins, and J. Smith. Cryptosporidiosis in a veterinary student. *J Am Vet Med Assoc* 180:408-409, 1982.

Anderson, B. C. Cryptosporidiosis: a review. *JAMA* 180:1455-1457, 1982.

Angus, K. W. Cryptosporidiosis in man, domestic animals and birds: a review. *J R Soc Med* 76:62-70, 1983.

Baxby, D., and C. S. Hart. The incidence of cryptosporidiosis: a two year prospective survey in a children's hospital. *J Hyg* 96:107-111, 1986.

Blagburn, B. L., and W. L. Current. Accidental infection of researcher with human *Cryptosporidium*. *J Infect Dis* 148:772-773, 1983.

Campbell, I., S. Tzipori, G. Hutchinson, and K. W. Angus. Effect of disinfectants on survival of *Cryptosporidium* oocysts. *Vet Rec* 111:414-415, 1982.

Campbell, P. N., and W. L. Current. Demonstration of serum antibodies to *Cryptosporidium* sp. in normal and immunodeficient humans with confirmed infection. *J Clin Microbiol* 18:165-169, 1983.

Centers for Disease Control of the USA. Cryptosporidiosis among children attending day-care centers, Georgia, Pennsylvania, Michigan, California, New Mexico. *Morb Mortal Wkly Rep* 33:599-601, 1984.

Current, W. L., N. C. Reese, J. V. Ernst, W. S. Bailey, M. B. Heyman, and W. M. Weinstein. Human cryptosporidiosis in immunocompetent and immunodeficient persons. *N Engl J Med* 308:1252-1257, 1983.

Current, W. L. Human cryptosporidiosis. *N Engl J Med* 309:1326-1327, 1983.

Current, W. L. Cryptosporidiosis. *J Am Vet Med Assoc* 187:1334-1338, 1985.

Dhillon, A. S., H. L. Thacker, A. V. Dietzel, and R. W. Winterfield. Respiratory cryptosporidiosis in broiler chickens. *Avian Dis* 25:747-751, 1981.

Guarda, L. A., S. A. Stein, K. A. Cleary, and N. G. Ordoñez. Human cryptosporidiosis in the acquired immunodeficiency syndrome. *Arch Pathol Lab Med* 107:562-566, 1983.

Heuschele, W. P., J. Oosterhuis, D. Janssen, P. T. Robinson, P. K. Ensley, J. E. Meier, T. Olson, M. P. Anderson, and K. Benirschke. Cryptosporidial infections in captive wild animals. *J Wildl Dis* 22:493-496, 1986.

Hoerr, F. J., F. M. Ranck, and T. F. Hastings. Respiratory cryptosporidiosis in turkeys. *J Am Vet Med Assoc* 173:1591-1593, 1978.

Højling, N., K. Molfack, and S. Jepsen. Cryptosporidiosis in human beings is not primarily a zoonosis. *J Infect* 11:270-272, 1985.

Jarrett, I. V., and D. R. Snodgrass. Cryptosporidia associated with outbreaks of neonatal calf diarrhoea. *Aust Vet J* 57:434-435, 1981.

Klesius, P. H., T. B. Haynes, and L. K. Malo. Infectivity of *Cryptosporidium* sp. isolated from wild mice for calves and mice. *J Am Vet Med Assoc* 189:192-193, 1986.

Mata, L., H. Bolaños, D. Pizarro, and M. Vives. Cryptosporidiosis in children from some highland Costa Rican and urban areas. *Am J Trop Med Hyg* 33:24-29, 1984.

Moon, H. W., and D. B. Woodmansee. Cryptosporidiosis, Update. *J Am Vet Med Assoc* 189: 643-646, 1986.

O'Donoghue, P. J. *Cryptosporidium* in man, animals, birds and fish (Review article). *Aust Vet J* 62:253-258, 1985.

Pohjola, S., E. Neuvonen, A. Niskanen, and A. Rantama. Rapid immunoassay for detection of *Cryptosporidium* oocysts. *Acta Vet Scand* 27:71-79, 1986.

Ryan, M. J., J. P. Sundberg, R. J. Sauerschell, and K. S. Tood, Jr. Cryptosporidium in a wild cottontail rabbit (*Sylvilagus floridanus*). *J Wildl Dis* 22:267.

Schultz, M. G. Emerging zoonoses. *N Engl J Med* 308:1285-1286, 1983.

Soave, R., and D. Armstrong. *Cryptosporidium* and cryptosporidiosis. *Rev Infect Dis* 8:1012-1023, 1986.

Tzipori, S., K. W. Angus, I. Campbell, and E. W. Gray. *Cryptosporidium:* evidence for a single-species genus. *Infect Immun* 30:884-886, 1980.

Tzipori, S., and I. Campbell. Prevalence of cryptosporidium antibodies in 10 animal species. *J Clin Microbiol* 14:455-456, 1981.

Tzipori, S. Cryptosporidiosis in animals and humans. *Microbiol Rev* 47:84-96, 1983.

Tzipori, S., M. Smith, C. Birch, G. Barnes, and R. Bishop. Cryptosporidiosis in hospital patients with gastroenteritis. *Am J Trop Med Hyg* 32:931-934, 1983.

Ungar, B. L. P., R. Soave, R. Fayer, and T. E. Nash. Enzyme immunoassay detection of immunoglobulin M and G antibodies to *Cryptosporidium* in immunocompetent and immunocompromised persons. *J Infect Dis* 153:570-578, 1986.

Upton, S. J., and W. L. Current. The species of *Cryptosporidium* (Apicomplexa: Cryptosporidiidae) infecting mammals. *J Parasitol* 71:625-629, 1985.

CUTANEOUS LEISHMANIASIS

(085.1 to 085.5)

Synonyms: Chiclero ulcer, espundia, pian-bois, uta, and buba (in the Americas); oriental sore, Aleppo boil, Bagdad sore, Delhi sore, and other local names (in the Old World).

Etiology: A flagellate protozoan of the genus *Leishmania*; it occurs in vertebrates, including man, in the aflagellate or amastigote form, and in vector insects (*Lutzomyia* spp. or *Phlebotomus* spp.) in the flagellate or promastigote form. Investigators disagree over the nomenclature to be used within the genus *Leishmania*, and the different schemes proposed have created confusion. The classification cannot be based on morphologic characteristics, since all the species of parasites in the genus, including *L. donovani* (visceral leishmaniasis), are almost identical in their morphology. The scheme adopted by Lainson and Shaw (1973) for the agents of American cutaneous leishmaniasis is followed here. These authors have proposed grouping New World leishmanias into two species complexes, one containing *L. mexicana* and its subspecies, and the other including *L. braziliensis* and its subspecies. This classification is based on such characteristics as vector, parasite localization in the insect's intestine, pathogenicity of the agent on hamster skin, and growth in culture media. The differential characteristics have been summarized by Bonfante-Garrido (1983) and are presented here: Vectors of the *L. mexicana* complex leishmanias are phlebotomines of the subgenus *Nyssomyia*; the leishmanias do not multiply in the hindgut of these insects (suprapylaria reproduction). *L. mexicana* inoculated in hamster skin reproduces rapidly and forms histiocytomas containing abundant amastigotes; metastasis is common. These leishmanias grow profusely in Novy, McNeal, and Nicolle (NNN) culture medium. *L. braziliensis* vectors are phlebotomines of the groups *Psychodopygus* and *Nyssomyia*; the parasites proliferate in the insect's hindgut triangle and the rest of the intestine (peripylaria reproduction). When inoculated in hamster skin, they very slowly produce small nodules or ulcers that contain few amastigotes and do not spread by metastasis; their development is slow or moderate in NNN culture medium.

In order to differentiate the numerous New World subspecies, many other characteristics are taken into account. Currently, the method most frequently used to characterize *Leishmania* is determination of its isozymic profile by electrophoresis. Other procedures in use are measurement of the buoyant density of DNA from the nucleus or kinetoplast, Adler serologic test, and monoclonal antibodies.

In the Old World, the causal agents of cutaneous leishmaniasis are *L. tropica*, *L. major*, and *L. aethiopica*. Cases of cutaneous lesions due to *L. donovani* (the agent of visceral leishmaniasis, or kala-azar) have been recorded in Africa and the Mediterranean basin. Post–kala-azar dermal leishmaniasis also occurs in India and sometimes in eastern Africa; it may appear up to several years after apparent recuperation from visceral leishmaniasis. Kala-azar cutaneous lesions are rare in the New World, but the presence of parasites in macroscopically normal skin of some visceral leishmaniasis patients has been confirmed. These and other findings indicate that the tissue tropisms of the different *Leishmania* species are not strict.

Geographic Distribution (Map 11): Human cutaneous leishmaniasis in the Americas occurs from southern Mexico to northern Argentina. In South America, only Chile and Uruguay are free of the parasite. Endemic areas in the Old World exist along the Mediterranean coast, in the Middle East, in several Asian Soviet Republics (Azerbaidzhan, Turkmenistan, Uzbekistan, Tadzhikistan, Kazakhstan), in northern China, and in northwestern India. In addition to foci on the Mediterranean coast of Africa, others exist in the west-central and east-central parts of that continent and some in the southern part. The *L. mexicana mexicana* subspecies is distributed in Mexico (Yucatan Peninsula and foci in Veracruz and Oaxaca), Guatemala, Belize, the state of São Paulo (Vale do Ribeira) in Brazil (Machado *et al.*, 1983), and perhaps in Texas, USA (Lainson, 1983); *L. m. amazonensis* is found in the Brazilian Amazon basin and Mato Grosso; *L. m. pifanoi* exists in Venezuela; and *L. m. venezuelensis* was described in 1980 and has been isolated on the banks of the Turbio River, Lara State, Venezuela (Bonfante-Garrido, 1983).

The main subspecies of *L. b. braziliensis* are *L. b. braziliensis*, *L. b. guyannensis*, *L. b. panamensis*, and *L. b. peruviana*. The distribution area of *L. b. braziliensis* encompasses eastern Bolivia, jungle regions of Brazil, Colombia, Ecuador, Paraguay, Peru, and Venezuela (Bonfante-Garrido, 1983). *L. b. guyannensis* is distributed to the north of the Amazon in Brazil, as well as in Guyana, Suriname, and French Guiana; *L. b. panamensis* exists in Panama, Costa Rica, Honduras, and perhaps in other Central American countries; and *L. b. peruviana* is limited to the Peruvian Andes and occurs at altitudes of 900 to 3,000 m.

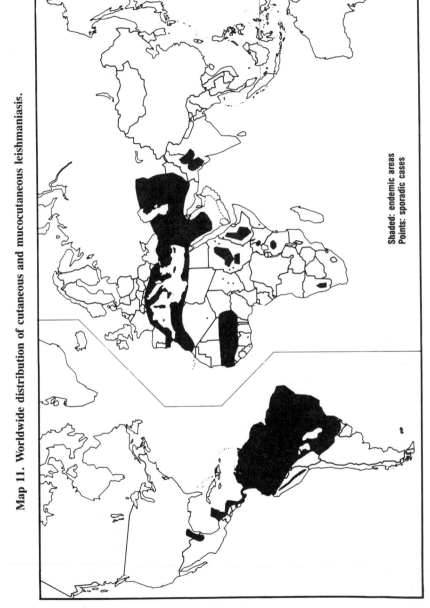

Map 11. Worldwide distribution of cutaneous and mucocutaneous leishmaniasis.

Shaded: endemic areas
Points: sporadic cases

Source: The Leishmaniases. WHO, 1984. (Tech. Rep. Ser. 701).

In several areas of the Americas, the ranges of *L. braziliensis* and *L. mexicana* overlap.

In the Old World, *L. tropica* (*L. tropica minor*) is found in some Mediterranean countries (Greece, Tunisia, Turkey), Israel, Kuwait, Iraq, Afghanistan, Iran, and Uganda. In other countries, its status is either unknown because of dubious identifications or lack of information over the last 15 years, or it has been eradicated, as in the USSR (World Health Organization, 1984). *Leishmania major* (*L. tropica major*) is present in the Arabian peninsula, Egypt, Israel, Iraq, Jordan, Syria, Turkey, Afghanistan, Iran, Pakistan, India, Libya, Algeria, Morocco, Mauritania, Mali, Senegal, Sudan, and Upper Volta. *L. aethiopica* is found in Ethiopia and Kenya (World Health Organization, 1984).

Occurrence: An estimated 400,000 new cases of cutaneous leishmaniasis occur every year. The World Health Organization ranks it among the six most important tropical diseases (Lainson, 1981). In 1972, 22,368 human cases of leishmaniasis (both cutaneous and visceral) were notified in the Americas (Pan American Health Organization, 1975), of which 20,348 occurred in Middle America, mainly Guatemala (for a rate of 29.6 per 100,000 inhabitants), and 2,020 occurred in South America (2.9 per 100,000 inhabitants).

In the Old World, as in Latin America, many cases are occasioned by the movement of people to endemic areas as a result of development projects. In the southern part of the Magreb in North Africa, several thousand cases occurred between 1976 and 1982. Of 87 Europeans living temporarily in an endemic area of Saudi Arabia, 47 were affected by cutaneous leishmaniasis (Bienzle *et al.*, 1978). Cases are sporadic in Africa, and the most important foci are found in the Saharan belt and in the eastern part of the continent. In Southeast Asia, the disease has declined so markedly that it has almost disappeared as a result of insecticide use in the campaign against malaria. With the exception of China, the countries of the Pacific coast of Asia are free of endemic leishmaniasis (World Health Organization, 1984).

A study in Panama (Herrer *et al.*, 1973) in which 2,947 wild animals of 42 species were examined found *L. braziliensis* in 16.9% of 396 two-toed sloths (*Choloepus hoffmanni*), with great variations in prevalence from one region to another; in one of the areas studied, infection rates were as high as 50%. Infection of the rice rat (*Oryzomys capito*) by *L. mexicana* was confirmed in 14.4% of 97 specimens studied in Panama and in 29.3% of 314 specimens examined in Trinidad.

The Disease in Man (Tables 10 and 11): The incubation period varies from several days to many months. In the Americas the disease occurs in several clinical forms, affecting only the skin or both the skin and mucous membranes. The descriptions below are provided inside the framework of the proposed nomenclature within the genus *Leishmania* to give a clearer picture of the different clinical forms associated with distinct geographic areas, especially in the Americas.

a) *L. mexicana mexicana*, predominant in southeastern Mexico and Central America, causes a benign infection with only one or a few skin ulcers (chiclero ulcer, chiclero ear, bay sore). The lesion is usually located on the earflap (chiclero ear) or, less frequently, on the face or extremities. The lesion begins with an erythematous papule that then ulcerates; when the scab falls off, the surface bleeds easily. Lesions localized on the earflap are deforming, tend to be chronic, and may last many years, while those on other parts of the body heal spontaneously in about

Table 10. Main reservoirs and vectors of cutaneous leishmaniasis in the New World.

Leishmania subspecies	Reservoirs	Vectors
L. mexicana mexicana	Sylvatic rodents: *Ototylomys phyllotis*[a] *Heteromys desmarestianus* *Sigmodon hispidus* *Nyctomys sumichrasti*	*Lutzomyia olmeca olmeca*[a]
L. m. amazonensis	*Proechymys guyannensis*[a] *Oryzomys* spp., *Neacomys spinosus*, *Nectomys squamipes*, and several marsupial species.	*L. flaviscutellata*[a]
L. m. venezuelensis	?	*L. olmeca bicolor*
L. m. pifanoi	Probably small sylvatic mammals	?
L. braziliensis braziliensis	Not well known; some wild animals are suspected.	*L. intermedia* and *L. pessoai* (southern Brazil) *Psychodopygus wellcomei* (northern Brazil) *P. panamensis* (Venezuela)
L. b. guyannensis	*Choloepus didactylus*[a] (sloth) and *Tamandua tetradactyla*[a] (anteater)	*L. umbratilis*[a] *L. anduzei* *L. whitmani*
L. b. panamensis	*Choloepus hoffmanni*[a]; *Bradypus infuscatus*; *Bassaricyon gabbii, Nasua nasua, Potos flavus*; *Aotus trivirgatus, Saguinus geoffroyi*	*L. trapidoi* *L. gomezi* *L. ylephiletor* *P. panamensis*
L. b. peruviana	*Canis familiaris*	*L. peruensis* and *L. verrucarum* (probable vectors)

[a] Confirmed main reservoir or vector.

Confirmed reservoir: Infected animal that has been demonstrated by ecologic studies to maintain the parasite in nature (WHO, 1984).

Confirmed vector: Anthropophilic, feeds on the animal reservoir; naturally infected with a parasite identical to that found in man and the reservoir (WHO, 1984).

Source: Table constructed on the basis of data from Lainson, 1982, and Bonfante-Garrido, 1983.

6 months. A salient feature of this form of cutaneous leishmaniasis is that it may very rarely disseminate to the lymph nodes. In Mexico, cases of mucocutaneous leishmaniasis have not been observed, but two or three cases of cutaneous lesions that invaded the contiguous mucosa have been reported. The main victims are gum tappers who work in the forest during the rainy season when phlebotomine flies are abundant.

b) *L. mexicana amazonensis* leishmaniasis occurs in the Brazilian Amazon basin. Human cases by this agent are rare. The infection causes single or multiple lesions that rarely heal spontaneously. About 30% of patients have diffuse cutaneous

Table 11. Main vectors of cutaneous leishmaniasis in the Old World.

Leishmania species	Vector	Main areas with endemic foci
L. major	Phlebotomus dubosqui P. papatasi P. salehi	Senegal and parts of western Africa, southeastern and northern Asia, USSR, India
L. tropica	Paraphlebotomus sergenti	Afghanistan, India, Iran, Iraq, Pakistan, USSR
L. aethiopica	Larrousius longipes L. pedifer	Ethiopia Ethiopia and Kenya

Source: Adapted from The Leishmaniases. WHO, 1984. (Tech. Rep. Ser. 701.)

leishmaniasis, which is characterized by thickening of the skin, especially on the face and legs, in the form of scattered plaques, papules, or nodules.

c) *L. mexicana pifanoi* causes a diffuse cutaneous leishmaniasis similar to lepromatous leprosy and is often confused with it. Diffuse leishmaniasis has been described in Venezuela, but also occurs in other areas. Outside the Americas, cases are known from Ethiopia and Kenya. This form appears in patients with immune system dysfunction; diffuse cutaneous leishmaniasis patients are anergic and do not respond to the Montenegro (intradermal) test. The lesions harbor a large number of parasites. Normal volunteers, inoculated with parasites from patients with diffuse leishmaniasis, developed a localized lesion at the inoculation site that healed without sequelae. For this reason, it is thought that this form is due more to a deficiency in the host's immune response than to some special property of the parasite. Human cases of diffuse cutaneous leishmaniasis are not very frequent.

d) *L. mexicana venezuelensis* causes ulcerous lesions and, less frequently, nodular or ulceronodular lesions.

e) *L. braziliensis braziliensis* causes the mucocutaneous form (espundia). The disease begins with a papular lesion on the face or extremities; it can develop into a painless ulcer that seldom heals spontaneously. A characteristic feature of this form is metastasis to the mucocutaneous areas of the body. In a significant proportion of untreated patients, lesions appear on the nasal septum, mouth, nasopharynx, and sometimes even the anorectal region, penis, scrotum, and vulva. These metastases can occur simultaneously with the primary lesion or, more frequently, much later, and can cause severe destruction of the affected tissue, disfiguring the patient. The secondary lesions can be ulcerous or indurated.

f) *L. braziliensis guyannensis* occurs in Guyana, French Guiana, Suriname, and northern Brazil. It causes single skin lesions that often spread along the lymphatic vessels and produce ulcers on the entire body ("pian-bois").

g) *L. braziliensis peruviana* exists in the villages of the Peruvian Andes and causes cutaneous leishmaniasis, or uta, characterized by a single lesion that tends not to metastasize and heals spontaneously. In 1972, 1,148 cases of uta were reported. It affects primarily children.

h) *L. braziliensis panamensis* causes ulcerous skin lesions and occasionally affects the mucosa.

In the Old World three main forms occur:

a) *L. major* causes the rural or wet form of leishmaniasis that occurs in semi-desert or desert regions. The lesion begins as a papule on the exposed parts of the body (face and extremities) and develops into a wet ulcer. Multiple lesions may follow by either direct spread or dissemination through the lymph system. The disease lasts about 2 to 8 months, and fibrosis during spontaneous healing leaves a permanent scar.

b) *L. tropica* causes the dry form of leishmaniasis, which occurs in urban and periurban areas primarily in the Middle East. The initial papule evolves slowly, and ulceration, when it occurs, is also slow to develop. The disease has a long course (a year or more) and leaves a permanent scar. In contrast to those of the wet form, the lesions contain a large number of parasites.

c) *L. aethiopica* causes three types of lesions: oriental button or furuncle, the mucocutaneous form, and diffuse cutaneous leishmaniasis. The lesion develops slowly and may or may not ulcerate later. Spontaneous healing occurs after 1 to 3 years or even longer (World Health Organization, 1984).

The Disease in Animals: With the exception of a form occurring in western Peru, leishmaniasis is a disease of wild animals.

Many infections in wild animals are inapparent. Some members of the *L. mexicana* complex produce apparent infections in rodents and other wild animals, causing skin alterations mainly at the tail root and occasionally on the ears and toes. Lesions consist of swellings, which exhibit hair loss or sometimes ulcerate, and in which the presence of amastigotes can be confirmed. Infection in these hosts is prolonged. *L. mexicana amazonensis* infection in rodents (*Proechimys guyannensis*) and other animals of the Amazon basin causes the skin to remain apparently normal and the parasites to be dispersed in the dermis.

The parasites of the *L. braziliensis* complex produce systemic infection in wild animals but rarely skin lesions. The parasites can be cultured from the blood, viscera (spleen, liver), and apparently normal skin.

In dogs, which are the only known animal hosts of uta on the western slope of the Peruvian Andes, lesions are absent or insignificant. However, dogs with cutaneous lesions have been found outside Peru in several endemic areas of the Americas. In Venezuela, nine (40.9%) of 22 dogs examined had skin lesions, and the presence of *Leishmania* was confirmed in Giemsa-stained smears. The single or multiple lesions were located on the scrotum, nose, ear, and extremities (Bonfante-Garrido *et al.*, 1981a). In endemic areas, equines with leishmaniasis can also be found. Of 116 burros studied in Venezuela, 28 had one or more ulcerous lesions and 17 had parasites, as revealed by microscopic examination. Based on its behavior in hamsters and culture media, the authors (Bonfante-Garrido *et al.*, 1981b) classified the agent as *L. braziliensis*.

Source of Infection and Mode of Transmission (Figure 62): The reservoirs of cutaneous leishmaniasis in the Americas are wild animals. The infection is transmitted from one animal to another by phlebotomine flies of the genera *Lutzomyia* and *Psychodopygus*. Man is infected accidentally by the bite of these phlebotomines when he enters enzootic areas in the jungle. Recent studies have shown that a large number of wild mammal species are infected, but not all of them can be considered primary hosts since they are either not very abundant or their infection rate is too low to enable them to fill this role. The reservoirs of American cutaneous leishmaniasis

Figure 62. Cutaneous leishmaniasis (*Leishmania mexicana*). Basic transmission cycle.

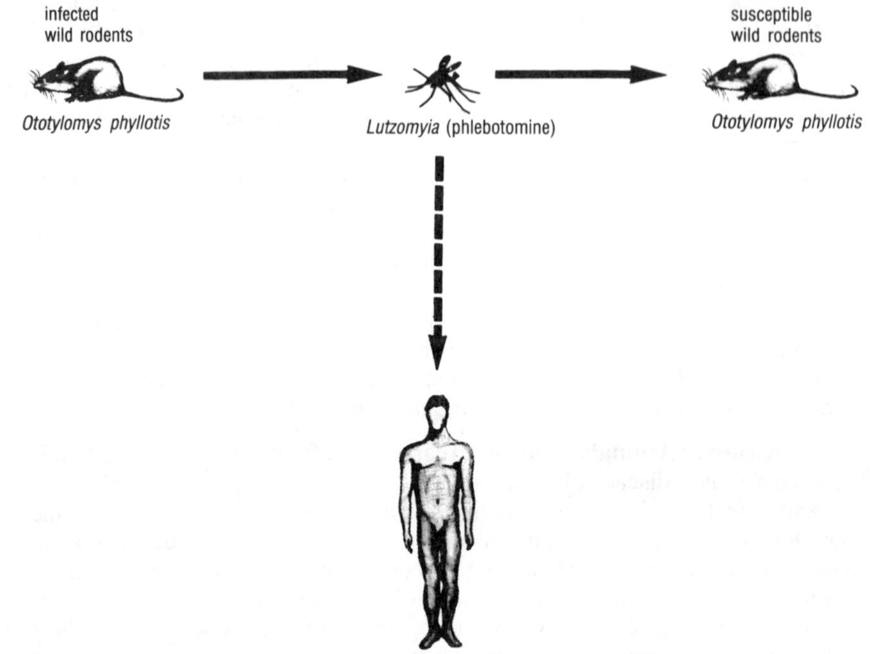

are thought to be sylvatic rodents or edentates. Dogs may also be a reservoir, since they are the only known host of *L. b. peruviana*, but it is suspected that they are merely a secondary host of this infection (uta) and that the primary host is a wild animal (Lainson, 1983). On the other hand, infected dogs have been found in other parts of the New World, and a growing role as a synanthropic secondary reservoir is attributed to them. Infected rats (*Rattus rattus*) have been found in Brazil. Opossums (*Didelphis marsupialis*) may also play a role as link between the wild enzootic cycle and the peridomestic one in Manaus, Brazil (World Health Organization, 1984). It is possible that infections produced by the *L. mexicana* complex are maintained in nature not by a single specific host, but by a variety of species associated with a particular habitat (World Health Organization, 1984). In several areas of the Americas, the relative roles of the different infected animal species have not yet been clarified.

The main reservoir of *L. major* in the USSR is the great gerbil, *Rhombomys opimus*. Infected colonies of this desert or semidesert rodent have been found from Iran, the southern USSR, and northern Afghanistan to Mongolia. In northwestern India, Israel, and Morocco the reservoirs are gerbils of the genus *Meriones*. Multiple skin lesions are found in many animals, on the ears, nape, and base of the tail. Lesions begin as nodules and can destroy part of the ear. Infection in these rodents is very prolonged. In Algeria, northwestern Libya, and Israel the reservoir is *Psammomys obesus*, and in Africa (Senegal and Ethiopia) it is species of *Mastomys*, *Tatera*, and *Arvicanthis*.

L. tropica has been isolated from dogs and *Rattus rattus*, but most researchers consider that the maintenance host is man himself. Lainson (1982) does not share this opinion and points out that interhuman transmission is unlikely since a limited number of amastigotes are contained in the few skin lesions this agent causes in humans.

Infection by *L. aethiopica* is maintained in Ethiopia and Kenya by hyracoid animals such as *Procavia capensis, Heterohyrax brucei*, and *Dendrohyrax arboreus*.

In the Americas, cutaneous leishmaniasis is a zoonosis and man is an accidental host. Man acquires the infection when he enters enzootic forest areas for occupational reasons (lumberjacks, gum tappers, petroleum workers, cattlemen, farmers, and others). In rural settlements within the jungle, cutaneous leishmaniasis can be an important, long-term problem. As people establish permanent settlements in enzootic areas, they create considerable ecologic changes, especially deforestation, the replacement of a wild mammalian fauna with domestic animals, and the consequent changes in the insect fauna as species better adapted to the new environment replace or dominate other species (Garnham, 1971). These ecologic changes also modify the epidemiology of cutaneous leishmaniasis. In Vale do Ribeira, São Paulo, Brazil, 80% of patients with cutaneous leishmaniasis worked near their homes and had no contact with the jungle. The devastation of the natural environment determined the species composition of phlebotomine flies in that region, and *Psychodopygus intermedius* came to predominate; it prefers secondary growth, enters human dwellings, and is anthropophilic (Tolezano *et al.*, 1980).

In west-central Venezuela, the disease used to occur exclusively in towns and villages located near mountainous areas with dense vegetation. In recent years, cases have been diagnosed in several neighborhoods on the perimeter of the city of Barquisimeto (Bonfante-Garrido *et al.*, 1984). It is not yet known whether this situation was brought about by some ecologic change, but the appearance of the disease in the urban environment illustrates that cutaneous leishmaniasis is not always sylvatic and rural and that its epidemiology is changing. Among the American cutaneous leishmaniases, uta in Peru is exceptional because no wild reservoirs of the parasite are known. In the Old World, *L. major* infection is a rural zoonosis, while infection due to *L. tropica* seems to be transmitted between humans in an urban environment.

Diagnosis: The most simple specific diagnosis consists of confirming the presence of the parasite in the lesions. For that purpose, material from the edge of the lesion (nodule or ulcer of the skin or mucosa) should be made into a film and stained using the Giemsa or Wright's technique. When the lesion is recent, abundant amastigotes can be found, but in chronic lesions it is difficult or impossible to demonstrate the presence of parasites by direct films or biopsies. Parasitologic diagnosis is especially difficult in the mucocutaneous form (Cuba *et al.*, 1981).

Isolation of the agent can be accomplished by culture in an appropriate medium, such as NNN. Another procedure is intracutaneous inoculation of the lesion material into hamsters. More reliable results are obtained by seeding a culture medium and inoculating hamsters simultaneously.

The parasites of the *L. mexicana* complex grow abundantly in laboratory media; when inoculated into the nose of a hamster, they cause a histiocytoma containing a great number of amastigotes to form in a few weeks, and the infection spreads by metastasis. By contrast, the parasites of the *L. braziliensis* complex grow more poorly in artificial culture media and when inoculated into hamsters produce a small nodule or ulcer containing few amastigotes that forms after 6 or more months; there is no metastasis of the initial lesion. Numerous serologic tests have been used for diagnosis of cutaneous leishmaniasis, among them immunofluorescence, direct agglutination, latex agglutination, immunodiffusion in gel, and ELISA. The indirect immunofluorescence test, which is widely used, gives better results with an amastigote antigen than with a promastigote antigen. However, there is no correlation between the reaction titer and clinical manifestations or duration or number of lesions (Cuba *et al.*, 1981). An IgA conjugate was superior to IgG when used in diagnosis of the mucocutaneous form (Lainson, 1983). In infection by *L. b. braziliensis*, the Montenegro test gives weak or negative reactions, and it is always negative in cases of diffuse cutaneous leishmaniasis (Lainson, 1983). Serology of Old World cutaneous leishmaniasis is generally negative (World Health Organization, 1984). The cutaneous or Montenegro test is group-specific and is useful for confirming parasitologic diagnosis, especially in epidemiologic studies.

Control: Patients infected by *L. braziliensis* should be treated early with pentavalent antimonials to prevent evolution of the infection to the mucocutaneous form. Patients infected by *L. mexicana amazonensis* should be treated in the same manner to prevent diffuse cutaneous leishmaniasis. Insecticides are difficult to apply in jungle or forest environments, but they should be used against the vectors in temporary camps or in domestic and peridomestic situations. The use of insecticides in antimalarial campaigns in Southeast Asia has led to the virtual disappearance of visceral and cutaneous leishmaniasis from that region, and the same happened with uta in several Andean villages in Peru. In the southern USSR, infection by *L. major* was controlled by eliminating colonies of the reservoir, *Rhombomys opimus*, from vast areas. Individual protection can be achieved by applying repellents to exposed parts of the body, especially after sunset. It is believed that uta could be prevented by destroying infected dogs in endemic areas of Peru. In the USSR, Israel, and Iran, immunization with virulent strains of *L. major* has been practiced against infection by that agent as well as *L. tropica*. Inoculation is done on a part of the skin where the scar will not be visible or unesthetic in order to prevent deforming lesions on the face. Inoculated individuals should remain outside endemic areas until immunity is established. This type of immunization is usually not recommended, but can be useful for persons who must enter high-risk areas.

Bibliography

Adler, S. Leishmania. *Adv Parasit* 2:35-96, 1964.

Biagi, F. *Enfermedades parasitarias*, 2nd ed. México, Prensa Médica Mexicana, 1974.

Bienzle, U., F. Ebert, and M. Dietrich. Cutaneous leishmaniasis in eastern Saudi Arabia. Epidemiological and clinical features in a non-immune population living in an endemic area. *Tropenmed Parasitol* 29:188-193, 1978.

Bonfante-Garrido, R., N. Morillo, and R. Torres. Leishmaniasis cutánea canina en Venezuela. *Bol Of Sanit Panam* 91:160-165, 1981a.

Bonfante-Garrido, R., E. Meléndez, R. Torres, N. Murillo, C. Arredondo, and I. Urdaneta. Enzootic equine cutaneous leishmaniasis in Venezuela. *Trans R Soc Trop Med Hyg* 75:471, 1981b.

Bonfante-Garrido, R. Leishmanias y leishmaniasis tegumentaria en América Latina. *Bol Of Sanit Panam* 95:418-426, 1983.

Bonfante-Garrido, R., S. Barroeta, M. A. Mejía de Alejos, E. Meléndez, C. Arredondo, R. Urdaneta, and I. Urdaneta. Urban cutaneous leishmaniasis in Barquisimeto, Venezuela. *Bull Pan Am Health Organ* 21:149-155, 1987.

Convit, J. J., and M. E. Pinardi. Cutaneous leishmaniasis. *In*: *Trypanosomiasis and Leishmaniasis*. *CIBA Foundation Symposium 20*. Amsterdam, Elsevier, 1974.

Cross, J. H., J. J. Gunning, D. J. Drutz, and J. C. Lien. Autochthonous cutaneous-subcutaneous leishmaniasis on Taiwan. *Am J Trop Med Hyg* 34:254-256, 1985.

Cuba, C. A. C., P. D. Marsden, A. C. Barreto, R. Rocha, R. R. Sampaio, and L. Patzlaff. Parasitologic and immunologic diagnosis of American (mucocutaneous) leishmaniasis. *Bull Pan Am Health Organ* 15:249-259, 1981.

Faust, E. C., P. F. Russell, and R. C. Jung. *Craig and Faust's Clinical Parasitology*, 8th ed. Philadelphia, Lea and Febiger, 1970.

Garnham, P. C. C. American leishmaniasis. *Bull WHO* 44:521-527, 1971.

Giannini, S. H., M. Schittini, J. S. Keithly, P. W. Warburton, C. R. Cantor, L. H. T. van der Ploeg. Karyotype analysis of *Leishmania* species and its use in classification and clinical diagnosis. *Science* 232:762-765, 1986.

Gustafson, T. L., C. M. Reed, P. B. McGreevy, M. G. Pappas, J. C. Fox, and P. G. Lawyer. Human cutaneous leishmaniasis acquired in Texas. *Am J Trop Med Hyg* 34:58-63, 1985.

Herrer, A., and S. R. Telford, Jr. *Leishmania braziliensis* isolated from sloths in Panama. *Science* 164:1419-1420, 1969.

Herrer, A., H. A. Christensen, and R. J. Beumer. Reservoir hosts of cutaneous leishmaniasis among Panamanian forest mammals. *Am J Trop Med Hyg* 22:585-591, 1973.

Killick-Kendrick, R., A. J. Leaney, W. Peters, J. A. Rioux, and R. S. Bray. Zoonotic cutaneous leishmaniasis in Saudi Arabia: the incrimination of *Phlebotomus papatasi* as the vector in the Al-Hassa oasis. *Trans R Soc Trop Med Hyg* 79:252-255, 1985.

Lainson, R., and J. Strangways-Dixon. The epidemiology of dermal leishmaniasis in British Honduras. Part II. *Trans R Soc Trop Med Hyg* 58:136-153, 1964.

Lainson, R., and J. J. Shaw. Leishmanias and leishmaniasis of the New World with particular reference to Brazil. *Bull Pan Am Health Organ* 7(4):1-19, 1973.

Lainson, R. Epidemiología e ecología de leishmaniose tegumentar na Amazonia. *Hileia Med (Belem)* 3:35-40, 1981.

Lainson, R. Leishmaniasis. *In*: Jacobs, L., and P. Arambulo (Section Eds.), CRC *Handbook Series in Zoonoses*. Section C, vol. 1. Boca Raton, Florida, CRC Press, 1982.

Lainson, R. The American leishmaniases: some observations on their ecology and epidemiology. *Tran R Soc Trop Med Hyg* 77:569-596, 1983.

Lumsden, W. H. R. Leishmaniasis and trypanosomiasis: the causative organisms compared and contrasted. *In*: *Trypanosomiasis and Leishmaniasis*. *CIBA Foundation Symposium 20*. Amsterdam, Netherlands, Elsevier, 1974.

Machado, M. I., R. V. Milder, G. Grimaldi, and H. Momen. Identification of *Leishmania mexicana mexicana* in the state of São Paulo, Brazil. *Rev Inst Med Trop S Paulo* 25:97, 1983.

Manson-Bahr, P. E. C. Leishmaniasis. *Int Rev Trop Med* 4:123-140, 1971.

Manson-Bahr, P. E. C., and D. J. Winslow. Cutaneous leishmaniasis. *In*: Marcial-Rojas, R. A. (Ed.), *Pathology of Protozoal and Helminthic Diseases*. Baltimore, Maryland, Williams and Wilkins, 1971.

Miles, M. A. Biochemical identification of the Leishmanias. *Bull Pan Am Health Organ* 19:343-353, 1985.

Pan American Health Organization. *Reported Cases of Notifiable Diseases in the Americas, 1970-1972*. Washington, D.C., PAHO, 1975. (Scientific Publication 308.)

Peters, W., S. Elbihari, C. Liu, S. M. Le Blaneg, D. A. Evans, R. Killick-Kendrick, V. Smith, and C. I. Baldwin. *Leishmania* infecting man and wild animals in Saudi Arabia, 1. General survey. *Trans R Soc Trop Med Hyg* 79:831-839, 1985.

Scorza, J. V., M. Valera, C. de Scorza, M. Carnevali, E. Moreno, and A. Lugo-Hernández. A new species of *Leishmania* parasite from the Venezuelan Andes region. *Trans R Soc Trop Med Hyg* 73:293-298, 1979.

Tikasingh, E. S. Enzootic rodent leishmaniasis in Trinidad, West Indies. *Bull Pan Am Health Organ* 8:232-242, 1974.

Tolezano, J. E., S. A. Macoris, and J. M. P. Diniz. Modificação na epidemiologia da leishmaniose tegumentar no Vale do Ribeira, Estado de São Paulo, Brasil. *Rev Inst A Lutz* 40:49-54, 1980.

World Health Organization. *The Leishmaniases.* Report of a WHO Expert Committee. Geneva, WHO, 1984. (Technical Report Series 701.)

GIARDIASIS

(007.1)

Synonym: Lambliasis.

Etiology: The taxonomy of species within the genus *Giardia* (*Lamblia*) is still being debated. Conventional criteria for differentiating species (such as animal host, some morphologic characters, and structural variations) have been considered, and, accordingly, the parasite found in dogs was named *G. canis*, the one in bovines *G. bovis*, and the one in humans *G. intestinalis* (*duodenalis, lamblia, enterica*). However, mammalian giardias are morphologically similar (with the exception of *G. muris*, found in mice, rats, and hamsters), and species specificity is not strict, as has been demonstrated by their transmission from one animal species to another. Consequently, the current tendency is to consider that *G. intestinalis* is common to man and several other mammalian species, such as dogs, cats, bovines, and guinea pigs. However, it is also possible that the differentiation of species of *G. intestinalis* and *G. muris* infecting mammals is only provisional. Now that *in vitro* culture of the parasite has been achieved, characterization of the species of *Giardia* by their antigenic and biochemical properties will be possible (Kulda and Nohýnková, 1978; Meyer and Radulescu, 1979; World Health Organization, 1981).

G. intestinalis is a flagellate protozoan whose life cycle includes trophozoite and cyst phases. The trophozoites vary greatly in size (from 9.5 to 21 microns in length and 5 to 15 microns in width), have four pairs of flagella and two nuclei, and cling to the mucosa of the host's small intestine by a disc-like structure. On the back of this disc is the median body, the shape of which has served as a basis for the taxonomic decision to classify mammalian *Giardia* into only two species: *G. intestinalis* and *G. muris*. This structure is basically identical in giardias from man, bovines, dogs, cats, guinea pigs, rabbits, and several other mammals, and has the hook shape of the claw of a hammer. Trophozoites multiply by binary fission and can reach considerable numbers. They encyst when the intestinal contents leave the jejunum and begin to lose moisture. The encysted trophozoite undergoes another division, and thus the mature cyst contains four nuclei. The cyst, ovoid and 7 to 10 microns in length, is passed to the environment with the feces. The cyst is the infective element and is very resistant to environmental factors; it can survive more than 2 months in water at 8°C and about 1 month at 21°C. Likewise, it is resistant to chlorinated disinfectants.

The cycle is repeated when a new host ingests the cysts: the parasite frees itself from the cyst in the duodenum and emerges as a tetranucleate trophozoite that quickly divides into two binucleate trophozoites.

Geographic Distribution: Worldwide.

Occurrence in Man: In developing countries, giardiasis is endemic and transmission is continuous. The disease mainly affects children, and their rate of infection is usually higher than the rate in adults. A study in Chile demonstrated prevalences of 29.9% in children under 10 years old, 18.6% in youths 10 to 19 years old, and 9.1% in persons over 20 years old (Ramírez *et al.*, 1972). Giardiasis can also occur epidemically. In the United States, 12 of 99 epidemics of water origin that occurred between 1971 and 1974 were caused by giardias, and more than 5,000 persons were affected. In 1974, 4,800 (10.4%) of 46,000 inhabitants in a town in New York State had clinical giardiasis due to contamination of the drinking water supply. Such epidemics affect all age groups equally. In populations that have not been exposed to the infection before, morbidity rates can reach 20% or more (Knight, 1980). Outbreaks are also common in institutions for children, such as orphanages and day-care centers. An outbreak in a day-care center in Chile affected nearly 60% of 111 children 3 months to 7 years old (Schenone *et al.*, 1976).

Giardiasis is the most common parasitic infection in the United States and Great Britain. In the United States, 3.8% of 414,800 fecal matter samples were positive for *G. intestinalis*; about 3,200 infections are recorded each year in Great Britain. Likewise, *G. intestinalis* is one of the agents of "tourist diarrhea." In a group of 21 persons whose feces were negative for *Giardia*, 15 out of 17 who became ill after visiting Leningrad were then positive for the protozoan's cysts (Kulda and Nohýnková, 1978).

Occurrence in Animals: Infection has been confirmed in a great variety of species of domestic and wild mammals. In the United States, 0.5% of dogs on a military base in Colorado and 36% of stray dogs in New Jersey were found to be infected. Studies carried out in Canada and Europe have also recorded significant proportions of infected dogs. In central New Jersey, the feces of 2.5% of stray cats contained cysts. Research in Colorado found the parasite's cysts in 10% of cattle, 18% of beavers, and 6% of coyotes.

An outbreak of giardiasis among nonhuman primates and zoo personnel was recorded in Kansas City, Missouri. High rates of infection have also been found in rats and other rodents, both synanthropic and wild, but whether the agent was *G. intestinalis* or *G. muris* has not been determined (Meyer and Jarroll, 1982).

The Disease in Man: The majority of infections are subclinical. In symptomatic individuals, the incubation period lasts 1 to 3 weeks. Symptomatology consists mainly of diarrhea and meteorism, frequently accompanied by abdominal pain. Less often there is nausea and vomiting. The acute phase of the disease lasts about 3 to 4 days.

In some patients giardiasis can be a prolonged illness, with episodes of recurring diarrhea and flatulence, urticaria, and intolerance for certain foods. These and other allergic manifestations associated with giardiasis disappear with specific treatment directed against the parasite.

The Disease in Animals: Infection and disease in animals follow the same patterns as in man. The disease is more frequent in young animals.

Source of Infection and Mode of Transmission: Man is the main reservoir of human giardiasis; the source of infection is feces containing the parasite's cysts. Although the infection cycle is usually extinguished in a few months, continuous transmission in endemic areas ensures the persistence of the agent. The existence of asymptomatic infected individuals and chronic patients and the resistance of cysts to environmental conditions are important factors in the epidemiology. As has been confirmed on volunteers, the median infective dose (ID_{50}) for man is 25 to 100 cysts. Some giardiasis patients shed up to 900 million cysts per day in their feces. Elimination of cysts can be intermittent and the quantity can vary greatly (Knight, 1980).

Direct transmission can occur, especially in children and groups of people with deficient hygiene practices, by hand-to-mouth transfer of cysts from the feces of infected persons. Another mode is transmission by contaminated drinking water and, to a lesser extent, food. Epidemics have occurred in several cities owing to contamination of the drinking-water supply. In that regard, it should be borne in mind that the chlorine concentration commonly used to treat water does not destroy the cysts.

An association between giardiasis, hypochlorhydria, and pancreatic disease has been described. These conditions appear in connection with protein-calorie malnutrition in children, which is so frequent in developing countries. Giardiasis and hypochlorhydria occur more commonly in persons of blood group A than in persons of other groups (Knight, 1980).

Animals probably constitute an additional reservoir of infection for humans. Giardias from man and those from domestic and wild animals are not only morphologically similar or identical, but several experiments have shown that they can cross the species barrier. *G. intestinalis* cysts of human origin have produced infection in several animal species, including dogs, raccoons (*Procyon lotor*), rats (*Rattus norvegicus*), gerbils (*Gerbillus gerbillus*), guinea pigs, mouflons (*Ovis musimon*), bighorn sheep (*Ovis canadensis*), and pronghorn antelope (*Antilocapra americana*). For some other species, results were negative. Likewise, it is interesting to note that *Giardia* cysts from beavers were infective for two of three human volunteers and four of four dogs, but not for hamsters, guinea pigs, mice, or rats. A human volunteer who ingested cysts from a black-tailed deer became infected, but dogs similarly exposed did not (World Health Organization, 1981). As has been pointed out (Meyer and Radulescu, 1979), the infective capacity depends as much on the number of cysts ingested as on factors inherent to the host, and even a homologous exposure can give negative results. A previous infection can confer resistance so that the exposed individual will not become infected. Conversely, positive results attributed to cross-species transmission may in reality be due to a recrudescence of a long-standing infection or to a recently acquired natural infection. The largest outbreak of human giardiasis attributed to an animal source occurred in 1976 in the town of Camas in Washington State, where 128 cases of giardiasis were confirmed among the 6,000 inhabitants. Part of the Camas water supply originated from two remote mountain streams. Epidemiologic investigation could not find any human source of contamination; on the other hand, several infected beavers were found in the area of the streams. It was possible to infect specific-pathogen–free (SPF) pups with *Giardia* cysts from the beavers. Another outbreak in which cross transmission was indicated occurred in 1978 in a zoo in the United States where six nonhuman primates and three female employees became ill. The index case was a gibbon that was placed in a special care unit where it spread the infection to other nonhuman primates and the three humans (Armstrong *et al.*, 1979).

Diagnosis: In acute diarrheic patients, both the trophozoite and the cyst phase of the parasite can be found in the feces. In some patients the examination must be repeated after several days in order to find evidence of the infection. Concentration methods are useful. However, in some cases it is necessary to resort to examination of duodenal fluid obtained by aspiration or biopsy to reveal the presence of trophozoites. This procedure is justified only in very serious cases. It must be taken into account that finding giardias in a patient does not always indicate a causal relationship to the person's symptoms, which may be caused by infection with other intestinal microorganisms (American Public Health Association, 1985).

Recently achieved *in vitro* culture of *G. intestinalis* allows the study of immunobiologic tests for diagnosis of the disease. One study demonstrated that the indirect immunofluorescence test was very specific but not very sensitive. Blastic transformation and macrophage migration inhibition tests have been reported to be very specific and sensitive (World Health Organization, 1981).

Control: Public water supply systems must be protected against contamination by human or animal feces. An adequate system of sedimentation, flocculation, and filtration can remove particles the size of *Giardia* from the water, allowing the use of surface water supply systems (Centers for Disease Control of the USA, 1977).

Sanitary elimination of feces is another important measure. In developing countries, prevailing socioeconomic conditions make it difficult to prevent infection in children. Instruction in personal hygiene is essential in institutions for children. Tourists should abstain from drinking tap water in places where its purity cannot be guaranteed. Dogs and cats with giardiasis should be treated (quinacrine, metronidazole) because of the close contact they may have with children (Meyer and Jarroll, 1982).

Bibliography

Armstrong, J., R. E. Hertzog, R. T. Hall, and G. L. Hoff. Giardiasis in apes and zoo attendants, Kansas City, Missouri. *CDC Vet Public Health Notes*, January 1979.

American Public Health Association. *Control of Communicable Diseases in Man*, 14th ed. (Ed. by A. S. Benenson). Washington, D.C., APHA, 1985.

Centers for Disease Control of the USA. Water-borne giardiasis outbreaks. Washington, New Hampshire. *Morb Mortal Wkly Rep* 26:169-170, 1977.

Georgi, M. E., M. S., Carlisle, and L. E. Smiley. Giardiasis in a great blue heron (*Ardea herodias*) in New York State: another potential source of waterborne giardiasis. *Am J Epidemiol* 123:916-917, 1986.

Knight, R. Epidemiology and transmission of giardiasis. *Trans R Soc Trop Med Hyg* 74:433-436, 1980.

Kulda, J., and E. Nohýnková. Flagellates of the human intestine and of intestines of other species. *In*: Kreier, J. P. (Ed.), *Parasitic Protozoa*, vol. 2. New York, Academic Press, 1978.

Meyer, E. A., and S. Radulescu. Giardia and giardiasis. *Adv Parasitol* 17:1-47, 1979.

Meyer, E. A., and E. L. Jarroll. Giardiasis. *In*: Jacobs, L., and P. Arambulo (Section Eds.), *CRC Handbook Series in Zoonoses*. Section C, vol. 1. Boca Raton, Florida, CRC Press, 1982.

Ramírez, R., H. Schenone, M. Galdames, E. Romero, E. Inzunza, A. Rojas, H. Palomino, and R. Székely. Frecuencia en Chile de las infecciones humanas por protozoos y helmintos intestinales (1962-1972). *Bol Chile Parasitol* 27:116-118, 1972.

Schenone, H., T. Saavedra, M. Galdames, E. Inzunza, M. Jiménez, and E. Romero. Epidemia de giardiasis en un jardín infantil y el uso de nimorazol en su control. *Bol Chile Parasitol* 31:12-15, 1976.

World Health Organization. *Intestinal Protozoan and Helminthic Infections.* Report of a WHO Scientific Group. Geneva, WHO, 1981. (Technical Report Series 666.)

MALARIA IN NONHUMAN PRIMATES

(084.4)

Synonyms: Monkey paludism, monkey malaria.

Etiology: More than 20 species of *Plasmodium* are known to occur in nonhuman primates. The taxonomy of some of these species is uncertain. The following plasmodia of nonhuman primates have been transmitted naturally or experimentally to man: *P. cynomolgi, P. knowlesi, P. inui, P. schwetzi, P. simium, P. brasilianum,* and *P. eylesi.* The plasmodium described in chimpanzees, which was given the name *P. rodhani,* is probably *P. malariae* (Collins and Aikawa, 1977).

The life cycle is divided into two phases, one in the mosquito vector and the other in the vertebrate host. The anopheline mosquito, when feeding on the blood of a primate, injects sporozoites into its bloodstream. In less than an hour the sporozoites disappear from the blood and enter the cells of the hepatic parenchyma, initiating the exoerythrocytic cycle. The parasites transform into schizonts and their nuclei divide by multiple fission; when mature, the schizonts free a large number of exo-erythrocytic merozoites. Seven to 10 days after the start of the infection, most of the merozoites break out of the hepatic cells into the bloodstream, infect the erythrocytes, and initiate the erythrocytic cycle. Some merozoites penetrate other liver cells and repeat the exoerythrocytic cycle. The erythrocytic parasites, or trophozoites, divide by mitosis to become mature schizonts, which form multiple erythrocytic merozoites by schizogony. When the red blood cell disintegrates, the merozoites are freed into the bloodstream and infect new red blood cells; thus, the erythrocytic cycle is repeated. The length of each cycle varies with the species of *Plasmodium.* The erythrocytic cycle is the phase that causes clinical manifestations, and it determines the periodicity of febrile attacks; different cycles are known as quotidian malaria (malarial attacks every 24 hours), tertian malaria (attacks at 48-hour intervals), and quartan malaria (attacks every 72 hours). After a series of asexual generations, some merozoites develop into macrogametocytes and micro-gametocytes. When ingested by anopheline mosquitoes, these cells mature and become macrogametes and microgametes; the sexual phase is completed by fertilization of the macrogametes by the microgametes. The process produces a motile egg, or ookinete, which lodges in the insect's stomach wall. There, it forms an oocyst that produces some 10,000 or more sporozoites, which migrate to the salivary glands. When injected into a new susceptible vertebrate host, the sporozoites reinitiate the cycle.

Geographic Distribution: The quartan species *P. brasilianum*, which is morphologically similar to *P. malariae* of man, is widely distributed among the neotropical monkeys of Brazil, Peru, Colombia, Venezuela, and Panama. *P. simium*, in southern and eastern Brazil, is a tertian species similar to *P. vivax* of man. *P. cynomolgi, P. inui, P. knowlesi,* and *P. eylesi* occur in nonhuman primates in several Asian countries. *P. schwetzi* is a parasite of anthropoid primates in Africa.

Occurrence in Man: Rare. Only three human infections acquired under natural field conditions are known: two cases caused by *P. knowlesi* in Malaysia and one by *P. simium* in Brazil.

Personnel in research laboratories have become infected accidentally with plasmodia of simian origin as a result of bites by infected anopheline mosquitoes. *P. knowlesi* has been transmitted from monkey to man by infected mosquitoes, as well as from one human to another and from man to monkey.

Out of 204 volunteers who received parasitized blood or were exposed to the bites of infected mosquitoes, 154 became infected with plasmodia of simian origin.

Occurrence in Nonhuman Primates: In the neotropics, *P. brasilianum* has been found in numerous species of monkeys of the family Cebidae. The infection rate is approximately 15% in monkeys of the genera *Alouatta* (howler monkey), *Ateles* (spider monkey), and *Cebus* (capuchin). Natural infection by *P. simium* has been found in approximately 30% of individuals of *Alouatta fusca* (brown howler monkey), and in *Brachyteles arachnoides* (wooly spider monkey). Among the nonhuman primates of Asia and Africa, the prevalence of infection is apparently high in areas with a large number of monkeys and appropriate anopheline vectors. On the other hand, there are areas in both the New and Old World with a sparse population of monkeys where the infection does not occur.

The Disease in Man: In general, human malaria caused by plasmodia of simian origin resembles a mild and benign infection caused by human plasmodia. The disease is of short duration, parasitemias are low, and relapses are rare. Recuperation is spontaneous, and very few patients require treatment. The pattern of malarial attacks depends on the species of parasite. *P. knowlesi* is a quotidian species, while *P. cynomolgi, P. schwetzi, P. simium,* and *P. eylesi* are tertian species, and *P. brasilianum* and *P. inui* are quartan species.

The Disease in Monkeys: In the natural hosts in Asia, the infection causes a mild and often clinically inapparent disease. Thus, *P. knowlesi* infection in *Macaca fascicularis* (cynomolgus monkey), the natural host in eastern Asia, is generally asymptomatic or characterized by mild and irregular fever, while in *Macaca mulatta* (rhesus monkey), experimental infection causes a serious and fatal disease. Infections caused by *P. inui* or *P. cynomolgi* are even less pathogenic for the natural hosts. *P. schwetzi* causes mild infection in chimpanzees, its natural hosts; *P. eylesi* causes high parasitemia in mandrills.

P. brasilianum appears to be more pathogenic for its natural hosts. Experimental infections, especially in *Cebus* and *Ateles*, can produce either an acute and fatal disease, or a disease with less serious symptomatology but a long duration and relapses.

Source of Infection and Mode of Transmission: Malaria of both humans and nonhuman primates is transmitted by anopheline mosquitoes, in which the parasite completes its sexual cycle. Which mosquito species transmit malaria of nonhuman primates in the forests of America, Africa, and a large part of Asia is not well known. In northwestern Malaysia, the vector of *P. cynomolgi* is *Anopheles balabacensis balabacensis*, which also transmits human malaria in this region. However, the transmission cycles of human malaria and nonhuman primate malaria are generally independent, since the vectors of human plasmodia feed at ground level, while those of simian plasmodia feed in the treetops (acrodendrophilic mosquitoes). In Brazil, the distribution of *P. simium* and *P. brasilianum* was found to be determined by the presence of acrodendrophilic mosquitoes (*A. cruzi* and *A. neivai*). This explains the rarity of human infection caused by plasmodia of simian origin. Nevertheless, in some regions of Brazil, such as the mountainous and wooded coast of Santa Catarina State, *A. cruzi* (which in other areas is exclusively acrodendrophilic) is the vector of human malaria and probably also of simian malaria. In this region *A. cruzi* has been found to feed at both ground and treetop level. Under such conditions, human infections caused by simian plasmodia may occur naturally. In western Malaysia a similar situation exists and can result in zoonotic infections, since both cycles (human and nonhuman) share the same vector. Risk is apparently limited to persons who live in or enter the jungle area, and it is unlikely that the infection can spread to human communities.

In tropical Africa, where chimpanzees are infected by *P. malariae* (*P. rodhani*) and *P. schwetzi*, the infection may be transmissible to humans entering the habitat of these primates. Malariologists point out, however, that plasmodia from nonhuman primates constitute little risk for the human population. *P. malariae* from chimpanzees cannot infect *Anopheles gambiae*, the vector of human malaria, and *P. schwetzi* does not develop fully in this mosquito. No cases are known of plasmodial transmission from chimpanzees to man by mosquitoes. It is not known which mosquitoes transmit plasmodia among these anthropoids, nor whether these plasmodia can survive in a human host.

The role nonhuman primates might play in maintaining a focus of infection is considered minimal if human malaria is eradicated from the area.

The true importance of monkey malaria can be better evaluated when methods become available to characterize simian plasmodia by their isozymes, DNA, or by immunologic techniques (World Health Organization, 1979).

Diagnosis: Routine diagnosis in man and monkeys is done by examination of thick films stained with Giemsa stain. Differentiation of the species of *Plasmodium* that infect nonhuman primates is based primarily on morphologic characteristics of the parasite's different developmental stages. Another criterion is host specificity. Specific diagnosis is very difficult, as in the case of *P. brasilianum* and *P. simium*, which are similar to the human plasmodia *P. malariae* and *P. vivax*, respectively. Some investigators maintain that New World monkeys acquired the plasmodia from man, possibly in recent times.

Because the routine diagnostic techniques for differentiating plasmodium species are imprecise, an undetermined number of human malaria cases caused by simian plasmodia may have been incorrectly diagnosed as being caused by human malarial agents.

Another difficulty in diagnosis by microscopic examination of blood preparations stems from the low parasitemia in nonhuman primates. To eliminate this difficulty, inoculation of blood into susceptible monkeys is recommended.

Control: Malariologists are in agreement that malaria of nonhuman primates does not present an obstacle, at least under present circumstances, to control and eradication programs for human malaria. The small number of confirmed cases of human infection caused by plasmodia of simian origin and the benign nature of the clinical manifestations do not justify special control measures.

To prevent the disease, nonimmune persons who have to go into the jungle should use repellents on exposed parts of the body and on clothing. The regular use of chemoprophylaxis would be justified only if the nonimmune person had to live in an area where human malaria is endemic.

Bibliography

Bruce-Chwatt, L. J. Malaria zoonosis in relation to malaria eradication. *Trop Geogr Med* 20:50-87, 1968.

Coatney, G. R. Simian malarias in man: facts, implications and predictions. *Am J Trop Med Hyg* 17:147-155, 1968.

Coatney, G. R. The simian malarias: zoonoses, anthroponoses, or both? *Am J Trop Med Hyg* 20:795-803, 1981.

Collins, W. E., and M. Aikawa. Plasmodia of nonhuman primates. *In*: Kreier, J. P. (Ed.), *Parasitic Protozoa*, vol. 3. New York, Academic Press, 1977.

Deane, L. M. Epidemiology of simian malaria in the American continent. *In: First Inter-American Conference on Conservation and Utilization of American Nonhuman Primates in Biomedical Research*. Washington, D.C., Pan American Health Organization, 1976. (Scientific Publication 317.)

Deane, L. M, M. P. Deane, J. A. Ferreira Neto, and F. B. Almeida. Studies on transmission of simian malaria and on a natural infection of man with *Plasmodium simium* in Brazil. *Bull WHO* 35:805-808, 1966.

Garnham, P. C. C. Recent research on malaria in mammals excluding man. *Adv Parasitol* 11:603-630, 1973.

Levine, N. D. *Protozoan Parasites of Domestic Animals and of Man*, 2nd ed. Minneapolis, Burgess, 1973.

Ristic, M., and R. D. Smith. Zoonoses caused by hemoprotozoa. *In*: Soulsby, E. J. L. (Ed.), *Parasitic Zoonoses*. New York, Academic Press, 1974.

Ruch, T. C. *Diseases of Laboratory Primates*. Philadelphia, Saunders, 1969.

Warren, McW. Simian and anthropoid malarias, their role in human disease. *Lab Anim Care* 20:368-376, 1970.

World Health Organization. *Parasitology of Malaria*. Report of a WHO Scientific Group. Geneva, WHO, 1969. (Technical Report Series 433.)

World Health Organization. *Parasitic Zoonoses*. Report of a WHO Expert Committee with the Participation of FAO. Geneva, WHO, 1979. (Technical Report Series 637.)

PNEUMOCYSTIS PNEUMONIA

(136.3)

Synonyms: Pneumocystosis, pneumocystic pneumonia, interstitial plasma-cell pneumonia.

Etiology: *Pneumocystis carinii*. The systematic classification of this agent is uncertain; most investigators consider it to be a sporozoon with schizogonic and sporogonic reproduction, while others think it is a yeast of the Ascomycetes group. *P. carinii* is an extracellular parasite found in the pulmonary alveoli and bronchioli; the cyst typically contains eight sporozoites. The cyst reacts positively to para-aminosalicylic acid (PAS) (Schiff's reaction) and stains well with Gomori's methenamine–silver nitrate method. Recently, *P. carinii* has been grown successfully in cell cultures of chick embryo pulmonary epithelium. It could be observed that the trophozoite adheres to cells by means of microtubules through which it feeds. When the trophozoite increases in size, it detaches from the cell and evolves into the cyst form. The liberation of sporozoites from the cyst results in new trophozoites (Hughes, 1977).

Geographic Distribution: Worldwide. Human infections caused by *P. carinii* have been described in numerous European countries and in several countries in Asia, Africa, Australia, North America, and Latin America.

Occurrence in Man: The disease occurs in two types of patients: debilitated children (infantile endemic pneumocystosis) and immunoincompetent adults or those treated with immunosuppressant drugs. The disease is seen primarily in children under 6 months of age who were born prematurely or are undernourished. During World War II and in the years immediately following it, several thousand cases of pneumocystosis, with a high case fatality rate, occurred in nursery homes in European countries. In a study carried out in a clinic for infants in Czechoslovakia, 216 of 364 cases of pneumonia were attributed to infection caused by *P. carinii* (Bommer, 1964). Among 2,671 Vietnamese orphans evacuated to the United States, there were seven cases of pneumocystis pneumonia, five of them fatal (Centers for Disease Control of the USA, 1976). In addition to this infantile form, the disease is seen in adults and children in association with both congenital and acquired immunodeficiency, as well as immunosuppression in cancer patients or organ transplant patients. Even though there were already several hundred cases occurring each year in the United States, interest in the disease has intensified since the emergence of the epidemic of acquired immunodeficiency syndrome (AIDS).[1] Approximately 50% of AIDS patients contract pneumocystis pneumonia, with highly fatal results.

---

[1] Acquired immunodeficiency syndrome was recognized for the first time in 1981; among other signs, it is characterized by acute immunosuppression, lymphopenia, anergy, reduction in the number of "helper" T-lymphocytes (or their decrease in relation to suppressor T-lymphocytes), hypergammaglobulinemia, and decrease of lymphocyte blastogenesis. The prodromal period of 2 to 8 months includes primarily fever, lymphadenopathy, diarrhea, weight loss, fatigue, and depression; later, there is onset of symptoms and signs related to the final illness, which can be an opportunistic infection, Kaposi's sarcoma, or both. Of the nearly 42,000 cases recorded in the United States up to October 1987, around

Asymptomatic infection is common in immunocompetent persons. Serologic studies have demonstrated that almost 100% of 2-year-old children in the Netherlands had antibodies for *P. carinii*, as did 75% of 4-year-olds in the United States (Hughes, 1982).

Occurrence in Animals: The infection is very widespread among rodents and lagomorphs and is latent; it can be activated by administering high doses of corticosteroids. *P. carinii* has also been found in various species of domestic and wild mammals.

The Disease in Man: In children, the incubation period is 1 to 2 months. Symptoms of the infantile endemic disease begin insidiously at 2 to 4 months of age. Anorexia and diarrhea are observed in the prodromal period. The afebrile disease is characterized by progressive interstitial pneumonia, with cyanosis, hypoxia, and tachypnea. In the hypoergic form, which occurs in immunoincompetent persons of any age, the disease is of sudden onset with fever, tachypnea, and cough. Radiography reveals a widespread increase in lung density and areas of emphysema; both lungs are almost always affected. The disease is generally fatal. In autopsy, the lungs are found to be enlarged, distended, and consolidated; the alveoli are filled with edematous and foamy fluid containing numerous parasites. Interstitial infiltration consists primarily of plasma cells in the infantile disease and of lymphocytes and histiocytes in the hypoergic disease.

The Disease in Animals: The asymptomatic infection has been found in rats, domestic and wild mice, lagomorphs, cats, and other animals. The latent infection can manifest itself clinically as pneumonia if the animal's resistance decreases. Several spontaneous cases of interstitial pneumonia due to this agent have been described in dogs, colts, pigs, marmosets, and one goat. Generally, clinical cases in animals are rare.

Source of Infection and Mode of Transmission: The epidemiology of the disease is not well known. Asymptomatic infection is common in man and animals. Clinical disease, on the other hand, occurs only in malnourished and premature children as well as immunologically compromised children and adults (persons with congenital or acquired immunodeficiency, or undergoing therapy with immunosuppressant medicine). Given these facts, the question is whether the disease is due to the activation of a latent infection, to a primary infection, or to reinfection. Some outbreaks in children in nurseries or among cancer or organ transplant patients seem to suggest a primary infection or reinfection, with the source of infection being patients with pneumocystis pneumonia. However, in other cases the disease is clearly a result of a latent infection activated by acquired immunodeficiency (AIDS, for example) or induced immunosuppression. Experimentally, latent infection can be activated in rats by treatment with corticosteroids. It has been demonstrated that

---

70% have occurred in homosexual or bisexual males, and almost all the rest in intravenous drug users (due to sharing contaminated needles), recipients of transfusions of contaminated blood or blood products, and heterosexual contacts of infected persons. The disease has been confirmed in at least 119 countries. A retrovirus first isolated from AIDS patients in the United States and France is the etiologic agent. The virus can be found in the blood, semen, and saliva of AIDS patients. See "Slow Viruses (Degenerative Encephalopathies) and Retroviruses of Man and Animals" for a further discussion of the virus.

axenic (germ-free) rats kept in sterilized isolation cages are free of infection, but become infected when exposed to the ambient air in open cages. On the other hand, it was not possible to infect them via the digestive route (Hughes, 1982). These studies indicate that primary infection is produced via the respiratory route and propagates from one animal to another (Hughes *et al.*, 1983). Congenital infection also occurs, as demonstrated by the few cases of pneumocystis pneumonia that have been seen in stillborn and 2- to 3-day-old babies.

There is some evidence suggesting that the infection can be transmitted between humans and also from rodents to man. The disease occurs mainly in institutions such as nurseries and orphanages, in which the infection is probably transmitted by aerosols containing the parasite. Higher titers have been found by the complement fixation test in personnel who cared for children with pneumocystosis than in persons who had no contact with these children, possibly indicating interhuman transmission of the agent. Transmission of the infection has also occurred between patients treated with immunosuppressant drugs who were kept in the same room and between children in the same family.

Evidence for the possibility of transmission from animals to man comes from observations in Czechoslovakia, where a high rate of pneumocystic infection of rodents was found in the houses of many index patients in outbreaks that occurred in children's institutions. In the same country, it was also pointed out that there is some relationship between the increase in the population density of the rodent *Microtus arvalis* and epidemic outbreaks. However, no proof yet exists that the infection can be transmitted from rodents to man, and some investigators even suggest that *Pneumocystis* of man and rodents may be different species or that there are species-specific strains of *P. carinii*.

Role of Animals in the Epidemiology of the Disease: Humans and animals could be infected from an unknown common source, for example soil, via airborne transmission. However, studies carried out on axenic and conventional rats have demonstrated that transmission occurs from one animal to another, and contaminated soil has not been confirmed to serve as a source of infection (Hughes *et al.*, 1983). Current knowledge does not permit definition of the role of animals in the epidemiology; more studies are needed to clarify intra- and interspecific transmission (World Health Organization, 1979).

Diagnosis: Diagnosis is based on demonstrating the parasite's presence in sputum, aspirated tracheal exudate, bronchial brushings, or histologic sections and impressions of affected pulmonary tissue. For diagnosis of a living child patient, exudate is extracted by inserting a catheter or bronchoscope in the hypopharynx. Biopsy of lung tissue by means of open lung surgery has also been used and provides the most satisfactory specimen for diagnostic purposes. The agent can be observed with the use of PAS, Gomori, and Giemsa stains. Serologic tests do not provide definitive results. According to some investigators, the complement fixation test, with lung material from infected children as antigen, has given excellent results, but other researchers disagree. Generally, results are less satisfactory in immunosuppressed individuals. The immunofluorescence test developed in recent years has not yet been evaluated sufficiently, but preliminary results indicate that it has good specificity but low sensitivity. The frequency of subclinical infection by *P. carinii* can make the results of serologic tests difficult to interpret (Hughes, 1977).

Control: Because of incomplete knowledge of the epidemiology of the disease, it is not possible to establish adequate control measures. Pneumocystis pneumonia patients in nurseries or rooms where other patients are being treated with immunosuppressant drugs should be removed and put in isolation. High-risk patients should be treated prophylactically with trimethoprim and sulphamethoxazole (a combination that is also the most indicated for treatment). This chemoprophylaxis has given good results in recipients of renal transplants, immunosuppressed by cyclosporine and steroids, among whom the occurrence of pneumocystosis is frequent (Hardy *et al.*, 1984). Given the possibility that rodents may be reservoirs of the agent and a source of infection for man, rodent control is advisable.

Bibliography

American Public Health Association. *Control of Communicable Diseases in Man*, 14th ed. (Ed. by A. S. Benenson). Washington, D.C., APHA, 1985.

Araujo, F. G., and J. S. Remington. *Pneumocystis carinii* infection. *In*: Hubbert, W. T., W. F. McCulloch, and P. R. Schnurrenberger (Eds.), *Diseases Transmitted from Animals to Man*, 6th ed. Springfield, Illinois, Thomas, 1975.

Areán, V. Pulmonary pneumocystosis. *In*: Marcial-Rojas, R. A. (Ed.), *Pathology of Protozoal and Helminthic Diseases*. Baltimore, Maryland, Williams and Wilkins, 1971.

Belding, D. I. *Textbook of Parasitology*, 3rd ed. New York, Appleton-Century-Crofts, 1965.

Biagi, F. *Enfermedades Parasitarias*, 2nd ed. Mexico, Prensa Médica Mexicana, 1974.

Bommer, W. Untersuchungen an *Pneumocystis carinii*. *Zentralbl Bakteriol [Orig]* 192:300-308, 1964.

Centers for Disease Control of the USA. *Pneumocystis carinii* pneumonia in Vietnamese orphans. *Morb Mortal Wkly Rep* 25:15, 1976.

Frenkel, J. K. Toxoplasmosis and pneumocystosis: clinical and laboratory aspects in immunocompetent and compromised hosts. *In*: Prier, J. E., and H. Friedman (Eds.), *Opportunistic Pathogens*. Baltimore, Maryland, University Park Press, 1974.

Hardy, A. M., C. P. Wajszczuk, A. F. Suffredini, T. R. Hakala, and M. Ho. *Pneumocystis carinii* pneumonia in renal-transplant recipients treated with cyclosporine and steroids. *J Infect Dis* 149:143-147, 1984.

Hofmann, B., N. Odum, P. Platz, L. P. Ryder, A. Svejgaard, P. B. Nielsen, W. Holten-Andersen, J. Gerstoft, J. O. Nielsen, and M. Hojon. Humoral response to *Pneumocystis carinii* in patients with acquired immunodeficiency syndrome and in immunocompromised homosexual men. *J Infect Dis* 152:838-840, 1985.

Hughes, W. T. *Pneumocystis carinii* pneumonia. *N Engl J Med* 297:1381-1383, 1977.

Hughes, W. T. Natural mode of acquisition for *de novo* infection with *Pneumocystis carinii*. *J Infect Dis* 145:842-848, 1982.

Hughes, W. T., D. L. Bartley, and B. M. Smith. A natural source of infection due to *Pneumocystis carinii*. *J Infect Dis* 147:595, 1983.

Kucera, K. Some new views on the epidemiology of infections caused by *Pneumocystis carinii*. *Proceedings, First International Congress of Parasitology*. Oxford, Pergamon Press, 1964.

Poelma, F. G. *Pneumocystis carinii* infection in 200 animals. *Z Parasitenkd* 46:61-68, 1975.

Ruskin, J., and J. S. Remington. The compromised host and infection. I. *Pneumocystis carinii* pneumonia. *JAMA* 202:1070-1074, 1967.

Shiota, T., H. Kurimoto, and Y. Yoshida. Prevalence of *Pneumocystis carinii* in wild rodents in Japan. *Zentralbl Bakteriol Mikrobiol Hyg [A]* 261:381-389, 1986.

Tanabe, K., T. Furuta, K. Ueda, H. Tanaka, and K. Shimada. Serological observations of *Pneumocystis carinii* infection in humans. *J Clin Microbiol* 22:1058-1060, 1985.

World Health Organization. *Parasitic Zoonoses*. Report of a WHO Expert Committee with the Participation of FAO. Geneva, WHO, 1979. (Technical Report Series 637.)

SARCOCYSTOSIS

(136.5)

Synonym: Sarcosporidiosis.

Etiology: Of the many species of *Sarcocystis*, the two of interest in the study of zoonoses are *S. hominis* (*S. bovihominis*) and *S. suihominis*.

The sarcocysts are coccidia whose life cycle requires two hosts, one definitive and one intermediate. The sexual cycle (gametogony) takes place in the definitive host and the asexual cycle (schizogony) in the intermediate host.

Man is the definitive host for both the species cited above. When cysts in muscle tissue (sarcocysts) are ingested with raw or insufficiently cooked beef (*S. hominis*) or pork (*S. suihominis*), the merozoites contained in the cysts are freed in the human intestine, penetrate the intestinal epithelium, and settle in the lamina propria. The merozoites quickly differentiate into microgametes and macrogametes and the latter, once fertilized, become oocysts which sporulate inside the intestine. After sporulation (formation of sporozoites), the oocysts contain two sporocysts, each of these with four sporozoites. The mature oocysts or, more frequently, the sporocysts (after rupture of the oocysts) are eliminated with the feces sporadically for several months. When a bovine ingests sporocysts of *S. hominis* or a swine ingests those of *S. suihominis* with its pasture, the combined action of bile and trypsin breaks the cyst wall and the sporozoites are freed. They are then transported from the intestinal wall, perhaps by the blood, to other organs. Schizogony occurs in the vascular endothelium; two generations of schizonts have been observed with up to 250 merozoites per schizont. The merozoites are transported in the bloodstream to muscle tissue, where they continue to multiply asexually and finally give rise to cysts containing thousands of merozoites. The life cycle is repeated when man ingests meat containing cysts filled with mature merozoites (Marcus, 1978; Tadros and Laarman, 1982).

Geographic Distribution: Worldwide.

Occurrence in Man: The intestinal infection in humans is found in most parts of the world, with an incidence between 6 and 10% (World Health Organization, 1981).

Muscular sarcocystosis also occurs in man but is rare. About 40 cases have been identified in different parts of the world. It has not been possible to determine the species of *Sarcocystis* that cause this infection (Beaver *et al.*, 1979).

Occurrence in Animals: The prevalence of infection by *Sarcocystis* spp. in bovines and swine is very high, sometimes reaching more than 90%. Information on muscular sarcocystosis in these animals usually refers to all *Sarcocystis* infections without differentiating between infecting species. In this regard, it should be noted that bovines, besides being intermediate hosts for *S. hominis*, are also hosts for *S. bovicanis* (*S. cruzi*) and *S. bovifelis* (*S. hirsuta*), whose definitive hosts are dogs and cats, respectively. In the same manner, swine, besides being intermediate hosts for *S. suihominis*, are also hosts for *S. suicanis* (*S. miescheriana*) and *S. porcifelis*. It is estimated that nearly half of the muscular cysts in bovines and swine are caused by *S. hominis* or *S. suihominis* (World Health Organization, 1981).

The Disease in Man: Intestinal sarcocystosis is usually asymptomatic. Experimentally infected volunteers experienced nausea, abdominal pain, and diarrhea 3 to 6 hours after eating beef (raw or undercooked) containing *S. hominis*. Abdominal pain and diarrhea recurred 14 to 18 days after the experimental ingestion, coinciding with the maximum elimination of sporocysts in the feces. Clinical symptoms are more pronounced when pork containing cysts of *S. suihominis* is ingested. Symptomatic infection is generally observed when the meat consumed contains a large number of merozoites. In Thailand, several cases of sarcocystosis included acute intestinal obstruction, which prompted resection of the affected segment of the small intestine. Histopathologic study of the resected segments revealed an eosinophilic or necrotizing enteritis. It is possible that a bacterial superinfection may also have been involved in the necrotizing enteritis (Bunyaratvej *et al.*, 1982).

In general, human muscular sarcocystosis is discovered fortuitously during examination of muscle tissue for other reasons. Although the infection is nearly always asymptomatic, in some cases muscular weakness, muscular pains, myositis, periarteritis, and subcutaneous tumefaction have been observed. However, in none of these cases was there conclusive proof that the muscular cysts were the definite cause of the clinical symptoms.

The Disease in Animals: *S. bovicanis* (*S. cruzi*) is pathogenic for bovines, whereas *S. hominis* and *S. bovifelis* are not.

In 29 suckling pigs given 50,000 to 500,000 sporocysts of *S. suihominis*, severe pathologic manifestations were observed 12 days after inoculation, and about half of the animals died.

Source of Infection and Mode of Transmission (Figure 63): Knowledge of the life cycle of *S. hominis* (see Etiology) indicates that the source of infection for man (definitive host) is raw or undercooked beef containing muscle cysts. Likewise, man acquires *S. suihominis* intestinal sarcocystosis from eating insufficiently cooked pork. In turn, humans contribute to perpetuating the cycle by defecating outdoors. Sporocysts in the feces are resistant to adverse environmental conditions, and intermediate hosts become infected by feeding on contaminated pasture or by coprophagy (swine). Specificity of these two species for the intermediate host is strict; thus, swine become infected only by sporocysts of *S. suihominis* and bovines by those of *S. hominis*.

The epidemiology of muscular sarcocystosis in man has not been clarified yet. It is believed that this infection could be due to accidental ingestion of sporocysts from an undetermined species of *Sarcocystis*, which has a carnivore as its definitive host and nonhuman primates on which the animal feeds as intermediate hosts (predator-prey relationship).

Figure 63. Sarcocystosis. Transmission cycle (*Sarcocystis suihominis* and *S. hominis*).

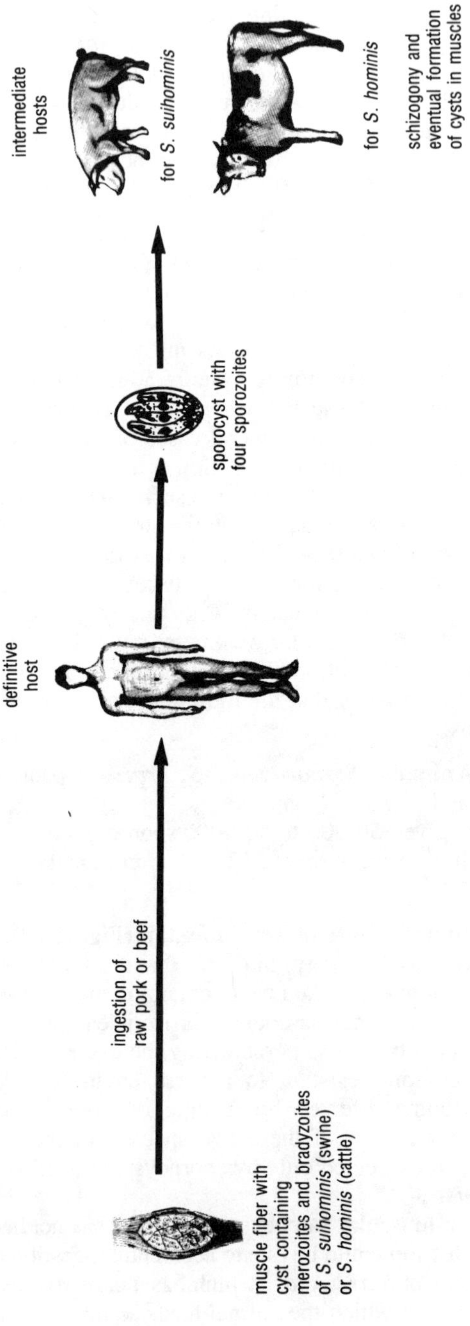

Diagnosis: Human intestinal sarcocystosis can be diagnosed by confirming the presence in the feces of mature sporocysts, which appear 9 to 10 days after the ingestion of raw meat. The most effective method is zinc sulfate flotation. *S. hominis* sporocysts measure 13 to 17 by 7.7 to 10.8 microns and those of *S. suihominis* 11.6 to 13.9 by 10 to 10.8 microns (Frenkel *et al.*, 1979).

Muscular cysts in bovines and swine are microscopic, have an elongated and cylindrical shape, and localize along the length of the muscle fiber. The cyst wall forms septa that separate the merozoites into partially curved compartments measuring 6 to 20 microns in length by 4 to 9 microns in width (Gorman, 1984). The cysts are most frequently found in the cardiac muscle, esophagus, and diaphragm of adult bovines and swine, they can be observed by trichinoscopy and, more efficiently, by tryptic digestion.

Serologic tests (indirect immunofluorescence, ELISA) are not considered useful (World Health Organization, 1981).

Control: Control is effected by interrupting the parasite's life cycle. Infection of bovines and swine can be prevented if environmental contamination by human feces is avoided. For prevention at the level of the definitive host, raw or undercooked beef or pork should not be consumed. Freezing of meat reduces the number of viable cysts.

Bibliography

Beaver, P. C., R. K. Gadgil, and P. Morera. *Sarcocystis* in man: a review and report of five cases. *Am J Trop Med Hyg* 28:819-844, 1979.

Bunyaratvej, S., P. Bunyawongwiroj, and P. Nitiyanant. Human intestinal sarcosporidiosis: report of 6 cases. *Am J Trop Med Hyg* 31:36-41, 1982.

Frenkel, J. K., A. O. Heydorn, H. Mehlhorn, and M. Rommel. Sarcocystinae: *Nomina dubia* and available names. *Z Parasitenkd* 58:115-139, 1979.

Gorman, T. Nuevos conceptos sobre sarcosporidiosis animal. *Monogr Med Vet* 6:5-23, 1984.

Marcus, M. B. *Sarcocystis* and sarcocystosis in domestic animals and man. *Adv Vet Sci Comp Med* 22:159-193, 1978.

Tadros, W., and J. J. Laarman. Current concepts on the biology, evolution and taxonomy of tissue cyst-forming eimeriid coccidia. *Adv Parasitol* 20:293-468, 1982.

World Health Organization. *Intestinal Protozoan and Helminthic Infections*. Report of a WHO Scientific Group. Geneva, WHO, 1981. (Technical Report Series 666.)

TOXOPLASMOSIS

(130)
(771.2) Congenital

Etiology: *Toxoplasma gondii*, a protozoan with a very complex developmental cycle; in light of new knowledge, it is classified as a sporozoon of the order Coccidia. *T. gondii* is found in three main forms: 1) tachyzoites or proliferative forms (also called trophozoites and endozoites), which occur in acute infection; 2) bradyzoites (merozoites, cystozoites), which encyst in the tissues (tissular cysts) and cause latent or chronic infection; and 3) oocysts, which form exclusively in the intestine of felines. The definitive hosts of *T. gondii* are domestic cats and several species of wild felids. In the cat intestine (enteroepithelial cycle), the parasite passes through five different asexual reproductive forms (A to E) and one gametogony ending in the formation of oocysts. Cats can become infected by any of the three forms listed above, in the following order of frequency: bradyzoites, oocysts, and, rarely, tachyzoites. In this host, the prepatent period (the time between the start of infection and the elimination of oocysts) differs according to the infective form, varying from 3 to 10 days with tissular cysts (bradyzoites) to 20 to 24 days with oocysts; the prepatent period with tachyzoites is 5 to 10 days or longer. Cats eliminate oocysts with their feces for only 3 to 15 days; upon acquiring immunity, they cease producing oocysts, but may start again if the acquired immunity weakens. The number of oocysts eliminated varies from a few thousand to millions. In recently eliminated fecal matter, the oocysts are not sporulated and are not infectious. Sporulation occurs after a day or more, depending on the ambient temperature, humidity, and aeration, and produces two sporocytes, each containing four sporozoites. The oocysts of *T. gondii* are morphologically similar to those of the genus *Isospora*. An important biological characteristic is that sporulated oocysts are very resistant to environmental factors and can survive in damp, shaded soil up to a year.

Cats occupy a singular place in the natural history of *T. gondii*, since in addition to being definitive hosts, with the parasite undergoing its sexual cycle in their intestine, they are also intermediate hosts for a tissular, extraenteric, and asexual cycle that occurs simultaneously with the enteroepithelial phase. Cats are thus complete hosts, both definitive and intermediate. All other animals, including man, are intermediate hosts in which the parasite has only an extraintestinal cycle.

The parasite begins the extraintestinal cycle when man or another intermediate host ingests a sporulated oocyst or animal tissue containing cysts filled with bradyzoites. Tachyzoites, or proliferative forms, develop and then multiply rapidly in the lamina propria of the intestine. The tachyzoites are carried via the lymph vessels and venous circulation to the lungs, and disseminate from there via the arterial circulation; they also spread from cell to cell by means of macrophages, lymphocytes, and granulocytes, in addition to circulating as free forms. *Toxoplasma* is an obligate intracellular parasite; the free forms disappear in a short while. Tachyzoites are found only in nucleated cells, where they proliferate rapidly until they destroy the cells. Tachyzoites can invade nucleated cells of any tissue, but they preferentially parasitize the muscular and nervous systems. They multiply in the cells by a peculiar form of schizogony (endodyogeny) and form cytoplasmic accumulations called terminal colonies or pseudocysts. When the parasitized cell bursts, the tachyzoites can infect new cells. This proliferative period corresponds to the acute phase of toxoplasmosis. As many as 100 parasites per cell can be found in this phase, and from the medical standpoint it is important to note that this is when the parasite is vulnerable to drugs.

As the host develops immunity, resistant forms of the parasite begin to appear, that is, true cysts encased in membranes. The cysts can be seen 1 or 2 weeks after infection. Each cyst, depending on its size, may contain hundreds or thousands of bradyzoites. The localization of the cysts is similar to that of the terminal colonies; they are found preferentially in the cells of the central nervous system, choroid and retina, and muscles (skeletal and myocardial). The cysts persist in the animal organism for years or for the entire lifetime of the host. The brain constitutes a special refuge for the cysts, possibly because it is protected against antibodies. The tissular cysts are resistant to environmental factors and are very important in the epidemiology of the disease. Encysted bradyzoites are not accessible to drugs now in use. The cycle is reinitiated when another intermediate or definitive host consumes meat or other tissue containing cysts.

The strains of *Toxoplasma* differ in their invasive power and multiplication rate, and thus in their virulence. Likewise, they differ in their pathogenicity for a given host; some strains are virulent for one animal species and not for another (Dubey, 1977).

Geographic Distribution: Worldwide; one of the most widespread zoonoses.

Occurrence in Man: The infection is very common, but the clinical disease is not. About one-third of the world's population is believed to possess antibodies for the parasite. The prevalence of seropositive persons or reactors to the intradermal test is generally higher in warm, humid climates than in cold or dry ones. Rates also differ with respect to altitude, higher rates being found at lower elevations.

As in other endemic diseases, the reactor rate is higher in older age groups since the chance of acquiring the infection increases with time. With a few exceptions, the seropositivity rate is low in children under 5 years of age; then it begins to increase and reaches a maximum in persons ranging between 20 and 50 years old, depending on the geographic area.

As a rule, the clinical disease occurs sporadically and has a low incidence. Its public health importance lies primarily in the severity of the congenital infection and its sequelae. In the United States, it is estimated that some 3,000 infants are born each year with congenital toxoplasmosis, and that the resultant annual cost is between US$31 and US$40 million. In Great Britain, only 37 cases occurred in 5 years (1976-1980), corresponding to an incidence of 12.2 congenital cases per million births (Bannister, 1982).

Although the disease occurs sporadically, some small epidemic outbreaks arising from a common source of infection have been described. Those reported in recent years have been associated with consumption of raw or undercooked meat, ingestion of raw goat's milk, or exposure to cat feces (Sacks, 1982, 1984; Luft and Remington, 1984; Coutinho *et al.*, 1982; Kean *et al.*, 1969). In 1979 an outbreak of acute toxoplasmosis affected 39 of 98 soldiers in a company that had been on maneuvers in the Panamanian jungle. The common source of infection was believed to be drinking-water taken from a brook that may have been contaminated by feces of wild felines (Benenson *et al.*, 1982).

Occurrence in Animals: The infection has been found in all zoogeographic areas and in some 200 species of mammals. Moreover, many species of birds also harbor the parasite, and thus almost all species of warm-blooded animals are susceptible, although to different degrees.

High reactor rates have been found among domestic animals. In certain areas, 25 to 45% of cats are seropositive. In Costa Rica, 237 cats from seven localities were examined, and the infection was confirmed in 60% by either serology or isolation of *T. gondii*. The parasite was isolated from 55 cats (23% of the total) by inoculation of feces in mice; 82% of these isolations were from cats under 6 months old. It is interesting to note that 60% of cats whose feces contained oocysts were serologically negative, indicating that they had a primary infection (Ruiz and Frenkel, 1980). Toxoplasmosis in wild felines is also of epidemiologic interest. In Córdoba, Argentina, 23 specimens of *Oncifelis geoffroyi*, *Felis colocolo*, and *F. eira* were studied serologically and parasitologically; oocysts were found in 37%, and 59% were serologic reactors (Pizzi *et al.*, 1978). Serologic studies carried out on sheep, goats, swine, equines, and cattle have confirmed that the infection is widespread among these animal species and that the reactor rate varies greatly according to geographic area, the serologic technique used, and its interpretation. In animals, as in man, the rate of seropositivity increases in older age groups.

Proof of the parasite's presence in the meat of food animals is of special interest in public health, since insufficiently cooked meat is one of the main sources of infection for man. In Europe, parasitism rates greater than 50% have been found in the meat of sheep and pigs killed in slaughterhouses. In other areas, such as Japan, the rates are much lower. As a general rule, cattle become infected less easily than other domestic mammals, and cysts occur in their muscles less frequently and persist for a shorter period of time; likewise, the serologic titers in cattle are not high and do not persist as in other species. Nonetheless, parasites have been isolated from in the retina and diaphragm of an appreciable proportion of cattle in several countries. In Argentina, the agent was present in the retina of 18.25% of 597 beef cattle and 7.7% of 65 newborn calves (Mayer and Boehringer, 1967). In Czechoslovakia, *Toxoplasma* was isolated from the diaphragm of eight of 85 bovines, and in Italy, from the retina of eight of 57 bovines. In contrast to these results from European countries, in New Zealand and the United States the presence of the parasite in the meat and viscera of cattle has not been demonstrated (Dubey and Streitel, 1976). The reasons for this difference are not yet clear.

Toxoplasmosis is also common in wild animals; humans have occasionally contracted the infection by eating insufficiently cooked meat from game animals, such as deer (Sacks *et al.*, 1983).

Most infections in animals are clinically inapparent. The clinical cases are similar to those in man; they occur sporadically, except in sheep, in which epizootic outbreaks have been observed in various parts of the world.

The Disease in Man: The infection is usually subclinical. Symptomatic toxoplasmosis can be congenital or acquired postnatally. Intrauterine infection is the most serious; its frequency varies from one area to another. In the United States, it is estimated that less than 0.1% of infected adults acquired the infection congenitally. Infection of the fetus takes place when the mother contracts a primary infection (symptomatic or asymptomatic) early in pregnancy. The severity of congenital infection varies with the duration of infection in the fetus, with the most severe lesions resulting from early infection, in the first trimester of pregnancy (World

Health Organization, 1979). The fetus is infected through the placenta as a consequence of maternal parasitemia. Prospective studies of women and experiments on rabbits show that a primary infection of the mother prior to pregnancy causes neither fetopathies nor congenital toxoplasmosis. Infection in the first trimester of pregnancy causes few acute cases of fetal infection, but the risk of severe fetopathies is great. Of children whose mothers become infected in the first trimester of pregnancy, an estimated 17% will become infected and 80% of those will suffer severe disease. Infections in the second trimester result in 25% of fetuses infected, of which 30% will have a severe disease. Infection in the third trimester of pregnancy results in a greater number of fetal infections, but their course is clinically inapparent. It is important to point out that a pregnant woman who becomes infected and transmits the infection to the fetus diaplacentally will acquire immunity, and the disease will present no risk to fetuses in subsequent pregnancies. The effects of congenital toxoplasmosis begin prenatally, with parasitemia and a generalized infection that can cause abortion or premature birth. The symptomatology of congenital toxoplasmosis varies considerably. Most congenital infections are not fatal, and clinical manifestations are observed in a maximum of 10 to 15% of the cases (World Health Organization, 1979).

Some congenitally infected children manifest only a decrease of visual acuity, while others are victims of severe disease. The illness is usually prolonged because of the immaturity of the newborn's immune system. The clinical picture can include retinochoroiditis, hydrocephaly, convulsions, and intracerebral calcification, especially in the occipital and parietal regions, as revealed by cranial radiography. Fever, eruptions, hepatomegaly, and splenomegaly may also be present. Some children are born with hydrocephaly, and some develop it later. Sequelae of prenatal infection may include convulsive attacks at the time of birth or shortly thereafter. Some sequelae, such as neuropsychic retardation, chorioretinitis, hydrocephaly, microcephaly, epilepsy, and deafness, may appear months or years later. In the classic disease picture, xanthochromia and mononuclear pleocytosis are found in the cerebrospinal fluid. Retinochoroiditis and signs of encephalitis are relatively frequent, while hydrocephaly occurs in 3 to 14% of children.

Toxoplasmosis acquired after birth is, in general, a less serious disease. Its manifestations are multiple, varying with the virulence of the strains and localization of the parasite. The most common clinical form is the lymphatic form, which may occur as an afebrile or febrile lymphadenopathy, with one or more lymph nodes affected. In general, the patient recovers spontaneously in a few weeks or months. Many cases do not require medical attention and go unnoticed. Lymphocytosis often occurs.

The serious form of acquired toxoplasmosis is not very common; it is manifested by fever, maculopapular eruption, malaise, myalgia, arthralgia, pneumonia, myocarditis, myositis, and meningoencephalitis. A patient may develop one or more of these visceral involvements and clinical manifestations.

Currently, more and more cases of toxoplasmosis are being seen in patients with immune system defects or those who are receiving immunosuppressive treatment. The disease in these patients is generally serious and often fatal. Encephalitis is very common in immunocompromised persons and is the most frequent cause of death. The disease is caused by reactivation of chronic infection, which the immunocompromised patient is not able to fight.

Ocular toxoplasmosis merits special mention. The most common manifestation of this form is retinochoroiditis (more than 80%), but other lesions and alterations may also occur, such as strabismus, nystagmus, and microphthalmia. Ocular lesions in toxoplasmosis of newborn infants are frequent and generally bilateral. When ocular manifestations occur later in life, the lesion is commonly unilateral. Chorioretinitis in adults is often a late sequela of congenital infection. The cause of recurrence of the disease is unknown.

The Disease in Animals: The disease in animals is similar to that in man. The infection is generally asymptomatic, but in some species, such as sheep, it can cause appreciable economic losses.

SHEEP: From the public health and economic standpoints, the most important species affected is sheep. The disease is economically significant in New Zealand, Australia, and Great Britain, and has also been confirmed in Denmark, Sweden, Norway, the USSR, Turkey, the United States, and perhaps in other countries with a developed sheep-raising industry. The prevalence of the infection is related to the abundance of cats (*Felis catus*) in pasture lands. A few cats are probably sufficient to contaminate a field in a short time, since one animal can eliminate millions of oocysts after ingesting just one infected mouse (Dubey, 1977). Consequently, sheep grazing in the vicinity have ample opportunity to ingest oocysts deposited with the feces of cats.

The disease is characterized by placentitis, abortions, encephalitis, and ocular lesions. Sheep with placentitis abort in the final month of pregnancy or give birth to dead or weakened lambs. Gray, necrotic foci can be found in the cotyledons. Congenitally infected lambs suffer from muscular incoordination, are physically weak, and are unable to feed themselves. As in humans, congenital toxoplasmosis in lambs occurs when the ewe is infected during pregnancy. When infection occurs between days 45 and 55 of gestation, the fetus generally dies; when infection occurs during the third month of pregnancy, the lamb is born alive but sick; and when infection occurs during the fourth month, the lamb may be born infected but asymptomatic. Disease in adult sheep is exceptional.

In New Zealand, toxoplasmosis is one of the main causes of perinatal mortality in sheep. In Tasmania, Australia, *T. gondii* is thought to have been the etiologic agent in 46% of the outbreaks of abortions and neonatal mortality in sheep between 1962 and 1968 (Munday, 1975).

SWINE: Several outbreaks of acquired toxoplasmosis have been described, causing pneumonia and encephalitis in suckling pigs and abortions in adults (Dubey, 1977). Swine toxoplasmosis seems to be economically important in Japan. Pork and mutton are often sources of infection for man.

CATTLE AND HORSES: Symptomatic toxoplasmosis is not frequent in bovines. There are descriptions of several outbreaks of the disease with an acute course, characterized by fever, dyspnea, and nervous signs.

In horses, asymptomatic infection is common, but the disease occurs only occasionally. Several cases of myelomalacia attributed to *T. gondii* have been described. Determination of the etiologic agent was based on the morphologic characteristics of the parasite, but the identification is in doubt.

CATS AND DOGS: Asymptomatic infection is quite common in cats, a species that plays an important role in the epidemiology of the disease. In Memphis, Tennessee, USA, the parasite was found in the brain of 24.3% of 140 cats examined, and in 11% in another US city (Dubey, 1973). Generalized, intestinal, encephalitic, and ocular forms of clinical toxoplasmosis have been described. Symptomatic infection occurs primarily in kittens. Diarrhea, hepatitis, myocarditis, myositis, pneumonia, and encephalitis have been observed in experimentally infected young animals.

In dogs, the rate of seropositive reactors is high. Symptomatic toxoplasmosis occurs primarily in puppies when their resistance is reduced by concurrent distemper or other illness.

RABBITS AND GUINEA PIGS: Toxoplasmosis occurs in domestic and wild rabbits worldwide. Several outbreaks of the acute disease with high mortality have been reported. The symptomatic disease occurs most frequently in young animals.

The disease has also been described in guinea pigs. High reactor rates have been found in some scientific institutes.

Recently, the importance of toxoplasmosis in laboratory animals has been recognized. *T. gondii* induces the production of interferon for about 4 days, which could invalidate the results of tests on experimental animals.

BIRDS: Clinical toxoplasmosis in birds is not common. The disease has been described in several species of domestic fowl (chickens, ducks, pigeons) and in wild birds kept in captivity. In acute cases, necrotic foci can be found in the liver, spleen, lungs, and lymph nodes. Asymptomatic infection in chickens can be very frequent, as has been demonstrated in Costa Rica. *T. gondii* was isolated from 54% of 50 chickens in which antibodies were not found. Birds may acquire the infection by pecking soil contaminated by oocysts from cat feces.

Source of Infection and Mode of Transmission (Figures 64 and 65): The definitive hosts of the parasite are domestic cats and some wild felines of the genera *Felis* and *Lynx*. Felids are fundamental in the epidemiology because their feces contain oocysts that sporulate in the external environment and are extremely resistant to physical and chemical factors. Cats become infected by eating raw meat, birds, or mice containing encysted bradyzoites. Cat feces are a source of infection for many mammals and birds. With confirmation of the sexual cycle of the parasite in the cat intestine and the formation of oocysts, the mechanism of infection of herbivores was at least partially explained; infection may occur by ingestion of forage or fodder contaminated with sporulated oocysts.

Carnivorous domestic animals, predators, and carrion-eaters contract the infection by consuming raw meat containing cysts (bradyzoites).

Man becomes infected by consuming raw or insufficiently cooked meat, primarily from sheep, swine, and, in some places, goats. The high rates of tissular cysts and seropositivity found in sheep and swine indicate that these animals constitute an important source of infection. The meat and eggs of fowl are much less important. In a children's tuberculosis sanatorium in France, seroconversion to the Sabin-Feldman dye test was found in a large number of persons who consumed rare mutton, but not in those who ate the meat cooked well done. A few years ago, a small outbreak of lymphadenitic toxoplasmosis was recorded among medical students who ate undercooked hamburgers at a university cafeteria. After an incubation period of 8 to 13 days, five students became ill with fever, cephalalgia, myalgia, lymphadenopathy, and splenomegaly, and they exhibited high and increasing titers to the Sabin-Feldman and complement fixation tests (Kean *et al.*, 1969). The beef used for the hamburgers may have been mixed with contaminated pork. Another episode occurred in the United States among four diners in a restaurant who ate a dish prepared with raw beef (Centers for Disease Control of the USA, 1975).

Figure 64. Toxoplasmosis. Transmission to domestic cats.

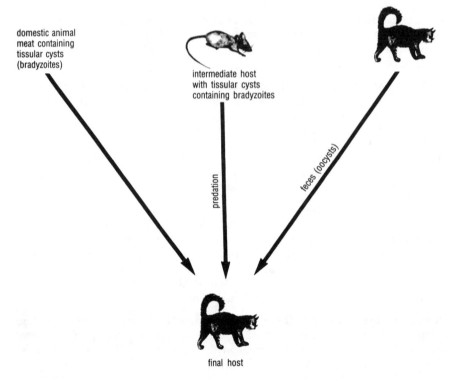

domestic animal
meat containing
tissular cysts
(bradyzoites)

intermediate host
with tissular cysts
containing bradyzoites

predation

feces (oocysts)

final host

[Transmission among wild felids occurs primarily by means of predation.]

It has been pointed out that a relationship exists between handling meat and seropositivity. In a serologic study among 144 workers in a slaughterhouse in Belo Horizonte, Brazil, the prevalence of reactors was 72%, with the highest rate (92%) among meat inspectors and the lowest (60%) among corral workers (Riemann *et al.*, 1975). A higher prevalence of reactors has also been found among housewives, who handle meat in the kitchen, than in the general population, which could be explained by contamination of the hands and subsequent infection via the mouth.

Another source of infection is food contaminated by cat fecal oocysts under deficient hygienic conditions. This may be the infection mechanism in some groups of vegetarians with high rates of serologic reactors, a situation that has been difficult to explain to date. There is also a relationship between cat ownership and the prevalence of seropositivity; the rate is at least twice as high among persons who have cats in their homes than among those who do not. However, this positive association has been refuted by some authors (Ganley and Comstock, 1980; Bannister, 1982). Recent studies have indicated that coprophilic flies and cockroaches might act as transport agents of cat fecal oocysts to foods.

Studies carried out on several atolls and islands corroborate that a relationship exists between cat fecal oocysts and the infection in humans and other animals. On one Pacific atoll where there are no cats, infection of humans and rats is almost nonexistent, while it has been confirmed on two neighboring atolls where there are cats. Similarly, the rate of toxoplasmosis infection in sheep on islands close to Australia was found to be related to the presence of cats and their population density.

Recent experiments have shed some light on the transmission mechanism of the infection in neotropical forests—where there are no domestic cats—among herbivores and among human inhabitants who do not consume raw meat. It has been found that several species of wild felids, among them ocelots (*Felis pardalis*) and jaguarundis (*Felis yagouaroundi*), can develop oocysts in their intestines. Contamination of the soil by fecal oocysts from wild felids could explain how the infection is transmitted to the Indians who live along the upper course of the Xingú River in Brazil; the reactor rate is high among these people although they do not keep cats or eat raw meat. The same mechanism could operate in the infection of insectivorous animals. The recent outbreak of toxoplasmosis among troops in the Panamanian

Figure 65. Toxoplasmosis. Transmission to domestic animals and man.

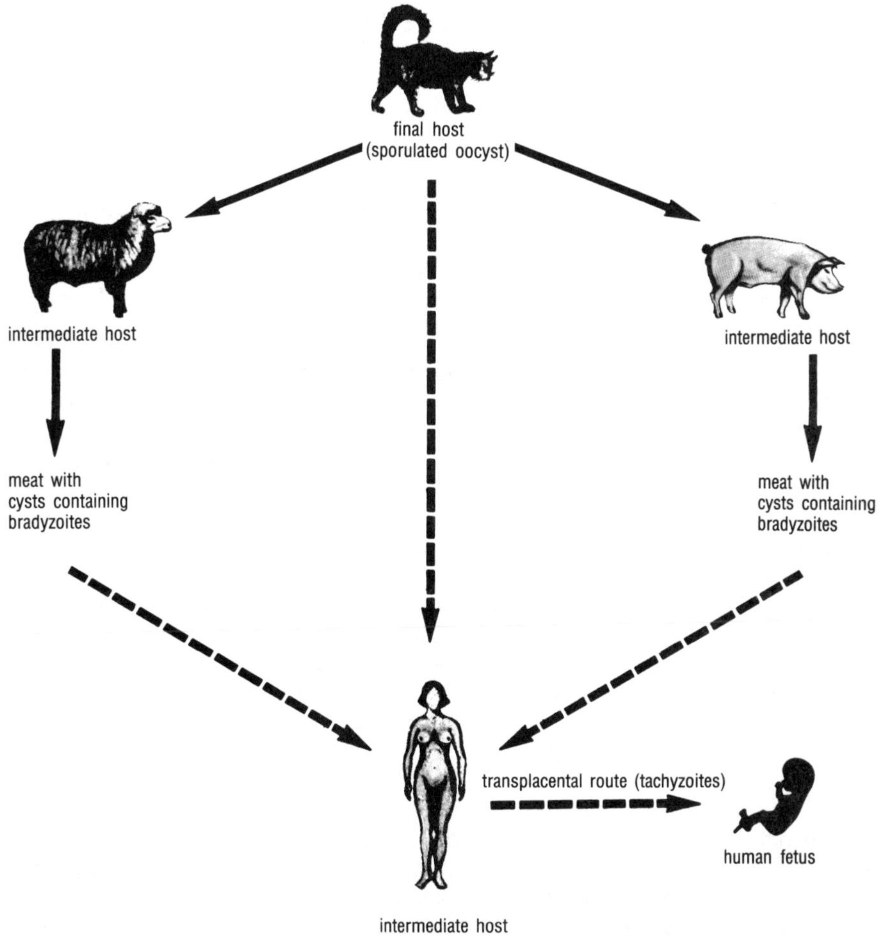

jungle has been associated with drinking the water from a brook presumably contaminated by feces of wild felids (Benenson *et al.*, 1982).

Over the years, proof has accumulated that humans can occasionally become infected by tachyzoites eliminated in milk. One such case has been described in a child in the United States (Riemann *et al.*, 1975); in Belo Horizonte, Brazil, three cases occurred in one family that drank raw goat's milk (Chiari and Neves, 1984). Since tachyzoites are destroyed by gastric juices, the parasite probably penetrated through the oral and pharyngeal mucosa.

In Costa Rica and England, oocysts of *T. gondii* have been isolated from soil samples, and a relationship has been shown to exist between the rate of positivity to the intradermal test and the degree of contact with the soil.

In laboratory personnel, infections have occurred by accidental inoculation with contaminated needles.

Transmission from mother to fetus through the placenta is of great medical interest, but is not important in maintaining the infection in nature. Congenital toxoplasmosis is seen in humans and several species of domestic animals.

The possibility of transmission of the infection by blood transfusions has been pointed out. Parasitemia occurs in the acute disease, but it has also been seen in chronic toxoplasmosis. The parasite was isolated from an asymptomatic mother 14 months after she gave birth to a congenitally infected infant, and from a patient who had recovered from toxoplasmic adenopathy 2 months earlier. Infection due to transfusion is rare but may occur. Four cases of toxoplasmosis transmitted by transfusion of leukocytes from two donors have been recorded.

Role of Animals in the Epidemiology of the Disease: Both cysts containing bradyzoites in the muscles and viscera of numerous animal species and oocysts in feline feces are important for maintaining the infection in nature. Tachyzoites play a role in intrauterine transmission in several animal species, including man. Man is an accidental host and does not play any role in maintaining the infection.

Diagnosis: Specific diagnosis can be made by demonstrating the presence of the agent and by means of serologic tests. The parasite can be isolated from tissues or body fluids by intraperitoneal inoculation in mice. Meat samples are subjected to peptic digestion prior to inoculation. In the first week after inoculation, the peritoneal exudate of the mice is examined for tachyzoites; after 6 weeks, serologic diagnosis is done on surviving animals, and mice that are positive are sacrificed to confirm the presence of cysts in the brain. Currently, detection of toxoplasmic antigens in tissues can be done by direct immunofluorescence or ELISA. The advantage of this latter method is that it allows discrimination between recent and chronic infection (Van Knapen and Paggabean, 1982).

In acute patients, the parasite can sometimes be seen by microscopic examination. For this purpose the direct immunofluorescence technique is very useful.

The following serologic tests are used: Sabin-Feldman dye test, indirect immunofluorescence, indirect hemagglutination, complement fixation, direct agglutination, and ELISA.

The Sabin-Feldman dye test is based on the failure of free tachyzoites (trophozoites) to be stained by basic methylene blue when placed in serum containing specific antibodies. It is a very sensitive test with satisfactory specificity, but it requires the use of mice and live toxoplasma parasites.

The indirect immunofluorescence test gives results comparable to Sabin-Feldman but without requiring the use of live parasites, and is currently in wide use.

The indirect hemagglutination test gives positive results at a later stage of infection; thus, its usefulness is limited in the acute phase of the infection. In addition, some difficulties have arisen in standardizing the antigen for this test.

The complement fixation test has limitations similar to the indirect hemagglutination test.

The indirect immunofluorescence and ELISA tests are of special interest since they allow detection of IgM antibodies, characteristic of the acute disease, for both congenital and acquired toxoplasmosis. Confirmation of the presence of IgM antibodies in the serum of a newborn baby is convincing proof that the fetus produced them *in utero* in response to infection, since maternal immunoglobulins of this type cannot cross the placental barrier except through a lesion in the placenta. In acute acquired toxoplasmosis, the M immunoglobulins reach maximum levels in the first month of the disease and persist an average of about 8 months. The ELISA test for specific IgM antibodies is estimated to have a sensitivity of 97% and a specificity of 100% (Wielaard *et al.*, 1983).

For all tests that do not discriminate between IgM and IgG antibodies, successive serologic examinations should be used to determine the increase in antibody titers.

The intradermal test with toxoplasmin is primarily useful in epidemiologic studies. The sensitivity reaction is delayed; the results become positive a few months after infection, and positivity may persist throughout life. The test does not indicate an active infection, but does show that the individual was exposed to the parasite and became infected.

Flotation procedures can be used to test for parasite oocysts in the feces of felines.

The ELISA test has been adapted for use in slaughterhouses for the purpose of detecting toxoplasmosis in swine (Waltman *et al.*, 1984).

Control: Cat fecal oocysts apparently constitute the main source of infection for herbivores and, in large part, for swine. In turn, insufficiently cooked meat is a main source of infection for humans. Therefore, reduced contamination of pastures by means of a decrease in the number of cats kept on farms would be an important measure.

Preventive measures should be taken by everyone, but especially by pregnant women since congenital toxoplasmosis, although not common, is often a serious clinical disease. Seronegative pregnant women are most vulnerable to infection. The main sources of infection are consumption of undercooked meat and handling of raw meat and cat feces. Consequently, to prevent materno-fetal infection, pregnant women should avoid eating undercooked meat and should wash their hands after handling raw meat, cat feces, or dirt or sand where these animals might have defecated. These preventive measures are also advised for immunocompromised patients.

Cat fecal matter should be disposed of in the toilet daily, before the oocysts can sporulate. Sandboxes used by cats should be treated with boiling water. Flies and cockroaches should be controlled to prevent those animals from acting as transport hosts for the fecal oocysts of cats.

Another prevention measure consists of only feeding cats meat that has been subjected to freezing[1] or cooking. Cats that eliminate oocysts in their feces should be removed from the household of a seronegative pregnant woman or an immu-

---

[1] Most tissular cysts die when meat is kept at $-15°C$ for more than 3 days or at $-20°C$ for more than 2 days.

nocompromised patient. In addition, cats belonging to these persons should be prevented from leaving the house to hunt rodents or birds. Experiments have demonstrated that the addition of monensin (a carboxylic ionophore produced by *Streptomyces cinnamonensis*) to dry cat food can suppress the excretion of oocysts in the feces (Frenkel and Smith, 1982).

Women who acquire a primary infection during pregnancy should be treated with a combination of sulfonamides and pyrimethamine. Toward that purpose, serologic testing is advisable for pregnant women at the beginning of gestation. Because pyrimethamine can be teratogenic, treatment in the first trimester of pregnancy should consist of sulfonamides only (Krick and Remington, 1978).

Bibliography

Bannister, B. Toxoplasmosis 1976-1980: review of laboratory reports to the Communicable Disease Surveillance Centre. *J Infect* 5:301-306, 1982.

Benenson, M. W., E. T. Takafuji, S. M. Lemon, R. L. Greenup, and A. J. Sulzer. Oocyst-transmitted toxoplasmosis associated with ingestion of contaminated water. *N Engl J Med* 307:666-669, 1982.

Beverley, J. K. A. Toxoplasmosis in animals. *Vet Rec* 99:123-127, 1976.

Bruner, D. W., and J. H. Gillespie. *Hagan's Infectious Diseases of Domestic Animals*, 6th ed. Ithaca and London, Cornell University Press, 1973.

Centers for Disease Control of the USA. Toxoplasmosis—Pennsylvania. *Morb Mortal Wkly Rep* 24:285-286, 1975.

Cordero del Campillo, M. Sobre la epidemiología de la toxoplasmosis. *Rev Vet Venez* 39:67-125, 1975.

Coutinho, S. G., M. A. Leite, M. R. Amendoeira, and M. C. Marzochi. Concomitant cases of acquired toxoplasmosis in children of a single family: evidence of reinfection. *J Infect Dis* 146:30-33, 1982.

Chiari, C. A., and D. P. Neves. Toxoplasmose adquirida através da ingestão de leite de cabra. *Mem Inst Oswaldo Cruz* 79:337-340, 1984.

Dubey, J. P. Feline toxoplasmosis and coccidiosis: a survey of domiciled and stray cats. *J Am Vet Med Assoc* 162:873-877, 1973.

Dubey, J. P. Toxoplasmosis. *J Am Vet Med Assoc* 189:166-170, 1986.

Dubey, J. P., and J. K. Frenkel. Immunity to feline toxoplasmosis: modifications by administration of corticosteroids. *Vet Pathol* 11:350-379, 1974.

Dubey, J. P., K. D. Murrell, R. D. Hanbury, W. R. Anderson, P. B. Doby, and H. O. Miller. Epidemiologic findings on a swine farm with enzootic toxoplasmosis. *J Am Vet Med Assoc* 189:55-56, 1986.

Dubey, J. P., and R. H. Streitel. Prevalence of *Toxoplasma* infection in cattle slaughtered at an Ohio abattoir. *J Am Vet Med Assoc* 169:1197-1199, 1976.

Dubey, J. P. *Toxoplasma, Hammondia, Besnoitia, Sarcocystis* and other tissue cyst-forming coccidia of man and animals. *In*: Kreier, J. P. (Ed.), *Parasitic Protozoa*, vol. 3. New York, Academic Press, 1977.

Frenkel, J. K. Toxoplasmosis. *In*: Marcial-Rojas, R. A. (Ed.), *Pathology of Protozoal and Helminthic Diseases*. Baltimore, Maryland, Williams and Wilkins, 1971.

Frenkel, J. K. Breaking the transmission chain of *Toxoplasma*: a program for the prevention of human toxoplasmosis. *Bull NY Acad Med* 50:228-235, 1974.

Frenkel, J. K., and D. D. Smith. Inhibitory effects of monesin on shedding of *Toxoplasma* oocysts by cats. *J Parasitol* 68:851-855, 1982.

Ganley, J. P., and G. W. Comstock. Association of cats and toxoplasmosis. *Am J Epidemiol* 111:238-246, 1980.

Hirt, J., E. J. Albesi, I. Di Bártolo, *et al. Toxoplasmosis.* Buenos Aires, El Ateneo, 1974.

Jacobs, L. New knowledge of *Toxoplasma* and toxoplasmosis. *Adv Parasitol* 11:631-669, 1973.

Jensen, R. *Diseases of Sheep.* Philadelphia, Lea and Febiger, 1974.

Jewell, M. L., J. K. Frenkel, K. M. Johnson, *et al.* Development of *Toxoplasma* oocyst in neotropical Felidae. *Am J Trop Med Hyg* 21:512-517, 1972.

Jones, S. R. Toxoplasmosis: a review. *J Am Vet Med Assoc* 163:1038-1042, 1973.

Kean, B. H., A. C. Kimball, and W. N. Christenson. An epidemic of acute toxoplasmosis. *JAMA* 208:1002-1004, 1969.

Krick, J. A., and J. S. Remington. Toxoplasmosis in the adult—an overview. *N Engl J Med* 298:550-553, 1978.

Levine, N. D. *Protozoan Parasites*, 2nd ed. Minneapolis, Burgess, 1973.

Luft, B. J., and J. S. Remington. Acute *Toxoplasma* infection among family members of patients with acute lymphadenopathic toxoplasmosis. *Arch Intern Med* 144:53-56, 1984.

Mayer, H. F., and I. K. de Boehringer. Nuevas comprobaciones sobre toxoplasmosis animal en la Argentina. *Rev Med Vet (B Aires)* 48:341-349, 1967.

McCabe, R. E., and J. S. Remington. Toxoplasmosis. *In*: Warren K. S., and A. A. F. Mahmoud (Eds.), *Tropical and Geographical Medicine.* New York, McGraw-Hill Book Company, 1984.

McCulloch, W. F., and J. S. Remington. Toxoplasmosis. *In*: Hubbert, W. T., W. F. McCulloch, and P. R. Schnurrenberger (Eds.), *Diseases Transmitted from Animals to Man*, 6th ed. Springfield, Illinois, Thomas, 1975.

Munday, B. L. Prevalence of toxoplasmosis in Tasmanian meat animals. *Aust Vet J* 51:315-316, 1975.

Nurse, G. H., and C. Lenghaus. An outbreak of *Toxoplasma gondii* abortion, mummification, and perinatal death in goats. *Aust Vet J* 63:27-29, 1986.

Pappas, M. G., M. N. Lunde, R. Hajkowski, and J. McMahon. Determination of IgM and IgG antibodies to *Toxoplasma* using the IFA test, ELISA and dot-ELISA procedures. *Vet Parasitol* 20:31-42, 1986.

Pizzi, H. L., C. M. Rico, and O. A. M. Pessat. Hallazgo del ciclo ontogénico selvático del *Toxoplasma gondii* en félidos salvajes (*Oncifelis geoffroyi, Felis colocolo y Felis eira*) de la Provincia de Córdoba. *Rev Milit Vet (B Aires)* 25:293-300, 1978.

Prickett, M. D., D. W. Dreesen, W. D. Waltman, J. L. Blue, and J. Brown. Correlation of tissue infection and serologic findings in pigs fed *Toxoplasma gondii* oocysts. *Am J Vet Res* 46:1130-1132, 1985.

Remington, J. S. Toxoplasmosis: recent developments. *Annu Rev Med* 21:201-218, 1970.

Riemann, H. P., P. C. Brant, D. E. Behymer, and C. E. Franti. *Toxoplasma gondii* and *Coxiella brunetti* antibodies among Brazilian slaughterhouse employees. *Am J Epidemiol* 102:386-393, 1975.

Riemann, H. P., A. T. Smith, C. Stormont, R. Ruppaner, D. E. Behymer, Y. Suzuki, C. E. Franti, and B. B. Verma. Equine toxoplasmosis: a survey for antibodies to *Toxoplasma gondii* in horses. *Am J Vet Res* 36:1797-1800, 1975.

Riemann, H. P., M. E. Meyer, J. H. Theis, G. Kelso, and B. S. Behymer. Toxoplasmosis in an infant fed unpasteurized goat milk. *J Pediatr* 84:573-576, 1975. Cited in Chiari and Neves, 1984.

Robertson, P. W., and V. Kertesz. Modified fluorescent antibody technique to detect immunoglobulin M antibodies to *Toxoplasma gondii* in congenital infection. *J Clin Microbiol* 2:461-462, 1975.

Ruiz, A., and J. K. Frenkel. Intermediate and transport hosts of *Toxoplasma gondii* in Costa Rica. *Am J Trop Med Hyg* 29:1161-1166, 1980.

Ruiz, A., and J. K. Frenkel. *Toxoplasma gondii* in Costa Rican cats. *Am J Trop Med Hyg* 29:1150-1160, 1980.

Sacks, J. J., R. R. Roberto, and N. F. Brooks. Toxoplasmosis infection associated with raw goat's milk. *JAMA* 248:1728-1732, 1982.

Sacks, J. J., D. G. Delgado, H. O. Lobel, and R. L. Parker. Toxoplasmosis infection associated with eating undercooked venison. *Am J Epidemiol* 118:832-838, 1983.

Sacks, J. J. Concurrent infection in families and patients with acute toxoplasmosis. *Arch Intern Med* 144:35-36, 1984.

Shadduck, J. A., and S. P. Pakes. Encephalitozoonosis (nosematosis) and toxoplasmosis. *Am J Pathol* 64:657-674, 1971.

Siim, J. C., U. Biering-Sorensen, and T. Moller. Toxoplasmosis in domestic animals. *Adv Vet Sci* 8:335-429, 1963.

Van Knapen, F., and S. O. Panggabean. Detection of *Toxoplasma* antigen in tissues by means of enzyme-linked immunosorbent assay (ELISA). *Am J Clin Pathol* 77:755-757, 1982.

Waltman, W. D., D. W. Dreesen, M. D. Prickett, J. L. Blue, and D. G. Oliver. Enzyme-linked immunosorbent assay for the detection of toxoplasmosis in swine: interpreting assay results and comparing with other serologic tests. *Am J Vet Res* 45:1719-1725, 1984.

Wielaard, F., H. van Gruijthuijsen, W. Duermeyer, A. W. L. Joss, L. Skinner, H. Williams, and E. H. van Elven. Diagnosis of acute toxoplasmosis by an enzyme immunoassay for specific immunoglobulin M antibodies. *J Clin Microbiol* 17:981-987, 1983.

World Health Organization. *Toxoplasmosis.* Report of a WHO Meeting of Investigators. Geneva, WHO, 1969. (Technical Report Series 431.)

World Health Organization. *Parasitic Zoonoses.* Report of a WHO Expert Committee with the Participation of FAO. Geneva, WHO, 1979. (Technical Report Series 637.)

VISCERAL LEISHMANIASIS

(085.0)

Synonyms: Kala-azar, Dumdum fever, infantile splenic fever, febrile tropical splenomegaly.

Etiology: *Leishmania donovani*, a viscerotropic flagellate protozoan, morphologically indistinguishable from the parasites that cause cutaneous leishmaniasis. In man and reservoir animals the parasite occurs in the aflagellate amastigote (leishmanial) form, while in the phlebotomine fly vector it has the flagellate promastigote (leptomonad) form. On the basis of biochemical differences (particularly the enzymatic profile) and serologic differences (Adler test,[1] excretion factor[2])

---

[1] The Adler or Noguchi-Adler test is based on the phenomenon that leishmanias cultured in homologous sera clump together and become immobilized, while this does not occur in heterologous sera. Using different serum dilutions it is possible to establish the lowest dilution at which the promastigotes do not become immobilized. By this test *L. d. donovani* can be distinguished from *L. d. infantum* and from the cutaneous leishmaniasis species of the Old and New World. However, *L. d. infantum* cannot be differentiated from *L. d. chagas* by this method, nor by their enzymatic profiles, but significant differences have been found by radiorespirometry and DNA analysis (Lainson, 1983).

[2] Promastigotes in a logarithmic growth phase in culture media excrete a substance called excretion factor (EF). With the use of homologous and heterologous antipromastigote sera, this factor or exoantigen can be characterized by immunodiffusion in gel. According to Lainson (1982), it is probable that this procedure measures the same antigens as the Adler test.

the species *Leishmania donovani* is classified into the following subspecies: *L. donovani donovani*, *L. d. infantum*, and *L. d. chagasi*. Some researchers consider these to be separate species making up a species complex. Classification into subspecies or species has the advantage of emphasizing the epidemiologic, ecologic, and clinical differences between disease forms in diverse zones.

It should also be pointed out that the division between cutaneous and visceral leishmaniasis is, for the most part, conventional and artificial, as indicated elsewhere (see "Cutaneous Leishmaniasis"). *L. donovani* very often causes cutaneous lesions in man, and the subspecies of *L. braziliensis* along with *L. major* are viscerotropic for lower animals. Recently, parasites identified as *L. tropica* have been isolated from patients with visceral leishmaniasis in India and Israel (Lainson, 1982). Notwithstanding, *L. donovani* stands out as the main agent of visceral leishmaniasis in man, which justifies its separate study.

Geographic Distribution and Occurrence in Man (Map 12): Endemic areas and foci of kala-azar exist in several places in the world (see map). *L. d. donovani* occurs in India, Bangladesh, and perhaps in Nepal and China. *L. d. infantum* is distributed on the European and African Mediterranean coast, in the Central Asian Soviet Republics, Iraq, Iran, Afghanistan, Egypt, Israel, Yemen, Saudi Arabia, northern and northwestern China, and eastern, western, and central Africa. *L. d. chagasi* occurs in the Americas. The main endemic zone of visceral leishmaniasis in the Americas is the northeastern and part of the eastern region of Brazil, although small foci have also been confirmed in the northern and west-central regions. Sporadic cases of the disease have been diagnosed in Mexico, Guatemala, El Salvador, Honduras, Martinique, Guadeloupe, Venezuela, Colombia, Ecuador, Suriname, Bolivia, Paraguay, and northern Argentina.

Although in most places the disease occurs sporadically, visceral leishmaniasis has on occasion reached epidemic proportions. In 1978, in northern Bihar, India, about 50,000 cases occurred; the infection extended to western Bengal, causing 7,500 cases in the first 8 months of 1982. The number of cases is declining in China. Prior to 1960, 600,000 cases were recorded in the northeastern and northwestern areas of the country; only 48 were notified in 1979, the majority in the northeast. A total of 1,969 clinical cases was registered in 1974 in Iraq, and the number fell to about 500 annual cases in subsequent years. In Sudan, 3,000 to 5,000 cases per year are recorded, but the estimated prevalence is much higher. In Brazil, the endemicity is highest in the states of Ceará and Bahia; 3,078 cases were notified in that country from 1971 to 1980, 44.6% of them occurring in Ceará State (World Health Organization, 1984).

In the Americas, the western Mediterranean region, and northern Africa, infants and young children are the most affected (infantile kala-azar), while in other areas morbidity is equally common in children over 5 years old and in young adults (Marinkele, 1981).

Transmission to man is seasonal and is related to the life cycle and fluctuations in density of the phlebotomine vectors and perhaps to the population dynamics of the animal reservoirs (World Health Organization, 1984).

Occurrence in Animals: Studies of the prevalence in animals have centered on dogs, which constitute the main source of infection for man in many zones.

In Ceará State, Brazil, a study carried out between 1953 and 1962 found the infection in 1.9% of 35,272 dogs with clinical symptomatology and in 1.5% of

Map 12. World distribution of visceral leishmaniasis.

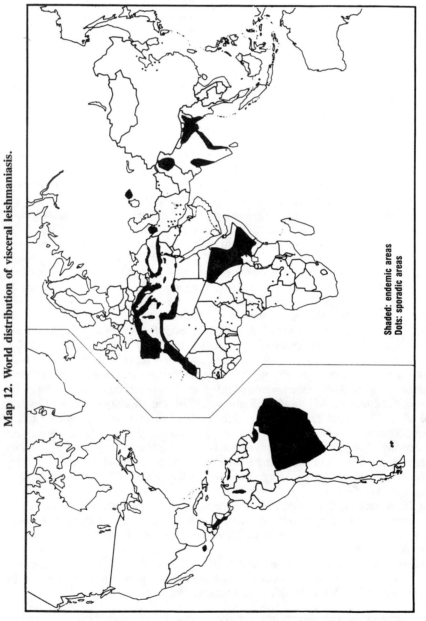

Shaded: endemic areas
Dots: sporadic areas

Source: The Leishmaniases. WHO, 1984. (Tech. Rep. Ser. 701.)

285,592 apparently healthy dogs (Deane and Deane, 1962). In the state of Bahia, 1.7% of 10,132 dogs examined from 1962 to 1969 were positive, and the prevalence rates reached 25% in the known foci of human kala-azar (Sherlock and Almeida, 1970). The highest rates were obtained with the complement fixation test. In Brazil, infection rates of 4 to 12% have been found in the fox *Lycalopex vetulus*.

In northern Iran, the viscera and skin of 161 jackals and 100 dogs were examined parasitologically; four and three of these animals, respectively, were found to be infected. Six of 48 jackals and six of 34 dogs gave positive results to a serologic test (immunofluorescence) (Hamidi *et al.*, 1982). In a leishmaniasis focus in Tuscany, Italy, 2.9% of 103 dogs were serologically positive and 1% of them had symptoms; in another focus, 23.9% of about 250 dogs examined were serologically positive, 10% had lesions, and 7% were positive to microscopic examination (Gradoni *et al.*, 1980).

The Disease in Man: The incubation period is generally from 2 to 6 months, but can vary from 10 days to several years. The promastigotes inoculated by a phlebotomine into human skin are engulfed by macrophages, where they become amastigotes. In some patients, especially in Africa, a primary leishmanioma forms several months before the other symptoms appear. Leishmanias multiply slowly by binary fission in the cytoplasm of the macrophages near the inoculation site. Some parasitized macrophages enter the bloodstream and reach the viscera, where the leishmanias multiply rapidly in the fixed macrophages, which they ultimately destroy.

Leishmanias invade the reticuloendothelial system, causing reticuloendotheliosis. Onset of the disease is insidious among people of endemic areas, and its course is chronic. In persons from areas free of the disease, the onset can be sudden. Fever is prolonged and irregular, frequently with two exacerbations per day. Some patients have coughing, diarrhea, and symptoms of intercurrent infections. The disease is characterized by splenomegaly and, later, by hepatomegaly; lymphadenopathy is common in some regions (Africa, the Mediterranean), and other symptoms include anemia with leukopenia, edema, increase of skin pigmentation, and emaciation. The abdomen sometimes becomes distended from the splenomegaly and hepatomegaly. Petechiae and hemorrhages of the mucous membranes are frequent. Secondary infections are common. Mortality is very high among untreated patients. Infection by *L. donovani* is not always accompanied by serious symptoms; it may occur asymptomatically or produce only mild symptoms, depending on the host's degree of resistance.

In the infection foci studied in Ceará, Brazil, 67% of the patients were 0 to 4 years old. A similar pattern of prevalence by age group is found for infections caused by *L. d. infantum* in the Mediterranean basin; by contrast, in India the infection is more prevalent in young adults.

In the Americas, cutaneous kala-azar lesions are very rarely seen, but the parasites have been found in macroscopically normal skin. In India, the skin often becomes gray, especially on feet, hands, and abdomen (kala-azar black fever). Nodular lesions can be observed in patients in Africa (Kenya, Sudan), the Mediterranean, and China. Another type of lesion appears a year or more after treatment with antimony and is called post–kala-azar dermal leishmanoid. These sequelae are rare in the endemic region of northeastern Brazil.

The Disease in Animals: Kala-azar of domestic dogs is focal in character, as it is in humans; the disease generally occurs in both species simultaneously, although there may be areas of canine infection where no human infection exists. The incubation period is 3 to 7 months. The severity of the disease varies. Cutaneous lesions are the most frequent and apparent symptom and consist of depilated areas with purpuric desquamation, mainly on joints and in skin folds. Sometimes, small ulcerations (which may or may not be covered with scabs) are seen on the nose, earflap, and back. Ulcerations can also be found on the nasal and oral mucosas. Conjunctivitis and keratitis are common. Exaggerated growth of the nails is often seen. The disease becomes chronic, and many animals manifest anorexia, irregular fever, apathy, polypnea, paleness of the mucous membranes, and emaciation. Some cases include edemas in different parts of the body and hemorrhages through the nasal orifices. The lesions seen in postmortem examination consist of disappearance of fatty tissue, splenomegaly, hepatomegaly, gelatinous and deep-red bone marrow, lymphadenopathy, and often ulcerations of the intestine.

The intensity of the parasitism apparently is not in direct proportion to the severity of the clinical picture, since highly parasitized dogs can display a mild symptomatology. In Brazil, more than 30% of infected dogs did not have any apparent clinical symptomatology (Hipólito *et al.*, 1965).

Infection in the fox *Lycalopex vetulus* in northeastern Brazil is similar to that in dogs. Some animals have clinically inapparent infections, while others manifest different forms of the disease, including very serious and fatal cases.

Source of Infection and Mode of Transmission (Figures 66 and 67): The epidemiology has unique features in each region and varies from one geographic area to another.

In the Americas, the reservoirs of kala-azar are dogs and wild canid species. Infection is spread among canids and from these animals to man by the bite of the phlebotomine fly *Lutzomyia longipalpis*. The most important endemic area in the Americas is in northeastern Brazil; principal foci are distributed in a semiarid region subject to prolonged drought. The disease is basically rural, with a few cases occurring in towns or on the outskirts of cities. The distribution of kala-azar is focal, and the greatest concentration of cases is around hills or in mountain valleys, where the disease is endemic with periodic epidemic outbreaks. In the flatlands, by contrast, cases are sporadic and occur primarily in humid areas, close to rivers. In Brazil, the geographic distribution of the disease coincides with that of the vector. The main, and possibly only, vector in the endemic area of northeastern Brazil is the phlebotomine *L. longipalpis*, an abundant insect that reaches its highest density some 2 months after the heaviest rains and is also resistant to drought. The vector feeds on dogs, wild animals, and, less frequently, man; it can be found both in the countryside and in dwellings.

Figure 66. Visceral leishmaniasis (*Leishmania donovani*). Basic transmission cycle in the Americas.

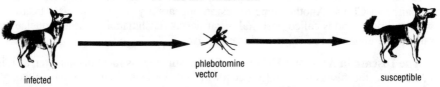

infected   phlebotomine
                            vector   susceptible

Figure 67. Visceral leishmaniasis. Basic cycle in India.

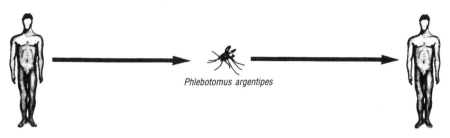

Phlebotomus argentipes

Dogs are an especially suitable reservoir because they offer the vector direct access to the parasitized macrophages of their cutaneous lesions. During the studies done in Ceará, parasites were found in the skin of 77.6% of 49 dogs with visceral leishmaniasis as opposed to only 16.3% of 43 human patients examined. In addition, the number of parasites encountered in human skin is less than in dog skin. Amastigotes are scarce in human skin and only rarely could serve as a source of infection for the vector.

A wild host of visceral leishmaniasis, the fox *Lycalopex vetulus*, is known in northeastern Brazil; it comes near houses to hunt chickens. Amastigotes are abundant in its skin and it is an important source of infection for the vectors (Garnham, 1971). In the tropical rain forest region of the lower Amazon, such as Pará State, where the number of cases in domestic dogs and humans is low, the reservoir of the parasite is suspected to be a wild canid. In this region, *L. donovani* has been isolated from the fox *Cerdocyon thous* (Lainson *et al.*, 1969; Silveira *et al.*, 1982).

In the Mediterranean basin, dogs are also the main reservoir, and the vectors are various species of the genus *Phlebotomus*. In the Middle East, jackals and dogs are the hosts and main sources of infection for phlebotomines. In India, by contrast, man himself is the main reservoir, and infected dogs or other animals have not been found (Bhattachayra and Gnosh, 1983). The disease was very common in the large cities of India, but its prevalence has been significantly reduced as a result of the antimalaria campaign. When the insect control campaign was interrupted, a resurgence of kala-azar to epidemic proportions occurred in Bihar (see Geographic Distribution and Occurrence in Man). In the absence of an animal reservoir, subclinical human infections may play an important role in maintaining the infection (Manson-Bahr and Apted, 1982). Interhuman transmission occurs by means of the vector *Phlebotomus argentipes*. In India, the number of parasites circulating in human blood was found to be sufficient to infect the vector. *P. argentipes* is eminently anthropophilic, feeding only on man. Transmission can take place inside houses, which constitute microfoci of infection (Manson-Bahr and Apted, 1982). In Sudan, infected wild rodents (*Arvicanthis niloticus*, *Acomys albigena*, and the domestic rat *Rattus rattus*) and carnivores (*Felis philippsi* and *Genetta sangalensis*) were found. It is believed that rodents are the primary hosts of the agent and carnivores are secondary reservoirs. The vector is *P. orientalis*. Humans develop parasitemia and, in epidemic situations, can be a source of infection for the vectors.

Numerous researchers believe that visceral leishmaniasis was originally an infection that circulated enzootically among wild animals (canids and perhaps rodents);

later, with the inclusion of domestic dogs in its cycle, the disease became synanthropic and eventually, like kala-azar in India, changed into an infection transmitted between humans (anthroponosis) without the intervention of an animal reservoir. An argument in favor of this hypothesis is dogs' low degree of adaptation to the parasite and their susceptibility to clinical disease, indicating that this species is a rather new host in the natural history of the disease. It has been suggested that the fox *Cerdocyon thous*, which becomes infected without becoming ill, could have been the original reservoir in the Americas. However, more research, especially concerning its rate of infection, is needed to confirm this animal as the original reservoir (Lainson, 1983).

Diagnosis: In the case of American visceral leishmaniasis, the parasite can rarely be observed in films of peripheral blood. By contrast, microscopic observations can give positive results for kala-azar in India. The most sensitive procedure (98% positive) is splenic aspiration, but this technique involves high risk, especially if the person conducting the aspiration does not have experience in the procedure. The presence of parasites can be confirmed in aspirated sternal or iliac bone marrow in 54 to 86% of cases and in material aspirated from lymph nodes in 64% (World Health Organization, 1984). At the start of the disease, when parasites are scarce, culture in NNN or another appropriate medium and intraperitoneal inoculation of hamsters can be used. In dogs and other canids, the parasites can be observed or can be isolated by culture or by hamster inoculation, using material from cutaneous lesions or the viscera of dead or destroyed animals.

In Brazil and other areas, the complement fixation test with antigen obtained from acid-resistant bacilli was used previously. However, this test was limited in sensitivity and impractical for the examination of a large number of samples; additional difficulties arose because a large proportion of anticomplementary sera was found. Currently, the indirect immunofluorescence test with *L. donovani* antigen is the most used. A drawback of this and other tests is cross-reactions with Chagas' disease, which can be a problem in areas where both diseases are endemic. However, it has been suggested (Badaró *et al.*, 1983) that this drawback can be surmounted by using promastigotes from *L. donovani chagasi* as antigen and establishing an adequate titer as significant. A simplified ELISA test has been evaluated in Kenya, with results of 98.4% sensitivity and 100% specificity. According to the authors (Ho *et al.*, 1983), this test could be used in the field to replace splenic aspiration.

The Montenegro intradermal test (leishmanine test) is not useful for epidemiologic studies of visceral leishmaniasis. This is a test of delayed sensitivity in cutaneous leishmaniasis and is group-specific but not species-specific; that is, it gives cross-reactions with other leishmaniases and trypanosomiases. The test continues to give positive results for 2 to 3 months after spontaneous or therapeutic cure. The leishmanine test gives false negative results in individuals who are anergic as a result of advanced age, generalized tuberculosis, leprosy, or terminal neoplasm.

Control: Control measures are directed against the vectors and reservoirs. Application of residual insecticides, such as DDT, in and around dwellings has given excellent results. The incidence of kala-azar in India has been significantly reduced by the antimalaria campaign, and the infection has almost disappeared from the districts that have been sprayed. Spraying should focus not only on dwellings but also on animal dens, rock walls, refuse dumps, and any other places where the vector breeds.

In regions where the infection has a zoonotic origin, important control measures are systematic elimination of infected dogs and, where possible, control of the fox population. In Crete, the incidence of the disease in humans was reduced significantly by the destruction of dogs. In northeastern Brazil, this measure has been applied systematically and tens of thousands of such dogs have been destroyed in Ceará State.

Human cases should be detected and treated with pentavalent antimony compounds; cases resistant to these drugs should be treated with diamidine compounds. Dogs are apparently resistant to treatment with drugs.

Bibliography

Araujo, F. G., and W. Mayrink. Fluorescent antibody test in visceral leishmaniasis. II. Studies on the specificity of the test. *Rev Inst Med Trop S Paulo* 10:41-45, 1968.

Badaró, R., S. G. Reed, and E. M. Carvalho. Immunofluorescent antibody test in American visceral leishmaniasis: sensitivity and specificity of different morphological forms of two *Leishmania* species. *Am J Trop Med Hyg* 32:480-484, 1983.

Bhattachayra, A., and T. N. Gnosh. A search for leishmania in vertebrates from kala-azar–affected areas of Bihar, India. *Trans R Soc Trop Med Hyg* 77:874-875, 1983.

Cahill, K. M. Field techniques in the diagnosis of kala-azar. *Trans R Soc Trop Med Hyg* 64:107-110, 1970.

Deane, L. M., and M. P. Deane. Visceral leishmaniasis in Brazil: geographical distribution and transmission. *Rev Inst Med Trop S Paulo* 4:198-212, 1962.

Delgado, O., and J. Romero. The use of counterimmunoelectrophoresis in leishmaniasis. *In*: *Third International Congress of Parasitology*. Munich, Facta, 1974.

Faust, E. C., P. F. Russell, and R. C. Jung. *Craig and Faust's Clinical Parasitology*, 8th ed. Philadelphia, Lea and Febiger, 1970.

Garnham, P. C. C. American leishmaniasis. *Bull WHO* 44:521-527, 1971.

Gradoni, L., E. Pozio, S. Bettini, and M. Gramiccia. Leishmaniasis in Tuscany (Italy). III. The prevalence of canine leishmaniasis in two foci of Grosseto Province. *Trans R Soc Trop Med Hyg* 74:421-422, 1980.

Hamidi, A. N., A. Nadim, G. H. Edrissian, G. Tahvildar-Bidruni, and E. Javadian. Visceral leishmaniasis of jackals and dogs in northern Iran. *Trans R Soc Trop Med Hyg* 76:756-757, 1982.

Hipólito, O., M. G. Freitas, and J. B. Figuereido. *Doenças Infeto-Contagiosas dos Animais Domésticos*, 4th ed. São Paulo, Melhoramentos, 1965.

Ho, M., J. Leeuwenburg, G. Mbugua, A. Wamachi, and A. Voller. An enzyme-linked immunosorbent assay (ELISA) for field diagnosis of visceral leishmaniasis. *Am J Trop Med Hyg* 32:943-946, 1983.

Lainson, R., J. J. Shaw, and Z. C. Lins. Leishmaniasis in Brazil. IV. The fox *Cardocyon thous* (L) as a reservoir of *Leishmania donovani* in Pará State, Brazil. *Trans R Soc Trop Med Hyg* 63:741-745, 1969.

Lainson, R. Leishmaniasis. *In*: Jacobs, L., and P. Arambulo (Section Eds.), CRC *Handbook Series in Zoonoses*. Section C, vol. 1. Boca Raton, Florida, CRC Press, 1982.

Lainson, R. The American leishmaniases: some observations on their ecology and epidemiology. *Trans R Soc Trop Med Hyg* 77:569-596, 1983.

Manson-Bahr, P. E. C. Leishmaniasis. *Int Rev Trop Med* 4:123-140, 1971.

Manson-Bahr, P. E. C., and F. I. C. Apted. *Manson's Tropical Diseases*, 8th ed. London, Baillière Tindall, 1982.

Marinkele, C. J. La lutte contre les leishmanioses. *Bull WHO* 59:189-203, 1981.

Mayrink, W., C. A. Chiari, P. A. Magalhaes, and C. A. da Costa. Teste do latex no diagnostico do calazar americano. *Rev Inst Med Trop S Paulo* 14:273-276, 1972.

Navin, T. R., M. Sierra, R. Custodio, F. Steurer, C. H. Porter, and T. K. Ruebush II. Epidemiologic study of visceral leishmaniasis in Honduras, 1975-1983. *Am J Trop Med Hyg* 34:1069-1075, 1985.

Sherlock, I. A., and S. P. de Almeida. Notas sobre leishmaniose canina no Estado de Bahia. *Rev Bras Malar* 22:231-242, 1970.

Silveira, F. T., R. Lainson, J. J. Shaw, and M. M. Povoa. Leishmaniasis in Brazil: XVIII. Further evidence incriminating the fox *Cardocyon thous* (L) as a reservoir of Amazonian visceral leishmaniasis. *Trans R Soc Trop Med Hyg* 76:830-832, 1982.

Theodor, O. Leishmaniases. *In*: Van der Hoeden, J. (Ed.), *Zoonoses*. Amsterdam, Netherlands, Elsevier, 1964.

Walton, B. C., M. G. Pappas, M. Sierra, Jr., R. Hajkowski, P. Jackson, and R. Custodio. Field use of the Dot-ELISA test for visceral leishmaniasis in Honduras. *Bull Pan Am Health Organ* 20:147-156, 1986.

Winslow, D. J. Kala-azar (visceral leishmaniasis). *In*: Marcial-Rojas, R. A. (Ed.), *Pathology of Protozoal and Helminthic Diseases*. Baltimore, Maryland, Williams and Wilkins, 1971.

World Health Organization. *The Leishmaniases*. Report of a WHO Expert Committee. Geneva, WHO, 1984. (Technical Report Series 701.)

SECTION B

HELMINTHIASES

1. Trematodiases
2. Cestodiases
3. Acanthocephaliasis and
   Nematodiases

1. Trematodiases

CLONORCHIASIS

(121.1)

Etiology: *Clonorchis sinensis*, a trematode 10 to 25 mm long by 3 to 5 mm wide that lives in the bile ducts of man, dogs, cats, swine, rats, and several species of wild mammals. The parasite requires two intermediate hosts for its development cycle. The first host is a gastropod mollusk of the family Bulimidae, *Parafossarulus manchouricus* being the most important of these snail species in several countries of the Far East. The second intermediate host is one of a large number of species of freshwater fish, belonging mainly to the family Cyprinidae. Several species of freshwater shrimp can also serve as a second intermediate host.

The definitive host, man or another animal, eliminates fully embryonated eggs with the feces. If the eggs reach water (river, lake, pond, reservoir) and are ingested by a suitable host, they hatch in the snail's intestine into a ciliated larva, or miracidium, which lodges in the intestinal wall or sometimes in another organ. Within the snail, the parasite passes through several stages of development and multiplication (sporocysts, rediae) before becoming a cercaria with a propulsive tail. Once mature, the cercaria emerges from the snail into the water and quickly attaches itself to an appropriate fish (second intermediate host); it then loses its tail, penetrates the skin, and enters muscle tissue, where it encysts and develops into a metacercaria. When man or another definitive host consumes raw, parasitized fish, the metacercariae lose their cystic envelopes in the intestine, enter the ampulla of Vater, and, moving against the bile flow, proceed toward the bile ducts. Egg-laying begins in approximately 1 month, reinitiating the cycle. The trematode is very long-lived, and egg-laying can last for several decades. The entire development cycle takes about 3 months.

Geographic Distribution and Occurrence: Endemic areas of clonorchiasis are limited to countries of the Far East: China, Taiwan, Hong Kong, Japan, South Korea, and Vietnam. Cases of clonorchiasis are also found in other parts of the world, in emigrants from the above-mentioned countries and in members of the indigenous population who eat raw fish imported from endemic areas. In spite of this, the parasitosis has never become established outside the area of the China Sea. In the Americas, cases have been recorded in persons who have lived in endemic areas, as well as in Asian immigrants. The infection rate was 26% among 150 Chinese immigrants in New York City, and 15.5% among 400 persons examined in Montreal, Canada (Sun, 1980). In Panama and Chile, several cases have occurred in Asians.

An estimated 20 million persons in China are infected by clonorchiasis in spite of efforts to improve environmental sanitation. In Japan and Taiwan, the incidence of infection in the under-40 age group has been markedly reduced in recent years (Bunnag and Harinasuta, 1984).

The parasitosis is declining, both in the absolute number of persons infected and in the intensity (number of parasites) per parasitized individual. This decrease is due to control measures that have been instituted and to the impact of industrialization, which brought with it pollution of rivers with wastes harmful to the intermediate host.

In some areas, the prevalence of infection in dogs, cats, and swine reaches very high rates. In the Canton region of China, where the prevalence of human clonorchiasis is high (40%), 44% of dogs and 72% of cats were found to be infected. The prevalence of infection in animals can greatly exceed that in man, as was confirmed in Shanghai, where 37% of dogs and 58% of cats were infected, while the rate of human infection was less than 3% (Rim, 1982). The parasite is abundant in nature in both these areas of China, and the difference in the rate of human infection is linked to the habit of eating raw fish. In some areas of Japan, 20.6% of dogs and 45.5% of cats have been found to be infected. In an area of high human endemicity in South Korea, 18.5% of swine and 10.9% of domestic rats were found to be parasitized by *C. sinensis* (Rim, 1982).

The Disease in Man and Animals: The acute phase of the disease can begin gradually or suddenly, with fever, chills, hepatomegaly, mild jaundice, and eosinophilia in 10 to 40% of the cases. In the chronic phase there may be cholecystitis and hepatitis.

Damage to liver function is related to the number of parasites and the occurrence of successive reinfections. When few parasites are present, the infection is asymptomatic; it passes unnoticed unless revealed by fecal examination. Such is the case in 60 to 80% of the infections in endemic areas of Japan. In other cases, anorexia, diarrhea, and hepatomegaly are observed. The disease is serious only when the parasite burden is large. These cases may include obstruction of the bile ducts, with consequent portal cirrhosis, catarrhal cholangitis, ascites, progressive edemas, and jaundice. Recurrent pyogenic cholangitis, due to partial obstruction of the bile ducts and secondary bacterial infection, is the most common complication of clonorchiasis. Pancreatitis is another frequent complication. It is usually mild, but acute episodes occur 1 to 3 hours after a heavy meal, occasioned perhaps by excessive secretion of pancreatic juices into a partially obstructed duct (Sun, 1980). The serious forms of the disease are now much less frequent.

A relationship is believed to exist between clonorchiasis and biliary lithiasis. Calculi form in the gall bladder around the eggs and dead trematodes. There are also indications that clonorchiasis is a predisposing factor for cholangiocarcinoma. The same relationship has been found in dogs and cats.

There is great disparity of opinion regarding the pathogenic role of *C. sinensis*, perhaps because most of those infected do not manifest clinical symptoms when the parasite burden is light. According to Manson-Bahr and Apted (1982), a mild infection is defined as 100 or less eggs per gram of feces; a moderate one, 100 to 1,000; and a massive one, over 1,000.

Source of Infection and Mode of Transmission: The epidemiologic chain successively involves mammals, aquatic snails, and freshwater fish. The most important host, by virtue of the parasite's specificity for it, is the snail (first intermediate host). The number of susceptible snail species is small. The species *Parafossarulus manchouricus* is the main host in China, Japan, South Korea, and Vietnam, but some other species in the genera *Bithynia* and *Alocinma* are also susceptible. This specificity of the parasite for the first intermediate host is the main reason for the geographic limitation of the parasitosis.

The parasite is less selective with regard to the second intermediate host. In the endemic region at least 80 species of naturally infected fish have been found.

In addition to humans, several species of mammals can serve as definitive hosts. Cats and dogs are important reservoirs. The definitive hosts are infected via the digestive tract by consuming raw freshwater fish containing metacercariae. For an area to become endemic, as has occurred in the Far East, the human population must customarily consume raw fish. The highest prevalence is found in adults, among whom this eating habit is more common. In southern China, an important contributing factor to the high prevalence of the infection is artificial cultivation of carp in ponds, an important industry in this region. Human fecal material is thrown into the ponds to promote the growth of plankton and feed the fish, facilitating the continued development of *Clonorchis* eggs by placing them in an environment in which snails abound.

Lower mammals, especially cats and dogs, can maintain the cycle of the parasite on their own. In central China, where eating raw fish is not a custom and where human cases are rare, a high proportion of cats and dogs are infected. The mode of infection for lower animals is similar to that for man.

Diagnosis: Specific diagnosis is made by finding the characteristic eggs in fecal matter or by a duodenal probe and the use of a strong solution of magnesium sulfate to produce a reflex contraction of the gallbladder. When the parasitosis is light, sedimentation methods must be used in the examination of feces. The parasite burden is evaluated by counting the eggs in the feces by means of the Stoll dilution method (Rim, 1982).

Use of several immunodiagnostic tests has been proposed, such as the intradermal test (immediate sensitivity), complement fixation, agglutination, and precipitation. These tests may give cross-reactions with several other parasitic diseases. The usefulness of these tests in clinical diagnosis is debatable, however, since the existence of the parasite's eggs can be demonstrated by fecal examination and constitutes irrefutable evidence.

Control: The infection can be prevented simply by not consuming raw fish. However, this ancestral habit is very difficult to change at the community level.

In China, the rate of human infection has been successfully reduced by preventing contamination of fish culture ponds. The use of seasoned and fermented manure instead of fresh human fecal matter has proved very helpful in reducing the infection of snails. In Japan, land drainage and the use of insecticides in agriculture, as well as industrialization and the resultant pollution of rivers with manufacturing wastes, have reduced the *Parafossarulus* population.

A biological control method that has been successful in tests involves introducing into the snails' habitat the cercariae of *Notocotylus attenuatus*, an intestinal trematode of ducks. This parasite affects the gonads of the snails.

Praziquantel is effective for treatment of clonorchiasis. Doses of 25 mg per kilogram of body weight three times a day for 1 day or 2 days have given cure rates of 86.8% and 100%, respectively (Rim, 1980).

Bibliography

Belding, D. L. *Textbook of Parasitology*, 3rd ed. New York, Appleton-Century-Crofts, 1965.

Bunnag, D., and T. Harinasuta. Opisthorchiasis, Clonorchiasis, and Paragonimiasis. *In*: Warren, S. K., and A. A. F. Mahmoud (Eds.), *Tropical and Geographical Medicine*, McGraw-Hill Book Company, New York, 1984.

Calero, M. C. Clonorchiasis in Chinese residents of Panama. *J Parasitol* 53:1150, 1967.

Faust, E. C., P. F. Russell, and R. C. Jung. *Craig and Faust's Clinical Parasitology*, 8th ed. Philadelphia, Lea and Febiger, 1970.

Gibson, J. B., and T. Sun. Clonorchiasis. *In*: Marcial-Rojas, R. A. (Ed.), *Pathology of Protozoal and Helminthic Diseases*. Baltimore, Maryland, Williams and Wilkins, 1971.

Komiya, Y. Clonorchis and clonorchiasis. *Adv Parasitol* 4:53-106, 1966.

Manson-Bahr, P. E. C., and F. I. C. Apted. *Manson's Tropical Diseases*, 18th ed. London, Baillière Tindall, 1982.

Purtilo, D. T. Clonorchiasis and hepatic neoplasms. *Trop Geogr Med* 28:21-27, 1976.

Rim, H. J. Modern therapy of human clonorchiasis. Abstract No. 305, *10th International Congress on Tropical Medicine and Malaria*, Manila, November 9-15, 1980.

Rim, H. J. Clonorchiasis. *In*: Hillyer, G. V., and C. E. Hopla (Section Eds.), *CRC Handbook Series in Zoonoses*. Section C, vol. 3. Boca Raton, Florida, CRC Press, 1982.

Sapunar, J., J. Faignenbaum, and F. Mora. Dos casos de clonorquiasis. *Bol Chile Parasitol* 18:45, 1963.

Sun, T. Clonorchiasis: A report of four cases and discussion of unusual manifestations. *Am J Trop Med Hyg* 29:1223-1227, 1980.

DICROCELIASIS

(121.8)

Synonym: Dicroceliosis.

Etiology: *Dicrocoelium dendriticum* (*D. lanceolatum*) and *D. hospes*, lancet-shaped trematodes, measuring 0.5 to 1 cm long and 1.5 to 2.5 mm wide, that live in the bile ducts of sheep, goats, cattle, and, less frequently, other domestic and wild herbivores.

D. dendriticum requires two intermediate hosts for its development, the first being a land snail and the second an ant. The adult trematodes deposit their eggs in the bile ducts of the definitive hosts; the eggs move with the bile and are eventually carried by the fecal matter to the exterior. The eggs contain a miracidium and are very resistant, capable of surviving many months in the environment. When ingested by a mollusk, the egg hatches and releases the miracidium. In the snail's tissues, the miracidium gives rise to two generations of sporocysts, the second of which produces large numbers of cercariae. Larval development within the mollusk takes about 4 months. The cercariae that escape from the snail are stuck together in a viscous mass ("slimeball") that adheres to vegetation. Each of the slimeballs, 1 to 3 mm in size, may contain 200 to 400 cercariae, which are released when ingested by an ant. They migrate through the ant's intestine to the abdomen and become encysted metacercariae, the infective form, in about 40 to 60 days. Herbivores consume ants containing the metacercariae along with their pasture, and in about 2 months the parasite reaches maturity and begins to lay eggs.

The life cycle of *D. hospes*, which has been determined more recently, follows the same general pattern as that of *D. dendriticum*. The first intermediate host is a pulmonate land snail of the genus *Limicolaria*, and the second is an ant of the genus *Camponotus*, in which the metacercariae develop. The definitive hosts are domestic herbivores (cattle, sheep, goats) and probably wild ruminants as well (Frank *et al.*, 1984).

Geographic Distribution and Occurrence: *D. dendriticum* is distributed throughout many countries of Europe, Asia, and possibly North Africa. The parasite is also found in Canada, the United States, Cuba, Colombia, and Brazil.

D. hospes is restricted to the sub-Saharan African savannah.

The few genuine human cases have occurred in several different European, Asian, and African countries. Numerous cases described in the USSR (*D. dendriticum*) and in Africa (*D. hospes*) are not due to actual infections but to consumption of liver from infected sheep or cows, and the consequent passage of eggs through the intestine.

The infection rates in sheep, goats, and cattle are high in many countries, especially those of Eastern Europe and some in Asia and Africa. Some recent prevalence data are available for two European and two African countries. In Switzerland, 46% of bovines were found to be infected by *D.* dendriticum, as were up to 100% of sheep in Yugoslavia (Malek, 1980). *D. hospes* infection was found in 50% of bovines and sheep in Ivory Coast, and in almost 94% of these animals in Nigeria (Frank *et al.*, 1984).

The Disease in Man and Animals: Dicroceliasis in animals and man is a less severe parasitosis than fascioliasis; it is generally asymptomatic or has a mild symptomatology.

In the majority of human cases the main symptoms are dyspepsia and flatulence. There may occasionally be constipation, diarrhea, and vomiting. Rarely, ectopic localizations of parasite eggs in the brain can cause neurologic symptoms. In domestic ruminants, heavy parasite loads can produce cirrhotic lesions and marked distension of the bile ducts. In such cases the symptomatology is similar to that of fascioliasis, consisting of weight loss, anemia, edemas, and digestive disorders.

Source of Infection and Mode of Transmission (Figure 68): The life cycle of the parasite requires a land snail and an ant as intermediate hosts. *D. dendriticum* uses many species of snails as the first intermediate host. In Yugoslavia (Rozman *et al.*, 1974), seven out of 17 species of snails examined were involved in the life cycle of the parasite. As in other parts of Europe, *Zebrina detrita* was the species with the highest infection rate. Besides this species, *Helicella candidula* and *H. ericitorum* are important hosts in Europe and parts of Asia. In the state of New York, USA, *Cionella lubrica* is the snail that serves as the first intermediate host.

Of eight species of ants (*Formica* spp.) studied in Yugoslavia, three were found to contain metacercariae of *D. dendriticum*. A significant difference has been found between the infection rates of ants attached to vegetation and those in ant hills. While ants attached to vegetation had infection rates over 70% (in two species of *Formica*), the others had infection rates of only 0.1 to 1%. Ants were found attached to vegetation most abundantly at the beginning of spring. Attachment of ants to plants facilitates their ingestion by definitive hosts (herbivores) and accidental hosts (man).

The main definitive hosts of the parasite are sheep, goats, and cattle. In some parts of the world, wild animals constitute an important reservoir. Herbivores become infected when they ingest parasitized ants with grass while grazing.

Figure 68. Dicroceliasis. Transmission cycle.

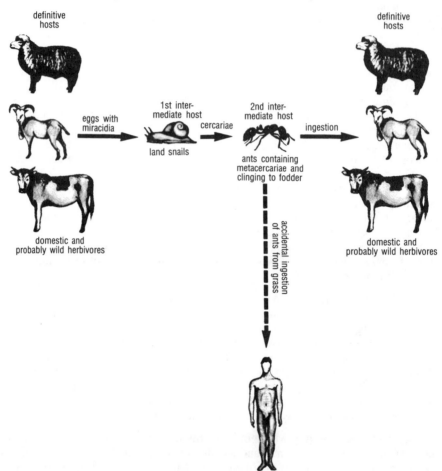

D. *hospes* uses snails of the genus *Limicolaria* as its first intermediate host and ants of the genus *Camponotus* as the second.

Man is an accidental host who is occasionally infected by nibbling on grass containing infected ants or by consuming vegetables or fruits contaminated with these insects.

Diagnosis: Diagnosis is based on examination of feces and identification of the characteristic eggs. The most appropriate procedure for finding *D. dendriticum* and other trematode eggs is sedimentation. In man, fecal examination can be combined with examination of bile obtained by a duodenal probe. It should be borne in mind that eggs of *Dicrocoelium* may appear in the feces as a result of consuming the liver of infected animals. To distinguish this mere passage of eggs from a true infection, the patient must be fed a controlled diet for several days and the feces reexamined periodically. Serologic tests (complement fixation, precipitation) can be of some help in detecting specific antibodies.

Control: The human parasitosis can be prevented by abstaining from consuming, nibbling, or sucking on blades of grass.

Some control of the infection in animals can be obtained by preventive doses of thiabendazole or diaphenethid, along with pasture rotation and application of molluscicides. In some areas of the USSR, chickens introduced into meadows have voraciously devoured snails, greatly reducing their population.

Bibliography

Frank, W., R. Lucius, and T. Romig. Studies on the biology, pathology, ecology and epidemiology of *Dicrocoelium hospes* (Looss, 1907) in West Africa (Ivory Coast). *In*: Markl, H., and A. Bittner (Eds.), *Recent German Research on Problems of Parasitology, Animal Health and Animal Breeding in the Tropics and Subtropics*. Tubingen, Institute for Scientific Cooperation, 1984.

Lapage, G. *Veterinary Parasitology*, 2nd ed. Edinburgh, Oliver and Boyd, 1968.

Malek, E. A. *Snail-transmitted Parasitic Diseases*, vol. 2. Boca Raton, Florida, CRC Press, 1980.

Price, D. L., and P. L. Child. Dicroceliasis (distomiasis, lancet fluke disease). *In*: Marcial-Rojas, R. A. (Ed.), *Pathology of Protozoal and Helminthic Disease*. Baltimore, Maryland, Williams and Wilkins, 1971.

Rozman, M., S. Gradjanin, and M. Cankovic. The transitory hosts of *Dicrocoelium dendriticum* in the mountain area of Vosnia and Herzegovina. *In*: *Third International Congress of Parasitology*. Munich, Facta Publication, 1974.

Soulsby, E. J. L. *Textbook of Veterinary Clinical Pathology*. Oxford, Blackwell, 1965.

ECHINOSTOMIASIS

(121.8)

Synonym: Echinostomatidosis.

Etiology: Species of several genera of the family Echinostomatidae, which are small trematodes living in the intestine (and sometimes other organs) of mammals, fowl, reptiles, and occasionally man. The nomenclature of some species is still uncertain. The species that most frequently invade the intestine of man are *Echinostoma ilocanum*, *E. lindoense*, *E. malayanum*, *E. revolutum*, and *Hypoderaeum conoideum*.

The development cycle varies in different species of echinostomes, but generally two intermediate hosts are required: the first of these is a freshwater snail, and the second may be another mollusk, a batrachian (tadpole or adult), or a fish. The definitive hosts, including man, are infected by consuming intermediate hosts in which metacercariae have developed.

Geographic Distribution and Occurrence: *Echinostoma* (*Euparyphium*) *ilocanum* is found in the Philippines, the islands of Java and Celebes (Indonesia), parts of southern China, and India. Parasitosis by this agent is rather common among the Ilocanos of Luzon, Philippines. In addition to man, it infects murid rodents, dogs, and cats. Cercariae encyst in any freshwater mollusk. The snails *Pila luzonica*, *P. conica*, and *Viviparus javanicus* play an important role in the epidemiology because the people customarily eat them raw.

E. lindoense is a parasite of anseriform fowl that appears to have adapted well to the human host. In 1940, infection rates of 24 to 96% were found in villages along the shore of Lake Lindu on Celebes. Owing to ecologic changes, no more human cases have been confirmed in recent years. The parasitosis has also been observed in India, Java, Malaysia, the Philippines, and Brazil.

E. malayanum occurs in dogs, cats, pigs, mongooses, and rarely man. The area of distribution of the parasite includes Malaysia, Thailand, India, and Sumatra (Indonesia).

E. revolutum is a parasite of ducks, geese, and other fowl. On Formosa (Taiwan), the estimated infection rate in these species varies between 2.8 and 6.5%. Human infections have been diagnosed in Java, Taiwan, and Mexico. The main source of infection for man is the clam *Corbicula fluminea* when it is consumed raw or undercooked.

Hypoderaeum conoideum is also a trematode parasite of fowl and is frequently found in the human population of northern Thailand, where the people habitually eat raw snails.

The Disease in Man and Animals: The clinical aspects have not been well studied. In general, echinostomes are not very pathogenic. When the number of parasites is large, there may be intestinal colic and diarrhea. Severe enteritis has been described in fowl due to *E. revolutum* and *H. conoideum*, more often the former.

Source of Infection and Mode of Transmission: The first intermediate hosts of *E. ilocanum* are planorbid snails of the genera *Gyraulus* and *Hippeutis*. The cercariae that emerge from these mollusks encyst and produce metacercariae in other snails, of which *Pila conica* and *P. luzonica* in the Philippines and *Viviparus javanicus* in Java are of special epidemiologic interest. These snails, when eaten raw, constitute the source of infection for humans. Several mammals in addition to man act as definitive hosts and maintain the chain of transmission.

E. lindoense also makes use of small planorbid snails as the first intermediate host and of other snails, such as *Viviparus*, and clams (*Corbicula* spp.) as the second intermediate host, in which the cercariae encyst. Man becomes infected by consuming raw clams. An interesting change occurred in the ecology of Lake Lindu (Celebes) and resulted in the disappearance of the human disease. A mullet, *Tilapia mossambica*, was introduced into the lake, and as this fish species multiplied, a reduction was seen in the population of the clam *Corbicula lindoensis*, which was the main source of human infection. The wildlife cycle, which develops between rodents as definitive hosts and freshwater snails as intermediate hosts, persists. In Brazil the trematode uses the snail *Biomphalaria glabrata* as an intermediate host. Rodents and anseriform fowl are the reservoirs of the parasite.

E. malayanum makes use of a snail of the genus *Lymnaea* as its first intermediate host; cercariae can encyst in both this and other snails, as well as in the fish *Barbus stigma*. Mammals are infected by ingesting the second intermediate host. Man is an accidental host. Maintenance of the cycle depends on other mammals, mainly dogs, cats, and pigs.

E. revolutum uses snails of several genera as the first intermediate host; metacercariae can form in the same host, other mollusks, clams (*Corbicula* spp.), or tadpoles. Man becomes infected by consuming the second intermediate host, especially clams, raw. The main reservoirs are many species of aquatic fowl, chickens, and pigeons.

The cercariae of *Hypoderaeum conoideum* develop in snails of the genera *Lymnaea* and *Planorbis*, and metacercariae develop in the same species or in other snails, as well as in frogs and tadpoles. Man is infected by consuming raw snails. The reservoir of the parasite is domestic and aquatic fowl.

Echinostomiasis occurs in ecologic regions where there are many bodies of water to support the intermediate hosts. The endemicity of the parasitosis is due to the habit of consuming raw mollusks, crustaceans, or fish.

Diagnosis: Diagnosis is based on the confirmation of the presence of eggs in fecal matter. The size of the eggs differs with the species of echinostome, and these eggs must be distinguished from unembryonated eggs of other intestinal or biliary trematodes.

Control: The slight clinical importance of the parasitosis does not justify the establishment of special control programs. In endemic areas, raw or undercooked mollusks, crustaceans, or fish should not be consumed; however, changes in this long-standing eating habit may be difficult to achieve.

Bibliography

Bandyopadhyay, A. K., and A. A. Nandy. A preliminary observation on the prevalence of echinostomes in a tribal community near Calcutta. *Ann Trop Med Parasitol* 80:373-375, 1986.

Carney, W. P., P. Purnomo, P. F. D. van Peenen, and J. S. Saroso. Echinostomiasis in Indonesia with special emphasis on *Echinostoma lindoense*. *In: Third International Congress of Parasitology*. Munich, Facta Publications, 1974.

Euzéby, J. *Les Zoonoses Helminthiques*. Paris, Vigot et Frères, 1964.

Faust, E. C., P. F. Russell, and R. C. Jung. *Craig and Faust's Clinical Parasitology*, 8th ed. Philadelphia, Lea and Febiger, 1970.

Swellengrebel, N. H., and M. M. Sterman. *Animal Parasites in Man*. Princeton, New Jersey, van Nostrand, 1961.

Ulmer, M. J. Other trematode infections. *In*: Hubbert, W. T., W. F. McCulloch, and P. R. Schnurrenberger (Eds.), *Diseases Transmitted from Animals to Man*, 6th ed. Springfield, Illinois, Thomas, 1975.

FASCIOLIASIS

(121.3)

Synonyms: Hepatic distomiasis, fasciolosis, and many local names.

Etiology: *Fasciola hepatica* and *F. gigantica,* trematodes that live in the bile ducts of domestic and wild herbivores and occasionally infect man. *F. hepatica* is flattened, about 2.5 to 3 cm long and 1.3 cm wide, brownish in color, and shaped like a laurel leaf. The adult parasites lay unembryonated eggs, which are carried by the bile to the intestine and evacuated with the feces. To mature, the eggs must have suitable moisture and temperature conditions. In summer, incubation is short and the miracidium (larva) emerges from the egg to the water in a few weeks; under conditions of low winter temperatures found in temperate climates, hatching takes several months. The eggs are resistant to environmental factors and can survive in fecal matter for approximately 1 year. The miracidia, by contrast, are very fragile and must find an appropriate host within 8 hours. The intermediate hosts are amphibious snails of the family Lymnaeidae. The most important of these snails in the different regions are *Lymnaea truncatula,* very widespread in Europe, Asia, and Africa; *L. humilis, L. bulimoides,* and *L. cubensis* in North America; *L. viator (L. viatrix)* and *L. diaphana* in a large part of South America; *L. tomentosa* in Australia and New Zealand; and *L. viridis* in Asia, Hawaii, and Papua New Guinea (Boray, 1982). *L. cubensis* and *L. columella* are the main intermediate hosts in the Caribbean, Colombia, and Venezuela (Malek, 1980). After penetrating the snail, the miracidia turn into sporocysts. In about 3 weeks the sporocysts produce rediae, which in turn can produce daughter rediae (second generation of rediae) or transform directly into cercariae. If the temperature is favorable, the cercariae may begin to emerge from the snails in about 6 weeks. When temperatures are under 10° C, the larval stages can survive for at least 100 days within the snail without completing their development, and can then begin to develop again when the temperature rises.

Upon leaving the snail, the cercariae swim actively in the water and encyst on vegetation. There they become metacercariae, which are characterized by their long survival in a wet environment but low resistance to desiccation. Cercariae have been shown to form metacercariae preferentially on certain species of plants, but they can also encyst on the surface of the water, enclosing small bubbles of air that allow them to float. The definitive hosts are infected by ingesting plants or water containing metacercariae. The larvae are released from the cystic envelope in the duodenum, pass through the intestinal wall to the abdominal cavity, perforate Glisson's capsule, and travel through the hepatic parenchyma to the bile ducts, where they mature. The prepatent period (from infection to the appearance of eggs in the host's feces) lasts about 2 months, but not all the young fasciolae mature at the same time and the process of maturation can extend another 2 months (Soulsby, 1982). The cycle is reinitiated by oviposition. *F. hepatica* can live in the bile ducts for several years.

F. gigantica has a life cycle similar to that of *F. hepatica.* Its intermediate hosts are aquatic snails belonging to the superspecies *Lymnaea auricularia.* The intermediate host in India and Pakistan is *L. rufescens;* in Malaysia, *L. rubiginosa;* in Iran, *L. geodrosiana;* and in Iraq, *L. euphratica.* The main intermediate host in Africa is *L. natalensis* (Malek, 1980). The development cycle of *F. gigantica* is more prolonged than that of *F. hepatica.* The occurrence of both trematodes in some countries, such as Pakistan, is determined by the presence of the appropriate intermediate hosts. *F. hepatica* cannot complete its larval cycle in *L. auricularia,* as *F. gigantica* cannot in *L. truncatula.* The definitive hosts of *F. gigantica* are sheep, goats, bovines, zebras, and occasionally man. This trematode is distinguished from *F. hepatica* by its larger size (2.5 to 7.5 cm by 1.2 cm).

Geographic Distribution: *F. hepatica* is distributed throughout the world, while *F. gigantica* occurs in Africa, several Asian countries, and Hawaii.

Occurrence in Man: Human fascioliasis occurs sporadically or in outbreaks and has been recorded in numerous countries in the Americas, Europe, Africa, and Asia. The most extensive epidemics have occurred in France, such as the one in Ain, Jura, Rhône, and Saône that affected nearly 500 people in 1956-1957 and included multiple familial cases, or the one in Lot valley in 1957 that affected almost 200 persons. The common source of infection was found to be watercress contaminated by metacercariae (Malek, 1980). In some departments in France, for example Haute-Vienne, fascioliasis cases occur in rural areas practically every year; from 1955 to 1979 there were 121 cases, 49 of them occurring within 24 families and 72 in other individuals (Rondelaud *et al.,* 1982). In addition to France, the infection is common in Italy, Poland, and England. The largest outbreak in this last country affected 40 persons in 1972 (Malek, 1980). The frequency of human infection in Latin America has been underestimated in the parasitologic literature. In Cuba alone, more than 100 cases were recorded up to 1944, and numerous later findings should be added to this total; in Chile, 82 cases were known up to 1959. Additionally, human infections have occurred in Argentina, Uruguay, Peru, Venezuela, Costa Rica, Puerto Rico, Dominican Republic, and Mexico. In 1978 in the canton of Turrialba, Costa Rica, 42 clinical cases were diagnosed (Mora *et al.,* 1980).

Human infection is often subclinical or has very mild symptomatology. The disease was studied in an endemic area in the Sierra Central of Peru. During 1968 and 1969 in 14 communities in Jauja Province, 1,557 fecal samples from schoolchildren 7 to 14 years old were examined, and trematode eggs were found in 15.6% (Bendezú, 1970). In the area near Atlixco in the state of Puebla, Mexico, fascioliasis was found in 0.6% of the population (Biagi, 1974). A coproparasitologic study was carried out in the mountainous region of Corozal, Puerto Rico, where bovine fascioliasis is hyperendemic, and eggs of *F. hepatica* were found in the feces of 12 of 100 individuals examined (Bendezú *et al.,* 1982).

More than 20 cases of infection by *F. gigantica* have been diagnosed in Hawaii. Likewise, isolated cases or small outbreaks have occurred in Asia and Africa.

Occurrence in Animals: Fascioliasis is a common disease of sheep, goats, and cattle in many parts of the world. Morbidity and mortality rates vary from one region to another. In endemic areas infection rates of more than 50% are commonly found. In the study carried out in the Sierra Central of Peru, infection rates were 18.6% in sheep in the "foci of origin" and 95.8% in the "foci of dissemination."

The losses caused by hepatic fascioliasis, like those occasioned by other chronic diseases, are difficult to determine. According to one estimate, the productive efficiency of cattle declines by 8% in mild infections and by more than 20% in severe infections; in sheep the loss in wool production can range from 20 to 39%. Losses are due to confiscation of livers, stunted growth, and reduction in wool, milk, and meat production. An additional cause is infectious necrotic hepatitis that may occur in sheep harboring spores of *Clostridium novyi* when young fasciolae invade the liver. In a study carried out in Australia, lambs were experimentally infected via the oral route with different doses of metacercariae, and the damage done by the parasitosis was analyzed 6 months after infection, using regression procedures. All the parasitized groups exhibited stunted growth as well as weight loss and decreased growth of wool. Similarly, a reduction in the efficiency of food conversion was observed in the groups with 45, 67, and 117 fasciolae (Hawkins and Morris, 1978).

Many other domestic and wild species are infected by *F. hepatica,* among them equines, camels, and wild herbivores.

The Disease in Man: The severity of the infection in man depends on the number of fasciolae and the duration of the infection. The migration of young fasciolae through the hepatic parenchyma can cause traumatic or necrotic lesions. In the bile ducts the adult *Fasciola* causes inflammatory, adenomatous, and fibrotic changes. Serious infections, with a large number of parasites, may produce biliary stasis, atrophy of the liver, and periportal cirrhosis. Cholecystitis and cholelithiasis occur with some frequency in chronic cases.

In the initial phase, which corresponds to the migration of the young fasciolae through the hepatic parenchyma, the clinical picture includes fever, malaise, hepatomegaly, pain in the right costal region, eosinophilia, and alterations in liver function tests.

In the chronic phase, the symptomatology is variable, with hepatobiliary manifestations, irregular fever, anemia, and eosinophilia. In a study of 47 patients in Chile, the main symptoms were abdominal pain, dyspepsia, weight loss, diarrhea, and fever. Ten of the 47 patients had jaundice. The eosinophil count was normal in nine and elevated in 38 cases (Faiguenbaum *et al.,* 1962).

During the larvae's migration into the peritoneal cavity, aberrant localizations can occur in different parts of the body; the symptomatology varies with the affected organ.

The Disease in Animals: Fascioliasis is a disease of herbivores. The most susceptible domestic species is sheep, followed by cattle. Two clinical forms of the disease, acute and chronic, can be distinguished.

The acute form occurs primarily in lambs and is caused by ingestion of a large number of metacercariae, with consequent sudden invasion and the migration of large numbers of young fasciolae into the hepatic parenchyma. The migrating parasites cause hemorrhages, hematomas and ruptures in the liver, inflammation of the organ and bile ducts, and destruction of hepatic tissue. Affected sheep may die suddenly without clinical manifestations, or 1 or 2 days prior to death may show debility, loss of appetite, and pain when palpated in the hepatic region. In less acute cases there may be weight loss and accumulation of fluid in the abdomen. Also common are eosinophilia, anemia, hypoalbuminemia, and a high level of serum glutamic-oxaloacetic transaminase. In older sheep (2 to 4 years) harboring latent spores of *Clostridium novyi* in the liver, invasion by the young fasciolae can give rise to infectious necrotic hepatitis, with fatal results. Bovines rarely suffer from acute fascioliasis.

The chronic form develops slowly and is characterized by weight loss, emaciation, submaxillary edema, anemia, debility, diarrhea, and ascites. The symptomatology depends on the number of parasites. Sheep that harbor a moderate number of *Fasciola* initially show loss of appetite, reduced weight gain, and progressive anemia. The condition of the animals deteriorates when food is scarce and improves when it is abundant, but they do not recover and the parsitosis has a cumulative effect over the years. Symptomatology includes cholangitis, biliary stasis, and destruction and fibrosis of hepatic tissue. Anemia and eosinophilia are persistent. Bovines are more resistant than sheep and can tolerate a larger number of parasites without significant clinical manifestations. Young bovines are more susceptible than adults.

In swine, fascioliasis is generally asymptomatic, becoming clinically apparent when debilitating factors, such as malnutrition or concurrent illnesses, are present.

The parasitosis has also been described in equines.

The pathogenesis, pathology, and symptomatology of the infection caused by *F. gigantica* are similar to those of the parasitosis caused by *F. hepatica*.

Source of Infection and Mode of Transmission (Figure 69): The ecology of fascioliasis is closely related to that of the snails that serve as intermediate hosts. Physiographic characteristics, soil composition, and climatic factors determine the reproduction rate of *Lymnaea* and thus the epidemiologic dynamics of the disease. *Lymnaea* and fascioliasis can be found in pastures in the most diverse areas of the world, from fields at sea level to Andean valleys at elevations above 3,700 meters. The different species of *Lymnaea* vary as to their physiologic characteristics, distribution, and survival time under adverse conditions. The best studied species are *L. truncatula* and *L. tomentosa*. From the ecologic standpoint, the habitat of

Figure 69. Fascioliasis. Transmission cycle.

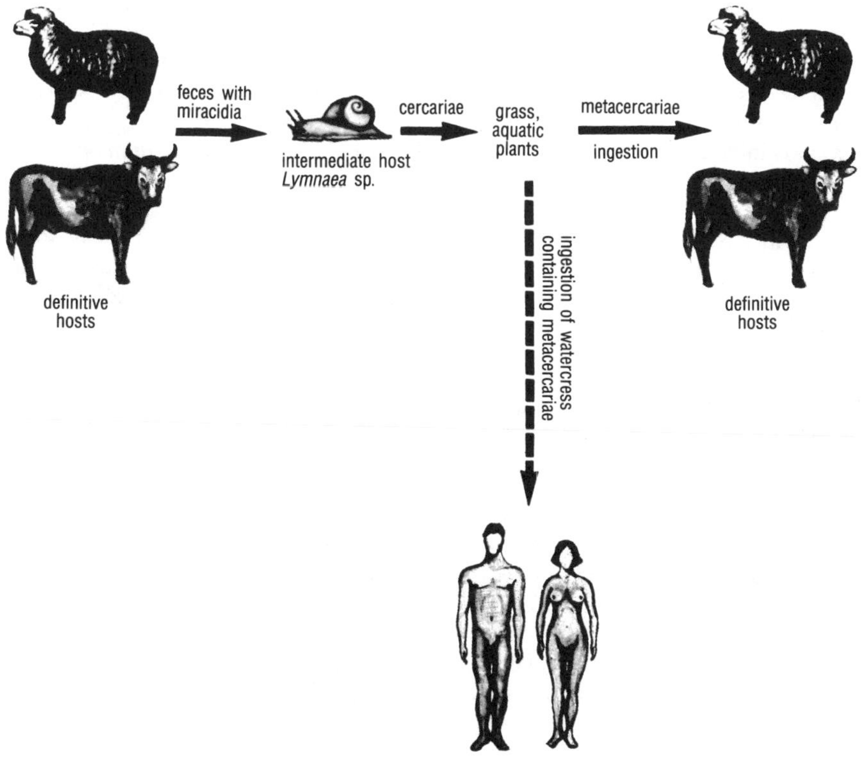

Lymnaea can be divided into two broad types: primary foci or reservoirs, and areas of dissemination. Primary foci are permanently moist areas such as small rivers, lakes, lagoons, and canals where the snails reproduce constantly. Wet fields with clayey soil constitute another type of reservoir. In the primary foci the snail population is uniform and generally at a low level. Areas that are alternately flooded and dried out are of special epidemiologic interest. The areas of dissemination of the original foci contain high concentrations of *Lymnaea*. The snails may come directly from the original foci, carried by the flooding, or they may be snails that were estivating during the dry season and are reactivated by the water. Rain (or irrigation) after a dry period creates favorable conditions in these fields for snail reproduction. The temporary or extension habitats in pastures constitute enzootic areas where serious outbreaks of fascioliasis occur. Outbreaks of acute fascioliasis are rare during winter in temperate climates; they generally occur when late summer or autumn rains follow a dry period. The effects of moisture and temperature cause many cercariae to leave the snails and encyst on the grass. Under these conditions, herbivores can become infected with a large number of metacercariae, and in 6 to 8 weeks they develop the acute form of the parasitosis due to liver damage. Chronic fascioliasis appears later, starting in late autumn. In rainy years, vast areas of pasture land may be contaminated with metacercariae, while in dry years the larvae are found only in low-lying, wet areas.

The most important definitive hosts are sheep. According to estimates, a sheep with a mild subclinical infection can contaminate a field with more than half a million eggs per day, and one with a moderate infection can spread 2.5 to 3 million. Sheep are followed in importance by cattle, but the latter's production of *Fasciola* eggs declines rapidly. Many other species of domestic and wild herbivores, among them lagomorphs, can serve as definitive hosts. Studies done in Australia indicate that some of these animals are only temporary hosts and cannot maintain the cycle by themselves for any length of time. Such would be the case with rabbits, whose contamination of pastures is insignificant.

Man is infected mainly by consuming salads of watercress (*Nasturtium officinale*) containing metacercariae. In France, where watercress salad is popular (each year 10,000 tons are consumed), human infection is more frequent than in other European countries. Contaminated lettuce or other plants that are eaten raw can sometimes serve as a source of infection, as can water from irrigation canals or other receptacles. Alfalfa juice has also been implicated in places where it is a customary drink.

Role of Animals in the Epidemiology of the Disease: Man is an accidental host. The infection in nature is maintained in a cycle between other animal species, mainly sheep and cattle, and snails of the family Lymnaeidae.

Diagnosis: During the acute phase of human fascioliasis, laboratory diagnosis cannot be accomplished by coprologic examination since no eggs are eliminated. This phase must be distinguished from other acute hepatic infections, and fascioliasis should be suspected given the appropriate epidemiologic antecedents and the presence of eosinophilia.

In animals, the diagnosis of acute fascioliasis is made at autopsy by examination of hepatic lesions and the discovery of immature parasites.

Diagnosis of chronic fascioliasis is based on coprologic examination and observation of parasite eggs. The most appropriate method is sedimentation.

Consumption of infected beef or sheep liver can give rise to trematode eggs in fecal matter and, consequently, a false positive result in the coprologic examination. By excluding liver from the patient's diet for several days, a correct diagnosis can be made. If the fecal examination is negative, the bile of human patients should be examined using a duodenal probe. In Latin America, there has sometimes been unnecessary and extended hospitalization and even surgery on patients with hepatic disorders when fascioliasis was not considered in the differential diagnosis.

For diagnosis of the infection during the prepatent period, numerous immunobiologic tests have been tried, among them a cutaneous test with fascioline (an extract of the parasite injected intradermally), complement fixation, immunofluorescence, immunoelectrophoresis, counterimmunoelectrophoresis, and, recently, ELISA. The tests can lack either sensitivity or specificity. The most sensitive test is ELISA. The advantage of serologic tests in man and animals during the prepatent period is early diagnosis, which would allow treatment (bithionol in man or the new anthelmintic triclabendazole in animals) before liver damage is too advanced.

Control: Human fascioliasis can be prevented by abstaining from the consumption of watercress of wild or unknown origin. This recommendation is especially valid for endemic areas. Watercress should be cultivated in controlled conditions that exclude animals or the possibility of snail infestation.

Control of animal infection consists primarily of administering fasciolicides to the definitive hosts, especially sheep and cattle, to reduce elimination of trematode eggs and to protect the health of the animals. Likewise, measures can be applied to reduce the population of the mollusks that serve as intermediate hosts.

A large number of chemical compounds active against *F. hepatica* are available (hexachloroethane, carbon tetrachloride, hexachlorophene bithionol, oxyclozanide, nitroxynil, and others). However, some of them, especially the older ones, have toxic effects or are not very active against immature fasciolae. Recently, a new benzimidazole compound (triclabendazole) has been tested and found very effective against both mature and immature fasciolae. Triclabendazole has been tried in sheep (Boray *et al.*, 1983) and cattle (Craig and Huey, 1984) with highly satisfactory results. Knowledge of the biology of the parasite and its snail hosts has permitted a strategic treatment plan to be established for sheep and bovine herds, with treatments two or three times a year. The time of year, or more precisely the months in which preventive treatment should be administered, varies with the ecologic conditions in each area, especially the climate. In addition to these strategic treatments, tactical doses may be required when climatic conditions (humidity and heat) favor rapid multiplication of mollusks.

Control of snails involves environmental modification or the use of chemical and biological measures. Drainage of the land, where this is technically and economically feasible, is the only permanent way to eliminate or control the mollusks. Chemical methods consist of applying molluscicides. Given the great capacity for reproduction and recuperation that species of *Lymnaea* have, molluscicides should be applied periodically to keep the snail population at a low level. This method is very costly and therefore cannot be applied on a large scale on most livestock establishments in developing countries; however, it could be used on small farms. In temperate climates, the molluscicides should be used in spring and early summer, and application should be repeated about 3 months later. In climates with only two seasons (dry and rainy), the molluscicides should be applied at the beginning and end of the rainy season. Biological control using the annelid *Chaetogaster limnaei,* which feeds on miracidia and cercariae, is being tried and could prove useful in certain areas.

Bibliography

Belding, D. L. *Textbook of Parasitology,* 3rd ed. New York, Appleton-Century-Crofts, 1965.

Bendezú, P. Algunos aspectos de la epidemiología de la distomatosis hepática y su control biológico en el Valle de Mantaro. *Bol Extr (IVITA)* 4:356-367, 1970.

Bendezú, P., and A. Landa. Distomatosis hepática. Epidemiología y control. *Bol IVITA,* 14:1-32, 1973.

Bendezú, P., A. Frame, and G. V. Hillyer. Human fascioliasis in Corozal, Puerto Rico. *J Parasitol* 68:297-299, 1982.

Biagi, F. *Enfermedades parasitarias,* 2nd ed. México, Prensa Médica Mexicana, 1974.

Blood, D. C., and J. A. Henderson. *Veterinary Medicine,* 4th ed. Baltimore, Maryland, Williams and Wilkins, 1974.

Boray, J. C. Experimental fascioliasis in Australia. *Adv Parasitol* 7:95-210, 1969.

Boray, J. C. Fascioliasis. *In:* Hillyer, G. V., and C. E. Hopla (Section Eds.), *CRC Handbook Series in Zoonoses,* Section C, vol. 3. Boca Raton, Florida, CRC Press, 1982.

Boray, J. C., P. D. Crowfoot, M. B. Strong, J. R. Allison, M. Schellenbaum, M. von Orelli, and G. Sarasin. Treatment of immature and mature *Fasciola hepatica* infections in sheep with triclabendazole. *Vet Rec* 113:315-317, 1983.

Cobas, J. M., L. Acosta, and R. Medina. Estudio clínico, epidemiológico y ecológico docente de fasciliasis hepática familiar. *Bol Hig Epidemiol (Habana)* 12:17-27, 1974.

Courtin, S., G. Ferriere, and J. Cerda. Primer estudio de *Fasciola hepatica* en el conejo silvestre (*Oryctolagus cuniculus*) de la precordillera de Nahuelbuta. *Bol Chile Parasitol* 30:65-67, 1975.

Craig, T. M., and R. L. Huey. Efficacy of triclabendazole against *Fasciola hepatica* and *Fascioloides magna* in naturally infected calves. *Am J Vet Res* 45:1644-1645, 1984.

Faiguenbaum, J., A. Feres, R. Doncaster, *et al.* Fascioliasis (distomatosis) hepática humana. *Bol Chile Parasitol* 17:7-12, 1962.

Faust, E. C., P. F. Russell, and R. C. Jung. *Craig and Faust's Clinical Parasitology,* 8th ed. Philadelphia, Lea and Febiger, 1970.

Hawkins, C. D., and R. S. Morris. Depression of productivity in sheep infected with *Fasciola hepatica. Vet Parasitol* 4:341-351, 1978.

Jensen, R. *Diseases of Sheep.* Philadelphia, Lea and Febiger, 1974.

Knobloch, J., E. Delgado, A. Alvarez, V. Reymann, and R. Bialek. Human fascioliasis in Cajamarca, Peru. I. Diagnostic methods and treatment with praziquantel. *Trop Med Parasitol* 36:88-90, 1985.

Malek, E. A. *Snail-transmitted Parasitic Diseases,* vol. 2. Boca Raton, Florida, CRC Press, 1980.

Mora, J. A., R. Arroyo, S. Molina, L. Troper, and E. Irías. Nuevos aportes sobre el valor de la fasciolina. Estudio en un área endémica de Costa Rica. *Bol Of Sanit Panam* 89:409-414, 1980.

Náquira-Vildoso, F., and R. A. Marcial-Rojas. Fascioliasis. *In:* Marcial-Rojas, R. A. (Ed.), *Pathology of Protozoal and Helminthic Diseases.* Baltimore, Maryland, Williams and Wilkins, 1971.

Rondclaud, D., E. Amat-Frut, and M. Pestre-Alexandre. La distomatose humaine à *Fasciola hepatica. Bull Soc Pathol Exot* 75:291-300, 1982.

Rubio, M., P. Olivos, and F. Puga. Nuevos casos de distomatosis o fascioliasis hepática en niños. *Bol Chile Parasitol* 16:38-41, 1961.

Soulsby, E. J. L. *Helminths, Arthropods and Protozoa of Domesticated Animals,* 7th ed. Philadelphia, Lea and Febiger, 1982.

Taylor, E. L. *La fascioliasis y el distoma hepático*. Rome, Food and Agriculture Organization of the United Nations, 1965. (Agricultural Studies 64.)

Ueno, H., R. Arandia, G. Morales, and G. Medina. Fascioliasis of livestock and snail host for *Fasciola* in the Altiplano Region of Bolivia. *Natl Inst Anim Health Q (Tokyo)* 15:61-67, 1975.

FASCIOLOPSIASIS

(121.4)

Etiology: *Fasciolopsis buski,* a trematode 2 to 7.5 cm long and 8 to 20 mm wide that lives attached to the mucosa of the duodenum and jejunum in humans and swine. The eggs eliminated with the feces must incubate for 3 to 7 weeks in still water at a temperature of 26 to 32° C. The miracidium (larva) that emerges from the embryonated egg penetrates the tissues of a small planorbid snail, mainly of one of three genera: *Segmentina, Hippeutis,* and *Polypylis.* In the mollusk it passes through the sporocyst stage and two generations of rediae. The second generation of rediae gives rise to large numbers of cercariae, which emerge from the snails to encyst (metacercariae) on aquatic plants. The definitive hosts, man or swine, become infected by consuming these aquatic plants with the attached metacercariae. In the intestine, the metacercaria is released from its envelope, and after about 3 months the parasite reaches maturity and reinitiates the cycle by oviposition.

Geographic Distribution and Occurrence: The parasitosis occurs in central and southern China, Taiwan, India, Bangladesh, the Indochina peninsula, and Indonesia. An estimated 100 million persons are parasitized. Prevalence is very variable. In some villages of Thailand, the infection affects up to 70% of the population. In various places in Chekiang (Zhejiang) and Kiansi (Jiangxi) Provinces, China, the prevalence can be as high as 85% of the population; on the other hand, in other areas of the country, infection rates vary from less than 1% to 5%. It is estimated that about half of all human infections occur in China (Malek, 1980). Children between the ages of 4 and 13 years are most affected.

In a study carried out in an endemic area of Thailand, similar prevalences were found in the human and swine populations. The swine were found to harbor a smaller number of parasites that produced fewer eggs than those lodged in the human intestine (Manning and Ratanarat, 1970). In some areas of China with high rates of human infection, the parasitosis in swine has not been confirmed.

The Disease in Man and Animals: To this parasite—the largest trematode that occurs in man—have been attributed traumatic, toxic, and obstructive effects, with epigastric pain, nausea, diarrhea, undigested food in the feces, and edemas of the face, abdomen, and legs. A recent clinical study in Thailand of a group of mostly young persons who eliminated eggs of *F. buski* and a similar control group showed that mild gastrointestinal symptoms occurred in both groups (Plaut *et al.,* 1969).

The severe disease described in the literature corresponds to cases in which the number of parasites is large.

Three to 12 parasites are usually found in naturally infected pigs. As a general rule, the health of the pig is not affected, and disease symptoms occur only in cases with a heavy parasite burden.

Source of Infection and Mode of Transmission: The source of infection for humans and swine is aquatic plants containing metacercariae.

Endemic areas have the ecologic conditions necessary for the growth of both the intermediate hosts and edible aquatic plants. In central Thailand, these conditions occur in flooded fields where edible aquatic plants are cultivated close to dwellings. These fields receive human excreta directly from the houses, which are built on posts.

Human and animal excreta promote the development of snails and plants, and provide the infective material (the parasite's eggs) for the intermediate hosts, the snails *Segmentina trochoideus, Hippeutis umbilicalis,* and *Polypylis haemisphaeru-la* in China, Thailand, and Taiwan, and the first two in Bangladesh (Gilman *et al.,* 1982). The epidemiologically important aquatic plants, whose fruits, pods, roots, bulbs, or stems are eaten by man, are water chestnuts (*Trapa* spp., *Eleocharis* spp.), lotus (*Nymphaea lotus*), and others of the genera *Ipomoea, Eichhornia, Neptunia,* and *Zizania*. Certain parts of these plants are eaten raw, and the teeth and lips are often used to peel the pods and bulbs. In areas where people habitually boil the plants or their "fruits" (water chestnuts) before eating them but give them raw to swine, the infection rate is much higher in these animals than in humans. In general, the prevalence of human infection is higher in areas where the aquatic plants are cultivated and lower in distant towns, since metacercariae attached to the plants are not resistant to desiccation that can occur when some time elapses between harvest and marketing.

The pig is considered a reservoir of the parasite that could maintain the infection in the human population even where facilities for sanitary elimination of human excreta are available. However, in Moslem countries, such as Bangladesh, swine do not play any role as a reservoir, man being basically the only reservoir and only source of infection for snails (Gilman *et al.,* 1982).

Diagnosis: Laboratory diagnosis is based on demonstration of the presence of eggs in fecal matter. The eggs are very similar to those of *Fasciola hepatica*. The parasite can easily be identified when found in vomit or feces.

Control: The simplest preventive measure for the human parasitosis would be to abstain from eating fresh or raw aquatic plants (or from peeling them with the teeth), but this recommendation requires a change of eating habits, which is difficult to achieve. Other measures to combat the parasitosis, in addition to health education, consist of the use of molluscicides, treatment of the affected population, processing of human excreta in septic tanks or with quicklime, and prohibition of swine raising in endemic areas.

Bibliography

Brown, H. W., and D. L. Belding. *Parasitología clínica,* 2nd ed. México, Interamericana, 1965.

Faust, E. C., P. C. Beaver, and R. C. Jung. *Animal Agents and Vectors of Human Disease,* 4th ed. Philadelphia, Lea and Febiger, 1975.

Faust, E. C., P. F. Russell, and R. C. Jung. *Craig and Faust's Clinical Parasitology,* 8th ed. Philadelphia, Lea and Febiger, 1970.

Gilman, R. H., G. Mondal, M. Maksud, K. Alam, E. Rutherford, J. B. Gilman, and M. U. Khan. Endemic focus of *Fasciolopsis buski* infection in Bangladesh. *Am J Trop Med Hyg* 31:796-802, 1982.

Malek, E. A. *Snail-transmitted Parasitic Diseases,* vol. 2. Boca Raton, Florida, CRC Press, 1980.

Manning, G. S., and C. Ratanarat. *Fasciolopsis buski* (Lancaster, 1857) in Thailand. *Am J Trop Med Hyg* 19:613-619, 1970.

Plaut, A. G., C. Kampanart-Sanyakorn, and G. S. Manning. A clinical study of *Fasciolopsis buski* infection in Thailand. *Trans R Soc Trop Med Hyg* 63:470-478, 1969.

Soulsby, E. J. L. *Textbook of Veterinary Clinical Parasitology.* Oxford, Blackweil, 1965.

GASTRODISCOIDIASIS

(121.8)

Synonym: Amphistomiasis.

Etiology: *Gastrodiscoides* (*Amphistomum*) *hominis*, a pear-shaped, bright-pink trematode, 9 to 15 mm long and 6 to 10 mm wide, usually found in the cecum and ascending colon of man and other definitive hosts, especially swine.

The development cycle of the parasite is not well known. The eggs, when deposited with feces, contain an embryo in an early stage of segmentation. The miracidium (larva) requires 9 to 16 days in the water to reach maturity. In experiments in India, miracidia produced infection in a planorbid snail, *Helicorbis coenosus*, which may be the natural intermediate host. Depending on the ambient temperature, the cercariae begin to emerge from the snails 28 to 152 days after infection. Like those of other species of the Gastrodiscidae, the cercariae of *G. hominis* are thought to encyst on aquatic plants and develop into metacercariae. The definitive hosts are infected by ingesting metacercariae.

It has been suggested that *G. hominis* from humans and swine may be different strains or varieties.

Geographic Distribution and Occurrence: The parasitosis occurs primarily in Bengal, Assam, Bihar, and Orissa (India) and in Bangladesh, but it has also been recorded in the Philippines, Indonesia, and in animals in Malaysia, Thailand, Java, and Burma. It has been reported in Indian immigrants in Guyana. The disease may be more widely distributed, since the parasite was found in a wild boar in Kazakhstan, USSR.

Human infection rates vary and may be very high, as in a village in Assam, India, where 40% of the population was affected.

In a slaughterhouse in India, the parasite was found in 27% of 233 pigs examined. The infection is also found in rodents and several species of nonhuman primates in Asia: rhesus monkeys (*Macaca mulatta*), cynomolgus monkeys (*M. fascicularis* and *M. philippinensis*), and *M. irus*. The rate of infection in 1,201 cynomolgus monkeys (*M. fascicularis*) was 21.4%.

The Disease in Man and Animals: The infection is clinically apparent only when the parasite burden is large. In these cases there may be alterations of the mucosa of the colon and cecum, colitis, and mucoid diarrhea.

Source of Infection and Mode of Transmission: The natural definitive host appears to be swine, in which high rates of infection have been found. The parasite has also been found in monkeys and rodents. In general, man is considered to be a secondary definitive host. However, the true relationship between the human and animal trematodes is not yet known, nor has it been determined if the animal parasites are transmissible to man. In some areas in India, the human infection occurs where infection in swine does not; the reverse situation has also been observed (Malek, 1980).

Definitive hosts acquire the infection through the digestive tract, probably by consuming raw aquatic plants containing metacercariae.

Diagnosis: Diagnosis is based on detection of eggs in fecal samples or, more easily, identification of the expelled trematode following administration of an anthelmintic to the affected person.

Control: For individual protection, people in endemic areas should refrain from eating raw aquatic plants.

Bibliography

Belding, D. L. *Textbook of Parasitology*, 3rd ed. New York, Appleton-Century-Crofts, 1965.

Dutt, S. C., and H. D. Srivastara. The life history of *Gastrodiscoides hominis* (Lewis and McConnel, 1876) Leiper, 1913, the amphistome parasite of man and pig. *J Helminthol* 46:35-46, 1972.

Faust, E. C., P. F. Russell, and R. C. Jung. *Craig and Faust's Clinical Parasitology*, 8th ed. Philadelphia, Lea and Febiger, 1970.

Faust, E. C., P. C. Beaver, and R. C. Jung. *Animal Agents and Vectors of Human Disease*, 4th ed. Philadelphia, Lea and Febiger, 1975.

Malek, E. A. *Snail-transmitted Parasitic Diseases*, vol. 2. Boca Raton, Florida, CRC Press, 1980.

Marcial-Rojas, R. A. Rare intestinal flukes. *In*: Marcial-Rojas, R. A. (Ed.), *Pathology of Protozoal and Helminthic Diseases*. Baltimore, Maryland, Williams and Wilkins, 1971.

Witenberg, G. G. Trematodiases. *In*: Van der Hoeden, J. (Ed.), *Zoonoses*. Amsterdam, Netherlands, Elsevier, 1964.

HETEROPHYIASIS

(121.6)

Synonym: Heterophydiasis.

Etiology: Intestinal trematodes of the family Heterophyidae, which comprises six genera and 10 species of parasites afflicting humans and other vertebrates. The most common species are *Heterophyes heterophyes, H. h. nocens* (possibly identical to the preceding species), *Metagonimus yokogawai*, and *Stellantchasmus falcatus*. The other species are *Haplorchis taichui, H. yokogawai, H. calderoni, H. vanissima, Stamnosoma armatum*, and *Cryptocotyle* (*Tocrotrema*) *lingua* (Malek, 1980). Any species in this family, all of which generally invade lower animals and birds, can infect man.

H. heterophyes is a very small, pear-shaped trematode, 1 to 1.7 mm long and 0.3 to 0.4 mm wide; it lives in the small intestine of man, cats, dogs, foxes, and other mammals and birds that feed on fish. Eggs found in the feces of definitive hosts contain fully developed miracidia, which must be ingested by an appropriate aquatic snail (first intermediate host) to continue their development. Inside the snail (*Pirenella* spp. in Egypt and *Cerithidea cingulata* and *Semisulcospira libertina* in Japan), the miracidia give rise to sporocysts, which in turn give rise to rediae, and finally to cercariae. The latter invade the second intermediate host, which may be one of several species of freshwater fish that customarily spawn in brackish or marine water. In these fish, the cercariae encyst and transform into metacercariae. In Egypt, metacercariae are found mainly in mullet (*Mugil*), *Tilapia*, and some other species; in Japan, they are found in several species of *Acanthogobius*. When man or another definitive host consumes raw fish containing metacercariae, the parasites are released from the cystic envelope; they develop in the intestine into adult trematodes, and produce mature eggs in 7 to 8 days.

M. yokogawai measures 1 to 2.5 mm long by 0.4 to 0.8 mm wide and lives in the small intestine of humans, dogs, cats, pigs, pelicans, and possibly other piscivorous birds. Its development cycle is similar to that of *H. heterophyes*. The first intermediate hosts are snails of the genera *Semisulcospira* and *Thiara*; the second are salmonoid and cyprinoid fish.

The life cycles of other members of the Heterophyidae are similar.

Geographic Distribution and Occurrence: *H. heterophyes* is found in Southeast Asia, the Far East, the Middle East, Turkey, the Balkans, and Spain. The largest endemic focus is located in the Nile Delta, where especially favorable conditions exist for the propagation of this parasitosis: enormous numbers of *Pirenella* snails live at the bottom of the brackish lagoons of the delta, mullets are abundant, people traditionally consume raw fish, and sanitary waste disposal is not available. Most mullets contain metacercariae, and nearly all cats and dogs are infected. In one town, an estimated 65% of the schoolchildren were parasitized.

In addition to the endemic and hyperendemic areas noted, *H. heterophyes* has also been recorded, at a very low prevalence, in western Africa.

A high prevalence of *H. heterophyes nocens* (probably synonymous with *H. heterophyes*) had been recorded in the prefecture of Yamaguchi, Japan. More recent studies in other prefectures indicate a prevalence of less than 1% (Malek, 1980).

M. yokogawai occurs primarily in the Far East and in the northern provinces of Siberia, and less frequently in central Europe; a few cases have been described in Spain. In some localities in the Far East, almost half of the population was found to be infected.

The distribution of *Stellantchasmus falcatus* encompasses Japan, the Philippines, Thailand, Indonesia, Hawaii, the Middle East, and Australia.

The Disease in Man and Animals: If the infection is mild, it is usually asymptomatic. A large parasite burden can cause irritation of the intestinal mucosa with excessive secretion of mucus, superficial necrosis of the epithelium, chronic diarrhea, colic, and nausea. Aberrant eggs of the parasite sometimes enter the bloodstream and produce granulomatous foci in various tissues and organs, including the myocardium and brain. Nevertheless, most human cases are benign. *Metagonimus* sometimes deeply invades the intestinal mucosa.

The clinical picture is similar in animals. The infection is clinically apparent only when the number of parasites is large.

Source of Infection and Mode of Transmission: The source of infection for man, other mammals, and birds is fish (from fresh, brackish, or sea water) infected with metacercariae of the parasite. Consumption of raw or undercooked fish is the main cause of human infection. The critical host, because of its specificity, is the melaniid snail; the parasite is less selective regarding the second intermediate host, which can be any of several species of freshwater, brackish water, or marine fish and even some shrimp. Contamination of the water with human or animal excreta is critical to the parasite's development cycle.

The primary definitive host varies with the species of the parasite: for some it is piscivorous birds; for others, dogs, cats, or even man. Secondary hosts are many species of wild birds and mammals that feed on fish.

Diagnosis: Diagnosis is based on microscopic observation of the eggs in fecal material. The eggs of *Heterophyes* and *Metagonimus* are difficult to distinguish from one another and from those of *Clonorchis* and *Opisthorchis*. The species can be identified by examining adult trematodes after the patient receives anthelmintic treatment.

Control: Human infection can be prevented by cooking fish adequately. Dogs and cats should not be fed raw fish or scraps containing raw fish.

Bibliography

Belding, D. L. *Textbook of Parasitology*, 3rd ed. New York, Appleton-Century-Crofts, 1965.

Faust, E. C., P. F. Russell, and R. C. Jung. *Craig and Faust's Clinical Parasitology*, 8th ed. Philadelphia, Lea and Febiger, 1970.

Malek, E. A. *Snail-transmitted Parasitic Diseases*, vol. 2. Boca Raton, Florida, CRC Press, 1980.

Spencer, H. Fascioliasis, heterophyiasis and other fluke diseases. *In*: Spencer, H. (Ed.), *Tropical Pathology*. New York, Springer Verlag, 1973.

Witenberg, G. G. Trematodiases. *In*: Van der Hoeden, J. (Ed.), *Zoonoses*. Amsterdam, Netherlands, Elsevier, 1964.

NANOPHYETIASIS

(121.9)

Synonyms: Salmon disease, salmon poisoning (animals).

Etiology: *Nanophyetus* (*Troglotrema*) *salmincola*, a small, digenetic intestinal trematode of canids and man. On the basis of some biological differences and their geographic distribution, two subspecies are recognized: *N. salmincola salmincola* and *N. salmincola schikhobalowi*.

The adult trematode measures 0.8 to 2.5 mm by 0.3 to 0.5 mm. Its life cycle requires two intermediate hosts, the first a snail of the family Pleuroceridae and the second a salmonid fish or, less frequently, a fish of another family. The eggs eliminated with the feces of the definitive hosts (canids, man) are not embryonated and must remain in water up to 200 days for the embryo to form completely. The miracidium released from the egg penetrates a snail, in which it undergoes several stages of transformation and multiplication (sporocysts and one or two generations of rediae) before finally giving rise to cercariae. These, in turn, penetrate an appropriate fish and encyst in its organs, where they transform into metacercariae and become infective after 11 days. When a definitive host eats raw fish containing metacercariae, the parasites mature and begin oviposition in 5 to 8 days.

Geographic Distribution and Occurrence: *Nanophyetus s. schikhobalowi* is distributed in the northern part of Sakhalin Island and along the mountain tributaries of the Amur river in eastern Siberia. The rate of human infection in some villages along the tributaries of the Amur can reach 98%.

Nanophyetus s. salmincola is distributed along the Pacific coast of the United States (Oregon, Washington, and northern California). Cases of naturally acquired human infection due to the American subspecies of the trematode are not known. However, this parasite is a vector for the agent of a severe disease of dogs and other canids, inappropriately called "salmon poisoning." In fact, *N. s. salmincola* in any of its developmental stages can act as a vector for *Neorickettsia helminthoeca* and another similar and as yet unclassified microorganism, known as the Elokomin agent of trematode fever. In contrast to the American trematode, *N. s. schikhobalowi* is not a host to these rickettsial agents.

The distribution of nanophyetiasis is determined by the presence of appropriate species of snails, the first intermediate host. In the endemic-enzootic area of Siberia these snails are *Semisulcospira laevigata* and *S. cancellata*, and in the United States, *Oxytrema silicula*.

The Disease in Man: Mild infections by *N. s. schikhobalowi* are asymptomatic. Patients with a parasite burden of 500 or more flukes experience diarrhea (43%), gastric pain (32%), constipation (16%), and nocturnal salivation (16%).

No natural infections by *N. s. salmincola* have been found in humans in the United States.

The Disease in Animals: Dogs, coyotes, and foxes are susceptible to "salmon poisoning," so named because the disease is associated with ingestion of salmon and trout from coastal streams in the Pacific Northwest region of the United States. Two microorganisms are known to cause the disease: *Neorickettsia helminthoeca* and the Elokomin agent of trematode fever. The two rickettsial agents are carried by *Nanophyetus s. salmincola. Neorickettsia helminthoeca* is the more virulent agent, and is blamed for high mortality in dogs as well as the low population levels of coyotes and foxes in the enzootic area of the United States. After an incubation period of 6 to 9 days, the disease has a sudden onset with fever and anorexia. Four to 5 days after the disease begins, the animals suffer persistent vomiting and, some time later, bloody diarrhea and rapid weight loss. Purulent ocular secretion and edema of the eyelids are common. Most of the animals die 6 to 10 days after the onset of the disease or 12 to 20 days after ingesting the infected fish. The Elokomin agent is less pathogenic and does not confer immunity against *N. helminthoeca*.

"Salmon poisoning" is unknown in eastern Siberia. The observations of Russian investigators indicate that the infection of dogs, cats, brown rats, and badgers by *N. s. schikhobalowi* can produce a severe and fatal disease.

Different species of salmonids experimentally exposed to *N. s. salmincola* cercariae showed different degrees of susceptibility or resistance, possibly determined by the duration of the host-parasite relationship. In general, species coming from enzootic areas were more resistant than those from other areas. Death occurred mainly in the first 24 hours, that is, during the period of penetration and migration of the cercariae.

In a short period of time (1 or 2 days) in their natural environment, it is doubtful that fish encounter a number of cercariae similar to the number that proved fatal in laboratory studies. It is believed, rather, that they acquire the infection in a gradual and cumulative manner. However, most researchers agree that the parasites are pathogenic for fish, especially if vital organs, such as the heart or gills, are affected by a large number of metacercariae. Additionally, stunted development of affected fish has been confirmed, as well as impairment of swimming ability (Millemann and Knapp, 1970).

Source of Infection and Mode of Transmission: The native human population and animals in eastern Siberia contract *N. s. schikhobalowi* infection by ingesting raw fish, especially salmonid fish, infected by metacercariae of the parasite.

Fish infected with metacercariae of *N. s. salmincola*, the vector of the agents of "salmon poisoning," constitute the source of infection for dogs and other canids in the enzootic region of the disease.

In the areas in both the USSR and the United States where the infection occurs, a high rate of infection by metacercariae is found in fish, especially salmonids.

Diagnosis: Diagnosis is confirmed by observation of the parasite's eggs in the feces of man or animals.

In "salmon poisoning," the existence of intracytoplasmic microorganisms similar to *Rickettsia* can be confirmed by microscopic examination of stained preparations of lymphatic tissue.

Control: In the endemic area of Siberia, the main prevention measure consists of educating the population, in an effort to change the habit of consuming raw fish.

Domestic animals should not be fed remains of raw fish and should be kept away from streams during the salmon migration period.

Bibliography

Baldwin, N. L., R. E. Millemann, and S. E. Knapp. "Salmon poisoning" disease. III. Effect of experimental *Nanophyetus salmincola* infection on the fish host. *J Parasitol* 53:556-564, 1967.

Gillespie, J. H., and J. F. Timoney. *Hagan and Bruner's Infectious Diseases of Domestic Animals*, 7th ed. Ithaca, New York, Cornell University Press, 1981.

Malek, E. A. *Snail-transmitted Parasitic Disease*, vol. 2. Boca Raton, Florida, CRC Press, 1980.

Millemann, R. E., and S. E. Knapp. Biology of *Nanophyetus salmincola* and "salmon poisoning" disease. *Adv Parasitol* 8:1-41, 1970.

OPISTHORCHIASIS

(121.0)

Etiology: *Opisthorchis felineus*, *O. viverrini*, and *Amphimerus* (*Opisthorchis*) *pseudofelineus*, trematodes that lodge in the bile ducts of man, cats, dogs, and other animals that feed on raw fish. The development cycle of *Opisthorchis* is similar to that of *Clonorchis* (see Clonorchiasis), requiring two intermediate hosts: the first, an aquatic snail, and the second, one of several species of freshwater fish.

O. felineus is 7 to 12 mm long and 2 to 3 mm wide. It produces eggs containing fully formed miracidia, which must reach the water to continue their development. Hatching occurs when the egg is ingested by a snail of a suitable species, such as *Bithynia* (*Bulimus*) *leachi* or *B. tentaculata*.

The sporocysts and rediae produced in these snails give rise to cercariae. About 2 months after infection of the mollusk, the cercariae mature, leave the host, and enter the water. When they come into contact with the second intermediate host, a fish of the family Cyprinidae, the cercariae lose their tails, penetrate the host's tissues, and encyst, transforming into metacercariae. After 6 weeks, the metacercariae reach maturity; when they are ingested along with the fish by a definitive host—man or another animal—they lose their cystic envelope in the duodenum. The parasites migrate through the ampulla of Vater and the network of bile ducts. In about a month, the trematode begins to lay eggs, reinitiating the cycle.

O. viverrini differs from *O. felineus* in only a few anatomical details. The first intermediate hosts of *O. viverrini* are the snails *Bithynia goniomphalus*, *B. funiculata*, and *B. laevis*; the second intermediate hosts are several species of cyprinid fish. The definitive hosts of this parasite are humans, dogs, cats, fishing cats (*Felis viverrina*), and other animals that frequently feed on fish or fish wastes.

Amphimerus pseudofelineus is about 4 mm long and 2 mm wide. The definitive hosts are man, dogs, coyotes (*Canis latrans*), domestic cats, and opossums; its intermediate hosts are not known.

Geographic Distribution and Occurrence: The main endemic areas of *O. felineus* are found in marshy land and river basins in the USSR, such as those of central Siberia, Kazakhstan, the lower Dnieper, and the Kama River. Smaller foci exist in eastern, southern, and central Europe, North Korea, and perhaps India, Japan, and the Philippines. It is estimated that more than 1 million persons are affected by this trematode. In some hyperendemic areas, such as Siberia, the infection rate is very high, not only among the nomadic population but also in some cities. Results of a study carried out a few years after World War II showed that an estimated 83% of the human population, 100% of the cats, and 90% of the dogs in the city of Tobolsk were infected. In Kazakhstan, 100% of some species of fish were found to have metacercariae. The snails that act as the first intermediate hosts are very abundant in some endemic regions, and their infection rate is high.

O. viverrini is found in Laos and northeastern Thailand. In the latter area, the prevalence of infection by *O. viverrini* has increased from 3.5 million cases in 1965 to 5.4 million in 1981 (Bunnag and Harinasuta, 1984). In some hyperendemic zones, the infection rate ranges between 72 and 87% of the population. The infection has been found in several animal species, even in regions where human opisthorchiasis has not been reported.

A. pseudofelineus was described in man under the name *Opisthorchis guayaquilensis* in Pedro P. Gómez Parish, Manabí Province, Ecuador. Eggs of the parasite were found in fecal samples of 7.3% of 245 persons in the area (with the rate varying from 4% in town to 32% in outlying localities). In this same parish, only three of 100 dogs and none of 80 pigs examined were found to be parasitized. The parasite has been found in several animal species in the United States, Brazil (Santa Catarina), Panama, and Ecuador (Artigas and Pérez, 1962).

The Disease in Man and Animals: The symptomatology of the disease is similar to that of the hepatic distomiasis caused by *Clonorchis siniensis* and depends on both the parasite burden and the duration of infection. In general, if only a few parasites are present, the infection will be asymptomatic, although some damage to the distal biliary passages may result. A parasitosis of medium intensity will include fever, diarrhea, flatulence, moderate jaundice, asthenia, cephalalgia, hepatomegaly, and passive congestion of the spleen. In chronic cases with a heavy parasite burden, the bile ducts become hypertrophic; mechanical obstruction and biliary stasis may occur, accompanied by secondary infections with cholangitis, cholangiohepatitis, and the formation of micro- and macroabscesses. In the case of a massive parasitosis, the pancreas may be invaded, causing catarrhal inflammation of the pancreatic ducts. Papulo-erythematous eruptions are frequent in infections by *O. fe-*

lineus. Opisthorchis is believed to play an etiologic role in the development of hepatic carcinomas, especially cholangiocarcinomas.

The pathology in animals is similar to that in man.

Source of Infection and Mode of Transmission: Man and other definitive hosts become infected by consuming raw or undercooked fish containing metacercariae. Human opisthorchiasis occurs only where suitable intermediate hosts are found (most importantly mollusks), and where people customarily eat raw, slightly salted, or sun-dried fish. In highly endemic areas, man is thought to be the main agent responsible for maintaining the cycle by contaminating rivers and lakes with feces containing parasite eggs. Under these conditions, animals contribute less to water contamination.

The main species of fish that transmit *O. felineus* infection to humans are *Idus melanotus*, *Tinca tinca*, and *T. vulgaris*, the species in which the parasite's metacercariae are most prevalent. In Thailand, the fish with the highest frequency of infection by the metacercariae of *O. viverrini* are *Hampala dispar, Puntius orphoides*, and *Cyclocheilichthys siaja*; rates of infection have been found to vary from 51% in the last species to 74% in the first.

Animals can maintain a natural cycle independent of man. In one area in the USSR, 85% of the cats examined were found to be infected, but no cases were detected in the human population, since the people there do not eat raw fish. The parasite's eggs contained in animal fecal matter deposited on riverbanks and shores can be washed into the water by rains.

Diagnosis: Laboratory diagnosis is based on discovery of the parasite's eggs, either in fecal material after sedimentation, or by duodenal probe.

Recently, the ELISA test has been tried with a soluble antigen extracted from adult *O. viverrini*. In the trial, 20 Laotian patients who were positive to parasitologic examination were also positive to the test. Groups infected by *Fasciola, Paragonimus*, and *Schistosoma* gave cross-reactions, generally with lower titers (Feldheim and Knobloch, 1982).

Control: The principal preventive measure consists of public health education to discourage the consumption of raw fish or the feeding of raw fish to animals. However, this is difficult to carry out in rural areas, where the level of education is low and where food habits are traditional. In cities, sanitary waste disposal is important in reducing pollution by the parasite's eggs in rivers and other bodies of water.

The use of 5-10% or 15% saline solution effectively destroys metacercariae in 10 and 3 days, respectively; freezing to $-10°C$ kills metacercariae in 5 days.

Praziquantel is the medicine of choice. One day of treatment with 25 mg per kilogram of body weight, taken three times after meals, achieved a 100% cure rate (Bunnag and Harinasuta, 1980).

Bibliography

Artigas, P. de T., and M. D. Pérez. Considerações sôbre *Opisthorchis pricei* Foster, 1939, *O. guayaquilensis* Rodríguez, Gómez e Montalván, 1949, e *O. psuedofelineus* Ward, 1901.

Descrição de *Amphimerus pseudofelineus minutus* n. subsp. *Mem Inst Butantan* 30:157-166, 1960-1962.

Borchert, A. *Parasitología Veterinaria*. Zaragoza, Acribia, 1964.

Bunnag, D., and T. Harinasuta. Studies on the chemotherapy of human opisthorchiasis in Thailand: I. Clinical trial of praziquantel. *Southeast Asian J Trop Med Public Health* 11:528-531, 1980.

Bunnang, D., and T. Harinasuta. Opisthorchiasis, clonorchiasis and paragonimiasis. *In*: Warren K. S., and A. A. F. Mahmoud, *Tropical and Geographical Medicine*. New York, McGraw-Hill Book Company, 1984.

Faust, E. C., P. F. Russell, and R. C. Jung. *Craig and Faust's Clinical Parasitology*, 8th ed. Philadelphia, Lea and Febiger, 1970.

Feldheim, W., and J. Knobloch. Serodiagnosis of *Opisthorchis viverrini* infestation by an enzyme immuno-assay. *Tropenmed Parasitol* 33:8-10, 1982.

Malek, E. A. *Snail-transmitted Parasitic Diseases*, vol. 2. Boca Raton, Florida, CRC Press, 1980.

Tansurat, P. Opisthorchiasis. *In*: Marcial-Rojas, R. A. (Ed.), *Pathology of Protozoal and Helminthic Diseases*. Baltimore, Maryland, Williams and Wilkins, 1971.

Witenberg, G. G. Trematodiases. *In*: Van der Hoeden, J. (Ed.), *Zoonoses*. Amsterdam, Netherlands, Elsevier, 1964.

PARAGONIMIASIS

(121.2)

Synonyms: Pulmonary distomiasis, endemic hemoptysis.

Etiology: About 40 species of the genus *Paragonimus* have been described, but the taxonomy of many of them is in doubt and only 28 are considered valid. The type species, which causes classic human paragonimiasis, is *P. westermani*. Several other species parasitize domestic and wild animals, but rarely affect humans.

Besides *P. westermani*, the main species that infect man are *P. pulmonalis*, *P. miyazakii*, *P. skryjabini* (*P. szechuanensis*), and *P. heterotrema* in Asia; *P. africanus* and *P. uterobilateralis* in Africa; and *P. mexicanus* (*P. peruvianus*, *P. ecuadoriensis*) in Latin America (Miyazaki, 1982). The validity of other species described from this last continent has not yet been determined.

The determination of isozymic profiles by means of electrophoresis will likely provide a better characterization of the species and subspecies of *Paragonimus* in the future, as this method has already for some protozoans (Zilmann and Voelker, 1980).

The development cycle of *P. westermani* requires two intermediate hosts: the first a gastropod mollusk and the second a freshwater crab or crayfish. Man and other mammals are the definitive hosts, in which the trematode mainly lodges in the lungs. The eggs of the trematode are eliminated to the exterior by expectoration or in the feces if the sputum is swallowed. The unembryonated eggs must reach water in order to complete their development. Hatching occurs after several weeks, and the egg releases a ciliated larva or miracidium that can swim freely in the water for only a short time before it must find an appropriate host. In eastern Asia, the main snail species that serve as the first intermediate host belong to the genera *Semisulcospira* and *Brotia* for *P. westermani* and *P. pulmonalis; Bythinella* and *Saganoa* for *P. miyazakii; Tricula* for *P. skryjabini* and *P. heterotrema*; probably *Potadoma* for *P. africanus* and probably *Potadoma* and *Afropomus* for *P. uterobilateralis*; and *Aroapyrgus costaricensis* in Costa Rica for *P. mexicanus* (Miyazaki, 1982). In the snail, the parasite goes through several stages of transformation and multiplication (sporocysts and two generations of rediae); at the end of 9 to 13 weeks, cercariae with a propulsive cauda are produced. In order to continue their development, the cercariae require a second intermediate host; this role can be filled by several species of freshwater crustaceans of the genera *Geothelphusa, Potamon, Sinopotamon, Potamiscus, Sundathelphusa, Eriocheir, Cambroides*, and several others in Asia; *Sudanonautes* and *Liberanautes* in Africa; and *Pseudothelphusa, Potamocarcinus, Ptychophallus*, and *Hypolobocera* in Latin America (Miyazaki, 1982). The second intermediate host becomes infected by feeding on infected snails or by ingesting free cercariae. In the crab or crayfish, the cercariae encyst (turning into metacercariae) in the gills, liver, and muscles.

The definitive hosts, such as man, various felids (tiger, leopard, lion, cat), wolves, foxes, different species of mustelids, wild rats, swine, dogs, and monkeys, are infected by ingesting freshwater crabs or crayfish containing metacercariae. In the intestine, the metacercariae are liberated from the cystic envelope and penetrate the intestinal wall; they remain in the peritoneal cavity for several days and then migrate through the diaphragm into the thoracic cavity and to the lungs, where the parasites lodge close to the bronchi and reach maturity. The parasite completes its development in the definitive host in about 10 weeks, reinitiating the cycle by oviposition. Recently, wild boars, rabbits, and mice have been discovered to be paratenic hosts, that is, intermediate transfer hosts in which the parasite does not mature and which are not essential to its life cycle. Human infection on the island of Kyushu, Japan, has been attributed to the ingestion of raw wild boar meat that contained larval forms of the parasite. The significance of this observation has not yet been completely evaluated (World Health Organization, 1979).

Geographic Distribution and Occurrence: The most important endemic areas are eastern and southeastern Asia, the maritime provinces of the USSR, Japan, Korea, China, Taiwan, the Philippines, Laos, Thailand, and isolated foci in Vietnam and India. The main etiologic agent is *P. westermani*, but in some countries other species are sympatric with it or occur alone. *P. pulmonalis*[1] exists in Japan, *P. miyazakii* in China, and *P. heterotrema* in China, Thailand, and Laos (Miyazaki, 1982). Several provinces in China contain areas of high endemicity of various *Paragonimus* species. In a study carried out in some provinces in Thailand, an infection rate of 6.5% was found in 503 persons examined. It is estimated that the infected population in Korea numbers between 1 and 1.5 million. In Taiwan the average rate of infection in schoolchildren is 1.6% (Malek, 1980). The rate of infection in Japan, which rose during and immediately after World War II, is declining. Much of the data available from various Asian countries is not current.

---

[1]*P. pulmonalis* is differentiated from *P. westermani* by being triploid and parthenogenetic instead of diploid and bisexual. The second intermediate host of *P. pulmonalis* is *Eriocheir japonicus*, while that of *P. westermani* in Japan is *Geothelphusa dahaani*.

In Africa, *P. africanus* occurs in Cameroon, and *P. uterobilateralis* in Cameroon, Liberia, Guinea, and Nigeria. A recent study carried out in an endemic region of Cameroon confirmed the presence of eggs of *P. africanus* in the sputum and/or feces of 5.6% of 900 persons examined, with the highest prevalence in the under-20-years age group (Kum and Nchinda, 1982). Paragonimiasis by *P. uterobilateralis* in the eastern part of Nigeria usually occurs as isolated cases. During and after the civil war in that country (1967-1970), there was a considerable increase in cases, and 100 cases were diagnosed in one university hospital (Nwokolo, 1972). Of the 69 patients whose sputum was examined, 66 had eggs of *P. uterobilateralis* and three had eggs of *P. africanus* (Voelker and Nwokolo, 1973). Isolated cases have been observed in Liberia and Guinea.

The main species that infects man in Latin America is *P. mexicanus*, of which *P. peruvianus* and *P. ecuadoriensis* are now considered synonyms. Human cases of the disease have occurred in Peru (Cajamarca and the coast north of Lima), Ecuador, Colombia, Costa Rica, Honduras, El Salvador, and Mexico. From 1921 to 1969, 511 cases were recorded in Ecuador; 316 cases were diagnosed from 1972 to 1976 in four of that country's provinces, the majority in Manabí (Arzube and Voelker, 1978). About 20 cases have been diagnosed in Cajamarca, Peru, and a few cases in Mexico.

The ratio of infection rates in males and females varies in different countries and may depend on local customs and habits related to eating or preparing crustaceans. The disease affects mainly young people.

The geographic distribution of the parasitosis in lower mammals is much broader than the corresponding human infection, since the latter depends on the eating habits of the population.

The Disease in Man: *P. westermani* localizes most frequently in the lungs and less frequently in other organs or tissues. The period between ingestion of the metacercariae and the appearance of symptoms is prolonged and variable. The prominent symptoms of pulmonary paragonimiasis consist of chronic coughing, thoracic pain, and blood-tinged, viscous sputum. Intense physical exercise can induce hemoptysis, which is usually not very abundant but is the most notable sign. Eosinophilia is common. A small number of parasites in the lungs does not significantly affect the health of the patient and does not interfere with routine activity. About two-thirds of the shadows revealed by radiography are located in the middle and lower portions of the lungs; they are rarely seen in the apex.

Ectopic localizations are fairly common. The most serious of these is cerebral paragonimiasis. An estimated 5,000 cases of cerebral paragonimiasis occur each year in South Korea, a hyperendemic area. Symptomatology is similar to that of cerebral cysticercosis, with cephalalgia, convulsions, jacksonian epilepsy, hemiplegia, paresis, and visual disorders. Abdominal paragonimiasis produces dull abdominal pain, and also causes mucosanguineous diarrhea when the intestinal mucosa is ulcerated. In other localizations, the symptomatology varies with the organ affected.

The predominant form of the infection caused by *P. skryjabini* in China or by *P. heterotrema* in Thailand is the subcutaneous nodular form, which is characterized by high eosinophilia and is clinically similar to cutaneous larva migrans. Besides migratory subcutaneous nodules, the most common manifestations caused by *P. skryjabini* in China consist of pleural, ocular, cerebral, pericardial, and hepatic lesions; pulmonary symptoms are relatively infrequent (Hu *et al.*, 1982). Cases of ectopic paragonimiasis of the brain, liver, and perivesical and cutaneous fat have also been observed in Latin America. Twelve cases of cutaneous paragonimiasis occurred in a single family in Ecuador; an isolated case also occurred in that country and another in Honduras (Brenes *et al.*, 1983).

The Disease in Animals: The lungs of animals parasitized by *P. westermani* frequently contain cysts, which pass to the respiratory tract and pleural cavity. The symptoms are similar to those of human pulmonary paragonimiasis, with coughing and bloody sputum.

The trematodes appear in the lungs of dogs between 23 and 35 days after experimental infection. The parasitosis begins as pneumonitis and catarrhal bronchitis, followed by interstitial pneumonia and cyst formation.

Source of Infection and Mode of Transmission (Figure 70): The source of *P. westermani* infection for man and other definitive hosts is freshwater crabs and crayfish containing metacercariae. The disease is transmitted by the ingestion of raw or undercooked crustaceans, crabs marinated in wine, or crustacean juices. Paragonimiasis is a public health problem only in countries where dishes prepared with raw crustaceans are eaten or where these animals are used for supposedly medicinal purposes. However, the problem also exists in Japan, where crustaceans are customarily eaten well cooked. The main sources of infection in that country were found to be hands and utensils that were contaminated when crustacean dishes were being prepared.

It is possible that man can also become infected by ingestion of animal meat containing immature parasites, as happened on the island of Kyushu, Japan, with raw meat from wild boars (*Sus scrofa leucomystax*). This hypothesis is reinforced by the fact that carnivores such as tigers and leopards, which feed on animals other than crustaceans, have been found infected, indicating the existence of paratenic hosts (Malek, 1980).

Wars and internal conflicts that force people to migrate and cause a scarcity of the usual protein sources can contribute to a pronounced increase in the prevalence of infection, as evidenced by the disease's history in Japan and Nigeria (see Geographic Distribution and Occurrence).

Transmission is always cyclic, that is, there cannot be direct infection from one definitive host to another. Consequently, the natural cycle can be maintained only where both appropriate intermediate hosts (snails and crustaceans) exist.

Man, domestic animals, and many species of wild animals constitute the reservoir of *Paragonimus* spp. (see Etiology). In endemic areas of eastern Asia, the infection rate in humans is high enough to maintain the cycle of infection through continual fecal contamination of freshwater courses. In these regions, the role of domestic and wild animals, which also serve as definitive hosts, may be of secondary importance. In certain areas of Japan, the mass administration of bithionol to the population was shown to produce a considerable reduction in the rate of infection of the second intermediate host (World Health Organization, 1979). In other parts of Asia, wild animals parasitized by *P. westermani* have been found where there are no known human cases, indicating the existence of a wild cycle independent of the domestic one. Both animals and man are infected by ingesting crustaceans containing metacercariae. In several parts of Asia, Africa, and Latin America, wild animals are more important than man or domestic animals in maintaining the infection cycle. For example, the main natural reservoir of *P. uterobilateralis* is the African civet

Figure 70. Paragonimiasis. Transmission cycle.

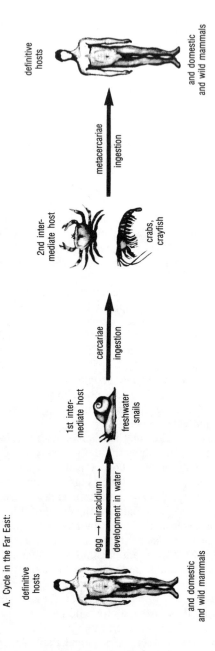

A. Cycle in the Far East:

definitive hosts

and domestic and wild mammals

egg → miracidium → development in water

1st intermediate host
freshwater snails

cercariae ingestion

2nd intermediate host
crabs, crayfish

metacercariae ingestion

definitive hosts

and domestic and wild mammals

Figure 70 (cont.)

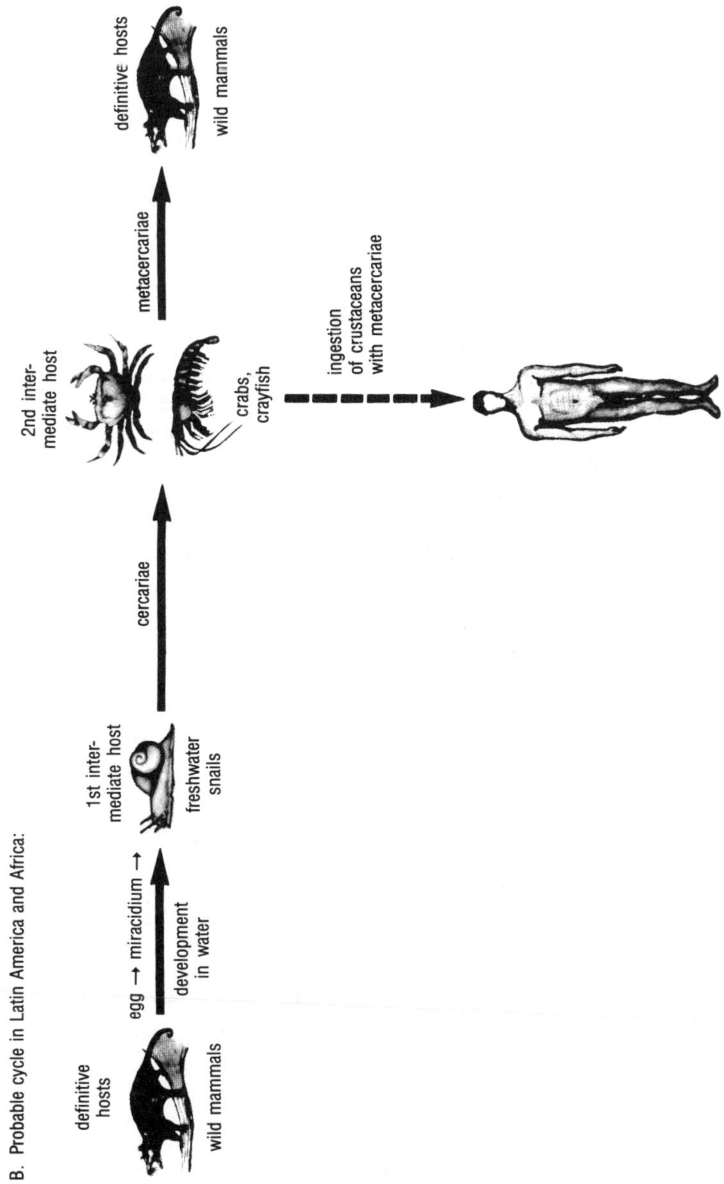

B. Probable cycle in Latin America and Africa:

definitive
hosts

wild mammals

egg → miracidium →

development
in water

1st inter-
mediate host

freshwater
snails

cercariae

2nd inter-
mediate host

crabs,
crayfish

ingestion
of crustaceans
with metacercariae

metacercariae

definitive hosts

wild mammals

(*Viverra civetta*); parasite eggs were found in the feces of 26 of 28 specimens examined (Sachs and Voelker, 1982).

Diagnosis: Radiographic examination is very useful for diagnosis, but interpretation of the results is not always easy in nonendemic areas, where paragonimiasis can be confused with tuberculosis.

Specific diagnosis of pulmonary paragonimiasis is based on identification of eggs found in the sputum or feces. The eggs are reddish brown in color, operculate, and enlarged at the opposite end; *P. westermani* eggs are 80 to 115 microns by 50 to 60 microns; the size varies in other species of *Paragonimus*.

Immunologic diagnosis is made by means of the complement fixation, indirect hemagglutination, precipitation, immunoelectrophoresis, and intradermal tests. Recently, an enzymatic immunoassay test using crude extracts of several species of *Paragonimus* as antigen has been tested in persons with paragonimiasis, as well as in groups infected by other helminths and groups without parasites. The most pronounced cross-reactions were observed with the sera of persons infected by *Fasciola hepatica*. Cross-reactions were not as notable when *P. westermani* antigen was used as compared to antigens of *P. africanus* and other species (Knobloch and Lederer, 1983). Likewise, a very purified antigen has been prepared by means of chromatography techniques; it does not give cross-reactions with other parasites and will allow a more specific diagnosis (World Health Organization, 1979). In Japan, all seropositive persons are treated with bithionol, including those in whose sputum or feces the trematode's eggs are not found. Immunobiologic diagnosis is especially useful in extrapulmonary paragonimiasis. The intradermal test is used in Japan for epidemiologic studies.

Control: In endemic areas, control measures should be directed at interrupting the cycle by the following means: a) education of the people to prevent consumption of raw or undercooked crabs and crayfish; b) mass treatment of the population with bithionol or praziquantel to reduce the reservoir of infection; c) elimination of stray dogs and cats for the same purpose; d) sanitary disposal of expectorations and fecal matter to prevent contamination of rivers; and e) control of snails with molluscicides where feasible.

To be effective, a control program should cover the entire watershed area and adjacent regions.

In Latin America, where the transmission cycle appears to exist predominantly among wildlife and where human cases are sporadic, the only practical control measure is public education regarding the dangers of consuming raw or undercooked crustaceans.

Praziquantel, niclofolan, and menichlopholan are effective drugs in the treatment of paragonimiasis. Recommended doses are 25 mg per kilogram of body weight three times a day (praziquantel) and one dose of 2 mg per kilogram of weight (niclofolan or menichlopholan) (Rim and Chang, 1980).

Bibliography

Alarcon de Noya, B., G. Abreu, and O. Noya G. Pathological and parasitological aspects of the first authochthonous case of human paragonimiasis in Venezuela. *Am J Trop Med Hyg* 34:761-765, 1985.

Alarcon de Noya, B., O. Noya G., J. Torres, and C. Botto. A field study of paragonimiasis in Venezuela. *Am J Trop Med Hyg* 34:766-769, 1985.

Arzube, M. E., and J. Voelker. Uber das Vorkommen menschlicher. Paragonimiasis in Ecuador (1972-1976). *Tropenmed Parasitol* 29:275-277, 1978.

Belding, D. L. *Textbook of Parasitology*, 3rd ed. New York, Appleton-Century-Crofts, 1965.

Borchert, A. *Parasitología veterinaria*. Zaragoza, Acribia, 1964.

Brenes, R. R., M. D. Little, O. Raudales, G. Muñoz, and C. Ponce. Cutaneous paragonimiasis in man in Honduras. *Am J Trop Med Hyg* 32:376-378, 1983.

Bunnang, D., and T. Harinasuta. Opisthorchiasis, Clonorchiasis and Paragonimiasis. *In:* Warren, K. S., and A. A. F. Mahmoud, *Tropical and Geographical Medicine*. New York, McGraw-Hill Book Company, 1984.

Davis, G. M., K. Hatano, T. Shimao, and M. Yokogawa. *X-ray Diagnosis of Paragonimiasis*. Tokyo, Keiso Shuppan Service Center, 1974.

Faust, E. C., P. F. Russell, and R. C. Jung. *Craig and Faust's Clinical Parasitology*, 8th ed. Philadelphia, Lea and Febiger, 1970.

Hu, X. S., R. Y. Feng, Z. R. Zheng, J. Z. Liang, H. X. Wang, and J. H. Lu. Hepatic damage in experimental and clinical paragonimiasis. *Am J Trop Med Hyg* 31:1148-1155, 1982.

Ibañez, N., H. Miranda, E. Fernández, and C. Cuba. *Paragonimus* y paragonimiasis en el norte peruano. Proceso del desarrollo de *Paragonimus peruvianus* Miyazaki, Ibañez y Miranda, 1969, en *Felis cati* L., gato doméstico infectado experimentalmente. *Rev Peru Biol* 1:31-56, 1974.

Knobloch, J., and I. Lederer. Immunodiagnosis of human paragonimiasis by an enzyme immunoassay. *Tropenmed Parasitol* 34:21-23, 1983.

Kum, P. N., and T. C. Nchinda. Pulmonary paragonimiasis in Cameroon. *Trans R Soc Trop Med Hyg* 76:768-772, 1982.

Little, M. D. *Paragonimus caliensis* sp. n. and paragonimiasis in Colombia. *J Parasitol* 54:738-746, 1968.

Malek, E. A. *Snail-transmitted Parasitic Diseases*, vol. 2. Boca Raton, Florida, CRC Press, 1980.

Miranda, H., P. Hernández, H. Montenegro, and F. Alva. Paragonimiasis. Nota sobre tres nuevas áreas de procedencia de portadores de la enfermedad. *Arch Peru Patol Clin* 21:215-222, 1967.

Miyazaki, I. *Paragonimus* and paragonimiasis in Latin American countries. *In: Third International Congress of Parasitology*. Munich, Facta Publications, 1974.

Miyazaki, I. Paragonimiasis. *In:* Hillyer, G. V., and C. E. Hopla (Section Eds.), *CRC Handbook Series in Zoonoses*. Section C, vol. 3. Boca Raton, Florida, CRC Press, 1982.

Nelson, G. S. Paragonimiasis. *In:* Hubbert, W. T., W. F. McCulloch, and P. R. Schnurrenberger (Eds.), *Diseases Transmitted from Animals to Man*, 6th ed. Springfield, Illinois, Thomas, 1975.

Nwokolo, C. Endemic paragonimiasis in Eastern Nigeria. *Trop Geogr Med* 24:138-147, 1972.

Rim, H. J., and Y. S. Chang. Chemotherapeutic effect of niclofolan and praziquantel in the treatment of paragonimiasis. *Korea Univ Med J* 17:113-126, 1980.

Sachs, R., and J. Voelker. Human paragonimiasis caused by *Paragonimus uterobilateralis* in Liberia and Guinea, West Africa. *Tropenmed Parasitol* 33:15-16, 1982.

Thatcher, V. E. *Paragonimus* in some wild and domestic animals of Panama. *Trans Am Microsc Soc* 86:335-336, 1967.

Voelker, J., and C. Nwokolo. Human paragonimiasis in Eastern Nigeria by *Paragonimus uterobilateralis*. *Z Tropenmed Parasitol* 24:323-328, 1973.

Yokogawa, M. *Paragonimus* and paragonimiasis. *Adv Parasitol* 3:99-153, 1965.

Yokogawa, M. *Paragonimus* and paragonimiasis. *Adv Parasitol* 7:375-387, 1969.

Zilmann, U., and J. Voelker. Zur Artcharakterisierung des lungenegels *Paragonimus ecuadoriensis* mit der Isoenzyme-Elektrophorese. *Tropenmed Parasitol* 31:15-20, 1980.

Zilman, U., and R. Sachs. Isoenzymes of South American *Paragonimus peruvianus* and *P. ecuadoriensis*. *Trop Med Parasitol* 37:153-154, 1986.

SCHISTOSOME DERMATITIS

(120.3)

Synonyms: Swimmer's itch or dermatitis, schistosoma cercarial dermatitis, bather's dermatitis.

Etiology: Cercariae (larvae) of avian schistosomes belonging mainly to the genera *Trichobilharzia, Gigantobilharzia, Ornithobilharzia, Microbilharzia,* and *Austrobilharzia;* and those of several species of the mammalian schistosomes *Schistosoma, Schistosomatium, Heterobilharzia,* and *Orientobilharzia.*

Man is an aberrant host for the schistosome parasites of birds and also for some species of the mammalian parasites.

The development cycles of nonhuman and human schistosomes are similar (see "Schistosomiasis"). The eggs of the trematodes, containing miracidia (first stage larvae), reach water with the fecal matter or urine of the definitive host. In the water the miracidium is released and swims in search of an appropriate intermediate host, which is usually a snail belonging to *Lymnaea, Stagnicola, Physa, Planorbis,* or another genus. The miracidia penetrate the hepatopancreas of the mollusks, where they pass through various stages of development and multiplication (sporocysts, rediae); then, after several weeks, cercariae with forked tails are released. The cercariae swim in the water until they find a definitive host; they then penetrate its skin, lose their tail, and turn into schistosomula. These immature schistosomes enter the venous or lymphatic circulation of the normal definitive host (bird or mammal) and travel to the liver where they reach maturity and mate; they then move to an egg-laying site.

The usual definitive hosts for avian schistosome species are wild and domestic ducks and geese, and other migratory waterfowl and birds. The hosts for mammalian schistosomes are bovines, sheep, goats, camels, equines, and swine (*Schistosoma bovis*); bovines (*Schistosoma spindale*); rodents (*Schistosomatium douthitti*); raccoons, several other wild species, and dogs (*Heterobilharzia americana*); and bovines, equines, and camels (*Orientobilharzia turkestanicum*).

In man, who is not the normal host, these parasites do not reach maturity, and the larvae remain in the skin and die.

Geographic Distribution and Occurrence: Swimmer's dermatitis has been described in America, Europe, Asia, Australia, New Zealand, and South Africa. In the Americas, cases have been diagnosed in Canada, the United States (including Hawaii), Mexico, El Salvador, Cuba, Haiti, and Argentina.

The disease occurs in persons who, for recreation (swimming) or occupational reasons, come into contact with contaminated water in rivers, lakes, flooded grounds, irrigation canals, and the ocean near the coast. Fishermen, clam diggers, rice-field workers, and washerwomen are the most exposed groups. In China, Vietnam, Malaysia, and Iran, important outbreaks of dermatitis have been recorded among rice field workers.

Dermatitis can also occur in persons exposed to the common species of human schistosomiasis (*Schistosoma mansoni*, *S. japonicum*, and *S. haematobium*), especially when they visit an endemic area for the first time.

The Disease in Man: Swimmer's dermatitis is basically a defense reaction to an aberrant parasite, which the host almost always successfully destroys but which causes allergic sensitization.

When man is exposed to cercariae for the first time, the symptomatology is mild and may pass unnoticed. Between 10 and 30 minutes after exposure, the affected person feels a transitory itching; macules appear, but vanish in 10 to 24 hours. After 5 to 14 days, small papules appear and are accompanied by temporary itching where the macules had been. The first signs and symptoms correspond to the migration of larvae in the skin. About 30 minutes after penetration, the cercariae are found in the malpighian layer of the epidermis, where they begin to disintegrate. The papules that appear later constitute an allergic reaction to the dead parasite.

The secondary response in individuals sensitized by previous exposures is accelerated and more intense than the primary reaction. The cercariae that have penetrated the epidermis are destroyed in less than 3 days. The symptomatology varies somewhat with the species of schistosome to which the cercariae belong, as well as with the response of the affected individual. Twenty minutes after penetration of the cercariae or when the skin dries, an intense itching may begin and then last an hour or more.

Macules appear along the penetration path of the cercariae; in 10 to 20 hours they are replaced by papules or, in some persons, by marked urticaria. Intense pruritis accompanies the papular eruption, which heals in approximately 1 week unless complicated by a secondary bacterial infection introduced when the affected person scratches with contaminated fingernails.

The Disease in Animals: Schistosomes of wild and domestic fowl, which belong to the subfamily Bilharziellinae, do not greatly compromise the health of their hosts. Growth and digestive disorders have occasionally been attributed to the infection.

The clinical picture of the parasitosis caused by *Schistosoma bovis* in its natural hosts (bovines, sheep, goats) is related to the lesions it causes in the liver, bladder, intestine, and sometimes in the genital organs. In the infection of bovines caused by *S. spindale*, hepatic cirrhosis is the predominant lesion.

Source of Infection and Mode of Transmission (Figure 71): The sources of infection for man are water courses (slow-moving rivers, lakes, irrigation canals) and flooded ground contaminated by avian or mammalian feces containing schistosome eggs; the miracidia develop in aquatic snails and give rise to cercariae. These larvae penetrate the skin of humans who come into contact with contaminated

Figure 71. Schistosome dermatitis. Mode of transmission.

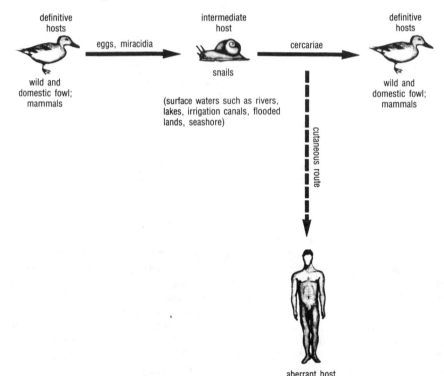

water, but they cannot continue their development in an aberrant host and disintegrate in the epidermis.

Diagnosis: Diagnosis is difficult and is based mainly on epidemiologic antecedents (contact with water that has previously caused cases of dermatitis, occupation of the patient) and clinical symptomatology. Infected mollusks found in the water to which the patient was exposed serve as support for the diagnosis.

In Sardinia, Italy, 34 persons who had suffered from dermatitis caused by cercariae of *S. bovis* were tested by indirect immunofluorescence using an antigen made from formalin-treated cercariae of *S. mansoni*. Of these individuals, 82% gave positive results; all of the controls were negative. Once the dynamics of the test are known, it could be useful in regions where "human" schistosomes do not exist.

Control: Molluscicides can be used in natural freshwater basins, irrigation canals, and rice fields to control the snail population.

In Japan, rice-field workers and other individuals have been protected with copper oleate, which is placed on the skin and allowed to evaporate. Dimethyl phthalate cream can also be used for the same purpose.

Bibliography

Belding, D. L. *Textbook of Parasitology*, 3rd ed. New York, Appleton-Century-Crofts, 1965.

Centers for Disease Control of the USA. Cercarial dermatitis among bathers in California; Katayama syndrome among travelers to Ethiopia. *Morb Mortal Wkly Rep* 31:435-438, 1982.

Faust, E. C., P. C. Beaver, and R. C. Jung. *Animal Agents and Vectors of Human Disease*, 4th ed. Philadelphia, Lea and Febiger, 1975.

Hunter, G. W. Schistosoma cercarial dermatitis and other rare schistosomes that may infect man. *In*: Marcial-Rojas, R. A. (Ed.), *Pathology of Protozoal and Helminthic Diseases*. Baltimore, Maryland, Williams and Wilkins, 1971.

Malek, E. A. *Snail-transmitted Parasitic Diseases*, vol. 1. Boca Raton, Florida, CRC Press, 1980.

Nelson, G. S. Schistosomiasis. *In*: Hubbert, W. T., W. F. McCulloch, and P. R. Schnurrenberger (Eds.), *Diseases Transmitted from Animals to Man*, 6th ed. Springfield, Illinois, Thomas, 1975.

Sadun, E. H., and E. Biocca. Intradermal and fluorescent antibody tests on humans exposed to *Schistosoma bovis* cercariae from Sardinia. *Bull WHO* 27:810-814, 1962.

Sahba, G. H., and E. A. Malek. Dermatitis caused by cercariae of *Orientobilharzia turkestanicum* in the Caspian Sea area of Iran. *Am J Trop Med Hyg* 28:912-913, 1979.

Soulsby, E. J. L. *Textbook of Veterinary Clinical Parasitology*. Oxford, Blackwell, 1965.

Yang, K. L., T. K. Tchou, C. C. T'ang, T. K. Ho, and H. C. Luo. A study on dermatitis in rice farmers. *Chin Med J* 84:144-159, 1965.

SCHISTOSOMIASIS

(120)

Synonyms: Bilharziasis, Katayama syndrome (acute schistosomiasis).

Etiology: The primary agents of human schistosomiasis are the three classic species of blood trematodes: *Schistosoma mansoni, S. japonicum*, and *S. haematobium*. Occasionally, man is invaded by species of *Schistosoma* that parasitize other animals. Because of their close relationship to the classic species, nonhuman schistosomes have been grouped with them into complexes. *S. rodhaini*, a parasite of dogs, cats, and rodents, belongs to the *mansoni* complex; the species *S. margrebowiei*, a parasite of antelopes, bovines, equines, and sheep, belongs to the *japonicum* complex, which also includes *S. mekongi*, a species that infects man and dogs in Kampuchea (Voge *et al.*, 1978); assigned to the *haematobium* complex are the species *S. bovis* (of bovines, camels, goats, sheep, and pigs), *S. mattheei* (of bovines, goats, sheep, rodents, and other animals), *S. leiperi* (of wild animals, buffaloes, goats, bovines, and sheep), and *S. intercalatum* (found in natural infections in domestic and wild ruminants of central Africa). Doubt still exists as to the taxonomic validity of some of these species.

Mixed infections by a "human" and "animal" species occur with some frequency in parts of the Old World. Natural hybridization has been confirmed between *S. mattheei* and *S. haematobium* in patients in eastern Transvaal, South Africa, and between *S. haematobium* and *S. intercalatum* in Cameroon (Wright and Ross, 1980). This hybridization of adult schistosomes in the definitive host of *S. haematobium* has raised doubt about the status of *S. intercalatum* and *S. mattheei* as true species (World Health Organization, 1980).

The different strains of *Schistosoma* vary in their infectivity for snails; and snail species, as well as populations within the species, vary in their susceptibility to the parasite.

Schistosomes live in the vascular system. They are digenetic trematodes with differentiated sexes in the definitive host. The life cycle is similar for each species, although they differ as to their intermediate hosts (species of snails) and the final localization of the adult trematodes in the circulatory system. *S. mansoni* is found primarily in the mesenteric veins that drain the large intestine and especially in the sigmoid branches; *S. japonicum* is found mainly in the mesenteric venules of the small intestine; and *S. haematobium* locates in the plexuses of the vena cava system that drains the bladder, pelvis, and uterus. The eggs are shed mainly with fecal matter in infections caused by *S. mansoni* and *S. japonicum*, and with the urine in the parasitosis caused by *S. haematobium*. The eggs hatch when they reach fresh water, and the released miracidia (larvae) swim in search of suitable intermediate hosts, which for *S. mansoni* and *S. japonicum* are snails of the genera *Biomphalaria* and *Oncomelania*, respectively, and for *S. haematobium* are snail species in the genus *Bulinus*, subgenus *Physopsis* (World Health Organization, 1980). Asexual multiplication in mollusks passes through the stages of mother sporocysts and daughter sporocysts, and ultimately gives rise to cercariae with a forked tail. Approximately 1 month elapses from penetration of the miracidium of *S. mansoni* into a suitable snail to the emergence of cercariae. A single miracidium can give rise to more than 100,000 cercariae. The cercaria pierces the epidermis of a definitive host that enters the water (man or other animal), loses its tail, and becomes a schistosomulum. The schistosomula enter the bloodstream via the lymphatic system and reach the lungs; they remain there for a short time and then localize in the liver, probably through the portal circulation. They reach sexual maturity in the liver, and then mate by means of the male trematode lodging the female in his gynecophoral canal (a longitudinal groove that runs almost the entire length of the male's ventral surface). Finally, traveling against the blood flow, the male carries the female to the venules where oviposition begins. In man, the prepatent period (from the time *S. mansoni* cercariae enter the body until oviposition) is some 40 to 60 days. The eggs are laid in venules close to the intestine (*S. mansoni* and *S. japonicum*) or the urinary bladder (*S. haematobium*) and, by a mechanism that is not yet well understood, they enter the intestine or urinary bladder and are transported outside by the feces or urine, thus reinitiating the cycle.

Geographic Distribution and Occurrence (Maps 13 and 14): Schistosomiasis occurs in 79 developing countries that together have a population of three billion inhabitants, approximately 600 million of whom are at risk of contracting the disease (Mahmoud, 1984). *S. mansoni* has the widest geographic distribution; it is found in 52 countries located in Africa, the eastern Mediterranean, the Caribbean, and South America. *S. mansoni* is the only species known in the Americas.

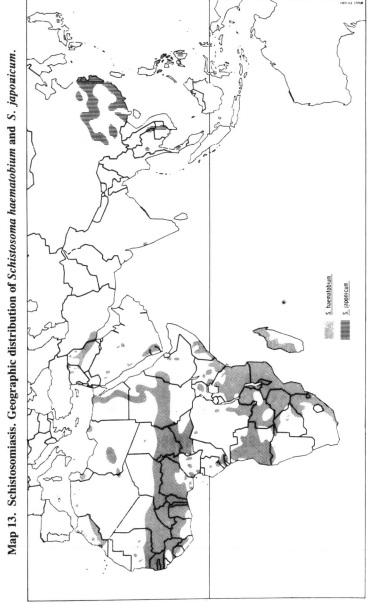

Map 13. Schistosomiasis. Geographic distribution of *Schistosoma haematobium* and *S. japonicum*.

Source: Bull WHO 59(1):117, 1981.

Map 14. Schistosomiasis. Geographic distribution of *Schistosoma mansoni and S. intercalatum.*

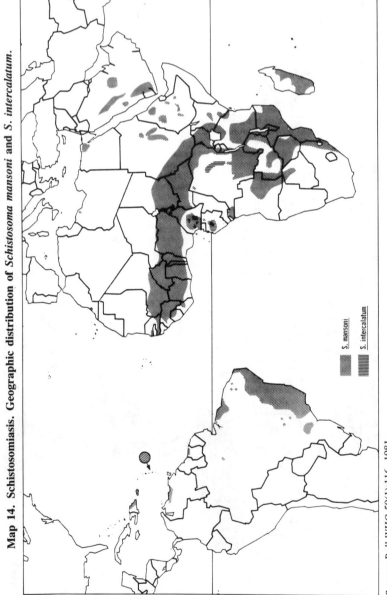

S. mansoni

S. intercalatum

Source: Bull WHO 59(1):116, 1981.

Infection caused by this species occurs in large areas of Brazil (where a hyperendemic region exists in the northeast), in northern and central Venezuela, on the coast of Suriname, in Puerto Rico, in the Dominican Republic, and on several islands of the Lesser Antilles. It is believed that schistosomiasis was introduced to the Americas as a consequence of the slave traffic from Africa. *S. mansoni* infection also occurs in most of the countries of sub-Saharan Africa, and is sympatric with *S. haematobium* in some areas. The Nile Delta is a hyperendemic area of *S. mansoni* infection. Autochthonous cases also occur in Yemen and Saudi Arabia.

S. haematobium, the agent of vesical schistosomiasis, is endemic in 53 countries in Africa, as well as in the Middle East.

The area of distribution of *S. japonicum* is limited to eight countries of Southeast Asia and the western Pacific (China, several small foci in Japan, the Philippines, Indonesia, Malaysia, Thailand, Laos, and Kampuchea).

Infections by *S. bovis* (*haematobium* complex) have been recorded in western and eastern Africa, the Middle East, and on the Mediterranean coast. *S. mattheei* is common in ruminants, solipeds, and baboons of central, southern, and eastern Africa. The eggs of this parasite are frequently found in human feces and urine, with rates of infection as high as 40% (World Health Organization, 1979).

S. intercalatum (*haematobium* complex) is found in jungle areas of central and western Africa. In an endemic population in Cameroon, eggs of this parasite were found in 54.2% of samples of rectal mucus from 500 schoolchildren. *S. rodhaini* is found in Zaire, Uganda, and Kenya; it infects a large number of animal species, including man, but has little importance in public health. *S. margrebowiei* is a parasite of domestic and wild animals in several African countries. It can infect man, but most infections are abortive (do not reach maturity) or spurious. This infection has been recorded after the ingestion of infected liver (World Health Organization, 1979).

According to various estimates, 100 to 300 million people in the world are infected by one or another species of *Schistosoma*. Little information is available on the present prevalence of the infection in the Americas. It is estimated that in Brazil alone there are 8 to 12 million infected persons. During the preparatory phase of the schistosomiasis control program in Brazil, a coproparasitologic study employing Kato's procedure was carried out in six endemic states (Ceará, Rio Grande do Norte, Paraíba, Pernambuco, Alagoas, and Sergipe). Feces samples from 739,995 schoolchildren from 7,900 different towns were examined, 22.8% were positive (Machado, 1982). In some localities of northeastern Minas Gerais, Brazil, 100% of the population was found to be infected. In addition, very high rates occur in the sugar-producing areas of Pernambuco, Alagoas, Sergipe, and Bahia and in some foci in the states of Minas Gerais, Rio Grande do Norte, and Paraíba. In the Caribbean region, the rates per 100,000 inhabitants in 1972 were as follows: Guadeloupe, 39.2; Puerto Rico, 1.3; Dominican Republic, 4.8; and Saint Lucia, 375.7. In the United States, an annual average of 170 cases was recorded between 1969 and 1972. None of the cases were autochthonous, and most were contracted in the Caribbean islands. It is estimated that some 400,000 infected persons currently live in that country, but there is no risk of the parasitosis becoming established because of the absence of specific snails necessary as intermediate hosts (Mahmoud, 1977).

Irrigation projects and population movement have extended the disease's range in some areas. In Brazil, schistosomiasis has spread to the states of São Paulo, Goiás,

Paraná, Santa Catarina, Pará, and Maranhão, where several isolated foci exist, and more recently to southern Minas Gerais (Katz and Carvalho, 1983). In Paraguay, where the disease has not been recorded, the construction of dams on the Paraná River in cooperation with neighboring countries has provided the potential for introducing the infection. A parasitologic survey found more than 100 Brazilian immigrants infected by *S. mansoni*. In the area of Yaciretá, the snail *Biomphalaria tenagophila*, although not yet infected, was found to be capable of serving as intermediate host for *S. mansoni* (Moreno González, 1981).

In Africa, the construction of dams has also contributed greatly to the infection's spread. In different areas of that continent, rates of infection by *S. mansoni* and *S. haematobium* vary from 10 to 80%.

It is estimated that there are close to a million infected persons in Yemen.

Infection by *S. japonicum* in China is localized in and to the south of the Yangtze River valley, an area with a population of 100 million inhabitants who work mainly in the rice fields. Before the control program began, the infected population was estimated at more than 10 million. In Japan, human infection has been reduced markedly on the two islands where foci exist, and only a few hundred carriers are left. An estimated 600,000 people are infected in the Philippines. High rates of infection have been found in two endemic areas on Celebes Island, Indonesia.

S. mansoni infection has been found in recent years in many animal species in Africa and South America. The infection has been confirmed in many species of rodents, other wild mammals, and bovines in Brazil; in baboons, rodents, and dogs in eastern Africa; and in gerbils of the genus *Gerbillus* and Nile rats in Egypt. The rates of infection are often high. In some areas of eastern Africa, more than 50% of baboons have been found infected (World Health Organization, 1979). Natural *S. japonicum* infection has been found in many animal species, and infection rates are high in some areas (see Source of Infection and Mode of Transmission). Rates of infection by *S. haematobium* in animals (nonhuman primates, rodents, swine) are always low (World Health Organization, 1979).

The Disease in Man: The severity of the disease varies with the parasite burden. The majority of infected persons harbor few parasites; it is estimated that less than 10% of those infected have a large number of parasites and suffer a severe, chronic disease of the liver or the urinary tract. School-age children and occupational groups such as fishermen, who enter the water frequently and stay a long time, have more intense infections due to the accumulation of parasites (Warren, 1982). Mild infections are often asymptomatic. The symptomatology of schistosomiasis as it develops is generally divided into four phases. The first phase corresponds to penetration by the cercariae, and is sometimes manifested by dermatitis. The second phase corresponds to invasion by the schistosomula; this stage may pass asymptomatically or may be evidenced by coughing and asthmatiform crises caused by the passage of the parasite through the pulmonary capillaries. The third phase, the acute or toxemic stage, corresponds to the maturation of the parasite and the beginning of oviposition; it is characterized by fever, prostration, anorexia, diarrhea, eosinophilia, and at times discrete hepatosplenomegaly. The fourth, or chronic, phase corresponds to proliferation of the parasites and tissular inflammation caused by egg deposition in different organs. The eggs of the parasite give rise to granulomas and nodules that provoke various disorders, depending on their number and location.

The infection caused by *S. mansoni* primarily gives rise to lesions in the intestinal wall; in time they spread to the liver and produce interlobular fibrosis and portal hypertension, ascites, and splenomegaly. In advanced stages there may be pulmonary lesions and respiratory symptoms. In the chronic phase, the intestinal, hepatointestinal, hepatosplenic, and pulmonary clinical forms can be distinguished.

The disease caused by *S. japonicum* is similar in its symptomatology to that caused by *S. mansoni*, but in general it is more serious. The incubation period is shorter, and the early lesions are located primarily in the small intestine instead of the colon, as in *S. mansoni* infection. The intestinal and hepatic fibrosis develops more rapidly because *S. japonicum* lays more eggs.

In infections caused by *S. haematobium*, the lesions and symptoms mainly involve the urogenital tract and, to a lesser extent, the intestine. Papillomatous folds, pseudoabscesses, and miliary pseudotubercles form in the wall of the bladder; on occasion, there is total fibrosis of this organ. Obstruction of the urethra and of the ureters is common. The main symptoms consist of hematuria and painful and frequent urination. In addition to cystitis, there may be hydronephrosis. The hepatopathies are less serious than in the infection caused by *S. mansoni*. The eggs may also be carried to the intestine, especially to the venules that drain the rectum, and may be eliminated with the feces. Evidence indicates that vesical schistosomiasis predisposes toward malignant tumors because of the continuous mechanical and toxic irritation produced by the eggs.

Acute schistosomiasis, called Katayama syndrome, occurs in primary infections by *S. mansoni* and *S. japonicum*, sometimes in intense secondary infections (those in which the parasite burden is large) by these species, and rarely in primary infections by *S. haematobium*. Symptomatology consists of intermittent fever, cough, lethargy, myalgia, and eosinophilia. This clinical picture can occur with light infections, in contrast to chronic schistosomiasis, which occurs only in heavily parasitized patients (Centers for Disease Control of the USA, 1982).

In human infection caused by *S. mattheei* or *S. intercalatum*, lesions and symptoms are generally mild. In general, *S. mattheei* is found in persons simultaneously infected by *S. mansoni* or *S. haematobium*. The infection caused by *S. intercalatum* occurs primarily in the young and disappears in older age groups as they acquire resistance to the parasite. About 90% of patients infected by *S. intercalatum* complain of intestinal disorders, and about 70% have bloody feces. Hepatomegaly occurs in approximately 50% of the cases, but portal hypertension is not seen. Other species of nonhuman schistosomes, such as *S. bovis*, *S. rodhaini*, and *S. margrebowiei*, produce an abortive infection in man (the parasite does not reach maturity).

The Disease in Animals: In animals infected by different schistosomes, two clinical syndromes are observed: acute intestinal and chronic hepatic. The intestinal syndrome occurs in heavily parasitized animals 7 to 9 weeks after infection, and is manifested by profuse diarrhea or dysentery, dehydration, anorexia, hypoalbuminemia, weight loss, and arrested development. The duration of the disease varies with the number of parasites, and recovery is spontaneous. The hepatic syndrome is considered to be a cell-mediated immune response by the host to the eggs of the parasite in its liver, which leads to granuloma formation, inflammation, fibrosis, and obstruction of the portal venous blood supply. Splenomegaly is frequent. The chronic disease occurs in animals exposed repeatedly to infection with a large number of cercariae, and is characterized mainly by emaciation, anemia, eosinophilia, and hypoalbuminemia. The most pathogenic schistosomes for bovines and sheep are *S. bovis* and *S. japonicum*. Infections by *S. mattheei* and *S. spindale* are cast off spontaneously, and thus the pathogenicity of these species is more limited (Soulsby, 1982).

Following experimental infection of six calves with 30,000 cercariae of *S. mansoni*, lesions similar to those occurring in man and other vertebrates were observed in autopsy. The eggs were viable and produced miracidia that were infective for *Biomphalaria glabrata*. The rate of natural *S. mansoni* infection in bovines in an endemic area of Minas Gerais, Brazil, was low (less than 3%) (Coelho *et al.*, 1982).

In Rwanda, Africa, a serious disease caused by *S. rodhaini* has been described in dogs.

Source of Infection and Mode of Transmission: Schistosomiasis is one of the principal human parasitoses and is very important in public health because of the debilitating effect it has on people throughout large areas of the world. It is likely that the geographic distribution of the disease will increase even more, since the susceptible species of snail live dispersed over a larger area than that in which the human disease is presently found. The opening of new agricultural areas by irrigation projects creates an environment favorable for snail reproduction, and the migration of parasitized individuals provides a source of infection for the mollusks. An example of the influence of environmental changes on the disease is the construction of the Aswan Dam in Egypt. This dam, which has benefited the national economy, has also wrought profound ecologic changes in the region and has favored the increase of populations of mollusks that serve as the intermediate hosts of *S. mansoni*, but not of *S. haematobium*. Before construction of the dam, *S. mansoni* schistosomiasis was common in the Nile Delta, but not very frequent in the region from Cairo to Khartoum (Sudan). The dam reduced the speed of the current of the Lower Nile and trapped the alluvial sediment. These changes favored both penetration of miracidia into snails and human contact with the cercariae that emerge from them. Furthermore, an increase occurred in human activity connected with the Nile, such as fishing and washing of clothes and utensils. All of these factors have contributed to an increased prevalence of schistosomiasis in Upper Egypt. The ecology of Lower Egypt (Nile Delta) also suffered modifications favorable to the parasite's intermediate hosts. The absence of alluvial sediment promoted the growth and spread of aquatic plants and enhanced the microflora that serves as food for snails, resulting in an increase in the snail population and greater possibility for transmission of the parasite to the human host (Malek, 1975).

The situation in Egypt, which has been repeated in several other countries of Africa, Asia, and America, demonstrates that knowledge of ecologic conditions is essential for understanding the changes in the human infection. The growing frequency of large dam construction in developing countries, sometimes without the ecologic and epidemiologic studies needed to establish preventive measures, brings with it the spread and intensification of schistosomiasis.

Snails of the genera *Biomphalaria* and *Bulinus*, intermediate hosts for *S. mansoni* and *S. haematobium*, respectively, are aquatic mollusks that flourish in irrigation canals, lagoons, river backwaters, and small natural pools of water. The relative permanence of the water is important. *Oncomelania*, the intermediate host for *S. japonicum*, is more amphibious and can survive several months in a relatively dry environment, maintaining the larval stages of the parasite. The snails become infected through contamination of the water by fecal matter (or urine in the case of *S. haematobium*) of the definitive hosts, mainly man.

Of the known species of snails in the Americas, only *Biomphalaria glabrata, B. straminea*, and *B. tenagophila* have been found naturally infected by *S. mansoni*; the first is the most efficient intermediate host. The populations of *B. glabrata* and *B. tenagophila* in different regions vary greatly in their susceptibility to infection. In Africa, all described species of *Biomphalaria* seem to be susceptible to some strains of *S. mansoni*. Intermediate hosts for *S. japonicum* are snails of the species *Oncomelania minima* and *O. hupensis*, including several subspecies of the latter. The snails that play a role in the transmission of *S. haematobium* all belong to the genus *Bulinus* (World Health Organization, 1980).

Hybridization between *S. haematobium* and "animal" schistosomes has important repercussions on control. Besides introducing the possibility of an animal reservoir, the hybridization provokes worry because the hybrids of *S. haematobium* and *S. mattheei* show greater infectivity for snails, mature more quickly, and produce more eggs (Wright and Ross, 1980).

Studies carried out in endemic areas have confirmed that the infectivity of most bodies of water is low; less than 5% of snails are infected, and cercariae are dispersed throughout a large volume of water, often with a concentration as low as one per liter of water. Likewise, cercariae do not survive more than a few hours if they do not find a suitable definitive host. These facts indicate that when contact with contaminated water is brief, the resulting human infection will usually be mild and asymptomatic (Warren, 1982). In general, it can be stated that the prevalence and intensity (parasite burden) of the infection depends on the population's or individual's length of exposure to water contaminated with cercariae.

Schistosomiasis is primarily a disease of rural areas. Man, or another definitive host, acquires the infection through the skin by entering contaminated water containing the appropriate mollusks in which the parasite has developed. The most frequently infected individuals are children and young adults (between the ages of 5 and 25), who in addition support the highest number of parasites. In some regions schistosomiasis is primarily a disease of farm laborers who work in irrigated fields (rice, sugarcane) and fishermen who work in fish culture ponds and rivers. Another exposed group is women who wash clothes or utensils along the banks of pools or streams. The infection can also be contracted while bathing, swimming, and playing in the water.

Man is the main definitive host for *S. mansoni* and can maintain the infection independently under favorable ecologic conditions. In the endemic areas of northeastern Brazil, several species of naturally infected wild rodents have been found, and a large proportion of them eliminated viable eggs in their feces. Some of these animals, by virtue of their large population and frequent contact with waterways, can contribute to the spread of the parasitosis. In Pernambuco, 16 (59%) of 27 rats (*Rattus rattus frugivorus*) were infected with *S. mansoni*; 15 of them eliminated viable eggs in their feces. In Alagoas, 737 animals of 12 species (11 rodents and one marsupial) were examined, and 8.5% proved to be infected. Eggs were found in the fecal matter of 79% of the infected rats of various species. In one locality, 54% of the human population was infected, as well as 23% of the rodents. In Minas Gerais, five species of rodents and one of marsupials were found to be naturally infected. Among rodents, *Nectomys squamipes* is of special interest because it is aquatic in its habits and eliminates a large percentage of fertile eggs (68.4%) (Ministry of Health of Brazil, 1968).

In spite of the high prevalence of the infection in rodents and the large proportion of viable eggs that they eliminate, doubt still exists as to whether these animals act as reservoirs for maintaining the parasite. In fact, in some areas of Brazil where the prevalence in humans has been reduced by chemotherapy, the rate of infection in rodents has also decreased.

In South America, the infection has been found in several species of marsupials, an edentate (*Myrmecophaga tridactyla*), and a squirrel monkey (*Saimiri*), in addition to rodents. In a village slaughterhouse in Pernambuco, Brazil, *S. mansoni* was found in four of 23 slaughtered cows; degenerated eggs of the parasite were found in the rectal mucosa of one of them.

In general, natural infection has been found in only a small proportion of African wild rodents, whose parasite loads have been small; thus, there is doubt that they could play any role in the epidemiology of the disease on that continent. By contrast, the infection rate is high among baboons (*Papio doguera* and *P. anubis*). In a national park in Tanzania, these primates (*P. anubis*) were found capable of maintaining the infection for 18 months in the absence of reinfection of snails by human hosts. In addition, the parasite from these primates gave rise to an outbreak (with 15 cases) among persons who visited the reserve and bathed in the river. It is probable that the monkeys originally contracted the infection from water contaminated by feces of parasitized humans; but it is significant that, once infected, the animals were able to maintain the parasitosis among themselves, independently of human hosts, and in turn cause infections in man.

In infections caused by *S. haematobium*, man is the only definitive host and important reservoir. It is thought that the few infections recorded in some primate species of the genera *Papio* and *Cercopithecus* were merely accidental and that the animals do not play any role as reservoirs.

In the infection caused by *S. japonicum*, many animal species in addition to man serve as reservoirs. The human parasite may be the source of infection for animals, and vice versa. In some parts of the Far East, dogs, cats, bovines, equines, swine, sheep, and goats, as well as rats, mice, felines, mustelids, and monkeys, have been found to be naturally infected. In China, natural infection has been found in 29 species of mammals. In some areas, microtine rodents support high parasite loads, and in others, rats are considered quite important in maintaining the infection, especially when the snail population is very low. A study carried out in an endemic area of Leyte Province, Philippines, found the following rates of infection among mammals: 48% in man, 38.2% in cows, 22.7% in rats, 18% in dogs, 13% in pigs, and 1.5% in water buffaloes. Dogs, cattle, and water buffaloes eliminated approximately 10 times more eggs per day than man. It was also found that cattle and goats eliminated the largest number of viable eggs, greatly surpassing humans in that regard. Nevertheless, by taking into consideration the relative numbers of each of these species of mammals (the human population far exceeds the others), the following relative index of transmission was established (% of total): man, 75.7%; dogs, 14.4%; and cows, 5.7%. If the size of each population were not taken into account, cattle (82.2%) and dogs (10.4%) would be more important than man (5.6%) in transmission of the infection.

A noteworthy situation exists in Taiwan, where the infection caused by *S. japonicum* is very widespread among rodents and domestic animals, but where there are no autochthonous human cases. The strain, which easily invades animals, produces an abortive infection in man (the parasite does not reach maturity). Strains distinguished by their adaptation to intermediate and definitive hosts are also found in other regions.

The infection of man by nonhuman schistosomes occasionally results in illness. *S. mattheei* is found in South Africa in mixed infections with *S. haematobium* and *S. mansoni*. The reservoirs of *S. mattheei* are mainly artiodactyls, but it has been pointed out that the parasite is adapting to man and that its importance may increase with the development of the cattle industry. Infection caused by *S. intercalatum*, a parasite of domestic and wild ruminants in central Africa, is spreading; in some villages in Zaire, it appears to have adapted to transmission between humans, independent of animals.

Other species of animal schistosomes only occasionally reach maturity in man, but they may cause dermatitis (see "Schistosome Dermatitis").

A very interesting aspect of infection by schistosomes is cross or heterologous immunity, for which the unsuitable name "zooprophylaxis" has been proposed. In many areas of Africa, man is exposed to cercariae of animal schistosomes, which are often more abundant than those of *S. haematobium* and *S. mansoni* and originate in the same mollusks. Experimental evidence shows that the infections caused by heterologous species confer partial immunity, consisting of attenuation of the severity of the natural disease and resistance against reinfection. Such protection can occur both in man infected with animal strains and in animals infected with human species (*S. mansoni* or *S. haematobium*). This phenomenon would explain why the human disease is less serious in some areas of Africa where the prevalence of animal schistosomiasis is high than it is in areas where the prevalence is lower. It is also believed that the diffusion in Taiwan of the autochthonous strain of *S. japonicum*, which in man produces only an abortive infection, could explain why pathogenic strains of the same species from China or Japan have not been able to establish themselves on that island.

It should be borne in mind that the infections caused by heterologous strains interfere with immunobiologic diagnosis by giving cross-reactions.

Role of Animals in the Epidemiology of the Disease: Man is the main reservoir of *S. haematobium, S. mansoni*, and *S. japonicum*. Domestic and wild animals play an important role as reservoirs only in schistosomiasis caused by *S. japonicum*. This disease can be considered as common to man and animals; the parasite can move freely between species through the intermediate hosts, except in a few situations of physiologic adaptation (geographic strains).

The only reservoir of *S. haematobium* is man; nonhuman primates are accidental hosts.

The role of animals in schistosomiasis caused by *S. mansoni* is more difficult to define. In Latin America, rodents are probably unable to maintain the infection for a lengthy period without the simultaneous existence of a human reservoir, and thus they would act only as temporary hosts. Nevertheless, these animals may contribute to the spread and prevalence of the parasitosis. Observations made in Africa indicate that baboons (*Papio* spp.) can maintain the parasitosis in their population and can give rise to human infections.

Man is an accidental host in infections caused by animal schistosomes, but evidence indicates that some species (*S. intercalatum* and *S. mattheei*) have a tendency to adapt to humans.

Diagnosis: Specific diagnosis is based on demonstrating the presence of eggs in fecal material (for *S. mansoni* and *S. japonicum*) or in both urine and feces (for *S. haematobium*). Nonoperculate eggs are characteristic of each species of human schistosome. Eggs of *S. mansoni* are yellowish brown, measure 110 to 180 microns in length by 40 to 70 microns in width, and have a characteristic lateral spine. The eggs of *S. haematobium* are approximately the same size and have a very pronounced terminal spine, while those of *S. japonicum* are smaller and have a rudimentary subterminal spine. In advanced chronic cases, eggs may be few and difficult to find; thus, if the fecal examination is negative, Kato's thick film method, concentration by formalin-ether or acid-ether, or examination of rectal scrapings (*S. mansoni* and *S. japonicum*) should be tried. The presence of the parasite's eggs is undeniable proof of infection, and examination of feces or urine should always be part of the diagnostic procedure. Proctoscopy may reveal small ulcerations and nodules.

The various immunobiologic tests (complement fixation, precipitation, circumoval radial immuno precipitation, flocculation, hemagglutination, immunofluorescence, and thin layer immunoassay) are useful, but they lack specificity and some lack sensitivity. The circumoval radial immuno precipitation test with fresh eggs of *S. mansoni* has proven very specific (96%) and sensitive (85%) when tried on individuals who were diagnosed by means of a series (three to six) of fecal examinations using the formalin-ether concentration technique. By comparison, the Ouchterlony and ELISA tests were less sensitive (Hillyer *et al.*, 1979). The recently introduced ELISA test has the advantage of allowing determination of the different types of antibodies (IgM, IgE, IgG) produced during the course of the infection, as well as the proportion of antibodies against different parasitic antigens (egg, cercaria, adult) in the acute and chronic disease (Lunde and Ottosen, 1980). Although many serologic methods are currently available, their limited specificity has restricted their wider use in diagnosis and epidemiologic studies (World Health Organization, 1980).

Control: The available control measures consist mainly of a) health education; b) prevention of contamination of bodies of water by human excreta; c) chemotherapy of the affected population; d) ecologic modifications; and e) application of molluscicides to control snails.

All these measures are valuable when realistically incorporated into a control program. Nevertheless, it should be borne in mind that schistosomiasis is mainly a disease of rural areas in developing countries and that the investments possible are necessarily limited. Efforts in public health education must take into account the high rate of illiteracy that persists in rural areas of many developing countries. Environmental sanitation (provision of safe drinking water and sanitary waste disposal) in a rural area involves high costs and, consequently, is difficult to implement quickly and on an adequate scale. The advent of new drugs that are much less toxic, orally administered, and more effective has made chemotherapy one of the principal control measures. This measure has two objectives: 1) to reduce the number of viable eggs eliminated by patients and thus interrupt the transmission of infection to snails and, ultimately, to man, and 2) to prevent the disease in those infected but not yet ill, as well as to allow recovery from reversible lesions in those already ill. Drugs recommended at present are metrifonate for *S. haematobium*, oxamniquine for *S. mansoni*, and praziquantel for all three common species of *Schistosoma*. On the other hand, hicantone and niridazole are no longer recommended because of their toxicity or carcinogenicity.

Clinical studies with praziquantel against *S. mansoni* in Brazil, *S. haematobium* in Zambia, and *S. japonicum* in Japan and the Philippines have given excellent results in both parasitologic cure and reduction of egg elimination (World Health Organization, 1980). In a recent field study in Gezira, Sudan, the "cure" rate was 63 to 96%, and the elimination of eggs was reduced over 95% (Kardaman *et al.*, 1983).

It is not recommended that the whole community be subjected to treatment, but instead that fecal examinations be carried out in the community and treatment given to those infected. In communities with a high prevalence of infection, treatment can be limited, for economic reasons, to the age group with the highest parasite burden, which would be children 7 to 14 years old.

Good results in mollusk control have been obtained in several areas by draining or filling swampy ground, eliminating vegetation in bodies of water, and improving irrigation systems. In Japan, lining irrigation canals with concrete gave excellent results. Control of snails with molluscicides is a fast and effective, although expensive, way to reduce transmission if it is combined with other prevention measures, especially chemotherapy. The cost-benefit relationship is more favorable when the volume of water to be treated is small, but can even be good in rivers and lakes when transmission is focal (limited to relatively small habitats). Selection of the molluscicide to be used depends on the nature of the snail's habitat, the cost of the chemical compound, and its possible harmful effects on fish and other forms of aquatic life. It must be borne in mind that some molluscicides, such as copper sulfate and sodium pentachlorophenate, are absorbed by mud and organic particles or inactivated by sunlight (Warren, 1982). Some compounds, such as niclosamide and N-tritylmorpholene, are active in doses of one part per million or less.

A pilot program carried out in Puerto Rico showed that the snail *Marisa cornuarietis* is useful in the biological control of *Biomphalaria glabrata*, intermediate host of *S. mansoni*. The introduction of that snail, together with chemical control, has almost eliminated *B. glabrata* on the nearby island of Vieques and, consequently, transmission of the parasitosis has been halted. *M. cornuarietis* is routinely used in Puerto Rico for that purpose. However, *M. cornuarietis* is not effective in ecosystems with dense vegetation or in swamps or rivers (World Health Organization, 1980). On Saint Lucia, in the Caribbean, the effect on *B. glabrata* of another snail, *Thiara granifera*, is being studied. In four field trials, *B. glabrata* was apparently eliminated from swampy areas and streams 6 to 22 months after the introduction of *T. granifera*. This snail is originally from Southeast Asia and it is spreading in the Caribbean. A great inconvenience and potential risk associated with *T. granifera* is that it can serve as intermediate host for *Paragonimus westermani* (Prentice, 1983). In Africa, tests using a fish that feeds on snails have given promising results.

Successful experiments have been carried out in the immunization of cattle and sheep against *S. bovis*, of sheep against *S. mattheei*, and of cattle against *S. japonicum* using irradiated homologous cercariae and schistosomula. This success has raised great interest among researchers because of the possible applications to human immunization (Bushara *et al.*, 1978; Bickle *et al.*, 1979; Majid *et al.*, 1980; Hsu *et al.*, 1983). All these experiments and a field study confirmed a great reduction in the parasite load and in the number of eggs eliminated, compared to control groups, when animals were exposed to a field strain. In general, better results have been obtained with highly irradiated cercariae than with less irradiated ones. It has been confirmed that irradiated cercariae only survive 2 to 4 days in the skin of mice and monkeys, and do not migrate to other tissues. Studies also indicate that irradiated schistosomula die in the skin of immunized laboratory animals (Hoffman *et al.*, 1981).

Bibliography

Bickle, Q. D., M. G. Taylor, E. R. James, G. Nelson, M. F. Hussein, B. J. Andrews, A. R. Robinson, and T. F. de C. Marshall. Further observations on immunization of sheep against *Schistosoma mansoni* and *S. bovis* using irradiation-attenuated schistosomula of homologous and heterologous species. *Parasitology* 78:185-193, 1979.

Brown, H. W., and D. L. Belding. *Parasitología Clínica*, 2nd ed. Mexico, Interamericana, 1965.

Burchard, G. D., and P. Kern. Probable hybridization between *S. intercalatum* and *S. haematobium* in western Gabun. *Trop Geogr Med* 37:119-123, 1985.

Bushara, H. O., M. F. Hussein, A. M. Saad, M. G. Taylor, J. D. Dargie, T. F. de C. Marshall, and G. S. Nelson. Immunization of calves against *Schistosoma bovis* using irradiated cercariae or schistosomula of *S. bovis*. *Parasitology* 77:303-311, 1978.

Centers for Disease Control of the USA. Cercarial dermatitis among bathers in California; Katayama syndrome among travelers to Ethiopia. *Morb Mortal Wkly Rep* 31:435-438, 1982.

Cheng, T. C. (Ed.). *Molluscicides in Schistosomiasis Control*. New York, Academic Press, 1974.

Coelho, P. M. Z., R. H. G. Nogueira, W. S. Lima, and M. C. Cunha. *Schistosoma mansoni*: experimental bovine schistosomiasis. *Rev Inst Med Trop S Paulo* 24:374-377, 1982.

Faust, E. C., P. C. Beaver, and R. C. Jung. *Animal Agents and Vectors of Human Disease*, 4th ed. Philadelphia, Lea and Febiger, 1975.

Faust, E. C., P. F. Russell, and R. C. Jung. *Craig and Faust's Clinical Parasitology*, 8th ed. Philadelphia, Lea and Febiger, 1970.

Fenwick, A. Baboons as reservoir hosts of *Schistosoma mansoni*. *Trans R Soc Trop Med Hyg* 63:557-567, 1969.

Hillyer, G. V., E. Ruiz Tiben, W. B. Knight, I. G. de Ríos, and R. P. Pelley. Immunodiagnosis of infection with *Schistosoma mansoni*: comparison of ELISA, radioimmunoassay, and precipitation tests performed with antigens from eggs. *Am J Trop Med Hyg* 28:661-669, 1979.

Hoffman, D. B., S. M. Phillips, and J. A. Cook. Vaccine development for schistosomiasis: report of a workshop. *Am J Trop Med Hyg* 30:1247-1251, 1981.

Hsu, S. Y. L., H. F. Hsu, Shou Tai Xu, Fu Hui Shi, Yi Xun He, W. R. Clarke, and S. C. Johnson. Vaccination against bovine schistosomiasis japonica with highly X-irradiated schistosomula. *Am J Trop Med Hyg* 32:367-370, 1983.

Hunter, G. W. Schistosome cercarial dermatitis and other rare schistosomes that may infect man. *In*: Marcial-Rojas, R. A. (Ed.), *Pathology of Protozoal and Helminthic Diseases*. Baltimore, Maryland, Williams and Wilkins, 1971.

Kardaman, M. W., M. A. Amin, A. Fenwick, A. K. Cheesmond, and H. G. Dixon. A field trial using praziquantel (Biltricide) to treat *Schistosoma mansoni* and *Schistosoma haematobium* in Gezira, Sudan. *Ann Trop Med Parasitol* 77:297-304, 1983.

Katz, N., and O. S. Carvalho. Introdução recente de esquistossomose mansoni no sul do Estado de Minas Gerais, Brasil. *Mem Inst Oswaldo Cruz* 78:281-284, 1983.

Lunde, M. N., and E. A. Ottosen. Enzyme-linked immunosorbent assay (ELISA) for detecting IgM and IgE antibodies in human schistosomiasis. *Am J Trop Med Hyg* 29:82-85, 1980.

Machado, P. H. The Brazilian program for schistosomiasis control, 1975-1979. *Am J Trop Med Hyg* 31:76-80, 1982.

Mahmoud, A. A. F. Schistosomiasis: *In*: Warren, K. S., and A. A. F. Mahmoud (Eds.), *Tropical and Geographical Medicine*, New York, McGraw-Hill Book Company, 1984.

Mahmoud, A. A. F. Schistosomiasis. *N Engl J Med* 297:1329-1331, 1977.

Majid, A. A., H. O. Bushara, A. M. Saad, M. F. Hussein, M. G. Taylor, J. D. Dargie, T. F. de C. Marshall, and G. Nelson. Observations on cattle schistosomiasis in the Sudan, a study in comparative medicine. *Am J Trop Med Hyg* 29:452-455, 1980.

Malek, E. A. Effect of the Aswan high dam on prevalence of schistosomiasis in Egypt. *Trop Geogr Med* 27:359-364, 1975.

Massoud, J., and G. S. Nelson. Studies on heterologous immunity in schistosomiasis 6 Observations on cross-immunity to *Ornithobilharzia turkestanicum, Schistosoma bovis, S. mansoni* and *S. haematobium* in mice, sheep, and cattle in Iran. *Bull WHO* 47:591-600, 1972.

Ministry of Health of Brazil. *Endemias rurais*. Rio de Janeiro, Departamento Nacional de Endemias Rurais, 1968.

Moreno González, F. Hallazgo de portadores de *Schistosoma mansoni* (Sambon, 1907) en el Paraguay. *Rev Parag Microbiol* 16:15-17, 1981.

Nelson, G. S. Schistosomiasis. *In*: Hubbert, W. T., W. F. McCulloch, and P. R. Schnurrenberger (Eds.), *Diseases Transmitted from Animals to Man*, 6th ed. Springfield, Illinois, Thomas, 1975.

Nelson, G. S. Zooprophylaxis with special reference to schistosomiasis and filariasis. *In*: Soulsby, E. J. L. (Ed.), *Parasitic Zoonoses*. New York, Academic Press, 1974.

Prentice, M. A. Displacement of *Biomphalaria glabrata* by the snail *Thiara granifera* in field habitats in St. Lucia, West Indies. *Ann Trop Med Parasitol* 77:51-59, 1983.

Soulsby, E. J. L. *Textbook of Veterinary Clinical Parasitology*. Oxford, Blackwell, 1965.

Soulsby, E. J. L. *Helminths, Arthropods and Protozoa of Domesticated Animals*, 7th ed. Philadelphia, Lea and Febiger. 1982.

Spencer, H., and J. B. Gibson. Schistosomiasis. *In*: Spencer, H. (Ed.), *Tropical Pathology*. New York, Springer Verlag, 1973.

Thomas, J. D. Schistosomiasis and the control of molluscan hosts of human schistosomes with particular reference to possible self-regulatory mechanisms. *Adv Parasitol* 11:307-394, 1973.

van Wijk, H. B., and E. A. Elias. Hepatic and rectal pathology in *Schistosoma intercalatum* infection. *Trop Geogr Med* 27:237-248, 1975.

Voge, M., D. Bruckner, and J. I. Bruce. *Schistosoma mekongi* sp. n. from man and animals, compared with four geographic strains of *Schistosoma japonicum*. *J Parasitol* 64:577-584, 1978.

Warren, K. S. *Schistosomiasis: The Evolution of a Medical Literature*. Cambridge, Massachusetts Institute of Technology, 1973.

Warren, K. S. Selective primary health care: strategies for control of disease in the developing world. I. Schistosomiasis. *Rev Infect Dis* 4:715-726, 1982.

World Health Organization. *Epidemiology and Control of Schistosomiasis*. Report of a WHO Expert Committee. Geneva, WHO, 1967. (Technical Report Series 372.)

World Health Organization. *Joint FAO/WHO Expert Committee on Zoonoses, Third Report*. Geneva, WHO, 1967. (Technical Report Series 378.)

World Health Organization. *Parasitic Zoonoses*. Report of a WHO Expert Committee with the Participation of FAO. Geneva, WHO, 1979. (Technical Report Series 637.)

World Health Organization. *Epidemiology and Control of Schistosomiasis*. Report of a WHO Expert Committee. Geneva, WHO, 1980. (Technical Report Series 643.)

Wright, C. A., and G. S. Ross. Hybrids between *Schistosoma haematobium* and *S. mattheei* and their identification by isoelectric focusing of enzymes. *Trans R Soc Trop Med Hyg* 74:326-332, 1980.

2. Cestodiases

BERTIELLIASIS

(123.9)

Etiology: *Bertiella* (*Bertia*) *studeri* and *B. mucronata*, anoplocephalid cestodes, or tapeworms, whose natural definitive hosts are nonhuman primates. Differentiation of the two species is based on the size of the glandular portion of the vagina, the size of the eggs and their pyriform apparatus, and the number of testes. Some parasitologists think that these differences are not sufficient to separate *B. mucronata* from *B. studeri*, and accept only the latter species name.

The body, or strobila, is 26 to 30 cm long and 1 cm wide. The gravid proglottids (segments) detach in groups of about 20 and are eliminated in the feces of the primates. The intermediate hosts, in which the cysticercoid larvae develop, are oribatid mites of the genera *Achipteria*, *Galumna*, *Scheloribates*, and *Scutovertex*. These oribatid mites are about 500 microns in size; they feed on organic matter in the dirt and become infected by ingesting cestode eggs found in fecal matter. When a primate accidentally ingests mites containing the cysticercoids, the larvae mature into adult cestodes in the primate's intestine.

Geographic Distribution and Occurrence: The parasitosis has been confirmed in many species of Old World nonhuman primates, as well as in *Alouatta*, *Cebus*, and *Callithrix* in South America (Feldman *et al.*, 1983) and green monkeys of African origin on St. Christopher Island in the Lesser Antilles. Parasitologists who accept the validity of the two species attribute infections in the Old World to *B. studeri* and those in the New World (except on St. Christopher) to *B. mucronata*.

The parasitosis rarely occurs in man; some 30 cases have been described worldwide, most of them in Asia. In the Americas, eight cases have been recorded: two in Argentina, two in Brazil, and one each in Paraguay, St. Christopher, Cuba, and the United States.

The Disease in Man and Animals: The infection is usually asymptomatic, but cases with recurrent abdominal pain, vomiting, anorexia, constipation, and intermittent diarrhea have been observed.

The parasitosis is asymptomatic in monkeys.

Source of Infection and Mode of Transmission: Nonhuman primates, which constitute the natural reservoir of the cestode, acquire the parasitosis by ingesting oribatid mites infected with the cysticercoid larvae. Man can become infected accidentally by the same mechanism (ingesting food containing oribatid mites) when in close contact with monkeys kept at home or in zoos.

Diagnosis: Diagnosis is based on microscopic observation of the proglottids eliminated in the feces, or discovery of the entire cestode after the patient has been treated. The eggs possess a characteristic pyriform apparatus.

Control: The disease in man can be prevented by avoiding close contact with monkeys.

Bibliography

Bolbol, A. S. *Bertiella* sp. infection in man in Saudi Arabia. *Ann Trop Med Parasitol* 79:643-644, 1985.

Costa, H. M. de A., L. Correa, and Z. Brener. Novo caso humano de parasitismo por *Bertiella mucronata* (Meyner, 1895), Stiles and Hassal, 1902 (Cestoda-Anoplocephalidae). *Rev Inst Med Trop S Paulo* 9:95-97, 1967.

D'Allesandro, B., P. C. Beaver, and R. M. Pallares. Bertiella infection in man in Paraguay. *Am J Trop Med Hyg* 12:193-198, 1963.

Denegri, G. M. Consideraciones sobre sistemática y distribución geográfica del género *Bertiella* (Cestoda-Anoplocephalidae) en el hombre y en primates no humanos. *Neotrópica* 31(85):55-63.

Faust, E. C., P. F. Russell, and R. C. Jung. *Craig and Faust's Clinical Parasitology*, 8th ed. Philadelphia, Lea and Febiger, 1970.

Feldman, R. E., G. M. Denegri, J. O. Avolio, and N. O. Cantu. Nuevo casos humanos de teniasis por *Bertiella mucronata* (Cestoda-Anoplocephalidae), Meyner 1895, en la Argentina. *Acta Bioquim Clin Lat-Am* (La Plata, Argentina) 17:571-578, 1983.

Richard-Lenoble, D., M. Kombila, M. L. Maganga, and G. Affre. *Bertiella* infection in a Gabon-born girl. *Am J Trop Med Hyg* 35:134, 1986.

Stunkard, H. W., T. Koivastik, and G. R. Healy. Infection of a child in Minnesota by *Bertiella studeri* (Cestoda-Anoplocephalidae). *Am J Trop Med Hyg* 13:402-409, 1964.

Turner, J. A. Other cestode infections. *In*: Hubbert, W. T., W. F. McCulloch, and P. R. Schnurrenberger (Eds.), *Diseases Transmitted from Animals to Man*, 6th ed. Springfield, Illinois, Thomas, 1975.

COENUROSIS

(123.9)

Synonyms: Coenuriasis, vertigo, gid, sturdy.

Etiology: *Coenurus cerebralis*, *C. serialis*, and *C. brauni*, larval stages of the cestodes *Taenia* (*Multiceps*) *multiceps*, *T. serialis*, and *T. brauni*, respectively. The validity of these species within the genus *Multiceps* is questioned by some parasitologists, who attribute the differences between them to factors inherent in the host rather than the parasite.

The definitive hosts, which harbor the tapeworms in their intestine, are domestic dogs and wild canids (coyotes, foxes, jackals). The intermediate hosts of *Taenia multiceps* are domestic herbivores, mainly sheep, in which the larval stage (*Coenurus cerebralis*) is found in the nervous system. The intermediate hosts of *T. serialis* are lagomorphs, especially the domestic rabbit and the hare; the coenurus (*C. serialis*) develops in their connective tissue. For *T. brauni*, the intermediate hosts are wild rodents, and in these animals likewise the coenurus (*C. brauni*) develops in the connective tissue.

The life cycle starts with the expulsion of gravid proglottids or eggs with the feces of the definitive host. Intermediate hosts are infected by ingesting the eggs with grass or water. The oncospheres (embryos) penetrate the wall of the small intestine and, through the blood vessels, are distributed to different tissues and organs. *C. cerebralis* reaches maturity only in the central nervous system, while the coenuri of the other two species develop in connective tissue. The coenurus reaches full development in the brain in 6 to 8 months and can reach a size of 5 cm or more; it forms a cyst that contains a considerable amount of liquid and has a germinal membrane with several hundred scolices. The cycle is completed when a dog or wild canid ingests tissue or an organ containing coenuri. Each coenurus can give rise to numerous tapeworms, which develop in the small intestine of the canids.

Geographic Distribution and Occurrence: *Taenia multiceps* and its larval stage (*C. cerebralis*) occur primarily in temperate climates. About 25 human cases of cerebral coenurosis have been recorded in the world. In the Americas, the disease has been reported only in Brazil, Mexico, and the United States (one case in each of those countries). Coenurosis in domestic herbivores has been observed in Europe, South Africa, New Zealand, and several countries in the Americas. The frequency of animal coenurosis is not well known; a prevalence of 0.78% was found in a study involving 85,300 sheep in an enzootic region of South Africa (Verster, 1966). *C. cerebralis* was diagnosed during autopsy in 182 (3%) of 6,210 sheep in northern Iraq (Karim, 1979). The infection is relatively common in Wales, United Kingdom (Greig and Holmes, 1977). The disease also occurs in small outbreaks, during which a number of sheep will become ill simultaneously.

Taenia serialis and its larval stage (*C. serialis*) have been recorded in Africa, the United States, and France. Human infection is rare; about 10 cases have been recognized, the majority in Africa (Faust *et al.*, 1974). In man the coenuri may invade the connective tissue and central nervous system. The frequency of coenurosis in leporids is not known.

Taenia brauni and its larval stage (*C. brauni*) occur in tropical Africa (central and eastern) and also in South Africa. In central Africa, where this is the only one of the three species found, about 25 human cases of coenurosis in connective tissue have been described, as well as one case with ocular localization. The frequency of coenurosis in wild rodents is not known.

The Disease in Man: The cerebral form is the most serious. Several years may pass between infection and the appearance of symptoms. The symptomatology varies with the neuroanatomic localization of the coenurus. Cerebral coenurosis is manifested by signs of intracranial hypertension, and the disease is very difficult to distinguish clinically from neurocysticercosis or cerebral hydatidosis. Symptoms that may be observed consist of headache, vomiting, paraplegia, hemiplegia, aphasia, and epileptiform seizures. The prognosis is always serious and the only treatment is surgery.

The coenurus can also develop in the vitreous humor and may affect the retina and choroid. The degree of visual damage depends on the size of the coenurus and the extent of the choroidoretinal lesion.

Coenurosis of the connective tissue (*C. brauni*), which is recorded primarily in tropical Africa, is the most benign form. The subcutaneous cysts resemble lipomas or sebaceous cysts.

The Disease in Animals: Cerebral coenurosis occurs primarily in sheep, although it may also occur in cattle, goats, and horses. Two phases can be distinguished in the symptomatology of cerebral coenurosis in sheep. The first phase is associated with the invasion and migration of the parasite. Massive invasion by oncospheres can cause meningoencephalitis and death of the animal. This acute form is not frequent and occurs principally in lambs. The second phase corresponds to the establishment of the coenuri in the cerebral tissue. In general, symptoms are not observed until the coenuri reach significant size and begin to exert pressure on the surrounding nervous tissue. Symptoms vary with the location of the parasite and may include circular movements, incoordination, paralysis, convulsions, excitability, and prostration. Mortality is high. Cranial softening was observed in 42% of 62 sheep with coenurosis (Skerritt and Stallbaumer, 1984). This softening occurs in young animals and those in which the coenuri are situated on the surface of the brain.

Source of Infection and Mode of Transmission (Figure 72): The transmission cycle of infection by *Taenia multiceps* takes place between dogs and domestic herbivores. Man is an accidental host and does not play any role in the epidemiology of the disease. The main factor in maintaining the parasitosis in nature is access by dogs to the brains of dead or slaughtered domestic herbivores that were infected with coenuri.

The transmission cycle of the other two species of *Taenia* depends on predation by dogs on leporids and rodents.

Figure 72. Coenurosis (*Taenia multiceps*). Transmission cycle.

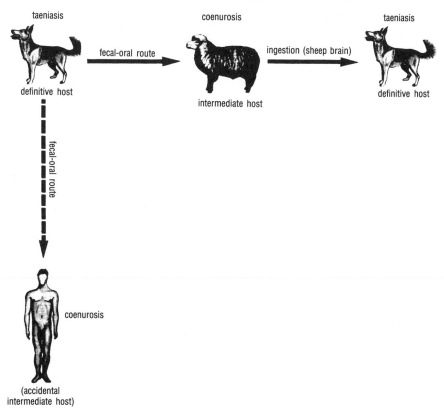

The source of infection for man as well as for the intermediate hosts is tapeworm eggs eliminated with the feces of dogs or other canids.

Diagnosis: Specific diagnosis can be made only by microscopic observation of the coenuri, which have multiple scolices within a single cyst. The coenuri rarely calcify, and thus radiography is not very helpful. Consequently, specific diagnosis is generally carried out following surgery or in autopsies. Immunobiologic tests (intradermal and hemagglutination tests) are of little use in the diagnosis of ovine coenurosis because of the frequency of cross-reactions with other cestodes (Dyson and Linklater, 1979).

Control: The disease in humans can be prevented by practicing good personal hygiene and preventing the contamination of food and water by dog feces.

To prevent coenurosis in domestic herbivores, dogs should be prevented from having access to dead animals and their offal. In enzootic areas, the number of dogs should be reduced and those remaining should be wormed periodically.

Bibliography

Dyson, D. A., and K. A. Linklater. Problems in the diagnosis of acute coenurosis in sheep. *Vet Rec* 104:528-529, 1979.

Euzeby, J. A. Zoonotic cestodes. *In*: Soulsby, E. J. L. (Ed.), *Parasitic Zoonoses*. New York, Academic Press, 1974.

Faust, E. C., P. F. Russell, and R. C. Jung. *Craig and Faust's Clinical Parasitology,* 8th ed. Philadelphia, Lea and Febiger, 1970.

Greig, A., and E. Holmes. Coenurosis in cattle. *Vet Rec* 100:266, 1977.

Jensen, R. *Diseases of Sheep*. Philadelphia, Lea and Febiger, 1974.

Karim, M. A. A survey of coenurosis in northern Iraq. *Trop Anim Health Prod* 11:157-158, 1979.

Lapage, G. *Parasitología veterinaria*. México, Continental, 1971.

Orihel, T. C., F. González, and P. C. Beaver. Coenurus from neck of Texas woman. *Am J Trop Med Hyg* 19:255-257, 1970.

Proctor, N. S. F. Coenurosis. *In*: Marcial-Rojas, R. A. (Ed.), *Pathology of Protozoal and Helminthic Diseases*. Baltimore, Maryland, Williams and Wilkins, 1971.

Skerritt, G. C., and M. F. Stallbaumer. Diagnosis and treatment of coenuriasis (gid) in sheep. *Vet Rec* 115:399-403, 1984.

Soulsby, E. J. L. *Textbook of Veterinary Clinical Parasitology*. Oxford, Blackwell, 1965.

Templeton, A. C. Human coenurus infection. A report of 14 cases from Uganda. *Trans R Soc Trop Med Hyg* 62:251-255, 1968.

Verster, A. Cysticercosis, hydatidosis and coenurosis in the Republic of South Africa. *J S Afr Vet Med Assoc* 37:37-45, 1966.

DIPHYLLOBOTHRIASIS

(123.4)

Etiology: Several species of the genus *Diphyllobothrium* (*Bothriocephalus*). Nomenclature within this genus is still imprecise because little is known as yet about the limits of intraspecific morphologic variations and the factors that cause them. In Alaska alone, six species of *Diphyllobothrium* have been described, five of which were found in man. The species *D. pacificum* has been described on the Pacific coast of South America. The type species, and most important one, is *D. latum*. It is hoped that chemotaxonomic studies of proteins and isozymic profiles can provide the basis for better classification of the diphyllobothriids (Von Bonsdorff, 1977).

The main definitive host of *D. latum* is man, but other mammals that feed on fish (dogs, cats, swine, wild canids and felines, as well as other wild species) can serve as hosts of this cestode. The life cycle of the parasite requires two intermediate hosts: the first of these is a copepod (small, planktonic crustacean) and the second, a freshwater fish from one of several species. The strobilar form, which lives in the intestine of man, dogs, cats, and various wild animals, measures 3 to 10 m and may have 3,000 or more proglottids. The gravid proglottids periodically expel eggs through the uterine pore. A single parasite can shed up to 1 million eggs per day. When eliminated with the host's feces, the eggs contain immature embryos, which must reach freshwater lakes, rivers, or reservoirs to develop further. After approximately 2 weeks in the water, a ciliated oncosphere (embryo), called a coracidium, emerges from the egg. To continue its development, the coracidium must be ingested within about 12 hours by a calanoid or cyclopoid copepod of the genus *Diaptomus* (the Americas), *Eudiaptomus* (Europe and Asia), *Acanthodiaptomus* (Scandinavia, the Alps, the Carpathians, Turkestan, and Tibet), *Arctodiaptomus* (the Urals), *Eurytemora* (North America), *Boeckella* (Australia), or *Cyclops* (Europe, Asia, and North Africa) (Von Bonsdorff, 1977). The coracidium crosses the mesogastrium of the copepod and lodges in the coelomic cavity, where it turns into a procercoid larva. Freshwater fish are infected by feeding on copepods. The larvae lodge in the musculature, gonads, coelom, liver, and other organs of the fish; there they transform into a second larval stage, the plerocercoid (also called "sparganum"). Large predatory fish can become infected with plerocercoids by feeding on smaller fish that contain the second larvae. The most important fish in the transmission of *D. latum* to man are pike (*Esox* spp.), perch (*Perca* spp. and *Stizostedion* spp.), burbot (*Lota* spp.), and acerina (*Acerina cernua*). In Chile, plerocercoids are found in salmonids introduced from Europe—rainbow trout (*Salmo gairdneri*) and brown trout (*Salmo trutta*)—but not found in autochthonous species of fish (Torres, 1982). Similarly, salmon of the genus *Oncorhynchus* are a source of infection in the United States, Japan, and Eurasia (Von Bonsdorff, 1977; Centers for Disease Control of the USA, 1981).

Man is also susceptible to *D. dendriticum*, whose life cycle is similar to that of *D. latum*. The most important definitive hosts of this diphyllobothriid are gulls, but other birds and mammals (dog, cat, rat) can play this role. Unlike *D. latum*, which can persist for many years in the human intestine, *D. dendriticum* is expelled after a few months.

D. pacificum is found on the Pacific coast of the Americas. Its natural definitive hosts are pinnipeds, such as the sea lion *Otaria byronia* (*O. flavescens*) on the Peruvian coast. The first intermediate host, as yet unidentified, would be a marine copepod, and the second, a marine fish (Miranda *et al.*, 1968). *D. pacificum* has been found in other pinnipeds of the family Otariidae along the northern Pacific coast and in fur seals (*Arctocephalus australis*) on San Juan Fernández Island. Plerocercoid larvae of *Diphyllobothrium* spp. have been found off the coast of Peru in the following species of marine fish: croakers (*Sciaena deliciosa*), cocos (*Paralonchurus peruanus*), *Trachinotus paitensis*, and others (Tantaleán, 1975; Escalante and Miranda, 1977).

Human infection due to consumption of marine fish also occurs in Greenland and southwestern Japan. The cestode responsible is *D. cordatum*, whose main definitive hosts are seals. This diphyllobothriid also occurs in dogs.

Human cases have been described in Alaska and in British Columbia, Canada, that were caused by *D. ursi* and resulted from consumption of salmon of the genus *Oncorhynchus*. The main definitive hosts of this diphyllobothriid are the bears *Ursus arctos* and *U. americanus*. Other human cases in Alaska and northeastern Siberia are due to *D. dalliae*, a diphyllobothriid of dogs, foxes, and gulls whose plerocercoids are found in blackfish (*Dallia pectoralis*).

Man and other mammals acquire diphyllobothriasis by eating raw or undercooked fish. In the intestine of man, the plerocercoid develops into an adult cestode in about 3 to 6 weeks; it then begins to release eggs, reinitiating the cycle.

Geographic Distribution and Occurrence: The principal endemic areas of *D. latum* are located in the subarctic and temperate regions of Eurasia. The most appropriate biotopes are lakes, river banks, and reservoirs. The areas of greatest prevalence of the parasitosis are eastern and northeastern Finland, northern Sweden, and northern Norway. Another endemic area is Karelia, Estonia, and the region around Leningrad, where lakes are abundant. Important foci are also found in Siberia. In the rest of Europe and Asia, the infection is also centered around lakes and rivers, but the prevalence is generally lower. In recent decades, the prevalence of the infection has decreased drastically in almost all the Eurasian countries. In Finland, where the prevalence was about 20% in the 1940s, a rate of 1.8% was found in the period 1969-1972. Notwithstanding, it was estimated in 1973 that more than nine million persons were infected worldwide (five million in Europe, four million in Asia, and 0.1 million in the Americas) (Von Bonsdorff, 1977; World Health Organization, 1979). Although *D. latum* could develop in many other biotopes in the world, human infection does not occur where people do not routinely consume raw fish.

D. latum appears to have been introduced into North and South America by European immigrants. In Australia, the cestode has been found only in European immigrants and, apparently, the parasite does not occur naturally in that country (Von Bonsdorff, 1977). In North America, the highest prevalence of diphyllobothriasis is found among Eskimos, with rates between 30 and 80% in some localities. The infection is probably caused by several species of *Diphyllobothrium*. Plerocercoids have been found in several species of fish in the Great Lakes in North America. The infection in man has been described in several areas of the United States and in Montreal and Toronto, Canada. In Chile, 44 cases of human infection by *D. latum* were reported among inhabitants of the endemic southern lake region of the country or in persons who had made extended visits to the region or consumed fish from the area. In northern Chile, between Santiago and Arica, 13 cases of infection by *D. pacificum* were diagnosed; in addition, plerocercoids of *D. dendriticum* were found in fish, and the adult parasite in gulls in the lake region of the south (Torres, 1982). In Peru, human infection is due to *D. pacificum*, which seems to be the most common cestode at present, since 136 of 314 patients diagnosed as having cestodiases between 1962 and 1976 were infected by *D. pacificum* (Lumbreras *et al.*, 1982).

The strobilar form, in addition to being found in humans, can also be found in dogs and cats, as well as wild mammals such as wolves, bears, and foxes. In Alaska, cestodes of the genus *Diphyllobothrium* were found in 57 out of 97 dogs autopsied. Studies carried out in some endemic areas indicate a high prevalence of plerocercoids in fish. The rate varies with the species and age of the fish. In the same body of water, parasites can be found in 100% of the individuals of one fish species, while other species are free of infection.

In Europe and Asia, the most important hosts of plerocercoids are pike (*Esox lucius*), perch (*Perca fluviatilis*), burbot (*Lota lota*), eel, and various salmonid species.

The Disease in Man: Man can harbor one or more parasites. *D. latum* attaches itself to the mucosa of the ileum and less frequently to that of the jejunum. In most cases, the parasitosis is asymptomatic. Some patients who harbor a large number of parasites may suffer mechanical obstruction of the intestine; others may have digestive disorders, debility, and loss of feeling in the extremities. The most serious complication of diphyllobothriasis is megaloblastic anemia, which occurs in approximately 2% of those parasitized. This complication has been observed in several countries, but especially in Finland, and it occurs mainly in individuals with parasites localized in the jejunum. The symptomatology is similar to that of pernicious anemia. It stems from the parasites blocking the absorption of vitamin B_{12} by interfering with its combination with the intrinsic factor (a normal component of the gastric juice), thus resulting in vitamin B_{12} deficiency. Patients frequently manifest slight jaundice, fever, glossitis, edema, hemorrhages, debility, and paresthesia in the legs. Megaloblastic anemia occurs mainly in persons 20 to 40 years old.

The Disease in Animals: Infection by *Diphyllobothrium* is not clinically apparent in dogs and cats. Several epizootics in trout have been described in Great Britain and Ireland; they were caused by infection with a large number of diphyllobothric plerocercoids that may not have been *D. latum*. In general, infection with a small number of larvae causes no major damage, but invasion by a large number of larvae may cause death.

Source of Infection and Mode of Transmission (Figure 73): The cycle of infection is maintained in nature by the contamination of rivers, lakes, and reservoirs by the feces of man and other mammals. Contamination of water with *D. latum* eggs allows the initial infection of copepods and subsequent infection of fish. Man becomes infected by eating fish or its roe or liver raw, lightly salted, or smoked without sufficient heat. An example of the relationship between eating habits and prevalence of the infection is provided by two linguistic groups in eastern and western Finland. While human diphyllobothriasis is common in eastern Finland, where consuming raw fish is an ancestral habit, in the western dialect group where this practice is not followed, infection is infrequent in spite of the existence of

Figure 73. Diphyllobothriasis (*Diphyllobothrium latum*). Transmission cycle.

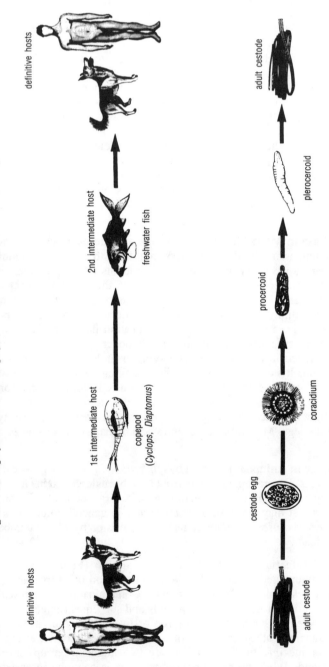

similar ecologic conditions (Von Bonsdorff, 1977). Human infection is not limited to the endemic areas but can be extended by the transport and consumption of infected frozen fish. "Seviche" (a popular dish made of fish with lemon juice, salt, and hot peppers), which is consumed in several countries on the Pacific coast of South America, can be a source of infection for man. The multiple cases of *D. pacificum* infection in Peru are attributed to seviche prepared with marine fish. The Japanese dish sushi, which is also made with raw fish, gave rise to four cases of diphyllobothriasis in California (Centers for Disease Control of the USA, 1981).

Man is the principal definitive host for *D. latum*, but in his absence other mammals can maintain the cycle by similar transmission mechanisms.

Pinnipeds are the main definitive hosts for *D. pacificum*, and gulls for *D. dendriticum*.

There are indications that species of anadromous fish (which migrate annually from the ocean to spawn in fresh water) could serve as a source of infection by various *Diphyllobothrium* species for both land and marine mammals. In this way freshwater fish that feed on anadromous fish could acquire larvae of marine origin, and land mammals could become infected by then eating these fish.

Diagnosis: Specific diagnosis is carried out by identifying the characteristic eggs of the cestode in fecal matter. Concentration of the eggs with formalin-ether sedimentation gives the best results.

Control: Prevention of the disease in man is based on the following: a) educating the population to abstain from eating raw or undercooked fish; b) treating cestode carriers with niclosamide or quinacrine (in Peru, excellent results were obtained by treating patients infected by *D. pacificum* with praziquantel—Lumbreras *et al.*, 1982); c) freezing fish from endemic areas to −10°C for 24 to 48 hours before shipping them to market; and d) controlling contamination of lakes and rivers.

Worming dogs may be useful. Domestic animals should not be fed raw fish.

Bibliography

Baer, J. C., C. H. Miranda, R. W. Fernández, and T. J. Medina. Human diphyllobothriasis in Peru. *Z Parasitenkd* 28:277-289, 1967.

Borchert, A. *Parasitología veterinaria*. Zaragoza, Acribia, 1964.

Centers for Disease Control of the USA. Diphyllobothriasis associated with salmon—United States. *Morb Mortal Wkly Rep* 30:331-332, and 337, 1981.

Escalante, H., and H. Miranda. Larvas plerocercoides de Diphyllobothridae: búsqueda en peces marinos e infección experimental. *In: Cuarto Congreso Peruano de Microbiología y Parasitología*, Abstract 109, 1977.

Escalante, H., and H. Miranda. *Diphyllobothrium pacificum*: hallazgo de larvas plerocercoides en peces marinos del Perú y desarrollo de formas adultas del parásito en *Canis familiaris. Bol Chile Parasitol* 41:7-13, 1986.

Faust, E. C., P. F. Russell, and R. C. Jung. *Craig and Faust's Clinical Parasitology*, 8th ed. Philadelphia, Lea and Febiger, 1970.

Lumbreras, H., A. Terashima, H. Alvarez, R. Tello, and H. Guerra. Single dose treatment with praziquantel (Cesol R. Embay 8440) of human cestodiasis caused by *Diphyllobothrium pacificum. Tropenmed Parasitol* 33:5-7, 1982.

Miranda, H., W. Fernández, and R. Bocanegra. Diphyllobothriasis. Estado actual en el Perú. Descripción de nuevos casos. *Arch Peru Patol Clin* 21:53-70, 1967.

Miranda, H., W. Fernández, and N. Ibañez. Diphyllobothriasis. Investigación de *Diphyllobothrium pacificum* (Nybelin, 1931) Margolis, 1956, en *Otaria byronia* (Sin. *Otaria flavescens*) y en peces marinos. *Arch Peru Patol Clin* 22:9-24, 1968.

Rausch, R. L., and D. K. Hilliard. Studies on the helminthic fauna of Alaska. XLIX. The occurrence of *Diphyllobothrium latum* (Linnaeus, 1758) (Cestoda-Dyphyllobothriidae) in Alaska, with notes on other species. *Can J Zool* 48:1201-1219, 1970.

Rees, G. Pathogenesis of adult cestodes. *Helminthol Abstr* 36:1-23, 1967.

Reyes, H., G. Doren, and E. Inzunza. Teniasis humana. Frecuencia actual de la infección por diferentes especies en Santiago de Chile. *Bol Chile Parasitol* 27:23-29, 1972.

Tantaleán, N. Hallazgo de larvas plerocercoides de Diphyllobothriidae Luhe, 1910 (Cestoda) en peces del mar peruano. *Bol Chile Parasitol* 30:18-20, 1975.

Torres, P. Estado actual de la investigación sobre cestodos del género *Diphyllobothrium* Cobbold en Chile. *Rev Med Chile* 110:463-470, 1982.

Turner, J. A. Other cestode infections. *In*: Hubbert, W. T., W. F. McCulloch, and P. R. Schnurrenberger (Eds.), *Diseases Transmitted from Animals to Man*, 6th ed. Springfield, Illinois, Thomas, 1975.

Vik, R. Diphyllobothriasis. *In*: Marcial-Rojas, R. A. (Ed.), *Pathology of Protozoal and Helminthic Diseases*. Baltimore, Maryland, Williams and Wilkins, 1971.

Von Bonsdorff, B. *Diphyllobothriasis in Man*. London, Academic Press, 1977.

Williams, H. H. Helminth diseases of fish. *Helminthol Abstr* 26:261-295, 1967.

World Health Organization. *Parasitic Zoonoses*. Report of a WHO Expert Committee, with the Participation of FAO. Geneva, WHO, 1979. (Technical Report Series 637.)

DIPYLIDIASIS

(123.8)

Etiology: *Dipylidium caninum*, a cestode 10 to 70 cm long whose definitive hosts are dogs, cats, and some wild felids and canids. The intermediate hosts are mainly dog fleas (*Ctenocephalides canis*) and cat fleas (*C. felis*). The flea of humans (*Pulex irritans*) and the dog louse (*Trichodectes canis*) can occasionally serve as intermediate hosts. The gravid proglottids detach singly or in groups from the strobila (the chain of segments or proglottids that make up the body of the cestode); they are motile and pass to the exterior on their own or with the feces. The proglottids disintegrate in the environment, releasing the eggs, which must be ingested by flea larvae in order to continue their development. The eggs hatch in the intestine of the flea larva, and the embryos (oncospheres) penetrate the coelomic cavity; there they turn into procercoids and, finally, cysticercoids, while the arthropod continues its own development. When a dog or cat ingests an infected flea, the cysticercoid develops into a mature tapeworm in the intestine of the definitive host, and the cycle is reinitiated.

Geographic Distribution: Worldwide.

Occurrence in Man: The literature records some 120 human cases of dipylidiasis worldwide, the majority in Europe and the United States. In Latin America, the disease has been observed in Chile (17 cases), Argentina, Uruguay, Brazil, Venezuela, Guatemala, Mexico, and Puerto Rico.

Occurrence in Animals: *D. caninum* is the most common cestode in dogs, with a high prevalence in almost all parts of the world. The infection rate in cats is much lower.

The Disease in Man: Dipylidiasis affects mainly infants and young children. The symptomatology consists of digestive disorders, such as diarrhea and colic, irritability, erratic appetite, and insomnia. In a series of patients studied in Chile (Belmar, 1963), abdominal distension was almost always seen. Elimination of motile proglottids is the sign usually noticed by the children's parents and is sometimes the only manifestation of the infection. In approximately 25% of the cases, more than one parasite has been found.

Niclosamide (Yomesan) is highly effective in the treatment of this parasitosis.

The Disease in Animals: Dipylidiasis, like other cestodiases of dogs and cats, rarely has clinical manifestations. Migration of gravid proglottids through the anus can produce irritation in that area. Presence of a large number of parasites may cause intestinal disorders of varying intensity.

Source of Infection and Mode of Transmission (Figure 74): The presence of fleas on dogs and cats ensures maintenance of the infection cycle. Man becomes infected accidentally by the same mechanism that results in infection of dogs and cats, that is, by ingesting fleas parasitized by larvae (cysticercoids) of *Dipylidium*.

Figure 74. Dipylidiasis (*Dipylidium caninum*). Transmission cycle.

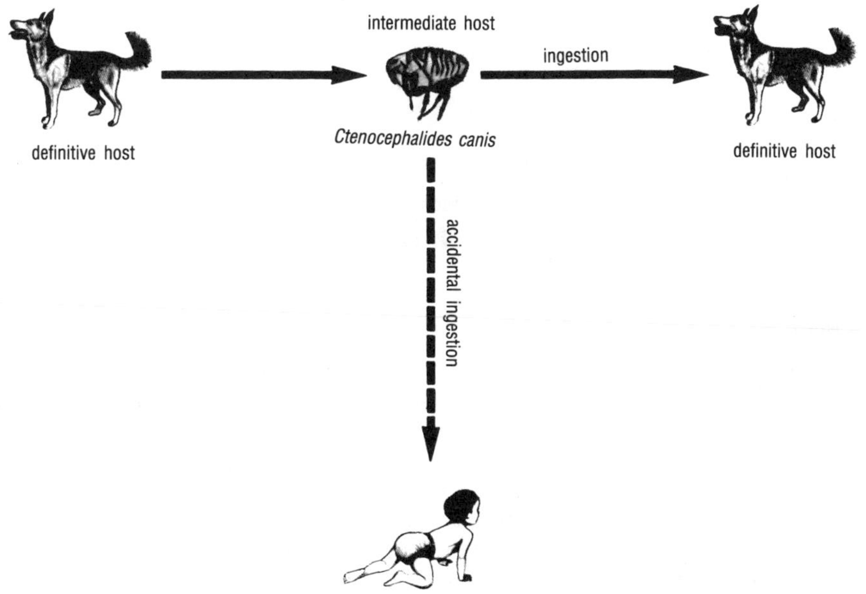

The human infection occurs most frequently in children in close contact with family pets and their ectoparasites. Man appears to be highly resistant to the infection, given the high frequency of the parasitosis in dogs and the relative rarity of the human disease.

Diagnosis: In man and animals, diagnosis is based on microscopic observation of the characteristic gravid proglottids. They resemble melon seeds and have two genital pores, one on each side; the eggs, five to 20 in number, are grouped in uterine capsules (oothecae). Because of their motility, the gravid proglottids attract the attention of parents of infected children; they can frequently be found on diapers. Material collected from the perianal region is more useful than fecal matter for diagnosis.

Control: Control measures consist of combating fleas on pets and administering taeniafuges or taeniacides to the definitive hosts. Rugs and other places in the house that may be infested with fleas should be cleaned and disinfected.

Bibliography

Belmar, R. *Dipylidium caninum* en niños. Comunicación de 13 casos y tratamiento con un derivado de salicilamida. *Bol Chile Parasitol* 18:63-67, 1963.

Faust, E. C., P. F. Russell, and R. C. Jung. *Craig and Faust's Clinical Parasitology*, 8th ed. Philadelphia, Lea and Febiger, 1970.

Soulsby, E. J. L. *Textbook of Veterinary Clinical Parasitology*. Oxford, Blackwell, 1965.

Turner, J. A. Human dipylidiasis (dog tapeworm infection) in the United States. *J Pediatr* 61:763-768, 1962.

HYDATIDOSIS

(122.0 to 122.4) Infection by *E. granulosus*
(122.5 to 122.7) Infection by *E. multilocularis*
(122.9) Others

Synonyms: Echinococcosis, echinococciasis, hydatid disease, hydatid cyst.

Etiology: The larval stage (hydatid) of the cestodes *Echinococcus granulosus*, *E. multilocularis*, *E. oligarthrus*, and *E. vogeli*. These are the only four species that are currently considered taxonomically valid. The taxonomic status of other species and subspecies of *Echinococcus* mentioned in the scientific literature is uncertain.

The definitive hosts of *E. granulosus* are domestic dogs and some wild canids. The adult cestode lives attached to the villi of the mucosa of the definitive host's small intestine, and is 3 to 6 mm long; it has three proglottids, of which only the last is gravid. The gravid proglottid, containing several hundred eggs, detaches from the strobila and disintegrates in the environment. Each egg contains an oncosphere with six hooks (hexacanth embryo), which must be ingested by an intermediate host to continue its development. Intermediate hosts are sheep, bovines, swine, goats, equines, camelids (Asian and American), cervids, and man. The oncosphere is released in the small intestine of the intermediate host, passes through the intestinal wall, and is carried by the bloodstream to various organs, where the larval stage, called the hydatid or hydatid cyst, develops. The most common localizations of these cysts are the liver and lungs, but they may become situated in any other organ. The hydatid cyst or larval form of *E. granulosus* is typically unilocular. The wall of the cyst is made up of two layers: a cuticular, laminated outer layer and a germinative or proligerous inner layer. The interior of the cyst is filled with liquid. Brood capsules or vesicles bud off from the germinative layer, and protoscolices, which constitute the infective agent, develop within them. These capsules either adhere to the cyst wall by means of a peduncle or float freely in the hydatid fluid. A large number of these brood capsules (endogenous daughter capsules) and free protoscolices float inside the hydatid, forming the so-called "hydatid sand." In sheep, the protoscolices form approximately 9 months after the eggs are ingested. The cycle is completed when a dog or other canid ingests the viscera of a sheep or other intermediate host in which there are hydatid cysts containing protoscolices (fertile cysts). The scolex attaches to the wall of the dog's small intestine and develops into an adult cestode that begins to produce infective eggs 47 to 61 days after the hydatid was ingested. A single visceral cyst can give rise to thousands or even tens of thousands of strobilae.

The species *E. granulosus* is polytypic, and morphological, biochemical, and biological variants have been found in different parts of the world. To avoid taxonomic confusion, their designation as "strains" has been proposed (Rausch, 1967) until their taxonomic and epidemiologic situation is completely clarified (World Health Organization, 1979). The situation in Great Britain provides an illustrative example. In this country two strains of *E. granulosus* occur: an equine strain whose development cycle involves horses and dogs, and an ovine strain that circulates between sheep and dogs. In addition to differences in morphology and in intermediate hosts, the two strains also differ in biochemical and physiological characteristics. Even though dogs are definitive hosts for both, it seems that the equine strain is not transmitted to sheep and vice versa. Doubts also exist about the equine strain's infectivity for man. In Latin America—except around Santa Maria, Rio Grande do Sul, Brazil—horses are rarely affected by the larval form of *E. granulosus*, in spite of their close contact with dogs. In the boreal region of the northern hemisphere, the strain of *E. granulosus* whose definitive hosts are wolves and intermediate hosts are the large members of the deer family (*Rangifer* and *Alces*) is transmitted with difficulty to domestic ungulates (Schantz, 1982). In Australia, three strains are distinguished; one circulates between the dingo and macropodid marsupials (wallabies, kangaroos), and the other two (one continental and the other from Tasmania) both develop between dogs and sheep, but differ in some biochemical, morphological, and biological properties (Thompson and Kumaratilake, 1982). Studies in the USSR have shown that the strain circulating between dogs and sheep is not infective for swine, and the strain circulating between dogs and swine is not transmitted to sheep.

The strobilar form of *E. multilocularis* (*E. alveolaris*, *E. sibiricensis*) is even smaller than that of *E. granulosus*, measuring 1.2 to 3.7 mm. The natural definitive hosts are foxes, chiefly the arctic fox (*Alopex lagopus*) and the red fox (*Vulpes vulpes*); the intermediate hosts are wild rodents, primarily species of the genera *Microtus* and *Clethrionomys*. Domestic dogs and cats may also serve as definitive hosts when they enter the cycle by feeding on infected wild rodents. The rodents develop the larval stage (hydatid) in the liver after ingesting eggs deposited with the fecal matter of definitive hosts; in about 60 days, the hydatid contains infective protoscolices. The hydatid has an alveolar, multilocular shape as a result of the continual formation of small, exogenous brood capsules that destroy the surrounding hepatic tissue. When a fox, dog, or cat preys on an infected rodent, the protoscolices it ingests give rise to the development of adult cestodes, and in 33 days the animal begins to eliminate infective eggs in its fecal matter.

The adult form of *E. oligarthrus* is about 2 to 3 mm long and consists of a scolex, an immature proglottid, a mature proglottid, and a terminal gravid proglottid. The definitive hosts are wild felids such as pumas, jaguars, and jaguarundis. The intermediate hosts are wild rodents. Polycystic hydatids have been found in the agouti (*Dasyprocta*) and possibly other rodents. However, some doubts exist as to whether all the infections found in rodents were due to *E. oligarthrus*, since these studies were done before the development cycle of *E. vogeli* was known; some animals could presumably have been infected by the latter species.

The strobilar form of *E. vogeli* is 3.9 to 5.6 mm long and has been found in a wild canid (*Speothos venaticus*). According to some findings (Rausch *et al.*, 1981), the main intermediate host is the paca (*Cuniculus paca*), but low rates of infection by larval forms have also been found in other rodents, including the agouti (*Dasyprocta punctata*) and the spiny rat (*Proechimys* spp.). The larval form in the intermediate hosts primarily affects the liver. The polycystic appearance is characteristic and is caused by the formation of numerous, often interconnected subdivisions produced by the endogenous proliferation of the cystic membranes; each of the multiple cysts gives rise to brood capsules (Rausch *et al.*, 1981).

Geographic Distribution: *E. granulosus* is the most widespread of the species, with areas of high endemicity in southern South America (Peru, Chile, Argentina, Uruguay, and southern Brazil), the Mediterranean coast (especially Greece, Cyprus, Yugoslavia, Rumania, Italy, southern France, Spain, and Portugal), the southern USSR, the Middle East, southwestern Asia (Turkey, Iraq, Iran), northern Africa (Algeria, Morocco, Tunisia), Uganda, Kenya, Australia, and New Zealand. In the latter two countries, the incidence has diminished notably because of control programs.

The distribution of *E. multilocularis* is limited to the northern hemisphere. The parasitosis occurs in central and eastern Europe, the USSR, Turkey, Iraq and northern India, some islands of Japan, several provinces of Canada, Alaska, and several north central states of the United States. The most important endemic areas are the northern tundra of Europe and Asia and its American extension, as well as central Siberia and the Central Asian Republics of the USSR.

E. oligarthrus and *E. vogeli* are present only in South and Central America. Infection by *E. oligarthrus* has been confirmed in animals, but not in man, in Argentina, Brazil, Panama, and Costa Rica. *E. vogeli* occurs in Ecuador, Colombia, Panama, and possibly Venezuela (D'Alessandro *et al.*, 1979).

The infections caused by *E. granulosus* and *E. multilocularis* can coexist in the same area, as they do, for example, in some parts of the USSR, Alaska, and Canada.

Occurrence in Man: The prevalence of classic unilocular hydatidosis caused by *E. granulosus* varies considerably between geographic areas. The highest infection rates are recorded in countries with livestock industries, especially sheep raising. It is essentially a rural infection, although cases also occur in periurban areas.

In human hydatidosis, as in other communicable diseases, a distinction must be made between rates of infection and rates of symptomatic illness.

The most common source of information on the incidence of the disease is hospital records of surgical operations. In Latin America, the highest concentration of cases occurs in the Southern Cone of South America (Chile, Argentina, Uruguay, and southern Brazil) and in the Peruvian sierra. The annual incidence per 100,000 inhabitants of cases involving surgery is approximately 1.0 in Peru, 2.0 in Argentina (1966), 7.8-7.9 in Chile (1969-1970), and about 20 in Uruguay. More recent information from Chile supports the previous data, since 8,028 new cases were diagnosed between 1969 and 1979, for an incidence of more than 7 per 100,000 inhabitants (Ramírez, 1982). However, these data give a false impression of the incidence because they do not pertain specifically to the rural population, where the problem exists, but to the total population of each country. The distribution of cases is very unequal, as is revealed by data from Uruguay, where the number of hospitalized hydatidosis cases per 100,000 inhabitants varies from 5 in the department of Montevideo to 105 in the department of Flores. While the annual rate of incidence in Argentina in 1966 was 2 per 100,000 inhabitants for the country as a whole, that for Neuquén Province was 52.4 in the same year, and that for Río Negro was 143 in 1969. A retrospective study of hospitalized cases in a hyperendemic region of Patagonia (Chubut Province, Argentina) found an annual incidence of between 13.4 and 75.8 new cases per 100,000 inhabitants from 1973 to 1979 (Varela-Díaz *et al.*, 1983). In 1973, the mortality rate per million inhabitants for hydatidosis was 9.6 in Uruguay, 5.8 in Chile, 2.7 in Argentina, and 1 in Peru. In Chile, the highest mortality rate was found among persons 15 to 44 years old.

Studies employing mass photofluorography (miniature-film radiography) of the populations of some countries provide an idea of the overall infection rate. In Uruguay, the Honorary Commission for Tuberculosis Control did five national radiographic surveys and found 30 presumptive hydatid cysts of the thorax per 100,000 inhabitants (in the final study, 78.4% were surgically confirmed). Assuming that for each intrathoracic cyst, four occur at other sites, the total prevalence can be estimated at 150 cysts per 100,000 persons, varying from 50 in the department of Montevideo to 580 in the department of Flores (Purriel *et al.*, 1973).

In Chile, a series of 115,819 autopsies performed between 1947 and 1970 in the Institute of Legal Medicine and in eight hospitals in Santiago uncovered 359 cases of hydatidosis. Of special interest are the 53,014 autopsies of individuals who died violent deaths in Santiago, among whom 108 cases of hydatidosis were found (for a rate of 204 per 100,000 inhabitants). This information is considered indicative of the prevalence of the infection in the country, since 40% of the population of Santiago comes from rural areas. In the cases discovered by this study, 79.4% of the cysts were located in the liver and 19.2% in the lungs (Schenone *et al.*, 1971).

Both the risk of contracting the infection and the risk of dying from hydatidosis increase with age.

New diagnostic techniques, especially the latex agglutination test, now make it possible to do extensive, low cost epidemiologic studies of the prevalence of the infection. With this test, which has high sensitivity and relatively good specificity, a large number of samples can be examined in a short time. For the purpose of eliminating false positive results, the positive sera can be retested with the immunoelectrophoresis test (Varela-Díaz *et al.*, 1976) or, preferably, the arc 5 double diffusion (DD5) test to confirm if they react with antigen 5.

Outside the Southern Cone of South America and the sierra of Peru, hydatidosis does not constitute a public health problem in Latin America. Sporadic cases occur in some countries, and the human disease is not recorded at all in others. In the United States, endemic areas have been found in California (among Basques who are involved in sheep raising and in contact with sheep dogs), Alaska (among Eskimos), and Arizona and New Mexico (among Indians). Similar foci probably exist in Idaho and Utah.

In Asia, the highest prevalences of infection are found in Turkey (300 annual cases), Iraq (more than 500 annual cases), and the southern Soviet Republics. In Africa, the largest centers of infection are located in Kenya and the northwestern part of the continent. The Mediterranean coast of Europe constitutes one of the areas of highest prevalence, comparable only to the Southern Cone of South America. The morbidity rate in Greece is estimated at 7.5 per 100,000 inhabitants; in Cyprus, 18.2 (currently declining); and in Dalmatia, Yugoslavia, 14. Oceania is another area of high prevalence; the morbidity rate in humans in Australia is estimated at 1.2 per 100,000 inhabitants (the rate was 9.3 in Tasmania before the control program was initiated), and in New Zealand, where the rate of infection is clearly declining, at 2.3 per 100,000.

Occurrence of the human infection caused by *E. multilocularis* is sporadic, and endemicity of the disease is low. From 1970 to 1980, 91 cases were diagnosed in France, equaling a prevalence rate comparable to the prevalences in Switzerland and Germany (Houin *et al.*, 1982). Annual incidence from 1965 to 1969 in Switzerland was estimated at 0.14 cases per 100,000 inhabitants. A high prevalence of this infection (1% of the population) was known only on Rebun Island, Japan, before control measures were established.

Up to now, no human infection by *E. oligarthrus* has been confirmed, and it has been demonstrated that the polycystic cases attributed to this parasite were caused by *E. vogeli*. Eight cases have been diagnosed in Colombia, one in Ecuador, and one in Panama, to which another five cases in Ecuador and two in Venezuela can probably be added. It is suspected that polycystic hydatid disease in man caused by *E. vogeli* also occurs in other South and Central American countries (D'Alessandro *et al.*, 1979).

Occurrence in Animals: In all the areas where the prevalence of human infection by *E. granulosus* is high, a similarly high rate of parasitism in both the intermediate and definitive hosts is to be expected. In dogs in endemic areas, infection rates greater than 30% are commonly found, by means of the arecoline test or in necropsy. In sheep, the most important intermediate hosts in many parts of the world, rates of infection are high. The rate of hydatid cysts found in slaughterhouses in hyperendemic areas of Latin America varies from 20 to 95% of sacrificed animals. The highest rates are found in rural slaughterhouses, where older animals are slaughtered. High prevalence rates are also found in cattle, swine, and goats. In Argentina and Uruguay, hydatid cysts have not been found in horses; in Chile, the prevalence in this species is low (0.29%), while in an area of Rio Grande do Sul, Brazil, it is about 20%. According to some parasitologists, the strain that parasitizes horses is a special biotype of *E. granulosus* that has adapted itself to this animal species (see Etiology).

In other parts of the world, such as the Middle East, high rates are found in camels in addition to sheep (intermediate hosts), and in dogs, jackals, and wolves (definitive hosts). Buffaloes are important intermediate hosts in some countries.

The prevalence of the infection caused by *E. multilocularis* in the natural definitive host (fox) can reach levels of 70% or more in some localities; in dogs in Alaska, it is around 6%. In rodents, the intermediate hosts of *E. multilocularis*, the infection rate is relatively low and varies from 2 to 10%.

Little is known of the prevalence of *E. oligarthrus* infection in wild felines (definitive hosts) and rodents (intermediate hosts). Infection by *E. vogeli* was found in 96 of 425 pacas (*Cuniculus paca*), the parasite's main intermediate host, caught in Colombia (Rausch *et al.*, 1981).

The Disease in Man: The cysts of *E. granulosus* may take many years to produce clinical symptoms. Many cysts are asymptomatic throughout the infected individual's life and are only discovered at autopsy, during surgery, or in radiographs taken for other reasons. The symptomatology depends on the location of the cyst and its size. The most common location is the liver, followed by the lungs. There are indications that the localization of the hydatids may depend on the strain of *E. granulosus*. Thus, in the case in wild *E. granulosus* of the boreal region, which circulates naturally between wild cervids and wolves, the lung localization predominates in humans, and the disease is generally more benign than that caused by the *E. granulosus* strain of the domestic cycle. In a small percentage of patients, the cysts localize in other organs or tissue. The hydatid causes an inflammatory reaction in the surrounding tissue, with formation of a fibrous, adventitious, encapsulating membrane. In locations where the growth of the cyst is not restricted by anatomical structures, it can reach a very large size and contain several liters of fluid. Rupture of the cyst presents the greatest danger for the patient and is often fatal, owing to the anaphylactic shock and pulmonary edema caused by rapid absorption of the released antigen. Slow absorption of the hydatid antigen causes the patient to become sensitized and manifest allergic reactions. Another serious consequence of cyst rupture is hydatid seeding within the abdominal or pleural cavity, and the formation of many new cysts. Rupture of a cyst can also cause arterial embolisms in the lungs and sometimes in other organs.

The symptomatology of hydatidosis is mainly a consequence of the pressure that the cyst exerts on the organ in which it is located and on surrounding tissues. In hepatic hydatidosis, most cysts (approximately 75%) are located in the right lobe; they may be situated either deep in the parenchyma or superficially, below Glisson's capsule. The intraparenchymatous cysts cause atrophy of the surrounding tissue and, through pressure on the veins and biliary passages, provoke congestion and biliary stasis, which may be complicated by a secondary infection. A subcapsular cyst may grow upward (anterosuperior cyst) and adhere to the diaphragm (the cyst may even cross the diaphragm and open into the thoracic cavity), or it may grow toward the peritoneal cavity, where it can adhere to and empty into the hollow abdominal viscera.

The second most common location is the lungs. The cyst is generally located in the lower lobe, and more frequently in the right lung than in the left. In the lung, as in the liver, a cyst's presence may be asymptomatic, or it may be manifested by symptoms such as pain in the affected side of the chest (especially if the cyst is peripheral), dry cough, hemoptysis, vomiting if the cyst ruptures, and sometimes deformation of the thorax. Expectoration of the cyst (hydatid vomica) occurs with some frequency and may be followed by recovery.

Bone hydatidosis causes destruction of the trabeculae, necrosis, and spontaneous fracture. This localization is estimated to occur in 1% of the cases.

Hydatidosis of vital organs, such as the central nervous system, heart, and kidneys has a grave prognosis.

The disease caused by *E. multilocularis*, or alveolar hydatidosis, is progressive and malignant. In the vast majority of cases, the multilocular cyst is located in the liver, and more rarely in other organs. In general, the cyst starts as a small vesicle, which, by exogenous and endogenous proliferation of the germinative membrane, forms multiple vesicles in all directions, producing its multilocular appearance. After a time, the center necroses and the cyst becomes a spongy mass consisting of small irregular cavities filled with a gelatinous substance. Metastasis can occur, giving rise to secondary cysts in different organs. The symptomatology is similar to that of a slowly developing mucinoid carcinoma of the liver. Alveolar hydatidosis is afebrile if there is no secondary infection, but causes hepatomegaly and often splenomegaly. In more advanced stages, ascites and jaundice appear as a consequence of intrahepatic portal hypertension. The course of the disease is always slow, and signs and symptoms appear after many years. The average age in a group of 33 cases in Alaskan Eskimos was 53 years, and the investigators (Wilson and Rausch, 1980) estimate that 30 years had passed from the time of infection to the appearance of symptoms. The most common objective signs were hepatomegaly and a palpable abdominal mass derived from the liver. By the time symptoms were apparent, the majority of the patients could not be operated on. The disease is usually fatal.

In the majority of cases of *E. vogeli* polycystic hydatidosis studied by other researchers (D'Alessandro *et al.*, 1979), a tumor-like mass was present in the hepatic region. In contrast to *E. multilocularis*, the cysts produced by *E. vogeli* are relatively large, full of liquid, and the brood capsules and protoscolices are numerous. The polycystic structure is usually visible on the surface of the liver, but it extends inside the parenchyma and sometimes to the biliary ducts. *E. vogeli* seems to be less organ-specific than *E. multilocularis*. Besides the liver, cysts can also be found in the mesenteries, omentum, pericardium, lungs, pleura, and other localizations. Focal necrosis is frequent, but large necrotic cavities are not observed.

To appreciate the importance of hydatidosis in public health, it should be borne in mind that the principal treatment is surgery, hospitalization is lengthy, about 60% of those operated on cannot return to work until about 4 months after leaving the hospital, and 40% are incapacitated for 6 or more months.

The Disease in Animals: Clinical symptoms are not seen in dogs parasitized by the adult form of *E. granulosus*. Infection with a large number of parasites probably causes enteritis. In the domestic intermediate hosts of *E. granulosus*, no definite clinical symptomatology has been found, even in cases of multiple cysts in the liver and lungs.

The most obvious economic losses are caused by the confiscation of viscera with hydatid cysts, especially livers. This procedure used to result in the loss of an estimated 1,500,000 pounds of viscera annually in New Zealand. Losses from confiscation of viscera are appreciable in southern South America. In Uruguay, approximately 60% of all beef livers are confiscated because of hydatidosis and fascioliasis. It has been estimated that the viscera of 2 million cattle and 3.5 million sheep are confiscated every year in the Southern Cone, causing losses estimated at US$6.3 million in Argentina and US$2.5 million in Chile.

The effect of hydatidosis on the production of meat, wool, and milk is not well known. Studies carried out in the USSR indicate that each cow with hydatidosis yields 4 kg less of meat and 2 kg less of fat; additionally, the meat is of poorer quality, all of which reduces the animal's value by 20%. Similar results have been estimated for swine. Chemical analyses have also shown an alteration in the composition of the meat of highly parasitized sheep and swine. The water content increases and the content of proteins, glycogen, lactic acid, and various vitamins decreases. Based on a limited experiment in sheep in Bulgaria, which requires further verification, it was concluded that the yield of wool, the weight of lambs at birth, and lambs' rate of development to maturity are 20 to 30% less in infected versus noninfected animals. However, studies carried out so far do not allow definite conclusions.

The costs of medical and surgical care of human patients must be added to the losses suffered by the livestock economy. Hospitalization is usually lengthy (about 7 weeks). The cost of hospitalization for a surgical case of hydatidosis, without complications, has been estimated to be US$1,500 to 2,000 in Argentina and Chile.

Foxes infected by the strobilar form of *E. multilocularis* do not manifest clinical symptoms, even when harboring an enormous number of parasites in their intestine. On the other hand, infection by the larval form in arvicoline rodents is often fatal when the cystic burden is large (Schantz, 1982).

Source of Infection and Mode of Transmission (Figures 75–79): The dog-sheep-dog cycle is the most important cycle in the endemic areas of the Southern Cone of South America and the Peruvian sierra, as well as in many other areas of the world. Sheep are the most important intermediate host of unilocular hydatidosis (*E. granulosus*) for several reasons: the infection rate is generally high among these animals, 90% or more of their cysts are fertile, they live in close association with dogs, and they are the animal most often slaughtered for household consumption on ranches.

The Southern Cone of South America is a region with a high concentration of sheep. Approximately 50% of the total sheep population lives on 10% of the total land area of the continent. The number of dogs on sheep ranches is high.

Sheep and other intermediate hosts contract hydatidosis by grazing on pastures contaminated with dog feces containing eggs of the cestode. The dogs in turn are infected by ingesting viscera that contain fertile cysts (with viable protoscolices). Man is an intermediate host, but does not play any role in the biological cycle. Nevertheless, he acts as the main agent responsible for perpetuating the infection by feeding dogs, either out of habit or necessity, viscera containing hydatid cysts. The strobilar form of *E. granulosus* can live in a dog's intestine for about a year, but it ceases to produce eggs after 6 to 10 months. Therefore, theoretically the infection would die out if man ceased reinfecting dogs by feeding them raw viscera. Domestic animals that serve as secondary hosts could still become infected for a time, since the eggs of *Echinococcus* are resistant to environmental factors, but the infection cycle would be halted if dogs were prevented access to the viscera of intermediate hosts.

A gravid proglottid of *E. granulosus* contains a very small number of eggs (from 200 to 800) compared to those of other tapeworms, which contain many thousands.

Figure 75. Hydatidosis (*Echinococcus granulosus*). Domestic transmission cycle.

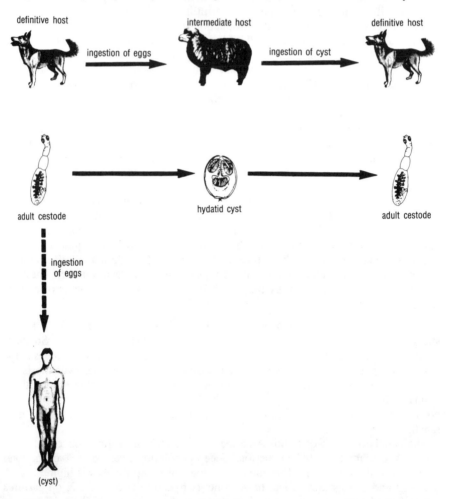

It is estimated that only one segment of *E. granulosus* is eliminated every two weeks (Lawson and Gemmell, 1983). This low biotic potential of *E. granulosus* is compensated for by the high rate of infection among dogs in endemic areas and by the large parasite burden of some of these hosts, two factors that assure contamination of the environment with a large number of eggs. It has also been observed that the eliminated segments can migrate some distance from fecal matter; they crawl over the grass and expel eggs that adhere to the vegetation.

The survival time and dispersion of the eggs have great epidemiologic importance. Eggs have little resistance to desiccation and extreme temperatures. According to the few laboratory studies that have been carried out, eggs of *E. granulosus* can survive in water or damp sand for 3 weeks at 30°C, 225 days at 6°C, and 32 days at 10 to 21°C (Lawson and Gemmell, 1983). After 10 days, radial dispersion up to 80 m from the place the feces were deposited has been confirmed for the eggs of other tapeworm species; they may be able to disperse even greater distances with the aid of mechanical vectors such as carrion birds and arthropods. The physical composition of the soil (its porosity) and the kind of vegetation cover also help determine the length of time that the eggs survive in the environment and are available to the intermediate hosts.

Man is an accidental host—except possibly among the Turkanas, a tribe in northwest Kenya (see below)—who contracts the infection by direct contact with

Figure 76. Hydatidosis *(Echinococcus granulosus).* **Wild transmission cycle and connection to the domestic cycle.**

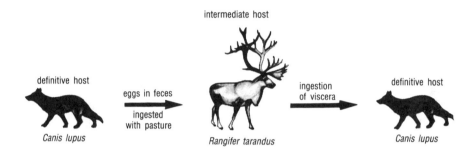

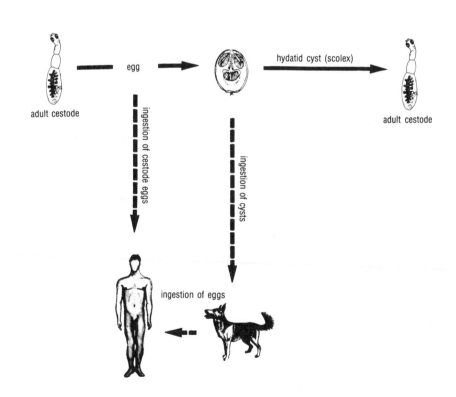

Figure 77. Hydatidosis (*Echinococcus multilocularis*). Transmission cycle.

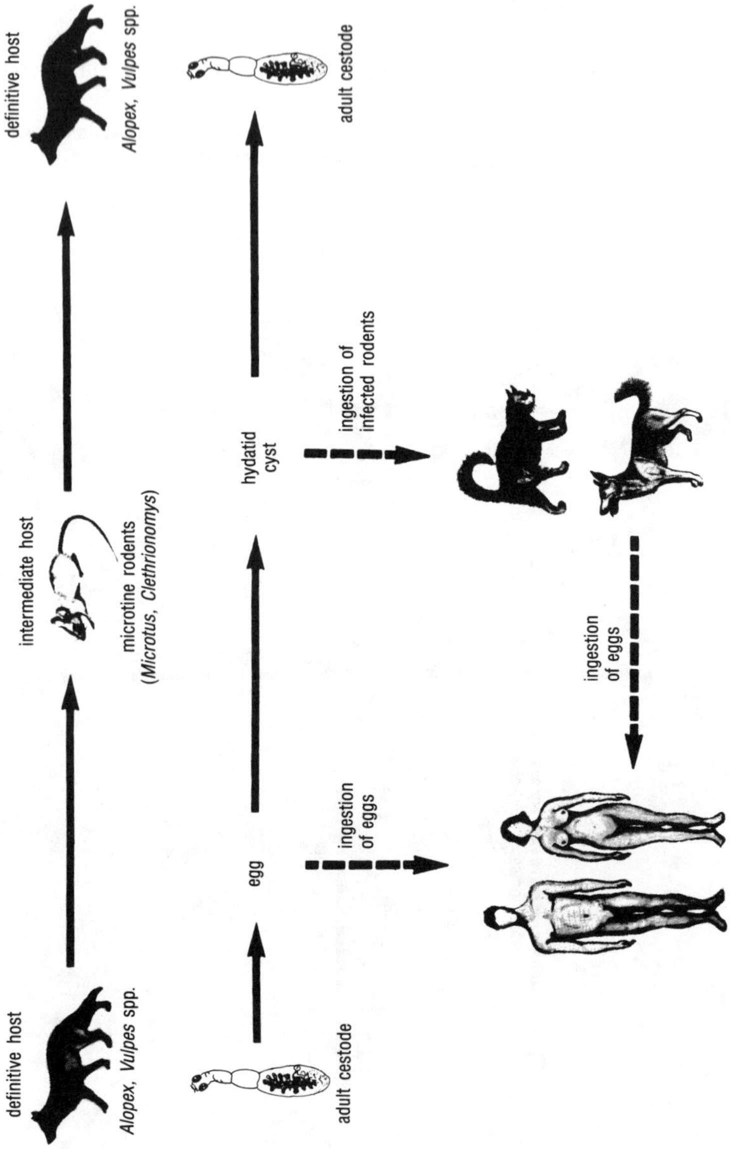

infected dogs, or indirectly through contaminated food, water, and objects. Direct contact is important. The gravid proglottids of *Echinococcus* are found primarily on the surface of fecal matter, and they can accumulate in the perianal region, where they disintegrate and release the eggs. The dog carries the eggs on its tongue and snout to different parts of its body, and a person's hands can become contaminated by touching the animal. Close contact with dogs and deficient personal hygiene practices are important factors in the transmission of the infection from dogs to humans. Another important source of human infection can be vegetables and water contaminated with the parasite's eggs. Coprophagic flies may serve as mechanical vectors of the eggs.

Although hydatidosis is usually an infection of the rural population, cases of the disease can occur in cities when dogs are fed raw viscera containing cysts.

The difference in infection rates between religious and ethnic groups is merely a reflection of their relationship with dogs. In Lebanon, for example, a higher prevalence of hydatidosis has been observed among Christians than among Moslems because the Koran asserts that dogs are "dirty" animals, and thus they are rarely kept as pets.

Figure 78. Hydatidosis (*Echinococcus vogeli*). Probable transmission cycle.

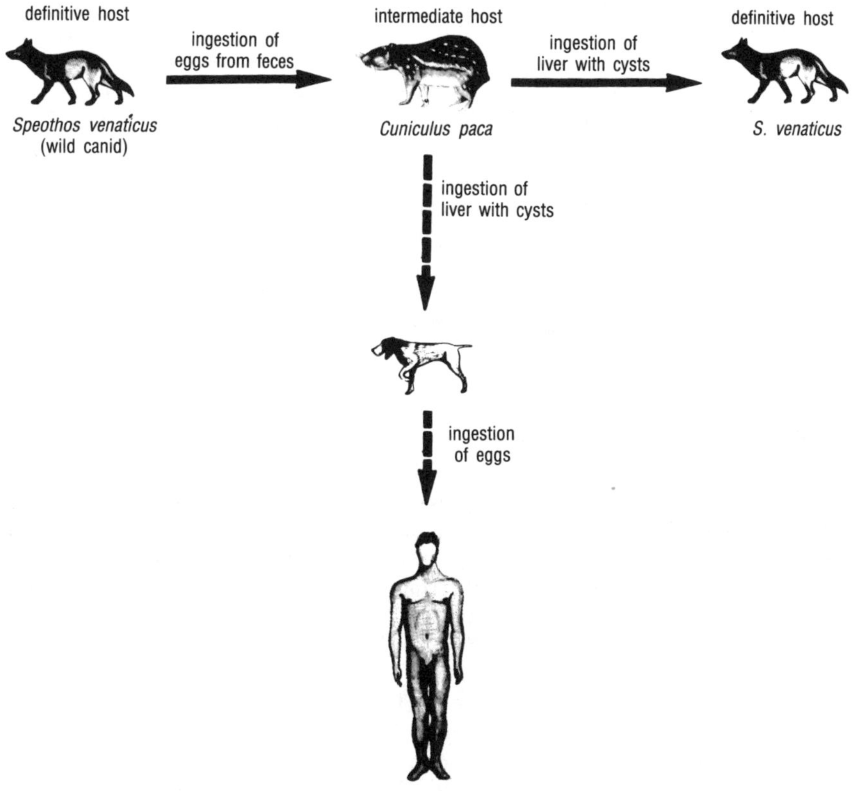

Figure 79. Hydatidosis (*Echinococcus oligarthrus*). Transmission cycle.

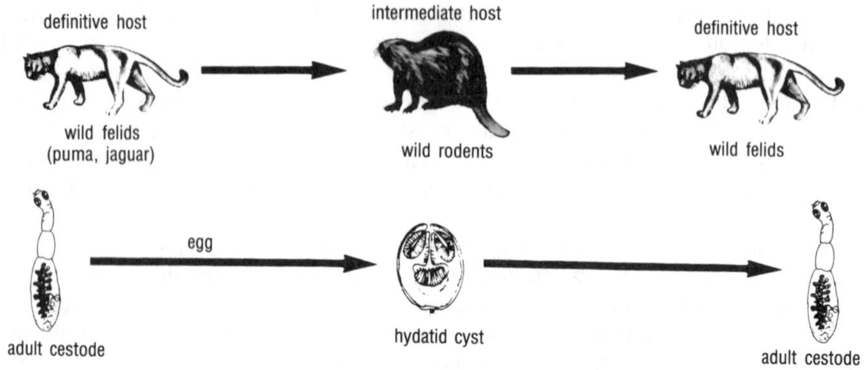

Note: Human cases have not been confirmed.

Long-standing cultural and religious habits account for the high and unusual incidence of hydatidosis among the members of the Turkana tribe of northwest Kenya, which has attracted the attention of researchers. A large number of dogs live with this pastoral tribe of about 150,000 persons, and the dogs have a high rate of infection; dog feces are used as a lubricant and medication. In addition, dead persons are either not buried or are covered with only a thin layer of earth. More than 1,500 tribal members with hydatidosis were operated on between 1965 and 1980; annual incidence, based on hospitalized cases of the disease, varies from 220 per 100,000 inhabitants in the northern part of the district to 18 per 100,000 in the southern part (French and Nelson, 1982). In contrast to findings in 111 patients with pulmonary hydatidosis in Uruguay (Yarzábal and Capron, 1971), whose cysts did not contain protoscolices, 60% of 154 cysts in Turkana patients were fertile and 79% of the larvae viable, comparable in this respect to cysts of camels (intermediate host with the highest rate of infection) and goats. Given the custom of not burying the dead, thereby permitting them to be devoured by dogs and jackals, it is thought (Macpherson, 1983) that man may serve as an intermediate host in the transmission cycle of *E. granulosus* in the Turkana district, which would make this situation unique in the world.

In the Holarctic region of North America (Alaska and Canada), unilocular hydatidosis (*E. granulosus*) exists in a wild cycle that develops between the wolf (*Canis lupus*) as definitive host and several cervid species as intermediate hosts. Another wild cycle independent of the domestic cycle has been described in Australia between dingoes and marsupials (wallabies and kangaroos). The strobilar form of *E. granulosus* has been found in three species of South American foxes of the genus *Dusicyon*, and the larval form in the European hare. In contrast to the disease in the boreal region of the Americas, the wildlife infection in Argentina appears to derive from the domestic cycle.

Alveolar hydatidosis (*E. multilocularis*) has many natural foci in the northern hemisphere; the parasite circulates between foxes of the genera *Alopex* and *Vulpes*, the definitive hosts, and arvicoline and microtine rodents. Man can come into accidental contact with the eggs of the cestode when skinning foxes. The major risk for humans occurs when domestic cats or dogs begin to prey on wild rodents; the eggs of *E. multilocularis* in the fecal matter of dogs and cats then provide the major source of infection for man. A community in which microtine rodents and dogs abound can become a hyperendemic focus, as has happened in some Eskimo villages of the North American boreal tundra. Contaminated food and water can serve as a source of infection, and coprophagous flies can act as mechanical transfer hosts of the eggs.

A study carried out in the mountainous region of Auvergne, France, found the infection in 23 (2.4%) out of 943 adult specimens of an intermediate host (*Arvicola terrestris scherman*). In the seven communes where the rodents were captured, prevalence varied from 0 to 4.65%, which indicates that the infection is focal in character. Only two (8.7%) of the 23 animals had fertile larvae. In the same region, 8.5% of 70 foxes (*Vulpes vulpes*) harbored the strobilar form, and five human cases occurred in 10 years, leading to the conclusion that the risk of human infection does exist, but is low (Pétavy and Deblock, 1983).

The cycles of *E. vogeli* and *E. oligarthrus* are exclusively sylvatic. Human cases caused by the former have been confirmed, but none by the latter. Man becomes infected accidentally by eggs of *E. vogeli*. The eggs probably reach the human environment through feces of dogs that are fed the viscera of the paca (*Cuniculus paca*) during hunts for this rodent, whose meat is very popular in some localities (D'Alessandro *et al.*, 1979).

Role of Animals in the Epidemiology of the Disease: With the possible exception of the situation in the Turkana district of Kenya (see above), hydatidosis is strictly a zoonosis. Man contracts the infection from canids; transmission is always cyclical, and neither interhuman transmission nor transmission from one intermediate host to another can occur.

Diagnosis: Radiography, computerized tomography, ultrasonography, and scintigraphy are very useful in the diagnosis of human hydatidosis. Specific diagnosis in man can be made by means of serologic tests or by identifying the larval stage of the parasite removed by surgery, which constitutes definitive proof.

Numerous immunobiologic tests have been used in the diagnosis of human hydatidosis by *E. granulosus*, among them Casoni's intradermal test, complement fixation, indirect hemagglutination, latex agglutination, immunoelectrophoresis, electrosyneresis, double diffusion to detect antibodies against antigen 5 (DD5), and, more recently, ELISA. Serologic tests are very valuable for diagnosis, but none is sensitive enough to discover all cases or specific enough not to give some cross-reactions with other parasitic diseases. Results of all the tests vary according to the location of the cyst and its physiopathologic state; all immunodiagnostic tests are less sensitive for detecting pulmonary than hepatic hydatidosis. The positivity rate also varies with the state of the cyst; hyaline cysts stimulate the immune system to a lesser degree than altered or recently broken cysts, thus inducing lower antibody levels and consequently a less marked response to the tests.

The most specific tests are immunoelectrophoresis and double diffusion based on the same principle (arc 5); the latter is preferable for its greater sensitivity (Coltorti and Varela-Díaz, 1978). The positivity criterion for this test is the formation of a characteristic precipitation band, called arc 5. Until recently, it was believed that tests based on reactivity to antigen 5 were species-specific, but cross-reactions have been found to occur with sera of patients infected by *E. multilocularis* and *E. vogeli*

(Varela-Díaz et al., 1977; Varela-Díaz et al., 1978); however, this fact does not affect diagnosis of generic hydatidosis. Likewise, it was found that these tests can give cross-reactions with sera from patients affected by multiple cysticercosis (Varela-Díaz et al., 1978; Schantz et al., 1980). The sensitivity of the double diffusion (DD5) test is generally between 50 and 75%, depending on the state of the cysts (hyaline or altered). Because of this low sensitivity, a negative result does not rule out the possibility of infection. In a study of a series of patients with a high proportion of hyaline cysts, the sensitivity was found to be only 51.6% in patients with intrathoracic hydatidosis and 46.3% in patients with hepatic hydatidosis. In spite of its low sensitivity, the advantage of the test is its high specificity; for example, in 1,539 patients who had a presumptive diagnosis of hydatidosis and who were in reality affected by three other diseases, the test gave negative results (Varela-Díaz and Coltorti, 1984).

The latex agglutination test is the simplest, fastest, and most economical. The sensitivity of this test is high and the specificity is relatively good (the rate of false positives is low). The latex test lends itself to screening large numbers of samples and is especially appropriate for seroepidemiologic studies (see Occurrence in Man). The indirect hemagglutination test is used worldwide, but with various techniques. Cross-reactions make it necessary to determine the diagnostic titer of the test for each region; for that purpose, hydatid disease samples must be compared to samples from other parasitic and nonparasitic diseases.

The complement fixation test is not very specific and has been practically abandoned. Reactivity to this test in patients who have undergone surgery disappears rapidly if no other cysts are present in the body, an advantage in the follow-up observation of these patients. Currently, this surveillance can be done better with the DD5 test.

In recent times, the ELISA test has become widely used for many communicable diseases and has been very useful in the diagnosis of various parasitoses. However, its usefulness for diagnosing hydatidosis is still being evaluated. According to some authors, ELISA does not have any advantages over classic tests, while others consider it more sensitive and specific (Ricard, 1979; Iacona et al., 1980; Guisantes et al., 1981). This test also makes it possible to measure different types of antibodies (IgM, IgG, IgE, and IgA), which justifies making every effort to standardize and evaluate it.

The M, G, and E immunoglobulins are present during active infection; M and E disappear soon after the cyst has been removed unbroken, while IgG persists for several years (Schantz, 1982).

The other species of Echinococcus share common antigens with E. granulosus and can be diagnosed with the same tests. However, the length of time it takes after infection for sera from patients with E. multilocularis to turn reactive is not known.

The techniques for performing the different serologic tests and the diagnostic criteria can be found in two documents produced by the Pan American Zoonoses Center of the Pan American Health Organization (Varela-Díaz and Coltorti, 1974; Pan American Zoonoses Center, 1979).

Casoni's intradermal test is still commonly used for diagnosing human hydatidosis; however, it has been shown that this allergenic test is not very reliable because of its marked lack of specificity.

While notable progress has been made in recent years in the immunodiagnosis of human hydatidosis, the same is not true for animal hydatidosis. None of the known serologic tests give reliable results in intermediate hosts other than man. In general, the tests in animals lack sensitivity or give a high rate of unspecific reactions. Postmortem examination of food animals in slaughterhouses and packing plants remains the only method for diagnosing hydatidosis in these species.

Intestinal echinococcosis in dogs can be diagnosed by administering arecoline hydrobromide and searching for the parasite in the feces. The maximum effectiveness of arecoline as a diagnostic tool is about 65%, if both the feces and vomit of treated dogs are examined. A negative diagnosis in a single dog is meaningless. The arecoline test should be reserved for diagnosing the infection in a group of dogs kept on a ranch, to find out if the owner is complying with sanitary rules.

Control: Control measures are directed at interrupting the transmission cycle at its most vulnerable point, that is, transmission from the intermediate to the definitive host. In theory, this measure should be very easy to accomplish and would consist of simply preventing dogs from eating the viscera of infected animals. However, such a measure requires a high degree of conscientiousness and responsibility on the part of rural inhabitants, which is difficult to achieve under present socioeconomic conditions in developing countries.

Conventional control measures consist of educating the rural population, centralizing the slaughtering of animals, ensuring sanitary conditions for slaughtering done on ranches, preventing dogs' access to raw viscera, registering dogs and reducing their number, and treating dogs with anthelmintics. These measures have given excellent results in various parts of the world. The infection has been eradicated in Iceland, and New Zealand and Tasmania have succeeded in markedly reducing prevalence rates in the definitive host, humans, and cattle. In these countries, the primary factors in the success of the control programs have been health education and a highly motivated population; even before control measures were established, health education had succeeded in notably reducing the problem. The main objective of these programs was to develop an understanding of the problem and a sense of responsibility in the rural community; a secondary measure was the administration of anthelmintics. By means of the program in Tasmania, the infection rate in dogs was reduced from 12.6% in 1965-1966 to 0.09% in 1981-1982, and the rate in sheep from 52.2% in 1966-1967 to 0.7% in 1981-1982. New cases of hydatidosis in man were reduced from 19 in 1966 to four in 1982, and the disease has practically disappeared in children and young adults (Tasmanian Hydatid Disease Newsletter, 1983). Great progress in the fight against hydatidosis has also been achieved in Cyprus by the application of classic control measures. The program in Cyprus is characterized by its special emphasis on reducing the dog population. Of an estimated 45,000 dogs, 30,000 were sacrificed in 2 years, and a large number of the females were sterilized. The remaining dogs are examined three or four times a year, and the infection rate has been reduced by more than 80%. The infection has been practically eliminated in food animals born after the start of the program (Polydorou, 1977).

The development of new drugs, of which praziquantel is the most effective, may make it possible to speed up control programs by means of systematic and repeated administration of these drugs to dogs in the prepatent period; the drugs must be given at sufficiently short intervals to prevent proglottids from developing to the gravid state and eliminating eggs to the external environment. The appropriate interval between doses is 6 weeks. It must be borne in mind, however, that praziquantel is not an ovicide (Thakur *et al.*, 1979a), and that at the beginning of such a control program there may be a massive elimination of cestode eggs. One way of avoiding the increase in eggs in the environment is to administer praziquantel and arecoline hydrobromide simultaneously, in addition to destroying eggs in feces (Thakur *et al.*, 1979b).

In Latin America and other developing areas where socioeconomic and cultural conditions differ from those in Iceland, New Zealand, and Tasmania, the relative effect of each of the known control procedures must be evaluated under prevailing field conditions and, where possible, adapted to the environment, or new procedures must be found. Regional programs for control of hydatidosis are being carried out in four Latin American countries: Uruguay, Argentina, Chile, and Peru. Programs have been organized in several provinces in Argentina. In the southern province of Neuquén, where treatment of dogs with praziquantel is used in conjunction with other measures, prevalence in domestic animals has been reduced, as has the annual incidence of new human cases, especially in children. A program was started in 1979 in the extreme south of Chile, the area of the country with the greatest concentration of sheep; praziquantel is administered to dogs every 45 days, and a rapid decrease of infection has been achieved in both dogs and lambs (Pan American Health Organization, 1983).

Currently, immunogenic products are not available to prevent infection in animals, but work is being carried out in this field and the results obtained have been encouraging. In a recent study, a group of lambs was inoculated with antigens secreted by oncospheres activated in a culture medium. The medium containing the antigens was later concentrated and emulsified with Freund's incomplete adjuvant, and was administered in two doses at a 6-week interval to eight lambs. Seven of these eight lambs completely resisted infection when exposed to 1,300 eggs of *E. granulosus* (Osborn and Heath, 1982). It has also been confirmed that treatment of sheep with mebendazole for 3 months can both damage the cysts and render the protoscolices of these cysts noninfective for dogs (Gemmell *et al.*, 1981).

For individual protection of humans, close contact with dogs should be avoided and correct personal and food hygiene maintained. Early diagnosis in man is important to avoid complications and to prevent rupture of the cyst, with the consequent seeding to multiple localizations. In cases that are no longer operable, prolonged treatment (for several years) with mebendazole is now used and in several incidences has produced regression of the cysts.

Control of the wild cycles of *E. multilocularis* and *E. vogeli* presents practically insolvable problems, as is the case with other diseases transmitted by wild animals.

More details about surveillance, prevention, and control of hydatidosis can be found in a guide prepared specifically on those subjects (Eckert *et al.*, 1981; World Health Organization, 1984.)

Bibliography

Araujo, F. P., C. W. Schwabe, J. C. Sawyer, and W. F. Davis. Hydatid disease transmission in California. A study of the Basque connection. *Am J Epidemiol* 102:291-302, 1975.

Belding, D. L. *Textbook of Parasitology*, 3rd ed. New York, Appleton-Century-Crofts, 1965.

Blood, B. D., and J. L. Lelijveld. Studies on sylvatic echinococcosis in southern South America. *Z Tropenmed Parasitol* 20:475-482, 1969.

Brown, H. W., and D. L. Belding. *Parasitología Clínica*, 2nd ed. Mexico, Interamericana, 1965.

Pan American Zoonoses Center. *Prueba de doble difusión arco 5 para el diagnóstico de la hidatidosis humana*. Buenos Aires, CEPANZO, 1979. (Technical Note 22.)

Coltorti, E. A. Standardization and evaluation of an enzyme immunoassay as a screening test for the seroepidemiology of human hydatidosis. *Am J Trop Med Hyg* 35:1000-1005, 1986.

Coltorti, E. A., and V. M. Varela-Díaz. Detection of antibodies against *Echinococcus granulosus* arc 5 antigens by double diffusion test. *Trans R Soc Trop Med Hyg* 72:226-299, 1978.

D'Alessandro, A., R. L. Rausch, C. Cuello, and N. Aristizábal. *Echinococcus vogeli* in man, with a review of polycystic hydatid disease in Colombia and neighboring countries. *Am J Trop Med Hyg* 28:303-317, 1979.

Eckert, J., M. A. Gemmel, and E. J. M. Soulsby. *Guidelines for Surveillance, Prevention and Control of Echinococcosis/Hydatidosis*. Geneva, World Health Oganization, 1981. (Mimeographed document.)

Faust, E. C., P. F. Russell, and R. C. Jung. *Craig and Faust's Clinical Parasitology*, 8th ed. Philadelphia, Lea and Febiger, 1970.

Ferro, A., P. L. Ceresto, J. L. Curuchet *et al*. Hidatidosis hepática. *Arch Int Hidatid* 24:173-221, 1970.

Fischman, A. Reactivity of latex and complement fixation tests in hydatid disease. *J Parasitol* 51:497-500, 1965.

French, C. M., and G. S. Nelson. Hydatid disease in the Turkana District of Kenya. II. A study in medical geography. *Ann Trop Med Parasitol* 76:439-457, 1982.

Gemmell, M. A. Screening of drugs and their assessment for use against the strobilate stage of *Echinococcus*. *Bull WHO* 39:57-65, 1968.

Gemmell, M. A., S. N. Parmeter, R. J. Sutton, and N. Khan. Effect of mebendazole against *Echinococcus granulosus* and *Taenia hydatigena* cyst in naturally infected sheep and relevance to larval tapeworm infections in man. *Z Parasitenkd* 64:135-147, 1981.

Guisantes, J. A., M. F. Rubio, and R. Díaz. Application of an enzyme-linked immunosorbent assay (ELISA) method to the diagnosis of human hydatidosis. *Bull Pan Am Health Organ* 15:260-266, 1981.

Houin, R., R. Deniau, M. Liance, and F. Puel. *Arvicola terrestris* an intermediate host of *Echinococcus multilocularis* in France: epidemiological consequences. *Int J Parasitol* 12:593-600, 1982.

Iacona, A., C. Pini, and G. Vicari. Enzyme-linked immunosorbent assay (ELISA) in the serodiagnosis of hydatid disease. *Am J Trop Med Hyg* 29:95-102, 1980.

Jenkins, D. J., and M. D. Rickard. Specific antibody response in dogs experimentally infected with *Echinococcus granulosus*. *Am J Trop Med Hyg* 35:345-349, 1986.

Jenkins, D. J., and M. D. Rickard. Specific antibody responses to *Taenia hydatigena*, *Taenia pisiformis* and *Echinococcus granulosus* infection in dogs. *Aust Vet J* 62:72-78, 1985.

Kagan, I. G. A review of serological tests for the diagnosis of hydatid disease. *Bull WHO* 39:25-37, 1968.

Lawson, J. R., and M. A. Gemmell. Hydatidosis and cysticercosis: the dynamics of transmission. *Adv Parasitol* 22:261-308, 1983.

Le Riche, P. D., and R. J. Jorgensen. Echinococcosis (Hydatidosis) and its Control. Nicosia, Food and Agriculture Organization of the United Nations. 1971. (N.E.A.H.I. Handbook 6.)

Macpherson, C. L. An active intermediate host role for man in the life cycle of *Echinococcus granulosus* in Turkane, Kenya. *Am J Trop Med Hyg* 32:397-404, 1983.

Macpherson, C. L. Epidemiology of hydatid disease in Kenya: a study of the dog intermediate hosts in Masailand. *Trans R Soc Trop Med Hyg* 79:209-217, 1985.

Medina, E. La hidatidosis, un problema de salud pública. *Bol Chile Parasitol* 30:83-86, 1975.

Mogillansky, P. Diagnóstico radiológico precoz del quiste hidatídico hepático. *Arch Int Hidatid* 24:223-229, 1970.

Osborn, P. J., and D. D. Heath. Immunization of lambs against *Echinococcus granulosus* using antigens obtained by incubation of oncospheres in vitro. *Res Vet Sci* 33:132-133, 1982.

Pan American Health Organization. *Hidatidosis.* Buenos Aires, Pan American Zoonoses Center, 1975. (News Bulletin 2.)

Pan American Health Organization. *Diagnosis of Animal Health in the Americas.* Washington, D.C., PAHO, 1983. (Scientific Publication 452.)

Pétavy, A. F., and S. Deblock. Connaissance du foyer Auvergnat d'echinococcose alvéolaire. *Ann Parasitol Hum Comp* 58:439-453, 1983.

Polydorou, K. The anti-echinococcosis campaign in Cyprus. *Trop Anim Health Prod* 9:141-146, 1977.

Purriel, P., P. M. Schantz, H. Boevide, and G. Mendoza. Human echinococcosis (hydatidosis) in Uruguay: a comparison of indices of morbidity and mortality, 1961-1962. *Bull WHO* 49:395-402, 1973.

Ramírez, R. Contribución al conocimiento de la epidemiología de la hidatidosis humana en Chile (1969-1979). *Rev Med Chile* 110:1125-1130, 1982.

Rausch, R. L. Taenidae. *In*: Hubbert, W. T., W. F. McCulloch, and P. R. Schnurrenberger (Eds.), *Diseases Transmitted from Animals to Man*, 6th ed. Springfield, Illinois, Thomas, 1975.

Rausch, R. L. A consideration of intraspecific categories in the genus *Echinococcus* Rudolphi, 1801 (Cestoda: Taeniidae.) *J Parasitol* 53:484-491, 1967.

Rausch, R. L., A. D'Alessandro, and V. R. Rausch. Characteristics of the larval *Echinococcus vogeli* (Rausch and Bernstein, 1972) in the natural intermediate host, the paca, *Cuniculus paca* L. (Rodentia: Dasyproctidae). *Am J Trop Med Hyg* 30:1043-1052, 1981.

Rausch, R. L., and S. H. Richards. Observation on parasite-host relationships of *Echinococcus multilocularis* (Leuckart, 1863) in North Dakota. *Can J Zool* 49:1317-1330, 1971.

Rausch, R. L., and J. J. Bernstein. *Echinococcus vogeli* ssp. (Cestoda: Taeniidae) from the bush dog, *Speothos venaticus* (Lund). *Z Tropenmed Parasit* 23:25-34, 1972.

Rickard, M. D. The immunological diagnosis of hydatid disease. *Aust Vet J* 55:99-104, 1979.

Schantz, P. M. Aspectos epidemiológicos de la hidatidosis quística en América del Sur. *Tórax* 22:222-231, 1973.

Schantz, P. M., and C. Colli. *Echinococcus oligarthrus* (Diesing, 1863) from Geoffroy's cat (*Felix geoffroyi* D'Urbigny and Gervais) in temperate South America. *J Parasitol* 59:1138-1140, 1973.

Schantz, P. M., C. Colli, A. Cruz-Reyes, and U. Prezioso. Sylvatic echinococcosis in Argentina. II. Susceptibility of wild carnivores to *Echinococcus granulosus* (Batsch, 1786) and host-induced morphological variation. *Z Tropenmed Parasit* 27:70-78, 1976.

Schantz, P. M., D. Shanks, and M. Wilson. Serologic cross-reactions with sera from patients with echinococcosis and cysticercosis. *Am J Trop Med Hyg* 29:609-612, 1980.

Schantz, P. M. Echinococcosis. *In*: Jacobs, L., and P. Arambulo III (Section Eds.), *CRC Handbook Series in Zoonoses.* Section C, vol. 1. Boca Raton, Florida, CRC Press, 1982.

Schenone, H., A. Rojas, and R. Ramírez. Frecuencia de hidatidosis en autopsias efectuadas en el Instituto de Medicina Legal y ocho hospitales de Santiago, Chile (1947-1970). *Bol Chile Parasitol* 26:98-103, 1971.

Schwabe, C. W. *Veterinary Medicine and Human Health*, 2nd ed. Baltimore, Maryland, Williams and Wilkins, 1969.

Sousa, O. E., and V. E. Thatcher. Observations on the life-cycle of *Echinococcus oligarthrus* (Diesing, 1863) in the Republic of Panama. *Ann Trop Med Parasitol* 63:165-175, 1969.

Szyfres, B. El control de las zoonosis. *In*: Sonis, A. (Ed.), *Medicina Sanitaria y Administración de Salud.* Buenos Aires, El Ateneo, 1971.

Szyfres, B., and I. G. Kagan. Prueba modificada de aglutinación látex como procedimiento tamiz para hidatidosis. *Bol Of Sanit Panam* 54:208-212, 1963.

Tasmanian Hydatid Disease Newsletter. November, 1973. Australia. Department of Health Services/Department of Agriculture.

Thakur, A. S. Análisis epizoótico y epidemiológico y control de la hidatidosis en América del Sur. *In: XIII Congreso Internacional de Hidatología* (Proceedings, pp. 25–29). Madrid, 1985.

Thakur, A. S., U. Prezioso, and N. Marchevsky. Ovicidal activity of praziquantel and bunamidine hydrochloride. *Exp Parasitol* 47:131-133, 1979a.

Thakur, A. S., C. S. Eddi, and U. Prezioso. Empleo del praziquantel solo y en combinación con el bromhidrato de arecolina para el tratamiento contra *Echinococcus granulosus* en perros. *Rev Med Vet (B Aires)* 60:154-157, 1979b.

Thatcher, V. E. Neotropical echinococcosis in Colombia. *Ann Trop Med Parasitol* 66:99-105, 1972.

Thompson, R. C. A., and L. M. Kumaratilake. Intraspecific variation in *Echinococcus granulosus*: the Australian situation and perspectives for the future. *Trans R Soc Trop Med Hyg* 76:13-16, 1982.

Touya, J. J., A. Osorio, E. F. Touya *et al*. Scintigraphy of the liver, lungs, spleen, kidneys, brains, heart and bones in the diagnosis of hydatid cysts. *In: Medical Radioisotope Scintigraphy*, vol. 2. Vienna, International Atomic Energy Agency, 1968.

Trejos, A., B. Szyfres, and N. Marchevsky. Comparative value of arecoline hydrobromide and bunamidine hydrochloride for the treatment of *Echinococcus granulosus* in dogs. *Res Vet Sci* 19:212-213, 1975.

Varela-Díaz, V. M., and E. A. Coltorti. *Técnicas para el diagnóstico immunológico de la hidatidosis humana*. Buenos Aries, Pan American Zoonoses Center, 1974. (Technical Scientific Monographs 7.)

Varela-Díaz, V. M., E. A. Coltorti, U. Prezioso *et al*. Evaluation of three immunodiagnostic tests for human hydatid disease. *Am J Trop Med Hyg* 24:312-319, 1975.

Varela-Díaz, V. M., E. A. Coltorti, M. I. Ricardes, U. Prezioso, P. M. Schantz, and R. García. Evaluation of immunodiagnostic techniques for the detection of human hydatid cyst carriers in field studies. *Am J Trop Med Hyg* 25:617-622, 1976.

Varela-Díaz, V. M., J. Eckert, R. L. Rausch, E. A. Coltorti, and U. Hess. Detection of the *Echinococcus granulosus* diagnostic arc 5 in sera from patients with surgically confirmed *E. multilocularis* infection. *Z Parasitenkd* 53:183-188, 1977.

Varela-Díaz, V. M., E. A. Coltorti, and A. D'Alessandro. Immunoelectrophoresis tests showing *Echinococcus granulosus* arc 5 in human cases of *Echinococcus vogeli* and cysticercosis-multiple myeloma. *Am J Trop Med Hyg* 27:554-557, 1978.

Varela-Díaz, V. M., E. A. Guarnera, N. Marchevsky, L. Rapoport, H. Conesa, and S. Espinola. Review of hospital cases in the assessment of hydatidosis as a health problem in the Argentine province of Chubut. *Z Parasitenkd* 69:507-515, 1983.

Varela-Díaz, V. M., and E. A. Coltorti. Immunodiagnostic confirmation of hydatid disease in patients with a presumptive diagnosis of infection. *Rev Inst Med Trop S Paulo* 26:87-96, 1984.

Wattal, C., N. Malla, I. A. Khan, and S. C. Agarwal. Comparative evaluation of enzyme-linked immunosorbent assay for the diagnosis of pulmonary echinococcosis. *J Clin Microbiol* 24:41-46, 1986.

Wilson, J. F., and R. L. Rausch. Alveolar hydatid disease. A review of clinical features of 33 indigenous cases of *Echinococcus multilocularis*. Infection in Alaskan Eskimos. *Am J Trop Med Hyg* 29:1340-1355, 1980.

Williams, J. F., H. López-Adaros, and A. Trejos. Current prevalence and distribution of hydatidosis with special reference to the Americas. *Am J Trop Med Hyg* 20:224-236, 1971.

Williams, J. F., and U. Prezioso. Latex agglutination test for hydatid disease using Boerner slides. *J Parasitol* 56:1253-1255, 1970.

Witenberg, G. G. Cestodiases. *In*: Van der Hoeden, J. (Ed.), *Zoonoses*. Amsterdam, Netherlands, Elsevier, 1964.

World Health Organization. *Parasitic Zoonoses*. Report of a WHO Expert Committee, with the Participation of FAO. Geneva, OMS, 1979. (Technical Report Series 637.)

World Health Oganization. *Guidelines for Surveillance, Prevention and Control of Echinococcosis/Hydatidosis*, 2nd ed. Geneva, 1984. (Document VPH/81.28.)

Yarzábal, L. A., and A. Capron. Aportes de la immunoelectroforesis al diagnóstico immunológico de la hidatidosis. *Tórax* 20:168-174, 1971.

HYMENOLEPIASIS

(123.6)

Etiology: The cestodes *Hymenolepis* (*Taenia*) *nana* and *H. diminuta*. Divergent opinions exist among parasitologists with respect to the nomenclature of *H. nana*, which infects man as well as rats, mice, and other rodents. Some consider that there are two subspecies of *H. nana*: *Hymenolepis nana fraterna* in rodents and *H. nana nana* in humans. Others maintain that the parasites are strains of a single species, physiologically adapted to particular hosts, but capable of causing cross-infections. Although children have been infected experimentally with the parasite of rodent origin and rodents with the one of human origin, human infection always occurs more easily with the human cestode. Currently, the single-species theory is more widely accepted; adaptive differences in the parasite have been found not only between the strains in man and rodents but also between strains in different rodent species, such as rats and mice.

The cycle of *H. nana* is direct in most cases, not requiring the intervention of an intermediate host. Man acts as both definitive and intermediate host for the vast majority of parasitoses caused by *H. nana*. The strobilar form of this parasite is very small (2.5 to 4 cm long and 1 mm wide); it has a filiform body made up of hundreds of trapezoidal proglottids, wider than they are long. The gravid proglottids disintegrate in the human intestine, and the completely embryonated eggs are carried with the feces to the external environment. When another human host ingests an embryonated egg, the oncosphere (hexacanth embryo) is released in the upper part of the small intestine and penetrates a villus, where in about 5 days it changes into a microscopic, oval, cysticeroid larva. The cysticercoid ruptures the villus, travels to the lumen of the intestine, and attaches itself to the lower small intestine; there it reaches the adult strobilar phase in 2 weeks and begins to release eggs, reinitiating the cycle. The adult *H. nana* dies in a few weeks, but the cestode population renews itself by new generations arising from the cysticercoids and by autoinfection. The strains of *H. nana* adapted to rodents have the same life cycle, with complete development in a single animal. The cysticercoid larva can also develop in coprophilic arthropods, as has been shown experimentally in coleopterans and flea larvae, and these insects can sometimes serve as intermediate hosts.

Another frequent mode of development is endogenous autoinfection, in which some cestode eggs hatch in the intestine, produce cysticercoids, and give rise to the adult form.

The other species, *Hymenolepis diminuta*, is a parasite of rodents and rarely of man. The strobilar form, which is found in the small intestine of rats or, more rarely, mice, is 20 to 60 mm long and about 4 mm wide in the distal portion. The embryonated eggs are eliminated with rodent fecal matter and must be ingested by an intermediate host for the oncosphere to develop further. The intermediate hosts are coprophilic arthropods, such as several species of coleopterans and lepidop-terans, myriapods, and the larvae of various fleas. The egg hatches in the intestine of these arthropods, and the oncosphere penetrates the coelomic cavity, where it changes into a cysticercoid larva. When the infected arthropod is ingested by a rodent, the cysticercoid develops into an adult cestode.

Geographic Distribution and Occurrence: The two species of *Hymenolepis* have worldwide distributions. The most frequent human cestodiasis is that caused by *H. nana*. Highest prevalence rates are found among infants in southern Europe, North Africa, several countries in the Middle East, India, and Latin America. High rates of infection have been found in children in Argentina, Brazil, Ecuador, Nicaragua, and Mexico. In Chile, 49.6% of 2,426 intestinal cestodiasis confirmed between 1961 and 1971 were due to *H. nana*. Evidence from Brazil indicates that the supposed relationship between a hot climate and a high prevalence of the parasitosis does not always hold true, since the highest rates are found in Brazil's southern states, while the lowest occur in 12 states from Amazonas to Rio de Janeiro. In general, the prevalence is higher in urban than in rural environments, and the highest concentrations of parasitized persons are found in children's institutions, such as orphanages, day-care centers, and schools.

The level of parasitism of rats by *H. nana* can be very high in some cities. In studies carried out in Santiago, Chile, 7.8% of 128 specimens examined were positive, and in Bombay, India, 14.5% of the rats tested were found to be infected.

H. diminuta is a common cestode in rodents but very infrequent in man. Reports of the total number of recorded human cases in the world vary, depending on the source, from 200 to more than 400. In the high plains of Papua New Guinea, eggs of *H. diminuta* were found in the feces of six (1.9%) of 316 children and adolescents, ages 6 to 15 years. Rates of infection of more than 1% were also found in Iran and Mexico. The infection has been confirmed in about 10 Latin American countries, in Italy and Belgium, and in some countries of Australasia and Africa.

The Disease in Man and Animals: Hymenolepiasis occurs primarily in children. The prepatent period lasts from 2 to 4 weeks. In many cases, the parasitosis is asymptomatic, but in patients with a large parasite burden, gastrointestinal disorders such as nausea, vomiting, abdominal pain, and diarrhea can occur. Also attributed to these infections, especially those caused by *H. nana*, are neurologic symptoms (irritability, uneasiness, and restless sleep) and allergic symptoms (anal and nasal pruritus). Eosinophilia greater than 5% has been observed in over 30% of cases. In general, *H. diminuta* appears to be less pathogenic than *H. nana*.

The parasitosis does not seem to markedly affect the health of rodents. A large number of parasites may cause catarrhal enteritis.

Source of Infection and Mode of Transmission (Figure 80): The reservoir of *H. nana* (human strains) is man himself, and transmission between humans occurs by

Figure 80. Hymenolepiasis (*Hymenolepis diminuta*). Transmission cycle.

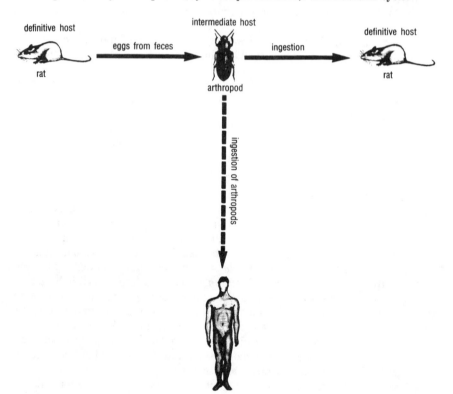

the fecal-oral route. Autoinfection is frequent. The role played by rodents in the epidemiology of the human parasitosis is not known. It has been shown experimentally that animal strains can infect humans and vice versa. Studies indicate that adaptation to a heterologous animal species requires multiple passages to be complete (Ferreti *et al.*, 1981). Consequently, it is believed that under natural conditions rodents play a very limited role in human infection. The limited importance of rodents is due in part to the short survival time of eggs in the environment, not exceeding 11 days even under optimal conditions. Rodents may play some role in the human parasitosis by contaminating foods with their feces. Another infrequent mechanism for human infection could be accidental ingestion of arthropods infected with cysticercoids (for example, cereal and flour beetles such as *Tenebrio molitor* or *Tribolium obscurus*). Deficient personal and environmental hygiene are important factors in the spread of the parasitosis.

H. nana is transmitted among rodents by the same mechanisms as in man. Coprophagia contributes significantly to the spread of the parasitosis. Ingestion of infected arthropods is probably a more important mechanism among rodents than among humans.

The natural reservoirs of *H. diminuta* are rodents, mainly rats. Man is infected only accidentally and interhuman transmission of the parasite does not occur. The life cycle of the parasite, which requires an intermediate host, explains the rarity of human infection. The necessary intermediate hosts of *H. diminuta* are several species of arthropods, which must be ingested by the definitive host for the parasite larva to develop into an adult cestode. Humans, especially children, ingest these arthropods only accidentally, for example, with contaminated precooked cereals.

The parasitosis can become established in laboratory rodent colonies, creating great difficulties in experimentation.

Diagnosis: Specific diagnosis is made by detecting the characteristic eggs in the feces. A negative result in a single fecal examination is not conclusive, and in that case the microscopic examination should be repeated one or more times. The eggs of *H. diminuta* can be distinguished from those of *H. nana* by their larger size (70 to 80 microns, or double that of *H. nana*) and the absence of filaments in the polar mamillae; moreover, the lanceolate hooks of the oncosphere are spread out like a fan in this species.

Control: Human disease can be prevented by the adoption of personal and environmental hygiene measures, control of rodents, and adequate protection of food against contamination by arthropods. One dose of praziquantel (25 mg/kg) was shown to cure the parasitosis in 23 of 30 schoolchildren (Pedro *et al.*, 1982), and similar results were obtained in other patients with the same single dose; tolerance was good, and an efficacy of over 90% was confirmed by fecal examination 1 month later (Baranski *et al.*, 1982). Thus, it would seem that the source of infection could be reduced with this medicine. However, even with its use, it was not possible to completely control the infection in an institution for children, although a high rate of recovery was recorded. New studies are needed to evaluate the effectiveness of repeated, spaced doses of praziquantel in controlling the parasitosis (Rocha *et al.*, 1981).

Bibliography

Andrade, R. M., and I. G. R. Campos. Prevalência de *Vampirolepis nana* en Belo Horizonte, M. G. (Brasil), com especial referencia a um foco isolado (Cestoda, Hymenolepididae). *Rev Bras Malar* 20:83-108, 1968.

Atias, A., and A. Neghme. *Parasitología Clínica*. Buenos Aires, Inter-Médica, 1979.

Baranski, M. C., N. R. Gomes, and O. F. de Godoy. Terapéutica da teniase e da Hymenolepsiase nana con dose oral única de praziquantel. Estudo eficácia, tolerância e segurança. *Rev Inst Med Trop São Paulo* 22:53-96, 1980.

Edelman, M. H., C. L. Spingarn, W. G. Naunberg, and C. Gregory. *Hymenolepis diminuta* (rat tapeworm) infection in man. *Am J Med* 38:951-953, 1965.

Faust, E. C., P. F. Russell, and R. C. Jung. *Craig and Faust's Clinical Parasitology*, 8th ed. Philadelphia, Lea and Febiger, 1970.

Ferreti, G., F. Gabriele, and C. Palmas. Development of human and mouse strains of *Hymenolepis nana* in mice. *Int J Parasitol* 11:425-430, 1981.

McMillan, B., A. Kelly, and J. C. Walker. Prevalence of *Hymenolepis diminuta* infection in man in the New Guinea Highlands. *Trop Geogr Med* 23:390-392, 1971.

Pedro, R. de J., E. R. Duberaldini, L. C. S. Dias, and M. M. Goto. Tratamento de escolares com *Hymenolepis nana* pelo praziquantel. *Rev Assoc Med Bras* 28:216-217, 1982.

Reyes, H., G. Doren, and E. Inzunza. Teniasis humana. Frecuencia actual de la infección por diferentes especies en Santiago de Chile. *Bol Chile Parasitol* 27:23-29, 1972.

Reyes, H., E. Inzunza, and G. Doren. Frecuencia de infección humana por *Hymenolepis diminuta* en Santiago de Chile, 1957-1971. *Bol Chile Parasitol* 27:29-33, 1972.

Rocha, R. S., O. S. Carvalho, J. S. Santos, and N. H. Katz. Tentativa de controle de *Hymenolepis nana* através de tratamentos clínicos repetidos com praziquantel, em uma comunidade fechada. *Rev Saúde Publica (S Paulo)* 15:364-370, 1981.

Tantaleán, Z. G. de, and I. E. Cáceres. Hospederos intermediarios de *Hymenolepis diminuta* en Lima (Perú). *Rev Peru Med Trop* 1:22-27, 1972.

Turner, J. A. Other cestoda infections. *In:* Hubbert, W. T., W. F. McCulloch, and P. R. Schnurenberger (Eds.), *Diseases Transmitted from Animals to Man*, 6th ed. Springfield, Illinois, Thomas, 1975.

Witenberg, G. G. Cestodiases. *In:* Van der Hoeden, J. (Ed.), *Zoonoses*. Amsterdam, Netherlands, Elsevier, 1964.

INERMICAPSIFERIASIS

(123.9)

Etiology: *Inermicapsifer madagascariensis* (*I. cubensis*), a tapeworm 24 to 42 cm long and a maximum of 2.6 mm wide. *Inermicapsifer* is distinguished from *Raillietina* (see "Raillietiniasis") by an unarmed scolex and sucker. The gravid segments, in which egg capsules take the place of a uterus, are longer than they are wide (in contrast to the nongravid segments, which are wider than they are long). Each gravid segment encloses 150 to 175 capsules that each contain six or more eggs. This cestode's life cycle is unknown, but by analogy to related parasites of the genus *Raillietina*, it is believed that an arthropod acts as intermediate host.

Geographic Distribution and Occurrence: *I. madagascariensis* is a parasite of rodents (*Arvicanthis*) in eastern Africa, where it very occasionally affects man. Outside Africa, it may be exclusively a human parasite. Human cases have been recorded in Madagascar, Zaire, Mauritius, Kenya, Thailand, and the Philippines. The highest number of cases (over 100) has been recorded in Cuba, mainly in children 1 to 2 years old. The parasitosis has also been recognized in Venezuela.

The Disease and Diagnosis: The parasitosis is generally unaccompanied by clinical symptoms. Specific diagnosis is based on microscopic examination of the proglottids. In order to differentiate *Inermicapsifer* from *Raillietina*, the scolex of the cestode, which may be expelled spontaneously or following treatment, must be examined.

Source of Infection and Mode of Transmission: The intermediate host is not known, but is probably an arthropod. The larval stage would develop in an arthropod that ingests cestode eggs deposited with the fecal matter of the definitive host (rodent or man). The cycle would be completed when the definitive host ingests an intermediate host infected with the larva. In Africa, the transmission cycle would be rodent-intermediate host-rodent and occasionally rodent-intermediate host-man. Outside the African continent, transmission would occur from human to intermediate host to human.

Control: Since the life cycle of the parasite and consequently the mode of transmission are unknown, the only preventive measures that can be recommended, based on the probable life cycle of the parasite, consist of rodent control and personal and environmental hygiene.

Bibliography

Belding, D. L. *Textbook of Parasitology*, 3rd ed. New York, Appleton-Century-Crofts, 1965.

Bisseru, B. *Diseases of Man Acquired from His Pets*. London, Heinemann, 1967.

Faust, E. C., P. F. Russell, and R. C. Jung. *Craig and Faust's Clinical Parasitology*, 8th ed. Philadelphia, Lea and Febiger, 1970.

Kouri, P., and J. G. Basnuevo. *Helmintología Humana*. La Habana, Siglo XX, 1949.

MESOCESTOIDIASIS

(123.9)

Etiology: *Mesocestoides lineatus* and *M. variabilis*. The life cycle of these cestodes is not well known yet. The definitive hosts are dogs, cats, and several species of wild carnivores. The first intermediate host is probably a coprophagous arthropod that ingests the eggs contained in the gravid proglottids eliminated by the definitive hosts. It has been possible to experimentally infect oribatid mites, in which cysticercoids developed. The second intermediate hosts, which harbor the plerocercoid larval form, or tetrathyridium, are amphibians, reptiles, birds, and mammals (rodents, dogs, cats). The tetrathyridium can lodge in the tissues or serous cavities of these animals, where it multiplies asexually. Some mammals, such as cats and dogs, can harbor both the adult cestode and the larval stage.

When a definitive host ingests meat of an animal infected by the larval form, the tetrathyridium develops into an adult cestode in the host's intestine in 16 to 20 days. The adult tapeworm can reach 40 cm in length and 2 mm in width.

Geographic Distribution and Occurrence: Mesocestoidiasis is rare in man. A few cases have been described, among them seven in Japan, two in the United States, two in Africa (in Rwanda and Burundi), one in Greenland, and one in Korea. In a study carried out in southern Malawi in Africa, *Mesocestoides* spp. were found in 34% of 120 native dogs autopsied.

The Disease and Diagnosis: In man the symptomatology consists primarily of digestive disorders, abdominal pain, and diarrhea.

In dogs and cats the adult parasite produces no apparent symptomatology. When the larval forms are abundant in serous cavities, they can cause peritonitis and dropsy in these animals.

Diagnosis is based on microscopic examination of the gravid proglottids. These segments are barrel-shaped and contain double-membrane eggs grouped in a central paruterine organ.

Source of Infection and Mode of Transmission: Dogs, cats, and wild carnivores contract the parasitosis by ingesting birds, amphibians, reptiles, and small mammals infected with the larval form (tetrathyridium). Man becomes infected occasionally through the same mechanism, that is, by ingesting raw meat of intermediate hosts. In Japan, several cases were attributed to eating raw snake liver, which may have been consumed because these animals are popularly believed to have curative properties for some sicknesses. The human case that occurred in Rwanda, Africa, was probably due to ingestion of raw partridge meat. In the same locality, infection with tetrathyridia was found in chickens, guinea hens, and partridges, and the adult cestode was found in a cat.

Control: Control measures should be directed toward interrupting transmission from the intermediate to the definitive host. To prevent human infection, raw or undercooked game meat should not be consumed.

Bibliography

Fitzsimmons, W. P. A survey of the parasites of native dogs in Southern Malawi with remarks on their medical and veterinary importance. *J Helminthol* 41:15-18, 1967.

Gleason, N. N., and G. R. Healy. Report of a case of *Mesocestoides* (Cestoda) in a child in Missouri. *J Parasitol* 53:83-84, 1967.

Soulsby, E. J. L. *Textbook of Veterinary Clinical Parasitology.* Oxford, Blackwell, 1965.

Turner, J. A. Other cestode infections. *In*: Hubbert, W. T., W. F. McCulloch, and P. R. Schnurrenberger (Eds.), *Diseases Transmitted from Animals to Man*, 6th ed. Springfield, Illinois, Thomas, 1975.

RAILLIETINIASIS

(123.9)

Etiology: *Raillietina demerariensis* and *R. celebensis* are the main species described in man. Many other species of the genus found in man are thought to be identical to these two. The definitive hosts of *R. celebensis* are mostly rodents. In the neotropical region, *R. demerariensis* has been found in both rodents and monkeys. The biological cycle is not known for either species, but the intermediate host is assumed to be an arthropod, as it is for other species of the genus. About 225 species of *Raillietina* parasitize birds and mammals. The intermediate hosts of various species for which the life cycle is known are beetles, flies, and ants, in whose tissues cysticercoids develop from the embryos contained in the eggs ingested with the feces of the definitive hosts. The cycle is reinitiated when the definitive host eats an arthropod infected with a cysticercoid.

The adult *R. demerariensis* measures 10 to 12 cm long by 3 mm wide and has many segments. The gravid proglottids are shaped like grains of rice; they contain 200 to 250 egg capsules with four to eight eggs each.

R. celebensis measures more than 40 cm in length. In the gravid proglottids, the uterus is replaced by 300 to 400 egg capsules containing up to four eggs each.

The species *R. asiatica*, *R. garrisoni*, and *R. siriraji* have been described in various Asian countries, but more detailed studies are needed to determine if they represent one or more than one valid species (Faust *et al.*, 1974).

Geographic Distribution and Occurrence: *R. demerariensis*, the neotropical species, has been found in human infections in Ecuador, Cuba, Guyana, and Honduras. *R. quitensis*, *R. equatoriensis*, *R. leoni*, and *R. luisaleoni* are considered to be synonymous with this species. The largest endemic focus is found in the parish of Tumbaco, near Quito, Ecuador, where the infection rate in school-age children varied from 4 to 12.5% during the period 1933 to 1961. The parasitosis was diagnosed in 0.14% of 8,148 children in the Children's Homes in Quito, and in 0.08% of the patients in another hospital in the same city. Outside of Ecuador, human infection is very rare, with only a few cases having been described in Cuba, Guyana, and Honduras.

The other species, *R. celebensis* (*R. formosana*), has been observed in children in Taiwan, Japan, Australia, and southeastern Africa. Infection by *R. garrisoni* has been diagnosed on the island of Mauritius and in the Philippines; in the latter country 20 cases have occurred. Eleven cases in Thailand are attributed to *R. siriraji* and this species also occurs in Turkestan, USSR. One case due to *R. asiatica* has been diagnosed in northern Iran (Jueco, 1982).

In Bombay, India, 5% of *Rattus rattus* and 7% of *Bandicota bengalensis* were found to be infected by the cestode in an examination of 200 specimens of each of the two murid rodent species. In other parts of eastern Asia, even higher rates of raillietiniasis have been found in rodents.

The Disease in Man: The infection occurs primarily in children. In Ecuador, the symptomatology attributed to this parasitosis consists of digestive upsets (nausea, vomiting, diarrhea, colic), nervous disorders (headaches, personality changes, convulsions), circulatory problems (tachycardia, arrhythmia, lipothymia), and general disorders (weight loss and retarded growth). Observations in the Philippines indicated that human infection is usually asymptomatic, and the parasite is expelled spontaneously by the affected individual.

Source of Infection and Mode of Transmission: Rodents are the reservoirs of the infection. By analogy with infections caused by *Raillietina* in other animal species, it is thought that man becomes infected by accidentally ingesting with his food an arthropod infected with cysticercoids.

Diagnosis: Proglottids can be observed in fecal matter; they resemble grains of rice and are frequently mistaken for such. The gravid proglottids of *R. demerariensis* contain over 200 egg capsules with four to eight eggs each. Free capsules can sometimes be found in the feces as a result of disintegration of the proglottid. The proglottids of *Raillietina* are similar to those of *Inermicapsifer*. The two genera are easily differentiated on the basis on their scolices, since that of *Raillietina* has hooks, while the scolex of specimens of the other genus is unarmed.

Control: Measures should be directed toward rodent control and personal and environmental hygiene.

Bibliography

Belding, D. L. *Textbook of Parasitology*, 3rd ed. New York, Appleton-Century-Crofts, 1965.

Faust, E. C., P. R. Russell, and R. C. Jung. *Craig and Faust's Clinical Parasitology*, 8th ed. Philadelphia, Lea and Febiger, 1970.

Jueco, N. L. *Raillietina* infection. *In*: Jacobs, L., and P. Arambulo III (Section Eds.), *CRC Handbook Series in Zoonoses*. Section C, vol. 1. Boca Raton, Florida, CRC Press, 1982.

León, L. A. Un foco endémico de raillietiniasis observado a través de treinta años. *Rev Medicina (México)* 44:342-348, 1964.

Niphadkar, S. M., and S. R. Rao. On the occurrence of *Raillietina* (R) *celebensis* (Jericki, 1902) in rats of Bombay with special reference to its zoonotic importance. *Indian Vet J* 46:816-818, 1969.

SPARGANOSIS

(123.5)

Synonym: Larval diphyllobothriasis.

Etiology: The second larval stage (plerocercoid or sparganum) of the pseudophyllidean cestode of the genus *Spirometra* (*Diphyllobothrium*, *Lueheela*). Several species of medical interest have been described: *Spirometra mansoni*, *S. mansonoides*, *S. erinacei-europaei*, *S. theileri*, and *S. proliferum*. These are the most commonly accepted species at the present time, but it should be noted that they are difficult to differentiate and that the taxonomy remains in doubt.

The definitive hosts are mainly domestic and wild canids and felids. The development cycle requires two intermediate hosts. The first is a copepod (planktonic crustacean) of the genus *Cyclops*, which ingests coracidia (free, ciliated embryos) that develop from *Spirometra* eggs when they reach the water with the feces of dogs or cats (definitive hosts). In the tissues of the copepod, the coracidium turns into the first larva, or procercoid. When a second intermediate host ingests an infected copepod, the procercoid develops into a second larval form, the plerocercoid or sparganum. The plerocercoid larva can be harbored by many vertebrates, including amphibians, reptiles, birds, small mammals (rodents and insectivores), man, non-human primates, and swine. Fish do not become infected. Some researchers believe that the second intermediate host is usually an amphibian, but can vary according to region. Numerous species of vertebrates become infected with plerocercoids by feeding on amphibians, but they may also develop plerocercoids after ingesting water containing copepods infected by procercoids (first larva). Several animal species that are not definitive hosts function as paratenic or transport hosts, since the larvae they acquire by feeding on animals infected with plerocercoids encyst again after passing through the intestinal wall and migrating to other tissues. This transfer process is undoubtedly important in the life cycle; but the fact that many species of secondary hosts can be infected directly by ingestion of copepods containing procercoids is probably no less important. When the sparganum reaches the intestine of the definitive host, it attaches to the mucosa; in 10 to 30 days, it matures into an adult cestode, completing the cycle.

The adult *S. mansonoides* reaches about 25 cm in length in the intestine of the definitive hosts (cat, dog). The sparganum found in the tissues of the secondary intermediate hosts and paratenic hosts, including man, varies from 4 to 10 cm in length.

Geographic Distribution and Occurrence: Sparganosis is found throughout the world, but human infection is not common. Just over 450 cases are known, mostly from Japan, China, Korea, and Southeast Asia. In the United States, about 60 cases have been described; in Latin America and the Caribbean, the disease has been recorded in Uruguay, Ecuador, Colombia, Venezuela, Guyana, Belize, and Puerto Rico; about 30 cases have been diagnosed in Africa. Infections in the Far East are attributed to plerocercoid larvae of *Spirometra mansoni*; in the United States, to *S. mansonoides*; in Europe, to *S. erinacei-europaei*; and in Africa, to *S. theileri*. However, as has already been mentioned, species identification can be difficult and therefore uncertain.

More recent research has indicated that both *S. mansoni* and *S. mansonoides* are widely distributed in the definitive hosts in North and South America. Consequently, it is uncertain which of the two species is the agent of human sparganosis in this region, since spargana isolated from humans generally do not reach sexual maturity when experimentally inoculated into definitive hosts (canines and felines) for the purpose of specific identification (Mueller *et al.*, 1975).

Infections caused by the adult cestode and by plerocercoid larvae are frequent in some areas. In some towns in Japan, 95% of the cats and 20% of the dogs are infected with *Spirometra*. Some time ago, a high infection rate was found in cats in Cuba. Studies carried out in Sydney, Australia, detected the parasite in 6% of domestic cats, 20.5% of stray cats, and 0.5% of dogs. High rates of infection in dogs, cats, and foxes were confirmed in the USSR. In Maracay, Venezuela, about 3% of the cats were found to be infected, and in other Latin American countries, the adult parasite has been recognized in domestic animals and several wild species (foxes, felids, and marsupials). Sparganosis (infection by the second larva) can be found in a great variety of animal species. In some localities of Florida, USA, infection with plerocercoids was found in 50 to 90% of the water snakes. On the outskirts of Brisbane, Australia, 25% of the frogs (*Hyla coeruela*) were found to be infected. Of special interest in Australia are data on wild pigs captured and fattened for human consumption. During the period 1971-1972, 100% of the pigs in a slaughterhouse in New South Wales were confiscated because they contained spargana. A high prevalence of sparganosis has also been found in Yugoslavia. Spargana were found in 49% of 37 *Leptodactylus ocellatus* frogs and in five of six *Philodryas patagoniense* snakes in Uruguay. Some of the snake specimens were intensely parasitized, owing to the fact that these snakes ingest parasitized frogs and thereby accumulate spargana (Dei-Cas *et al.*, 1976). High rates of infection in frogs and snakes have been confirmed in Asian countries where parasitologic studies have been carried out.

The Disease in Man: The incubation period, determined in a study of 10 patients who ate raw frog meat, lasts from 20 days to 14 months (Bi *et al.*, 1983). The most common localizations of the sparganum are subcutaneous connective tissue and superficial muscles. The lesion is nodular, develops slowly, and can be found on any part of the body. The main symptom is pruritus, sometimes accompanied by urticaria. The lesion is painful when there is inflammation. The patient may feel discomfort when the larva migrates from one location to another. In a recent clinical study of 22 cases of sparganosis in the province of Hunan, China, half the patients suffered from migratory subcutaneous nodules, which disappeared and reappeared as the sparganum migrated (Bi *et al.*, 1983). The subcutaneous lesion resembles a lipoma, fibroma, or sebaceous cyst. Ocular sparganosis occurs mainly in Vietnam, Thailand, and parts of China. Its main symptoms consist of a painful edema of the eyelids, with lacrimation and pruritus. A nodule measuring 1 to 3 cm forms after 3 to 5 months, usually on the upper eyelid.

Migration of the sparganum to internal organs can give rise to the visceral form of the disease. The preferred localizations are the intestinal wall, perirenal fat, and mesentery; vital organs are rarely affected. When the plerocercoid invades the lymphatic system, it produces a clinical picture similar to that of elephantiasis. Eosinophils are abundant in the areas near the parasite; examination of blood samples reveals mild leukocytosis and increased eosinophilia.

An infrequent but serious form is proliferative sparganosis caused by *Spirometra proliferum*. The sparganum of *S. proliferum* is pleomorphic, with irregular branches and proliferative buds that detach from the larva and migrate to different tissues in the host, where they repeat the process and invade other organs. The life cycle of *S. proliferum* is not known. Seven of 10 described cases of this clinical form are known to have been caused by *S. proliferum*, five in Japan, one in the United States, and one in Venezuela; in the remaining three cases the larvae were too undifferentiated for positive identification (Beaver and Rolon, 1981; Moulinier *et al.*, 1982).

The Disease in Animals: The adult cestode, which lodges in the intestine of the definitive host, generally does not affect the health of the animal. In cats, however, it may produce weight loss, irritability, and emaciation, together with an abnormal or exaggerated appetite. Infection by the larvae or spargana can be clinically apparent when their number is large and especially when they invade vital organs. In the intermediate host, the disease is almost always asymptomatic if the number of parasites is relatively small.

Source of Infection and Mode of Transmission (Figure 81): Sparganosis is maintained in nature primarily by contamination of natural or artificial bodies of water (lagoons, marshes, lakes, and others) with feces from felids and canids infected with *Spirometra* spp. Contamination of water with eggs of *Spirometra* spp. leads to the infection of copepods and, consequently, of the second intermediate hosts that ingest these crustaceans. An important means of infection is the transfer of

Figure 81. Sparganosis. Probable transmission cycle.

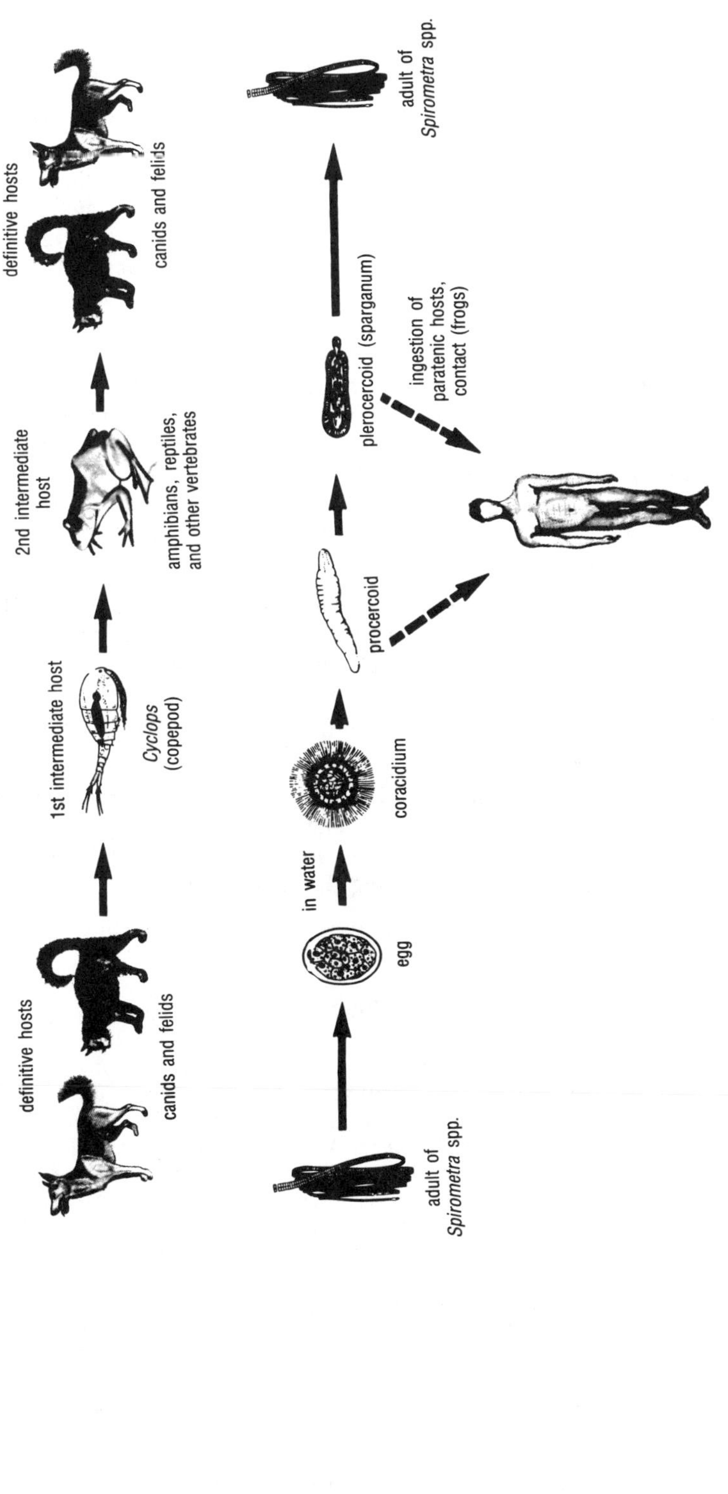

the second larva (sparganum, plerocercoid) from one secondary host to another, which increases the number of animal species and individuals infected. The common route of infection is ingestion; various mammal and bird species become infected by feeding on parasitized frogs or snakes. The high rate of infection in wild pigs in Australia may be due to this mechanism, although it may also stem from ingestion of copepods with drinking-water from lagoons. In any case, contamination of the water by wild canids (definitive hosts) that share the habitat assures that the cycle is perpetuated.

The infection rate in man is low, compared to the rate in other animals. Man acquires sparganosis mainly by ingesting larvae contained in raw or undercooked meat of animals infected with spargana, such as amphibians, reptiles, birds, and wild mammals. Another mode of infection, also by larval transfer, is by contact. In Vietnam and Thailand, frogs are popularly believed to have an antiphlogistic effect, and their muscles are applied as poultices. This custom is responsible for ocular sparganosis. It is also probable that man can acquire sparganosis via drinking-water, by ingesting copepods infected with procercoids (first larvae).

Man is an accidental host and does not usually play any role in the life cycle of the parasite. However, under ecologic conditions in some regions of central Africa, it is suspected that man acts as an intermediate host. In this region, hyenas are the definitive hosts of *Spirometra*, and man is apparently the only host infected with spargana. In these circumstances, the infection cycle is maintained as a result of a tribal custom of letting hyenas devour human corpses.

Diagnosis: Specific diagnosis can be made only by removing the nodular lesion and confirming the presence of the plerocercoid. Attempts have been made to identify the species of *Spirometra* larvae by infecting dogs and cats via the digestive route. For reasons already mentioned, differentiation of species has proven difficult. Diagnosis in definitive hosts infected with adult cestodes can be made by coprologic examination or autopsy.

Control: Human sparganosis can be prevented by avoiding ingestion of contaminated water that has not been treated, and by making sure that meat that might contain spargana is sufficiently cooked. In the Far East, public health education should emphasize the danger of using the tissue of frogs or other cold-blooded animals for medicinal purposes.

Bibliography

Beaver, P. C., and F. A. Rolon. Proliferating larval cestode in a man in Paraguay. A case report and review. *Am J Trop Med Hyg* 30:625-637, 1981.

Bi, W. T. *et al.* (A report of 22 cases of sparganosis mansoni in Hunan Province). *Chin J Pediatr* 21:355, 1983. Summary Document WHO/HELM/85.17., p. 4, 1985.

Daly, J. J. Sparganosis. *In*: Jacobs, L., and P. Arambulo III (Section Eds.), *CRC Handbook Series in Zoonoses*. Section C, vol. 1. Boca Raton, Florida, CRC Press, 1982.

Dei-Cas, E., N. Rodríguez, C. Bott, and J. J. Osimani. Larvas plerocercoides de *Spirometra* (Dibothriocephalidae) en el hombre y en animales silvestres de Uruguay. *Rev Inst Med Trop S Paulo* 18:165-172, 1976.

Euzeby, J. A. Zoonotic cestodes. *In*: Soulsby, E. J. L. (Ed.), *Parasitic Zoonoses*. New York, Academic Press, 1974.

Faust, E. C., P. F. Russell, and R. C. Jung. *Craig and Faust's Clinical Parasitology*, 8th ed. Philadelphia, Lea and Febiger, 1970.

Kelly, J. D. Anthropozoonotic helminthiases in Australia. *Int J Zoonoses* 1:1-12, 1974.

Moulinier, R., E. Martínez, J. Torres, O. Noya, B. A. de Noya, and O. Royes. Human proliferative sparganosis in Venezuela: Report of a case. *Am J Trop Med Hyg* 31:358-363, 1982.

Mueller, J. F. The biology of *Spirometra*. *J Parasitol* 60:3-14, 1974.

Mueller, J. F., O. M. Fróes, and T. Fernández R. On the occurrence of *Spirometra mansonoides* in South America. *J Parasitol* 61:774-775, 1975.

Smyth, J. D., and D. D. Heath. Pathogenesis of larval cestodes in mammals. *Helminthol Abstr* 39:1-23, 1970.

Strauss, W. G., and J. H. Manwaring. Sparganosis. A new case in the United States and review of the literature. *Dermatol Trop* 3:73-78, 1964.

Turner, J. A. Other cestode infections: *In*: Hubbert, W. T., W. F. McCulloch, and P. R. Schnurrenberger (Eds.), *Diseases Transmitted from Animals to Man*, 6th ed. Springfield, Illinois, Thomas, 1975.

Witenberg, G. G. Cestodiases. *In*: Van der Hoeden, J. (Ed.), *Zoonoses*. Amsterdam, Netherlands, Elsevier, 1964.

TAENIASIS AND CYSTICERCOSIS

(123.0) Infection by *Taenia solium* (intestinal form)
(123.1) Infection by *Cysticercus cellulosae*
(123.2) Infection by *T. saginata*

Etiology: The cestodes *Taenia solium* and *T. saginata* and their respective larval stages *Cysticercus cellulosae* and *C. bovis*. The definitive host of both taeniae is man, in whose small intestine they lodge. The intermediate hosts of *T. solium* are the domestic pig and wild boar; those of *T. saginata* are bovines, mainly domestic cattle.

The strobila (chain of segments) of *T. solium* measures 2 to 4 m in length and is made up of 800 to 1,000 proglottids (segments). The gravid proglottids contain from 30,000 to 50,000 eggs; they detach from the strobila in groups of five or six and are expelled with the feces. Pigs, because of their coprophagic habits, may ingest a large number of eggs, both those contained in the proglottids and those existing free in fecal matter. The embryos (oncospheres) are released from the eggs in the pig's intestine, penetrate the intestinal wall, and within 24 to 72 hours spread from there via the circulatory system to different tissues and organs of the body. Complete development of the cysticercus (*C. cellulosae*) takes place in 9 to 10 weeks. It is 8 to 15 by 5 by 10 mm in size, and looks like a fluid-filled bladder; it holds the invaginated scolex equipped with suckers and hooks. When a human consumes undercooked pork that contains a cysticercus, the scolex of the larva evaginates in the small intestine and it attaches to the intestinal wall, usually in the jejunum. After

62 to 72 days, the larva has developed into an adult taenia and the first proglottids are expelled in the feces, thus renewing the cycle. *T. solium* can survive in the human intestine for a long time; cases have been observed in which the tapeworm persisted for 25 years.

The public health significance of *T. solium* lies in the fact that man can also be infected by the eggs of the taenia and can develop cysticerci in his tissues.

The existence of different strains or subspecies has been proposed as an explanation for the differences in size of the hooks of the cysticerci found in pigs, cats, dogs, man, and baboons. A multilobular cysticercus without a scolex has frequently been observed in human cysticercosis in Mexico; it has been designated *Cysticercus racemosus* and may or may not be a *T. solium* larva. Most investigators are inclined to believe that it is a degenerative state of *T. solium*.

The strobila of *T. saginata* is longer than that of *T. solium*; it is composed of 1,000 to 2,000 proglottids and is 4 to 10 m long. The gravid proglottids, which can contain more than 100,000 eggs, detach from the strobila one by one; they are motile and seek exit via the anal sphincter. Eggs are either expelled from the proglottid or released when it disintegrates, but only about half contain mature and infective oncospheres. Some oncospheres can mature in the environment. Viable eggs that are ingested by grazing cattle develop into cysticerci (*C. bovis*) in a manner similar to the eggs of *T. solium* in swine. Development takes 60 to 75 days. Cysticerci begin to degenerate in a few weeks, and after 9 months, many of them are dead and calcified. Man is infected by ingesting raw beef containing viable cysticerci. The adult taenia develops in his intestine in 10 to 12 weeks and renews the cycle.

Human cysticercosis caused by ingestion of the eggs of *T. saginata* either does not occur or is very rare.

T. saginata eggs can survive several weeks or months in waste water, bodies of water, or on grass.

In addition to *T. solium*, *T. saginata*, and the species of the genus *Taenia* covered elsewhere (see "Coenurosis"), other species can occasionally infect man. Among them are the larval phase of *T. crassiceps*, which has caused a human intraocular cysticercosis in Canada; the cysticercus of *T. ovis*, found in the spinal cord of man in the USSR; and cysticerci of *T. hydatigena* and *T. taeniaeformis*, found in human hepatic tissue.

Geographic Distribution: Both these species of *Taenia* are distributed throughout the world. *T. solium* is much more common in developing countries, while *T. saginata* is more universally distributed.

Occurrence in Man: It was estimated in 1947 that nearly 39 million people in the world were infected by *T. saginata* and 2.5 million by *T. solium*. Some authors think that the number of infected persons must have increased since that time, along with the increase in human and animal populations. However, the prevalence of taeniasis in man is not well known. It is not a notifiable disease, and the available information is based on isolated studies of specific sectors of the population, such as school-age children and recruits. Widespread studies and mass treatment have been carried out in the USSR. In that country, a general prevalence rate of *T. saginata* infection of 600 per 100,000 inhabitants was obtained in 1950 by fecal examinations of 14,200,000 persons. In 1966, the rate of positivity was 75 per 100,000 inhabitants based on 65,800,000 examinations; the reduction is attributed to mass treatment of the population. These studies have identified areas of high endemicity in the republics south of the Caucasus, with prevalence rates as high as 45,200 per 100,000 inhabitants in Azerbaidzhan.

The distribution and prevalence rates of the two taeniases vary considerably in different geographic areas of the world. Several socioeconomic and cultural factors influence the prevalence. Taeniasis caused by *T. solium* is much more prevalent in developing countries than in industrialized ones because of differences in environmental and personal hygiene standards as well as in swine-raising technology. Taeniasis by *T. solium* is absent from Moslem and Jewish population groups that adhere to the dietary restrictions of the religions. Eating habits and a preference for dishes made with raw meat are important factors in the prevalence of both taeniases in some populations. Infection caused by *T. saginata* is probably on the increase in Europe because of a growing predilection for eating rare steaks. Another factor that has acted to raise the incidence of taeniasis in recent years is the increasing use of detergents that impede the natural destruction of the parasite's eggs in sewer systems.

The countries with the highest endemicity (more than 10% of the population) of *T. saginata* infection are Ethiopia, Kenya, and Zaire. The Caucasus region and the Soviet Republics in south central Asia, as well as some countries on the Mediterranean (Syria, Lebanon, and Yugoslavia), are also endemic areas. In some parts of Yugoslavia, up to 65% of the children were found to be infected. Southwest Asia, Japan, Europe, and South America are regions of moderate prevalence, and Canada, the United States, Australia, and some countries of the western Pacific have low prevalence rates.

Infection by *T. solium* is endemic in Latin America, southern Africa (especially among the Bantu), and in the non-Islamic countries of Southeast Asia.

Little information is available on the prevalence of taeniasis in the Americas. Studies carried out during the last 10 years have recorded the following rates of infection by *T. saginata*: 0.02% in the United States, 0.1% in Cuba, 1.7% in Guatemala, 1 to 2% in Brazil, 1.6% in Chile, and 0.6% in Argentina.

A problem of special public health importance is human infection caused by *Cysticercus cellulosae*, which is often a very serious illness. Human cysticercosis exists throughout the world, but it is especially important in rural areas of developing countries, including those in Latin America. Neurocysticercosis, the most serious form, has been observed in 17 Latin American countries. A 0.43% rate of neurocysticercosis was found in the course of 123,826 autopsies in nine countries that account for two-thirds of the population of Latin America. It has been estimated that out of every 100,000 inhabitants, 100 suffer from neurocysticercosis and as many as 30 from ocular or periocular cysticercosis. The highest morbidity rates are found in Brazil, Chile, Peru, El Salvador, Guatemala, and Mexico (World Health Organization, 1979). The prevalence of neurocysticercosis seems to be especially high in Mexico and Central America. It was estimated that cysticercosis was the cause of 1% of all deaths in the general hospitals of Mexico City and 25% of the intracranial tumors. Autopsies carried out from 1946 to 1979 on 21,597 individuals who died in general hospitals in Mexico found cerebral cysticercosis in 2.9%, leading to the conclusion that about 3% of the general population was affected by this parasitosis, with or without clinical manifestations (Mateos, 1982). In the Triângulo Mineiro, Minas Gerais, Brazil, a rate of 2.4% of cysticercosis was found in 2,306 autopsies; 66% of these individuals had cysts in the central nervous system,

26.8% had cardiac localization, 25% had musculoskeletal cysts, and 7.1% had cutaneous cysts (Gobbi *et al.*, 1980).

In India, cerebral cysticercosis is second in importance, after tuberculosis, as a cause of expansive diseases of the skull, and is one of the principal causes of epilepsy. Neurocysticercosis is also common in Indonesia.

On the other hand, human cysticercosis has disappeared in western and central Europe; it is also disappearing in eastern and southern Europe.

Occurrence in Animals: Information on swine and bovine cysticercosis comes from meat inspection records at slaughterhouses and packing plants. However, it must be borne in mind that usual inspection methods, which consist of cutting the meat at sites where the parasite preferentially locates, reveal only a portion of infected carcasses. It is also important to point out that swine raised on small rural farms, where they often have an opportunity to ingest human feces, are generally slaughtered by their owners without veterinary inspection or are sold without restrictions at market.

In all areas where human taeniasis exists, animal cysticercosis is also found, with variations in prevalence from region to region. In the Americas, only some countries and islands in the Caribbean have not recorded this parasitosis. In Brazil, which accounts for more than 65% of the total swine population in Latin America, 0.83% of 12 million pigs slaughtered in 10 states in the 3-year period 1970-1972 were found to be infected with *C. cellulosae*. Similar rates have been observed in Mexico and several South American countries, such as Chile (0.7%) and Colombia. In Central America, infection rates vary from 1.37% (Panama) to 2.57% (Honduras). Information on bovine cysticercosis is more limited. In four South American countries, the rates vary from 0.01% (Colombia), 0.04% (Chile), and 0.5% (Uruguay) to 2.65% (Brazil). In Mexico the rate is 0.01%, in Nicaragua 0.14%, in El Salvador 3.07%, and in Cuba it varies from 0.13 (public sector) to 0.22% (private sector).

In South Africa, the only African country with an appreciable number of swine (more than one million), the infection rate found in slaughterhouses was under 1.5%. In Zaire, the rate varies in different regions from 0.1% to 8.1%. The highest levels of bovine cysticercosis are found in Botswana and Kenya, with rates of 8% and 20%, respectively, according to records from export slaughterhouses.

Few data are available about the prevalence of the animal infection in Asia.

Swine cysticercosis is disappearing in Europe. In the USSR, the rate of cysticercosis in swine was 0.14% in 1962 and only 0.004% in 1970. Similar figures have been reported from Hungary and other countries of eastern Europe. At present, very few endemic foci are found on that continent, as a consequence of improved and modernized swine-raising practices. Conversely, bovine cysticercosis is increasing as a result of the large concentrations of cattle raised together on modern ranches and the increase in human infection due to consumption of rare beef. In some areas of western Europe, prevalence rates of 5 to 10% are found in cattle, and in some endemic foci in eastern Europe, the rate is much higher.

Economic losses due to the confiscation of bovine and swine carcasses infected by cysticercosis can be significant. In 1963, swine cysticercosis was the reason for 68% of all confiscations in six slaughterhouses in Central America and Panama, causing an estimated loss of one-half million dollars. During 1980, 264,000 swine carcasses were confiscated in Mexico, and total losses due to swine cysticercosis were estimated at about US$43 million. Losses due to bovine cysticercosis in Latin

America are possibly even greater than those due to swine cysticercosis. It is estimated that the loss of one infected bovine amounts to US$25 in developing countries and US$75 in industrialized countries (Pawlowski and Schultz, 1972). The economic impact consists of not only the losses caused by the animal parasitosis, but also the cost of treating human neurocysticercosis, which involves large expenses for surgery, hospitalization, and work days lost. The cost of medical care in Mexico for a patient with neurocysticercosis has been estimated at more than US$2,000.

The Disease in Man: Taeniasis by *T. saginata* is often subclinical and is only revealed by fecal examination or when the infected person consults a physician after feeling the movement of the proglottids in the anal region. In clinical cases, the most common symptomatology consists of abdominal pains, nausea, debility, weight loss, flatulence, and diarrhea or constipation. A patient may have only one of these symptoms, or several. The gravid proglottids of *T. saginata* sometimes travel to different organs (appendix, uterus, bile ducts, nasopharyngeal pathways), causing disorders related to the site in which they settle. A high percentage of patients experience a decrease in gastric secretion. Individual reactions to the infection differ and may be influenced by psychogenic factors, since patients often notice symptoms only after they see the proglottids (Pawlowski, 1982). Taeniasis caused by *T. solium* is more rarely clinically apparent than that caused by *T. saginata*, and is usually benign and mild. In addition, complications like appendicitis and cholangitis have not been recorded in *T. solium* taeniasis; this is explained by the fact that proglottids of *T. solium* lack motility.

Cysticercosis is a much more serious disease. The incubation period is quite variable; symptoms may appear from 15 days to many years after infection takes place. Man can harbor from one to several hundred cysticerci in various tissues and organs. The localization that most often prompts a medical consultation is the central nervous system (neurocysticercosis), and in second place is localization in the eye and its surrounding tissues (ocular and periocular cysticercosis). Localization in muscles and subcutaneous connective tissue is generally not clinically apparent unless large numbers of cysticerci are involved, causing muscular pain, cramps, and fatigue. The symptomatology of neurocysticercosis varies with the number of cysticerci, their stage of development (young, mature, intact, degenerate), their morphologic strain (vesicular or racemose), their location in the central nervous system, and the reaction of the patient. The cysticerci locate most frequently in the meninges, cerebral cortex, and ventricles, and less frequently in the parenchyma. The symptoms generally appear several years after the infection, when death of the larva causes inflammatory toxic reactions. The symptoms are often not well defined and may resemble those of a cerebral tumor, basal meningitis, encephalitis, intracranial hypertension, and hysteria. The most prominent symptom in many patients is epileptiform attacks that recur at irregular intervals.

The presence of cysticerci in the central nervous system does not always give rise to clinical symptoms. Data from several Latin American countries show that in 46.8% of the cases in which cysticerci were found in the central nervous system during autopsy, the individual had had no clinical manifestations of the parasitosis during his life.

Ocular and periocular cysticercosis is less frequent (about 20% of the cases). The cysticerci locate primarily in the vitreous humor, subretinal tissue, and the anterior chamber of the eye. The parasitosis may cause uveitis, iritis, and retinitis, as well as palpebral conjunctivitis, and may affect the motor muscles of the eye.

Taeniasis can be treated with niclosamide (Yomesan) or praziquantel, but until recently no effective chemotherapy was available for cysticercosis. Surgery was the only treatment, and it presented serious risks in the case of neurocysticercosis. An estimated 30% of such patients die during the operation or in the postoperative period. The advent of new drugs, especially praziquantel, opens promising perspectives for treatment, but important questions such as indications and contraindications, dosages, and duration of chemotherapy are yet to be resolved. In clinical studies carried out thus far, tolerance to the drug was good in 80% of the cases, and the symptoms observed in the rest were attributed to the patient's reaction to cysticerci altered (degenerated or killed) by the praziquantel. Satisfactory results were obtained with praziquantel in about 60% of neurocysticercosis cases. However, it should be borne in mind, first, that the drug has no effect on calcified cysticerci, and second, that asymptomatic cases can become symptomatic, either by natural changes in the parasite, or by alterations in the cysticerci or reactions of the host induced by the drug. For all these reasons and also because emergency situations may arise, treatment should be carried out only in neurologic institutions under strict medical supervision. In a recent study in Mexico, praziquantel was administered for 15 days to 26 patients with cysticercosis of the cerebral parenchyma who were otherwise in good general health and did not have intracranial hypertension. During treatment, a strong inflammatory reaction was observed, as evidenced by an increase in proteins and cells in the cerebrospinal fluid; concurrently, cephalalgia and exacerbation of neurologic symptoms were observed. After 3 months, all the patients improved and 50% became asymptomatic. Computerized tomography showed that the total number of cysts was reduced from 152 to 51; the diameter of the cysts was reduced about 72%, and nine of the 26 patients no longer showed any cysts in radiographs (Sotelo et al., 1984). Praziquantel was 100% effective in the treatment of subcutaneous cysticercosis (Baranski, 1984). Clinical trials on 178 patients proved that daily doses of 20 to 75 mg of praziquantel per kilogram of weight for 6 to 21 days resulted in significant clinical improvement (Groll, 1982).

The Disease in Animals: Cysticercosis does not usually manifest itself clinically in animals. Experimental infection of cattle with a high dose of *T. saginata* eggs can produce fever, debility, sialorrhea, anorexia, and muscular stiffness. Death may occur as a result of degenerative myocarditis. In isolated cases, infected swine may experience hypersensitivity of the snout, paralysis of the tongue, and epileptiform convulsions, but the useful life of swine is usually too short for neurologic manifestations to appear.

Dogs that ingest human feces and become infected with the eggs of *T. solium* sometimes show symptoms of cerebral cysticercosis, which may be confused with those of rabies.

Source of Infection and Mode of Transmission (Figures 82 and 83): In contrast to his role in most zoonotic diseases, man constitutes an essential link in the epidemiology of taeniasis and cysticercosis. Humans are the definitive hosts of both species of *Taenia*; their feces contaminate cow pastures and infect coprophagous swine. Taeniae can live for many years in the human small intestine, and the number of eggs in the gravid proglottids eliminated with the feces can reach hundreds of thousands in just one day, although not all are mature. Sometimes just one human carrier of *T. saginata* can be a source of infection for several hundred cattle in a feedlot. Epizootic outbreaks of cysticercosis (*C. bovis*) have been described in

Figure 82. Taeniasis and cysticercosis (*Taenia saginata*). Transmission cycle.

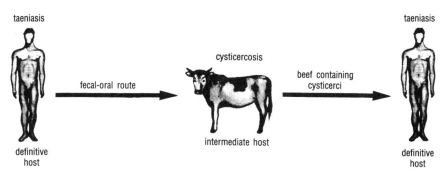

Figure 83. Taeniasis and cysticercosis (*Taenia solium*). Transmission cycle.

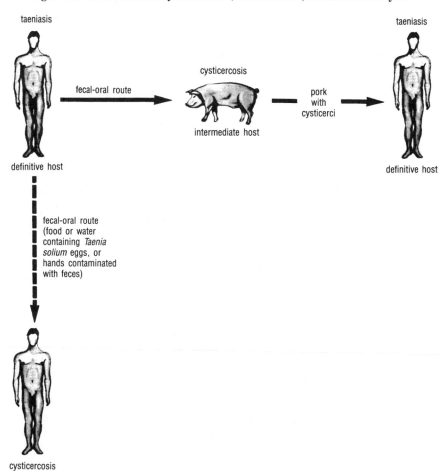

Canada, the United States, and Czechoslovakia. Survival of the eggs in pastures depends on the ambient temperature and humidity: in summer, eggs can survive for about 2 months in the environmental conditions found in Europe, while they may survive more than 5 months in winter; in the highlands of Kenya, eggs of *T. saginata* have been found to remain viable up to a year. In developing countries, where people often defecate in open fields, both swine and cattle have easy access to taeniae eggs. The use of sewer water for irrigation or of contaminated water from a river or other source for watering animals contributes to the spread of cysticercosis. Taeniae eggs can be carried several kilometers by river water, and they may be transported over long distances by gulls and other birds. A role in the dissemination of taeniae eggs is also attributed to coprophagous insects.

The intermediate hosts (bovines, swine) develop cysticerci in their tissues after ingesting taeniae eggs. *C. bovis* can remain viable for about 9 months in live bovines and for about 2 weeks in the carcass, while *C. cellulosae* can survive several years in swine and more than 1 month in the carcass.

Humans acquire *T. solium* taeniasis by eating raw or undercooked pork containing cysticerci (*C. cellulosae*). In this regard, it should be remembered that only a fraction of the pigs butchered in Latin America and other developing countries are subject to veterinary inspection in slaughterhouses.

Man acquires cysticercosis mainly by the following routes: a) ingestion of *T. solium* eggs with food (vegetables, fruits) and water contaminated by feces of a taenia carrier; and b) ingestion of eggs introduced to the mouth by the contaminated hands of an individual with poor hygienic habits, or of oncospheres from the intestine that are transferred from the anal region to the mouth (anus-hand-mouth). Likewise, it has been suggested that the gravid proglottids of the taenia could be carried to the stomach by reversed peristalsis and from there once again into the intestine, where the oncosphere would be liberated and give rise to cysticercosis; however, this mechanism of autoinfection has not yet been confirmed.

The great contrast between the prevalence rates of *T. solium* taeniasis and swine and human cysticercosis in developing countries and the rates in industrialized countries is attributable mainly to different systems of swine husbandry. Infection by *T. solium* has almost disappeared from developed countries because modern swine-raising practices do not permit access to human feces; the opposite is the case on the family farms where swine are raised in developing countries. Differences in environmental sanitation, education, and adherence to the rules of personal hygiene also help explain the contrast. Furthermore, human taeniasis only occurs among populations that habitually consume undercooked meat and/or organs.

Man acquires *T. saginata* taeniasis by consuming raw or undercooked beef containing cysticerci (*C. bovis*). Human infection is closely related to the habit of eating dishes containing raw or insufficiently cooked meat. The infection can also be contracted by tasting meat dishes during their preparation. The risk of contracting the infection is five times greater in a family in which there is a carrier of *T. saginata* than in the general population, and 14 times greater among workers involved in processing and marketing raw meat.

Diagnosis: Diagnosis of human intestinal taeniasis is made by identifying gravid proglottids in the feces. In the case of infection by *T. saginata*, anal swabs should be used rather than direct examination of fecal samples. Proglottids are not eliminated on a daily basis, so the examination must be repeated if results are negative.

Differential diagnosis between *T. saginata* and *T. solium* is based on the number of lateral branches of the uterus in the proglottid, which usually number 16 to 30 in the first species and 7 to 12 in the second. Such differentiation is not possible with proglottids in which the uterus has 12 to 16 branches. When the scolex or scolices are expelled (spontaneously or because of treatment), *T. saginata* can be identified by microscopy, since its scolex lacks hooks but that of *T. solium* has them. The new taeniacidal drugs cause the scolices to disintegrate, removing them as a basis for the differential diagnosis.

Diagnosis of subcutaneous cysticercosis can be made by biopsy of the nodules or by radiography. Ocular cysticerci can be discovered by ophthalmoscopy. Computerized axial tomography (CAT) is very useful in the diagnosis of neurocysticercosis because this procedure allows lesions of various densities to be distinguished and absorption coefficients of different tissues to be quantified. Lesions in the brain caused by *C. cellulosae* have very different absorption coefficients from normal cerebral tissue. CAT makes visible the characteristics and localization of the lesions (Lombardo, 1982). The cerebrospinal fluid of those affected by neurocysticercosis shows an increase in the level of proteins, especially the gammaglobulin fraction, and a marked cellular reaction with a high percentage of plasmacytes and eosinophils. Eosinophilia in the blood is also generally present. When used together with other diagnostic procedures, serologic tests can be valuable, but their sensitivity and specificity are not altogether satisfactory.

The tests of choice for human cysticercosis are ELISA, immunoelectrophoresis, indirect hemagglutination, and complement fixation.

Diagnosis of bovine and swine cysticercosis is made during postmortem examination in slaughterhouses and packing plants. In some swine with intense infections, cysticercosis can be diagnosed antemortem by examination of the tongue. The current inspection method based on cutting into sites where the cysticerci commonly locate is not very effective, and many cases of mild infection may pass unnoticed. Reliable serologic methods are not available at present.

Control: Control measures consist of interrupting the epidemiologic chain at the level of the definitive host (man) and of the intermediate hosts (swine and bovines). In the USSR, rates of infection caused by *T. saginata* have been reduced by means of public health education and mass therapeutic treatment of the population in endemic areas. Between 1964 and 1972, the rate of infected bovine carcasses fell from 1.09% to 0.38%.

An important factor in preventing the human disease is improvement of environmental and personal hygiene levels in rural areas, which is closely tied to education and economic development. Health education should be continual and the danger of eating raw or undercooked meat should be stressed.

In advanced countries, improved techniques and the concentration of swine-raising operations in large units under hygienic conditions (where the animals do not have access to human feces) have brought about drastic reductions in the rate of taeniasis caused by *T. solium* and the rate of cysticercosis. Meat inspection, in spite of its limitations, is a very important measure in controlling the diseases. Unfortunately, in some regions of Latin America and many other developing countries, only a small proportion of the swine are subject to veterinary inspection. In Central America, many of the swine raised by peasants are sacrificed by their owners or in small municipal slaughterhouses lacking veterinary inspection. A priority objective where it is feasible should be to concentrate the slaughter, not only for the economic benefits that would result, but also for the protection of human health. However, this and other measures, such as environmental sanitation in rural areas, education and personal hygiene, and hygienic raising of swine, are difficult to carry out in the foreseeable future in economically depressed countries while current socioeconomic conditions prevail.

Studies carried out in the last two decades have demonstrated that bovines acquire strong immunity against reinfection by *T. saginata* and that resistance can be conferred on them by inoculation with viable oncospheres (parenteral route), oncospheres attenuated by radiation (oral route), or the excretions of oncospheres in culture medium. Likewise, vaccination with a heterologous species such as *T. hydatigena* or other taenia has been shown to increase resistance against *T. saginata*. Investigations have centered on providing passive protection to newborns through the colostrum by immunizing the mothers. Antigens secreted in culture medium by activated oncospheres of *T. taeniaeformis* as well as those of *T. saginata* have proven to be effective for immunizing pregnant cows, by intramuscular or intramammarial inoculation, and for the subsequent passive transference of immunity to calves via the colostrum (Soulsby and Lloyd, 1982). Protection of the newborn is important, since it has been confirmed that in a calf with a developed immune system, the cysticercus survives no more than 9 months after initial infection; on the other hand, if the infection occurs in the neonatal period, the cysticerci can survive several years. After this critical period, the calves can be actively immunized by vaccination at 2 or 3 months of age. In a field trial carried out in Australia (Rickard *et al.*, 1982) with a large number of animals that grazed on pasture land irrigated with waste water, a reduction in both the rate of infection and the level of infection (number of cysticerci) was confirmed in animals immunized with antigens of *T. hydatigena*. It was concluded that although this method significantly reduced infection rates, it might not be practical for common use, and that homologous vaccination with antigens of *T. saginata* should perhaps be used. However, the use of homologous antigens has the drawback of requiring human carriers of the parasite as donors.

Similar tests have not been carried out on swine.

Praziquantel has been tested extensively against bovine cysticercosis, and has been shown to be effective in a single dose of 50 mg/kg of body weight against 3-month-old cysticerci, but not against 1-month-old cysticerci (Gallie and Sewell, 1978). Praziquantel was also tested in Mexico against swine cysticercosis, and was proven effective (Chavarría and Díaz-Gonzalez, 1978).

The World Health Organization has prepared a guide on the surveillance, prevention, and control of taeniasis/cysticercosis that contains an excellent update on various aspects of the disease (World Health Organization, 1983).

Bibliography

Abdussalam, M. The problem of taeniasis-cysticercosis. *In: VII Inter-American Meeting on Foot-and-Mouth Disease and Zoonoses Control.* Washington, D.C., Pan American Health Organization, 1975. (Scientific Publication 295.)

Acha, P. N., and F. J. Aguilar. Studies on cysticercosis in Central America and Panama. *Am J Trop Med Hyg* 13:48-53, 1964.

Almeida, G. L. G. de. Cisticercose suina no Brasil. *Bol Def Sanit Anim (Brasilia)* 7:41-50, 1973.

Atias, A., and A. Neghme. *Parasitología Clínica*. Buenos Aires, Inter-Médica, 1979.

Baranski, M. C. Treatment of dermal cysticercosis with praziquantel. A new cestocidal agent. *Rev Inst Med Trop S Paulo* 26:259-266, 1984.

Belding, D. L. *Textbook of Parasitology*, 3rd ed. New York, Appleton-Century-Crofts, 1965.

Bessonov, A. S. Perspectives on the eradication of several helminthozoonotic diseases in the USSR. *In*: Soulsby, E. J. L. (Ed.), *Parasitic Zoonoses*, New York, Academic Press, 1974.

Biagi, F. *Enfermedades parasitarias*. México, D. F., La Prensa Médica Mexicana, 1974.

Chavarría, M., and D. Díaz-González. Droncit en el tratamiento de la cisticercosis porcina. *Espec Vet (México)* 1:159-165, 1978.

Flisser, A., K. Willms, J. P. Laclette, C. Larralde, C. Ridaura, and F. Beltrán (Eds.), *Cysticercosis: Present State of Knowledge and Perspectives*. New York, Academic Press, 1982.

Gallie, G. J., and M. M. H. Sewell. The efficacy of praziquantel against the cysticerci of *Taenia saginata* in calves. *Trop Anim Health Prod* 10:36-38, 1978.

Gemmell, M., Z. Matyas, Z. Pawlowski, and E. J. L. Soulsby (Eds.). *Guidelines for Surveillance, Prevention and Control of Taeniasis/Cysticercosis*. Geneva, WHO, 1983. (Document VPH/83.49.)

Gobbi, H., S. J. Adad, R. R. Neves, and H. O. Almeida. Ocorrência de cisticercose (*Cysticercus cellulosae*) em Uberaba, M. G. *Rev Patol Trop* (Goiana, Brasil) 9:51-59, 1980.

Groll, E. Chemotherapy of human cysticercosis with praziquantel. *In*: Flisser, A. *et al.*, (Eds.), *Cysticercosis: Present State of Knowledge and Perspectives*. New York, Academic Press, 1982.

Lombardo, L. La cisticercosis cerebral en México. III. Diagnóstico. *Gac Med Méx* 118:4-16, 1982.

Mateos, J. H. *La cisticercosis cerebral en México*. II. Frecuencia. *Gac Med Méx* 118:2-4, 1982.

Mitchell, J. R. Meat-borne zoonoses in East Africa. *Vet Bull* 38:829-833, 1968.

Mosienyane, M. G. A survey of *Cysticercus bovis* (measles) infestation in cattle sent for slaughter to Botswana Meat Commission (BMC). A ten-year retrospective study, 1974-1983. *Int J Zoonoses* 13:124-130, 1986.

Okolo, M. I. O. Studies on *Taenia saginata* cysticercosis in Eastern Nigeria. *Int J Zoonoses* 13:98-103, 1986.

Pawlowski, Z., and M. G. Schultz. Taeniasis and cysticercosis (*Taenia saginata*). *Adv Parasitol* 10:269-343, 1972.

Pawlowski, Z. S. Clinical expression of *Taenia saginata* infection in man. *In*: Prokopic, J. (Ed.), *First International Symposium of Human Taeniasis and Cattle Cysticercosis*. Ceské Budejovice, Czechoslovakia, 20-24 September 1982.

Pawlowski, Z. S. Cestodiases. Taeniasis, Diphyllobothriasis, Hymenolepiasis, and Others. *In*: Warren, S., and A. A. F. Mahmoud, *Tropical and Geographical Medicine*. New York, McGraw-Hill Book Co., 1984.

Rausch, R. L. Taeniidae. *In*: Hubbert, W. T., W. F. McCulloch, and P. R. Schnurrenberger (Eds.), *Diseases Transmitted from Animals to Man*, 5th ed. Springfield, Illinois, Thomas, 1975.

Rickard, M. D., L. Brumley, and G. A. Anderson. Field trial to evaluate the use of antigens from *Taenia hydatigena* oncosphere to prevent infection with *Taenia saginata* in cattle grazing on sewage-irrigated pasture. *Res Vet Sci* 32:189-193, 1982.

Schenone, H., and T. Letonja. Cisticercosis porcina y bovina en Latinoamérica. *Bol Chile Parasitol* 29:90-98, 1974.

Schenone, H. Cysticercosis as a Public Health and Animal Health Problem. *In*: *VII Inter-American Meeting on Foot-and-Mouth Disease and Zoonoses Control*. Washington, D.C., Pan American Health Organization, 1975. (Scientific Publication 295.)

Shulman Ye, S. Biology and taxonomy of *Taenia saginata* and *Taenia solium*. *In*: Lysenko, A. (Ed.), *Zoonoses Control*, vol. 2. Moscow, Centre of International Projects GKNT, 1982.

Slais, J. *The Morphology and Pathogenicity of the Bladder Worms*. The Hague, W. Junk, 1970.

Slonka, G. F. An epizootic of bovine cysticercosis. *J Am Vet Med Assoc* 166:678-681, 1975.

Sotelo, J., F. Escobedo, J. Rodríguez-Carbajal, B. Torres, and F. Rubio-Donnadieu. Therapy of parenchymal brain cysticercosis with praziquantel. *N Engl J Med* 310:1001-1007, 1984.

Soulsby, E. J. L. *Textbook of Veterinary Clinical Parasitology*. Oxford, Blackwell, 1965.

Soulsby, E. J. L. Taeniasis and Cysticercosis: The Problem in the Old World. *In*: *VII Inter-American Meeting on Foot-and-Mouth Disease and Zoonoses Control*. Washington, D.C., Pan American Health Organization, 1975. (Scientific Publication 295.)

Soulsby, E. J. L., and S. Lloyd. Active and passive immunization of cattle against infection with *Taenia saginata*. *In*: Prokopic, J. (Ed.), *First International Symposium on Human Taeniasis and Cattle Cysticercosis*. Ceské Budejovice, Czechoslovakia, 20-24 September 1982.

World Health Organization. *Parasitic Zoonoses*. Report of a WHO Expert Committee, with the Participation of FAO. Geneva, WHO, 1979. (Technical Report Series 637.)

3. Acanthocephaliasis and Nematodiases

ACANTHOCEPHALIASIS

(127.7)

Synonyms: Macracanthorhynchosis.

Etiology: The acanthocephalans, or thorn-headed helminths, which had previously been included among the Nematoda, but have been reclassified as a separate class, Acanthocephala.

Several acanthocephalans cause human infection, and *Macracanthorhynchus hirudinaceus* (*Gigantorhynchus hirudinaceus*, *G. gigas*, *Echinorhynchus gigas*) is the species of greatest interest. Other species are *Moniliformis moniliformis*, *Acanthocephalus rauschi*, *A. bufonis* (*A. sinensis*), and *Corynosoma strumosum*.

The definitive hosts of *M. hirudinaceus* are swine and wild boars, in which the parasite lives in the small intestine. The parasites are milky white or slightly pink, cylindrical, and somewhat flattened; females measure 35 cm or more in length by 4 to 10 mm in width, and males are about 10 cm long by 3 to 5 mm wide. The proboscis has five or six sets of curved spines, arranged in alternate rows. The eggs are ovoid and about 70 to 110 microns long; they are already embryonated when expelled with the feces of the definitive host. To continue their development, the eggs must be ingested by beetle grubs, usually those of dung beetles of the family Scarabaeidae. Once inside these intermediate hosts, the eggs hatch in the midgut and the free larvae penetrate the body cavity of the coleopteran, where they continue their development and encyst. When a swine or another definitive host (peccary, squirrel, muskrat, man) ingests a parasitized coleopteran, the larva sheds its cystic envelope and, after 2 to 3 months, reaches maturity and begins oviposition; the cycle is thus renewed. A female can produce more than 250,000 eggs per day for almost 10 months. The eggs are very resistant to environmental factors and can survive in the soil for several years.

Definitive hosts of *M. moniliformis* are several species of rats, and intermediate hosts are beetles and cockroaches. The vertebrate hosts of *Corynosoma strumosum* are the arctic fox (*Alopex lagopus*), dog, sea otter (*Enhydra lutris*), and several species of cetaceans and pinnipeds; the intermediate host is probably an amphipod crustacean, *Pontoporeia affinis*. Many species of fish serve as paratenic hosts.

Geographic Distribution and Occurrence: *M. hirudinaceus* is found in swine throughout much of the world. Western Europe seems to be free of the infection. In some areas, the infection is common in swine and can reach high rates; in Byelorussia, USSR, 17 to 32% of the herds were found to be infected, and the prevalence rate ranged from 0.9 to 5% and occasionally up to 23% (Soulsby, 1982). Rates found in China varied from 3 to 7.4% in one province and from 50 to 60% in another (Leng *et al.*, 1983).

Human infection was said to be common during the last century in the region of the Volga in Russia, owing to consumption of raw *Melolontha* beetles. However, more recent studies have not confirmed human cases (Leng *et al.*, 1983), with the exception of one case in a 5-year-old child recorded in 1958 (Faust *et al.*, 1974).

Isolated cases have also been described in Czechoslovakia, Bulgaria, Madagascar, and Thailand. Since 1970, human infection has necessitated emergency surgery on children in three provinces in northern China and one in southern China. A study of hospital records demonstrated that in one province (Liaoning), more than 200 surgical interventions were required for intestinal perforations; in one hospital in that province, 115 cases of abdominal colic caused by macracanthorhynchosis were treated (Leng *et al.*, 1983).

Isolated cases of human infection by *Moniliformis moniliformis* have been described in Italy, Sudan, Java, Israel, and the United States of America (Faust *et al.*, 1974). A case of human infection by *Acanthocephalus bufonis* was described in Indonesia, one by *A. rauschi* in Alaska, and one by *Corynosoma strumosum*, also in Alaska (Schmidt, 1971).

The Disease in Man: The pathologic effects and symptomatology of the human infection have not been well studied. The case histories recorded in China, which are the most numerous, refer to extreme cases with acute abdominal colic and perforation of the intestine. The two most recent cases in children required resection of part of the jejunum, which had multiple perforations (Leng *et al.*, 1983).

In an experimental autoinfection by *Moniliformis moniliformis*, a researcher experienced acute gastrointestinal pain, diarrhea, somnolence, and general debility.

The Disease in Animals: *M. hirudinaceus*, which attaches with its proboscis to the wall of the swine's small intestine (usually the jejunum, but in some cases the duodenum and ileum), produces an inflammatory reaction that can progress to necrosis and the formation of small, sometimes caseous nodules. Clinical manifestations depend on the intensity of infection (number of parasites), the degree of penetration of the parasite into the intestinal wall, and, especially, the presence of a secondary bacterial infection. The most severe cases are due to perforation of the intestine, leading to peritonitis and death.

In mink, which are accidental hosts, *C. strumosum* has caused bloody diarrhea and anemia.

Source of Infection and Mode of Transmission: The development of the parasite is cyclical and requires an intermediate host. Although swine and boars are the reservoir and main hosts of *M. hirudinaceus*, the species specificity of the parasite is not strict, and it can infect more than a dozen different species of vertebrates, including man (DeGiusti, 1971). Swine are infected by ingesting scarabaeid coleopterans, which serve as intermediate hosts. In China, besides scarabaeids, members of the beetle family Cerambycidae were found infected with the last immature stage larva (cystacanth) (Lenz *et al.*, 1983).

Man becomes infected in a manner similar to swine, by accidental or deliberate ingestion of coleopterans.

Most infections occur in children from rural areas, who catch beetles for play; sometimes they toast them (insufficiently) to sample their strange taste. In southern China, some rural residents believe that coleopterans are effective against nocturia and administer them to children for that reason.

Diagnosis: Diagnosis can be done by confirming the presence in the feces of thick-shelled eggs containing the first larval stage (acanthor). The eggs are easier to see after centrifugal concentration. The adult parasite can be examined after the patient is treated with piperazine citrate or another drug and expels it from the intestine.

However, in many if not most cases, such as the ones in China, diagnosis is made after emergency surgery.

Control: Human infection can be prevented by avoiding the ingestion of coleopterans. To control the parasitosis in swine, the animals should be kept under hygienic conditions and provided with abundant food to discourage rooting and ingestion of coleopterans.

Bibliography

DeGiusti, D. L. Acanthocephala. *In*: Davis, J. W., and R. C. Anderson (Eds.), *Parasitic Diseases of Wild Mammals*, Ames, Iowa State University Press, 1971.

Faust, E. C., P. F. Russell, and R. C. Jung. *Craig and Faust's Clinical Parasitology*, 8th ed. Philadelphia, Lea and Febiger, 1970.

Leng, Y. J., W. D. Huang, and P. N. Liang. Human infection with *Macracanthorhynchus hirudinaceus* (Travassos, 1916) in Guangdong province, with notes on its prevalence in China. *Ann Trop Med Parasitol* 77:107-109, 1983.

Schmidt, G. D. Acanthocephalan infections of man, with two new records. *J Parasitol* 57:582-584, 1971.

Soulsby, E. J. L. *Helminths, Arthropods and Protozoa of Domesticated Animals*, 7th ed. Philadelphia, Lea and Febiger, 1982.

ANGIOSTRONGYLIASIS

(128.8)

Synonyms: Angiostrongylosis, eosinophilic meningitis or meningoencephalitis (*A. cantonensis*), abdominal angiostrongylosis (*A. costaricensis*).

Etiology: Two metastrongylids, *Angiostrongylus* (*Morerastrongylus*) *costaricensis* and *A. cantonensis*, are the etiologic agents. The first species is responsible for abdominal angiostrongyliasis, and the second one for eosinophilic meningitis or meningoencephalitis.

The definitive hosts of both species are rodents; man is an accidental host. Both species require mollusks as intermediate hosts for the completion of their life cycle.

The main definitive host of *A. costaricensis* is the cotton rat, *Sigmodon hispidus*, in which the adult nematode lodges in the mesenteric arteries and their branches on the intestinal wall. The first-stage larva emerges from eggs laid in the arteries, penetrates the intestinal wall, and is then carried with the fecal matter to the exterior. In order to continue their development, the first-stage larvae have to be ingested by a slug, *Vaginulus ameghini*,[1] in which they change successively into second- and third-stage larvae. When the infective third-stage larva is ingested by a rodent, it seeks the ileocecal region, where it penetrates the intestinal wall and locates in the lymphatic vessels (both inside and outside the abdominal lymph nodes). In this location the larvae undergo two molts before migrating to their final habitat, the mesenteric arteries of the cecal region. Oviposition begins after about 18 days, and the first-stage larvae appear in the feces 24 days after infection (prepatent period). In man, an accidental host, the parasite can reach sexual maturity and produce eggs, but the eggs usually degenerate, causing a granulomatous tissue reaction.

The development cycle of *A. cantonensis* is similar to that of *A. costaricensis*. The intermediate hosts are various species of land snails, slugs, and freshwater snails. The definitive hosts can become infected by ingesting infected snails, or plants and water contaminated by them with the third larvae. In addition, infection can occur as a result of consuming transfer hosts (paratenic hosts), such as crustaceans, fish, amphibians, and reptiles, which in turn have eaten infected mollusks (primary intermediate hosts). The definitive hosts of *A. cantonensis* are primarily various species of the genus *Rattus*. When they enter a rat's body, the third-stage larvae (which developed in a mollusk) penetrate the intestine and are carried by the circulatory system to the brain, where they undergo two more molts and become young adult parasites. From the cerebral parenchyma they migrate to the surface of the brain. They remain for a time in the subarachnoid space and later migrate to the pulmonary arteries, where they reach sexual maturity and begin oviposition. The eggs hatch in the pulmonary arterioles, releasing the first larva, which migrates up the trachea, is swallowed, and is eliminated with the feces. Mollusks are infected by ingesting fecal matter of infected rodents.

---

[1] "*V. ameghini* is a natural host of *Angiostrongylus costaricensis* in Costa Rica and Panama. It should be noted that this Neotropical slug can be confused with the Pacific Islands and Southeast Asian *Vaginulus plebeuis*. It has actually been misidentified as *V. plebeuis* by Morena and Ash (1970) in Costa Rica and by Tesh *et al.* (1973) in Panama" (Malek, 1985, p. 227).

In man, who is an accidental host, the larvae and young adults of *A. cantonensis* generally die in the brain, meninges, or medulla oblongata. The nematode can occasionally be found in the lungs.

Geographic Distribution and Occurrence: Abdominal angiostrongyliasis, caused by *A. costaricensis* (Morera and Cespedes, 1971), is a parasitosis described a few years ago in Costa Rica; it is one of the most recently recognized zoonoses. More than 130 human cases, mostly in children, have been diagnosed in Costa Rica. Human disease has also been confirmed in Honduras, El Salvador, and Brazil. Suspected clinical cases have occurred in Nicaragua and Venezuela. In Panama, the adult parasite was found in five species of rodents belonging to three different families. In the past few years, the parasite has been found in several specimens of *Sigmodon hispidus* in Texas, USA (Uberlaker and Hall, 1979); *Oryzomys caliginosus* in Colombia (Malek, 1981); and slugs (*Vaginulus* spp.) in Guayaquil, Ecuador (Morera *et al.*, 1983). The parasitosis is probably much more widespread than is currently recognized. *A. costaricensis* has not been recorded outside the Americas.

Human cases of parasitism by *A. cantonensis* have occurred in Thailand, Vietnam, Kampuchea, the Philippines, Indonesia, Taiwan, Japan, Australia, and several Pacific islands. The parasite is much more widely distributed, and its existence in rats has been confirmed in southern China, India, Malaysia, Sri Lanka, Madagascar, Mauritius, and Egypt. Until recently, the geographic distribution of *A. cantonensis* was thought to be limited to Asia, Australia, the Pacific islands, and Africa. However, in recent years its presence has been confirmed in Cuba, where infected rats (*Rattus norvegicus*) and mollusks have been found (Aguiar *et al.*, 1981); likewise, five human cases of meningoencephalitis have been attributed to *A. cantonensis* in that country (Pascual *et al.*, 1981). It is believed that the parasite was introduced to the island some years ago by rats from a ship from Asia. In a study carried out on rat species (*R. norvegicus*, *R. rattus*, and *R. exulans*) on the Hawaiian and Society Islands, the parasite was found in more than 40% of the specimens captured. In Egypt, 32.7% of 55 specimens of *R. norvegicus* harbored the parasite (Yousif and Ibrahim, 1978). In the province of Havana, Cuba, 12 out of 20 captured *R. norvegicus* were infected (Aguiar *et al.*, 1981). In view of the worldwide distribution of *R. norvegicus* and *R. rattus*, these rodents were examined for the parasite in Puerto Rico, London, and New Orleans, but the results were negative.

Eosinophilic meningitis associated with infection by *A. cantonensis* has been recorded in several hundred patients in endemic areas.

The Disease in Man: The clinical manifestations of abdominal angiostrongyliasis caused by *A. cantonensis* are moderate but prolonged fever, abdominal pain on the right side, and, frequently, anorexia, diarrhea, and vomiting. Leukocytosis is characteristic (20,000 to 50,000 per mm^3), with marked eosinophilia (11 to 82%). Palpation sometimes reveals tumoral masses or abscesses. Rectal examination is painful, and a tumor can occasionally be palpated. Lesions are located primarily in the ileocecal region, the ascending colon, appendix, and regional lymph nodes, but they are also found in the small intestine. Granulomatous inflammation of the intestinal wall can cause partial or complete obstruction. Out of 116 children with intestinal eosinophilic granulomas studied from 1966 to 1975 in the National Children's Hospital in Costa Rica, 90 had surgery (appendectomy, ileocolonic resection, or hemicolectomy). Appendicitis was the preoperative diagnosis in 34 cases. All but two of the children survived and recovered. The highest prevalence (53%) was found in children 6 to 13 years old, and twice as many boys as girls were affected (Loría-Cortés and Lobo-Sanahuja, 1980). Ectopic localizations may occur; when the liver was affected in some Costa Rican patients, the syndrome resembled visceral larva migrans (Morera et al., 1982).

The symptomatology of eosinophilic meningitis and meningoencephalitis was studied in 1968 and 1969 in 125 patients from southern Taiwan. Most patients had a mild or moderate symptomatology, and only a few suffered serious manifestations; four of the patients died and another three had permanent sequelae. Young specimens of A. cantonensis were found in the cerebrospinal fluid of eight patients, and the parasite was found during autopsy in another. In 78% of the patients, the disease has a sudden onset, with intense headaches, vomiting, and moderate intermittent fever. More than 50% of the patients experienced coughing, anorexia, malaise, constipation, and somnolence, and less than half had stiffness of the neck. Pleocytosis was particularly pronounced during the second and third weeks of the disease. The percentage of eosinophils was generally high and was directly related to the number of leukocytes in the cerebrospinal fluid. Leukocytosis and eosinophilia in the blood were also high. The disease occurs mainly in children in Taiwan, while in other endemic areas it occurs mainly in adults. Angiostrongyliasis caused by A. cantonensis is not always expressed as simple meningitis; there have been outbreaks or isolated cases in which the spinal cord, spinal nerves, and brain were extensively affected. The reason for the different clinical pictures is not known, but it may be due to the number of parasites present (intensity of infection). Eosinophilic meningitis, which is the most common clinical form, usually occurs after the ingestion of paratenic hosts (such as shrimp) or contaminated vegetables, either of which generally contain few larvae, while the more serious forms of the disease are due to direct consumption of intermediate hosts, such as infected mollusks (Kliks et al., 1982). In American Samoa, an outbreak of radiculomyeloencephalitis was described in 16 fishermen who had consumed raw or undercooked Achatina fulica (giant African snail), a known intermediate host of A. cantonensis. The incubation period was 1 to 6 days, and the disease lasted 10 weeks. In addition to eosinophilia in the spinal fluid and blood, the disease was characterized by acute abdominal pain, generalized pruritus, and later by pain, debility, paresthesia in the legs, and dysfunction of the bladder (urinary retention or incontinence) and the intestines. Half of the patients suffered transitory hypertension and/or lethargy; three entered a coma and one died. Of the 12 hospitalized patients, 10 had to use wheelchairs to move around (Kliks et al., 1982).

Serologic studies carried out in Australia, in human populations living in localities where the infection occurs in rats and those living in other places where it does not, indicate that many human infections are asymptomatic (Welch et al., 1980).

The Disease in Animals: In rodents, A. costaricensis produces lesions that are located primarily in the cecum, as well as focal or diffuse edema of the subserosa, a reduction in mesenteric fat, and swelling of the regional lymph nodes. In highly parasitized animals, eggs and larvae may be found in various viscera of the body. No significant difference in weight between parasitized and nonparasitized animals has been confirmed.

Rats infected by *A. cantonensis* may show consolidation and fibrosis in the lungs. However, the physical appearance of the animals does not reflect the degree of pathologic changes.

For both parasites, the prevalence of the infection is greater in adult than in young rodents.

Source of Infection and Mode of Transmission (Figures 84 and 85): Several species of rodents are known to serve as definitive hosts of *A. costaricensis*: *Sigmodon hispidus*, *Rattus rattus*, *Zygodontomys microtinus*, *Liomys adspersus*, *Oryzomys fulvescens*, and *O. caliginosus*; also, natural infection has been found in a coati (*Nasua narica*) and marmosets (*Saguinus mystax*). In a study carried out in Panama (Tesh *et al.*, 1973), the highest prevalence of the infection was found in the cotton rat (*S. hispidus*), which was also the most abundant rodent in the six localities studied. The cotton rat inhabits areas close to dwellings in both tropical and temperate America; it is omnivorous, feeding on both plants and small vertebrate and invertebrate animals, including slugs (*V. ameghini*). All these facts indicate that the cotton rat is a prime reservoir and that it plays an important role in the epidemiology of the parasitosis. Rodents are infected by ingesting infected mollusks. Another probable source of infection is plants contaminated with mollusk secretions ("slime") containing third-stage infective larvae of the parasite.

The manner in which man contracts the infection is not well known. Infection probably occurs by ingestion of poorly washed vegetables containing small slugs or their secretions. It is believed that children can become infected while playing in

Figure 84. Angiostrongyliasis (*Angiostrongylus costaricensis*). Transmission cycle.

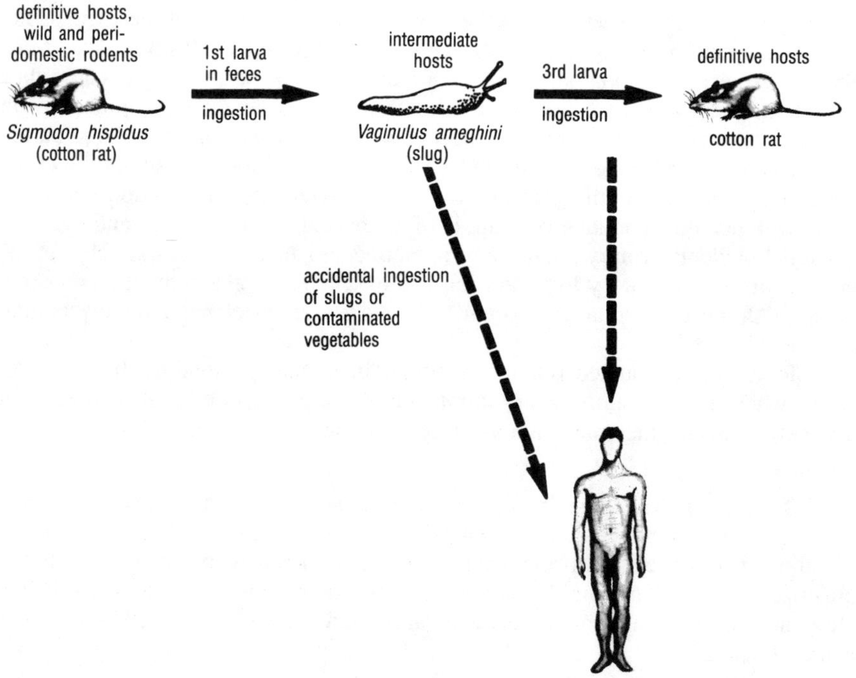

definitive hosts, wild and peri-domestic rodents

Sigmodon hispidus (cotton rat)

1st larva in feces → ingestion

intermediate hosts

Vaginulus ameghini (slug)

3rd larva → ingestion

definitive hosts

cotton rat

accidental ingestion of slugs or contaminated vegetables

Figure 85. Angiostrongyliasis (*Angiostrongylus cantonensis*). Transmission cycle.

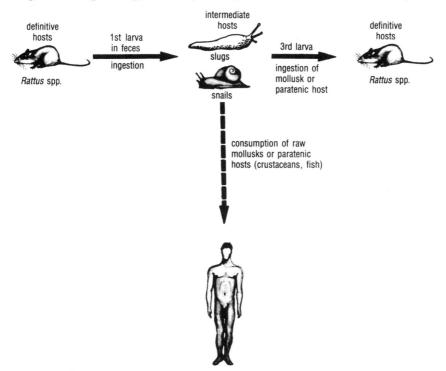

areas where slugs are abundant by transferring snail secretions found on vegetation to their mouths. An increase in cases in children occurs in Costa Rica during the rainy season, when slugs are most plentiful. Humidity is an important factor in the survival of both the first- and third-stage larvae in the environment, since they are susceptible to desiccation.

The parasite species in the Far East (*A. cantonensis*) has been found in at least ten different species of the genus *Rattus* and in *Bandicota indica* and *Melomys littoralis*. These rodents, natural definitive hosts, are infected by consuming mollusks or paratenic hosts that harbor third-stage larvae. The infection rate of the mollusks is usually high; both the prevalence and the number of larvae an individual mollusk can harbor vary according to the species. Man, who is an accidental host, is infected by consuming raw mollusks and also paratenic hosts such as crustaceans or fish.

The ecology of angiostrongyliasis is closely related to the plant community, since it ultimately supports the appropriate mollusks and rodents. The frequency of the human parasitosis depends on the abundance of these hosts and the degree to which they are infected, and, also, in the case of *A. cantonensis*, on eating habits (consumption of raw mollusks, crustaceans, and fish).

Diagnosis: Diagnosis of the human infection caused by *A. costaricensis* can be made by examining surgical specimens and confirming the presence of parasites and their eggs. Immunobiologic methods for diagnosis are not available at present.

No laboratory method exists for confirming infection by *A. cantonensis*. Only in a few cases has it been possible to detect the presence of the parasite in cerebrospinal fluid or the eye of patients. In endemic areas, the disease should be suspected in cases of meningitis or meningoencephalitis with eosinophilia in the blood and cerebrospinal fluid.

Recent studies have indicated that immunobiologic tests can be useful. In American Samoa, both in a previous outbreak of eosinophilic meningitis and the radiculomyeloencephalitis outbreak, serologic titers that were considered significant were revealed using the ELISA test (Kliks *et al.*, 1982). Other tests that have been studied and that could be used after a better evaluation of their sensitivity and specificity are indirect immunofluorescence, immunoelectrophoresis, gel diffusion, and latex agglutination.

Control: At least theoretically, angiostrongyliasis could be controlled by reducing rodent and mollusk populations. Preventive measures at the individual level consist of washing vegetables thoroughly, washing hands after garden or field work, not eating raw or undercooked mollusks and crustaceans, and not drinking water that may be unhygienic.

Bibliography

Aguiar, P. H., P. Morera, and J. Pascual. First record of *Angiostrongylus cantonensis* in Cuba. *Am J Trop Med Hyg* 30:963-965, 1981.

Andersen, E., D. J. Gubler, K. Sorensen, J. Beddard, and L. R. Ash. First report of *Angiostrongylus cantonensis* in Puerto Rico. *Am J Trop Med Hyg* 35:319-322, 1986.

Chen, S. N. Enzyme-linked immunosorbent assay (ELISA) for the detection of antibodies to *Angiostrongylus cantonensis*. *Trans R Soc Trop Med Hyg* 80:398-405, 1986.

Kliks, M. M., K. Kroenke, and J. M. Hardman. Eosinophilic radiculomyeloencephalitis: an angiostrongyliasis outbreak in American Samoa related to ingestion of *Achatina fulica* snails. *Am J Trop Med Hyg* 31:1114-1122, 1982.

Loría-Cortés, R., and J. F. Lobo-Sanahuja. Clinical abdominal angiostrongylosis. A study of 116 children with intestinal eosinophilic granuloma caused by *Angiostrongylus costaricensis*. *Am J Trop Med Hyg* 29:538-544, 1980.

Malek, E. A. *Snail-transmitted Parasitic Diseases*, vol. 2. Boca Raton, Florida, CRC Press, 1980.

Malek, E. A. Presence of *Angiostrongylus costaricensis* Morera and Cespedes, 1971, in Colombia. *Am J Trop Med Hyg* 30:81-83, 1981.

Malek, E. A. *Snail Hosts of Schistosomiasis and Other Snail-transmitted Diseases in Tropical America: A Manual*. Washington, D.C., Pan American Health Organization, 1985. (Scientific Publication 478.)

Morera, P. Life history and redescription of *Angiostrongylus costaricensis* Morera and Cespedes, 1971. *Am J Trop Med Hyg* 22:613-621, 1973.

Morera, P., F. Pérez, F. Mora, and L. Castro. Visceral larva migrans-like syndrome caused by *Angiostrongylus costaricensis*. *Am J Trop Med Hyg* 31:67-70, 1982.

Morera, P., R. Lazo, J. Urquizo, and M. Llaguno. First record of *Angiostrongylus costaricensis* (Morera and Cespedes, 1971) in Ecuador. *Am J Trop Med Hyg* 32:1460-1461, 1983.

Pascual, J. E., R. P. Bouli, and H. Aguiar. Eosinophilic meningoencephalitis in Cuba, caused by *Angiostrongylus cantonensis*. *Am J Trop Med Hyg* 30:960-962, 1981.

Rosen, L. Angiostrongyliasis. *In*: Hubbert, W. T., W. F. McCulloch, and P. R. Schnurrenberger (Eds.), *Diseases Transmitted from Animals to Man*, 6th ed. Springfield, Illinois, Thomas, 1975.

Tesh, R. B., L. J. Ackerman, W. H. Dietz, and J. A. Williams. *Angiostrongylus costaricensis* in Panama: report of the prevalence and pathologic finding in wild rodents infected with the parasite. *Am J Trop Med Hyg* 22:348-356, 1973.

Uberlaker, J. E., and N. M. Hall. First report of *Angiostrongylus costaricensis* (Morera and Cespedes, 1971) in the United States. *J Parasitol* 65:307, 1979.

Wallace, G. D., and L. Rosen. Studies on eosinophilic meningitis. I. Observations on its prevalence in wild rats. *Am J Epidemiol* 81:52-62, 1965.

Welch, J. S., C. Dobson, and G. Campbell. Immunodiagnosis and seroepidemiology of *Angiostrongylus cantonensis* zoonoses in man. *Trans R Soc Trop Med Hyg* 74:614-623, 1980.

Yii, Chin-Yun. Clinical observations on eosinophilic meningitis and meningoencephalitis caused by *Angiostrongylus cantonensis* on Taiwan. *Am J Trop Med Hyg* 25:233-249, 1976.

Yousif, F., and A. Ibrahim. The first record of *Angiostrongylus cantonensis* from Egypt. *Z Parasitenkd* 56:73-80, 1978.

ANISAKIASIS

(127.1)

Etiology: The etiologic agent of human anisakiasis is the larval stage of ascaridoid nematodes of the family Anisakidae, belonging to the genera (or groups) *Anisakis*, *Phocanema* (*Terranova*), and *Contracaecum*. The adult parasites lodge in the stomach and small intestine of piscivorous marine animals. Although several species of *Anisakis* (type species *A. simplex*) are recognized as valid, the larvae found in fish or in man lack many of the diagnostic characters of the adult parasites and, therefore, the species to which they belong cannot be determined. On the basis of some morphologic characteristics, investigators classify the larvae into three types, type I being the most common. Type I larvae of *Anisakis* spp. have been found in 123 different species of fish and one species of squid in Japanese waters. The larvae identified in man are also type I (Myers, 1975; Smith and Wootten, 1978).

The basic life cycle and its variations in the numerous species of the family are not yet well known, but it is recognized that marine anisakids generally require at least one and more commonly two intermediate hosts. The feces of the definitive hosts—mainly ichthyophagous marine mammals such as dolphins, porpoises, whales, and seals—contain the parasite's eggs, which require an incubation period in water in order to release a microscopic second-stage larva. This larva must be ingested by an intermediate host in order to continue its development cycle. The first intermediate hosts are marine invertebrates; larvae have been found in crustaceans, but it has not been possible to determine whether these were second-stage larvae. For this reason, some researchers think that marine invertebrates may be the only intermediate hosts, and that the larvae they harbor (third stage) could be infective for the definitive host and for man. In one species of fish (*Fundulus heteroclitus*) fed experimentally with second-stage larvae, the second larval molt was confirmed, and thus this fish can be considered a true intermediate host. In other species, however, for example *Lebistes reticulatus*, the second molt does not occur, and such a fish should be considered a paratenic (transfer) host. Consequently, fish may act as a second intermediate host or paratenic host, depending on the species. With respect to *Contracaecum* spp., fourth-stage larvae and adults have been found in fish, which can therefore be considered definitive hosts. Marine mammals would be infected by third-stage larvae, which go through two molts before they become adult anisakids and begin to lay eggs, thus reinitiating the cycle.

Because of the difficulty of maintaining marine vertebrates in the laboratory, much of the information on anisakids pertains to species that infect land and freshwater vertebrates. It is hoped that artificial culture of the parasites in the laboratory, using eggs of various genera and species of anisakids found in different definitive hosts, can help to clarify their life cycle and resolve current questions.

Man is an aberrant host in whom the larva ingested with raw fish or squid does not reach maturity. An exception occurred when the existence of a young adult *Phocanema decipiens* was confirmed in a California patient (Kliks, 1983). The large majority of symptomatic human cases are due to species of the genus *Anisakis*, which are the most invasive for man.

Geographic Distribution and Occurrence: Parasites of the genus *Anisakis* are found in most oceans and seas, but some species have a more restricted distribution. Human infection occurs in countries where marine fish are eaten raw, lightly salted, or smoked. From 1955, when human infection was described for the first time in the Netherlands, to 1968, 160 cases occurred in that country. Since 1969, when freezing fish for 24 hours before marketing became mandatory, only a few cases have occurred. The country with the highest frequency of human anisakiasis is Japan, where 487 cases occurred up to 1976. Isolated cases have been recorded in Denmark, England, Germany, Belgium, France, and Korea. In the western hemisphere, one case of anisakiasis was recorded in Chile (Sapunar *et al.*, 1976) and 23 cases in North America, of which 11 occurred in California and five in Alaska (Kliks, 1983). Most of the American cases were due to *Phocanema decipiens*, and the others to *Anisakis* spp.

Both in Japan and the Netherlands, the recorded prevalence was higher in males than in females. In Japan the highest rate of infection is found in persons between 20 and 50 years old.

Many species of fish have been found to be naturally infected. The prevalence of infection in fish can be very high. A study of Baltic herring found that up to 95% of the fish were infected at certain times of the year, with an average of 14 larvae each.

In Peru, larvae of *Anisakis* spp. have been found in three species of marine fish caught close to the port of Callao. Larvae were found in 48.6% of 222 specimens of jacks (*Trachurus murphyi*); 1.5% of 381 croakers (*Sciaena deliciosa*); 1.6% of 180 "cocos" (*Polyclemus peruanus*); and none of 250 "cojinobas" (*Seriolella violacea*). The highest rates of infection were found between December and March (Tantalean, 1972). In Chile, 27% of 311 *Trachurus murphyi* harbored larvae of *Anisakis* spp.; likewise, infection by other species of Anisakidae has been confirmed in *Merluccius gayi* (hake), *Cilus montti* (corbina), and *Thyrsites atun* (sierra), all fish that are consumed regularly (Torres *et al.*, 1978).

The Disease in Man: Anisakiasis can occur clinically in several forms. The larvae may remain in the cavity of the stomach or intestine without penetrating the tissues, causing an infection that is often asymptomatic. In general, asymptomatic or mild cases are caused by *Phocanema* spp. These infections are discovered when live larvae are expelled by means of coughing, vomiting, or defecating. In laboratory examinations of two recent cases of infection by *Phocanema* spp., only light and transitory eosinophilia was found.

In the invasive forms, the larvae penetrate into the gastric or intestinal submucosa. Symptoms of gastric anisakiasis appear 4 to 6 hours after the consumption of raw fish, and consist of sudden epigastric pain, often with nausea and vomiting. Eosinophilia is present in about half of the patients, but not leukocytosis. The gastric form of the disease is seldom diagnosed correctly; it can become chronic, lasting more than a year. In Japanese patients, where gastric anisakiasis is more prevalent than intestinal anisakiasis, occult blood has been found in the gastric juice, as well as hypoacidity or anacidity. The clinical picture of gastric anisakiasis is similar to and has been confused with that of peptic ulcer, gastric tumor, acute gastritis, cholecystitis, and other gastrointestinal pathologies.

Intestinal anisakiasis has an incubation period of about 7 days and is manisfested by severe pain in the lower abdomen, nausea, vomiting, fever, diarrhea, and occult blood in the feces. There is leukocytosis but seldom eosinophilia (Smith and Wootten, 1978). This form can be confused with appendicitis and peritonitis.

Sometimes the parasites perforate the intestinal wall and lodge in the mesenteric veins or various organs. In these invasive forms, the larvae are found in eosinophilic granulomas, phlegmons, or abscesses. The clinical picture of mesenteric anisakiasis varies with the organ affected.

The anatomopathologic examination of cases of invasive anisakiasis reveals ulcerations and hemorrhagic foci in the mucosa as well as localized and diffuse tumors in the intestinal or stomach wall. Histopathologic sections reveal intense eosinophilic infiltration, with edema, histiocytes, lymphocytes, neutrophils, plasmocytes, and sometimes giant cells. These eosinophilic abscesses or phlegmons contain anisakid larvae. Experiments indicate that the eosinophilic granulomas arise as a consequence of allergic reaction to local sensitization, but this pathogenic mechanism has not yet been confirmed.

In a clinicopathologic study of 92 cases in Japan, anisakiasis was localized in the stomach of 65% of the patients and in the intestine (large or small) of 30%. In the Netherlands, intestinal anisakiasis was more prevalent than gastric anisakiasis. Most cases in the United States were a noninvasive transitory anisakiasis caused by larvae of *Phocanema* spp., which were located in the lumen of the digestive tract. The main symptoms consisted of mild epigastric pain and nausea beginning when the infected fish was ingested and lasting up to 20 hours; in about 2 weeks, the parasite was expelled by coughing or vomiting, or was found in the mouth (Kliks, 1983).

The Disease in Animals: The larvae of anisakids can cause serious pathologic changes in many species of marine fish. The parasitosis can affect various organs, and the number of larvae may reach several hundred per fish. The most commonly affected organ is the liver, and atrophy frequently occurs. A cod parasitized by *Contracaecum* spp. weighs less than a healthy fish, and if the number of larvae is large, the fat content of its liver may be significantly reduced. In young fish, the larvae of *Contracaecum* can cause death when invading the cardiac region. In addition to the liver, anisakid larvae can encapsulate in other organs, causing alterations such as perforations of the stomach wall, visceral adhesions, and muscle damage. In spite of these observations by several researchers, knowledge of the pathologic effects of the parasitosis in fish is still incomplete, and experimental infection studies will be necessary to determine precisely the pathology originated by anisakids in these animals (Smith and Wootten, 1978).

In marine mammals, 100 or more of the parasites (larvae and adults) are sometimes found deeply inserted into tumors in the gastric mucosa; it can thus be assumed that parasitic invasion affects the health of these animals. Lesions are usually observed when the parasite burden is large, and especially when large numbers of these nematodes are inserted in one spot of the gastric mucosa or submucosa. The parasites that are free in the lumen of the digestive tract do not cause any apparent pathology. A study of experimental infection by *Phocanema decipiens* was carried out on two species of seals, *Phoca vitulina* and *Halichoerus grypus*. In *Phoca vitulina*, stomach ulcers were associated with clusters of adult *P. decipiens* in the mucosa, and inflammatory lesions were observed when individual nematodes were inserted in the stomach wall. Raised, inflammatory lesions occurred in *H. grypus* when the parasites were inserted in clusters or individually in the mucosa. Histologic examination of the lesions confirmed that they were eosinophilic granulomas (McClelland, 1980).

Source of Infection and Mode of Transmission (Figure 86): The main source of infection for man is marine fish, many species of which are highly parasitized by anisakid larvae. The larvae are killed by heating to 60°C for 1 minute or freezing to −20°C for 24 hours, with the exception of some North American species that can survive such freezing for 52 hours. Human cases are caused by consuming raw, lightly salted, or smoked fish, whether or not it has been refrigerated. In the Netherlands, the occurrence of the disease was due to the habit of consuming raw or lightly salted herring ("green herring"). Although the habit persists, the incidence of human anisakiasis has been drastically reduced by the requirement that fish be frozen before it is sent to market. In recent years, the highest incidence of the disease has been recorded in Japan, where many fish dishes are eaten raw or pickled in vinegar. In the United States, at least two cases were linked to eating seviche (pieces of raw fish seasoned in lemon juice for several hours), and others to eating Japanese raw fish dishes.

The conditions necessary for transmission to humans exist on the Pacific coast of Latin American countries. In Peru and Chile, anisakid larvae have been found in the stomach wall, intestinal wall, mesentery, and on the surface of the gonads of several species of commercial marine fish; in addition, in those countries and others along the Pacific coast, seviche is a very popular dish. One case of human infection was recorded in Chile (Sapunar *et al.*, 1976).

According to Japanese parasitologists, anisakid larvae found in cephalopods such as cuttlefish and octopus are third-stage larvae and thus would be infective for man (and for the natural definitive hosts) when those invertebrates are consumed raw or undercooked. Marine fish can become second intermediate hosts by eating infected invertebrates; they can also ingest other infected fish and become paratenic hosts. Occasionally, if the fish is a compatible host, the larvae can develop to maturity; otherwise, they are evacuated with the feces or they penetrate the tissues and survive, encapsulated or free, in the liver and other locations.

Cleaning fish immediately after they are caught not only prevents them from spoiling, but also prevents *Anisakis* larvae from migrating from the intestine to the muscles. With the installation of refrigeration facilities on ships, this practice has been abandoned and currently fish are not eviscerated until their arrival at the

Figure 86. Anisakiasis. Possible mode of transmission to man.

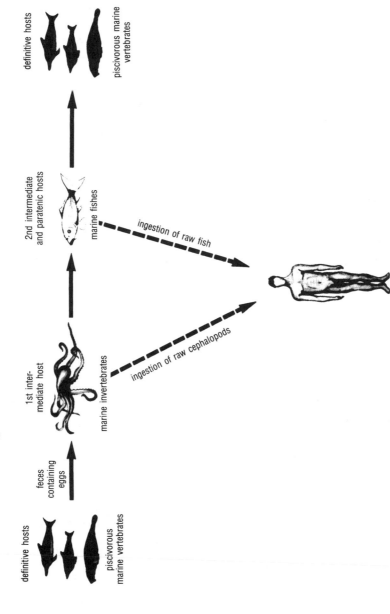

Note: The development cycle of marine anisakids is still not well clarified.

processing plant. The risk of human infection thus increases in countries where fish are eaten raw, because of the increased number of larvae found in the muscles (World Health Organization, 1979).

It has been observed that some fourth-stage larvae and adult parasites of *Contracaecum* spp. emigrate from dead fish to the exterior through the gills or anus, while others penetrate the intestinal wall and enter the mesentery and muscles. To prevent migration to the musculature, fish should be eviscerated immediately after being caught; it should be borne in mind, however, that if the wastes are thrown into the sea they could serve as a source of infection for marine mammals and possibly some fish.

Diagnosis: Diagnosis of the infection has very rarely been made prior to surgery. The presence of larvae or their remains can be confirmed in the lesions. Intact larvae can be identified to genus (or group) but not to species. When infection is caused by *Anisakis* spp., the type of larva can be determined (see Etiology).

The complement fixation, diffusion in agar gel, indirect immunofluorescence, and cutaneous tests have so far been of limited use owing to a lack of sensitivity or specificity. More studies are needed in this respect.

Control: The disease in humans can be prevented by not eating raw fish.

Control at the community level can be achieved by freezing fish at − 20°C for at least 24 hours. Salting is also effective when concentrated salt solutions that reach all parts of the fish are used. Prohibiting the sale of fish that has not undergone these processes is the most effective measure that can be applied. It is also important to eviscerate fish immediately after they are caught.

Bibliography

Arean, V. M. Anisakiasis. *In*: Marcial-Rojas, R. A. (Ed.), *Pathology of Protozoal and Helminthic Diseases*. Baltimore, Maryland, Williams and Wilkins, 1971.

Bier, J. W. Experimental anisakiasis: cultivation and temperature tolerance determinations. *J Milk Food Technol* 39:132-137, 1976.

Cheng, T. C. The natural history of anisakiasis in animals. *J Milk Food Technol* 39:32-46, 1976.

Chitwood, M. Nematodes of medical importance found in market fish. *Am J Trop Med Hyg* 19:599-602, 1970.

Faust, E. C., P. C. Beaver, and R. C. Jung. *Animal Agents and Vectors of Human Diseases*. Philadelphia, Lea and Febiger, 1975.

Grabda, J. Apparition saisonniere des larves d'*Anisakis simplex* chez le hareng de la Baltique du sud-ouest. *In*: *Proceedings, Third International Congress of Parasitology*. Munich, Facta Publications, 1974.

Kates, S., K. A. Wright, and R. Wright. A case of human infection with the cod nematode *Phocanema* spp. *Am J Trop Med Hyg* 22:606-608, 1973.

Kliks, M. M. Anisakiasis in the western United States: four new case reports from California. *Am J Trop Med Hyg* 32:526-532, 1983.

Little, M. D., and H. Most. Anisakid larva from the throat of a woman in New York. *Am J Trop Med Hyg* 22:609-612, 1973.

McClelland, G. *Phocanema decipiens*: pathology in seals. *Exp Parasitol* 49:405-419, 1980.

Myers, B. J. The nematodes that cause anisakiasis. *In: Proceedings, Third International Congress of Parasitology*. Munich, Facta Publications, 1974.

Myers, B. J. The nematodes that cause anisakiasis. *J Milk Food Technol* 38:774-782, 1975.

Oishi, K., K. Nagano, and M. Suzuki. Pathogenic capacity of Anisakinae larvae from cod and Alaska pollack. *In: Proceedings, Third International Congress of Parasitology*. Munich, Facta Publications, 1974.

Sapunar, J., E. Doerr, and T. Letonja. Anisakiasis humana en Chile. *Bol Chile Parasitol* 31:79-83, 1976.

Smith, J. W., and R. Wootten. Anisakis and anisakiasis. *Adv Parasitol* 16:93-163, 1978.

Sugimachi, K., K. Inokuchi, T. Ooiwa, T. Fujino, and Y. Ishii. Acute gastric Anisakiasis. *JAMA* 253:1012-1013, 1985.

Tantalean, M. La presencia de larvas de *Anisakis* spp. en algunos peces comerciales del mar peruano. *Rev Peru Med Trop* 1:38-43, 1972.

Torres, P., G. Pequeño, and L. Figueroa. Nota preliminar sobre Anisakidae (Railliet and Henry, 1912, Skrjabin and Korokhin, 1945) en algunos peces de consumo habitual por la población humana de Valdivia (Chile). *Bol Chile Parasitol* 33:39-46, 1978.

Van Thiel, P. H. The final hosts of herringworm *Anisakis* marina. *Trop Geogr Med* 18:310-328, 1966.

World Health Organization. *Parasitic Zoonoses*. Report of a WHO Expert Committee, with the Participation of the FAO. Geneva, WHO, 1979. (Technical Report Series 637.)

Yokogawa, M., and H. Yoshimura. Clinicopathologic studies on larval anisakiasis in Japan. *Am J Trop Med Hyg* 16:723-728, 1967.

ASCARIASIS

(127.0)

Synonyms: Ascaridiasis, ascaridosis.

Etiology: The agent of human ascariasis is the nematode *Ascaris lumbricoides*, and that of the disease in swine, *A. suum*. The two species are closely related and show only small morphologic and physiologic differences. Both species can occasionally infect the heterologous host and reach a certain degree of development. Experimentally, it has been possible to infect suckling pigs with *A. lumbricoides*, which reached maturity and produced eggs. In man, *A. suum* rarely reaches maturity; it usually does not go beyond the larval stage and only rarely advances to the intestinal phase.

A. lumbricoides is the largest intestinal nematode. The female is 20 to 35 cm long and 3 to 6 mm thick. The males are smaller and have a curved distal portion. No intermediate host is involved in the development cycle of *Ascaris*. The eggs, which are eliminated with feces, are not segmented; they require an incubation period in the external environment to permit development of the third-stage larvae. Under favorable temperature and moisture conditions, the infective larva develops within the egg in about 20 days. Humans or swine are infected by ingesting eggs containing the third-stage larvae, picked up from the soil or grass. The larvae emerge from the eggs in the duodenum and penetrate the intestinal wall. Most of them reach the liver through the portal circulation about 24 hours after the eggs were ingested. The larvae are then carried by the blood from the liver to the heart, and from there to the lungs. After a period of time they break out of the pulmonary capillaries, enter the alveoli, and migrate through the bronchial tubes and trachea to the pharynx, from whence they are swallowed and reach the intestine. In the intestine, the larvae mature and develop into male and female adults. In man, the prepatent period (from infection with eggs of *A. lumbricoides* to oviposition) lasts 60 to 75 days, while in swine infected by *A. suum*, eggs appear in the feces in a shorter period of time.

From the epidemiologic point of view, it should be noted that the eggs are very resistant to environmental factors and can remain viable for several years if protected from direct sunlight and desiccation in sandy soil.

Geographic Distribution and Occurrence: Both *A. lumbricoides* and *A. suum* have worldwide distribution; ascariasis is one of the most widespread parasitoses. It has been estimated that between 644 million and 1 billion persons are infected worldwide, 42 million of whom are in Central and South America. The estimated worldwide mortality by ascariasis is 20,000 cases per year due to intestinal complications, and estimated annual morbidity is a million cases, mainly due to pulmonary manifestations and malnutrition (Walsh and Warren, 1979). The parasitosis is most prevalent in rural areas and in hot, humid climates. The highest rate of infection is found in children. Prevalence rates vary considerably according to differences in environmental sanitation, health education of the population, personal and food hygiene, type of soil and climate, and perhaps some other factors.

A. suum is found everywhere where swine are raised. Studies carried out in slaughterhouses have shown that the prevalence rate is high, ranging from 20% to more than 70%. The highest rate is found in piglets 2 to 5 months old; the rate declines with age.

It is not known to what extent *A. suum* is involved in human infection, but it is probably not very important. Suckling pigs have been infected experimentally with embryonated eggs of *A. lumbricoides*, resulting in a patent infection with egg-laying adult parasites. Cases caused by accidental ingestion of *A. suum* eggs have been seen in a laboratory worker and some students, and one case occurred in a child who ingested swine fecal matter. Intestinal infection was verified in seven of 17 volunteers after each one was administered 25 eggs of *A. suum* containing infective larvae. These facts indicate that human intestinal ascariasis by *A. suum* can occur, but it is probably seldom recognized. A WHO Expert Committee on the Control of Ascariasis has stressed a different aspect: "When infective eggs are ingested the larvae of *Ascaris suum* unquestionably hatch in the intestine and migrate to the lungs in man as they do in many other mammals. It is a reasonable assumption that a significant proportion of respiratory illness experienced by people having contact with pigs is caused by *A. suum* as well as by *A. lumbricoides*" (World Health Organization, 1967). In developing countries where man and swine are in close contact and personal and environmental hygiene are deficient, it could be anticipated that the larval phase of *A. suum* might participate together with *A. lumbricoides* in the pulmonary alterations caused by the parasite's migration, and that a small fraction of human intestinal ascariases might be due to the porcine parasite.

The Disease in Man and Animals: The course of the disease and the symptomatology are similar in both humans and swine. Children and suckling pigs are most affected. In the early age group, not only is the infection rate higher, but the number of parasites is larger. Two phases are distinguished: the initial phase produced by migrating larvae, and the later phase caused by adult parasites.

The initial phase is characterized by respiratory symptoms attributable to the damage produced by the larvae during pulmonary migration. In intense and repeated larval invasions, the symptomatology consists of fever, irregular and asthmatic breathing, and spasmodic coughing. Aberrant larvae located in the brain, eyes, and kidneys usually give rise to serious symptoms. When newborn suckling pigs are infected by a large number of larvae, they may exhibit pneumonia with coughing and pulmonary exudate.

The symptomatology in the intestinal phase also depends on the number of adult ascarides present. Mild infections are generally asymptomatic; when the parasite burden is large, there may be vague abdominal discomfort, colic, diarrhea, and vomiting. The most serious complications in children include intestinal obstruction by a large mass of parasites and complications resulting from the aberrant migration of adult parasites to various organs.

Large numbers of ascarides in the intestines can cause diarrhea and stunted development in swine.

No information is available on the frequency and seriousness of the disease caused by the larval phase of *A. suum* in humans. Four students who involuntarily ingested a large number of *A. suum* eggs with their food manifested, after 10 to 14 days, pulmonary infiltration, eosinophilia, asthmatiform symptoms, and an increase in circulating IgE globulins, indicating the allergic nature of the disease. The adult of *A. suum* remains in the human intestine a relatively short time, judging from experimental infections induced in volunteers.

Source of Infection and Mode of Transmission (Figure 87): Humans are the reservoir of *A. lumbricoides*, as swine are for *A. suum*. The source of infection is soil (geohelminthiasis) and vegetation on which fecal matter containing eggs of *Ascaris* has been deposited. Transmission to man can occur directly from the soil or indirectly, by means of dust, water, vegetables, or objects to which the parasite's eggs have adhered. The infection is almost always acquired by ingestion, but there are unconfirmed indications that in some areas it may occur by inhalation of eggs.

The main factor in maintaining human ascariasis is fecal contamination of the soil around dwellings. Clay soils are particularly suited for the survival of *Ascaris* eggs. To have some idea of the degree of soil contamination possible, it should be borne in mind that a single female *Ascaris* can produce 200,000 eggs per day and that it is not rare to find 100 eggs per gram in the feces of children. The higher rates of infection in preschool children are explained by their more frequent contact with soil and their lack of personal hygiene.

The epidemiology of swine ascariasis is similar to that of human ascariasis.

Role of Animals in the Epidemiology of the Disease: The role played by swine in the epidemiology of human ascariasis is not well defined. It has been confirmed experimentally that cross-infections can occur between swine and humans or humans and swine. However, the frequency of heterologous infections is unknown, given the difficulty of distinguishing between the two agents.

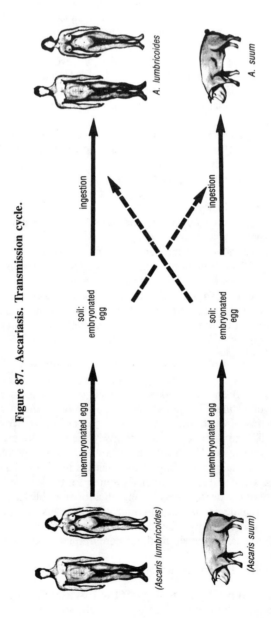

Figure 87. Ascariasis. Transmission cycle.

Ascaris of swine differs in several respects from the human parasite. Its development in both the lungs and intestine of the pig requires less time than the human parasite's development in the homologous host. In man, *A. suum* rarely achieves oviposition and stays a relatively short time in the intestine. Consequently, human infection by adult *A. suum* is probably rare or infrequent, but the rate is essentially unknown because the human intestinal parasitosis is usually assumed to be due to *A. lumbricoides*. The ascarides expelled by man are rarely studied to identify the species. There is no doubt that intestinal infections by *A. suum* occur in humans, as illustrated by the case in a child in Great Britain who ingested dirt from a garden that had been fertilized with swine excreta. Study of the dentate edge on the oral border of the lips of the expelled parasite confirmed that it was *A. suum* (Crewe and Smith, 1971). Later, a case of intestinal obstruction by multiple specimens of *A. suum* was described in a 9-year-old girl in Zimbabwe (Davies and Goldsmid, 1978).

An investigation of the role of swine in the epidemiology of *A. lumbricoides* ascariasis was carried out in a village in southwestern Nigeria where the inhabitants lived in close contact with swine. The study identified the intestinal infection caused by *A. lumbricoides* in both swine and the human population. However, an effort to experimentally infect pigs with eggs of *A. lumbricoides* was unsuccessful (Kofie and Dipeolu, 1983). An interpretation of the results of the study should take into account that experimental infection of swine, even with the homologous parasite, does not always result in patent parasitosis, with elimination of eggs in the feces. Studies have indicated that repeated exposure to small doses, as occurs in nature, is more effective in producing infection than one-time exposure to a large number of eggs.

Occasionally, *A. lumbricoides* has been found in the intestine of nonhuman primates, and its larvae in the lungs of several other species of animals. *A. suum* can infect cattle, sheep, and goats and can reach sexual maturity in these animals. In some described cases, doubt exists about the identity of the parasite.

Diagnosis: In the pulmonary migration phase, diagnosis is difficult or impossible to confirm by means of laboratory tests. Sometimes larvae can be found in the sputum of both humans and suckling pigs.

In the intestinal phase, the characteristic eggs are found in the feces.

In swine infection, a count greater than 1,000 eggs per gram of fecal matter is considered indicative of clinical ascariasis.

Control: Human ascariasis is a problem primarily found in areas with a low economic level, deficient environmental sanitation, and low standards of personal hygiene. In several industrialized countries, the prevalence rates of the parasitosis have been significantly reduced without the adoption of specific control measures, as a result of an improved standard of living.

The principal measures that should be included in a control program consist of massive and periodic treatment of the population with anthelmintics (pyrantel pamoate, mebendazole, flubendazole, or albendazole), sanitary waste disposal and provision of clean drinking-water, and public health education for the purpose of instilling good personal hygiene habits in the population. In some countries (Japan, Korea, and Israel), human ascariasis has been practically eradicated.

The effective drugs now available make it possible to establish programs in swine-raising operations to reduce the economic losses caused by this parasitosis. The most practical method is the use of drugs (fenbendazole, cambendazole, dichlorvos) administered in feed.

Bibliography

Arean, V. M., and C. A. Crandall. Ascariasis. *In*: Marcial-Rojas, R. A. (Ed.), *Pathology of Protozoal and Helminthic Diseases*. Baltimore, Maryland, Williams and Wilkins, 1971.

Crewe, W., and D. H. Smith. Human infection with pig *Ascaris* (*A. suum*). *Ann Trop Med Parasitol* 65:85, 1971.

Davies, N. J., and J. M. Goldsmid. Intestinal obstruction due to *Ascaris suum* infection. *Trans R Soc Trop Med Hyg* 72:107, 1978.

Faust, E. C., P. F. Russell, and R. C. Jung. *Craig and Faust's Clinical Parasitology*, 8th ed. Philadelphia, Lea and Febiger, 1970.

Galvin, T. J. Development of human and pig *Ascaris* in the pig and rabbit. *J Parasitol* 54:1085-1091, 1968.

Jaskoski, B. J. An apparent swine *Ascaris* infection of man. *J Am Vet Med Assoc* 138:504, 1961.

Kofie, B. A. K., and O. O. Dipeolu. A study of human and porcine ascariasis in a rural area of south-west Nigeria. *Int J Zoonoses* 10:66-70, 1983.

Lindquist, W. D. Nematodes, Acanthocephalids, Trematodes, and Cestodes. *In*: Dunne, H. W. (Ed.), *Diseases of Swine*, 3rd ed. Ames, Iowa State University Press, 1970.

Pawlowski, Z. S., and F. Arfaa. Ascariasis. *In*: Warren, K. S., and A. A. F. Mahmoud (Eds.), *Tropical and Geographical Medicine*. New York, McGraw-Hill Book Co., 1984.

Philipson, R. F., and J. W. Race. Human infection with porcine *Ascaris*. *Br Med J* 3:865, 1967.

Phills, J., A. J. Harrold, G. V. Whiteman, and L. Perelmutter. Pulmonary infiltrates, asthma and eosinophilia due to *Ascaris suum* infestation in man. *N Engl J Med* 286:965-970, 1972.

Soulsby, E. J. L. *Textbook of Veterinary Clinical Parasitology*. Oxford, Blackwell, 1965.

Soulsby, E. J. L. *Helminths, Arthropods and Protozoa of Domesticated Animals*, 7th ed. Philadelphia, Lea and Febiger, 1982.

Walsh, J. A., and K. S. Warren. Selective primary health care. An interim strategy for disease control in developing countries. *N Engl J Med* 301:967-974, 1979.

World Health Organization. *Soil-transmitted Helminths*. Report of a WHO Expert Committee on Helminthiases. Geneva, WHO, 1964. (Technical Report Series 277.)

World Health Organization. *Control of Ascariasis*. Report of a WHO Expert Committee. Geneva, WHO, 1967. (Technical Report Series 379.)

World Health Organization. *Intestinal Protozoan and Helminthic Infections*. Report of a WHO Scientific Group. Geneva, WHO, 1981. (Technical Report Series 666.)

CAPILLARIASIS

(127.5) *C. philippinensis*
(128.8) *C. hepatica* and *C. aerophila*

Synonym: Capillariosis.

Etiology: The etiologic agent of hepatic capillariasis is *Capillaria hepatica*, that of intestinal capillariasis is *C. philippinensis*, and that of pulmonary capillariasis is *C. aerophila*. The three species have different development cycles.

C. hepatica is a common parasite of rodents and several other species of mammals. The adult female measures around 5 to 8 cm long and 0.1 mm wide, and the male is about half as long. The adult parasite lodges in the hepatic parenchyma, where it lays eggs that remain trapped in the tissue of the organ. In order for *C. hepatica* to continue its development, the infected rodent must be eaten by a carnivore (intercalated host). This animal frees the eggs enclosed in the hepatic tissue, and eliminates and disseminates them with its fecal matter. The eggs require a long incubation period in the external environment, estimated at 1 to 2 months under favorable conditions of temperature, aeration, and moisture. When rodents ingest the eggs, the infective larvae are released in their intestine, enter the intestinal wall, and are carried by the bloodstream to the liver, where they mature in approximately a month. *C. hepatica* belongs to the group of helminths transmitted via the soil (geohelminthiasis). In moist soils the eggs can remain viable for many months.

The adult stage of *C. philippinensis* lodges in the small intestine of man. The female measures only 2.5 to 4.3 cm long, and the male is even smaller. The development cycle has recently been clarified. Some females of the parasite are oviparous; others are both oviparous and larviparous. The parasite has two life cycles, one consisting of internal reproduction and the other of external development. The internal autoinfection cycle gives rise to a large number of larvae and adult parasites; the external cycle requires an intermediate host, which is one of several species of freshwater fish. When the eggs contained in human fecal matter enter streams, ponds, or rivers and are ingested by appropriate fish, they hatch in the fish's intestine, releasing larvae that become infective in 3 weeks. When man eats infected fish, the larvae continue their development and the parasites reach sexual maturity in the human intestine.

C. aerophila is a parasite of the trachea and bronchi of foxes, dogs, coyotes, and, rarely, other wild animals or cats. The female is about 3 cm long, and the male about 2.5 cm. The eggs are deposited in the lungs and carried by coughing to the pharynx; they are then swallowed and eliminated in the feces. After an incubation period of 5 to 7 weeks in the external environment, the larvae inside the eggs reach the infective stage. When eggs containing infective larvae are ingested by an appropriate host (dog, fox), the larvae are freed in the intestine and migrate to the lungs where, after 40 days, the parasites reach maturity and reinitiate the cycle with oviposition.

Geographic Distribution and Occurrence: *C. hepatica* is found on all continents among synanthropic and wild rodents, with a prevalence rate that varies from 0.7 to more than 85%. Besides rodents, the parasite has occasionally been found in other species of domestic and wild mammals. The infection is very rare in man; 11

cases of hepatic infection have been confirmed in Europe (nine in Czechoslovakia and two in Italy) and another 14 in the rest of the world (among them, one in Brazil, one in Mexico, five in the United States, and three in South Africa).

Intestinal capillariasis caused by *C. philippinensis* was recognized for the first time in 1963 on Luzon Island in the Philippines. More than 1,000 cases were recorded in 1967 with a 10% case fatality rate. From 1963 to the present, an estimated 2,000 cases have occurred in seven provinces of Luzon. However, the prevalence of the infection seems relatively low, since less than 3% of 4,000 inhabitants of the endemic area examined during the epidemic outbreak of 1967 had eggs of the parasite in their feces (Banzón, 1982). Outside the endemic area of the Philippines, two cases were diagnosed in Thailand.

C. aerophila has been diagnosed in animals in North and South America, Europe, Asia, and Australia. In New York State, 37% of wild foxes were found to be infected. The prevalence rate is usually high in colonies of silver foxes raised for fur. Research carried out in several areas of the central United States found 38% of 395 coyotes (*Canis latrans*) to be parasitized (Morrison and Gier, 1978). Up to the present, only nine cases of human infection are known; seven of them occurred in the USSR, one in Morocco, and the other in Iran (Aftandelians *et al.*, 1977).

The Disease in Man: Clinical cases of hepatic capillariasis are due to a massive invasion of the liver by *C. hepatica*, which reaches maturity and begins to produce eggs in that organ, as is the case in the animal parasitosis. The disease is serious and frequently fatal. A prominent sign is hepatomegaly; the other most common symptoms are high morning fever, nausea and vomiting, diarrhea or constipation, abdominal distension, edema of the extremities, splenomegaly, and sometimes pneumonitis. A large part of the symptomatology is due to secondary infections in weakened patients, mostly children. In a recent case in an adult from Nigeria, the most prominent pathologic feature was severe hepatic fibrosis and functional disorders related to these lesions (Attah *et al.*, 1983). Laboratory examinations reveal hyperleukocytosis with eosinophilia, hypochromic anemia, and abnormal values in liver function tests. Postmortem examination discovers the presence of white to grayish nodules on the surface of the liver. Histologically, the principal lesions consist of necrotic foci and granulomas. The adult parasites and eggs are found in the necrotic masses. Subclinical human infections undoubtedly occur, as attested to by solitary hepatic granulomas found in nine individuals autopsied during a study carried out in Czechoslovakia. In seven of the nine cases, only one parasite larva was found in the lesion (Slais, 1973).

Intestinal capillariasis caused by *C. philippinensis* is a serious and fatal disease if not treated (thiabendazole) in time. Most patients range in age from 20 to 45 years old, and males predominate. The disease begins with insignificant symptoms such as borborygmus and vague abdominal pain. Intermittent diarrhea and weight loss begin after 2 or 3 weeks and become persistent as the illness advances; these are the most prominent symptoms. Gastrointestinal function is seriously affected; in addition, malabsorption and the loss of large quantities of protein, fat, and minerals have been confirmed. Death occurs as a result of heart failure or an intercurrent infection a few weeks or months after the onset of the symptomatology.

Asthmatiform symptoms occur in pulmonary capillariasis caused by *C. aerophila*, with coughing, mucoid or sometimes blood-tinged expectoration, fever, dyspnea, and moderate eosinophilia. Biopsy reveals granulomatous lesions produced by cellular reaction to a foreign body (Aftandelians *et al.*, 1977).

The Disease in Animals: Infections by *C. hepatica* in animals have the same characteristics as those in man. Mild infections are subclinical, while intense infections can cause hepatitis, splenomegaly, ascites, and eosinophilia.

C. philippinensis has not been found in land animals, but the existence of an animal reservoir is suspected, given the poor adaptation of the parasite to man. Experimental infection in primates of the genus *Macaca* and in wild rats is asymptomatic. In gerbils, on the other hand, the infection is manifested by a symptomatology similar to that in man (Banzón, 1982). Intense infections by *C. aerophila* in animals can cause rhinitis, tracheitis, and bronchitis, which may end in bronchopneumonia caused by a secondary bacterial infection.

Source of Infection and Mode of Transmission (Figures 88–90): The main reservoir of *C. hepatica* is rodents. The infection is contracted by ingestion of embryonated eggs picked up from the soil, which were disseminated by carnivores (see Etiology). In the domestic and peridomestic environment, the disseminating or temporary hosts can be cats and dogs that hunt rodents. Other possible mechanisms for releasing the eggs from the liver of rodents are cannibalism and death and decomposition of the infected animals. For man, the source of infection is the soil, either directly or indirectly, and penetration is via the oral route. There are more than 30 described cases of spurious infections due to the ingestion of raw liver of rodents or other mammals (squirrels, monkeys, wild boars) infected with unembryonated

Figure 88. Hepatic capillariasis (*Capillaria hepatica*). Transmission cycle.

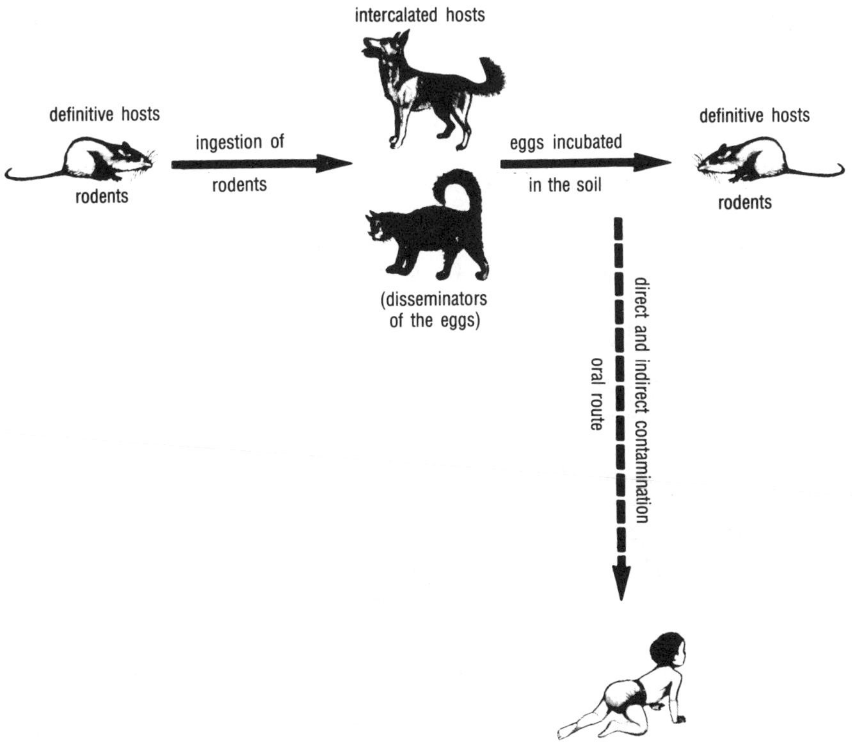

Figure 89. Intestinal capillariasis (*Capillaria philippinensis*). Transmission cycle.

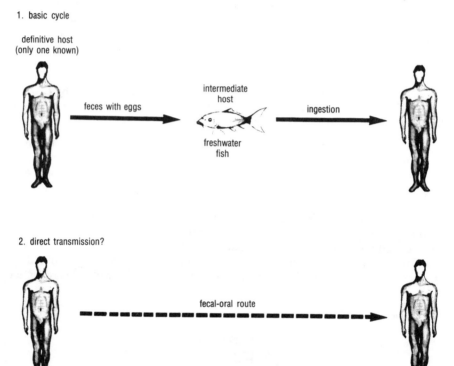

1. basic cycle

definitive host
(only one known)

feces with eggs

intermediate host

freshwater fish

ingestion

2. direct transmission?

fecal-oral route

eggs. In such cases, the eggs of the parasite pass through the human digestive tract and are eliminated with the feces.

Man is the only known definitive host of *C. philippinensis*. Because of the serious pathologic effects it produces in this host, the parasite-human relationship is believed to be fairly recent. It is suspected that another animal may act as definitive host, but it has not yet been identified if it exists. The main source and manner of infection is through ingestion of raw fish (intermediate host) containing the infective larvae. Contamination of bodies of water with human excreta ensures perpetuation of the cycle. Direct interhuman transmission may also occur, as suggested by the fact that the infection can be transmitted experimentally from one gerbil to another, using different intestinal stages of the parasite (Banzón, 1982).

The source of *C. aerophila* infection for man and animals is soil, where the eggs deposited with the feces of animals continue their incubation and the larvae reach the infective stage. Larvae can remain viable inside the eggs for a year or more. Children probably acquire the infection by ingesting dirt or water and food contaminated with eggs.

Diagnosis: While the patient is alive, specific diagnosis of hepatic capillariasis can only be made by hepatic biopsy and identification of the parasite or its eggs. The discovery of *C. hepatica* eggs in human feces does not signify infection, but rather

Figure 90. Pulmonary capillariasis (*Capillaria aerophila*). Transmission cycle.

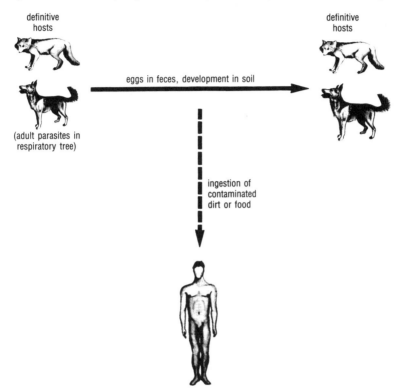

definitive
hosts

definitive
hosts

eggs in feces, development in soil

(adult parasites in
respiratory tree)

ingestion of
contaminated
dirt or food

the passage of eggs through the intestine after ingestion of the liver of infected animals, such as monkeys, wild boars, or squirrels.

Diagnosis of intestinal capillariasis (*C. philippinensis*) usually presents no difficulties, and is made by means of coprologic examination; in some cases, however, a series of examinations is necessary to confirm diagnosis. Serologic tests are not sufficiently specific for routine use.

Diagnosis of pulmonary capillariasis can be done by confirmation of the presence of the typical eggs or eosinophils in the sputum, or by biopsy of pulmonary tissue.

Control: Since hepatic capillariasis occurs primarily in young children, in whom geophagy is common, and in environments with an abundance of rats, the principal preventive measures are rodent control and improved attention to children's hygiene.

In endemic areas, intestinal capillariasis can be prevented by abstaining from eating raw or undercooked fish. Patients should be treated with thiabendazole, not only for therapeutic reasons but also to decrease the dissemination of parasite eggs. Hygienic elimination of human excreta is very important.

To prevent pulmonary capillariasis in silver foxes and, consequently, in the personnel on breeding farms, the animals must be kept in clean and dry installations. Every case of infection should be treated (with thiabendazole) as soon as possible.

Bibliography

Aftandelians, R., F. Raafat, M. Taffazoli, and P. C. Beaver. Pulmonary capillariasis in a child in Iran. *Am J Trop Med Hyg* 26:64-71, 1977.

Arean, V. M. Capillariasis. *In*: Marcial-Rojas, R. A. (Ed.), *Pathology of Protozoal and Helminthic Diseases*. Baltimore, Maryland, Williams and Wilkins, 1971.

Attah, E. B., S. Nagarajan, E. N. Obineche, and S. C. Gera. Hepatic capillariasis. *Am J Clin Pathol* 79:127-130, 1983.

Banzón, T. Human intestinal capillariasis (*Capillaria philippinensis*). *In*: Schultz, M. G. (Ed.), *CRC Handbook Series in Zoonoses*. Section C, vol. 2. Boca Raton, Florida, CRC Press, 1982.

Chitwood, M. B., C. Velázquez, and N. G. Salazar. *Capillaria philippinensis* sp. n. (Nematoda: Trichinellidae), from the intestine of man in the Philippines. *J Parasitol* 54:368-371, 1972.

Cross, J. H., T. Banzón, M. D. Clarke *et al.* Experimental transmission of *Capillaria philippinensis* in monkeys. *Trans R Soc Trop Med Hyg* 66:819-827, 1972.

Fresh, J. W., J. H. Cross, V. Reyes *et al.* Necropsy findings in intestinal capillariasis. *Am J Trop Med Hyg* 21:169-173, 1972.

Morrison, E. E., and H. T. Gier. Lungworms in coyotes on the Great Plains. *J Wildl Dis* 14:314-316, 1978.

Slais, J. The finding and identification of solitary *Capillaria hepatica* (Bancroft, 1893) in man in Europe. *Folia Parasitol* (*Praha*) 20:149-161, 1973.

Soulsby, E. J. L. *Helminths, Arthropods and Protozoa of Domesticated Animals*, 7th ed. Philadelphia, Lea and Febiger, 1982.

Watten, R. H., W. M. Beckner, J. H. Cross *et al.* Clinical studies of *Capillariasis philippinensis*. *Trans R Soc Trop Med Hyg* 66:828-834, 1972.

CUTANEOUS LARVA MIGRANS

(126.2) by *Ancylostoma braziliense*
(126.8) by other ancylostomes

Synonyms: Creeping verminous dermatitis, serpiginous eruption, larva currens (infection by larvae of *Strongyloides* spp.).

Etiology: The main etiologic agent is the third-stage larva of *Ancylostoma braziliense*, an intestinal nematode of dogs, cats, and several species of wild carnivores. More rarely, cutaneous larva migrans may be due to other animal ancylostomatids, such as *A. caninum* of dogs and wild carnivores; *Uncinaria stenophala* of dogs, cats, and several species of wild carnivores; and *Bunostomum phlebotomum* of bovids.

Man is an aberrant host; the larvae of *A. braziliense* cannot complete their development cycle and do not produce an intestinal infection in humans. The species of animal ancylostomatids that occasionally cause human intestinal an-cylostomiasis are discussed under "Zoonotic Ancylostomiasis." *A. braziliense* is a small species of ancylostome, the female of which measures about 1 cm long and 0.37 mm wide. Its life cycle is similar to that of other ancylostomes (see "Zoonotic Ancylostomiasis").

The name larva currens has been given to the rapidly moving pruriginous and urticant cutaneous eruption originated by penetration of filariform larvae of *Strongyloides stercoralis*, especially in cases of external autoinfection. Man, dogs, and cats are the main hosts of the parasite (see "Strongyloidiasis"). Strongyloids of rodents can produce similar lesions.

Geographic Distribution and Occurrence: Cutaneous larva migrans is usually found in tropical and subtropical countries. Among the places where the disease has occurred are Argentina, Uruguay, southern Brazil, Mexico (especially the Gulf coast), the Caribbean islands, the southeastern United States, several countries in Europe, South Africa, Australia, India, and the Philippines.

The infection caused by *A. braziliense* in cats and dogs is widespread in tropical and subtropical areas.

The Disease in Man: Upon penetrating the skin, the filariform larva produces a pruriginous papule at the entry site. In the following days, the larva migrates through the germinal layer producing sinuous tunnels. The larva advances in the skin several millimeters to several centimeters per day. Vesicles form on the skin along the tunnels. The migration of the larvae and the corresponding tissue reaction cause strong pruritus, which is particularly intense at night and may keep the patient awake (especially if the larvae are numerous). Secondary bacterial infections are frequent, since the pruritus induces the patient to scratch. The lesion is most often located on the feet, legs, and hands, but can occur on any part of the skin exposed to contaminated soil, and can be single or multiple. Lesions on the palms of the hands or soles of the feet are painful.

The larvae can remain alive and travel in the skin for several weeks or months. The levels of IgE immunoglobulins are elevated during the infection. Cure is spontaneous and can be accelerated by administration of thiabendazole (50 mg per kilogram of body weight orally for 3 days; topical application of the same drug on the anterior part of the tunnels can be used in addition to oral medication).

Some patients suffer a temporary pneumonitis with eosinophilia (Loeffler syndrome) when the larvae invade the lungs. In these cases, larvae can be found in the sputum. Recently, larvae of *Ancylostoma* have also been found in the cornea. This finding confirmed that the larvae of animal ancylostomes can occasionally produce visceral forms of the parasitosis.

In larva currens, caused by *Strongyloides stercoralis*, the lesion is less well defined than in cutaneous larva migrans and is characterized by intense erythema, rapid progression, and quick disappearance.

The Disease in Animals: The disease caused by ancylostomes in carnivores, which are their principal hosts, is mainly intestinal; it is expressed as diarrhea, anemia, malabsorption, and degeneration of the parenchyma of different organs. Invasion of the skin by the larval parasites can cause dermatitis, generally of short duration. The lesions are limited to the parts of the animal's body that are in contact with the soil. The most prominent signs consist of erythema and papules that disappear about 5 days after the beginning of the infection. Experiments have demonstrated that repeated percutaneous exposures to *Ancylostoma caninum* exacerbate the symptomatology and provoke more intense reactions (Buelke, 1971).

Source of Infection and Mode of Transmission (Figure 91): The eggs of the parasite are eliminated with the fecal matter of dogs or cats, and release the infective filariform larvae when environmental conditions (especially moisture and temperature) are favorable. Humid soils are the most suitable for the development of the larvae. In countries with a temperate climate, human infections occur in summer, and in tropical climates they occur in seasons with sufficient humidity. Man is infected by contact with soil contaminated with feces of dogs and cats. Children are the group most exposed to risk, especially when they play in sand. Likewise, workers in close contact with the soil, such as gardeners, farmers, and construction and mine workers, are exposed.

Diagnosis: Clinical diagnosis is made on the basis of the nature of the lesions and the symptomatology, such as serpiginous tunnels and intense pruritus. Diagnosis can be confirmed by biopsy of the affected skin to confirm the presence of larvae, but this is rarely done and larvae may not be found even when it is. Identification of the parasite on the basis of the larva is very difficult. Infection by *A. braziliense* has been well studied, but the difficulty of identifying larvae in the lesions has made it impossible to clarify the relative prevalence of other ancylostomes of animal origin in the infection.

In differential diagnosis, cutaneous lesions caused by larvae of *Gnathostoma spinigerum* as well as cutaneous dirofilariasis, myiases, and dermatitis by schistosome cercariae should be taken into account.

Figure 91. Cutaneous larva migrans. Transmission cycle.

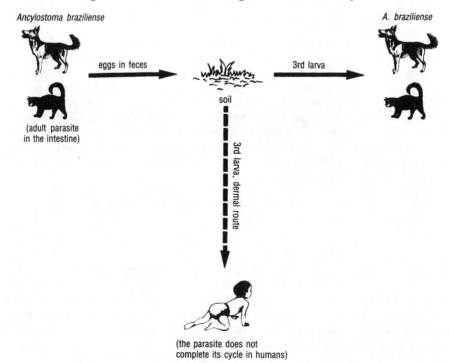

In addition, when the larvae of human ancylostomes (*Ancylostoma duodenale* and *Necator americanus*), invade the skin of man, they can produce macules, papules, and localized erythema, sometimes with intense pruritus ("ground itch" or "dew itch").

Control: The principal measures consist of periodic anthelmintic treatment of dogs and cats and the elimination of stray animals. Dogs and cats should not be allowed on beaches or in places where children play in sand.

Bibliography

Brown, H. W. Diseases caused by metazoa. *In:* Beeson, P. B., W. McDermott, and J. B. Wyngaarden (Eds.), *Cecil Textbook of Medicine,* 15th ed. Philadelphia, Saunders, 1979.

Brown, H. W., and D. L. Belding. *Parasitología Clínica,* 2nd ed. Mexico, Interamericana, 1965.

Buelke, D. L. Hookworm dermatitis. *J Am Vet Med Assoc* 158:735-739, 1971.

Faust, E. C., P. C. Beaver, and R. C. Jung. *Animal Agents and Vectors of Human Disease,* 4th ed. Philadelphia, Lea and Febiger, 1975.

Faust, E. C., P. F. Russell, and R. C. Jung. *Craig and Faust's Clinical Parasitology,* 8th ed. Philadelphia, Lea and Febiger, 1970.

Fuller, C. E. A common source outbreak of cutaneous larva migrans. *Public Health Rep* 81:186-190, 1966.

Marcial-Rojas, R. A. Cutaneous larva migrans of hookworm origin. *In:* Marcial-Rojas, R. A. (Ed.), *Pathology of Protozoal and Helminthic Diseases.* Baltimore, Maryland, Williams and Wilkins, 1971.

Meyers, W. M., and R. C. Neafie. Creeping eruption. *In:* Binford, C. H., and D. H. Connor (Eds.), *Pathology of Tropical and Extraordinary Diseases.* Washington, D.C., Armed Forces Institute of Pathology, 1976.

DIOCTOPHYMOSIS

(128.8)

Synonym: Dioctophymiasis.

Etiology: The etiologic agent is a very large, blood-red nematode, *Dioctophyma* (*Dioctophyme*) *renale*, which in the adult stage lodges in the kidneys of carnivores, such as mustelids and wild and domestic canids. In dogs, the adult female of the parasite can reach up to 1 m in length and 5 to 12 mm in width, and thus is known as the giant kidney worm; the male is much smaller. The size of the parasite depends on the size of the host species; for example, in ferrets the parasite is only a few centimeters long.

The definitive host eliminates the eggs of the parasite via the urine. To continue their development cycle, the eggs require a long period of incubation in water, its exact length being determined by environmental conditions. At the end of this period, when they contain the first-stage larvae, the eggs must be ingested by an intermediate host. This host is a free-living, aquatic oligochaete annelid (limicoline worm), *Lumbriculus variegatus*. In the intermediate host, the larva is quickly released from the egg and develops to the second and eventually the third stage, which is infective to the definitive hosts. If a fish (*Ictalurus nebulosus* or *Esox lucius* in North America, *Idus* spp. in Europe) or a frog (*Rana pipiens*, *R. clamitans*, *R. septentrionalis*) ingests an infected oligochaete, the larva encysts in its mesentery or liver. Recent experimental data suggest that fish and frogs act as paratenic or transport hosts and might not be essential to the development cycle. The infective larvae ingested by the carnivorous definitive host, either with the intermediate host (aquatic oligochaete) or with the paratenic host (fish or frogs), penetrate the gastric submucosa where they undergo a molt. From the stomach the larvae move to the liver, then to the peritoneal cavity, and finally to the kidneys. Some of the parasites complete their development cycle in the peritoneal cavity, in which case their eggs are not carried to the exterior. Likewise, when *D. renale* of only one sex lodge in the kidneys of a definitive host, that animal plays no role in the life cycle. The prepatent period (from ingestion of the infective larva to appearance of eggs in the urine) lasts from 3½ to 6 months.

Geographic Distribution and Occurrence: With the possible exception of Africa and Oceania, the geographic distribution of the parasite encompasses all the continents. It has been found in many species of carnivorous animals. The most frequently reported form is canine dioctophymosis. In the Americas, the animal parasitosis has been described in Canada, the United States, Brazil, Paraguay, Uruguay, and Argentina, among other countries. The highest prevalence has been found in wild mink (*Mustela vison*) in Canada. In one study carried out in Ontario, 18% of 700 mink were parasitized, and in another, 39% of 1,072 specimens examined over a 7-year period were infected. In Michigan, USA, the infection rates found in two studies in wild mink were 2.5% and 8.6%, respectively. The high prevalence rates found in mustelids lead researchers to believe that these animals are the main reservoir and principal definitive hosts of *D. renale* in North America.

In northern Iran, 13% of stray dogs and 35% of jackals were found to be infected. Cases in bovines, equines, and swine are recorded infrequently.

The disease is very rare in man. Just over a dozen cases worldwide have been reported in the literature.

The Disease in Man and Animals: In humans and dogs, the nematode usually locates in only one kidney, most often the right one, and in most cases only one parasite is found. *Dioctophyma* destroys the renal parenchyma and in extreme cases leaves only the capsule of the organ.

The most prominent symptoms consist of renal colic and hematuria. In some cases, the parasite or parasites migrate to the ureter or urethra and obstruct the flow of urine.

In dogs, the parasite is frequently found only in the peritoneal cavity, where it sometimes causes peritonitis, but more commonly provokes no symptoms. Even renal infection in dogs, when limited to a single kidney, can be asymptomatic. The healthy kidney compensates for the loss of renal function and usually becomes hypertrophic.

Human cases described to date have all been renal.

Source of Infection and Mode of Transmission (Figure 92): In North America, mustelids, especially mink, appear to be the main reservoir. Several facts support this assumption. The rate of infection in wild mink is sufficiently high and the number of parasites of both sexes that they harbor is sufficiently large to maintain the cycle in nature. In other areas, it is likely that other species of mustelids or wild canids serve as main definitive hosts. There are indications that in northern Iran this role is fulfilled by the jackal, in which an infection rate of 35% has been found.

The wild definitive hosts are infected by ingestion of frogs or fish (paratenic hosts) and aquatic oligochaetes (intermediate hosts) that contain the third larvae.

Dogs and humans are accidental hosts, and almost always harbor only one parasite; when more than one nematode is present, they are frequently of the same sex. These two host species are infected by ingestion of raw fish and frogs. The rarity of human infection can be explained by the fact that larvae are located in the mesentery and liver of fish and frogs, organs that are generally not consumed by man.

Figure 92. Dioctophymosis (*Dioctophyma renale*). Transmission cycle.

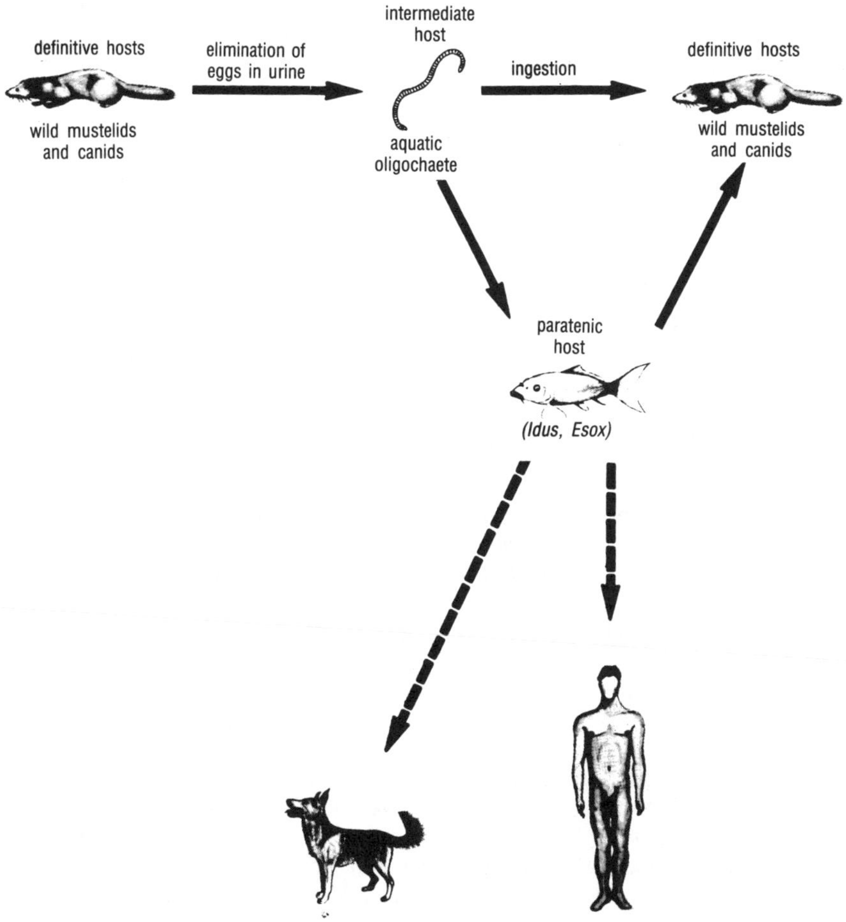

Diagnosis: When the parasite infecting man or dog is a female, the parasitosis can be diagnosed by examining the eggs in the urinary sediment. Renal infections caused by a male parasite or located in the peritoneum can only be diagnosed by laparotomy or at autopsy.

Control: The infection can be prevented, both in humans and dogs, by avoiding the consumption of raw or undercooked fish and frogs.

Bibliography

Barriga, O. O. Dioctophymiasis. *In*: Schultz, M. G. (Ed.), *CRC Handbook Series in Zoonoses*. Section C, vol. 2. Boca Raton, Florida, CRC Press, 1982.

Fyvie, A. *Dioctophyma renale*. *In*: Davis, J. W., and R. C. Anderson (Eds.), *Parasitic Diseases of Wild Mammals*. Ames, Iowa State University Press, 1971.

Hanjan, F. A., A. Sadighian, B. Mikakhtar, and F. Arfaa. The first report of human infection with *Dioctophyma renale* in Iran. *Trans R Soc Trop Med Hyg* 62:647-648, 1968.

Karmanova, E. M. The life cycle of *Dioctophyme renale*. *Helminthol Abstr* 33:394, 1964.

Osborne, C. A., J. B. Stevens, G. F. Hanlon *et al*. *Dioctophyme renale* in the dog. *J Am Vet Med Assoc* 155:605-620, 1969.

Soulsby, E. J. L. *Helminths, Arthropods and Protozoa of Domesticated Animals*, 7th ed. Philadelphia, Lea and Febiger, 1982.

DRACUNCULIASIS

(125.7)

Synonyms: Dracontiasis, dracunculosis, guinea-worm disease.

Etiology: *Dracunculus medinensis*, one of the longest nematodes, the female measuring from 55 to more than 100 cm in length and about 2 mm in width. The male is rarely found in patients, as it dies soon after copulation. Judging from a specimen found in India in a natural infection, the male measures about 4 cm in length. In its adult state, *D. medinensis* parasitizes man and a large variety of domestic and wild animals. A very closely related species, *D. insignis*, is found in raccoons (*Procyon lotor*) and other mammals in the United States and Canada.

In the definitive host, the gravid female is found in the subcutaneous tissue, especially of the legs, feet, and knees, and rarely of other parts of the body. At the end of the prepatent period, which lasts many months, the female introduces her anterior end into the skin, giving rise to first a papule and then a vesicle. When man or another infected animal enters water, the vesicle bursts and leaves part of the parasite exposed, and its prolapsed uterus releases a large number of rhabditoid first-stage larvae (some 500,000 larvae are deposited the first time the patient enters the water and lesser numbers thereafter). Many of the adult parasites die and are expelled spontaneously; others are extracted still alive by the patients. To continue its development the larva must be ingested by an intermediate host, which is a copepod of the genus *Cyclops*. Some 15 species of *Cyclops* are known to be able to serve as intermediate hosts. If the larva is ingested by a suitable species of copepod, it will continue its development in the coelomic cavity of this host for 3 to 6 weeks, until it becomes an infective, third-stage larva. When a definitive host—man, dog, or another mammal—ingests the infected copepod, the larva is released, penetrates the intestinal wall, and travels to the connective tissue, possibly via the lymphatic system, where it embeds itself. The female is fertilized in the subcutaneous connective tissue and then penetrates deeply into the tissue, remaining there for months until the uterus is filled with first-stage larvae. The mature female emerges to the surface of the skin 10 to 14 months after infection, and reinitiates the cycle by releasing larvae from her uterus when the definitive host enters water.

Geographic Distribution and Occurrence (Map 15): Dracunculiasis is endemic in large areas of western Africa, some parts of eastern Africa, and in western India. Some relatively unimportant endemic foci persist in Pakistan, Iran, Saudi Arabia, Yemen, and possibly Iraq. The distribution of the parasitosis is limited to tropical and subtropical regions, since the larva of *D. medinensis* develops best at a temperature between 25 and 30°C and does not develop completely at temperatures under 19°C (Muller, 1979).

The World Health Organization estimated the prevalence in 1976 at about 10 million parasitized persons. However, only 26,980 cases were reported in 1978. There is obvious underreporting, as was demonstrated in a study carried out in Togo in 1977, where less than 4% of observed cases had been reported to the public health authorities (World Health Organization, 1982).

In some endemic foci, a high proportion of the population is infected. In some small villages of Ghana and southern India, the infection has been found in 50% of the inhabitants. The most affected age group is the 20-to-40-year-old group. Reinfection is common (Johnson and Joshi, 1982).

In the Western Hemisphere, foci used to exist in some parts of the Antilles, the Guiana region, and in Bahia, Brazil, but all died out spontaneously. The infection seems to have been introduced from Africa with the slave traffic.

D. medinensis has been found in domestic animals, mainly dogs but also cats, bovines, and equines. In addition, cases have been recorded in primates, wild carnivores, and gazelles.

There are indications that species of *Dracunculus* that parasitize other animals can occasionally infect man. Some sporadic cases of human dracunculiasis in the eastern United States have been attributed to *D. insignis*, a parasite of wild carnivores and dogs in North America (World Health Organization, 1979).

The Disease in Man: The prepatent period, from infection to the emergence of the parasite in the skin, lasts about a year. The symptoms appear when the parasite begins its migration to the skin surface. Shortly before or simultaneous with the formation of the vesicle on the skin, allergic manifestations appear, such as urticaria, pruritus, dyspnea, vomiting, mild fever, and occasionally fainting. These symptoms are believed to be due to a diffusible toxin produced by the parasite. Once the vesicle is formed and before the parasite emerges, the patient feels a strong burning sensation, which he may try to alleviate by submerging the affected area in cold water. Symptoms disappear when the vesicle breaks and the parasite emerges.

Map 15. Areas where cases of dracunculiasis have been notified or probably exist.

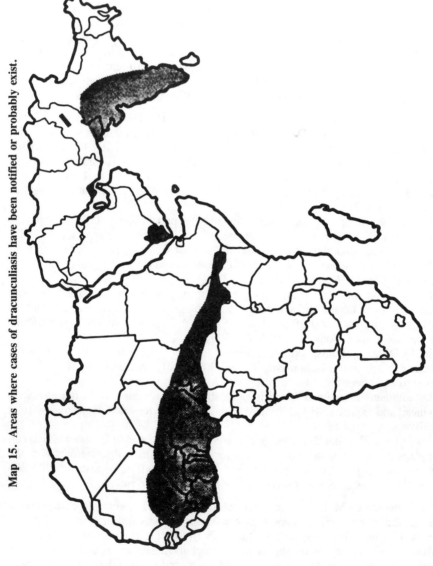

Source: WHO. Dracunculiasis surveillance. *Wkly Epidemiol Rec* 57:65, 1982.

The vesicle and the subsequent skin ulceration generally appear on the feet, legs, and knees, and less frequently on the upper part of the body. The ulcer heals about a month after the patient is rid of the parasite.

The most serious complications result from secondary bacterial infections through the open lesion, which can spread along the tunnel excavated by the parasite. These secondary infections often occur as a result of failed attempts to extract the parasite. If the adult nematode breaks during attempts at extraction, the larvae may remain trapped in the subcutaneous tissue and give rise to cellulitis and abscesses. Chronic ulcers, arthritis, and tendon contractions are other frequent sequelae.

Even if complications do not occur, many patients remain incapacitated for several weeks or months. A study carried out in the district of Ibadan, Nigeria, determined that the duration of the disability averaged 100 days. The degree of incapacity was related to the number of parasites and their location; localization in the ankles and feet affected the patients most seriously (Kale, 1977).

The Disease in Animals: The course of animal dracunculiasis and the clinical manifestations are very similar to those in man.

Source of Infection and Mode of Transmission (Figure 93): The disease is found in rural areas and is directly related to a lack of clean water in poor areas in arid regions or in parts of the tropics and subtropics with prolonged dry seasons. In the latter areas, maximum transmission occurs in the dry season when lagoons, ponds, and other bodies of water are at a low level and the density of infected copepods increases. In addition, the scarcity of water usually forces the inhabitants to resort to any source available. In desert climates, however, transmission of the infection is more frequent in the rainy season. The main sources of infection for man are shallow lagoons, ponds, wells dug in dry river beds, cisterns, and wells that people must enter by means of access steps to obtain water. Copepods harboring the third-stage larva constitute the infective element; they can only live in still water. The human host contaminates water with the larvae that escape from the emerging parasite, and in turn becomes infected by ingesting copepods, the intermediate hosts of *D. medinensis*, with water. The infection has a markedly seasonal character for two reasons: a) the influence of climate on the water supply, and b) the development cycle of the parasite (Muller, 1979). As pointed out previously, the time of maximum transmission varies in different areas and under different ecologic conditions. In the Sahel region of Africa, where the annual rainfall is less than 75 cm^3, infection occurs in the rainy season and for a few months afterwards, until the lagoons dry up. However, in the desert foci of southern Iran, where rainwater is collected in large, protected cisterns, which rarely dry out, the incidence is higher in the dry season when the density of copepods is greater. In each endemic area, one or two species of *Cyclops*, generally the largest and most carnivorous species, act as intermediate hosts. In an endemic region of Nigeria, it has been estimated that each inhabitant ingests some 75 infected copepods per year.

Man is undoubtedly the main definitive host and reservoir of the parasite. The role of animals in the epidemiology of human dracunculiasis is not clear and is open to debate. Domestic animals, especially dogs, may constitute an additional reservoir of secondary importance in areas where rates of human infection are high. Indications exist that these animals can maintain the infection in nature on their own, without human involvement, although it has not yet been completely clarified what proportion of these hosts are infected by *D. medinensis* as opposed to another

Figure 93. Dracunculiasis (*Dracunculus medinensis*). Transmission cycle.

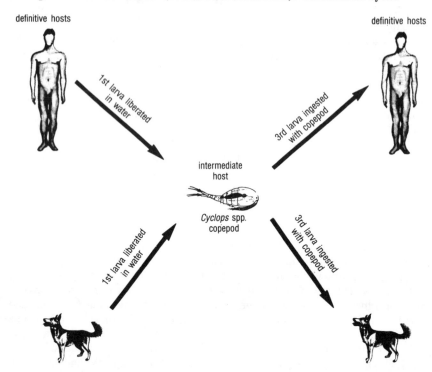

Note: The role of animal reservoirs in the transmission of the parasite to man is controversial.

species of *Dracunculus*. *D. medinensis* occurs in some places where the human infection has not been recorded, such as Malaysia and Tanzania. Moreover, in Kazakhstan, USSR, after human dracunculiasis was eradicated from an endemic focus, 11.7% of 213 dogs examined were found to be infected.

Several researchers attribute little or no importance to any host other than man, since no proof yet exists that any other animal participates in the cycle of transmission to humans. In principle, the animal reservoirs do not constitute a barrier to dracunculiasis control plans, since these plans almost always consist of preventing the population's water supply from becoming contaminated with larvae eliminated by the definitive hosts, whether man or animals.

Diagnosis: Diagnosis presents no difficulties once the cephalic end of the parasite emerges. Diagnosis can be confirmed, if thought necessary, by throwing some cold water on the ulcer and examining one drop for the presence of first-stage larvae. Dead and calcified parasites can be seen in radiologic examination.

Several immunologic tests have been described for patients with patent infections, but for now they have little practical application (Muller, 1979). The indirect immunofluorescence test gave positive reactions in experimentally infected monkeys 4 to 8 months before the emergence of the parasite, and the antibodies disappeared 2 to 9 months after the emergence. This test could prove useful for early diagnosis of the disease, once it is adequately evaluated on human patients.

Control: The main preventive measure consists of providing the population with a potable water supply. In large populations, excellent results have been obtained after systems with running water were introduced. In rural areas, water sources can be protected by the use of cement curbstones to prevent direct human contact with the water. Another possible measure, still little used, is chemical treatment of the water (with temefos) to kill copepods.

By piping water to a city of 30,000 inhabitants in Nigeria, the incidence was reduced from 60% to zero in the course of 2 years. In Tashkent and Samarkand, USSR, the disease was eradicated more than 40 years ago by eliminating wells with steps, and substituting for them extraction wells with curbstones. These procedures have also made it possible to reduce the prevalence in several villages in India, where a national program to eradicate the disease was undertaken a few years ago. As a first step, a study was carried out in every village in the endemic areas to find out the magnitude of the problem. This survey confirmed that more than 7,500 villages (or nearly 1.26% of all the villages in the country), with a population of nearly six million inhabitants, were affected by dracunculiasis. With the problem defined, the strategy consists mainly of visiting the affected areas every 6 months, establishing priorities for improving the water supply sources, and educating the population about safe drinking-water. At the individual level, the infection can be prevented by boiling or filtering water; copepods can be removed simply by pouring water through a cloth.

Bibliography

Beverley-Burton, M., and V. F. Y. Crichton. Identification of Guinea-worm species. *Trans R Soc Trop Med Hyg* 67:151, 1973.

Brown, H. W., and D. L. Belding. *Parasitología Clínica*, 2nd ed. México, Interamericana, 1965.

Faust, E. C., P. F. Russell, and R. C. Jung. *Craig and Faust's Clinical Parasitology*, 8th ed. Philadelphia, Lea and Febiger, 1970.

Johnson, S., and V. Joshi. Dracontiasis in western Rajasthan, India. *Trans R Soc Trop Med Hyg* 76:36-40, 1982.

Kale, O. O. The clinico-epidemiological profile of guinea-worm in the Ibadan District of Nigeria. *Am J Trop Med Hyg* 26:208-214, 1977.

Muller, R. *Dracunculus* and dracunculiasis. *Adv Parasitol* 9:73-151, 1971.

Muller, R. Guinea-worm disease: epidemiology, control, and treatment. *Bull WHO* 57:683-689, 1979.

Muller, R. Dracunculiasis. *In*: Warren, K. S., and A. A. F. Mahmoud (Eds.), *Tropical and Geographical Medicine*. New York, McGraw-Hill Book Co., 1984.

Price, D. L., and P. L. Child. Dracontiasis (dracunculiasis, dracunculosis, Medina worm, Guinea worm). *In*: Marcial-Rojas, R. A. (Ed.), *Pathology of Protozoal and Helminthic Diseases*. Baltimore, Maryland, Williams and Wilkins, 1971.

World Health Organization. *Parasitic Zoonoses*. Report of a WHO Expert Committee, with the Participation of the FAO. Geneva, WHO, 1979. (Technical Report Series 637.)

World Health Organization. Dracunculiasis surveillance. *Wkly Epidemiol Rec* 57:65-72, 1982.

World Health Organization. Dracunculiasis. Global surveillance summary—1985. *Wkly Epidemiol Rec* 61:29-32, 1986.

ESOPHAGOSTOMIASIS AND TERNIDENSIASIS

(127.7)

Synonyms: Helminthoma, helminthic abscesses, nodular worm infection.

Etiology: *Oesophagostomum stephanostomum*, *O. bifurcum*, *O. aculeatum* (*O. apiostomum*), and *Ternidens diminutus*, strongylid nematodes that live in the intestine of nonhuman primates and sometimes in man, causing the formation of nodules in the intestinal wall.

The life cycles of the species of *Oesophagostomum* that occur in primates are not well known, but it is assumed that they follow patterns similar to those of other species of the genus, which are common parasites of domestic animals. The adult females, which measure 8.5 to 13 mm in length (*O. aculeatum*) and live in the large intestine, deposit eggs resembling those of human ancylostomids. Eggs carried to the exterior with fecal matter release a first-stage larva which, after undergoing several molts, is transformed into a third-stage infective larva. The infection of primates (nonhuman and human) occurs via the oral route. In the stomach and small intestine, the larva frees itself from its cuticular sheath; it then penetrates the intestinal mucosa, especially in the large intestine, where it forms nodules (thus the name "nodular worm"). Within these nodules it is transformed into a fourth-stage larva that migrates to the lumen of the large intestine, where it undergoes another molt and matures sexually; females begin oviposition and thus the cycle is renewed. Eggs appear in the feces 30 to 40 days after ingestion of third-stage larvae. Most of the parasites found in man are immature or nongravid.

The females of *Ternidens diminutus* measure 8 to 16 mm long. *T. diminutus* lives mainly in the large intestine, but sometimes has been found in the small intestine. Its life cycle has not been completely clarified yet. Its development is known from the time the eggs are eliminated with the feces up to the development of the third larva in the soil, but what happens to the parasite from then on is not known. Attempts to infect human volunteers and several species of nonhuman primates with third-stage larvae have failed. Consequently, it is suspected that *T. diminutus* requires an intermediate host for its subsequent development.

Both the adults of *Oesophagostomum* spp. and *T. deminutus* and their eggs resemble the ancylostomids, with which they have often been confused.

Geographic Distribution and Occurrence: *O. stephanostomum* has been found in man in Africa and South America (Brazil), *O. bifurcum* in Africa, and *O. aculeatum* in Asia. Human esophagostomiasis is rare. Most of the cases (about 50) have occurred in Africa, especially in Uganda and Ghana. It was also reported that 4% of the prisoners in jails in northern Nigeria were infected. In Asia one case occurred in Indonesia, and the one known case in South America was diagnosed in Brazil.

Infection by *Oesophagostomum* in nonhuman primates is common. Rates of infection are especially high in captive animals.

Human infection by *T. diminutus* has been observed in the southern half of Africa, and it is very frequent in Zimbabwe, where rates of infection varying from 0 to 87% of the population have been found in the different districts. A coprologic study that included 5,545 patients in a hospital in Zimbabwe discovered that *T. diminutus* was the second most common parasite (3.75% versus 5.75% for ancylostomids), but the intensity of infection was almost always low. *T. diminutus* is found in nonhuman primates in Africa and Asia; apparently, it is less frequent in these animals than *Oesophagostomum* spp.

The Disease in Man and Animals: Mild infections by *Oesophagostomum* spp. in man go unnoticed. In clinical cases, the symptomatology varies from vague abdominal malaise to intestinal obstruction caused by tumors. The lesions consist of nodules in the intestinal wall, primarily in the large intestine, which contain necrotic material and the larva or immature parasite. Abscesses, fistulas, and tumors can also occur in the intestinal wall. The disease may be confused with ameboma, carcinoma of the colon, appendicitis, and ileocecal tuberculosis.

Dysenteric diarrhea occurs in intensely parasitized monkeys. Several authors think that *Oesophagostomum* spp. are important pathogenic agents in nonhuman primates that can sometimes cause the death of the animal. However, on the basis of case descriptions, it is difficult to determine if the parasitosis was really the main cause of death.

T. diminutus is relatively slightly pathogenic, and the large majority of infections that it produces are asymptomatic. The adult parasites cause small crateriform ulcerations in the intestinal wall; very occasionally, they can give rise to perforations and peritonitis. In the larval phase, nodules are formed in the intestinal wall.

Source of Infection and Mode of Transmission: Nonhuman primates constitute the main reservoir of the infection. In esophagostomiasis the source of infection is the soil, where the parasite's eggs, deposited with the feces of nonhuman primates, release the larvae that develop to the infective stage. The infection occurs by the oral route. Man is an accidental host in whom the parasite seldom reaches maturity and oviposition.

The life cycle of *T. diminutus* and the epidemiology of the infection have not yet been clarified. Some investigators recognize the possibility that, in addition to the cycle between monkeys and man, a human-to-human cycle may exist.

Diagnosis: In man, parasitologic diagnosis of esophagostomiasis presents difficulties. The patient rarely eliminates eggs in the feces; when some eggs are found, they can be easily confused with those of ancylostomids, which, moreover, may be present in the same individual. Most diagnoses have been made after surgery, when the larva has been found in the thick, yellowish pus in the nodule. Specific identification of the parasite is very difficult.

Diagnosis of the parasitosis by *T. diminutus* does not present major difficulties and is done by coprologic examination. The eggs of *T. diminutus* are slightly larger than those of ancylostomids and *Oesophagostomum* spp. To differentiate them, it may be necessary to culture them in feces and obtain the first-stage larva. In preliminary studies, the immunofluorescence test has given promising results. Cross-reactions have been observed in persons infected by *Necator americanus*, but with a lower titer.

Control: Both esophagostomiasis and ternidensiasis are caused by helminths transmitted from the soil. Human protection consists of observing the rules of personal hygiene.

Bibliography

Dooley, J. R., and R. C. Neafie. Oesophagostomiasis. *In*: Binford, C. H., and D. H. Connor (Eds.), *Pathology of Tropical and Extraordinary Diseases*, vol. 2. Washington, D.C., Armed Forces Institute of Pathology, 1976.

Faust, E. C., P. C. Beaver, and R. C. Jung. *Animal Agents and Vectors of Human Disease*, 4th ed. Philadelphia, Lea and Febiger, 1975.

Goldsmid, J. M. Studies on intestinal helminths in African patients at Harari Central Hospital, Rhodesia. *Trans R Soc Trop Med Hyg* 62:619-629, 1968.

Goldsmid, J. M. Studies on the life cycle and biology of *Ternidens diminutus* (Railliet and Henry, 1905), (Nematoda: Strongylidae). *J Helminthol* 45:341-352, 1971.

Goldsmid, J. M. *Ternidens diminutus* (Railliet and Henry, 1909) and hookworm in Rhodesia and a review of the treatment of human infection with *T. diminutus*. *Cent Afr J Med* (Suppl) 18:14-26, 1972.

Haag, E., and A. H. Van Soest. Oesophagostomiasis in man in North Ghana. *Trop Geogr Med* 16:743-756, 1964.

Kilala, C. P. *Ternidens diminutus* infecting man in southern Tanzania. *East Afr Med J* 48:636-645, 1971.

Rogers, S., and J. M. Goldsmid. Preliminary studies using the indirect fluorescent antibody test for the serological diagnosis of *Ternidens diminutus* infection in man. *Ann Trop Med Parasitol* 71:503-504, 1977.

Ruch, T. C. *Diseases of Laboratory Primates*. Philadelphia, Saunders, 1959.

Spencer, H. Nematode Diseases. *In*: Spencer, H. (Ed.), *Tropical Pathology*. New York, Springer, 1973.

GNATHOSTOMIASIS

(128.1)

Synonyms: Gnathostomosis, larva migrans caused by *Gnathostoma*.

Etiology: The main agent of the human disease is the larva of *Gnathostoma spinigerum* and, rarely, that of *G. hispidum*.

G. spinigerum is a spiruroid nematode which, in the adult stage, lodges in the stomach wall of cats, wild felids, and dogs. The female of the parasite measures 2.5 to 5 cm and the male is approximately half as large. The eggs are eliminated with the fecal matter of the definitive hosts; they hatch in the water after a week of incubation, releasing a first-stage larva. This larva actively penetrates a copepod of the genus *Cyclops*, reaches its hemocoel, and in 10 to 15 days transforms into a second-stage larva. When an appropriate freshwater fish ingests the infected copepod, the larva continues its development; it passes from the fish's intestine to the musculature, where at the end of a month it encysts as a third-stage larva. This infective larva measures about 4 mm and is coiled in a spiral inside a fibrous cyst about 1 mm in size. Experimental infection has shown that fish, amphibians, and rodents can serve as second intermediate hosts or as transport hosts. Many animal species, such as snakes, birds, and some mammals, can serve as transport hosts, in which the third-stage larva ingested with infected fish does not continue its development but encysts again and serves as a source of infection for the definitive hosts. Cats, dogs, and all other natural definitive hosts are infected by consuming fish or paratenic (transport) hosts that contain the third-stage larvae. In the stomach of the definitive hosts, the larvae are released from their cysts, penetrate the stomach wall, migrate to the liver, and from there go to other organs and tissues (muscular and connective); then, from the peritoneal cavity they again penetrate the stomach and lodge in the mucosa. After about 6 months in the gastric mucosa, they mature and begin oviposition.

The adult stage of *G. hispidum* parasitizes the stomach mucosa of pigs and wild boars. Its development cycle requires only one intermediate host. The eggs of the parasite hatch in water and release a second-stage larva. The larva continues its development when ingested by a *Cyclops* spp. copepod, and becomes a third-stage infective larva in its coelom. If an infected copepod is ingested with water by a pig, the larva develops to the adult stage in a manner similar to *G. spinigerum*.

Geographic Distribution and Occurrence: *G. spinigerum* is distributed among animals in a much more widespread area than it is among humans. In an endemic area of southern Japan, 35% of cats and 4% of dogs were parasitized by *G. spinigerum*; between 60 and 100% of one species of freshwater fish contained larvae. In the markets of Thailand, larvae were found in 37% of the fish, 80% of the eels, and 90% of the frogs (Daengsvang, 1973). An infection rate of 60 to 100% was found in the fish *Ophiocephalus argus* in Japan.

The largest concentrations of human cases have been recorded in Thailand and Japan, where hundreds of cases have been reported each year. Human infection is less frequent or rare in Malaysia, Indochina, China, Indonesia, and India. Sporadic cases have also been registered in Australia and Israel. Two human cases by larvae similar to *G. spinigerum* have been described in Mexico (Peláez and Pérez Reyes, 1970), but the species was not identified; in California, USA, an ocular case was described (Tudor and Blair, 1971).

G. hispidum is relatively common in pigs in Europe, Asia, and Australia, but is not important in public health. A few human cases have been described; however, the identity of the parasite was uncertain (Daengsvang, 1982).

The Disease in Man: Man is an aberrant host in which the larva of the parasite only exceptionally reaches sexual maturity. The larva migrates from one site to another and does not become established in the host's stomach. In most cases, a single larva is responsible for the clinical picture. The first symptoms appear 1 or 2 days after the ingestion of infected raw fish (or the meat of paratenic hosts, such as chickens and ducks) and consist of nausea, salivation, urticaria, pruritus, and stomach discomfort; mild leukocytosis and marked eosinophilia are common. Later symptoms are due to the migration of the larva into the liver and other organs. The movements of the larva inside the abdominal or thoracic organs can cause acute pain of limited duration. The symptoms resemble cholecystitis, appendicitis, cystitis, or other diseases, depending on the organ affected by the larva (internal or visceral gnathostomiasis). Approximately 1 month after the infective food was eaten, the larva locates in the subcutaneous tissue, usually of the chest, abdomen, extremities, and head, initiating the chronic phase in which the organic symptoms abate and disappear and eosinophilia gradually decreases. The most prominent symptom is an intermittent subcutaneous edema that changes location each time the larva moves. The edema is pruriginous but not painful, and initially lasts a week or more; its duration then becomes progressively shorter with each recurrence. In older infections the edemas recur at longer intervals. The larva can survive in the human body for a long time, and one case lasting 16 years has been recorded.

In its erratic migration the larva can affect a variety of organs and tissues. The clinical picture it produces in the skin is similar to that of cutaneous larva migrans (see the section on that disease). The most serious localizations, fortunately rare, are in the brain and eyes.

The Disease in Animals: In the natural definitive hosts (cats and dogs) the larvae can cause tissue destruction as a result of their migration through different organs. The adult parasite locates in the stomach wall, where it produces cavities full of serosanguineous fluid and hyperplasia of the wall, with the formation of nodules. In cats, the cavities created in the stomach wall by the parasite can open onto the peritoneum, leading to peritonitis and death.

Source of Infection and Mode of Transmission: The reservoirs of the parasite are cats, dogs, and several species of wild mammals. These definitive hosts become infected primarily by consuming infected fish or other animals that serve as paratenic hosts.

Man is infected in a similar manner. The habit of eating fish or fowl raw and only seasoned with vinegar is an essential factor in the occurrence of the human disease and its endemicity in Thailand and Japan. The parasitosis in animals is much more widespread than the human infection, since the latter is closely related to eating habits.

In each endemic area, one or two species of fish serve as the main source of infection for man. Very high infection rates were found in two species of *Ophiocephalus* in Japan (*O. argus* and *O. tadianus*), and each fish contained hundreds of larvae. In Thailand, besides several species of *Ophiocephalus*, sources of infection include catfish (*Clarias batrachus*), eels, frogs, freshwater snakes, chickens, and ducks (Daengsvang, 1982).

Diagnosis: In endemic areas, migratory and recurrent subcutaneous edemas accompanied by leukocytosis and high eosinophilia can be considered pathognomonic. Specific diagnosis can be made only by identifying the larva in surgically obtained specimens. The intradermal test (which has a low specificity) and the precipitation test are among the immunobiologic tests used.

In dogs and cats, diagnosis can be made by detecting eggs in the feces, but it must be borne in mind that the eggs are sometimes few in number or are eliminated irregularly.

Control: In enzootic areas the best way to prevent human disease is by abstaining from eating raw or undercooked fish and fowl.

Bibliography

Daengsvang, S. An experimental study on the life cycle of *Gnathostoma hispidum* (Fedchenko, 1872) in Thailand with special reference to the incidence and some significant morphological characters of the adult and larval stages. *Southeast Asian J Trop Med Public Health* 3:376-389, 1972. (Summarized in *Helminthol Abstr* 42:410, 1973.)

Daengsvang, S. Gnathostomiasis. *In*: Schultz, M. G. (Ed.), *CRC Handbook Series in Zoonoses*. Section C, vol. 2. Boca Raton, Florida. CRC Press, 1982.

Faust, E. C., P. C. Beaver, and R. C. Jung. *Animal Agents and Vectors of Human Disease*, 4th ed. Philadelphia, Lea and Febiger, 1975.

Peláez, D., and R. Pérez Reyes. Gnatostomiasis humana en América. *Rev Latinoam Microbiol* 12:83-91, 1970.

Soulsby, E. J. L. *Textbook of Veterinary Clinical Parasitology*. Oxford, Blackwell, 1965.

Soulsby, E. J. L. *Helminths, Arthropods and Protozoa of Domesticated Animals*, 7th ed. Philadelphia, Lea and Febiger, 1982.

Swanson, V. L. Gnathostomiasis. *In*: Marcial-Rojas, R. A. (Ed.), *Pathology of Protozoal and Helminthic Diseases*. Baltimore, Maryland, Williams and Wilkins, 1971.

Swanson, V. L. Gnathostomiasis. *In*: Binford, C. H., and D. H. Connor (Eds.), *Pathology of Tropical and Extraordinary Diseases*. Washington, D.C., Armed Forces Institutes of Pathology, 1976.

Tudor, R. C., and E. Blair. *Gnathostoma spinigerum*. An unusual cause of ocular nematodiasis in the Western Hemisphere. *Am J Ophthalmol* 72:185, 1971. Cited in Daengsvang, 1982.

Witenberg, G. G. Helminthozoonoses. *In*: Van der Hoeden, J. (Ed.), *Zoonoses*. Amsterdam, Netherlands, Elsevier, 1964.

GONGYLONEMIASIS

(128.8)

Synonym: Gongylonematosis.

Etiology: *Gongylonema pulchrum* (*G. ransomi*, *G. scutatum*), a spiruroid nematode of the family Thelaziidae, whose main hosts are ruminants, swine, and wild boars. The adult parasite lives in the esophageal mucosa and submucosa of the definitive hosts, but can also be found in the rumen and the oral cavity. It is filiform and its size varies according to the host. In ruminants, the male can reach about 62 mm in length and 0.15 to 0.3 mm in diameter, and the females up to 145 mm by 0.2 to 0.5 mm; in man or swine the parasite is smaller.

The females of *G. pulchrum* deposit completely embryonated eggs in the esophagus and rumen of the definitive host. The eggs are eliminated to the exterior with the feces, and must be ingested by an intermediate host for the life cycle to continue. These hosts are several species of coprophagic beetles of the genera *Aphodius*, *Ontophagus*, *Blaps*, and others. Experimental infection of a small cockroach, *Blatella germanica*, was also possible. The egg hatches in the beetle's intestine, and the larva penetrates its hemocoel, where in about a month it develops to the third (infective) stage and encysts. Ruminants acquire the parasitosis upon ingesting the small beetles with grass or other infested food, and swine become infected by coprophagia. The migration route of the larva in the definitive host is still not well known, but experimental infections in guinea pigs provide evidence that the larva frees itself from the coleopteran in the stomach and migrates through the stomach wall to the esophagus, where it matures in about 2 months and reinitiates the cycle with oviposition.

Geographic Distribution and Occurrence: *G. pulchrum* is widely distributed geographically. In addition to domestic and wild ruminants, swine, and wild boars, the parasite has been found—although less frequently—in other animal species, such as equines, canines, felines, rodents, and primates (human and nonhuman). The prevalence of the infection in domestic ruminants varies with the area. In surveys carried out in the United States, the parasite was detected in 10% of 29 bovines in Georgia and 5% of 20 bovines in Florida; the rate was 5.9% in 1,518 pigs, varying from 0 to 21% according to geographic origin. In slaughterhouses of the Ukraine, USSR, the parasite was found in 32 to 94% of adult cattle, 39 to 95% of sheep, and 0 to 37% of swine (Cebotarev and Poliscuk, 1959). A study in a slaughterhouse in Tehran, Iran, found *G. pulchrum* in the esophagus of 49.7% of the cattle examined (Anwar *et al.*, 1979).

Human infection by *G. pulchrum* is rare, and only 46 cases have been recorded. (Cappucci *et al.*, 1982). Among the countries where the infection has been diagnosed are the United States, the USSR, Italy, Federal Republic of Germany (in a Greek immigrant), Hungary, Yugoslavia, Bulgaria, Turkey, China, Sri Lanka, Morocco, and New Zealand.

The Disease in Man: In human cases, parasites have been found actively moving in the submucosa of lips, gums, hard palate, soft palate, and tonsils. The lesions are irritated areas produced by the parasite's movement through the mucosa and submucosa. Pharyngitis and stomatitis have sometimes been confirmed. Two cases described in China included bloody sialorrhea and eroded and bleeding patches on the esophageal mucosa.

The Disease in Animals: In ruminants, *G. pulchrum* is found mainly in the mucosa and submucosa of the esophagus, but the mature parasite can move in any of several directions and invade the pharynx, oral cavity, or rumen. In swine, it is found in the stratified squamous epithelium of the tongue mucosa.

According to observations in Iran, the infection did not produce lesions indicative of a significant pathologic condition (Anwar *et al.*, 1979). Histologic examination of swine tongues in the United States revealed a mild and chronic inflammatory process (Zinter and Migaki, 1970). On the other hand, in the USSR, important lesions of the esophagus of infected bovines have sometimes been found, with hyperemia, edema, and deformations of the organ among the effects cited; likewise, the infection is blamed for occlusions of the esophagus due to a reflex reaction caused by nerve irritation (Cebotarev and Poliscuk, 1959).

Source of Infection and Mode of Transmission: Ruminants and other animals become infected by ingesting coleopterans containing third-stage larvae. Man is an accidental host who does not play any role in the maintenance of the parasite in nature and probably is infected by the same mechanism. Salads and raw vegetables are thought to be the vehicles by means of which man ingests the small beetles. It has also been suggested that the species of *Aphodius*, because of their size (4 to 6 mm) and capacity for flight, could be accidentally inhaled and then swallowed (Weber and Mache, 1973).

The maintenance of the parasite in nature is assured by its broad diffusion and prevalence among herbivores, swine, and other animals (definitive hosts), and the large number of susceptible species of beetles (intermediate hosts). In the Ukraine, USSR, 60 to 90% of the beetles were found to be infected. The highest rates corresponded to several species of *Aphodius* and *Geotrupes*, and the number of larvae per beetle ranged between one and 193 (Cebotarev and Poliscuk, 1959).

Diagnosis: Most of the human cases were diagnosed because the patient felt something moving in the submucosa of the oral cavity or observed the parasite emerging from the mouth. Specific diagnosis is done by extracting the parasite and identifying it under the microscope.

Diagnosis in live animals is rarely attempted or achieved. The eggs are not always found by fecal examination, even when flotation or sedimentation methods are used (Cebotarev and Poliscuk, 1959). The parasites can be detected by postmortem examination of the esophagus (ruminants) or the tongue (swine).

Control: Because of the rarity and mildness of human infection, special control measures are not justified. Individual protection can be obtained by observing the rules of personal, food, and environmental hygiene.

Most helminthologists agree that *G. pulchrum* does not cause major damage to animals. Moreover, it would not be feasible to adopt measures aimed at preventing animals at pasture from ingesting beetles.

Bibliography

Anwar, M., H. Rak, and T. W. Gyorkos. The incidence of *Gongylonema pulchrum* from cattle in Tehran, Iran. *Vet Parasitol* 5:271-274, 1979.

Cappucci, D. T., J. K. Augsburg, and P. C. Klinck. Gongylonemiasis. *In*: Schultz, M. G. (Ed.), *CRC Handbook Series in Zoonoses*. Section C, vol. 2. Boca Raton, Florida, CRC Press, 1982.

Cebotarev, R. S., and V. P. Poliscuk. Gongylonematosis of domestic animals under conditions of Ukrainian Polesie and forest-steppe areas. *Acta Parasitol Pol* 7:549-557, 1959.

Faust, E. C., P. C. Beaver, and R. C. Jung. *Animal Agents and Vectors of Human Disease*. Philadelphia, Lea and Febiger, 1975.

Soulsby, E. J. L. *Helminths, Arthropods and Protozoa of Domesticated Animals*, 7th ed. Philadelphia, Lea and Febiger, 1982.

Weber, G., and K. Mache. Uber Hauterscheinungen bei *Gongylonema pulchrum*, sein Erste Beobachtung in Deutschland beim Menschen. *Hautarzt* 24:286-288, 1973.

Zinter, D. E., and G. Migaki. *Gongylonema pulchrum* in tongues of slaughtered pigs. *J Am Vet Med Assoc* 157:301-303, 1970.

LAGOCHILASCARIASIS

(128.8)

Etiology: *Lagochilascaris minor*, a small ascarid, the female of which measures 6 to 20 mm in length by 0.20 to 0.80 mm in width; the male is smaller. So far, it has been identified only in man, and its natural host and development cycle are unknown.

In the lesions it causes in man, the ascarid has been found in various degrees of development, from second-stage larvae to adults, including gravid females (Moraes *et al.*, 1983).

Geographic Distribution and Occurrence: The distribution of the disease is limited and its occurrence extremely rare. Only 19 human cases are known (seven in Brazil, five in Suriname, five in Trinidad and Tobago, one in Costa Rica, and one in Venezuela) (Volcan *et al.*, 1982; Moraes *et al.*, 1983). All the patients were black; they ranged in age from 5 to 39 years, and most lived in jungle regions.

The Disease in Man: The disease is characterized by fistulous abscesses in the subcutaneous tissue of the neck region, but it can also affect the mastoid apophysis, tonsils, maxillae, and paranasal sinuses. The process begins with a tumor that eventually opens to the surface of the skin, releasing pus in which adult parasites, larvae, and eggs are intermittently found. The fistulas may also open in the nasopharynx, in which case purulent material and parasites are eliminated through the nose and mouth. The process is chronic and may last for years.

Source of Infection and Mode of Transmission: The natural reservoir is unknown. The rarity of the human infection would indicate that man is an accidental host and is unable by himself to maintain the parasite in nature.

It is not known how humans become infected. In a recent revision of the genus *Lagochilascaris*, the possibility was suggested that man is infected by ingesting embryonated eggs (possibly eliminated by another animal species), and that the larvae are released in his intestine and migrate to the lungs to continue their development. The third-stage larva would then ascend to the trachea, but instead of being swallowed, as occurs with the larva of *Ascaris lumbricoides*, it would become established in the retropharyngeal region.

Diagnosis: Specific diagnosis is made by identifying the parasite found in lesions. The eggs are also characteristic and resemble those of *Toxocara cati* or *Ascaris lumbricoides*. In a recent case described in Venezuela, eggs of *L. minor* were found in the feces of the patient (an occurrence that had not been observed before) and were at first confused with those of *A. lumbricoides* (Volcan *et al.*, 1982).

Control: Lack of knowledge about the transmission of the parasite to man prevents determination of effective control measures.

Bibliography

Arean, V. M. Lagochilascariasis. *In:* Marcial-Rojas, R. A. (Ed.), *Pathology of Protozoal and Helminthic Diseases.* Baltimore, Maryland, Williams and Wilkins, 1971.

Artigas, P. de T., P. Araujo, N. Romiti, and M. Rubio. Sôbre um caso de parasitismo humano por *Lagochilascaris minor* Leiper, 1909, no Estado de São Paulo, Brasil. *Rev Inst Med Trop S Paulo* 10:78-82, 1968.

Costa, H. M. de A., A. V. M. Da Silva, P. Rabelo Costa, and S. F. Assis. *Lagochilascaris minor* Leiper, 1909 (Nematoda-Ascaridae) de origen humana. *Rev Inst Med Trop São Paulo* 28:126-130, 1986.

Moraes, M. A. P., M. V. C. Arnaud, and P. E. Lima. Novos casos de infecção humana por *Lagochilascaris minor* (Leiper, 1909) encontrados no estado de Pará, Brasil. *Rev Inst Med Trop São Paulo* 25:139-146, 1983.

Oostburg, B. F. J., and A. A. O. Varma. *Lagochilascaris minor* infection in Suriname. *Am J Trop Med Hyg* 17:548-550, 1968.

Oostburg, B. F. J. Thiabendazole therapy of *Lagochilascaris minor* infection in Suriname. Report of a case. *Am J Trop Med Hyg* 20:580-583, 1971.

Rosemberg, S., M. B. S. Lopes, S. Mazuda, R. Campos, and M.C. R. Vieira Bressan. Fatal encephalopathy due to *Lagochilascaris minor* infection. *Am J Trop Med Hyg* 35:575-578, 1986.

Sprent, J. F. A. Speciation and development in the genus *Lagochilascaris*. *Parasitology* 62:71-112, 1971.

Volcan, G. S., F. Rojas Ochoa, C. E. Medrano, and Y. de Valera. *Lagochilascaris minor* infection in Venezuela. *Am J Trop Med Hyg* 31:1111-1113, 1982.

MAMMOMONOGAMIASIS

(128.8)

Synonyms: Syngamosis, syngamiasis.

Etiology: Two species of the family Syngamidae, *Mammomonogamus* (*Syngamus*) *laryngeus* and *M. nasicola*, the former a parasite of the laryngotracheal region, and the latter a parasite of the nasal fossae of bovines, bubalines, and occasionally sheep, goats, and deer. The taxonomy of *Mammomonogamus* is not yet well defined (Macko *et al.*, 1981). Some helminthologists consider *M. nasicola* and *M. laryngeus* to be synonymous. The male and female parasites are found permanently coupled in a Y formation in the locations mentioned.

The development cycle of these syngamids in mammals is not well known; it is believed to be similar to that of the fowl parasite *Syngamus trachea*. The eggs deposited by the parasite in the tracheal mucus are coughed up, swallowed, and eliminated with the feces. In the external environment the infective larva (third-stage) develops within the egg; it may be released from the egg and continue its development in the soil. Herbivores are infected by ingesting eggs containing the infective larvae or by ingesting the free larvae. The infection can also probably be produced by ingestion of paratenic hosts, such as earthworms, snails, and several types of arthropods, as happens in avian syngamosis (*S. trachea*). In an herbivore's digestive tract, the larvae are released from their protective membranes, cross the intestinal wall to the mesenteric veins, and migrate to their final location (tracheolaryngeal or nasal), where the adult parasites couple and remain in permanent union. The cycle is reinitiated with oviposition.

Geographic Distribution and Occurrence: *M. laryngeus* is found in ruminants in tropical America and in India, Malaysia, Vietnam, and the Philippines. *M. nasicola* occurs in Africa, Brazil, the eastern USSR, and the Caribbean. However, information is still lacking on the full geographic distribution of the two nematode species.

Some studies were carried out a few years ago in slaughterhouses in Brazil to find out the prevalence of the infection in bovines. In the state of São Paulo, 27 (45%) of 60 slaughtered cows were found to be infected (Santos and Fukuda, 1977), as were 18 (37.5%) of 48 young bulls in the state of Rio de Janeiro (Freire and Biachin,

1979). In Honduras, only 2.8% of 70 bovines examined were parasitized (Secretariat of Natural Resources of Honduras, 1980).

Human infection is rare, and only 80 cases have been recorded (Gardiner and Schantz, 1983). With the exception of one case in the Philippines, the rest of the cases occurred in the Caribbean region and Brazil. The majority of the cases (51) occurred in inhabitants of Martinique or in persons who visited the island (Mornex et al., 1980).

The Disease in Man and Animals: In man, the symptomatology consists of tracheolaryngeal irritation, with stubborn cough but without fever. In some patients there is hemoptysis. A case was reported (Birrel, 1977) in an Australian woman who lived in Guyana for 10 months; she had respiratory symptoms consisting of a chronic cough and hemoptysis, and experienced loss of weight. In April 1977, she was admitted to Brisbane Hospital, Queensland, Australia, where bronchoscopy revealed larvae of a parasite that was identified as *M. laryngeus*. Extraction of the parasites resulted in disappearance of the symptoms. A similar case was recently described in the United States of America. A woman who spent 2 weeks vacation in Martinique and Saint Lucia developed a chronic cough and mild fever the day after returning to her country. A cyst was discovered by bronchoscopy, and it was found to contain nematodes identified as *M. laryngeus*. With the removal of the cyst the cough stopped (Gardiner and Schantz, 1983).

The animal infection is rarely symptomatic, and large numbers of *M. laryngeus* are required to produce an afebrile laryngitis or tracheitis. No symptoms have been observed in nasal infections (*M. nasicola*).

Source of Infection and Mode of Transmission (Figure 94): The reservoirs of *M. laryngeus* and *M. nasicola* are ruminants. Man is infected only accidentally. The sources of infection for ruminants are soil, pasture, and water; for humans, they are probably plant foods and water contaminated with eggs or free larvae of the parasite.

The exogenous development of these parasites is not well known, but it is thought to be similar to that of *Syngamus trachea* of fowl. In the life cycle of the latter parasite, paratenic hosts are very important (see Etiology), since the infective third-stage larvae encyst in the coelom of these hosts and can survive a year or more.

Diagnosis: The eggs of the parasite can be observed in feces and, more rarely, in sputum. Coughing fits may expel these parasites, which are easy to identify. Animal mammomonogamiasis is most often found in necropsy.

Diagnosis in humans is usually effected by bronchoscopy and detection of the parasite.

Control: Prevention consists of observing the basic rules of food hygiene.

Bibliography

Birrell, D. J. Thoracic Medical Registrar, The Prince Charles Hospital, Cherside, Brisbane, Queensland, Australia. Personal communication, May 1977.

Borchert, A. *Parasitología Veterinaria*. Zaragoza, Spain, Acribia, 1964.

Euzéby, J. *Les Zoonoses Helmintiques*. Paris, Vigot Frères, 1964.

Faust, E. C., P. C. Beaver, and R. C. Jung. *Animal Agents and Vectors of Human Disease*, 4th ed. Philadelphia, Lea and Febiger, 1975.

**Figure 94. Mammomonogamiasis (*Mammomonogamus laryngeus*).
Probable transmission cycle.**

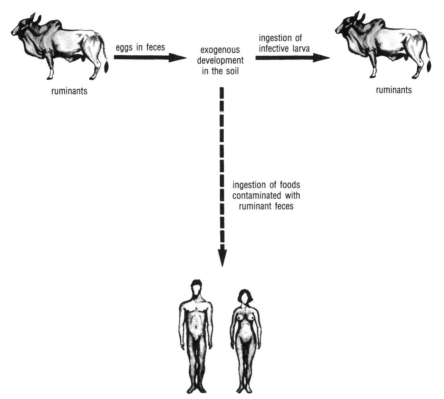

Freire, N. M. S., and I. Biachin. Prevalencia de *Mammomonogamus laryngeus* (Railliet, 1899) em bovinos no Rio de Janeiro. *Arq Esc Vet UFMG (Minas Gerais)* 31:23-24, 1979.

Gardiner, C. H., and P. M. Schantz. *Mammomonogamus* infection in a human. *Am J Trop Med Hyg* 32:995-997, 1983.

Macko, J. K., V. Birova, and R. Flores. Deliberations on the problems of *Mammomonogamus* species (Nematoda, Syngamidae) in ruminants. *Folia Parasitol (Praha)* 28:43-49, 1981.

Mornex, J. F., J. Magdeleine, and J. de Thore. La syngamose humaine (*Mammomonogamus nasicola*) cause de toux chronique en Martinique. 37 observations récentes. *Nouv Presse Med* 9:3628, 1980.

Pessôa, S. B. *Parasitologia Médica,* 6th ed. Rio de Janeiro, Koogan, 1963.

Santos, I. F., and R. T. Fukuda. Ocorrência de *Syngamus laryngeus* em bovinos do Município de Novo Horizonte. *S P Científica (São Paulo)* 5:391-393, 1977.

Secretariat of Natural Resources of Honduras. *Muestreo Patológico de Honduras.* Tegucigalpa, 1980.

Soulsby, E. J. L. *Textbook of Veterinary Clinical Parasitology.* Oxford, Blackwell, 1965.

MICRONEMIASIS

(128.8)

Etiology: *Micronema deletrix*, a very small, saprophytic nematode, the female measuring barely 250 to 445 microns. It is a free-living, rhabditiform species, whose habitat is soil rich in decomposing organic matter. All developmental stages are found in the external environment—eggs, larvae, and the female and male adult forms (Shadduck *et al.*, 1979).

M. deletrix is a facultative parasite of humans and equines. Males have not been found in animal tissue; therefore, it has been deduced that the nematode reproduces parthenogenetically in the animal organism. Eggs, larvae, and mature females are all observed in the lesions the nematode causes in tissues. Generally, a female contains only one egg.

It has been pointed out that it may be erroneous to attribute all cases of infection to *M. deletrix* since greater knowledge is needed about the other species of the genus *Micronema* (Gardiner *et al.*, 1981).

Geographic Distribution and Occurrence: The distribution of the nematode in its natural habitat has been studied very little.

Only three human cases are known, and all of them were fatal. One occurred in Canada (Hoogstraten and Young, 1975) and the other two in the United States (Shadduck *et al.*, 1979; Gardiner *et al.*, 1981).

Cases of micronemiasis in equines have been diagnosed in the United States and in Egypt. Its occurrence is rare and only seven cases have been recognized. However, the infection may occur more frequently in equines and go undiagnosed. An illustrative example in this respect is a study carried out in Egypt, in which *M. deletrix* was found in two of 28 dead equines that had shown symptoms of encephalitis (Ferris *et al.*, 1972).

The Disease in Man and Animals: The three known human cases died after manifesting symptoms of meningoencephalitis. In two cases the lesions and nematodes were limited to the brain, but in the third one micronemes were also found in the liver and heart.

The disease in equines is similar to that in man. The symptomatology resembles that of viral encephalitides, with lethargy, ataxia, lateral or ventral recumbency, incoordination, kicking, and death. A nasal tumor was described in one horse, and in another, granulomas in the maxillae and the respective sinuses. In this last case, up to 87,500 parasites per gram were extracted from the granulomatous mass (Johnson and Johnson, 1966). In two equine cases, other organs were affected in addition to the brain (Alstad *et al.*, 1979).

In both humans and equines, the lesions consist of numerous foci of encephalomalacia, especially in areas adjacent to the larger blood vessels. Generally, the lesions are less extensive and the necrosis less intense in animals than in man. The nematodes are found in the walls of the vessels and the perivascular spaces, and they are abundant in the malacic foci (Shadduck *et al.*, 1979).

Source of Infection and Mode of Transmission: The source of infection is soil rich in humus and decomposing organic matter, which is the natural habitat of *M.*

deletrix. Neither the mode of transmission nor the route of penetration of the nematode into the animal body is known. In one case (a Canadian child), the nematode could have entered through multiple lacerations the child received in an accident, which were probably contaminated with equine feces. In another case, infection is suspected to have occurred through decubitus ulcers. The portal of penetration in the equine cases was probably sores in the mouth.

Diagnosis: In all of the cases, diagnosis was made postmortem by histopathology and confirmation of the nematode in the tissues.

Control: Special control measures are not justified.

Bibliography

Alstad, A. D., I. E. Berg, and C. Samuel. Disseminated *Micronema deletrix* infection in the horse. *J Am Vet Med Assoc* 174:264-266, 1979.

Ferris, D. H., N. D. Levine, and P. D. Beamer. *Micronema deletrix* in equine brain. *Am J Vet Res* 33:33-38, 1972.

Gardiner, C. H., D. S. Koh, and T. A. Cardella. *Micronema* in man: third fatal infection. *Am J Trop Med Hyg* 30:586-589, 1981.

Hoogstraten, J., and W. G. Young. Meningo-encephalomyelitis due to the saprophagous nematode, *Micronema deletrix*. *J Can Sci Neurol* 2:121-126, 1975.

Hoogstraten, J., D. H. Connor, and R. C. Neafie. Micronemiasis. *In:* Binford, C. H., and D. H. Connor (Eds.), *Pathology of Tropical and Extraordinary Diseases,* vol. 2. Washington, D.C., Armed Forces Institute of Pathology, 1976.

Johnson, K. H., and D. W. Johnson. Granulomas associated with *Micronema deletrix* in the maxillae of a horse. *J Am Vet Med Assoc* 149:155-159, 1966.

Shadduck, J. A., J. Ubelaker, and V. O. Telford. *Micronema deletrix* meningoencephalitis in an adult man. *Am J Clin Pathol* 72:640-643, 1979.

STRONGYLOIDIASIS

(127.2)

Synonym: Strongyloidosis.

Etiology: The etiologic agents of human strongyloidiasis are *Strongyloides stercoralis* and *S. fuelleborni*. A prominent characteristic of these nematodes is that free-living generations alternate with parasitic ones. The free-living adults are sexually differentiated into males and females.

The adult female of *S. stercoralis* is filariform, measures almost 2.2 mm in length by 50 microns in diameter, and lives in the intestinal mucosa of the duodenum and jejunum of man, other primates, dogs, cats, and foxes. Males are not found in the parasitic phase of the cycle, and reproduction is parthenogenetic. Oviposition occurs in the epithelium or even in the submucosa; the eggs release rhabditiform (first-stage) larvae that migrate to the intestinal lumen. The rhabditiform larvae, which are evacuated with the feces to the exterior, can follow two courses of development: a direct cycle (homogonic) or an indirect one (heterogonic). In the direct cycle, the larva undergoes two molts (later it will undergo two more molts in the host's body) to become a filariform or strongyloid larva, which is infective. In the indirect cycle, considered by many investigators to be the basic cycle, the rhabditiform larvae undergo four molts and in 2 to 5 days metamorphose into free-living male and female adults. The fertilized female deposits eggs in the soil that complete their development in a few hours and release rhabditiform larvae; these in turn develop into filariform larvae infective for man and animals. There is evidence that the free-living parasites originate only one generation of larvae. The homogonic and heterogonic cycles are genetically determined and, moreover, the heterogonic development depends on environmental conditions (humidity and temperature).

The filariform larvae produced by either cycle enter the host's body through the skin (occasionally through the mouth), localize in small blood vessels, and are carried by the venous circulation to the heart and from there to the lungs. From the pulmonary capillaries they enter the alveoli and ascend to the trachea; they then descend through the esophagus to the intestine, where they are transformed into parthenogenetic females that quickly begin oviposition, thus repeating the life cycle. The prepatent period in man lasts 2 to 4 weeks; it is shorter in dogs.

Hyperinfection and autoinfection are also known in man. In hyperinfection, the rhabditiform larvae are transformed into filariform larvae in the intestine, penetrate the mucosa of the lower part of the ileum or colon, and migrate via the bloodstream to the lungs; from there they pass to the trachea, esophagus, and finally the intestine, where they mature. In autoinfection, the filariform larvae are originated in the same way as above, are eliminated with the fecal matter, and reinfect man by penetration of the perianal or perineal skin. It is not known if these forms of infection occur in dogs, but strongyloidiases have been observed in experimentally infected dogs, and it is probable that persistent cases result from autoinfections. Nearly a third of the experimentally exposed dogs are not capable of eliminating the infection spontaneously, a finding that parallels the situation in man in certain respects. Persistent, chronic human infection was still present after 35 years in 30% of the United States veterans who had been prisoners of war in southeastern Asia (Grove and Northern, 1982).

S. stercoralis, which infects dogs and cats, is similar both morphologically and physiologically to the human parasite. However, susceptibility of the animals to different geographic strains or biotypes varies. Studies by several researchers have demonstrated that dogs are susceptible to strains of *S. stercoralis* of human origin from one part of the world but not another (Grove and Northern, 1982).

S. fuelleborni inhabits the intestine of primates (human and nonhuman). Its development cycle is similar to that of *S. stercoralis*, with the difference that the eggs do not hatch in the intestine but in the environment, and thus can usually be found in fresh feces.

Other species of *Strongyloides* of animal origin can also infect man. However, they do not develop beyond the larval forms, which remain in the skin and cause symptoms of cutaneous larva migrans (World Health Organization, 1979).

Geographic Distribution and Occurrence: *S. stercoralis* is cosmopolitan, but it is more common in the tropics and subtropics than in temperate climates. The prevalence of the infection is not well known. In 1947 it was estimated that approximately 35 million people were parasitized (among them, 21 million in Asia, 8.5 million in tropical America, and 400,000 in the United States). The infection has been observed in Mexico, in all of the countries of Central America, and in some of the countries of South America. Within the last 20 years, the following rates have been reported: Panama, 20%; Colombia, 16%; French Guiana, 23.6%; Uruguay, 4.3%; and Argentina, 7.6%. In Iquitos, Peru, a rate of 60% was found. In Brazil, the rates vary from 4.1 to 58.3% in different areas (Rio Doce, Minas Gerais). The infection rate can reach 85% among poor socioeconomic groups in the hot and humid regions of the tropics. By contrast, in hot, semiarid areas, the infection rate rarely exceeds 3%.

The infection in dogs also seems to have cosmopolitan distribution. In Malaysia, 6.3% of dogs and 4.8% of cats were found to be infected, and in Canada and the United States, 2% and 1.5% of dogs, respectively. In a recent study in Australia, only two dogs among 646 examined were found to be infected.

S. fuelleborni is a common parasite of Old World nonhuman primates. It is frequent in these animals in the wild as well as in colonies. In the humid jungle regions of central Africa (Central African Republic, Cameroon, and Ethiopia), this species is more prevalent than *S. stercoralis* in the human population. Human infection by *S. fuelleborni* also has a high prevalence in the African savannah, for example in Zambia, where 9.9% of strongyloidiases was due to *S. fuelleborni* (Hira and Patel, 1977). A study carried out in a village in Zaire found prevalence rates of 34% in 76 children and 48% in 185 persons from the general population (Brown and Girardeau, 1977). In a jungle area in southern Cameroon, 154 Pygmies were examined; *S. fuelleborni* was found in 31% of them and *S. stercoralis* in only 1%. In another area, the prevalences were 7% and 2%, respectively, for the two species.

The Disease in Man: Infection by *S. stercoralis* is of very long duration in a high proportion of persons. Mild infections are usually well tolerated and produce no symptomatology or only vague and variable intestinal disorders. In persons with a heavy parasite burden or with decreased resistance, however, the clinical picture can vary from mild to very serious, and the infection may even prove fatal.

Penetration of the skin by the filariform larva produces only a small papule at the invasion site, or allergic reactions with urticaria and pruritus if the patient has been sensitized by prior exposure. In some patients, urticaria appears periodically, coinciding with attacks of diarrhea and reappearance of larvae in the feces. Skin lesions can be caused not only by *S. stercoralis* but also by other species of *Strongyloides*. Based on experimental infections in a volunteer, it is suspected that the cases of dermatitis with serpiginous eruption seen in hunters in the swampy areas of Louisiana, USA, are due to *S. procyonis*, a parasite of raccoons, or to *S. myopotami* from otters.

During the larvae's pulmonary migration phase, the symptomatology can vary from an irritating cough to full-blown pneumonitis and bronchopneumonia. The serious pulmonary symptoms are generally due to autoinfection. However, most often the bronchopulmonary manifestations are discrete and disappear in a few days.

Intestinal symptoms dominate the clinical picture. Depending on the severity of the lesions caused by the parasites in the intestinal mucosa, the symptomatology may correspond to either edematous catarrhal enteritis (with thickening of the intestinal wall) or ulcerative enteritis. Among other symptoms, epigastric pain, diarrhea, dyspepsia, nausea, and vomiting are frequent. Both the abdominal pain and the diarrhea occur intermittently. Leukocytosis and eosinophilia are common.

Although 50% or more of the infected individuals do not have symptoms, it should be borne in mind that asymptomatic individuals can suddenly develop a serious clinical form of the illness if their resistance decreases. This phenomenon may be due to endogenous hyperinfection causing a rapid increase in the number of infective larvae. This disturbance in the equilibrium of the host-parasite relationship may occur in individuals weakened by concurrent illnesses, malnutrition, or therapy with immunosuppressant drugs. Several fatal cases of strongyloidiasis have occurred in patients treated with corticosteroid or cytotoxic drugs. The clinical picture consists of ulcerative enteritis with abdominal pain, intense diarrhea, vomiting, malabsorption, dehydration, hypoproteinemia, and hypokalemia, and sometimes results in death. Disseminated or invasive strongyloidiasis can affect any organ, but the lungs are most frequently exposed. Clinical pulmonary strongyloidiasis is manifested as asthma, cavitation, opacities, consolidation, and infiltrations. Secondary bacterial infections often occur, giving rise to bacteremia, peritonitis, meningitis, endocarditis, and formation of abscesses in different locations. It is believed that the filariform larvae spread bacteria from the intestine to different parts of the body (Boram *et al.*, 1981; Igra-Siegman *et al.*, 1981; Ramos *et al.*, 1984).

The pathogenicity of *S. fuelleborni* has been studied very little. Because simultaneous parasitoses occur so frequently in the tropics, it is difficult to relate a particular symptom to a specific parasite. The most common complaints attributable to this agent are abdominal pain and occasional diarrhea, as was observed in patients in Zambia and also in an experimentally infected volunteer (Hira and Patel, 1977). Generally, infections by *S. fuelleborni* are not intense enough to cause illness. Superinfections are not observed.

The Disease in Animals: Age is an important factor in the infection of dogs and cats. Infection by *S. stercoralis* is manifested clinically only in young animals; as the skin thickens with age, the larva has more difficulty penetrating it. In addition, it has been shown that dogs and cats that have gotten rid of the parasite are resistant to reinfection for more than 6 months. In contrast to human infection, which is generally very prolonged if untreated, the disease in animals is of limited duration.

The infection can occur subclinically or symptomatically. In symptomatic cases, the first signs to appear in puppies are loss of appetite, purulent conjunctivitis, coughing, and sometimes bronchopneumonia. In the larval penetration phase, there may be violent pruritus, erythema, and alopecia. The intestinal phase begins a week to 10 days later, with diarrhea, abdominal pains, and vomiting. Serious cases can include dehydration, emaciation, bloody diarrhea, and anemia, and can result in death.

Although strongyloidiasis produced by experimental infection has been observed to take a chronic course in some adult dogs, the disease seen in veterinary practice is limited to puppies.

In nonhuman primates infected with *S. fuelleborni*, the most prominent symptom is diarrhea, which can vary from mild and benign to intense and hemorrhagic.

Eosinophilia is less intense in animals than in humans; in dogs, for example, it rarely surpasses 14%.

Source of Infection and Mode of Transmission (Figures 95 and 96): Man is the principal reservoir of *S. stercoralis*. The main source of infection for humans and animals is soil contaminated by feces. The route of infection is most commonly cutaneous (rarely oral), when the host comes into contact with third-stage or

Figure 95. Strongyloidiasis (*Strongyloides stercoralis*). Transmission cycle.

1. human strain of *S. stercoralis*

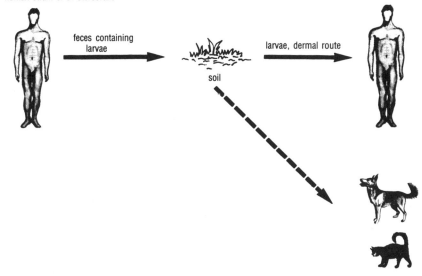

feces containing larvae

soil

larvae, dermal route

2. animal strain of *S. stercoralis*

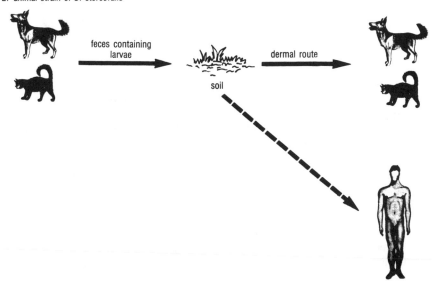

feces containing larvae

soil

dermal route

Note: The participation of animals in the human infection cycle is poorly understood.

filariform larvae. Warm, moist soils favor the exogenic and heterogonic (indirect) cycle that produces free-living nematodes, allowing rapid multiplication of the infective larvae. This fact explains why the infection is more common in the tropics and subtropics.

Figure 96. Strongyloidiasis (*Strongyloides fuelleborni*). Transmission cycle.

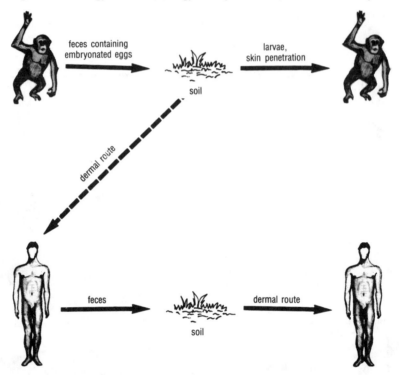

The role of dogs and cats in the epidemiology of the disease has not been well evaluated yet. The susceptibility of dogs to certain biotypes or geographic strains would indicate that, at least in some areas of the world, they could contribute to human infection by contaminating the soil. However, only one case in which the source of human infection is attributed to dog fecal matter is recorded in the literature (Georgi and Sprinkle, 1974). On the other hand, the frequency of cross-infections between humans and animals is difficult to determine because both the adult parasites and the larvae of *S. stercoralis* from different animal species and from man lack distinctive characteristics.

Nonhuman primates are the reservoir of *S. fuelleborni*. The source of infection is primate feces (nonhuman and human). Originally, the infection was zoonotic (from nonhuman to human primates), but evidence is increasing that *S. fuelleborni* infection in several regions of Africa occurs by interhuman transmission. Recent studies carried out in Zambia have confirmed that the parasitosis occurs among the populations of periurban and urban areas, environments where nonhuman primates are generally absent, and in very young children (34% of 76 children under 200 days old) (Hira and Patel, 1980; Brown and Girardeau, 1977). Consequently, in these situations it is undoubtedly man who maintains the cycle of the parasite in nature. Likewise, the high prevalence of infection in some communities, such as among the Pygmies, would indicate a tendency on the part of the parasite to adapt to humans.

Other species of *Strongyloides* of animal origin rarely manage to complete their life cycle in man. In an experimental infection of a volunteer with infective larvae of *S. procyonis*, very few specimens reached maturity and oviposition. Most species of animal *Strongyloides* can invade the skin of man and cause transitory dermatitis.

Role of Animals in the Epidemiology of the Disease: Strongyloidiasis caused by *S. stercoralis* is a common disease and apparently intercommunicable between man, dogs, and cats. It is thought that in certain areas the infection can be transmitted from one species to another by means of contaminated soil.

Intestinal strongyloidiasis caused by *S. fuelleborni* is an infection of both zoonotic and interhuman transmission. Dermatitis in man caused by other species of *Strongyloides* is zoonotic.

Diagnosis: Laboratory confirmation consists of finding rhabditiform larvae (*S. stercoralis*) in human or dog feces. Elimination of larvae with the feces may be intermittent and, therefore, examinations should be repeated. Duodenal aspiration also varies in its effectiveness, but this method is recommended as a supplement to coprologic examination. Occasionally, larvae can be observed in the sputum.

When the infection is due to *S. fuelleborni*, embryonated eggs instead of larvae can be found in fresh fecal samples.

Control: The most important control measure consists of reducing the source of infection; soil contamination should be prevented by means of sanitary disposal of human feces. All infected persons, even those without symptoms, should be treated (with thiabendazole). The use of footwear provides good protection in endemic areas. Likewise, good personal hygiene habits are important.

Before beginning treatment of a patient with immunosuppressants, it should be ascertained whether he is infected by *S. stercoralis*, and if so, he should be treated first with thiabendazole to prevent hyperinfection.

Dogs, cats, and monkeys in contact with man should be examined, and treated if found to be infected.

Bibliography

Adam, M., O. Morgan, C. Persaud, and W. N. Gibbs. Hyperinfection syndrome with *Strongyloides stercoralis* in malignant lymphoma. *Br Med J* 1:264-266, 1973.

Bisseru, B. Strongyloidiasis and anisakiasis. *In*: Hubbert, W. T., W. F. McCulloch, and P. R. Schnurrenberger (Eds.), *Diseases Transmitted from Animals to Man*, 6th ed. Springfield, Illinois, Thomas, 1975.

Boram, L. H., K. F. Keller, D. E. Justus, and J. P. Collins. Strongyloidiasis in immunosuppressed patients. *Am J Clin Pathol* 76:778-781, 1981.

Brown, R. C., and M. H. Girardeau. Transmammary passage of *Strongyloides* spp. larvae in the human host. *Am J Trop Med Hyg* 26:215-219, 1977.

Cruz, T., G. Reboucas, and H. Rocha. Fatal strongyloidiasis in patients receiving corticosteroids. *N Engl J Med* 20:1093-1096, 1966.

Dancescu, P. Observations concerning the parasitic load, duration of infection and clinical manifestations of strongyloidiasis. *Trans R Soc Trop Med Hyg* 70:162, 1976.

Faust, E. C., P. C. Beaver, and R. C. Jung. *Animal Agents and Vectors of Human Disease*, 4th ed. Philadelphia, Lea and Febiger, 1975.

Georgi, J. R., and C. L. Sprinkle. A case of human strongyloidiasis apparently contracted from asymptomatic colony dogs. *Am J Trop Med Hyg* 23:899-901, 1974.

Gilliard, H. Pathogenesis of *Strongyloides*. Review article. *Helminthol Abstr* 36:247-260, 1967.

Grove, D. I., and C. Northern. Infection and immunity in dogs infected with a human strain of *Strongyloides stercoralis*. *Trans R Soc Trop Med Hyg* 76:833-838, 1982.

Grove, D. I. Strongyloidiasis. *In*: Warren, K. S., and A. A. F. Mahmoud (Eds.), *Tropical and Geographical Medicine*. New York, McGraw-Hill Book Co., 1984.

Hira, P. R., and B. G. Patel. *Strongyloides fuelleborni* infections in man in Zambia. *Am J Trop Med Hyg* 26:640-643, 1977.

Hira, P. R., and B. G. Patel. Human strongyloidiasis due to the primate species *Strongyloides fuelleborni*. *Trop Geogr Med* 32:23-29, 1980.

Igra-Siegman, Y., R. Kapila, P. Sen, Z. C. Kaminski, and D. B. Louria. Syndrome of hyperinfection with *Strongyloides stercoralis*. *Rev Infect Dis* 3:397-407, 1981.

Marcial-Rojas, R. A. Strongyloidiasis. *In*: Marcial-Rojas, R. A. (Ed.), *Pathology of Protozoal and Helminthic Diseases*. Baltimore, Maryland, Williams and Wilkins, 1971.

Pampiglione, S., and M. L. Ricciardi. Parasitological survey among Bayaka and Badhelli pygmies (Cameroon). *In*: *Proceedings, Third International Congress of Parasitology*. Munich, Facta Publications, 1974.

Pessôa, S. B. *Parasitología Médica*, 6th ed. Rio de Janeiro, Koogan, 1963.

Ramos, M. C., R. J. Pedro, L. J. Silva, M. L. Branchinni, and F. L. Gonçalves, Jr. Estrongiloidiase maciça. A propósito de quatro casos. *Rev Inst Med Trop São Paulo* 26:218-221, 1984.

Soulsby, E. J. L. *Textbook of Veterinary Clinical Parasitology*. Oxford, Blackwell, 1965.

World Health Organization. *Parasitic Zoonoses*. Report of a WHO Expert Committee, with the Participation of FAO. Geneva, WHO, 1979. (Technical Report Series 637.)

THELAZIASIS

(128.8)

Synonyms: Conjunctival spirurosis, thelaziosis, eyeworm.

Etiology: *Thelazia callipaeda*, *T. californiensis*, and *T. rhodesii*, spiruroid nematodes whose adult stage lodges in the conjunctiva of domestic and wild mammals and, occasionally, of man. Other species of the genus *Thelazia* have not been found in humans; the identification is doubtful in the only human case attributed to *T. rhodesii*, which was reported in Spain (Weinmann, 1982).

The female of *T. callipaeda*, a parasite of dogs and other canids, measures 7 to 17 mm, and the male is 7 to 11.5 mm long. The adult nematode lays completely embryonated eggs that release a first-stage larva. To continue their development, thelaziae require an intermediate host, which is one of several species of Muscidae. The flies, by sucking the secretions at the inside corner of the eye, ingest the larvae (or eggs containing them), which after several weeks develop inside the insect into infective third-stage larvae and then migrate to the proboscis. When the infected arthropod feeds on a new vertebrate host, it releases the infective larvae into the ocular secretion. In 2 to 6 weeks the parasites mature and begin to produce eggs; thus the cycle is completed.

The intermediate hosts of *T. rhodesii* are several species of *Musca* (*M. autumnalis*, *M. convexifrons*, *M. larvipara*), *Morellia simplex*, and *Stomoxys calcitrans*. The intermediate host of *T. callipaeda* is not known for certain. In the Soviet Far East, larvae of the parasite have been found in the drosophilid fly *Phortina variegata*, and it is believed that this species could be the vector. The intermediate host of *T. californiensis* is the fly *Fannia thelaziae*, a member of the *F. benjamini* complex (Wienmann, 1982). The development cycles of *T. callipaeda* and *T. californiensis* are thought to be similar to those of other species in the genus.

Geographic Distribution and Occurrence: *T. callipaeda* is found in dogs and wild canids in the Far East. Human cases total more than 20 and have occurred in China, Thailand, Korea, Japan, India, and the eastern region of the USSR.

T. californiensis occurs in the western United States, where it parasitizes the black-tailed jackrabbit (*Lepus californicus*), deer, coyotes, foxes, raccoons, bears, dogs, and less frequently cats and sheep. About 10 human cases have been recognized, all of them in California.

T. rhodesii parasitizes bovines, bubalines, goats, sheep, and deer in Europe, North Africa, and the Middle East. One human case was described in Spain, but the parasite's correct identification has been doubted (Weinmann, 1982).

The Disease in Man and Animals: In man, thelaziae lodge in the conjunctival sac, where they cause irritation, lacrimation, conjunctivitis, and sometimes corneal scarring and opacity. Some infections are manifested only by the bothersome sensation of a foreign body in the affected eye.

In animals, the parasite is found under the nictitating membrane. The symptomatology is similar to that of human thelaziasis. Conjunctivitis is often aggravated by pruritus, which causes the animal to rub its eye against objects. Corneal lesions are more common in animals than in humans, but it has not been established whether they are due to the parasites or to other, concurrent causes. The intensity of symptoms is quite variable and may depend on the species of *Thelazia* affecting the animal; *T. rhodesii* is considered to be the most pathogenic.

Source of Infection and Mode of Transmission: The reservoirs are several species of domestic and wild mammals. In a village in Thailand, where one human case caused by *T. callipaeda* occurred, five of seven dogs examined were infected. The infection is transmitted from one animal to another and from animal to man by various species of Muscidae.

Some species of *Thelazia* are very particular about their intermediate hosts, the first-stage larva only developing to infective larva in certain species of flies. This particularity largely determines the geographic distribution of both *T. californiensis* and *T. callipaeda*. The predilection of the different vectors for feeding on one or another animal species is of great importance in the epidemiology and is a factor that limits the number of human cases.

Transmission is seasonal and occurs when vector flies are abundant.

Diagnosis: After local anesthetic is administered to the patient, the parasites can be extracted with ophthalmic forceps and identified.

Control: The rarity of human infection does not justify special control measures.

In areas of the USSR where the infection of livestock by *T. rhodesii* and *Trichostrongylus skryjabini* is frequent and recurs every year, bovines are usually treated in winter to reduce the number of adult parasites in summer.

Bibliography

Bhaibulaya, M., S. Prasertsilpa, and S. Vajrasthira. *Thelazia callipaeda* (Railliet and Henry, 1910) in man and dog in Thailand. *Am J Trop Med Hyg* 19:476-479, 1970.

Marcial-Rojas, R. A. Other rare spirurids which infect man. *In*: Marcial-Rojas, R. A. (Ed.), *Pathology of Protozoal and Helminthic Diseases*. Baltimore, Maryland, Williams and Wilkins, 1971.

Smith, T. A., and M. I. Knudsen. Eye worms of the genus *Thelazia* in man, with a selected bibliography. *Calif Vect Views* 17:85-94, 1970.

Soulsby, E. J. L. *Textbook of Veterinary Clinical Parasitology*. Oxford, Blackwell, 1965.

Soulsby, E. J. L. *Helminths, Arthropods and Protozoa of Domesticated Animals*, 7th ed. Philadelphia, Lea and Febiger, 1982.

Weinmann, C. J. Thelaziasis. *In*: Schultz, M. G. (Section Ed.), *CRC Handbook Series in Zoonoses*. Section C, vol. 2. Boca Raton, Florida, CRC Press, 1982.

TRICHINOSIS

(124)

Synonyms: Trichiniasis, trichinellosis, trichinelliasis.

Etiology: The agent is a small filiform nematode, *Trichinella spiralis*, which in the adult stage lives a few weeks in the small intestine of a large number of mammal species, and in the larval stage forms a cyst in the musculature of these hosts, where it can remain viable for years. The adult female parasite is 3 to 5 mm long and 0.06 mm wide, and the male is about half that size.

When a carnivore or omnivore ingests meat containing the encapsulated infective larva, the larva frees itself in the stomach from both the capsule and the muscle tissue; it then lodges in the villi and glandular crypts of the small intestine where it continues its development, reaching the adult stage in 2 to 3 days. A short time after copulation, the males die and the females begin to deposit larvae that hatched from eggs in their uterus. Larvae appear 4 to 7 days after ingestion of the infected meat and may continue to be released for several weeks. The larvae cross the intestinal wall, enter the lymphatic vessels, and travel via the thoracic duct to the superior vena cava. From there they go to the heart and are spread by the arterial circulation to other organs and tissues, in which they can remain for a limited time. They again enter the circulatory system, but then leave the capillaries and lodge in striated muscles, where they finally encapsulate. The larvae that remain in other organs and tissues, including the smooth muscles, die in a short time. From the fifth day of infection larvae can be found penetrating the sarcolemma of the muscle fibers. The parasite prefers the most active muscle groups, especially the pillars of the diaphragm, the masseter, lingual, ocular, back, and lumbar muscles. About 2 weeks after infection, the host's tissues begin to surround the larvae with a capsule, which is finished in about 4 or 5 weeks and is shaped like a lemon. The larva continues growing in the muscle fiber until encapsulation is completed and reaches a maximum size of 1 mm. Fully formed, sexually differentiated infective larvae are found curled into a spiral inside the capsule. Thus, the entire cycle develops within a single host. In order to initiate a new cycle, the larvae encapsulated within the muscle tissue must be ingested by a new host, of either the same or a different animal species, which may be man.

The intestinal phase of development is generally short and varies from 10 days to several weeks, depending on the host species. The encapsulated larvae can survive for years in the host's muscle tissue. In time, the fibrous capsule thickens and the cyst begins to calcify. It is estimated that larvae can remain alive in human muscle tissue for 5 to 10 years. The encysted larva is very resistant to physical and chemical factors. Its resistance to rotting is very important from the epidemiologic standpoint; larvae have been found to remain alive and often infective for at least 4 months in meats in advanced states of decomposition. The larvae in muscle tissue are also resistant to desiccation, salting, and smoking.

Several geographic strains have been identified, which differ in some of their physiologic properties, including their invasiveness and pathogenicity for swine and laboratory animals. Some morphologic differences have also been found. The strains of *T. spiralis* found in eastern Africa and in the Arctic region are much less infective for swine and rats than those prevalent in Europe or America. This characteristic of the African and Arctic strains is pronounced, and it is undoubtedly very important in the epidemiology of the disease in those regions. The opinions of helminthologists are divided with respect to the taxonomic rank that should be given these variant strains. Some propose to recognize them as simply variants, strains, or isolates, while others give them the rank of species or subspecies.

The studies carried out so far do not provide a taxonomic basis sufficient for the designation of new species (Madsen, 1976). Recent studies have demonstrated that strains of *Trichinella* isolated from swine, those from wild canids from the Arctic regions, and the strain *T. spiralis* var. *pseudospiralis* are reproductively compatible; the porcine strain and *pseudospiralis* are the most different (Belosevic and Dick, 1980; Dick and Chadee, 1983). Although the objections to establishing different species within the genus *Trichinella* may be valid, the existence of intraspecific variation is undeniable and has epidemiologic importance. The main variants are the following: 1) *T. spiralis* var. *domestica* (*T. spiralis* var. *spiralis*), which is the agent of both the domestic and peridomestic cycle and has as its main hosts swine, rats, and mice; 2) *T. spiralis* var. *nativa*, which circulates among wild carnivores (bears, foxes) in the Arctic region; 3) *T. spiralis* var. *nelsoni*, which circulates among wild carnivores and pigs in eastern and southern Africa, but has also been found in the southern USSR, Bulgaria, and Switzerland; and 4) *T. spiralis* var. *pseudospiralis*, which was originally isolated from a raccoon (*Procyon lotor*) in the northern Caucasus and is characterized by not provoking formation of capsules around muscular larvae, by the smaller size of the larvae, and by infecting birds in addition to mammals. Natural infections in birds have been confirmed in the USSR, Asia, North America, and possibly Spain (Wheeldon *et al.*, 1983).

Geographic Distribution: *T. spiralis* is cosmopolitan. Its presence has not been confirmed in Australia, nor in several Latin American, Asian, and African countries. However, it should be borne in mind that research has been limited for the most part to the domestic cycle, especially the cycle in swine, rats, and man, and that the infection can exist in wild animals without cases being recorded in humans or synanthropic animals. For the geographic distribution of the different variants of *T. spiralis*, see Etiology.

Occurrence in Man: As with many other communicable diseases, there is a great difference between the proportion of persons infected and those with clinical symptoms. At present, the rates of both infection and morbidity are clearly decreasing in the developed countries of Europe and the Americas.

In the Americas, the disease has occurred in Canada, the United States, Mexico, Venezuela, Chile, Argentina, and Uruguay. In some other countries or territories, isolated cases have been recorded, but it is not clear whether they were autochthonous or imported cases.

Few outbreaks of trichinosis have been recorded in Canada. In 1974, 1975, and 1976, there were 49, 3, and 31 clinical cases, respectively. Examination of diaphragms of persons dead from other causes revealed percentages of infection ranging from 1.5% in Toronto to 4 to 6% in British Columbia. Infection among indigenous peoples is frequent in northern Canada, but clinical cases are sporadic or affect only small groups. In that region the source of infection is wild mammals, both terrestrial and marine (*T. spiralis* var. *nativa*).

In the United States, 1,428 cases were recorded in the 10 years from 1972 to 1981, for an annual average of 143 cases. Of the 188 cases that occurred in 1981, 81.3% originated in five northeastern states and Alaska. The rate per million inhabitants was 0.8 for the whole country, 36.7 for Rhode Island, and 33.9 for Alaska (Centers for Disease Control of the USA, 1982). The rate of clinical cases has declined substantially compared to the rate in the 10-year period 1947-1956, during which an average of 358 annual cases was recorded. There is also a clear reduction in the intensity of infections, as evidenced by the decrease in deaths by trichinosis, both in absolute numbers and as a proportion of total cases. In the period 1947-1956, 84 deaths occurred (annual average of 8.4) and the case fatality rate was 2.3%, while in the period 1972-1981 there were seven deaths and a case fatality rate of 0.49%. The prevalence of infection has declined sharply, as confirmed by postmortem examinations. Between 1936 and 1941, an estimated 12% of the population was infected, while in 1970 the adjusted rate of infection was 2.2%. A good indicator of the reduction in the rate of infection is data on live larvae (proof of infection that is recent or not more than 10 years old) found in diaphragms. According to estimates for 1940, 7.3% of the population had live trichinae in their diaphragms, while in 1970 the rate was 0.7%.

In Mexico, studies done between 1939 and 1953 by various investigators discovered trichinae in 4 to 15% of autopsies; a study in 1972-1973 found the larvae in 4.2% of 1,000 bodies examined. Data obtained by the Pan American Health Organization (PAHO) show that there were only three diagnosed cases in Mexico in 1975. However, the disease is apparently not as rare as was presumed, as indicated by data from Zacatecas, where between 1978 and July 1983 there were 17 outbreaks with a total of 108 cases (Fragoso *et al.*, 1984).

Outbreaks of trichinosis occur periodically in Argentina and Chile, which are the only South American countries where the disease is important from the public health standpoint. In Argentina 129 cases occurred in 1981, 151 in 1982, and 87 in 1983 (Argentine Ministry of Health and Social Action, 1982 and 1983). In Chile there were 167 cases in 1975 and 66 (with one death) in 1981; in the province of Concepción, 79 patients were treated during 1979 and 1980 (Cabrera *et al.*, 1982). According to PAHO, the rate per 100,000 inhabitants in 1976 was 0.1 in Argentina and 0.5 in Chile. In the city of Santiago, Chile, several studies have been carried out by examination of persons dead by accidents or other violence. A 1982 study found a prevalence of infection of 2.8%, which is comparable to the rates determined by previous studies in 1966-1967 and 1972. However, all the larvae were calcified and the highest prevalence rates had shifted to older age groups, which could be interpreted as a decrease in new infections (Escobar *et al.*, 1982).

No cases have been reported in Uruguay since 1948. The parasite was found in three of 100 cadavers in a study carried out in 1943.

In Venezuela, 15 cases were recorded in 1972 and one in 1974. Previous reports had indicated that autochthonous cases do not occur in that country.

In Europe, the morbidity rate has declined in recent decades, both in western and eastern countries. In Poland, where previously more than 500 cases occurred per year, the incidence has diminished notably and no major outbreaks have been notified in recent years. In the USSR, the endemic area with the highest prevalence is found in Byelorussia, where 90% of all cases have occurred. The sporadic cases recorded in the northern and central Asian regions of the USSR resulted from consumption of meat of wild animals.

In most of Asia, human trichinosis is not important, but epidemics have been recorded in Lebanon, the last one in 1970. In Thailand, the first outbreak occurred in 1962 in the northern part of the country, and from that year to 1973, 975 cases and 58 deaths were recorded. The first outbreak in Japan occurred in 1974 (Ruitenberg *et al.*, 1983). The situation in China was unknown, but some reports have appeared in recent years. One of them (Li *et al.*, 1983) described an outbreak of 86 cases in Harbin, Heilongjiang Province, during which epidemiologic investigation found encysted larvae in the remains of meat from swine, dogs, and sheep; an earlier publication (Wang and Luo, 1981) gave information about 58 cases due to consumption of bear meat.

No cases are known in man in Australia. The first human case in New Zealand was diagnosed in 1964. The Hawaiian Islands constitute the only endemic area in the Pacific; a study done there in 1964 found the parasite in the diaphragms of 7.4% of the cadavers examined.

The situation in Africa is peculiar. In the countries of northern Africa bordering the Mediterranean, some outbreaks of human trichinosis were known (in Algeria and more recently in Egypt among Copts and tourists), but it was believed that the disease did not exist south of the Sahara. The first outbreak elsewhere on the continent was diagnosed in 1959 in Kenya, East Africa, but trichinosis was not found in domestic swine there. The investigation demonstrated that the human infection originated as a result of consumption of meat from the bush pig (*Potamochoerus porcus*). Later research in Africa discovered that the parasite is widely distributed in the wild fauna, including warthogs (*Phacochoerus aethiopicus*), hyenas, jackals, and some felids. Several subsequent outbreaks of human trichinosis have occurred in Kenya and also in Senegal. *T. spiralis* isolated in Kenya has the peculiarity of being weakly invasive for domestic swine and laboratory animals; it is currently known as *T. spiralis* var. *nelsoni*. An outbreak that affected 89 persons in 1975 in Bagnolo-in-Piano, Reggio nell'Emilia, Italy, was attributed to the same variant of *T. spiralis*. The outbreak was due to consumption of raw meat from a horse imported from eastern Europe. As an herbivore, the horse is an odd host for *Trichinella*, and it is presumed that the animal may have accidentally ingested remains of an infected rodent along with its feed. A similar outbreak occurred in France (Bellani *et al.*, 1978). Recently, in the area around Paris, an outbreak of more than 250 human cases of trichinosis was discovered. It was linked to consumption of raw or semi-raw meat from a horse imported from the United States (Ancelle and Dupouy-Camet, 1985).

The infection is frequent in the Arctic regions and is mainly due to consumption of bear meat. Cases linked to walrus meat were first described in Greenland and then in northern Alaska (Margolis *et al.*, 1979). The variant of trichina that circulates at these latitudes is *T. spiralis* var. *nativa*, which is characterized by greater resistance to freezing temperatures than *T. spiralis* var. *domestica*.

Human infection by *T. spiralis* var. *pseudospiralis* has not been confirmed.

In summary, it can be stated that human trichinosis is widespread in many parts of the world, but that morbidity rates are low.

Occurrence in Animals: *T. spiralis* has a wide range of hosts among domestic and wild animals. The infection has been confirmed in 104 species of mammals (58 species of carnivores, 27 rodents, 7 insectivores, and 12 species in other orders). Of special interest among domestic animals are swine, whose meat and by-products are the main source of infection for man. The infection rate in swine depends on how they are managed and, in particular, how they are fed. There is a marked difference in the rates of infection of swine fed grains and those fed raw wastes from either the home or from slaughterhouses, as has been clearly demonstrated by data from the United States: In 1950 the prevalence of trichinosis in swine fed wastes was 11%, while it was only 0.63% in those fed grain. When mandatory cooking of wastes was established, the prevalence in waste-fed swine decreased rapidly between 1954 and 1959 to 2.2%; currently, it is only 0.5%, whereas in grain-fed swine it is about 0.12%. High rates such as those found in Lebanon (25%) are not frequent.

In many European countries, the parasitosis is no longer found in swine; the highest frequency encountered is about 0.1%, usually on small farms. In 1976 in the Federal Republic of Germany, only one infected pig was found out of 32 million examined by trichinoscopy. In the Netherlands, not a single infected pig was discovered by trichinoscopic examinations between 1926 and 1962. However, use of the digestion method demonstrated that some pigs had very low intensity infections, with 0.025 larvae per gram of meat (Ruitenberg *et al.*, 1983).

In Brazil, Paraguay, Ecuador, Colombia, and Venezuela, the parasite has not been found by trichinoscopic examination. In Argentina and Chile, trichinoscopy records indicate a general prevalence of 0.14 to 0.33%. Of course, the prevalence is much higher in selected groups of animals, such as pigs that roam around garbage dumps or pigs fed kitchen wastes on small farms, and it is these animals that frequently give rise to epidemic outbreaks in the Southern Cone of South America.

Dogs and cats are involved in the domestic cycle because, as carnivores, they have ample opportunity to become infected; for this reason, the prevalence in these animals is generally higher than in pigs. Studies of street dogs in different neighborhoods of Santiago, Chile (Letonja and Ernst, 1974) found rates that varied from 1.2 to 4%, while 72% of 36 dogs captured in 1955 in the municipal slaughterhouse were infected. In a later study in the community of Máfil, Valdivia Province, Chile, 30 urban dogs and 30 rural dogs were examined, and 6.6% and 16.6%, respectively, were found infected (Oberg *et al.*, 1979). Trichinae were found in 3.3% of 150 dogs studied in Mexico City, but in none of 600 dogs examined in the city of Maracay, Venezuela. Infection rates of 45 to 60% have been found in dogs in Alaska, Greenland, and Siberia.

The parasite was discovered in seven of 12 cats examined in San Luís, Argentina, in 2% of 50 cats in Santiago, Chile, and in 25% of 300 cats in Mexico. By contrast, in Maracay, Venezuela, none of 120 cats examined gave a positive result.

In the United States, Europe, and the USSR, the infection in dogs and cats is relatively frequent, with prevalence rates higher than those in pigs.

Rats also participate in the synanthropic cycle. In the United States, rural rats are not infected, but a high rate of infection has been found among rats living in garbage dumps (5.3% of 1,268 specimens). A similar situation exists in Europe. In the USSR, 1.6% of 8,037 rats were found to be infected. High rates of infection have been found in Lebanon (36% in a study in 1952) and in British Columbia, Canada (25% in 1951). Studies carried out in Ecuador, Venezuela, Panama, Costa Rica, Puerto Rico, and more recently in Santos, São Paulo, Brazil (Paim and Cortes, 1979) yielded negative results. Almost all of these studies employed trichinoscopy, so the presence of very low levels of infection cannot be discounted. Numerous studies have been done in Chile, where an important role in the epizootiology is attributed to rats. Of rats captured in garbage dumps in Santiago and Antofagasta, 8% and 28.6%, respectively, were found to be infected. Studies done in 1951 and 1967 in the municipal slaughterhouse of Santiago revealed infection rates in *Rattus norvegicus* of 10% and 25%, respectively. A high rate of infection (8%) was also found in rats captured in 1938 in several sectors of the city of Concepción. In an epidemiologic study of an outbreak that affected 60 persons, 12.3% of swine and 30.7% of *R. norvegicus* were found to be infected. Infection in rats has also been found in Uruguay, Argentina, Peru, and Mexico, but most of these studies are only of historical value.

The main reservoirs of *T. spiralis* in nature are wild carnivores. The fox (*Vulpes vulpes*) is an important reservoir in Europe because of its population density and high infection rates. Trichinosis is also frequent among Old World badgers (*Meles meles*), wolves (*Canis lupus*), lynxes (*Lynx lynx*), and wild boars (*Sus scrofa*). In Alaska and other areas of the Arctic and Subarctic, high rates of infection have been found in the polar bear (*Thalarctos maritimus*), with an average of 45% parasitized, as well as in other bears, foxes (arctic and red), and several species of mustelids. Among marine mammals, the infection has been confirmed in walruses (*Odobenus rosmarus*), with a prevalence of 0.6 to 9%, and low rates have been found in other pinnipeds and cetaceans. In Iowa, USA, the parasite was discovered in 5% of minks and 6.4% of foxes. Low-intensity infection was found in wild rodents (*Microtus pennsylvanicus*, *Sigmodon hispidus*, and others) in Virginia, USA (Holliman and Meade, 1980).

In sub-Saharan Africa, only a wild cycle is known (see Occurrence in Man). The parasite is widely distributed among wild carnivores. The infection has been confirmed in the hyena, jackal, leopard, lion, serval (*Felis serval*), and wild pigs.

Hyenas (*Crocuta crocuta* and *Hyaena hyaena*) seem to be the main reservoirs. Of 23 spotted hyenas (*C. crocuta*), 10 were positive (Nelson and Guggisberg, 1963).

Except in Chile and Argentina, studies have not been done on the wild fauna of Latin America, and thus the status of the disease in these animals has not been determined. In central Chile, 2,063 wild animals were examined, of which 301 were carnivores (usually highly parasitized) and 1,762 were rodents (generally not very highly parasitized), and the infection was not found in any of them. Out of 20 animals examined in the provinces of San Luís and Mendoza, Argentina, a fox (*Pseudalopex gracilis*), an armadillo (*Chaetophractus villosus*), and a rodent (*Graomys griseoflavus*) were found to be infected.

The Disease in Man: Only a small proportion of infections are manifested clinically. Symptomatic cases result from the ingestion of a large number of larvae. Many sporadic cases pass unnoticed or are confused with other diseases because of the variability of the symptoms.

The incubation period lasts about 10 days, but can vary greatly—from 1 to 43 days—and seems to be related to the number of larvae ingested.

Three phases of the disease are described: intestinal, larval migration, and convalescence. The intestinal phase is generally expressed as a nonspecific gastroenteritis, with anorexia, nausea, vomiting, abdominal pain, and diarrhea. Seven to 11 days after the contaminated food was ingested, signs of the muscular invasion phase begin, with edema of the upper eyelids (a very common and prominent sign), myalgias (which may be pronounced and in diverse locations), cephalalgia, fever lasting several days, sweating, and chills. There may also be urticarial or scarlatiniform eruptions, and respiratory and neurologic symptoms. Most patients have leukocytosis and eosinophilia. In 95.9% of 47 Chilean patients, eosinophilia with values greater than 6% was found. The clinical disease lasts about 10 days in moderate infections, but may persist a month or more in massive infections. Muscular pains can sometimes persist for several months.

In epidemic outbreaks, mortality varies from 0 to 35%, but is usually under 1%.

The Disease in Animals: Trichinosis in swine rarely is diagnosed during the life of the animal. In massive infections, pigs manifest anorexia, emaciation, and muscular pain, especially in the hind legs. Experimental doses of 100,000 larvae produced a fatal infection in 10 to 20 days.

The symptoms of massive infections in dogs and cats are similar to those in pigs.

Source of Infection and Mode of Transmission (Figures 97 and 98): Two cycles can be distinguished, domestic (synanthropic) and wild.

The domestic and peridomestic cycle centers around the pig and includes other animals such as dogs, cats, and rats. The parasite is transmitted from pig to pig mainly by the ingestion of garbage containing swine muscle fibers. For that reason, the incidence in swine is particularly high when they are fed kitchen, restaurant, and slaughterhouse scraps, or when they feed in town garbage dumps. The encysted larva is very resistant to putrefaction, and thus another source of infection for swine can be dead infected animals, including rats, that are sometimes found in garbage dumps. It has also been shown that the pig can acquire the infection from another pig by coprophagia, since encysted larvae are eliminated in fecal matter during the first 24 hours after a pig ingests infective meat. This mode of infection, however, seems to be rare.

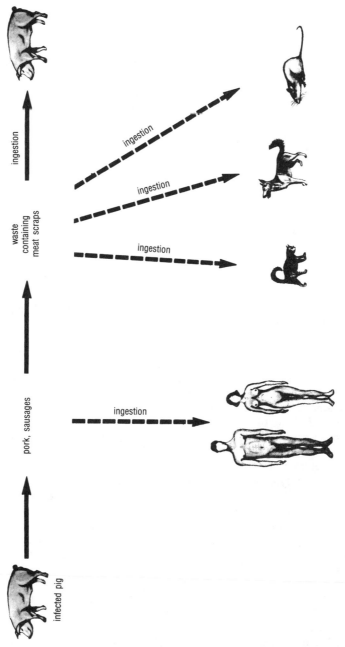

Figure 97. Trichinosis. Synanthropic transmission cycle.

Figure 98. Trichinosis. Wild transmission cycle.

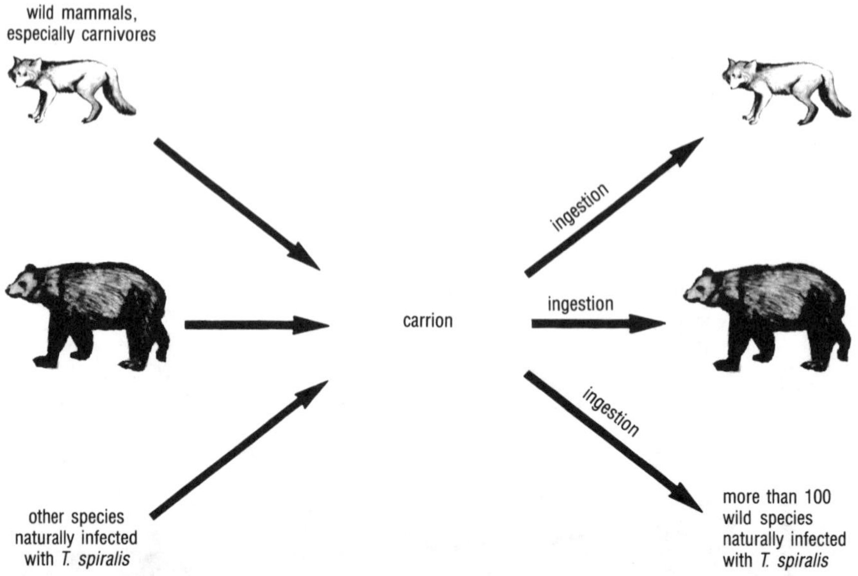

Dogs, cats, and rats are infected from the same sources as pigs and are included in the cycle, but most researchers believe that their epidemiologic role is secondary. An aspect that merits more study is the association between rats and swine, to which some epidemiologists attribute great importance and others none or very little; it is hoped that future studies will resolve this controversy. Sled dogs in the Arctic are infected by eating wild animal meat fed to them by man or by consuming carrion they find in their habitat. This explains the extremely high rates (50% or more) found among dogs in that region.

Man is a victim of the cycle he himself creates by feeding pigs with raw remains from other parasitized pigs. However, man is an accidental host in whom the parasite finds a dead end. Humans contribute biologically to the cycle only under exceptional circumstances, such as occur in eastern Africa where some tribes abandon the bodies of the dying or dead to hyenas. The human infection occurs as a result of consuming pork and especially pork by-products that are raw or insufficiently cooked or treated. In spite of the low prevalence of the infection in swine, the human disease often occurs in the form of epidemic outbreaks. It is estimated that the meat of a single parasitized pig weighing some 100 kg can be a potential source of infection for 360 persons. Since pork is frequently added to beef in the manufacture of sausage, the potential numbers affected are even greater. In Argentina and Chile, outbreaks most commonly occur in rural areas, the source of infection being a pig killed by its owner and thus not subjected to sanitary inspection. The sources of infection are almost always pigs fed kitchen, restaurant, and slaughterhouse wastes, and, in small towns, animals kept at garbage dumps. However, it should be borne in mind that an inspected pig can sometimes give rise to an outbreak, since trichinoscopy cannot discover low-level parasitoses. The United States is one of the few developed countries in which trichinosis is still a public health problem, although on a much smaller scale than it used to be. Of 947 human cases for which the source of infection could be ascertained, 79.1% were attributable to pork products, 6% were due to ground beef (probably contaminated with pork), and 13.9% were linked to wild animal meat, especially bear. In Alaska, half the cases were due to bear meat and the other half to walrus meat. In contrast to the epidemiologic pattern in Latin America, where the infection often results from slaughter of pigs and preparation of sausage at home, 81% of the cases in the United States were linked to pork products acquired in supermarkets, butcher shops, and similar outlets. Products acquired directly from farms originated only 13.8% of the cases recorded between 1975 and 1981 (Schantz, 1983).

In man, as in animals, the frequency of the infection and its intensity increase with age, as a result of longer opportunity for infection and reinfection. The infection rates found in the United States between 1966 and 1970 by examination of 8,071 diaphragms were 1.8% in persons under 45 years of age and 4.8% in individuals over that age. The same study found the average intensity in the bodies of those under 45 years old to be 2.4 trichinae per gram of diaphragm material, while for older persons it was 12.2 per gram.

Religion and ethnic origin have a great influence on the prevalence of the infection. The prevalence of trichinosis is very low among Muslims, Jews, and Seventh Day Adventists, whose religious beliefs prohibit the consumption of pork. In the Middle East, the disease occurs in Lebanon, where the Christian population is large, but is very rare in the predominantly Muslim countries. On the other hand, prevalence rates in the United States are higher in some ethnic groups, such as Italians, Germans, and Poles, because of their preference for pork products processed at a temperature insufficient to destroy the larvae. In the USSR, the habit of consuming raw salt pork (which contains muscle fibers) explains why this product is one of the main sources of infection.

Food preservation technology and the peculiarities of the different variants of *Trichina* also influence the occurrence and prevalence of trichinosis. The reduction in the incidence and intensity of human infection observed in the United States in the last decades is due in large part to the generalized practice of freezing pork products, both commercially and at home. Freezing is an effective means of killing the trichina larvae (*T. spiralis* var. *domestica*) found in pork and pork products. Regulations in Canada and the United States establish that pork products less than 15 cm thick must be frozen at −15°C for 20 days or −30°C for 6 days. The trichinae (*T. spiralis* var. *nativa*) found in terrestrial and marine mammals of the Arctic region resist low temperatures for a long time. For example, viable larvae have been found in bear meat frozen at an ambient temperature of −32°C for several weeks. A similar observation was confirmed in walrus meat kept in a home freezer at −12°C for a month. This resistance to low temperatures of the Arctic trichinae would explain why human cases of trichinosis occur in that region in spite of the inhabitants' custom of freezing their meats.

Most outbreaks in Argentina and Chile occur in winter or early spring when home slaughter of pigs is more frequent. Neighbors usually participate in sausage-making and eat the recently made products at community meals.

The wild cycle is independent of the domestic cycle. Wild carnivores are the main reservoirs and primary hosts of *T. spiralis*. The chief mode of transmission is by consumption of carrion, which generally consists of the bodies of older and thus more intensely parasitized animals.

In some parts of the world, such as the Arctic and Subarctic and eastern Africa, the meat of wild animals constitutes the main source for human infection. In Africa, three outbreaks are known to have been caused by consumption of bush pig (*Potamochoerus porcus*) meat. Although the immediate source of human infection was the meat of wild pigs, the main reservoirs seem to be wild carnivores, especially hyenas.

The strains of *Trichina* isolated in Africa (*T. spiralis* var. *nelsoni*) are not very virulent for swine and laboratory animals. An outbreak of human trichinosis in Italy and another in France were attributed to that variant. No trichinae are found in domestic and synanthropic animals in these areas, and the suspected source of infection was meat from imported horses, which was eaten raw. Although trichinosis is rare in herbivores, the infection can be reproduced experimentally. The horses are thought to have become infected by eating feed accidentally contaminated by the remains of an infected rodent or other animal.

Outbreaks in the Arctic region usually affect only a few persons. Nevertheless, an epidemic was recorded in Greenland in 1947 that caused 300 cases and 33 deaths. The origin of that epidemic was not discovered, but in a later outbreak the source of infection was found to be walrus meat. Two more outbreaks due to consumption of walrus meat were subsequently described in Alaska (Margolis *et al.*, 1979). The relative rarity of clinical cases at these latitudes is explained by the low intensity of parasitism in wild animals. Both inside and outside the Arctic region, cases of human trichinosis linked to bear meat have occurred. Since 1967, 5% of the human cases in the United States have resulted from ingestion of that meat (Schantz, 1983). In several European countries, infection due to bear or wild boar meat is playing an increasing role in the epidemiology of the disease, and outbreaks of this nature have been described in Czechoslovakia and the USSR (Ruitenberg *et al.*, 1983). A report published in China attributes 58 cases of trichinosis to consumption of bear meat (Wang and Luo, 1981).

Dogs have significant contact with wild ecosystems and might serve as hosts linking both cycles.

Role of Animals in the Epidemiology of the Disease: Trichinosis is a disease of wild and domestic animals that is accidentally transmitted to man by the ingestion of raw or undercooked meat or meat products. It is a food-originated zoonosis.

Diagnosis: In an outbreak, the clinical diagnosis of patients presents no major difficulties, but because of the variable symptomatology of trichinosis, sporadic cases are often confused with other diseases. Confirmation of eosinophilia, an increase in muscular enzymes, and erythrosedimentation are of great help in the diagnosis.

Specific diagnosis can be made by muscle biopsy and observation of larvae. The most useful method is the digestion technique. The biopsy is generally done 3 or 4 weeks after infection. The operation is painful, and larvae are not always found in mild infections because of the necessarily small size of the tissue sample.

Numerous immunobiologic tests are presently available, such as bentonite floc-culation, Suessenguth-Kline cholesterol flocculation, latex agglutination, complement fixation, indirect immunofluorescence, indirect hemagglutination, and, lately, ELISA. The different tests and antigens vary both in sensitivity and specificity. At present, the ELISA test is considered the most sensitive and versatile (it allows detection of the different classes of immunoglobulins). In a recent study of an outbreak caused by bear meat in which 58 persons were affected (92% confirmed by muscle biopsy), the ELISA test detected IgG specific antibodies in 100% of the cases in the first month of the disease and IgM antibodies in 86% of the cases. In a high percentage of cases, these antibodies persisted up to 11 months. It was also possible to detect IgA antibodies, which were presumed to have been of intestinal origin, in 62% of the patients in the first month of the disease; their detection is important, since patients can be treated with anthelmintics at that stage. The indirect immunofluorescence test was somewhat less sensitive (95% sensitivity) and became negative faster (Knapen *et al.*, 1982).

Most of the serologic tests do not give positive results until the third week of infection. As with other diseases, two blood samples should be obtained in order to confirm serologic conversion.

The intradermal test is not useful for diagnosis because of its lack of specificity and sensitivity. In endemic areas, a reactor rate of up to 38% has been found, and thus a positive reaction in a patient does not always indicate a recent infection. On the other hand, in many confirmed cases of infection the intradermal test turns out negative.

Diagnosis of swine trichinosis is of great interest from the standpoint of control. Two main procedures are available for postmortem diagnosis: trichinoscopy and artificial digestion. Trichinoscopy is used in the veterinary inspection of pork in slaughterhouses and meat-packing houses in many countries. It is a rapid process, but is not very sensitive and does not reveal light infections. Trichinoscopy has rendered great service in public health protection, but it has serious limitations because of its low sensitivity. In Sweden in 1961 and in West Germany in 1967, epidemic outbreaks involving several hundred cases occurred following consumption of pork and pork products that had previously passed trichinoscopic examination. Some experts estimate that trichinoscopy can detect infection when there are three or more larvae per gram of muscle; according to others, the figure is 10 or more larvae per gram.

The artificial digestion method is much more efficient, but it is slow and does not lend itself to the rhythm of processing hogs in slaughterhouses and packing plants. Its sensitivity is primarily attributable to the use of a sample that is 50 to 100 times larger than that used in trichinoscopy. A practical modification of this method has recently been proposed, which consists of mixing diaphragm samples of 20 to 25 hogs from the same source. If trichinae are found in the composite sample, a 50 to 100 g sample of diaphragm muscle tissue from each individual pig is examined. However, this method has not been widely accepted in the industry in some countries.

In the last few years, great progress has been achieved in perfecting the ELISA test, which can be automated for use in slaughterhouses with substantial savings of resources and time. One of the biggest drawbacks of the test was the high proportion of false positives (15%). This drawback has been surmounted by the availability of antigens purified by various methods (Seawright *et al.*, 1983; Gamble *et al.*, 1983; Gamble and Graham, 1984).

Control: A rational approach for control programs is to focus on reducing and eventually eradicating the infection in swine, whose meat is the main source of human infection. The law requiring kitchen or slaughterhouse wastes to be heat-treated (100°C), introduced as part of the campaign to eradicate vesicular exanthema in swine and hog cholera, has proven most beneficial in the United States. However, compliance with this regulation is very difficult to ensure and, therefore, the results are not always satisfactory.

The trichinosis problem in some Latin American countries is centered on the small rural farms raising a few pigs fed with household or restaurant scraps. These farms are very difficult to supervise, and pigs are slaughtered by the farmers without veterinary inspection. Continuous education of the population could at least partially remedy the situation. Another source of human infection is swine kept in town or village garbage dumps. In these cases, municipal and health authorities should take measures to prohibit this practice.

Trichinoscopy, which is practiced in slaughterhouses in Argentina, Chile, and other countries, has been shown to be effective in protecting the population. Although the technique leaves much to be desired, when correctly executed it protects the consumer at least against massive infections. The digestion method is much more efficient, but is costly for developing countries. Currently, hopes are founded on implementing the automated ELISA test.

At the individual level, humans can avoid the infection by abstaining from eating pork or pork products derived from animals that may not have been subjected to veterinary inspection.

Pork or pork products that have not been inspected can be submitted to several processes to destroy the trichinae. Cooking at 77°C is more than sufficient to inactivate the parasite. Special care should be taken with rib roasts, pork chops, and pork sausages, which are not always sufficiently cooked. Most trichinae are also destroyed by freezing the meat at -15°C for 20 days or at -30°C for 6 days. This process is effective as long as the piece is no thicker than 15 cm. Smoking, salting, or drying of pork are not sure methods of killing larvae. The meat of wild animals should be cooked; this is the only sure method of destroying the larvae of the *Trichinella* variant found in the Arctic.

Open garbage dumps to which pigs could gain access should be eliminated both in towns and on farms.

Under epidemiologic conditions in Latin America, rodent control is advisable.

Bibliography

Alvarez, V., G. Rivera, A. Neghme, and H. Schenone. Triquinosis en animales de Chile. *Bol Chile Parasitol* 25:83-86, 1970.

Ambia, J., and H. Quiroz. Incidencia de *Trichinella spiralis* en perros de la ciudad de México. *Veterinaria Méx* 7:17-19, 1976.

Ancelle, T., and J. Dupouy-Camet. L'Épidémie de Trichinose en Région Parisienne. Le Vecteur cheval. Communication Médecine. *Le Monde*, 17 September 1985, p. 18.

Argentine Ministry of Health and Social Action. *Bol Epidemiol Nac* 13, 1982 and 13, 1983.

Belding, D. L. *Textbook of Parasitology*, 3rd ed. New York, Appleton-Century-Crofts, 1965.

Bellani, L., A. Mantovani, S. Pampilione, and I. Filippini. Observations on an outbreak of human trichinellosis in Northern Italy. *In:* Kim, C. W., and Z. S. Pawlowski (Eds.), *Trichinellosis*. Hanover, New Hampshire, University Press of New England, 1978. Cited in Ruitenberg *et al.*, 1983.

Belosevic, M., and T. A. Dick. *Trichinella spiralis:* comparison with an Arctic isolate. *Exp Parasitol* 49:266-276, 1980.

Cabrera, G., N. Pinilla, L. M. Dall'Orso, and G. Parra. Brote epidémico de triquinosis en Concepción, Chile. Estudio serológico. *Bol Chile Parasitol* 37:47-49, 1982.

Centers for Disease Control of the USA. *Trichinosis Surveillance. Annual Summary, 1975.* Atlanta, Georgia, 1976. (DHEW Publ. CDC 76-8256.)

Centers for Disease Control of the USA. *Trichinosis Surveillance. Annual Summary, 1981.* Atlanta, Georgia, CDC 1982.

Dick, T. A., and K. Chadee. Interbreeding and gene flow in the genus *Trichinella. J Parasitol* 69:176-180, 1983.

Dick, T. A., B. Kingscote, M. A. Strickland, and C. W. Douglas. Sylvatic trichinosis in Ontario, Canada. *J Wildl Dis* 22:42-47, 1986.

Escobar, A., M. Saldaña, and H. Schenone. Prevalencia de la triquinosis humana en Santiago, Chile (1982). *Bol Chile Parasitol* 37:66-67, 1982.

Taubert, G. M., P. Viens, and P. Magluilo. Superiority of the ELISA technique over parasitological methods for detection of trichinellosis in slaughtered pigs. *Can J Comp Med* 49:75-78, 1985.

Fragoso, R., P. Tavizón, and H. Villacaña. Universidad Autónoma de Zacatecas. Personal communication, 1984.

Gamble, H. R., W. R. Anderson, C. E. Graham, and K. D. Murrell. Diagnosis of swine trichinosis by enzyme-linked immunosorbent assay (ELISA) using an excretory-secretory antigen. *Vet Parasitol* 13:349-361, 1983.

Gamble, H. R., and C. E. Graham. Monoclonal antibody-purified antigen for immunodiagnosis of trichinosis. *Am J Vet Res* 45:67-74, 1984.

Gould, S. E. Clinical manifestations. *In*: Gould, S. E. (Ed.), *Trichinosis in Man and Animals.* Springfield, Illinois, Thomas, 1970.

Holliman, R. B., and B. J. Meade. Native trichinosis in wild rodents in Henrico County, Virginia. *J Wildl Dis* 16:205-207, 1980.

Kagan, I. G., and L. G. Normann. The serology of trichinosis. *In*: Gould, S. E. (Ed.), *Trichinosis in Man and Animals.* Springfield, Illinois, Thomas, 1970.

Kohler, G., and E. J. Ruitenberg. Comparison of three methods for the detection of *Trichinella spiralis* infections in pigs by five European laboratories. *Bull WHO* 50:413-419, 1974.

Leighty, J. C. The role of meat inspection in preventing trichinosis in man. *J Am Vet Med Assoc* 165:994-995, 1974.

Li, J. *et al.* (An outbreak of trichinosis in Harbin, Heilongjian Province: report of 86 cases). *Chin J Infect Dis* 1:260, 1983. Summary in *WHO/HELM/85.17*.

Letonja, T., and S. Ernst. Triquinosis en perros de Santiago, Chile. *Bol Chile Parasitol* 29:51, 1974.

MacDonald, K. Trichinosis. *In*: Top, F. H., and P. F. Wehrle (Eds.), *Communicable and Infectious Diseases*, 7th ed. St. Louis, Mosby, 1972.

Madsen, H. The principles of the epidemiology of trichinelliasis with a new view on the life cycle. *In*: Kim, C. W. (Ed.), *Trichinellosis*. New York, Intext, 1974.

Madsen, H. The life cycle of *Trichinella spiralis* (Owen, 1835) Railliet, 1896 (Syns: *T. nativa* Britov and Boev, 1972, *T. nelsoni* Britov and Boev, 1972, *T. pseudospiralis* Garkavi, 1972), with remarks on epidemiology, and a new diagram. *Acta Parasitol Pol* 24:143-158, 1976.

Margolis, H. S., J. P. Middaugh, and R. D. Burgess. Arctic trichinosis. Two Alaskan outbreaks from walrus meat. *J Infect Dis* 139:102-105, 1979.

Martínez-Marañón, R., J. Trejo, and B. Delgado. Frecuencia de la infección por *Trichinella spiralis* en 1.000 diafragmas de cadáveres de la ciudad de México en 1972-1973. *Rev Invest Salud Pública* (México) 34:95-105, 1974.

Merkushev, A. V. Trichinosis in the Union of Soviet Socialist Republics. *In*: Gould, S. E. (Ed.), *Trichinosis in Man and Animals.* Springfield, Illinois, Thomas, 1970.

Neghme, A., and H. Schenone. Trichinosis in Latin America. *In*: Gould, S. E. (Ed.), *Trichinosis in Man and Animals.* Springfield, Illinois, Thomas, 1970.

Nelson, G. S. Trichinosis in Africa. *In*: Gould, S. E. (Ed.), *Trichinosis in Man and Animals*. Springfield, Illinois, Thomas, 1970.

Nelson, G. S., C. W. A. Guggisberg, and J. J. Mukundii. Animal hosts of *Trichinella spiralis* in East Africa. *Ann Trop Med Parasitol* 57:332-346, 1963.

Oberg, C., S. Ernst, P. Linfati, and P. Martin. Triquinosis en perros de la comuna de Máfil, Provincia de Valdivia, Chile. *Bol Chile Parasitol* 34:46-47, 1979.

Ooi, H. K., M. Kamiya, M. Ohbayashi, and M. Nakazawa. Infectivity in rodents and cold resistance of *Trichinella spiralis* isolated from pig and polar bear, and *T. pseudospiralis*. *Jap J Vet Res* 34:105-110, 1986.

Paim, G. V., and V. A. Cortes. Pesquisa de *Trichinella spiralis* em roedores capturados na zona portuária de Santos. *Rev Saúde Publica* 13:54-55, 1979.

Pan American Health Organization. *Annual Report of the Director, 1975*, and *Annual Report of the Director, 1976*. Washington, D.C., PAHO, 1976 (Official Document 143), and 1977 (Official Document 150).

Rausch, R. L. Trichinosis in the Arctic. *In*: Gould, S. E. (Ed.), *Trichinosis in Man and Animals*, Springfield, Illinois, Thomas, 1970.

Ruitenberg, E. J., F. van Knapen, and A. Elgersma. Incidence and control of *Trichinella spiralis* throughout the world. *Food Technol* 37:98-100, 1983.

Schad, G. A., D. A. Leiby, C. H. Duffy, K. D. Murrell, and G. L. Alt. *Trichinella spiralis* in the black bear (*Ursus americanus*) of Pennsylvania: distribution, prevalence and intensity of infection. *J Wildl Dis* 22:36-41, 1986.

Schantz, P. M. Trichinosis in the United States, 1947-1981. *Food Technol* 37:83-86, 1983.

Seawright, G. L., D. Despommier, W. Zimmermann, and R. S. Isenstein. Enzyme immunoassay for swine trichinellosis using antigens purified by immunoaffinity chromatography. *Am J Trop Med Hyg* 32:1275-1284, 1983.

Soulsby, E. J. L. *Textbook of Veterinary Clinical Parasitology*. Oxford, Blackwell, 1965.

Steele, J. H., and P. V. Arambulo. Trichinosis. A world problem with extensive sylvatic reservoirs. *Int J Zoonoses* 2:55-75, 1975.

Szekely, R., J. Sapunar, F. Rodríguez *et al*. Brote epidémico de triquinosis en la zona central de Chile. *Bol Chile Parasitol* 30:87-88, 1975.

van Knapen, F., J. H. Franchimont, A. R. Verdonk, J. Stumpf, and K. Undeutsch. Detection of specific immunoglobulins (IgG, IgM, IgA, IgE) and total IgE levels in human trichinosis by means of the enzyme-linked immunosorbent assay (ELISA). *Am J Trop Med Hyg* 31:973-976, 1982.

Wang, B. K., and X. P. Luo. (A report of 58 cases of human trichinosis caused by eating raw bear meat). Translation by the authors. *Chung Hua Yu Fang I Hsueh Tsa Chi* 15:143-144, 1981. Summary in *WHO/HELM/82.6*.

Wheeldon, E. B., T. A. Dick, and T. A. Schultz. First report of *Trichinella spiralis* var. *pseudospiralis* in North America. *J Parasitol* 69:781-782, 1983.

Zimmermann, W. J. Trichinosis in wildlife. *In*: Davis, J. W., and R. C. Anderson (Eds.), *Parasitic Diseases of Wild Mammals*. Ames, Iowa State University Press, 1971.

Zimmermann, W. J. Trichinosis. *In*: Hubbert, W. T., W. F. McCulloch, and P. R. Schnurrenberger (Eds.), *Diseases Transmitted from Animals to Man*, 6th ed. Springfield, Illinois, Thomas, 1975.

Zimmermann, W. J., J. H. Steele, and I. G. Kagan. Trichiniasis in the US population, 1966-70. *Health Serv Rep* 88:606-623, 1973.

TRICHOSTRONGYLIASIS

(127.6)

Synonyms: Trichostrongylosis, trichostrongylidosis.

Etiology: Several species of *Trichostrongylus*, short, slender nematodes that inhabit the small intestine and stomach of sheep, goats, and bovines, and sometimes of other domestic and wild animals. The following species of *Trichostrongylus* have been identified in man: *T. axei, T. colubriformis, T. orientalis, T. skryjabini, T. vitrinus, T. probolurus, T. capricola, T. brevis, T. affinis,* and *T. calcaratus*. The species are difficult to differentiate, and human case histories often indicate only the genus and not the species. Other trichostrongylids have very occasionally been found in man. Among these are *Haemonchus contortus* (one case in Brazil, one in Iran, and three in Australia), *Ostertagia ostertagi,* and *O. circumcincta* (two cases by the former in Iran, one case by each in Azerbaidzhan, USSR).

The developmental cycle of trichostrongylids is direct. The eggs of the parasite are eliminated with the feces of the hosts, and under favorable conditions of temperature, moisture, and aeration they release the first-stage larva in 1 or 2 days. This larva goes through several molts, and in a few more days develops into an infective pseudofilariform larva. When ingested by a host, the larva continues its development directly (without pulmonary migration) in the digestive tract, where it reaches maturity and begins oviposition. The prepatent period for *T. colubriformis* and *T. axei* in bovines lasts about 20 days.

Geographic Distribution and Occurrence: Trichostrongylids are very common parasites in domestic ruminants and their distribution is worldwide.

Human trichostrongyliasis occurs sporadically, but in some geographic areas it is highly endemic. Prevalence rates found in Iran were 7.5% in the northern part of the country and 69 to 85% in Isfahan. Endemic areas are dispersed throughout southern Asia, from the Mediterranean to the Pacific, including the Asian areas of the USSR. In some localities in Iraq, up to 25% of the population has been found to be infected. The infection is very common in some areas of Korea and Japan, as well as in parts of Africa (Zaire and Zimbabwe). Human infection has also been described in Europe (Hungary and German Democratic Republic) and in Australia. In the Americas, the infection has been confirmed in Brazil, Chile, Peru, Uruguay, and the United States. In Brazil, 75 cases of infection by *Trichostrongylus* spp. were found in 46,951 persons examined. In Chile, 45 cases were diagnosed between 1938 and 1967, and 17 cases were found among 3,712 persons examined in the province of Valdivia between 1966 and 1971.

The Disease in Man: The parasites lodge in the duodenum and jejunum. Infections are usually asymptomatic or mild and are discovered in coprologic examinations carried out for the diagnosis of other parasitoses. In intense infections with several hundred parasites, there may be transitory eosinophilia, digestive disorders, diarrhea, abdominal pain, weight loss, and slight anemia. The infection can last several years. The clinical picture in man has not been studied very much and is difficult to define, since other species of parasites are generally found in an individual infected with trichostrongylids.

The Disease in Animals: The different species of *Trichostrongylus*, together with other gastrointestinal parasites of several genera and species, constitute the etiologic complex of parasitic gastroenteritis of ruminants (trichostrongylidosis, verminous gastroenteritis), an important disease in terms of its economic impact. Verminous gastroenteritis is the cause of stunted growth in lambs and calves, and may result in illness and death of young animals and, occasionally, adults.

The various gastrointestinal parasites differ in their pathogenicity. The tri- chostrongylids *T. axei, T. colubriformis,* and *T. vitrinus* and many other species of the genus, which lodge in the small intestine, are among the most pathogenic parasites of the ruminant digestive tract. Lambs up to 1 year and calves 3 to 6 months old are the animals most affected by trichostrongyliasis. Although several species of *Trichostrongylus* affect both sheep and cattle, their transmission between the two domestic species is rare, probably because different biotypes of the parasite are physiologically adapted to different animal species. This characteristic may be useful for control purposes.

Although naturally occurring verminous gastroenteritis is always a mixed infec- tion, trichostrongylids are the most important pathogens for sheep. The losses caused by gastroenteritis in sheep are substantial, especially in recently weaned lambs and in young sheep about 1 year old. The disease rarely occurs in adult sheep or cattle, since the animals acquire resistance as a result of continuous exposure. The most important factors that determine whether the disease becomes clinically appar- ent are the number of parasites and the nutritional state of the animal. In temperate climates, the most severe infections occur during winter and autumn, when moisture and cold favor the survival of the larvae. About 6 to 8 weeks after lambing, pasture lands become heavily infested due to increased oviposition, which is probably associated with the stress experienced by the nursing ewes. Overloading pastures with excessive numbers of animals causes a pronounced increase in outbreaks of gastroenteritis, as a consequence of both the increased contamination of pastures with parasite eggs and the lower nutritional state of the animals. Lambs and calves are more resistant to the infection when they are well fed, and thus the disease is most often seen in recently weaned animals or at times of the year when pasture is scarce. Prematurely weaned lambs or lambs of mothers with defective udders are especially susceptible to clinical trichostrongyliasis.

The infection is manifested clinically by weight loss and profuse diarrhea (when *Trichostrongylus* spp. predominates), which dirties the wool of the hind legs. Acute cases of trichostrongyliasis may end in death in 2 to 3 weeks. The disease is seen simultaneously in many animals in a flock.

Haemonchosis (*Haemonchus contortus*) of domestic ruminants causes pro- nounced anemia and debility.

Source of Infection and Mode of Transmission (Figure 99): The reservoirs of most of the species of *Trichostrongylus* are, with few exceptions, domestic and wild herbivores. However, *T. orientalis* is a parasite of man and only occasionally of sheep. This species occurs in Asia and is transmitted indirectly between humans, especially in areas where human fecal matter is used as fertilizer in agriculture. *T. orientalis* is the predominant species in human infections. *T. brevis* is another human species that has been described in Japan. The species of animal origin produce rather sporadic cases in man, although areas of high prevalence are known. The number of species of *Trichostrongylus* that infect man varies in different areas.

Figure 99. Trichostrongyliasis. Transmission cycle.

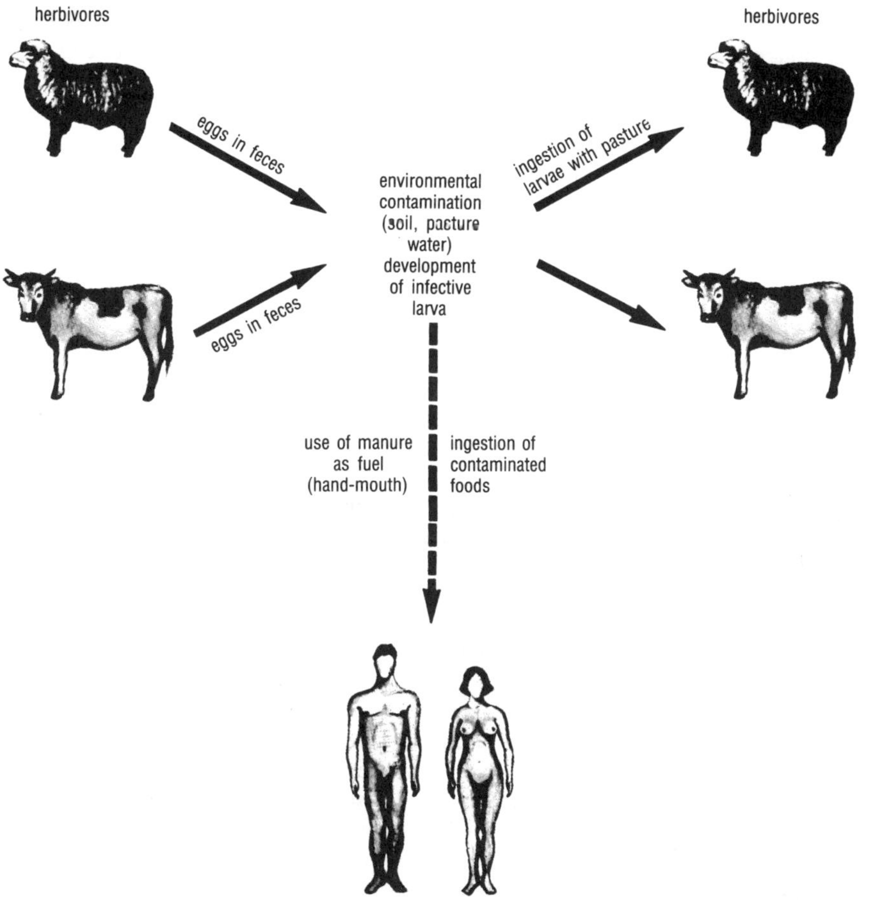

In Isfahan, Iran, seven different species of *Trichostrongylus* have been found in the rural inhabitants of the region.

The sources of infection are soil and vegetation, in which the eggs deposited with the animal host's feces develop in a few days to the infective larval stage. Man and animals are infected orally. Man acquires the infection mainly by consuming raw vegetables contaminated with the infective larvae. The rapid development of the infective larva after hatching favors contamination of human foods. A lack of personal and environmental hygiene, as well as proximity to animals—conditions that are common among populations at a low socioeconomic level in endemic areas—are important factors in transmission of the infection. Another important factor in transmission is the preparation and use of animal manure as fuel.

Diagnosis: Laboratory diagnosis of human trichostrongyliasis is made by identifying the eggs in the feces or by coproculture. It is important to distinguish the eggs of trichostrongylids from those of ancylostomids.

The best method for diagnosing parasitic gastroenteritis of domestic animals is necropsy and a parasite count, which reveals the intensity of the infection. Coprologic examination and egg counts are very useful, but it should be borne in mind that many larvae do not develop to maturity, and thus the number of eggs does not necessarily indicate the true number of parasites. Therefore, best results are obtained when coprologic examinations are supplemented by necropsies. A count of more than 1,000 eggs per gram of fecal matter indicates a heavy parasite load, which in most cases will be manifested clinically.

The eggs of *Trichostrongylus* are difficult to distinguish from those of *Cooperia* and *Ostertagia*. Coproculture can be used to determine which species predominates. However, this differentiation is not important from the practical standpoint, since the treatment and control measures are similar for the different species of gastrointestinal parasites.

Control: Preventive measures for the human infection consist of improved food, environmental, and personal hygiene. In endemic areas, raw vegetables or other foods likely to be contaminated with the larvae of the parasite should not be eaten.

In animals, control measures are directed toward keeping both pasture contamination and animal infections at low levels. To attain this objective, the animals must be kept in a good nutritional state; similarly, anthelmintics should be administered at appropriate times and pastures should be properly managed. Above all, pastures should not be overburdened, so that the animals are not deprived of sufficient food. It is also important to provide animals with mineral supplements, especially cobalt, copper, and phosphorus.

From autumn to spring lambs should be given anthelmintics every 4 to 6 weeks. If climatic conditions do not favor persistence of larvae in the fields, treatments can be spaced farther apart. The most strategically important doses are those given to ewes 1 month before lambing and to lambs on the day of weaning. The preferred medicines for these treatments are thiabendazole and other benzimidazoles, organic phosphates, levamisole, and ivermectin. These drugs are also indicated when outbreaks of gastroenteritis occur. An important problem in control is the development of resistance to anthelmintics. Such resistance can be measured by making an egg count in the coprologic examination or a parasite count during necropsy after the anthelmintic was administered. The use of reduced-spectrum anthelmintics is recommended, along with spaced rotation of different drugs. For repeated preventive doses, such as those given to lambs under 1 year of age, phenothiazine can be used, in deference to the high cost of thiabendazole.

Pasture management is important. Most of the larvae die in a field left ungrazed for about a month, and for this reason pasture rotation can be effective in controlling the disease. On livestock operations where both sheep and cattle are raised, these species can be alternated on pastures, since neither host is very susceptible to the strains of trichostrongylids affecting the other.

Bibliography

Blood, S. C., and J. A. Henderson. *Veterinary Medicine*, 4th ed. Baltimore, Maryland, Williams and Wilkins, 1974.

Euzéby, J. *Les Zoonoses Helminthiques*. Paris, Vigot Frères, 1964.

Ghadirian, E., and F. Arfaa. First report of human infection with *Haemonchus contortus, Ostertagia ostergagi*, and *Marshallagia marshalli* (Family Trichostrongylidae) in Iran. *J Parasitol* 59:1144-1145, 1973.

Ghadirian, E., F. Arfaa, and A. Sadighian. Human infection with *Trichostrongylus capricola* in Iran. *Am J Trop Med Hyg* 23:1002-1003, 1974.

Marcial-Rojas, R. A. Trichostrongyliasis. *In*: Marcial-Rojas, R. A. (Ed.), *Pathology of Protozoal and Helminthic Diseases*. Baltimore, Maryland, Williams and Wilkins, 1971.

Soulsby, E. J. L. *Helminths, Arthropods and Protozoa of Domesticated Animals*, 7th ed. Philadelphia, Lea and Febiger, 1982.

Tongston, M. S., and S. L. Eduardo. Trichostrongylidosis. *In*: Schultz, M. G. (Section Ed.), *CRC Handbook Series In Zoonoses*. Section C, vol. 2. Boca Raton, Florida, CRC Press, 1982.

Torres, P., L. Figueroa, and N. Navarrette. Trichostrongylosis en la provincia de Valdivia, Chile. *Bol Chile Parasitol* 27:52-55, 1972.

Witenberg, G. G. Helminthozoonoses. *In*: Van der Hoeden, J. (Ed.), *Zoonoses*. Amsterdam, Netherlands, Elsevier, 1964.

World Health Organization. *Parasitic Zoonoses*. Report of a WHO Expert Committee with the Participation of FAO. Geneva, WHO, 1979. (Technical Report Series 637.)

World Health Organization. *Intestinal Protozoan and Helminthic Infections*. Report of a WHO Scientific Group. Geneva, WHO, 1981. (Technical Report Series 666.)

TRICHURIASIS OF ANIMAL ORIGIN

(127.3)

Synonyms: Trichocephaliasis, trichocephalosis, whipworm.

Etiology: The main agent of human trichuriasis is *Trichuris trichiura* (*Trichocephalus trichiurus*); the animal parasites *T. vulpis* and *T. suis* only rarely affect man.

T. trichiura inhabits the cecum, appendix, and colon of man and other primates; *T. vulpis* parasitizes the large intestine of dogs and foxes, and *T. suis* that of domestic swine and wild boars. Nematodes of the genus *Trichuris* are characterized by a long and thin anterior part of the body, and a posterior part that is much thicker and shorter. *T. vulpis* has some morphologic characteristics (absence of caudal papillae and longer cloaca in males) that distinguish it from *T. trichiura* and other species, while *T. suis* is morphologically identical to *T. trichiura*, for which reason some helminthologists consider them synonymous.

The males of *T. trichiura* and *T. suis* measure about 30 to 45 mm, and the females from 35 to 50 mm; *T. vulpis* measures 45 to 75 mm. The development cycle is similar in all the species. The female parasite lays eggs that are eliminated to the exterior with the feces. In the soil, under favorable conditions of humidity and temperature, the larvae develop inside the eggs to the infective stage. The animal host contracts the infection by ingesting the embryonated eggs. The larvae are released in the small intestine and lodge in the crypts for 2 to 10 days; the parasites then move to the large intestine, where they mature and begin oviposition in about 3 months. The prepatent period of *T. suis* is a little shorter (from 6 to 7 weeks).

Geographic Distribution and Occurrence: The three species have worldwide distribution. *T. trichiura* is one of the most common human parasites; it is most prevalent in tropical and subtropical regions. As has been demonstrated in Chile (Atías and Neghme, 1979), a close relationship exists between soil humidity and the prevalence of human infection. A parasitologic study found a 1.2% infection rate in the arid and hot northern area of that country, while in the south, which has high humidity and abundant vegetation, the proportion of infected persons was as high as 60%. *T. trichiura* is also common among nonhuman primates.

T. vulpis is very common in dogs, as some studies have demonstrated. For example, in New Jersey, USA, 38% of 2,737 dogs examined were infected; in New York, the prevalence was 31%, and in Detroit, 52%. Infection of swine by *T. suis* is especially high among suckling pigs and less so in adult animals.

Infection of man by *T. vulpis* has been recognized on a few occasions in the United States, Italy, and Romania. A few years ago, 100 human appendixes were examined in New York State; *T. trichiura* was found in six of them, and a trichurid identified as *T. vulpis* was discovered in another (Kenney and Yermakov, 1980).

Naturally occurring human infection by *T. suis* would not be recognizable in routine parasitologic examinations. In addition, it is unknown if *T. trichiura* of nonhuman primates is transmitted to man.

The Disease in Man: The symptomatology is related to the intensity of infection. Many infections are not sufficiently intense to provoke a pathologic effect. Infection by a large number of parasites can cause abdominal pain and distension as well as diarrhea, which is sometimes bloody. In very heavy infections in children (hundreds or thousands of parasites), there can be strong tenesmus and rectal prolapse. Massive parasitoses occur mainly in tropical regions in children 2 to 5 years old who are usually malnourished and often infected by other intestinal parasites and microorganisms. Pica and anemia are common signs among these children.

The Disease in Animals: The infection in animals is similar to that in man. Young dogs infected by hundreds or thousands of *T. vulpis* usually suffer profuse diarrhea and weight loss; in very severe infections there can be hemorrhagic diarrhea, anemia, jaundice, and death.

Epidemic outbreaks caused by *T. suis* have occurred in suckling pigs, with manifestations of anorexia, dysentery, dehydration, anemia, and death.

Source of Infection and Mode of Transmission: The reservoir of *T. trichiura* is man. Maintenance of the parasite in nature is assured by the ample human reservoir, the abundance of eggs the parasite produces (between 200 and 300 per gm of feces and per female), and the long survival of the eggs in soil. The source of infection for man is the soil and food contaminated by embryonated eggs. The parasite of nonhuman primates is similar or identical to human *T. trichiura* and cross-infection is believed to be possible (Flynn, 1973). However, it is not known whether there are strains of *T. trichiura* adapted to different animal species, or whether the parasites are interchangeable between human and nonhuman primates. *T. vulpis* has been recognized as the agent in a few cases of human infection; although the actual number of human cases due to this agent may be greater, dogs do not seem to have an important role in the epidemiology of human trichuriasis.

Controversy exists over whether or not *T. trichiura* and *T. suis* are identical. Nevertheless, some facts demonstrate that these two species are different, although very similar. The oocyte of *T. trichiura* has four diploid chromosomes, while that of *T. suis* has six. It has also been confirmed recently that the sizes of the eggs and the infective larvae differ, as do the time required to reach the infective stage in the exterior environment and the time needed for development in suckling pigs.

After several failed attempts at cross-infection, humans were successfully infected with embryonated eggs of *T. suis* and suckling pigs with *T. trichiura*. In addition, infection was confirmed in a laboratory technician who had handled eggs of *T. suis* (Beer, 1976). These findings would indicate that in certain situations of close contact between pigs and man, swine feces could serve as a source of infection. However, it is not known how frequently, if at all, natural human infection by *T. suis* occurs. According to a report by a Scientific Group of the World Health Organization (1981), "infections of zoonotic origin probably play a minor role, if any, in the epidemiology of human trichuriasis."

Diagnosis: Diagnosis is based on confirmation of the presence in the feces of the typical eggs (barrel-shaped, brownish in color, and with a prominent plug at each end). The size of *T. trichiura* eggs is 50 to 54 microns by 22 to 23 microns. The eggs of *T. vulpis* are much larger (from 70 to 89 microns), while those of *T. suis* are slightly larger than those of *T. trichiura*. However, it would be inadvisable to identify the species only on the basis of egg size.

Control: Prevention of human infection requires improvement of environmental hygiene, and especially the adequate disposal of excreta to avoid contamination of the soil. Personal and food hygiene (washing of vegetables and some fruits) are also important.

Bibliography

Atías, A., and A. Neghme. *Parasitología Clínica*. Buenos Aires, Inter-Médica, 1979.

Beer, R. J. S. The relationship between *Trichuris trichiura* (Linnaeus, 1758) and *T. suis* of the pig. *Res Vet Sci* 20:47-54, 1976.

Flynn, R. J. *Parasites of Laboratory Animals*. Ames, Iowa State University Press, 1973.

Kenney, M., and V. Yermakov. Infection of man with *Trichuris vulpis*, the whipworm of dogs. *Am J Trop Med Hyg* 29:1205-1208, 1980.

Neafie, R. C., and D. H. Connor. Trichuriasis. *In*: Binford, C. H., and D. H. Connor (Eds.), *Pathology of Tropical and Extraordinary Diseases*, vol. 2. Washington, D.C., Armed Forces Institute of Pathology, 1976.

Soulsby, E. J. L. *Helminths, Arthropods and Protozoa of Domesticated Animals*, 7th ed. Philadelphia, Lea & Febiger, 1982.

World Health Organization. *Intestinal Protozoan and Helminthic Infections*. Report of a WHO Scientific Group. Geneva, WHO, 1981. (Technical Report Series 666.)

VISCERAL LARVA MIGRANS AND TOXOCARIASIS

(128.0)

Synonym: Larval granulomatosis.

Etiology: The term visceral larva migrans is currently reserved for visceral, extraintestinal infections caused mainly by *Toxocara canis* and, to a lesser extent, by *T. cati* (*T. mystax*).

T. canis is an ascarid that lives in its adult stage in the small intestine of dogs and several wild canids. The female measures 9 to 18 cm in length, and the male 4 to 10 cm. Eggs deposited with fecal matter are very resistant to environmental factors and can remain viable for many months or even several years. Under favorable environmental conditions of moisture, temperature, and aeration, the egg, which is unsegmented when deposited with the feces, develops into a second-stage or perhaps third-stage (infective) larva in about 15 days (Araujo, 1972). When a puppy less than 3 weeks old ingests eggs containing infective larvae, they emerge in the intestine, pass through the intestinal wall, and enter the bloodstream, migrating to the liver and then the lungs. After reaching the lungs, the larvae pass through the pulmonary capillaries and travel by means of the bronchial tree to the trachea and pharynx. They are swallowed, pass through the stomach, where they undergo a molt, and eventually arrive in the intestine; there they molt a final time, reaching the adult stage and oviposition. The prepatent period (from infection to the appearance of eggs) usually lasts 4 to 5 weeks. The average life span of *T. canis* in the intestine is 4 months, and most of the parasites are expelled 6 months after the infection was contracted. One female can produce up to 200,000 eggs per day and, taking into account that a puppy can harbor several hundred parasites, it can be assumed that the host's surroundings are seeded with millions of eggs (Schantz and Glickman, 1983).

In puppies, almost all the larvae follow the tracheal migration and reach the intestine. In dogs older than 6 months, the larvae also travel to the lungs, but instead of then migrating to the trachea, they proceed to the heart through the pulmonary vein and from there to different organs and tissues (somatic migration), where they encyst and do not continue their development.

Besides the age factor, the destination of the larvae (tracheal or somatic migration) is determined by the infective dose. It has been demonstrated experimentally (Dubey, 1978) that puppies infected orally with 10,000 eggs did not develop a parasitosis with a patent period (elimination of eggs in the feces), but those that received 1,000 eggs or less developed intestinal toxocariasis and shed eggs. Three of six adult dogs that received 100 eggs manifested a patent infection.

Prenatal transmission is very important in the infection of dogs by *T. canis*. When an adult bitch is infected, the larvae can be harbored alive in her tissues for months or even years; if she becomes pregnant, the larvae migrate through the placenta to the liver of the fetus. In newborn puppies, the larvae migrate from the liver to the lungs and then to the intestine, where they mature; eggs can be found in the feces after 3 weeks. A mobilization of the larvae to the mammary glands of the bitch may also occur, and the puppies are then infected when suckling (transmammary or lactational route).

When embryonated eggs are ingested by man and other nonspecific hosts, such as rodents, pigs, and lambs, somatic migration is the rule; migration of the larvae from the lungs via the trachea to the intestine is rare. Some prey species, such as rodents, act as transport or paratenic hosts.

T. cati is a smaller ascarid than *T. canis* and its natural hosts are cats and wild felids. The life cycle of *T. cati* is similar to that of *T. canis*. Cats can be infected at any age; prenatal infection has not been observed in these animals, but transmammary infection has.

Geographic Distribution and Occurrence: *T. canis* and *T. cati* are found throughout the world in dogs and cats, respectively. Several investigators maintain that virtually all puppies are born infected by *T. canis* and that less than 20% of adult dogs eliminate eggs in the feces. In a review of the literature, Schantz and Glickman (1983) found that the prevalence of intestinal toxocariasis in nearly 42,000 dogs of all ages averaged 15.2%, with reported rates varying from 0 to 93%.

The prevalence of human infection is not well known since the disease is not notifiable, the clinical signs are unspecific, and the diagnosis is difficult to confirm in the laboratory (Glickman and Schantz, 1981).

The clinical disease has been diagnosed in a total of more than 1,900 human cases from 48 different countries (Ehrhard and Kernbaum, 1979). Of 780 well documented cases, 56% occurred in patients less than 3 years old. Most clinical cases have been recorded in industrialized countries, since these countries possess better diagnostic facilities, but the disease undoubtedly occurs with the same or greater frequency in developing countries. Patients with ocular invasion are those who most often seek medical assistance, but for each ophthalmic case there may be several with larval infections in other organs, such as the heart, liver, lungs, and brain.

In a serologic study carried out with 8,457 sera representative of the population of the United States, 2.8% gave positive results to the ELISA test. The highest rates were found in children under 12 years old and among persons at the lower socioeconomic levels (Schantz and Glickman, 1983). Similar rates have been found in Great Britain. In a study in western Japan, 3.1% of children and 3.7% of women tested positive to ELISA, and serologic prevalence was observed to increase with age (Matsumura and Endo, 1983). These studies indicate that human infection is often asymptomatic.

Intestinal infection with adult parasites is very rare in man. Two cases caused by *T. canis* and a larger number due to *T. cati* have been described, but the accuracy of the diagnosis has been questioned in several of the reports.

The Disease in Man: Human infection is caused by *Toxocara* larvae, and the localization is extraintestinal (visceral larva migrans). The larvae released from ingested eggs migrate from the intestine to different organs and tissues, where they can remain for a long time. The syndrome occurs primarily in children between the ages of 18 months and 3 years (the age group most likely to ingest *Toxocara* eggs), but it also occurs in adults. In the organs the larvae produce multiple abscesses and allergic-type eosinophilic granulomas. Clinical manifestations depend on the number of larvae and their anatomic location. For the most part, infections are mild and asymptomatic, with the exception of persistent eosinophilia. In symptomatic cases, the seriousness of the clinical picture varies, but those with a mild symptomatology predominate. The most prominent sign is persistent eosinophilia. The percentage of eosinophils may reach more than 50% of the total leukocyte count. Hepatomegaly and pneumonitis with hypergammaglobulinemia are common in the first stages of the disease. Frequent reinfections affect the liver and lungs simultaneously, weakening the patient. In older children and adolescents, a syndrome with fever, fits of coughing, nausea, vomiting, and dyspnea is common in the first week. The symptoms may recur for several months. In young children the disease can be more severe, with asthmatic attacks, high fever, anorexia, arthralgia, myalgia, nausea, vomiting, hepatomegaly, lymphadenopathy, and sometimes urticaria and angioneurotic edema.

Larva migrans can also affect the eyes (ocular larva migrans); this form occurs in older children and sometimes in adults. Ocular infection is occasionally preceded by or concurrent with the visceral form. The presence of the larva in the eye can cause progressive deterioration and sudden loss of vision. Strabismus is common. The infection is unilateral and generally without systemic symptoms or eosinophilia. The single granulomatous lesion is located close to the optic disk and the macula retinae. Endophthalmias caused by *Toxocara* larvae have often been confused with retinoblastomas, and have resulted in enucleation of the eyeball.

The larvae can locate in the central nervous system, but their precise etiologic role in cerebral affections has not been determined. It is possible that an association exists between cerebral invasion by *Toxocara* larvae and some cases of epilepsy.

Fatalities caused by visceral larva migrans are rare.

The Disease in Animals: Acute infection is seen in puppies and kittens a few weeks old. The symptomatology consists primarily of digestive disorders, diarrhea, vomiting, flatulence, and loss of vitality. Dogs infected with a large number of parasites in the prenatal period die at 2 or 3 weeks of age. Sudden death is often due to obstruction and rupture of the small intestine, with consequent peritonitis. In puppies that were infected prenatally, signs of pneumonia are sometimes present due to large-scale pulmonary invasion by larvae that became mobilized in the mother. Intestinal infections with few parasites are generally asymptomatic, as is common in adult animals. Dogs and cats that survive the critical period of infection recover completely and expel the parasites from their intestine in the first 6 months of life.

Source of Infection and Mode of Transmission (Figure 100): The reservoir of *T. canis* is the domestic dog and also wild canids. It has been estimated that one gram of fecal matter from an infected puppy can contain up to 15,000 *Toxocara* eggs. The high degree of resistance of the eggs to physical and chemical factors leads to a high level of soil contamination and makes soil an important source of infection. Dogs are infected via the placenta, by ingestion of embryonated eggs, or by the transmammary route (lactational). The disease can also be contracted by ingesting paratenic hosts, such as rodents, that contain encysted larvae (extraintestinal somatic infection). Occasionally, bitches can become infected by licking their pups and ingesting larvae that migrate from the lungs to the intestine and are eliminated directly with fecal matter or expelled with vomitus.

Cats of any age can be infected by ingesting eggs of *T. cati* eliminated with the feces of other cats, or by eating rodents that contain larvae in their organs and tissues (transport hosts). Cats in the neonatal period can also be infected by their mother's milk (transmammary route).

The extensive distribution and high prevalence of *Toxocara* in dogs and cats, the large number of eggs that these animals eliminate, and the resistance of the eggs are

Figure 100. Visceral larva migrans and toxocariasis. Transmission cycle.

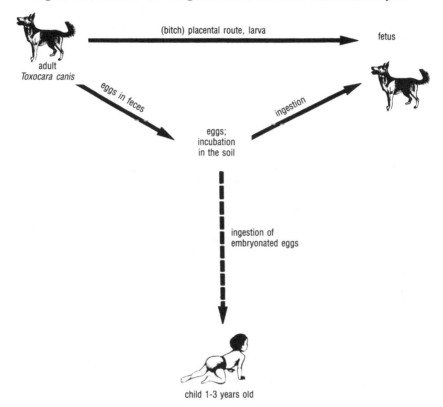

contributory factors to contamination of the soil, which is the source of infection for man. Humid soils are the most favorable for survival of the eggs. The infection is not spread directly from person to person, but is instead transmitted by means of soil contaminated with dog or cat feces. Children are the most exposed group because they commonly play on the ground and put dirt and contaminated objects in their mouths. Moreover, since pica is not rare in children, geophagia plays an important role in the transmission of the infection. Adults can acquire the infection if they do not observe the basic rules of personal hygiene; dirty hands are almost always the vehicle for the parasite's eggs.

In Great Britain, the infection has been found both in dog and cat owners and in persons who do not have these animals in their homes. A recent study demonstrated that the source of infection can be public recreation areas. In that country, *Toxocara* eggs were found in 24.4% of 800 soil samples from 10 parks in six cities (Borg and Woodruff, 1973). The experience is different in the United States, where a close association has been found between owning dogs, especially puppies, and contracting visceral larva migrans. However, not all cases originate in the family home or yard; as was confirmed in Great Britain, public parks constitute a source of infection for children. In the United States, between 10 and 32% of soil samples from public places contained *Toxocara* eggs. Similar results have been obtained in the Federal

Republic of Germany, Brazil, and Czechoslovakia (Schantz and Glickman, 1983). In Londrina, Parana State, Brazil, the soil from 15 public squares and other urban tracts was examined, and nine (60%) of the samples were found to be contaminated by *Toxocara* eggs. In addition, when soil samples from 10 squares in the same city were examined over a 15-month period, great variation was found in the viability of the eggs during different times of the year (Chieffi and Mueller, 1978).

Diagnosis: The diagnosis of human larval toxocariasis presents great difficulties. The infection may be suspected based on the presence of leukocytes and persistent eosinophilia, hypergammaglobulinemia, and hepatomegaly, together with the symptomatology described earlier or evidence from ophthalmoscopic examinations in the case of ocular toxocariasis. A history of pica and exposure to dogs are other risk factors to consider.

Diagnosis is confirmed by histopathologic examination of hepatic tissue obtained by biopsy, or of the eyeball in cases of enucleation. Detection of granulomatous foci is not sufficient to establish specific diagnosis; it is necessary to find the larva. This is a laborious process requiring serial sections of the pathologic specimen. Even in an organ as small as the eyeball, more than 100 sections may have to be made in order to locate the larva. In several extraocular cases, definitive diagnosis was obtained by laparotomy and resection of a granuloma visible as white plaques on the surface of the liver.

In light of the difficulty of basing the diagnosis on clinical signs or of finding the larvae, immunobiologic tests acquire special importance. Several tests have been used, among them complement fixation, indirect immunofluorescence, indirect hemagglutination, double gel diffusion, and cutaneous hypersensitivity, but all of them lack sensitivity or specificity. The ELISA test has now replaced the others (Cypess *et al.*, 1977; Ruitenberg and van Knapen, 1977) because it is superior both in sensitivity and specificity. Lately, excretor-secretor (ES) antigens obtained from the larva in culture media are being used for this test, which is estimated to have a sensitivity of 78% and a specificity of 92%.

Differential diagnosis between ocular larva migrans and retinoblastoma is of special interest. In ocular larva migrans, examination of the aqueous humor usually reveals numerous eosinophils and a normal proportion of lactate dehydrogenase. In diagnosis of the ocular form, the ELISA test has a sensitivity of 73% and a specificity of 95% (Schantz and Glickman, 1983).

Diagnosis of intestinal toxocariasis in dogs and cats does not present any difficulties and is done by identifying the parasite's eggs in fecal matter.

Control: The primary control measure consists of periodic worming of dogs and cats. Treatment of newborn dogs with prenatal infection is especially important in prophylaxis. Puppies should be treated 2 weeks after birth with piperazine adipate or with one of the new anthelmintics (pyrantel pamoate, levamisole, or mebendazole), and the medication repeated at 4, 6, and 8 weeks of age. The mothers should be treated at the same time. The feces of other dogs and cats should be examined, and the animals wormed if *Toxocara* eggs are found.

Experiments with different compounds indicate that some act against somatic larvae in bitches. The most effective compound seems to be fenbendazole. In a recent study (Burke and Roberson, 1983), daily treatment of bitches with fenbendazole from day 40 of gestation to 14 days after parturition reduced by 89% the number of *T. canis* in their pups, compared to those of untreated mothers.

The disease in humans can be prevented by observing the rules of personal hygiene and teaching them to children at the earliest possible age.

Dogs should not be allowed in parks or other public recreation areas; stray dogs should be eliminated.

Bibliography

Araujo, P. Observações pertinentes as primeiras ecdises de larvas de *Ascaris lumbricoides, A. suum e Toxocara canis*. *Rev Inst Med Trop São Paulo* 14:83-90, 1972.

Arean, V. M., and C. A. Crandall. Toxocariasis. *In:* Marcial-Rojas, R. A. (Ed.), *Pathology of Protozoal and Helminthic Diseases*. Baltimore, Maryland, Williams and Wilkins, 1971.

Beaver, P. C. Zoonoses, with particular reference to parasites of veterinary importance. *In:* Souslby, E. J. L. (Ed.), *Biology of Parasites*. New York, Academic Press, 1966.

Beaver, P. C. The nature of visceral larva migrans. *J Parasitol* 53:3-12, 1969.

Bisseru, B. Toxocara infection. *In:* Graham-Jones. O. (Ed.), *Some Diseases of Animals Communicable to Man in Britain*. Oxford and New York, Pergamon Press, 1968.

Bisseru, B., A. W. Woodruff, and R. I. Hutchinson. Infection with adult *Toxocara canis*. *Br Med J* 1:1583-1584, 1966.

Borchert, A. *Parasitología Veterinaria*. Zaragoza, Spain, Acribia, 1964.

Borg, O. A., and A. W. Woodruff. Prevalence of infective ova of *Toxocara* species in public places. *Br Med J* 4:470-472, 1973.

Buchwalder, R. Probleme des Spulwurmbefalles beim Hund und seine Bedeutung als Zoonose. *Monatsh Veterinarmed* 28:98-103, 1973.

Burke, T. M., and E. L. Roberson. Fenbendazole treatment of pregnant bitches to reduce prenatal and lactogenic infections of *Toxocara canis* and *Ancylostoma caninum* in pups. *J Am Vet Med Assoc* 183:987-990, 1983.

Cypess, R. H., M. H. Karol, J. L. Zidian, L. T. Glickman, and D. Gitlin. Larva-specific antibodies in patients with visceral larva migrans. *J Infect Dis* 135:633-640, 1977.

Chieffi, P. P., and E. E. Mueller. Estudo da variação mensal na contaminação do solo por ôvos de *Toxocara* sp. (Nematoda, Ascaroidea), na zona urbana do município de Londrina, Estado do Paraná, Brasil. *Rev Inst Lutz* 38:13-16, 1978.

Dubey, J. P. Patent *Toxocara canis* infection in ascarid-naive dogs. *J Parasitol* 64:1021-1023, 1978.

Ehrhard, T., and S. Kernbaum. *Toxocara canis* et toxocarose humaine. *Bull Inst Pasteur* 77:225-227, 1979. Cited in Glickman and Schantz, 1981.

Faust, E. C., P. C. Beaver, and R. C. Jung. *Animal Agents and Vectors of Human Disease*, 4th ed. Philadelphia, Lea and Febiger, 1975.

Glickman, L. T., and P. M. Schantz. Epidemiology and pathogenesis of zoonotic toxocariasis. *Epidemiol Rev* 3:230-250, 1981.

Lamina, J. Immunodiagnosis of visceral larva migrans in man. *In:* Soulsby, E. J. L. (Ed.), *Parasitic Zoonoses*. New York, Academic Press, 1974.

Matsumura, K., and R. Endo. Seroepidemiological study on toxocaral infection in man by enzyme-linked immunosorbent assay. *J Hyg (Camb)* 90:61-65, 1983.

Olsen, O. W. *Animal Parasites, Their Life Cycles and Ecology*, 3rd ed. Baltimore, Maryland, University Park Press, 1974.

Ruitenberg, E. J., and F. van Knapen. The enzyme-linked immunosorbent assay and its application to parasitic infections. *J Infect Dis* 136:267-273, 1977.

Schantz, P. M., and L. T. Glickman. Ascáridos de perros y gatos: un problema de salud pública y de medicina veterinaria. *Bol Of Sanit Panam* 94:571-586, 1983.

Tagle, I. *Enfermedades Parasitarias de los Animales Domésticos*. Santiago de Chile, Andrés Bello, 1970.

Taylor, J. H. Toxocara infections in man and animals. *Vet Bull* 34:634-637, 1964.

Woodruff, A. W. Toxocariasis. *Br Med J* 3:663-669, 1970.
World Health Organization. *Joint FAO/WHO Expert Committee on Zoonoses, Third Report*. Geneva, WHO, 1967. (Technical Report Series 378.)

ZOONOTIC ANCYLOSTOMIASIS

(126.3 and 126.8)

Synonyms: Uncinariasis, ankylostomiasis, necatoriasis, hookworm disease.

Etiology: The main agents of human ancylostomiasis are the nematodes *Ancylostoma duodenale* and *Necator americanus*. Occasionally, larvae of *A. ceylanicum*, *A. caninum*, and, more rarely, other specific animal ancylostomes (*Necator suillus*, *N. argentinus*, *Ancylostoma malayanum*) infect man and reach maturity in the human intestine.

For a long time, confusion existed with respect to the taxonomy of *A. ceylanicum* and *A. braziliense*, which were considered to be synonymous. *A. ceylanicum* has now been established as a distinct species and the main etiologic agent of zoonotic cases of human intestinal ancylostomiasis; likewise, research has confirmed that *A. braziliense* does not reach the adult state in humans.

The life cycles of the different species of ancylostomes are similar. The adult parasites, cylindrical and 5 to 20 mm long (depending on sex and species), live in the small intestine of the host. Each female lays thousands of eggs per day, which are eliminated to the exterior with fecal matter. Under favorable environmental conditions, such as moist soil, temperatures between 23 and 30°C, and protection from direct sunlight, embryogeny is rapid, and the first-stage larva (rhabditiform larva) can hatch from the egg in 24 to 48 hours. These larvae are not resistant to low temperatures or desiccation. In the course of a week, the larva undergoes two molts and develops into a third-stage larva, which is infective. The third-stage larva is filariform; it encysts in its cuticular envelope, does not feed, and can survive in the soil for several weeks.

Animal hosts can be infected through the skin or digestive tract, the route being dependent on the species of parasite. When the infection route is through the skin, as in classic human ancylostomiasis caused by *A. duodenale* or *N. americanus*, the parasites penetrate the lymphatic vessels and blood capillaries and travel to the lungs. Once in the lungs they pass through the capillaries and advance up the bronchial tree; they eventually reach the epiglottis and are then swallowed. In the intestine they undergo another molt and reach maturity; 1 or 2 months after infection, the females begin to lay eggs. In infections via the oral route, which are frequent with *A. caninum*, all the parasite's development takes place in the gastrointestinal tract.

Although rarely, infections can also occur in the opposite direction, that is, infection of animals with human ancylostomes. *A. duodenale* has been found in swine and dogs in Europe, Asia (China), and Australia, and also in zoo animals. *N. americanus*, or a very similar species, has been found in the intestines of several species of monkeys and other wild animals. *N. suillus*, which is adapted to the pig, is a species very closely related or identical to *N. americanus*; it is a common parasite of swine in Trinidad.

Geographic Distribution and Occurrence: *A. ceylanicum* is a common parasite of domestic cats, wild felids, and dogs. Its geographic distribution is difficult to determine because it was formerly confused with *A. braziliense*. Infections of man by *A. ceylanicum* are not frequent, but they are important in some areas, such as Taiwan, Southeast Asia, and Suriname (World Health Organization, 1981). Cases have also occurred in Japan, India, Sri Lanka, eastern Africa, Zimbabwe, Liberia, Madagascar, Brazil, and Guyana.

In a study of 175 residents of a village close to Calcutta, India, and of eight inhabitants of that city treated with anthelmintics, *A. ceylanicum* was found in 16 persons (8.7%). Nearly all of the cases of this infection occurred simultaneously with infection by *A. duodenale* or *N. americanus*. The infection caused by *A. ceylanicum* was not very intense; only one parasite was found in 14 individuals, and two specimens each in the other two (Chitwood and Schad, 1972).

Infection by *A. ceylanicum* occurs sporadically, and generally involves few specimens of the parasite. An exception was the situation discovered among Dutch sailors returning from the former colony of West New Guinea. *A. ceylanicum* (originally identified as *A. braziliense*) was found in the feces of nine out of 11 individuals treated with anthelmintics, three of whom expelled between 97 and 291 specimens. In some individuals, *A. ceylanicum* was the only species found, while in others *N. americanus* was also present, although in smaller numbers. *A. ceylanicum* was also found in Dutch soldiers returning from Suriname, and it is not infrequent among immigrants from that country in Amsterdam, especially children. It is presumed that the parasite was introduced into Suriname by immigrants from India (Zuidema *et al.*, 1972).

In India, Malaysia, Taiwan, and Japan, high rates of infection by *A. ceylanicum* have been found in dogs and cats. To determine the prevalence of the infection in Suriname, necropsies were performed on 102 stray dogs and 58 stray cats in five different localities. *A. ceylanicum* was found in 80% of the dogs and 60% of the cats (Rep, 1968).

A. caninum is a cosmopolitan parasite, common in dogs, foxes, and other wild carnivores. Human intestinal ancylostomiasis by this species is rare, with only six cases recorded in the literature. Human infection by other animal ancylostomes is even rarer; one case has been recorded by each one of the following species: *N. suillus*, *N. argentinus*, and *A. malayanum* (Barriga, 1982).

The Disease in Man: In general, intestinal infections caused by *A. ceylanicum* have very little effect on human health, mainly because, as mentioned above, the number of parasites is very limited. Most often, this species occurs in concurrent infections with *A. duodenale*, *N. americanus*, or both. In the few confirmed cases of intense infection by *A. ceylanicum*, the symptomatology was similar to that caused by human ancylostomes, and anemia was the main sign.

Eight volunteers who received 50 to 150 larvae of *A. ceylanicum* by the percutaneous route developed papules at the site of inoculation; 15 to 20 days later they complained of epigastric discomfort, headache, and fatigue, and had eosinophilia.

The prepatent period lasted 3 to 5 weeks. The early symptoms described were similar to those observed in volunteers who received the human ancylostomes *N. americanus* and *A. duodenale* (Wijers *et al.*, 1966).

The Disease in Animals: The symptomatology of ancylostomiasis in dogs and cats depends on several factors, such as number of parasites, nutritional state of the animal, age, and history of previous infection by these nematodes. Young animals are the most affected. Loss of blood caused by the ancylostomes, together with malnutrition, which very frequently accompanies the pathologic picture, produces hypochromic microcytic anemia. In intense infections, enteritis (sometimes with hemorrhagic diarrhea) and deficiencies in intestinal absorption are frequent. Eosinophilia, generally 10 to 15%, is lower than in human patients, in whom it can reach very high levels.

Prenatal infection is seen with some frequency in dogs. When many of the parasites mature suddenly, the death of the pup often results. These infections are due to third-stage larvae that have remained immobilized and inactive, but viable, in various organs and tissues of the mother; the larvae then mobilize during gestation and infect the progeny, either during the prenatal period via the placenta or via the milk in the first weeks of life.

Mild infections are generally asymptomatic.

Source of Infection and Mode of Transmission (Figure 101): The source of infection for man is soil contaminated with the feces of infected dogs or cats. Soils

Figure 101. Zoonotic ancylostomiasis. Transmission cycle.

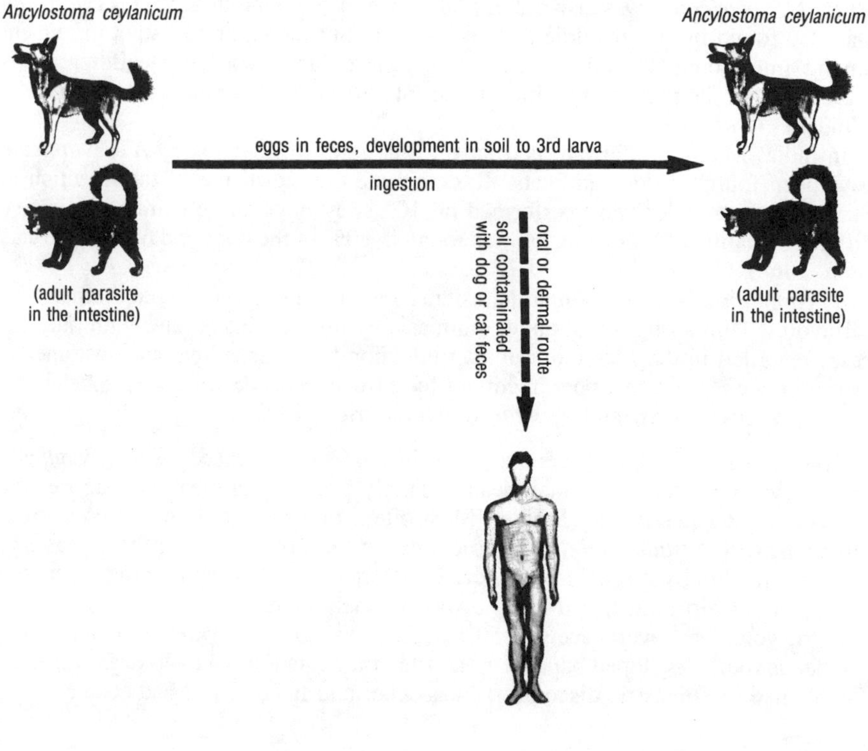

Ancylostoma ceylanicum

Ancylostoma ceylanicum

eggs in feces, development in soil to 3rd larva

ingestion

oral or dermal route

soil contaminated with dog or cat feces

(adult parasite in the intestine)

(adult parasite in the intestine)

that retain moisture are the most favorable. Survival of the larvae depends on moisture and temperature conditions. The larvae can invade the human host orally or through the skin.

Diagnosis: The infection can be confirmed by discovery of the eggs in fecal matter. Counting the number of eggs (Stoll or Kato-Katz method) indicates the intensity of the infection. When less than 2,000 eggs per gram of fecal matter are found, which would correspond to less than 50 parasites, the infection is rarely clinically apparent; 5,000 eggs per gram are found in infections with clinical significance; and more than 11,000 eggs per gram are found in cases with marked anemia (Barriga, 1982). For specific diagnosis, the patient should be given an anthelmintic (bephenium hydroxynaphthoate, pyrantel pamoate, mebendazole, thiabendazole), and the expelled parasites identified.

Control: Since its importance in humans is limited, ancylostomiasis of zoonotic origin does not require special control measures.

Bibliography

Anten, J. F. G., and P. J. Zuidema. Hookworm infection in Dutch servicemen returning from West New Guinea. *Trop Geogr Med* 16:216-224, 1964.

Barriga, O. O. Ancylostomiasis. *In*: Schultz, M. G. (Ed.), *CRC Handbook Series in Zoonoses*. Section C, vol. 2. Boca Raton, Florida, 1982.

Carroll, S. M., and D. I. Grove. Experimental infection of humans with *Ancylostoma ceylanicum*: clinical, parasitological, haematological and immunological findings. *Trop Geogr Med* 38:38-45, 1986.

Chitwood, A. B., and G. A. Schad. *Ancylostoma ceylanicum*: a parasite of man in Calcutta and environs. *Am J Trop Med Hyg* 21:300-301, 1972.

Faust, E. C., P. C. Beaver, and R. C. Jung. *Animal Agents and Vectors of Human Disease*. Philadelphia, Lea and Febiger, 1975.

León, E. de, and J. F. Maldonado. Uncinariasis (Ancylostomiasis). *In*: Marcial-Rojas, R. A. (Ed.), *Pathology of Protozoal and Helminthic Diseases*. Baltimore, Maryland, Williams and Wilkins, 1971.

Rep, B. H. Hookworms and other helminths in dogs, cats and man in Surinam. *Trop Geogr Med* 20:262-270, 1968.

Soulsby, E. J. L. *Textbook of Veterinary Clinical Parasitology*. Oxford, Blackwell, 1965.

Tagle, I. *Enfermedades parasitarias de los animales domésticos*. Santiago, Chile, Andrés Bello, 1970.

Velásquez, C. C., and B. C. Cabrera. *Ancylostoma ceylanicum* (Looss, 1911) in a Filipino woman. *J Parasitol* 54:430-431, 1968.

Wijers, D. J. B., and A. M. Smith. Early symptoms after experimental infection of man with *Ancylostoma braziliense* var. *ceylanicum*. *Trop Geogr Med* 18:48-52, 1966.

Witenberg, G. G. Nematodiases. *In*: Van der Hoeden, J. (Ed.), *Zoonoses*. Amsterdam, Netherlands, Elsevier, 1964.

World Health Organization. *Intestinal Protozoan and Helminthic Infections*. Report of a WHO Scientific Group. Geneva, WHO, 1981. (Technical Report Series 666.)

Yoshida, Y., K. Okamoto, and J. C. Chin. *Ancylostoma ceylanicum* infection in dogs, cats and man in Taiwan. *Am J Trop Med Hyg* 17:378-381, 1968.

Zuidema, P. J., B. H. Rep, and H. C. L. Meuzelaar. Ancylostomiasis in Dutch servicemen returning from Surinam. *Trop Geogr Med* 24:68-72, 1972.

ZOONOTIC FILARIASES

(125.1 and 125.6)

Etiology: The etiologic agents of zoonotic filariases are *Brugia malayi* (subperiodic form) and possibly *B. pahangi*, *Dirofilaria immitis*, *D.* (*Nochtiella*) *tenuis*, *D.* (*Nochtiella*) *repens*, and several species of unidentified animal filariae, some of which are described as "similar to *Dipetalonema*" (Beaver *et al.*, 1984).

According to present knowledge, animals do not participate in the epidemiology of human filariases caused by *Wuchereria bancrofti*, *Brugia malayi* (periodic form), *B. timori*, *Onchocerca volvulus*, *Loa loa*, *Mansonella ozzardi*, *Tetrapetalonema* (*Dipetalonema*) *perstans*, and *T.* (*Dipetalonema*) *streptocerca*, which are all considered to be parasites specific to humans (Dissanaike, 1979). For several of these species, natural infection has never been demonstrated in lower animals. There are also doubts that infections by *Loa loa* occasionally found in mandrills (*Mandrillus leucophaeus*) are really due to the human parasite. It is thought that the common parasite of the mandrill is a different subspecies, *L. loa papionis*, and that it is transmitted by a different vector species in the genus *Chrysops*. The only natural animal infections by *Onchocerca volvulus* were found in a gorilla from Zaire and in a spider monkey, *Ateles geoffroyi*, in Mexico (Dissanaike, 1979). Several human cases due to onchocercas of animal origin (*O. gutturosa*, *O. cervicalis*) have been described (Ali-Khan, 1977). *Tetrapetalonema perstans* and *T. streptocerca* have been found in anthropoid apes, but not enough is known about their biology to determine their epidemiologic importance (World Health Organization, 1979). Some human cases caused by dipetalonemas have occurred (Green *et al.*, 1978; Beaver *et al.*, 1980). Parasites similar to *Mansonella ozzardi* have been observed in neotropical monkeys, but uncertainty exists as to whether they are the same species as the parasite of man (Dissanaike, 1979).

One of the prominent features in the epidemiology of filariases and the biology of filariae is that their life cycle requires an arthropod host. The adult parasites, females and males, live in a vertebrate host's tissues or body cavities. The females are viviparous, incubating their eggs *in utero* and releasing embryos called microfilariae, which circulate in the bloodstream or lodge in the skin. The microfilariae are ingested by an arthropod that feeds on the host. Inside a mosquito or other arthropod, the microfilaria continues its development into a third-stage larva that migrates to the invertebrate host's mouthparts. When the latter feeds again, it releases the infective larva, which enters the body of the vertebrate animal and continues its development, reaching sexual maturity and producing microfilariae. The parasite's localization differs with the species of filaria; for example, adult parasites of *Wuchereria bancrofti* and *Brugia malayi* lodge in the lymphatic system in humans; *Dirofilaria immitis*, in the right side of the heart in dogs; and *D. tenuis* and *D. repens*, in the subcutaneous tissue of raccoons and dogs, respectively.

The microfilariae of some species appear in the blood with a marked nocturnal or diurnal periodicity. Other species do not display this phenomenon to as great a degree, and are called subperiodic for this reason. *B. malayi* has a nocturnal periodic form in which the microfilariae disappear or are very rare during the day, and a nocturnal subperiodic form with maximum filaremia during the night but filariae also present during the day. *D. repens* is of diurnal periodicity, while *D. immitis* has a nocturnal subperiodicity, with filaremia five to 10 times greater in the afternoon or at night than in the morning or at midday. This phenomenon, which is interpreted as an adaptation of the filariae to the feeding habits of the vectors, is important in the epidemiology and diagnosis.

Geographic Distribution and Occurrence: Periodic *Brugia malayi* is the cause of most of the human cases of Malaysian filariasis that occur in Southeast Asia, India, Korea, and China. Periodic strains of the parasite are transmitted from person to person by mosquito bites and are not found naturally in animals, although they can be transmitted experimentally to cats and monkeys.

Subperiodic *B. malayi* is limited to wooded and swampy regions. It is found in Indonesia, peninsular Malaysia and Thailand, southern Vietnam, and three foci in the Philippines. Transmission occurs between jungle animals and man by means of mosquitoes, primarily those of the genus *Mansonia*. The parasite has been found in several species of nonhuman primates, domestic cats, wild felids, and pangolins (*Manis javanica*). Likewise, the vectors feed on other domestic animals and man. *B. pahangi*, whose microfilariae are not easily distinguishable from those of *B. malayi*, is a parasite of dogs, cats, wild felids, and sometimes primates. Its area of distribution in Malaysia coincides with that of *B. malayi*, and it probably also infects man. Experimentally, the infection was transmitted from cat to man, but it is not known if human infection occurs naturally, given the difficulty in distinguishing *B. pahangi* from *B. malayi*. The vectors of *B. pahangi* are *Armigeres subalbatus* and *Mansonia* spp. In the United States, six cases of human infection by *Brugia* spp. of animal origin have been described, but it was not possible to determine the species of the filariae. Although only one species of *Brugia* is known in that country (*B. beaveri* from raccoons), the human cases have occurred in places geographically distant from its known area of distribution, and therefore it is believed that there could be another species as yet undescribed (Gutiérrez and Petras, 1982). Two cases of human infection by a zoonotic species of *Brugia* have been described in Colombia (Kozek *et al.*, 1984).

Dirofilaria immitis is widespread among dogs throughout the world, although the prevalence varies greatly in different areas. About 80 human cases of pulmonary dirofilariasis have been diagnosed, most of them due to *D. immitis*. The majority occurred in the United States, mainly in the southeast; 20 cases were recorded in Australia and 10 cases in Japan (Takeuchi *et al.*, 1981).

Subcutaneous human dirofilariasis is usually due to *D. tenuis*, a parasite of raccoons (*Procyon lotor*) in the United States, and to *D. repens*, a parasite of dogs and felids in other countries. More than 100 cases of subcutaneous human dirofilariasis have been diagnosed in numerous countries of Europe, Asia, Africa, and the Americas (Argentina, Brazil, the United States, and Canada). The greatest numbers of cases have been recorded in the USSR, Italy, and Sri Lanka (Dissanaike, 1979).

The few cases of zoonotic onchocerciasis have been diagnosed in Canada, the United States, the USSR, and Switzerland (Ali-Khan, 1977). Human cases of cutaneous or ocular infection by filariae "similar to *Dipetalonema*" have been recognized in the United States (three in Oregon and one in Alabama) and in Costa Rica (one case) (Green *et al.*, 1978; Beaver *et al.*, 1980; Beaver *et al.*, 1984).

The Disease in Man: The main symptomatology of filariases caused by *B. malayi* (brugiasis), both periodic and subperiodic (zoonotic), consists of lymphadenopathies, lymphangitis, and high eosinophilia. Attacks of lymphadenopathy lasting several days occur at irregular intervals, with fever, malaise, cephalalgia, nausea, tumefaction of one leg, and sterile abscesses. In advanced cases, elephantiasis of the lower extremities may occur due to obstruction of the lymphatic circulation. Elephantiasis of the scrotum, such as is seen in Bancroft's filariasis (*Wuchereria bancrofti*), is rare in brugiasis. Many infections among the natives of endemic regions occur asymptomatically in spite of the presence of filaremia.

In the six cases of human infection by *Brugia* spp. of animal origin in the United States, the parasite was unexpectedly found in an infarcted lymph node in patients who had no other symptomatology related to this infection (Gutiérrez and Petras, 1982). The two Colombian cases were also characterized by lymphadenopathy (Kozek *et al.*, 1984).

Two types of human dirofilariasis can be distinguished: pulmonary and subcutaneous. Man is an aberrant host for animal dirofilariae, and the parasites rarely manage to produce microfilariae. In fact, adult dirofilariae, in some cases even females with microfilariae in their uterus, have been observed in human patients in whom dirofilaremia could not be detected. For reasons still unknown, all patients have been adults, in spite of the fact that children are equally exposed to the vector mosquitoes.

Pulmonary dirofilariasis is due to *D. immitis*. Most persons infected are asymptomatic, and the pulmonary lesion is discovered when a radiologic examination is performed for other reasons, or by pulmonary lobectomy done because a malignant tumor is suspected. In symptomatic cases, there is coughing and thoracic pain for a month or more, and occasionally hemoptysis, fever, malaise, chills, and myalgia. A round and circumscribed ("coin-shaped") nodular lesion 1 to 4 cm in diameter is observed in the radiologic examination. Eosinophilia is rarely confirmed. Only in two cases in the United States and one in Brazil has the parasite been found in the heart (right side), while in almost all other cases the dirofilaria was lodged in a lobe of the right lung, partially occluding a small artery and forming a thrombus. The parasites are found dead and usually in some stage of degeneration in all pulmonary cases. Human infections are caused by only one parasite or, exceptionally, by two. The lesion may be confused with a neoplasm in the radiologic examination.

Subcutaneous dirofilariasis is due to *D. tenuis* (United States), *D. repens* (Africa, Asia, Europe, South America), and sometimes other species of animal dirofilariae. The lesion consists of a nodule or subcutaneous swelling around the parasite. The lesion can be located on different exposed parts of the body; the original name of *D. conjunctivae* (currently invalid) derived from the parasite's frequent localization in the eyelids. The nodules and tumefactions may or may not be painful, and some are migratory. In general, a single parasite is responsible for the lesion, and on some occasions it has been retrieved alive. In a few cases microfilariae have been observed in the uterus of the parasite, but they have never been found in the bloodstream of the patient. The lesion is inflammatory, with accompanying histiocytes, plasmocytes, lymphocytes, and abundant eosinophils. Blood eosinophilia is present with some frequency.

The cases of zoonotic onchocerciasis in North America were manifested as fibrotic nodules of the wrist tendon.

In Oregon, USA, three cases of ocular involvement occurred, with actively motile filariae present in the anterior chamber of the eye. The causal agent was classified as *Dipetalonema* sp., with morphology similar to *D. arbuta* from porcupines

(*Erethizon dorsatum*) or *D. sprenti* from beavers (*Castor canadensis*). In a case that occurred in a Costa Rican child, the filaria was found in a subcutaneous artery.

The Disease in Animals: Subperiodic *B. malayi* occurs in monkeys, wild felids, and other wild mammals, as well as in the domestic cat. In cats, as in man, the parasite is found in the lymphatic vessels, and microfilariae appear in the blood 75 to 140 days after infection. The effect of the infection on animal health has not been studied very much.

D. immitis is found in the right ventricle and pulmonary artery in dogs, usually in a mass that includes both sexes of the parasite. When the number of parasites is small, the infection is asymptomatic. In cases of symptomatic dirofilariasis of long duration, the most prominent signs are chronic cough, loss of vitality, and, in serious forms, cardiac insufficiency. Chronic passive congestion can develop in several organs and produce ascites; thromboses may cause pulmonary infarctions, resulting in sudden death. The acute hepatic syndrome (inferior vena cava syndrome) consists of the obstruction of the inferior vena cava by a large number of adult parasites that matured simultaneously, with consequent acute congestion of the liver and kidneys, hemoglobinuria, and death in 24 to 72 hours.

D. repens lodges in the subcutaneous connective tissue of dogs and cats; it may cause pruritus and eczema leading to loss of hair and scab formation. However, in many cases it does not produce any disorders in the animal.

Source of Infection and Mode of Transmission (Figures 102–104): The reservoirs of subperiodic brugiasis, which occurs in the swampy forest regions of Southeast Asia, are monkeys, cats, and wild carnivores. High rates of infection have been found in the monkeys *Presbytis obscurus* and *Macaca irus*. The relative importance of wild and domestic animals as reservoirs is unknown, but it is probable that the latter serve more frequently as a source of infection for man (Denham and McGreevy, 1977). The infection is transmitted by mosquitoes of the genus *Mansonia* from animal to animal, from animal to human, and from human to human. The maximum concentration of microfilariae in the blood occurs at night to coincide with the nocturnal feeding habits of the vectors. Although *Mansonia* mosquitoes usually feed outside houses, they have also been found inside them, as is demonstrated by the fact that the infection occurs in young children.

In other zoonotic human infections by *Brugia* spp., *Onchocerca* spp., and *Dipetalonema* spp. (or other similar filariae), the source of infection is wild animals of undetermined species.

The main reservoir of *D. immitis* is the dog, and the disease is transmitted by mosquitoes; man is infected only accidentally. When a person is inoculated with third-stage larvae by a mosquito, most of the larvae die in the subcutaneous connective tissue. A few, however, may escape from this tissue (especially in repeated infections), continue their development, and migrate to the lungs. Microfilariae can develop to the infective (third-stage) larva in many species of mosquitoes, not all of which have the same efficiency as vectors. The reservoir of *D. repens* is dogs and that of *D. tenuis* is raccoons.

Man is an accidental host of zoonotic filariae (with the exception of subperiodic *B. malayi*) and does not play any role in the epidemiology.

Role of Animals in the Epidemiology of the Disease: Of the large number of filariae species that exist in nature, only eight have adapted to man, and their

Figure 102. Zoonotic filariasis (pulmonary dirofilariasis). Transmission cycle.

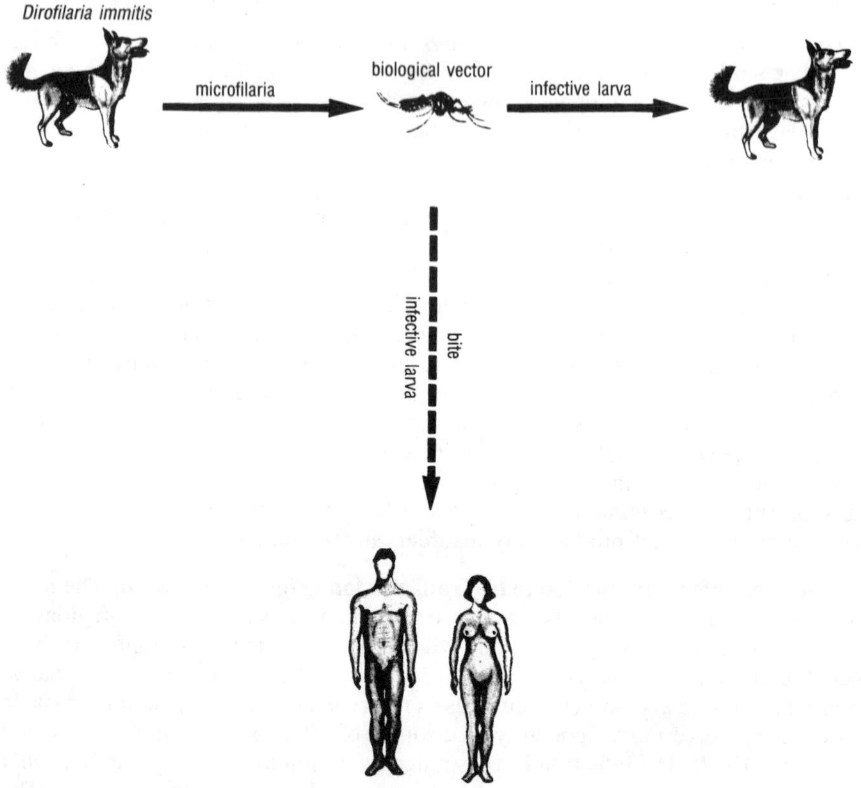

transmission is interhuman (see Etiology). The other species of filariae are parasites of animals, affecting man only occasionally and thus not constituting a public health problem. One exception is subperiodic *Brugia malayi*, which is an important pathogen for man.

Diagnosis: Specific diagnosis of filariasis caused by *B. malayi* is possible when microfilariae are detected in the patient's blood by examining thick films stained with Giemsa or, preferably, by using the Knott concentration method or Millipore filters. Since microfilaremia takes several months to appear after infection, lymph node biopsy can be useful for early diagnosis. Complement fixation, hemagglutination, immunofluorescence, bentonite flocculation, double gel diffusion, immunoelectrophoresis, and counterimmunoelectrophoresis are among the immunobiologic tests used. Problems of both sensitivity and specificity occur in the serology of filariasis. For the time being, purified antigens for the different species of filariae are not available. With the improvement of culture methods, it is hoped that specific homologous antigens will be obtained for each species as well as for each developmental stage of the parasite, allowing a more specific serologic diagnosis. Another difficulty is the lack of correlation between the serologic titer and the intensity of infection. Occasionally, a low or negative titer is found in the presence

Figure 103. Zoonotic filariasis (subcutaneous dirofilariasis). Transmission cycle.

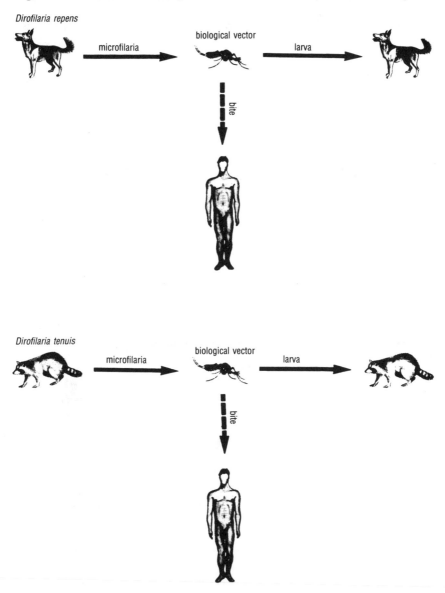

of appreciable microfilaremia, which could be explained by an excess of circulating antigen and the absorption or neutralization of the antibodies. Procedures for measuring circulating antigens in the blood, either free or bonded to immune complexes, would perhaps provide a more useful indication of active infection and the parasite burden (WHO Scientific Working Group on Filariasis, 1981). In a recent study, counterimmunoelectrophoresis was very satisfactory for detecting both circulating antigens and antibodies in dogs experimentally infected with *Dirofilaria immitis* (Tagawa *et al.*, 1983).

Specific diagnosis of human dirofilariasis (pulmonary and subcutaneous) is always done postoperatively, when the parasite is found in surgical specimens.

Figure 104. Zoonotic filariasis (subperiodic *Brugia malayi*).
Probable transmission cycle.

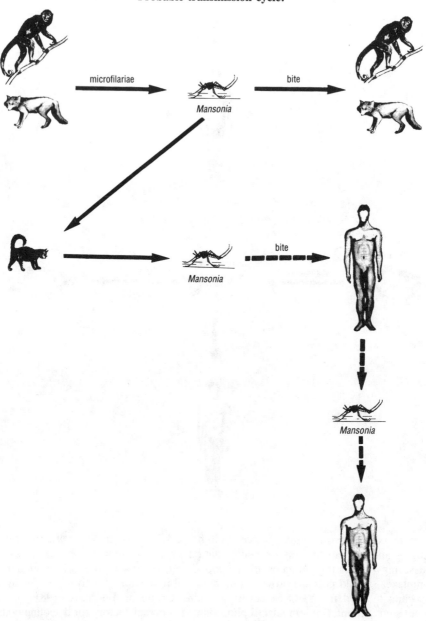

Diagnosis of canine filariasis is made by identifying microfilariae in the blood, using the Knott concentration method or Millipore filters. In the case of *D. immitis*, a blood sample should preferably be obtained during the nocturnal hours when the microfilaremia reaches its maximum level. It is necessary to differentiate *D. immitis* from *D. repens* and *Dipetalonema reconditum*. Microfilaremia by *D. immitis* appears in dogs 6 months after infection. Microfilaremia is not detectable (occult dirofilariasis) in approximately 15% of dogs infected by *D. immitis*.

Control: Human filariasis is combated by controlling the vector arthropods with insecticides. Mass therapeutic treatment with diethylcarbamazine has been employed successfully in some communities. Control of subperiodic brugiasis is difficult because of the ecologic characteristics of the endemic area and because of the abundance of wildlife reservoirs. In India and Sri Lanka, population levels of the intermediate hosts and vectors of subperiodic *B. malayi*, which are mosquitoes of the genus *Mansonia*, were reduced by eliminating several species of floating aquatic plants to which the mosquito larvae attached.

In highly enzootic areas, *D. immitis* infection in dogs can be prevented by destroying the infective larvae with diethylcarbamazine administered in daily oral doses, starting before the mosquito season begins and continuing for 2 months. The drug should not be given to dogs with microfilaremia, as it can produce anaphylactoid shock.

Bibliography

Ali-Khan, Z. Tissue pathology and comparative microanatomy of *Onchocerca* from a resident of Ontario and other enzootic *Onchocerca* species from Canada and the USA. *Ann Trop Med Parasitol* 71:469-482, 1977.

Ando, K., P. C. Beaver, T. Soga, T. Maehara, and S. Kitamura. Zoonotic subcutaneous filaria of undetermined classification. *Am J Trop Med Hyg* 34:1138-1141, 1985.

Beaver, P. C. Filariasis without microfilaremia. *Am J Trop Med Hyg* 19:181-189, 1970.

Beaver, P. C., R. Brenes, and G. Vargas Solano. Zoonotic filaria in a subcutaneous artery of a child in Costa Rica. *Am J Trop Med Hyg* 33:583-585, 1984.

Beaver, P. C., E. A. Meyer, E. L. Jarroll, and R. C. Rosenquist. *Dipetalonema* from the eye of a man in Oregon, USA. *Am J Trop Med Hyg* 29:369-372, 1980.

Beaver, P. C., and T. C. Orihel. Human infection with filariae of animals in the United States. *Am J Trop Med Hyg* 14:1010-1029, 1965.

Buckley, J. J. C. Occult filarial infections of animal origin as a cause of tropical pulmonary eosinophilia. *East Afr Med J* 335:493-500, 1958.

Centers for Disease Control of the USA. Human *Dirofilaria immitis* infection—Texas. *Morb Mortal Wkly Rep* 23:379, 1974.

Denham, D. A., and P. B. McGreevy. Brugian filariasis: epidemiological and experimental studies. *Adv Parasit* 15:243-309, 1977.

Dissanaike, A. S. Zoonotic aspects of filarial infections in man. *Bull WHO* 57:349-357, 1979.

Faust, E. C., P. C. Beaver, and R. C. Jung. *Animal Agents and Vectors of Human Disease*, 4th ed. Philadelphia, Lea and Febiger, 1975.

Faust, E. C., P. F. Russell, and R. C. Jung. *Craig and Faust's Clinical Parasitology*, 8th ed. Philadelphia, Lea and Febiger, 1970.

Green, B. M., G. F. Otto, and W. B. Greenough III. Circulating non-human microfilaria in a patient with systemic lupus erythematosus. *Am J Trop Med Hyg* 27:905-909, 1978.

Gutiérrez, Y., and R. E. Petras. *Brugia* infection in northern Ohio. *Am J Trop Med Hyg* 31:1128-1130, 1982.

Harrison, F. G., and J. H. Thompson. Dirofilariasis. *In*: Marcial-Rojas, R. A. (Ed.), *Pathology of Protozoal and Helminthic Diseases*. Baltimore, Maryland, Williams and Wilkins, 1971.

Jackson, R. F. Thiacertasimide for preventive treatment of *Dirofilaria immitis*. *J Am Vet Med Assoc* 154:395-396, 1969.

Jung, R. C., and P. H. Espenan. A case of infection in man with *Dirofilaria*. *Am J Trop Med Hyg* 16:172-174, 1967.

Kelly, J. D. Anthropozoonotic helminthiases in Australia. The role of animals in disease transmission. *Int J Zoonoses* 1:13-24, 1974.

Kozek, W. J., M. A. Reyes, J. Ehrman, F. Garrido, and M. Nieto. Enzootic *Brugia* infection in a two-year-old Colombian girl. *Am J Trop Med Hyg* 33:65-69, 1984.

Ludlam, K. W., L. A. Jachowski, and G. F. Otto. Potential vectors of *Dirofilaria immitis*. *J Am Vet Med Assoc* 157:1354-1359, 1970.

Melvin, D. M., K. W. Walls, and J. W. Smith. Blood and tissue parasites. *In*: Balows, A., and W. J. Hausler, Jr. (Eds.), *Diagnostic Procedures for Bacterial, Mycotic and Parasitic Infections*, 6th ed. Washington, D.C., American Public Health Association, 1981.

Orihel, T. C., and P. C. Beaver. Morphology and relationship of *Dirofilaria tenuis* and *Dirofilaria conjunctivae*. *Am J Trop Med Hyg* 14:1030-1043, 1965.

Ottesen, E. A. Filariases and Tropical Eosinophilia. *In*: Warren K.S., and A. A. F. Mahmoud (Eds.), *Tropical and Geographical Medicine*. New York, McGraw-Hill Book Co., 1984.

Otto, G. F. Geographical distribution, vectors and life cycle of *Dirofilaria immitis*. *J Am Vet Med Assoc* 154:370-373, 1969.

Pacheco, G., and H. L. Schofield. *Dirofilaria tenuis* containing microfilariae in man. *Am J Trop Med Hyg* 17:180-182, 1968.

Palmieri, J. R., S. Ratiwayanto, S. Masbar, S. Tirtokusomo, J. Rusch, and H. A. Marwoto. Evidence of possible natural infection of man with *Brugia pahangi* in South Kalimantan (Borneo), Indonesia. *Trop Geogr Med* 37:239, 1985.

Pendergraft, G. E., L. D. Evert, M. J. Morrell, and V. Jonsson. The dog heartworm: a possible problem in man. *Mo Med* 66:731-736, 1969.

Soulsby, E. J. L. *Textbook of Veterinary Clinical Parasitology*. Oxford, Blackwell, 1965.

Tagawa, M., K. Uematsu, K. Kurokowa, and H. Tanaka. Circulating antigens and antibodies of *Dirofilaria immitis* in the dog detected by counterimmunoelectrophoresis. *Jpn J Vet Sci* 45:323-329, 1983.

Takeuchi, T., K. Asami, S. Kobayashi, M. Masuda, M. Tanabe, S. Miura, M. Asakawa, and T. Murai. *Dirofilaria immitis* infection in man: report of a case of the infection in heart and inferior vena cava from Japan. *Am J Trop Med Hyg* 30:966-969, 1981.

Witenberg, G. G. Helminthozoonoses. *In*: Van der Hoeden, J. (Ed.), *Zoonoses*. Amsterdam, Netherlands, Elsevier, 1964.

WHO Scientific Working Group on Filariasis. The immunology of filariasis. *Bull WHO* 59:1-8, 1981.

World Health Organization. *Joint FAO/WHO Expert Committee on Zoonoses, Third Report*. Geneva, WHO, 1967. (Technical Report Series 378.)

World Health Organization. *WHO Expert Committee on Filariasis, Third Report*. Geneva, WHO, 1974. (Technical Report Series 542.)

World Health Organization. *Parasitic Zoonoses*. Report of a WHO Expert Committee, with the Participation of FAO. Geneva, WHO, 1979. (Technical Report Series 637.)

Section C

ARTHROPODS

DERMATITIS CAUSED BY MITES OF ANIMAL ORIGIN

(133.9)

Etiology: In addition to the mite that causes sarcoptic scabies (see "Zoonotic Scabies"), there are several other species that occasionally infest human skin and cause a temporary dermatitis, although they are incapable of establishing themselves on this aberrant host. These animal parasites belong to the families Cheyletidae, Dermanyssidae, and Macronyssidae. The mites of the genus *Cheyletiella* are obligate parasites of lagomorphs, dogs, and cats. The species transmissible to man are *C. parasitovorax*, *C. yasguri*, and *C. blakei*. These mites measure 386 by 266 microns and are characterized by a transverse line halfway along their body; the palpi end in hooks turned towards the face and the legs have feathery appendages. The limited attempts so far at transmission between different animal species indicate that the mite is not very species-specific.

The life cycle is completed in its entirety on the host in about 35 days. The larvae, which go through two nymphal stages before becoming adults, hatch from eggs adhering to the hair. The adult female and the eggs can survive 10 days off the animal body, but the larvae, nymphs, and adult males are not very resistant and die in about 2 days in the environment.

Mites of the genus *Cheyletiella* are external parasites of the skin and hair and do not excavate tunnels or furrows in the skin.

The family Dermanyssidae includes the mite *Dermanyssus gallinae*, a parasite of chickens and other domestic and wild fowl. During the day this mite hides in cracks in hen houses, under boards, or in other places, where the female mite lays eggs. At night, the mites come out of their hiding places and feed on birds. Females begin oviposition 12 to 24 hours after feeding on a host's blood. The eggs can hatch in 2 to 3 days, releasing a six-legged larva that undergoes a molt to become a first-stage nymph and then a second and third molt to become an adult parasite. The whole life cycle can be completed in 1 week under favorable environmental conditions.

The species *Ornithonyssus bacoti*, *O. bursa*, and *O. sylviarum* belong to the family Macronyssidae. The first species parasitizes rodents, especially *Rattus norvegicus*, and the other two are found on birds. *O. sylviarum* and *O. bursa* can complete their entire life cycle on the birds, sometimes in less than a week. *O. bacoti* lays its eggs in the burrows or nests of rodents or in the cracks of the cages of laboratory animals (mice, rats, and hamsters).

Geographic Distribution and Occurrence: *Dermanyssus gallinae*, *Ornithonyssus bacoti*, and mites of the genus *Cheyletiella* have worldwide distribution. *O. bursa* is found mainly in tropical and subtropical regions, and *O. sylviarum* lives in temperate regions of the northern hemisphere and also in Australia and New Zealand.

The frequency of these infestations on man and other animals is difficult to determine because records of their incidence are not available.

Cheyletiella yasguri has been found in some dog kennels. Many cases of infestations on cats (attributed mainly to *C. blakei*) have been detected because their owners were also affected and required medical attention. Sometimes, the infestation is discovered as a consequence of a coprologic examination, as happened in a laboratory in the United States when very large eggs (230 by 110 microns) were found in the feces of a cat. This finding prompted the examination of another 41 cats from the same supplier and 10 of them were found to be infested. On the other hand, 28 cats from two other suppliers were negative (Fox and Hewes, 1976). *C. parasitovorax* is found on rabbits. The infestation affects a large number of animals in some laboratory colonies.

Dermanyssus gallinae is rarely present in modern establishments where fowl are raised in cages, but it is more frequent on rural poultry farms and in hen houses. The main hosts are chickens; however, the mite is also found on turkeys, pigeons, canaries, and several species of wild fowl. Houses can be invaded by mites from nearby hen houses or pigeon nests. In Rotterdam, the Netherlands, 23 persons from eight families were found to be infested.

Ornithonyssus sylviarum is a very common parasite in modern fowl breeding establishments, both in the United States and in other countries of the northern hemisphere with temperate climates. Infestation of fowl by *O. bursa* is especially important in Australia, where, besides chickens, it affects pigeons, sparrows, and other birds. The rodent mite *O. bacoti* is frequent wherever *Rattus norvegicus* is abundant. This mite is fairly common in laboratory rodent colonies in some areas and rare in others.

The Disease in Man: Infestation of man by *Cheyletiella* spp. is produced by close contact with infested animals. The disease consists of a papular and pruriginous eruption on the arms, thorax, waist, and thighs. Human infestation is transitory and disappears spontaneously when the reservoir animals living with man (mainly cats and dogs) are treated.

Infestation by *Dermanyssus gallinae* is painful and may produce a papular urticaria. *Ornithonyssus bacoti* causes a similar condition, with painful bites and, sometimes, allergic dermatitis. Infestation can be a particular problem when rodenticides are applied without previous application of insecticides, which forces the mites to seek alternate hosts. *O. sylviarum* attacks man in the absence of its natural hosts; sometimes it causes immediate irritation and then erythema, edematization, and pruritus. The other bird mite, *O. bursa*, also frequently attacks man and causes a mild skin irritation.

The Disease in Animals: The symptomatology of infestation by *Cheyletiella* spp. in dogs and cats is very variable. In many or perhaps the majority of cats, the infestation occurs asymptomatically; dogs and some cats display a localized or generalized furfuraceous dermatitis, which is sometimes pruriginous. Alopecic areas, erythroderma, and a papular eruption can also be found.

Dermanyssus gallinae produces anemia and irritation in birds, and can cause the interruption of egg laying when the infestation is very intense; the loss of blood can be so severe that the birds die of anemia. In Australia, *D. gallinae* is a vector of *Borrelia anserina*, the agent of fowl spirochetosis. An intense infestation by *Ornithonyssus sylviarum* or *O. bursa* gives the plumage a dirty appearance. Large concentrations of mites around the cloaca can cause the skin to crack and form scabs. The economic importance of these mites is still in doubt. It has been claimed that *O. sylviarum* does not affect egg laying (Loomis, 1978). Infestation by *O. bacoti* causes debility, anemia, reduced reproduction, and death of laboratory rodents (Flynn, 1973).

Source of Infection: Man is an accidental host of these animal mites, they do not reproduce on human skin and they abandon it after a short time. The infestation of man by *Cheyletiella* spp. is very similar to that caused by the animal variants of *Sarcoptes scabiei* (see "Zoonotic Scabies").

Man becomes infested with *Cheyletiella* spp. by close contact with cats and dogs carrying this mite. Human infestation can also be produced indirectly, since the adult mites can survive off the animal body for about 10 days. This latter mode of transmission can occur when cats are allowed to sleep on beds.

Dermanyssus gallinae can enter dwellings and attack man when pigeons or other birds nest on the exterior of houses. Hen houses located near human dwellings are another source of infestation for man.

Transmission of *Ornithonyssus bacoti* from rodents to man occurs in houses where rats are abundant. Human infestations become especially intense when the mites must search for an alternate host because rodents were poisoned before insecticides were used.

Human infestation by *O. sylviarum* and *O. bursa* occurs mainly by handling birds.

Diagnosis: Mites of the genus *Cheyletiella* can be detected on dogs and cats by microscopic examination of superficial skin scrapings, or by coprologic examination since these animals frequently ingest the mites. On the other hand, skin scrapings from humans do not reveal the mites, possibly because man dislodges them by scratching and bathing (Miller, 1983), and because they are few in number since they do not reproduce on human skin. *Dermanyssus gallinae* can be observed on birds at night with the unaided eye; during the day, it can be found by searching in its hiding places. The red color of the engorged mite helps make it visible.

The species of *Ornithonyssus* that infest birds can be detected day or night on the feathers and skin.

Control: To prevent human infestation by *Cheyletiella*, dogs and cats that harbor mites should be treated with insecticides (organophosphates, methyl carbamate, or calcium sulfide) for 3 to 4 weeks at 3 to 7 day intervals. It is also important to adequately clean the environment and objects with which the animals were in contact.

Control of the other mites is based on the same principles.

Bibliography

Ewing, S. A., J. E. Mosier, and T. S. Fox. Occurrence of *Cheyletiella* spp. on dogs with skin lesions. *J Am Vet Med Assoc* 151:64-67, 1967.

Flynn, R. J. *Parasites of Laboratory Animals*. Ames, Iowa State University Press, 1973.

Faust, E. C., P. F. Russell, and R. C. Jung. *Parasitología Clínica*. México, Salvat, 1974.

Fox, J. G., and K. Hewes. *Cheyletiella* infestation in cats. *J Am Vet Med Assoc* 169:332-333, 1976.

Harwood, R. F., and M. T. James. *Entomology in Human and Animal Health*, 7th ed. New York, Macmillan, 1979.

Loomis, E. C. External parasites. *In*: Hofstad, M. S., B. W. Calnek, C. F. Helmboldt, W. M. Reid, and H. W. Yoder, Jr. (Eds.), *Diseases of Poultry*, 7th ed. Ames, Iowa State University Press, 1978.

McKeevar, P. J., and S. K. Allen. Dermatitis associated with *Cheyletiella* infestation in cats. *J Am Vet Med Assoc* 147:718-720, 1979.

Miller, W. H. Cheyletiella infestation. *In*: Parish, L. C., W. B. Nutting, and R. B. Schwartzman (Eds.), *Cutaneous Infestations of Man and Animals*. New York, Praeger, 1983.

Pecheur, M., and H. Wissocq. Un cas de gale due à *Cheyletiella parasitovorax* chez un chat. *Ann Méd Vét* 125:191-192, 1981.

Soulsby, E. J. L. *Helminths, Arthropods and Protozoa of Domesticated Animals*, 7th ed. Philadelphia, Lea and Febiger, 1982.

Tika Ram, S. M., K. C. Satija, and R. K. Kaushik. *Ornithonyssus bacoti* infestation in laboratory personnel and veterinary students. *Int J Zoonoses* 13:138-140, 1986.

MYIASES

(134.0)

Definition: Myiases are diseases caused by the invasion of the tissues or open cavities of animals by dipteran larvae.

Classification: Myiases are classified as follows: a) specific, caused by fly larvae that are obligate parasites and feed on the live tissues of animals or man; b) semi-specific, due to dipteran larvae that usually develop in carcasses and decaying animal or vegetable matter, but can facultatively invade necrotic tissues of live animals (these flies are generally secondary invaders, attracted by the fetid odors of purulent or contaminated wounds); and c) accidental, caused by numerous fly species of several genera that normally deposit their eggs in excreta, decomposing organic matter, or foods, and only occasionally invade wounds and the gastrointestinal or urinary tracts.

Etiology: Numerous species of flies can cause myiasis. Only the most important ones are considered here.

1. Myiasis Caused by Larvae of *Cochliomyia hominivorax*

Synonym: Screwworm.

Cochliomyia hominivorax (*Callitroga americana*) is a bluish green fly of the family Calliphoridae. It measures about 12 to 15 mm long, has three dark bands on the back, and is found only in the Americas. The larva of this fly ("screwworm") is an obligate parasite that can invade the tissues of any warm-blooded animal. It is one of the main agents of myiases from the southern United States to Argentina and Chile. Myiases by *C. hominivorax* cause great economic losses in cattle, sheep, goats, and equines. Before the eradication campaign was begun in the southern United States, annual losses in that country due to animal myiases were estimated to be between US$50 million and US$100 million. This species is also responsible for the majority and most serious forms of human myiases in the Americas.

The female of *C. hominivorax* mates only once. On the skin, close to a wound, she deposits packets containing from a dozen to 400 eggs, overlapped like roof tiles. A single female can produce up to 4,000 eggs. The larvae emerge from the eggs after 11 to 21 hours and penetrate deeply into the tissues of the wound, where they feed and develop. Four to 8 days later, they fall to the ground, bury themselves, and pupate. In hot and humid weather, the adult fly emerges from the pupa in a little less than a week; a longer time is required when the climate is cooler. The flies mate 3 to 4 days after emergence, and in a few more days the fertilized females begin to lay eggs. In summer the entire development cycle can be completed in just over 3 weeks, so that several generations of flies can be born in a single season. Adult flies live about 2 weeks and feed on plant juices. Females can travel about 50 km under their own power and are also carried considerable distances by automobiles on which they alight. These facts suggest that eradication programs in which sterilized males are released should cover extensive areas to achieve a lasting effect.

Myiases occur in the hot season, from late spring to early autumn. The larvae, which are screw-shaped and measure some 12 mm in length, destroy the tissue where they lodge, and are concealed by the exudate of the wound. The profuse reddish brown exudate from the wound stains the skin or wool and attracts other flies, both of the same and of other species, which deposit more eggs (or larvae).

All types of accidental wounds (large or small), surgical incisions (castration, dehorning, docking), shearing cuts, umbilical wounds, and even skin abrasions and tick bites can give rise to invasion by larvae of *C. hominivorax* and resultant myiasis.

It has been shown experimentally that the larvae can penetrate intact skin of guinea pigs and rabbits.

Secondary bacterial infections of wounds invaded by larvae of *C. hominivorax* are common. The secondary infections aggravate the picture because of their own action and because they attract many species of semispecific flies, which, in turn, deposit more eggs and larvae in the lesion.

The larvae invade not only skin wounds, but can also become established in open body cavities, such as the nasal fossae, mouth, orbit, external ear, and vagina.

Clinical manifestations consist of severe pain in the affected region and intense pruritus that causes the animal or human host to scratch. If the animals are not treated, continuous tissue destruction and toxemia produce restlessness, depression, weight loss, prostration, and finally death. Occasionally, when flies are very abundant, mortality may reach 20% of the affected animals. The most serious clinical pictures generally appear in sheep, goats, and horses, species which most frequently develop secondary infections.

Human myiases occur among rural populations, especially where and when there is a great abundance of *C. hominivorax* flies, whose reproduction depends mainly on domestic animal hosts. As a result, when myiases are abundant in animals, many cases can occur in man. Human myiasis is clinically similar to that of animals. In addition to the invasion of wounds and ulcers (varicose ulcers of the legs), myiasis also occurs in a furuncular form, characterized by a nonmigratory cutaneous nodule. Most myiases of the natural cavities are also due to larvae of *C. hominivorax*. Invasion of the nasal fossae (rhinomyiasis) is the most frequent and generally occurs as a complication of ozena. The larvae of *C. hominivorax* often destroy the cartilage and palatine vault and can penetrate into the nasal sinuses and even reach the cranial cavity.

To prevent invasion by *C. hominivorax* larvae—the principal myiasis in the Americas—parturition in domestic animals should not coincide with the season when flies are abundant. The navels of animals born during the hot season should be treated with repellent preparations. During such seasons, castrations, dehorning, docking, branding, or other operations that leave tegumentary lesions should be avoided. All accidental wounds, whether affected by myiases or not, should be cleaned and adequately treated as soon as possible and covered with an insecticidal preparation (ronnel, lindane, coumaphos, or others).

Good results have been obtained in regional fly eradication programs in the Americas by releasing large numbers (1,000 per square mile per week) of artificially bred males sterilized with gamma rays. The sterile males compete in the mating process with the fertile males of the natural fly population. Since females mate only once in their lives, they are rendered functionally sterile if they mate with the sterilized specimens. The program began with a pilot project in Curaçao; the infestation was eradicated in 1954 and the island remained free of the fly until 1975. In the first 9 months of that year, however, 261 cases of myiasis occurred on the island, including 14 in humans. Dogs were the most frequently affected species, with 179 cases.

The southeastern United States was freed of *C. hominivorax* in 1959, as were Puerto Rico and the Virgin Islands in 1974. On the other hand, the southwestern United States remained infested in spite of implementation of the same measures, mainly because of the prevalence of the fly on the other side of the border. For that reason, a joint program with Mexico was formulated in 1972 to establish a barrier of sterile males in the isthmus of Tehuantepec after the infestation was eradicated in the north. For that same purpose, a laboratory was set up in the state of Chiapas for the production of sterile males (Miller, 1982). Later, an additional element was introduced into the fight, consisting of bait containing an insecticide (dichlorvos) deadly to the fly (Miller, 1982). This program has allowed the eradication of the screwworm in the United States and two-thirds of Mexico, and there are plans to extend it to Central America, Panama, and the rest of Latin America.

2. Myiasis Caused by Larvae of *Chrysomyia bezziana*

The fly *Chrysomyia bezziana* is a species similar to the previous one and causes similar lesions. Its distribution covers the tropical areas of Asia (India, Indonesia, Taiwan, the Philippines), islands of the Pacific, Papua New Guinea, and tropical Africa. The animals most often attacked are cattle, but it also infests sheep, goats, buffaloes, equines, swine, and dogs. Human myiasis is more frequent in India and other parts of Asia than in Africa. Like *Cochliomyia hominivorax*, it deposits eggs near wounds, ulcers, and natural openings (genitals, nose, commissure of the lips, eyes) (Harwood and James, 1979). The lesions produced by this myiasis on the face are sometimes very deforming, have a fetid odor, and frequently are invaded by secondary infections.

3. Furuncular Myiasis Caused by Larvae of *Cordylobia anthropophaga*

Cordylobia anthropophaga ("tumbu fly") is another fly of the family Calliphoridae and is found in sub-Saharan Africa. *C. anthropophaga* is yellow and measures 9.5 mm in length; the female deposits eggs in dry sand, straw, and even clothes that have been contaminated with urine or feces. The larva can survive without eating for 1 or 2 weeks after hatching, if it does not find a host sooner. The larvae penetrate through intact skin of the host to the subcutaneous tissue, generally in the feet. The lesion is pruriginous and furunculoid and exudes a serous liquid. The larvae mature in about 1 week; they abandon the host and pupate for 3 or 4 weeks before emerging as adult flies.

All the human cases described in Europe and the United States were contracted in Africa, where the disease is widespread. The most affected domestic animal is the dog, but the fly can infest many other domestic and wild species. Another African dipteran that attacks man more rarely but produces more intense and severe infestations is *C. rodhaini* (Harwood and James, 1979). Its main hosts are antelopes and the giant rat (Soulsby, 1982).

4. Myiasis Caused by Larvae of *Dermatobia hominis*

Synonyms: Torsalo (Central America), moyocuil (Mexico), berne (Brazil), mucha (Colombia), mirunta (Peru), and ura (Argentina, Paraguay, and Uruguay).

Dermatobia hominis is a large fly, about 12 to 18 mm in length, of the family Cuterebridae; it has a dark blue, hairy thorax that contrasts with its brilliant blue abdomen. *D. hominis* is widely distributed in tropical America, from Mexico south to Paraguay and northeastern Argentina. It attacks all kinds of domestic and wild mammals and causes great economic damage, especially in cattle.

The fly lives in humid forested areas and in underbrush. Its life cycle begins when the female lays her eggs on the abdomen of another insect (from any of about 50 zoophilic species), which she captures in flight. This nonparasitic transport relationship is known as phoresy. The number of eggs deposited in this way varies from 15 to 20, and the incubation period lasts 7 to 10 days. When the vector transporting the incubated eggs comes into contact with an animal, the larvae penetrate the animal's skin—often through the lesion created by the bite of the vector—and enter subcutaneous tissue, producing a furuncular myiasis. The larvae live in the animal for a period of 5 to 12 weeks, at the end of which they leave the furuncles and fall to the ground to pupate. The pupae remain in the ground for 15 to 60 days before metamorphosing into adult flies. After emerging from the pupae, the flies mate and the female proceeds to lay eggs, apparently only once in her life (Faust *et al.*, 1975). Adult flies do not feed and possess vestigial mouthparts.

Each lesion generally contains only one larva, but there may be multiple furuncles, depending on the number of larvae deposited. In cattle, the preferred localizations are the forequarters and back. In man, the lesions are found primarily on the exposed parts of the body, such as the scalp, legs, arms, hands, face, and neck. Besides causing skin myiasis, the larva of *D. hominis* can invade the eyelids, orbits, and mouth. These cavity myiases are seen primarily in children. The furuncular nodule is characterized by a small orifice through which the posterior spiracles of the larva can frequently be seen.

A large number of parasitic furuncles can afflict cattle and dogs. Often, these nodules are invaded by larvae of other flies and by bacteria, causing abscesses. The hides of intensely parasitized animals lose much of their value. It has been estimated that Brazil loses about US$200 million per year from the decrease in production of meat and milk and the damage to hides caused by this myiasis (Steelman, 1976).

In man, the pain in the affected region is intermittent; it is especially intense in furuncular myiasis of the scalp. In some regions, myiasis caused by *D. hominis* can be very frequent. On a eucalyptus plantation in Brazil, 41.3% of 363 inhabitants had parasitic nodules. In Venezuela, 104 cases of myiasis by this fly have been described, and in Panama, there have been palpebral cases and one cerebral case, in which the larvae in the scalp penetrated through the fontanelle of a child. The number of larvae per person is variable.

The objective of a control program should be to prevent larvae from reaching the ground and subsequently transforming into pupae. The systemic organophosphate insecticides now in use make it possible to destroy the larvae on the animals. However, it should be borne in mind that a control program must cover a wide area to have an effect on the fly population. Important factors in the success of a program are the collaboration of cattlemen and control of animal movement. Studies of mass fly breeding have been done with the aim of using the sterilized male technique for this species' control and eradication. A possible obstacle to the use of this technique is the finding observed in the laboratory by several investigators that the female may mate several times before oviposition (Marin-Rojas, 1975).

5. Myiasis Caused by Larvae of *Cuterebra* spp.

The flies of the genus *Cuterebra* resemble bees and measure 20 mm or more in length. Their larvae are obligate parasites of rodents and lagomorphs in North America.

The adult females deposit eggs on vegetation in the habitat of their hosts. The larvae are born at intervals, invade the subcutaneous tissue of the animals through intact skin, and form furunculoid nodules. They can also invade natural apertures. Inside the skin the larvae mature in about 1 month, and then they abandon the host to pupate in the ground.

The larvae of *Cuterebra* spp. cause subcutaneous cysts in rodents and lagomorphs. *C. emasculator* frequently parasitizes the scrotum of mice and chipmunks, destroying their testicles.

In addition to their natural hosts, the larvae of *Cuterebra* spp. can occasionally invade man, cats, dogs, and domestic rabbits. Lesions found on the nape or in the submandibular region in cats often cause pruritus and induce the animal to scratch, leading to bacterial infections. Cases of orchitis have also been described in both dogs and cats (Soulsby, 1982). More than a dozen cases have been reported in man, most of them producing subcutaneous lesions (Magnarelli and Andreadis, 1981).

6. Myiasis Caused by Larvae of *Hypoderma* spp.

This myiasis is caused by larvae of two species of flies of the family Oestridae: *Hypoderma lineatum* and *H. bovis*. Both flies are found in the northern hemisphere—in the United States and Canada as well as in Europe and some parts of Asia and northern Africa. Parasitized cattle have occasionally been introduced into several South American countries, Australia, and South Africa, but the fly has not established itself permanently in these places.

The flies, which resemble bees, deposit their eggs on hair on the lower part of an animal's body, preferentially the feet. *H. lineatum* deposits a row of eggs and *H. bovis* lays isolated eggs. The larvae are born in 2 to 6 days and primarily invade the subcutaneous connective tissue, through which they migrate. First-stage larvae of *H. bovis* migrate along the nerves and gather in the epidural fat along the spinal cord. The larvae of *H. lineatum* concentrate primarily in the submucosa of the esophagus. The larvae remain in these places for some time, and in January and February they finally migrate to the subcutaneous tissue of the dorsolumbar region, where they remain in the second and third larval stages for 10 to 11 weeks.

The flies spend about 10 of the approximately 11 to 12 months of their entire life cycle as larvae inside the animal body. Each larva in the dorsolumbar region is surrounded by a cyst about 3 cm in diameter that contains a pore through which the parasite breathes. The final-stage larva emerges from the hole in the cyst, falls to the ground, and pupates. Depending on climatic conditions, the pupal stage lasts 1 to 3 months; when the flies emerge, they mate very quickly and the females begin to lay eggs. The adult flies live 8 days or less.

In some regions, the larvae of *Hypoderma* cause substantial economic losses. In France, losses due to bovine hypodermiasis have been estimated to be more than US$35 million annually; in the United States (in 1956), losses were US$192 million, and in Great Britain, £13 million (Soulsby, 1982).

The economic losses are due mainly to stunted growth, decrease in the production of milk and meat, and deterioration of the hides.

The most affected animals are calves. Adult animals are less vulnerable, since some resistance is established with age. The number of furuncles can vary from one to several hundred. Secondary infection usually leads to the formation of abscesses. Migration of *H. bovis* larvae through the epidural fat of the spinal canal may cause inflammation and necrosis of the adipose tissue and sometimes of the periosteum. The larvae of *H. lineatum* can cause stenosis and inflammation of the tissues underlying the esophageal mucosa. Adult flies, when abundant, cause restlessness in cattle, provoke stampedes, and interfere with feeding.

Man is an accidental and aberrant host of the larvae of *H. bovis*, *H. lineatum*, and rarely *H. diana* (whose larvae parasitize European deer). The development of the parasite in humans is generally arrested in the first larval stage and rarely reaches the third, mature stage. A serologic study (immunoelectrophoresis) of more than 100 cases in France concluded that the species that most frequently affects man is *H. bovis* (Doby and Deunff, 1982). The myiasis it causes is subcutaneous and only occasionally does a conjunctival or conjunctivo-palpebral invasion occur. Endophthalmias are rare. The cutaneous invasion may be manifested as a serpiginous myiasis similar to cutaneous larva migrans or as a subcutaneous myiasis with moving furuncles that appear and disappear. The parasitism may cause pruritus, restlessness, pain, and stomachal disorders (Harwood and James, 1979). Children are affected more frequently than adults.

Most of the life cycle of *Hypoderma* takes place in the animal (10 months out of 12); consequently, the larval phase is the best point to attack the fly. The basic control procedure consists of treating bovines with larvicides. Early treatment with organophosphate insecticides is carried out at the beginning of autumn in order to prevent the larva from completing its development and establishing itself under the skin. This procedure prevents economic losses and obstructs further development of the fly. To reduce the risk of nerve damage caused by the destruction of intraspinal larvae after application of the larvicide, it is best not to administer the treatment in late autumn when larval migration is well advanced.

When an animal is treated for hypodermiasis or dermatobiasis in the manner described above, its milk should not be consumed for 48 hours, and the animal should not be slaughtered for food for 7 days or more, depending on the insecticide employed.

Late treatment is done in spring, when the first manifestations of the subcutaneous localization of the larvae are noted. Skin lotions or powders containing active ingredients such as dichlorobenzene, rotenone, or organophosphorus compounds are used to kill the larvae in situ through the furuncular orifice.

This myiasis has been eradicated in several European countries, including Sweden, Denmark, the Netherlands, Cyprus, and Bavaria, West Germany. Good results were also obtained in Ireland, where the infestation rate was reduced to very low levels.

7. Myiasis Caused by Larvae of *Oestrus ovis* and *Rhinoestrus purpurensis*

The adult of *Oestrus ovis*, a gray fly 10 to 12 mm in length, is larviparous, depositing larvae in the nostrils of sheep, goats, and, occasionally, man. Its distribution is worldwide, and it is found in all areas where sheep are raised. *Rhinoestrus purpurensis* (*R. purpureus*) is similar to *O. ovis* in its morphology and development cycle. The larval forms are obligate parasites of equines and develop in their nasal sinuses and larynx. The fly is found in Europe, Asia, and Africa.

The first larvae enter the nasal fossae and feed on mucus and desquamated cells; then they penetrate the frontal or maxillary sinuses where they mature. At the end of 2 to 10 months, the mature larva migrates again to the nasal fossae where it is expelled by sneezing, falls to the ground, and pupates for 4 to 5 weeks. The fly that emerges from the pupa lives 2 to 28 days.

The adult fly is annoying to animals, and when it is abundant it provokes restlessness. The larva causes chronic rhinitis and sinusitis. The morbidity rate in a flock may be very high, but mortality is nil. The most prominent symptom is a mucopurulent nasal discharge. Breathing is sometimes made difficult because of swelling of the nasal mucosa.

Man is an accidental and aberrant host in which the larva does not develop beyond the first stage. Human cases of myiasis by *O. ovis* have been described in several parts of the world, including the United States, Ecuador, Chile, and Uruguay. In Benghazi, Libya, 80 cases of external ophthalmomyiasis were diagnosed in 2 years, representing an estimated incidence of 10 per 100,000 inhabitants. The parasitosis occurs mostly among shepherds, but in that area cases also occur in urban inhabitants since sheep are maintained in residential zones (Dar *et al.*, 1980). The most common form in man is conjunctival invasion, evidenced by lacrimation and the sensation of a foreign body in the eye. In general, it is a benign disease that lasts only a few days since the larva cannot develop beyond the first stage. Serious cases, with destruction of the eye and perforation of the orbital walls, are rare. In Africa, cases of oral and nasal myiasis have occurred, in which the larvae penetrate the nasal fossae and frontal sinuses and produce local pain, frontal headache, and insomnia. The course is usually 3 to 10 days. Cases of external auditory canal invasion (otomyiasis) have also been described.

Treatment with organophosphorus compounds is effective against all larval phases and, if carried out annually, can substantially reduce the fly population in a livestock establishment.

8. Myiasis Caused by Larvae of *Gasterophilus* spp.

The three most important species are *Gasterophilus intestinalis*, *G. nasalis*, and *G. haemorrhoidalis*. These species are widely distributed on all continents. Other species (*G. inermis*, *G. pecorum*, and *G. nigricornis*) are limited to the Old World. The normal hosts of the larvae of these flies are horses and other equines, in which the larvae lodge in the stomach. The rates of larval infection in equines are high in many parts of the world. The site of oviposition depends on the species of fly; *G. intestinalis*, which is the most common, deposits its eggs mainly on the lower part of the horse's front legs, *G. nasalis* on the skin of the submaxillary region, and *G. haemorrhoidalis* on the lip hairs. Depending on the species of fly, the larva emerges from the eggs in 3 to 7 days. It is carried to the mouth by the animal licking or biting itself, invades the oral mucosa, and after 1 month moves to the pharynx and finally to the cardiac of the stomach, where it completes its growth in 8 to 10 months. It has been estimated that less than 1% of the larvae lodge in the glandular part of the stomach. In the spring, when the larvae are mature, they are eliminated with the feces, pupate in the ground for about a month, and give rise to the adult fly, which reinitiates the cycle.

Little is known about the effect of stomach infection by *Gasterophilus* spp. larvae on the health of equines. According to some observations, the infection can cause anorexia and mild colic. Ulceration of the nonglandular portion of the stomach is the most frequent lesion. Abscesses, rupture of the stomach, and peritonitis may occasionally occur (Soulsby, 1982). Adult flies frighten and disturb the animals.

In man, the larvae rarely develop beyond the first stage and only exceptionally reach the stomach. The most common clinical form is a dermal affliction similar to cutaneous larva migrans (see that disease), with superficial serpiginous tunnels in the skin that stand out as red stripes on the skin surface. The lesion is accompanied by intense itching. The species that most frequently attacks man is *G. intestinalis*, and the lesions are generally located on the extremities. Persons most affected are those in close contact with equines.

Since the larvae remain for a long time in the horse's stomach, this stage presents a good point of attack for interrupting the fly's life cycle and reducing its population. All horses in an establishment should be given two doses of dichlorvos or metrifonate, one at the end of autumn and the other at the end of winter or in early spring.

9. Myiasis Caused by Larvae of *Wohlfahrtia* spp.

Specific myiases are also caused by larvae of *Wohlfahrtia vigil* and *W. magnifica*, flies of the family Sarcophagidae. Both species are larviparous. *W. vigil* occurs in Canada and the United States, where its larvae parasitize rodents, lagomorphs, foxes, mink, dogs, other carnivores, and occasionally man. The adult flies feed on plant nectar. The larvae are deposited in packets, either on the animals or in their environment, and penetrate intact skin to produce a furuncular lesion. The larvae mature in 7 to 9 days, abandon the animal, and pupate for 10 to 12 days. Eleven to 17 days after the adults emerge, they begin larviposition and the cycle is completed (Faust *et al.*, 1975).

W. vigil is a major pest on mink and fox breeding farms in Canada and the northern United States. Newborn and young animals are the most exposed. In rodents, this fly can cause severe tissue destruction. In humans, the infestation is limited to children who spend time outdoors, in whom it causes small subcutaneous abscesses, irritability, fever, and dehydration.

W. magnifica occurs in the European and African Mediterranean area, the Middle East, the USSR, and China. The fly is attracted to skin wounds; it deposits its larvae in these wounds and also in natural orifices of humans, sheep, bovines, and other domestic animals, including geese and other birds (Harwood and James, 1979). *W. magnifica* myiasis is an important disease of sheep in the southern part of the USSR. The larvae are large and can cause serious deformities in man if they are not extirpated in time.

10. Semispecific Myiases

A large number of dipterans of various species, genera, and families are facultative parasites of animals and man. These flies, which normally lay their eggs or larvae on decomposing meat or dead animals, occasionally invade necrotic tissue of wounds on live animals. The larvae of these dipterans do not penetrate healthy skin and rarely invade recent, clean wounds. Their medical importance lies in the fact that the larvae of some species do not always restrict themselves to feeding on necrotic tissues, but can occasionally penetrate deeply and damage healthy tissues. One such species is *Lucilia* (*Phaenicia*) *sericata*, whose larvae do not usually cause major damage, but do sometimes destroy healthy tissue in wounds and can invade the human nasal fossae in large numbers.

Most of the dipterans that cause semispecific myiases belong to the families Sarcophagidae and Calliphoridae. In the myiases that occur in the Americas, *Cochliomyia hominivorax*, whose larva is a primary agent, must be distinguished from *C. macellaria*, which is a secondary invader. The larvae of several of these dipteran species are the agents of "calliphorine myiasis" ("blowfly" or "fleece-fly strike" in Australia), which causes great economic losses in sheep in certain areas. The most susceptible breed is the merino, and the highest incidence of the disease occurs in Australia, South Africa, and Great Britain. In hot, humid summers when the population of calliphorine flies is large, sheep suffer in their development, and losses occur in both wool and meat production. Invasion by larvae of these flies may also cause high mortality. In Australia, the most important flies are *Lucilia cuprina*, *L. sericata*, and various species of the genus *Calliphora*; in Canada and the United States, *Phormia regina* and *Protophormia terraenovae*. The most common site of larval invasion is the anal-vulvar or anal-preputial region, where the skin often becomes excoriate by soft feces and urine whose odor attracts the flies. Any accidental or surgical wound (docking, castration) may be the seat of calliphorine myiasis. According to some authors, a lesion is not essential for invasion to occur, since in hot summers with abundant rains followed by sunshine, tufts of wool may rot close to their base and attract swarms of flies.

When the density of calliphorine flies is low, the larvae are deposited in dead animals. The situation changes when climatic conditions favor a rapid increase in the fly population; this leads to invasion of contaminated wounds, especially around wet and dirty wool. The life cycle of these flies can be completed in a few weeks or, under particularly favorable conditions, in only one week, allowing many generations of flies to be born in a single season.

In areas where calliphorine flies are a problem, wool should be sheared between the hind legs and around the tail, and dips or sprays containing larvicides and insecticides (ronnel, coumaphos, diazinon) should be used. All wounds, whether new or already invaded, should be treated immediately and protected with larvicides. The bodies of dead animals, on which these flies multiply, should be removed by incineration or burial. Studies carried out in Australia with a drying agent (mixture of zinc and aluminum oxides with sterols and several fatty acids) have confirmed that its application to sheep wool can prevent 75% of calliphorine myiases (Hall *et al.*, 1980).

11. Accidental Myiases

Accidental myiases are due to flies of numerous families that normally deposit their eggs or larvae in fecal matter, decomposing plants, or other substances suitable for their development. These flies can lay eggs or larvae accidentally on human or animal foods, giving rise to an intestinal myiasis. Most eggs or larvae ingested in this way are destroyed in the digestive tract, but some survive and continue their larval development. The fly *Sarcophaga haemorrhoidalis* has been found on several occasions to be responsible for intestinal myiasis. Larvae of other flies, such as *Musca domestica*, *Fannia canicularis*, *F. scalaris*, *Muscina stabulans*, and several species of Calliphoridae and Sarcophagidae can also cause intestinal myiasis (Harwood and James, 1979). Many times the ingested larvae are eliminated with the feces without causing any damage or symptoms. In other cases there may be abdominal pain, nausea, and, in intense infestations, bloody diarrhea and damage to the intestinal mucosa. Myiases of the urinary tract (cystomyiasis) have also been described, but are rare. Recently, a case was described in India of urethral myiasis caused by larvae of the domestic fly in a patient immobilized in a hospital bed; part of the glans was necrotic (Gupta *et al.*, 1983). Cases of urogenital myiasis are also known from other parts of the world. These infestations have usually occurred in immobilized elderly patients suffering from incontinence. In rural areas some cases have been originated by larvae of the fly *Fannia* spp., which is abundant in privies (Pospisil and Povolny, 1980). In some of the urogenital myiases, as in the enteric ones, the larvae did not go beyond the first stage, that is, they could not feed and develop ("pseudomyiasis"), but in other cases second and third-stage larvae were found in the bladder.

Role of Animals in the Epidemiology of the Disease: Animals play an essential role in the life cycle of the flies whose larvae cause specific myiases. Man is only an accidental host of these larvae, and in some myiases, such as those due to *Oestrus ovis* or *Gasterophilus* spp., an aberrant host in which the larvae cannot complete their development.

Larval invasions of human skin or natural cavities occur when there is a high incidence of animal myiasis. The victims are persons in rural areas where the flies and the natural hosts of their larvae are abundant.

Control: Specific myiases of animals are controlled mainly with the measures described above for each fly species. The same measures apply to prevention of human myiases. In man, any wound should be treated as soon as possible and taken care of until it heals. Personal and environmental hygiene measures are important to prevent the disease in man.

Bibliography

Atias, A., R. Donckaster, H. Schenone, and M. Olivares. Myiasis ocular producida por larvas de *Oestrus ovis*. *Bol Chile Parasitol* 25:37-38, 1960.

Beesley, W. N. Arthropods–Oestridae, myiases and acarines. *In*: Soulsby, E. J. L. (Ed.), *Parasitic Zoonoses*. New York, Academic Press, 1974.

Blood, D. C., and J. A. Henderson. *Veterinary Medicine*, 4th ed. Baltimore, Maryland, Williams and Wilkins, 1974.

Brown, H. W., and D. L. Belding. *Parasitología Clínica*, 2nd ed. México, Interamericana, 1965.

Dar, M. S., M. Ben Amer, F. K. Dar, and V. Papazotos. Ophthalmomyiasis caused by the sheep nasal bot, *Oestrus ovis* (Oestridae) larvae, in the Benghazi area of eastern Libya. *Trans R Soc Trop Med Hyg* 74:303-306, 1980.

Doby, J. M., and J. Deunff. Considerations sur le fréquence respective des espèces d'hypodermes (Insecta, Diptera, Oestroidea) à l'origine des cas humains d'hyperdermose en France. *Ann Parasitol Hum Comp* 57:497-505, 1982.

Del Ponte, E. *Manual de Entomología Médica y Veterinaria Argentinas*. Buenos Aires, Librería del Colegio, 1958.

Euzéby, J. Traitement et prophylaxie d'hypodermose des bovins: données actuelles. *Rev Méd Vét* 127:187-235, 1976.

Faust, E. C., P. F. Russell, and R. C. Jung. *Parasitología Clínica*. México, Salvat, 1974.

Faust, E. C., P. C. Beaver, and R. C. Jung. *Animal Agents and Vectors of Human Disease*, 4th ed. Philadelphia, Lea and Febiger, 1975.

Gupta, S. C., S. Kumar, and A. Srivastava. Urethral myiasis. *Trop Geogr Med* 35:73-74, 1983.

Hall, C. A., I. C. A. Martin, and P. A. McDonnell. The effect of a drying agent (B26) on wool moisture and blowfly strike. *Res Vet Sci* 29:186-189, 1980.

Harwood, R. F., and M. T. James. *Entomology in Human and Animal Health*, 7th ed. New York, Macmillan, 1979.

Hevia, H., H. Schenone, F. Pescetto, and H. Reyes. Myiasis tegumentarias. *Bol Chile Parasitol* 16:96-98, 1961.

James, M. T. *The Flies That Cause Myiasis in Man*. Washington, D.C., Bureau of Entomology and Plant Quarantine. US Department of Agriculture, 1948. (Publication 631.)

Jensen, R. *Diseases of Sheep*. Philadelphia, Lea and Febiger, 1974.

Magnarelli, L. A., and T. G. Andreadis. Human cases of furuncular, traumatic, and nasal myiasis in Connecticut. *Am J Trop Med Hyg* 30:894-896, 1981.

Marin-Rojas, R. Control inmunológico del tórsalo (*Dermatobia hominis* L. Jr.) Notas preliminares. *Rev Latinoamer Microbiol* 17:21-24, 1975.

Miller, R. B. Screwworms. *In*: Hillyer, C. V., and C. E. Hopla (Section Eds.), *CRC Handbook Series in Zoonoses*. Section C, vol. 3. Boca Raton, Florida, CRC Press, 1982.

Pessôa, S. B. *Parasitología Médica*, 6th ed. Rio de Janeiro, Koogan, 1963.

Pospisil, L., and D. Povolny. Ein einwandfrer Nachweis der urogenitalen Myiasis in Mitteleuropa, verursacht von der Fleischfliége *Thyrsocnema incisilobata* (Pandellé, 1896) (Diptera, Sarcophagidae). *Zentralbl Bakteriol Mikrobiol Hyg* [A] 247:418-423, 1980.

Rawlins, S. C. Current trends in screwworm myiasis in the Caribbean region. *Vet Parasitol* 18:241-250, 1985.

Readshaw, J. L. Screwworm eradication a grand delusion? *Nature* 320:407-410, 1986.

Sharman, R. Myiases as Zoonoses of Importance in the Americas. *In*: *II Inter-American Meeting on Foot-and-Mouth Disease and Zoonoses Control*. Washington, D.C., Pan American Health Organization, 1970. (Scientific Publication 196.)

Smith, D. R., and R. R. Clevenger. Nosocomial nasal myiasis. *Arch Pathol Lab Med* 110:439-440, 1986.

Soulsby, E. J. L. *Helminths, Arthropods and Protozoa of Domesticated Animals*, 7th ed. Philadelphia, Lea and Febiger, 1982.

Steelman, C. D. Effects of external and internal arthropod parasites on domestic livestock production. *Ann Rev Entomol* 21:155-178, 1976. Cited in Harwood and James, 1979.

PENTASTOMIASES

(136.9)

Neither the taxonomy of the pentastomids nor their phylogenetic status is yet well defined. Some researchers assign them an intermediate position between Arthropoda and Annelida and have proposed placing them in a separate phylum. However, on the basis of ultrastructural, embryologic, and genetic studies they are currently considered to constitute a class, Pentastomida, within the Arthropoda (Self, 1982). The class Pentastomida contains two genera of medical interest, Linguatula *and* Armillifer.

1. Linguatuliasis

Etiology: *Linguatula serrata*, a linguiform parasite; the adult female measures about 10 cm long, and the male barely 2 cm. The adults lodge in the nasal passages, frontal sinuses, and tympanic cavities of dogs, other canids, and felids.

The development cycle of the parasite requires an intermediate host. This role is fulfilled by herbivores, mainly sheep, goats, and lagomorphs, but also bovines, deer, equines, swine, and several other species of mammals. Man is an accidental and aberrant intermediate host.

The embryonated eggs laid by linguatulae in the upper respiratory passages of the host are expelled to the exterior by sneezing and spitting, or with the feces if the eggs are swallowed. The eggs ingested by the intermediate host with food or water release the first-stage larvae in the intestine; they possess four clawed feet and an apparatus that allows them to perforate the intestinal wall. The first larvae migrate to the thoracic and abdominal cavities and encyst in different organs, such as the lymph glands, liver, spleen, and lungs, where they form small pentastomid nodules that are discovered in the veterinary inspection of meat. About 250 to 300 days after the infection and after a series of molts within the cyst, the larva reaches the infective or nymph stage. The nymph is about 5 mm long and resembles the adult parasite. It can break the cystic envelope, migrate through the peritoneal cavity, and penetrate different tissues. When a carnivore ingests the parasite along with tissues or organs of an infected intermediate host, the infective nymph migrates through the stomach and esophagus to the nasopharynx, where it undergoes several molts, reaches maturity, and begins oviposition, thus renewing the cycle.

Geographic Distribution and Occurrence: *L. serrata* is widely distributed throughout the world. Human infection is infrequent and most cases have been recorded in several countries of Europe, the Middle East, and North Africa. In the Americas, human linguatuliasis has been diagnosed in Brazil, Chile, Colombia, Panama, Cuba, the United States, and Canada.

The infection rate in dogs is very high in some areas. *L. serrata* was found in 43.3% of stray dogs in Beirut, Lebanon, 38% in parts of India, and a high percentage in Mexico City. The highest rates are seen in areas where dogs are fed raw viscera from sheep and goats. Infected dogs have been found in the Midwest and in Georgia, USA, but the prevalence rate obtained by coprologic examination was very low (Ehrenford and Newberne, 1981). Data on the frequency of larvonymphal infection in domestic herbivores are not available. In Lebanon, four of 10 goat livers acquired in 10 randomly selected butcher shops had larvae in the hepatic lymph nodes; of an equal number of sheep livers, two were parasitized. In the United States, the principal intermediate hosts seem to be wild rabbits, which have been found infected in several southern states (Gardiner *et al.*, 1984). A study carried out in eight southeastern states found 2% of 260 *Sylvilagus floridanus* rabbits to harbor nymphs of *L. serrata*, but the infections were not intense (Andrews *et al.*, 1980).

The Disease in Man: Man can become infected by ingesting either eggs or nymphs.

When the infection occurs by ingesting eggs, the larvae that hatch become encapsulated in various organs and can survive for about 2 years. Upon dying, the larvae are absorbed or the cyst calcifies. The larvae mainly locate in the liver, either beneath Glisson's capsule or in the parenchyma and, to a lesser extent, in the mesentery and intestinal wall. The encysted nymphs generally do not produce clinical symptoms, and the infection is almost always discovered by surgery, radiologic examination, or autopsy. Described clinical cases have included prostatitis, ocular infection (anterior chamber of the eye), and acute abdomen due to a parasitized and inflamed lymph node adhering to the intestinal wall.

The "halzoun" and "marrara" syndromes are currently attributed to infection caused by ingestion of the nymph of *L. serrata* with raw or undercooked liver or lymph nodes from goats and sheep. Halzoun occurs in Lebanon, Turkey, and Greece, and marrara, a similar syndrome, in Sudan. The symptoms appear a few minutes to a half hour after the infective food is eaten. The variation in the incubation period probably depends on the place where the nymphs are released from their cysts, since those that are swallowed require more time to migrate to the tonsils and nasopharyngeal mucosa than those that become free in the mouth. The most prominent symptoms are irritation and pain in the throat. Sometimes there is congestion and intense edema of the region, which may extend to the larynx, eustachian tube, conjunctiva, nose, and lips. Lacrimation and a runny nose are frequent. Sometimes there is also dyspnea, dysphagia, vomiting, headaches, photophobia, and exophthalmia. The most serious symptomatology is believed to occur in persons sensitized by visceral infections with *L. serrata*. The course of the disease is rapid and benign. About 50% of the patients recuperate in less than 1 day; in others the illness may last 1 or 2 weeks.

The Disease in Animals: The adult parasite causes a mucopurulent nasal catarrh, with sneezing, copious nasal discharge, and sometimes epistaxis. However, in mild infections no lesion is found in the nasal conchae.

Larval infection in domestic herbivores and omnivores (intermediate hosts) is asymptomatic. The parasites only cause damage to the affected organs when they are present in large numbers.

Source of Infection and Mode of Transmission (Figure 105): The natural reservoirs are wild and domestic canids and felids. Carnivores acquire the infection by ingesting viscera and tissues of the intermediate hosts. In endemic areas, the cycles between dogs and goats and dogs and sheep are of special interest. Hunting dogs become infected when they capture infected lagomorphs. In the wild cycle the infection circulates between wild herbivores and their carnivore predators.

Herbivores become infected by ingesting pasture contaminated with feces or secretions of the definitive hosts.

Figure 105. Pentastomiasis (*Linguatula serrata*). Transmission cycle.

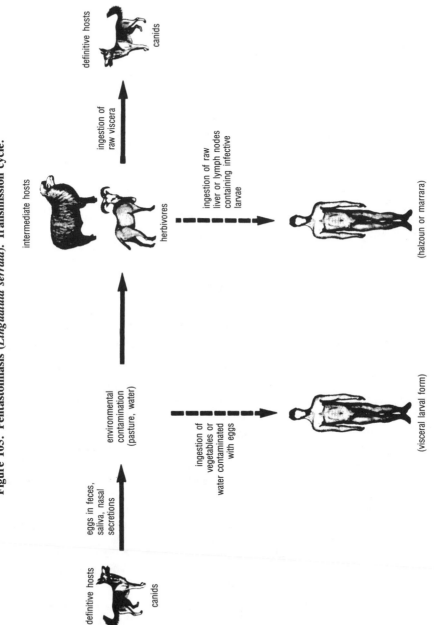

Man acquires the visceral form by consuming vegetables or water contaminated with parasite eggs that were shed with fecal material, saliva, or the nasal discharge of dogs or other definitive hosts. Man contracts halzoun or marrara by consuming raw liver or lymph nodes from sheep or goats (or other domestic herbivores) parasitized by the infective nymphs.

Diagnosis: The visceral form (small pentastomid nodules) caused by the nymphs is rarely diagnosed in living persons (unless found during surgery) or living domestic animals. Radiographs showing calcified cysts may arouse suspicion of the infection's presence. Specific diagnosis is effected by identification of the nymph in a biopsy specimen. Histopathologic examination reveals a granulomatous tissue reaction with multiple eosinophilic abscesses, at the center of which degenerated nymphs are found (Ali-Khan and Bowmer, 1972).

In cases of halzoun or marrara, the larva should be obtained for identification.

In dogs with suspicious nasal catarrh, diagnosis can be confirmed by detecting eggs in the feces.

Control: Prevention of the visceral infection consists of observing the rules of food hygiene. To avoid halzoun or marrara, organs of domestic animals should not be eaten raw or undercooked.

Dogs should not be fed raw viscera of goats, sheep, or other animals.

2. Armilliferiasis

Etiology: *Armillifer armillatus*, *A. moniliformis*, and *A. grandis* are cylindrical, vermiform pentastomids of the family Porocephalidae which in the adult state live in the respiratory tract of snakes.

The life cycle of *Armillifer* is similar to that of *Linguatula* (see Linguatuliasis) with the difference that the definitive hosts are snakes and the intermediate hosts are mainly wild rodents on which snakes feed. The female of *Armillifer* deposits eggs in the respiratory cavities of the reptiles, and the eggs are expectorated or swallowed and then eliminated with the feces. The life cycles of the different species are not yet well known.

Geographic Distribution and Occurrence: *A. armillatus* and *A. grandis* are African species. *A. moniliformis* is found in Asia.

Armilliferiasis occurs mainly in southeastern and southern Asia and western Africa (Nigeria, Zaire); it seems to be infrequent in eastern and southern Africa. No cases of armilliferiasis have been diagnosed in the Americas.

Encysted larvae were found in 22.5% of adults autopsied in a hospital in Kinshasa, Zaire, and in 8% of the autopsies in Cameroon; they were also discovered in 1.4% of the radiographs taken in a university hospital in Ibadan, Nigeria. A high infection rate (45.4%) was found by postmortem examination of Senoi natives in Malaysia. The most frequent locations are the liver and lungs.

The Disease in Man: It is similar to the visceral form of linguatuliasis and generally asymptomatic. The infected person usually harbors few nymphs (from 1 to 12). A high parasite load can give rise to a serious disease, especially if the larvae lodge in vital organs, where they can produce multifocal abscesses, tumors, or obstruction of ducts (Self *et al.*, 1975).

Figure 106. Pentastomiasis (*Armillifer* spp.). Transmission cycle.

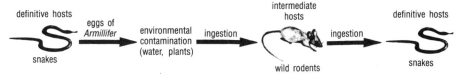

The Disease in Animals: Nonhuman primates also are accidental hosts of the infection. The larvae of *Armillifer* spp. are found mainly in Old World primates and less commonly in those of the Americas. The infection is usually asymptomatic.

Source of Infection and Mode of Transmission (Figure 106): The reservoirs and definitive hosts of *Armillifer* spp. are snakes, probably including all members of the families Boidae and Viperidae (Self, 1982). Snakes become infected by swallowing wild mammals containing the nymph.

Man contracts the infection by consuming water or vegetables contaminated with eggs eliminated in the feces or saliva of snakes, by consuming raw or undercooked snake meat, or by handling these reptiles and placing contaminated hands to the mouth. Other intermediate hosts are infected in a similar manner. It should be noted that the eggs of *Armillifer* are resistant to environmental factors.

Diagnosis: Some cases can be diagnosed by radiographic examination, which reveals the calcified, half-moon-shaped larvae. In most cases, however, the encapsulated larvae of pentastomids are found during autopsy or by laparotomies performed for other reasons.

Control: Preventive measures consist of observing the rules of food hygiene.

Bibliography

Ali-Khan, Z., and E. J. Bowmer. Pentastomiasis in western Canada: a case report. *Am J Trop Med Hyg* 21:58-61, 1972.

Andrews, C. L., W. R. Davidson, and E. E. Provost. Endoparasites of selected populations of cottontail rabbits (*Sylvilagus floridanus*) in the southeastern United States. *J Wildl Dis* 16:395-401, 1980.

Borchert, A. *Parasitología Veterinaria*. Zaragoza, Spain, Acribia, 1964.

Ehrenford, F. A., and J. W. Newberne. An aid to clinical diagnosis of tongue worms (*Linguatula serrata*) in dogs. *Lab Anim Sci* 31:74-76, 1981.

Faust, E. C., P. F. Russell, and R. C. Jung. *Craig and Faust's Clinical Parasitology*, 8th ed. Philadelphia, Lea and Febiger, 1970.

Gardiner, C. H., J. W. Dyke, and S. F. Shirley. Hepatic granuloma due to a nymph of *Linguatula serrata* in a woman from Michigan: a case report and review of the literature. *Am J Trop Med Hyg* 33:187-189, 1984.

Gill, H. S., B. V. Rao, and R. C. Chhabra. A note on the occurrence of *Linguatula serrata* (Frohlich 1789) in domesticated animals. *Trans R Soc Trop Med Hyg* 62:506-508, 1968.

Hopps, H. C., H. L. Keegan, S. L. Price, and J. T. Self. Pentastomiasis. *In*: Marcial-Rojas, R. A. (Ed.), *Pathology of Protozoal and Helminthic Diseases*. Baltimore, Maryland, Williams and Wilkins, 1971.

Khalil, G. M., and J. F. Schacher. *Linguatula serrata* in relation to halzoun and the marrara syndrome. *Am J Trop Med Hyg* 14:736-746, 1965.

Kuntz, R. E. Biology of pentastome parasites: pentastomiasis in nonhuman primates. *In*: *Proceedings, Third International Congress of Parasitology*. Munich, Facta Publications, 1974.

Meyers, W. M., R. C. Neafie, and D. H. Connor. Pentastomiasis. *In*: Binford, C. H., and D. H. Connor (Eds.), *Pathology of Tropical and Extraordinary Diseases*, vol. 2. Washington, D.C., Armed Forces Institute of Pathology, 1976.

Prathap, K., K. S. Lau, and J. M. Bolton. Pentastomiasis: A common finding at autopsy among Malaysian aborigenes. *Am J Trop Med Hyg* 18:20-27, 1969.

Self, J. T., and R. E. Kuntz. Host-parasite relations in some Pentastomida. *J Parasitol* 53:202-206, 1970.

Self, J. T., H. C. Hopps, and A. O. Williams. Pentastomiasis in Africans. *Trop Geogr Med* 27:1-13, 1975.

Self, J. T. Pentastomiasis. *In*: Hillyer, G. V., and C. E. Hopla (Section Eds.), *CRC Handbook Series in Zoonoses*. Section C, vol. 3. Boca Raton, Florida, CRC Press, 1982.

TUNGIASIS

(134.1)

Synonyms: Chigoe, jigger flea, burrowing flea, sand flea, nigua, pique, bicho de pé, bicho de porco.

Etiology: A small flea, *Tunga* (*Sarcopsylla*) *penetrans*. The ovigerous female is an obligate parasite of warm-blooded animals, including swine, man, and non-human primates.

The pregnant female penetrates the skin of man or another animal, where she feeds continuously on blood and deposits her eggs. After entering the host, the flea enlarges to a spherical form about 5 mm in diameter, approximately five times its size before skin penetration. The eggs are expelled through the opening in the skin, and if they fall on sandy soil the larvae hatch in 3 to 4 days. The larvae molt twice and then bury themselves in the ground to pupate. Under favorable conditions, the larval and pupal stages last no more than 10 to 14 days each (Harwood and James, 1979). Both males and females of the young adult fleas that emerge at the end of the pupal stage feed on the blood of animals. After mating, the male dies and the female penetrates the skin of an animal and reinitiates the cycle with oviposition.

Geographic Distribution and Occurrence: *Tunga penetrans* is believed to be native to the tropical and subtropical regions of Central America, the Caribbean, and South America. Currently, human and animal tungiasis is infrequent in the Americas, due perhaps to the use of insecticides in the antimalarial campaigns.

Indications exist that *T. penetrans* was introduced or reintroduced into Africa in 1872 by a British ship that arrived from South America and unloaded its sand ballast on the beaches of Angola. Whether by this means or by means of infested members of the crew, *T. penetrans* was introduced into Angola and spread from there to the whole western coast of Africa; it later reached eastern Africa and Madagascar.

Outside Africa and the Americas, *T. penetrans* is present in western India and in Pakistan, where it was probably introduced by workers returning home from Africa (Connor, 1976; Harwood and James, 1979).

In some parts of Africa, human infestation by *T. penetrans* can reach very high rates. In a village in the state of Lagos, Nigeria, 373 children 6 to 14 years old were examined and 41.5% were found to harbor the flea in their toes. Prevalence declines with age, a fact that is attributed to the greater thickness of the skin of older persons as well as their more frequent use of footwear (Ade-Serrano and Ejezie, 1981).

Little information is available about the frequency of infestation in animals. Outbreaks in swine have been described in Tanzania and Zaire (Cooper, 1967; Verhulst, 1976).

The Disease in Man and Animals: The flea usually penetrates the human epidermis in the instep, toes, interdigital spaces, or under the edge of a toenail, but it can lodge in any exposed part of the body. Upon penetration, the insect produces a mild but persistent pruritus; later, as it increases in size, it causes swelling of the surrounding tissue and localized pain. The pain is particularly intense when the flea penetrates under a nail. The female of *T. penetrans* reaches its maximum size in about 2 weeks; then it expels the eggs, collapses, dies, and is eliminated, leaving behind a crateriform ulceration. Purulent secondary infections occur frequently. The lesions originated by *Tunga* also offer favorable conditions for tetanus, gas gangrene, and blastomycosis. Only one or two lesions are usually found in an individual, but there can be hundreds.

In the outbreak that occurred in swine in Tanzania, the infestation affected the scrotum, feet, snout, and teats, but did not cause marked inflammation, pruritus, or pain (Cooper, 1967). The outbreak in Zaire was characterized mainly by agalactia of sows, resulting in the death of suckling pigs who could not feed because fleas infesting the maternal nipples obstructed or compressed the lactiferous ducts (Verhulst, 1976).

Source of Infection and Mode of Transmission *T. penetrans* is found primarily in dry and sandy places, inside and outside poorly constructed human dwellings, and in pigsties, stables, and chicken houses. Humans contract the infection by going barefoot in soil containing fleas that originated from swine or dogs infested with tungiasis. Dogs and sometimes swine can carry the infestation to huts with dirt floors. Conversely, man can introduce the fleas into the animals' environment.

Diagnosis: In areas where *T. penetrans* is common, diagnosis does not present any difficulties. Specific diagnosis can be made by extracting the flea from the skin for identification.

Control: Application of DDT or other insecticides eliminates the larvae and adult fleas from the environment and also from animals.

The use of shoes, especially boots, confers good protection. However, this simple preventive measure is difficult to apply in infested areas because of the low economic level of the population and the tropical climate.

Tungiasis by itself is innocuous, but secondary infections should be prevented. For that purpose, the flea should be extracted and the wound treated with an antiseptic and bandaged until it heals. One study (Ade-Serrano *et al.*, 1982) found treatment with niridazole to be useful; however, side effects were observed in 15.6% of the children treated (abdominal pain, nausea, and vomiting).

Bibliography

Ade-Serrano, M. A., and G. C. Ejezie. The prevalence of tungiasis in Oto-Ijanikin village of Badagry, Lagos State of Nigeria. *Ann Trop Med Parasitol* 75:471-472, 1981.

Ade-Serrano, M. A., O. G. Olomolehin, and A. Adewunmi. Treatment of human tungiasis with niridazole (Ambilhar), a double-blind placebo-controlled trial. *Ann Trop Med Parasitol* 76:89-92, 1982.

Connor, D. H. Tungiasis. *In*: Binford, C. H., and D. H. Connor (Eds.), *Pathology of Tropical and Extraordinary Diseases*, vol. 2. Washington, D.C., Armed Forces Institute of Pathology, 1976.

Cooper, J. E. An outbreak of *Tunga penetrans* in a pig herd. *Vet Rec* 80:365-366, 1967.

Del Ponte, E. *Manual de Entomología Médica y Veterinaria Argentinas*. Buenos Aires, Librería del Colegio, 1958.

Faust, E. C., P. F. Russell, and R. C. Jung. *Craig and Faust's Clinical Parasitology*, 8th ed. Philadelphia, Lea and Febiger, 1970.

Harwood, R. F., and M. T. James. *Entomology in Human and Animal Health*, 7th ed. New York, Macmillan, 1979.

Pessôa, S. B. *Parasitologia Médica*, 6th ed. Rio de Janeiro, Koogan, 1963.

Swellengrebel, N. H., and M. M. Sterman. *Animal Parasites in Man*. Princeton, Van Nostrand, 1961.

Verhulst, A. *Tunga penetrans* (*Sarcopsylla penetrans*) as a cause of agalactia in sows in the Republic of Zaire. *Vet Rec* 98:384, 1976.

ZOONOTIC SCABIES

(133.0)

Synonyms: Scabiosis, mange, sarcoptic acariasis.

Etiology: The agent of human scabies is the mite *Sarcoptes scabiei*. The female measures about 350 to 450 by 250 to 350 microns, and the male is about half that size. The mites of sarcoptic scabies lodge in furrows that they excavate in the epidermis of man or animals and lay their eggs there. The six-legged larvae emerge from the eggs after 3 to 8 days, and they excavate lateral tunnels or migrate below the epidermal scales. Some 4 to 6 days later the larvae give rise to eight-legged, first-stage nymphs, or protonymphs, which in turn transform into tritonymphs, and finally reach the adult stage. The ovigerous females that live (and die) in the tunnels reinitiate the cycle with oviposition. The entire life cycle can take 10 to 14 days.

Sarcoptic scabies affects man and a large number of domestic and wild animals. Some authors assign specific names to the mites of each animal species, such as *Sarcoptes scabiei* for the human parasite, *S. equi* for the horse parasite, *S. ovis* for the sheep parasite, etc. Others recognize only one species, *S. scabiei*, and regard the mites of different animal species as subspecies, varieties, or biological strains. Disregarding the taxonomic question, the fact is that the mites are not strictly species-specific and a mite of one animal species can live, at least temporarily, on other animal species, including man. For example, *S. equi* or *S. scabiei* var. *equi*, which is adapted to horses, can infect bovines and man, although generally for a short time. *Notoedres cati*, the agent of head scabies in cats, occasionally causes temporary dermatitis in humans (see also "Dermatitis Caused by Mites of Animal Origin").

Geographic Distribution and Occurrence: The mite is distributed worldwide. Human scabies is prevalent primarily among poor and undernourished persons in socioeconomic classes with low levels of hygiene. However, in the last few years a wave of human infestations unrelated to socioeconomic stratum, hygienic level, age, sex, or race occurred in Europe and the United States.

All animals raised by man for food and transportation are susceptible to *Sarcoptes* spp. Among pets and laboratory animals, dogs, rabbits, hamsters, and some non-human primates are afflicted by the mite. The infection is also seen in zoo animals.

Dog scabies is the variety most frequently transferred to man, but other sarcoptic scabies mites can also be transmitted when humans have close contact with animals (see Source of Infection and Mode of Transmission). It is believed that many cases diagnosed as insect bites or papular urticaria are really scabies of zoonotic origin (Smith and Claypole, 1967).

The Disease in Man: The disease due to the homologous (human) variety of *S. scabiei* is characterized by tunnels in the skin that may be a few millimeters to 2 cm long. These furrows are very thin and sinuous and are difficult to observe without the aid of a magnifying glass; they are generally not very abundant and are situated primarily in the skin of the interdigital spaces, back of the hand, elbows, axillae, torso, inguinal region, chest, penis, and navel. The most prominent symptom is itching, which is especially intense at night; the patient's scratching can give rise to new foci of scabies and, often, purulent secondary infections. The irritation and pruritus are manifested 1 or 2 weeks after infection occurs and may be an allergic reaction. Scabies can persist for a long time if not treated (lindane, tetraethylthiuram monosulfide, benzyl benzoate ointment).

The disease caused by animal sarcoptes is much more benign. The animal mites generally do not excavate tunnels in human skin, and the infection is superficial. However, a researcher who experimentally infested herself with canine sarcoptes was able to confirm by histopathologic examination the existence of mite tunnels in her skin (Kummel, cited in Schwartzman, 1983). The lesion can vary from an irritating papular eruption, which is the most frequent form, to an intense allergic sensitization with the appearance of vesicles. Excoriations are also frequent. The location of lesions in 22 patients infested by *S. scabiei* var. *canis* corresponded to the places most exposed to infested dogs, such as forearms, hands, torso, and thighs (Smith and Claypole, 1967). In 35 patients who were in contact with water buffaloes infested with *S. scabiei* var. *bubalis*, the lesions were distributed on the face, fingers, hands, thighs, and legs (Chakrabarti *et al.*, 1981). The interdigital folds and the external genital organs, which are frequently affected by the human mite, are places almost never attacked by sarcoptes of animal origin. The infection heals by itself in about 3 weeks. Spontaneous healing is attributed to the fact that the parasites either do not reproduce at all or do so only for a short time on the heterologous host. An infection lasting for a longer period of time is usually due to new exposures.

The Disease in Animals: Sarcoptic scabies in animals generally starts on the head and on areas of the body with delicate skin. In equines, the lesions are observed on the head and neck; in dogs, on the ear flaps, snout, and elbows. Like the human parasites, the mites of animals produce an allergic sensitization with intense itching and the formation of papules and vesicles. The vesicles open and become covered with scales and scabby plaques. There is proliferation of the connective tissue and keratinization, causing the skin to thicken and form creases. Hair loss in the affected regions is also frequent.

Scabies restricted to a small area does not particularly affect an animal's condition, but when it spreads to large areas of the body it can have an adverse impact on the animal's health.

Source of Infection and Mode of Transmission: The mite is transmitted mainly by very close contact with animals and, less frequently, by contaminated objects. The parasite can survive for several days off the animal's body—on clothing, towels, bedclothes, animal bedding, harnesses, and horse blankets—and thus these objects can serve as sources of infection.

Each animal species is a reservoir of the mite that attacks its own kind, but cross-transmission occurs occasionally between species.

Human scabies is transmitted mainly from person to person. Many animal species—such as equines, dogs, bovines, buffaloes, sheep, goats, swine, camels, and zoo animals—can occasionally transmit scabies to man. One of the main sources of zoonotic scabies is the dog. Infestation by *S. scabiei* var. *canis* occurs through close contact with scabietic dogs and can appear in several members of the family at the same time. It has been estimated that approximately 1% of the dogs in Great Britain have scabies; a study of 65 persons who had been in contact with 28 dogs with scabies confirmed the presence of scabietic lesions in 34 of them. In the US Army dermatology clinic at Fort Benning, Georgia, 20 cases of scabies acquired from dogs were observed in the course of 1 year (Smith and Claypole, 1967). Research at the University of Pennsylvania confirmed that approximately 33% of dogs with scabies originated infestations in members of their owners' families (Schwartzman, 1983). A study at the School of Veterinary Medicine of São Paulo, Brazil, traced the human contacts of 27 dogs with sarcoptic scabies; out of 143 exposed persons, cutaneous lesions compatible with scabies were found in 58 (40.6%) (Larsson, 1978). When scabies was still frequent in domestic animals in the Netherlands, about 25% of the veterinarians in rural areas were affected by sarcoptes of zoonotic origin. Scabies of animal origin is also seen elsewhere among rural inhabitants. Transmission of sarcoptic scabies (*S. scabiei* var. *bubalis*) from water buffaloes to man was described in India. Of 52 persons who had been in contact with scabietic buffaloes, 35 (67.3%) had symptoms of scabies, and the presence of the mite was confirmed in 22 (42.3%). All the persons who contracted the infestation (people in charge of handling and milking the buffaloes), had intense pruritus a few hours after their initial contact with the affected animals (Chakrabarti *et al.*, 1981).

Zoonotic scabies, although a nuisance, is not an important public health problem because it heals spontaneously and is not transmitted from person to person.

Diagnosis: Specific diagnosis of homologous infections does not present any difficulties. The parasite can be found in one or more of its developmental stages by microscopic examination of skin lesion scrapings treated with a potassium hydroxide solution.

Human scabies of zoonotic origin is more difficult to diagnose by laboratory methods. The mites are hard to find because they are usually few in number, due to the fact that they reproduce little or not at all on man.

Control: In order to prevent human scabies of zoonotic origin, animals must be treated with dips or sprays. Lindane, benzyl benzoate, and other scabicides have given excellent results in both human and animal cases. Lindane should also be applied to the places where animals are kept.

Bibliography

Borchert, A. *Parasitología Veterinaria*. Zaragoza, Spain, Acribia, 1964.

Chakrabarti, A. Some epidemiological aspects of animal scabies in human populations. *Int J Zoonoses* 12:39-52, 1985.

Chakrabarti, A., A. Chatterjee, K. Chakrabarti, and D. N. Sengupta. Human scabies from contact with water buffaloes infested with *Sarcoptes scabiei* var. *bubalis*. *Ann Trop Med Parasitol* 75:353-357, 1981.

Faust, E. C., P. F. Russell, and R. C. Jung. *Craig and Faust's Clinical Parasitology*, 8th ed. Philadelphia, Lea and Febiger, 1970.

Lapage, G. *Veterinary Parasitology*, 2nd ed. Edinburgh and London, Oliver and Boyd, 1968.

Larsson, M. H. Evidências epidemiológicas da ocorrência de escabiose em humanos, causada pelo *Sarcoptes scabiei* (Degeer, 1778) var. *canis* (Bourguignon, 1853). *Rev Saúde Pública* 12:333-339, 1978.

Schmitt, S. M., T. M. Cooley, P. D. Friedrich, and T. W. Schillhorn van Veen. Clinical mange of the black bear (*Ursus americanus*) caused by *Sarcoptes scabiei* (Acarina, Sarcoptidae). *J Wildl Dis* 23:162-164, 1987.

Schwartzman, R. M. Scabies in animals. *In*: Parish, L. C., W. B. Nutting, and R. M. Schwartzman (Eds.) *Cutaneous Infestations of Man and Animals*. New York, Praeger, 1983.

Smith, M. E., and C. T. Claypole. Canine scabies in dogs and in humans. *JAMA* 199:59-64, 1967.

Tas, J., and J. Van der Hoeden. Scabies. *In*: Van der Hoeden, J. (Ed.), *Zoonoses*. Amsterdam, Netherlands, Elsevier, 1964.

Thomsett, L. R. Mite infestations of man contracted from dogs and cats. *Br Med J* 3:93-95, 1968.

Yunker, C. E. Mites. *In*: Flynn, R. J., *Parasites of Laboratory Animals*. Ames, Iowa State University Press, 1973.

SUMMARY OF PARASITIC ZOONOSES

Below is reprinted the partial list of parasitic zoonoses from the Report of the
WHO Expert Committee, with the participation of FAO (*Parasitic Zoonoses*, Geneva, WHO, Technical Report Series 637, 1979), which can serve as a quick
reference for some characteristics of these infections.

This list is not comprehensive and is confined to those diseases in which the
animal link in the chain of infection to man is considered to be important, although
not always essential.

Diseases or causative organisms of particular importance over large areas have
been marked with an asterisk (*).

Disease in man	Causative organism	Principal vertebrate animals involved
1. PROTOZOAN INFECTIONS		
Amoebiasis	*Entamoeba histolytica*	Nonhuman primates, dogs
Babesiosis	*Babesia divergens*	Cattle
	Babesia microti	Voles, mice
Balantidiasis	*Balantidium coli*	Swine, rats, nonhuman primates
Giardiasis	*Giardia* species	Beavers
Leishmaniasis*		
Visceral	*Leishmania donovani*	Dogs, foxes, rodents
Cutaneous	*Leishmania tropica*	Dogs, rodents
Mucocutaneous	*Leishmania* species	Dogs, wild mammals
Malaria	*Plasmodium knowlesi*	Monkeys
	Plasmodium simium	Monkeys
	Plasmodium cynomolgi	Monkeys
Pneumocystis infection	*Pneumocystis carinii*	Dogs, rats
Sarcosporidiosis		
Intestinal	*Sarcocystis miesheriana* (syn. *S. suihominis*; = *Isospora hominis* proparte)	Pigs
	Sarcocystis hominis (syn. *S. bovihominis*; = *Isospora hominis* proparte)	Cattle
Muscle	*Sarcocystis* species (*S. lindemanni*)	Unknown
Toxoplasmosis*	*Toxoplasma gondii*	Cats, mammals, birds
Trypanosomiasis*		
African	*Trypanosoma rhodesiense*	Game animals, cattle
American	*Trypanosoma cruzi*	Dogs, cats, pigs, other small mammals
2. HELMINTHIC INFECTIONS		
TREMATODE INFECTIONS:		
Amphistomiasis	*Gastrodiscoides hominis*	Swine
Cercarial dermatitis	Schistosomatids	Birds, mammals
Clonorchiasis*	*Clonorchis sinensis*	Dogs, cats, swine, wild mammals, fish

Dicrocoeliasis	*Dicrocoelium dendriticum*	Ruminants
	Dicrocoelium hospes	Ruminants
Echinostomiasis	*Echinostoma ilocanum* and other *Echinostoma* species	Cats, dogs, rodents
Fascioliasis	*Fasciola hepatica*	Ruminants
	Fasciola gigantica	Ruminants
Fasciolopsiasis*	*Fasciolopsis buski*	Swine, dogs
Heterophyiasis	*Heterophyes heterophyes* and other heterophids	Cats, dogs, fish
Metagonimiasis	*Metagonimus yokogawai*	Cats, dogs, fish
Opisthorchiasis*	*Opisthorchis felineus*	Cats, dogs
	Opisthorchis viverrini and occasionally other *Opisthorchis* species	Cats, wildlife, fish
Paragonimiasis*	*Paragonimus westermani* and other *Paragonimus* species	Cats, dogs, wild felidae and suidae, rodents
Schistosomiasis	*Schistosoma japonicum**	Wild and domestic mammals
	Schistosoma haematobium	Rodents
	Schistosoma mansoni	Baboons, rodents
	Schistosoma mekongi	Dogs, monkeys
	Schistosoma mattheei and occasionally other schistosomes	Cattle, sheep, antelopes

CESTODE INFECTIONS:

Bertiella infection	*Bertiella studeri*	Primates
Coenuriasis	*Taenia multiceps*	Sheep, ruminants, pigs
	Taenia brauni	Dogs, rodents, wild carnivores
Diphyllobothriasis*	*Diphyllobothrium latum*	Fish, carnivores
Dipylidiasis	*Dipylidium caninum*	Dogs, cats
Echinococcosis*	*Echinococcus granulosus*	Dogs, wild carnivores, domestic and wild ungulates
	Echinococcus multilocularis	Foxes, cats, dogs, rodents
	Echinococcus vogeli	Dogs, bush dogs, pacas
Hymenolepiasis	*Hymenolepis diminuta*	Rats, mice
	Hymenolepis nana	Rats, mice
Inermicapsifer infection	*Inermicapsifer madagascariensis*	Rodents
Raillietina infection	*Raillietina madagascariensis*	Rodents
Sparganosis	Pseudophyllidean tapeworms	Cats, carnivores, mice, other vertebrates, amphibians
Taeniasis*	*Taenia saginata*	Cattle
Taeniasis-cysticercosis*	*Taenia solium*	Swine

NEMATODE INFECTIONS:

Ancylostomiasis	*Ancylostoma ceylanicum* and other *Ancylostoma* species	Dogs
Ascariasis	*Ascaris suum*	Swine
Capillariasis		
Hepatic	*Capillaria hepatica*	Rodents
Intestinal	*Capillaria philippinensis*	Fish
Dioctophymiasis	*Dioctophyme renale*	Fish, dogs, mustelids
Dracunculiasis*	*Dracunculus medinensis*	Dogs, other carnivores

Filariasis	*Brugia malayi* (subperiodic strain)	Primates, cats, dogs, wild carnivores
	Dirofilaria immitis	Dogs, cats, other mammals
	Dirofilaria repens	Dogs, cats, other mammals
	Dirofilaria tenuis	Dogs, cats, other mammals
Gongylonemiasis	*Gongylonema* species	Ruminants, rats
Lagochilascariasis	*Lagochilascaris minor*	Wild felidae
Larva migrans, cutaneous	*Ancylostoma brasiliense* and other *Ancylostoma* species	Cats, dogs
		Cats, dogs, sheep, swine, etc.
	Strongyloides species	
Larva migrans, visceral:		
Angiostrongyliasis	*Angiostrongylus cantonensis*	Rats
	Angiostrongylus costaricensis	Rats, coatimundi
Anisakiasis	Anisakine species	Fish, marine mammals
Gnathostomiasis	*Gnathostoma spinigerum*	Cats, dogs, other vertebrates (fish)
Toxocariasis	*Toxocara canis* and other *Toxocara* species	Dogs, cats
Mammomonogamiasis	*Mammomonogamus laryngeus*	Ruminants
Oesophagostomiasis	*Oesophagostomum apiostomum* and other *Oesophagostomum* species	Primates
Strongyloidiasis	*Strongyloides stercoralis*	Dogs, monkeys
	Strongyloides fuelleborni	Dogs, monkeys
Ternidens infection	*Ternidens diminutus*	Primates
Thelaziasis	*Thelazia* species	Dogs, ruminants
Trichinellosis*	*Trichinella spiralis* and other *Trichinella* species	Swine, rodents, wild carnivores, marine mammals
Trichostrongyliasis	*Trichostrongylus colubriformis* and other *Trichostrongylus* species	Ruminants

3. INFECTIONS CAUSED BY ARTHROPODS AND PENTASTOMID PARASITES

Myiasis*	*Calliphora, Cochliomyia, Cordylobia, Dermatobia, Gastrophilus, Chrysomyia, Hypoderma, Oestrus, Wohlfahrtia,* other genera	Mammals
Pentastomid infections	*Linguatula* species	Dogs, snakes, other vertebrates
	Armillifer species	Dogs, snakes, other vertebrates
Pneumoacariasis	*Pneumonyssus simicola*	Monkeys
Scabies	*Sarcoptes* species	Domestic animals
Tungiasis	*Tunga penetrans*	Domestic and wild mammals

APPENDIXES

APPENDIX I

Zoonoses and Diseases Common to Man and Animals Transmitted by Foods[1]

Diseases of food origin can be classified as intoxications or infections. Intoxications are caused by ingesting toxins or toxicants with food, while infections are caused by the reaction of the human or animal host to the development or multiplication of an infectious agent in its body or to the toxins the agent produces once established in the host's intestine or other tissue.

The diseases in this Appendix are grouped according to the type of agent. Only those that are considered zoonoses or communicable diseases common to man and animals are included, with the addition of a few in which animal feces and foods of animal origin are implicated as sources of infection for man. Readers with a greater interest in diseases transmitted by foods are directed to the original publication from which this Appendix was adapted (Bryan, 1982); that publication includes a very wide range of human infections and poisonings acquired through foods.

The diseases are discussed in their order of importance, based on criteria established by Bryan, although the relative damage caused by each disease may vary with the geographic area and time. Symptoms are listed according to their order of occurrence or their predominance, but it should be borne in mind that a given case may not manifest all of them or may present additional symptoms. No attempt has been made to enumerate here all the foods implicated, only those of greatest public health importance. The authors are responsible for modifications or additions introduced to the original publication by Bryan.

---

[1] Adapted with the permission of the author from F. L. Bryan, *Diseases Transmitted by Foods (A Classification and Summary)*, 2nd ed. Atlanta, Georgia, Centers for Disease Control of the USA, 1982. (HHS Publ. (CDC) 83-8237.)

1. Bacterial Diseases

Disease	Etiologic agent	Nature of organism/toxin	Incubation period/ signs and symptoms	Source, reservoir, and epidemiology	Foods involved	Specimens/ laboratory tests	Control measures
Salmonellosis	*Salmonella cholerae-suis*, *S. enteritidis* serotypes Typhimurium, Heidelberg, Derby, Java, Infantis, Agona, Enteritidis, Montevideo, Newport, Panama, Stanley, etc. Over 1,600 serotypes known, but only about 50 commonly occur.	Gram-negative, non-spore-forming, (mostly motile) rod. Aerobic, facultatively anaerobic. Possesses O (somatic) and two phases of H (flagellar) antigens. Usually more than 10^5 cells required to cause illness.	5 to 72 hours, usually 12 to 36 hours. Diarrhea, abdominal pain, chills, fever, vomiting, dehydration, prostration, anorexia, headache, malaise. Duration of several days. Septicemia or focal infection may also occur.	Feces of infected domestic or wild animals and man. Infants, aged, and malnourished persons and those with concomitant diseases are more susceptible. Carrier state usually lasts a few days to a few weeks, but is sometimes months. Fifty percent of infected persons carry salmonellae for 2–4 weeks. Occasionally waterborne.	Meat, poultry, and eggs, and their products. Other incriminated foods have included coconut, yeast, cottonseed protein, smoked fish, dry milk, chocolate candy.	Feces (stools, fecal swabs, filter paper wipes). Suspect foods; environmental swabs (if serotype). Preenrichment, selective enrichment, plating, screening, serotyping. Phagetyping for Typhimurium, Panama, Enteritidis, Infantis, and Thompson.	Chill foods rapidly in small quantities. Cook foods thoroughly. Pasteurize egg products and milk. Avoid cross-contamination from raw to cooked foods. Wash hands after touching raw meat. Sanitize equipment. Heat-treat feed and feed ingredients. Process meat and poultry in sanitary manner. Maintain farm sanitation. Practice personal hygiene. Protect food and feed from animal, human, bird, insect, and rodent excreta.
Arizonosis infection	*Arizona hinshawii*	Gram-negative, non-spore-forming motile rod. Similar to salmonellae. Delayed fermentation of lactose. Over 300 serotypes.	2 to 46 hours, usually 12 hours. Abdominal pain, diarrhea, nausea, chills, headache, weakness, fever. Lasts a few days.	Feces of infected persons and animals. Reptiles and turkeys are frequently infected.	Eggs, turkey, chicken, cream-filled pastry, ice cream, custard containing eggs.	Feces, suspect food. Selective enrichment, plating, biochemical identification, serotyping.	Chill foods rapidly in small quantities. Cook foods thoroughly. Avoid cross-contamination from raw to cooked food. Clean and sanitize equipment. Reheat leftover food thoroughly.

Disease	Etiologic agent	Nature of organism/toxin	Incubation period/ signs and symptoms	Source, reservoir, and epidemiology	Foods involved	Specimens/ laboratory tests	Control measures
Staphylococcal in- toxication (Staphylo- enterotoxicosis, sta- phylococcal food poisoning)	Toxins A, B, C, D, E, or F Staphylococ- cus aureus. Toxins elaborated in foods.	Gram-positive, non- spore-forming, non- motile cocci occur- ring in irregular, grape-like clusters. Aerobic, faculta- tively anaerobic; coagulase-positive; ferments mannitol; grows well in 10% salt media; produces lipase and hemoly- sin; often produces orange or yellow pig- ments. Frequently lysed by phage type group III. Resistant to many antibiotics. Toxin is protein (18 amino acids), heat stable. Less than 1 μg can cause illness.	1 to 7 hours, usually 2 to 4 hours. Sudden onset of nau- sea, excessive sali- vation, vomiting, retching, diarrhea, abdominal cramps, dehydration, sweat- ing, weakness, pros- tration. Fever usually does not occur. Short duration of not more than a day or two.	Nose and throat dis- charges; hands and skin, infected cuts, wounds, burns; boils; pimples; acne; feces. Anterior nares of man are the pri- mary reservoirs. Mastitic udders of cows and ewes. Arthritic and bruised tissues of poultry. Foods are usually contaminated after cooking when han- dled by infected per- sons and then kept at room temperature several hours or stored in large con- tainers.	Cooked ham, meat products; poultry and dressing; sauces and gravy; cream-filled pastry; potato, ham, poultry, and fish salad; milk, cheese, bread pudding. Left- over foods that are high in protein.	Vomitus, feces from sick persons. Nasal swab, pus from in- fected sores from food workers. Sus- pect food. Organism: selective enumeration, isola- tion, lipase (egg yolk) reaction, coag- ulase reaction, phage- typing. Toxin: extraction, concentration, gel diffusion.	Chill foods rapidly in small quantities. Pre- pare foods the day of serving, whenever possible. Restrict persons with diar- rhea, colds, infected cuts from food work. Sanitize equipment. Thorough cooking, reheating, pasteuriz- ing destroys the orga- nism but not the toxin.
Clostridium perfrin- gens gastroenteritis	Clostridium perfrin- gens (welchii) type A. Large numbers of vegetative cells must be ingested to cause illness. Enterotoxin (protein) released during sporulation in the gut.	Gram-positive, spore-forming, non- motile, encapsulated, short rod. Anaero- bic. Produces leci- thinase. Strains form either heat-resistant (some survive boil- ing for 1 to 5 hours) or heat-sensitive spo- res. Heating encour- ages spores to germi- nate. Approximately 90 known serotypes. Usually more than 10^6 bacterial cells re- quired to cause ill- ness.	8 to 24 hours, me- dian 12 hours. Acute abdominal pain, diarrhea. Occa- sionally dehydration and prostration. Nau- sea, vomiting, fever, and chills are rare. Short duration of 1 day or less.	Feces of infected per- sons and animals. Soil, dust, sewage. Both raw and cooked foods are frequently contaminated with C. perfringens. Im- plicated foods are usually those kept at room temperature, held warm (but not hot) for several hours, or stored in large containers in refrigerators.	Cooked meat or poultry, gravy, stew, and meat pies.	Feces, suspect food; environmental swabs (if serotype). Anaerobic isolation, selective enumera- tion, blood and egg yolk reaction, bio- chemical and micro- biological identifica- tion, heat resistance evaluations, serotyp- ing.	Chill food rapidly in small quantities. Pre- pare foods the day of serving whenever possible. Use clean pans for storage. Hold hot foods at 60°C or above. Prac- tice personal hy- giene. Cure meats adequately. Dispose of sewage in sanitary manner. Thorough cooking will destroy vegetative cells but not heat-resistant spores. Reheat left- over food to 70°C or above.

895

Disease	Etiologic agent	Nature of organism/toxin	Incubation period/ signs and symptoms	Source, reservoir, and epidemiology	Foods involved	Specimens/ laboratory tests	Control measures
Enteritis necrotican (Pig bel, darmbrand)	Clostridium perfringens type C (formerly typ: F). Necrotoxin released during growth in gut.	Gram-positive, spore-forming, non-motile rod. Anaerobic. Produces lecithinase and necrotoxin. Strains differ in minor antigens.	6 hours to 6 days, usually 24 hours. Diarrhea, prolonged abdominal pain, gangrene of small intestine, shock, toxemia. Case fatality rate: 40%.	Animal feces. Malnutrition and diet may predispose people to attack. Cooked meat held without refrigeration for many hours. Only two reported outbreaks.	Pork, other meat, fish.	Feces, bowel contents, blood, suspect food. Anaerobic isolation, identification, toxin testing.	Eat balanced diet. Chill foods rapidly in small quantities. Thorough cooking will destroy vegetative cells but not heat-resistant spores. Reheat leftover food to >70°C. Hold hot food at >60°C.
Botulism	Toxins A, B, E, F, or G of Clostridium botulinum. Toxins C and D cause botulism in animals. Most outbreaks in humans are caused by toxins A, B, and E. Toxin elaborated in foods, wounds, or infant gut.	Gram-positive, spore-forming, motile rod. Anaerobic. Produces neurotoxins that interfere with acetylcholine at peripheral nerve endings. Spores are among the most heat resistant. Toxins are simple proteins and are heat-labile.	2 hours to 6 days, usually 12 to 36 hours. Nausea, vomiting, abdominal pain, and diarrhea may appear early. Headache, vertigo or dizziness, lassitude, double vision, loss of reflex to light, dysphagia, dysphonia, ataxia, dry mouth, weakness, constipation, respiratory distress, respiratory paralysis. Partial paralysis may persist 6 to 8 months. Sensorium usually clear. Case fatality rate: 35 to 65%; death usually occurs in 3 to 10 days.	Soil, mud, water, intestinal tract of animals. Spores widely distributed in soil, but type varies with location.	Improperly canned low-acid food (green beans, corn, beets, asparagus, chili peppers, mushrooms, spinach, figs, olives, tuna). Smoked fish. Fermented foods (seal flippers, salmon eggs). Food stored in oil or vacuum-packed also involved. Improperly home-cured hams.	Blood serum, feces, stomach contents, autopsy tissue. Suspect food. Food: (Toxin) extraction, mouse neutralization. Serum and feces: Mouse neutralization. History of eating canned or vacuum-packed food useful in diagnosis.	Heat containers of low-acid food at high temperatures under pressure for sufficient time. Cook home-canned food thoroughly (boil and stir for 15 min.). Acidify food. Keep food refrigerated. Cure in sufficient concentration of salt. Add sufficient nitrite to pasteurized meat products. Discard swollen cans. Bivalent A-B and monovalent E antitoxins and polyvalent A-B-C-D-E-F and A-B-C-D-E-F antitoxin available for treatment.

Disease	Etiologic agent	Nature of organism/toxin	Incubation period/signs and symptoms	Source, reservoir, and epidemiology	Foods involved	Specimens/laboratory tests	Control measures
Campylobacteriosis (*Campylobacter jejuni* enteritis)	*Campylobacter jejuni* (*Vibrio fetus*)	Gram-negative, motile, comma- to S-shaped organism. Forms spirals. Microaerophilic. 10^6 bacterial cells required to cause illness in single volunteer trial.	1 to 7 days, usually 3 to 5 days. Diarrhea (stools often foul-smelling, bile-stained, watery, mucoid or bloody), abdominal pain, fever, anorexia, malaise, headache, myalgia, nausea, vomiting, arthralgias. Duration 1 to 5 days.	Intestine, liver, and gallbladder of cattle, sheep, pigs, poultry, and other animals. Contact with infected animals or their tissues another mode of transmission. Waterborne outbreaks documented.	Raw milk, raw beef liver and meat, poultry (?), water.	Blood, feces, suspect food. Isolation (10% CO_2), identification, serology.	Cook meat thoroughly. Pasteurize milk. Chill foods rapidly in small quantities. Avoid cross-contamination from raw foods of animal origin.
Shigellosis (Bacillary dysentery)	*Shigella sonnei, S. flexneri, S. dysenteriae, S. boydii*	Gram-negative, nonmotile rod. Aerobic, facultatively anaerobic. Similar to *Escherichia coli* but does not ferment lactose. Relatively fragile. More than 30 serotypes. As few as 10 *S. dysenteriae* and 100 *S. flexneri* have caused illness in human volunteers.	1 to 7 days, usually less than 4 days. Extremely variable, mild to severe symptoms: Abdominal cramps, fever, chills, diarrhea, watery stools (frequently containing blood, mucus, or pus), tenesmus, lassitude, prostration, nausea, vomiting, dehydration.	Feces of infected persons. Main mode of transmission: person-to-person. Also waterborne. Carriers shed organism for a few weeks to 2 months or longer.	Moist, mixed food. Potato, tuna, shrimp, turkey, and macaroni salads; milk, beans, apple cider, and poi reported as vehicles.	Feces, suspect food. Enrichment (foods), selective isolation, biochemical identification, serotyping of groups other than *sonnei*.	Practice personal hygiene. Dispose of sewage in sanitary manner. Chill foods rapidly in small quantities. Prepare food in sanitary manner; avoid touching foods which are not to be subsequently cooked. Cook foods thoroughly. Protect and treat water. Control flies.

Disease	Etiologic agent	Nature of organism/toxin	Incubation period/ signs and symptoms	Source, reservoir, and epidemiology	Foods involved	Specimens/ laboratory tests	Control measures
Escherichia coli diarrheas	*Escherichia coli.*[2] Both enterotoxigenic and invasive strains cause illness. Both heat-stable and heat-labile enterotoxins produced.	Gram-negative, non-spore-forming rod. Aerobic, facultatively anaerobic. Ferments lactose. Indole positive, methyl red positive, Voges-Proskauer negative, citrate negative. Possesses O, 90 K, and 50 H antigens. Usually more than 10^6 bacterial cells required to cause illness.	8 to 24 hours, mean 11 hours (invasive type). Fever, chills, headache, myalgia, abdominal cramps, profuse watery diarrhea. Similar to shigellosis. 8 to 44 hours, mean 26 hours (enterotoxigenic type). Diarrhea (rice-water stools), vomiting, dehydration, shock. Similar to cholera. The classic enteropathogenic serotypes cause outbreaks in nurseries.	Feces of infected persons. Modes of transmission: contaminated food and water, person-to-person. Infants are more susceptible. Possibly important cause of travelers' diarrhea. The same pathogenic serotypes of *E. coli* have been found in children and animals. Dogs and cats have been indicated as sources of infection.	Cheese, coffee substitute, salmon (?), or any food contaminated by feces.	Feces, throat swabs, blood from patients, suspect food. Selective enrichment, plating, biochemical identification. Toxin testing of ligated ileum, suckling infant mice, and adrenal tumor cells. Invasiveness tested by inoculation in guinea pig eye and observation for keratoconjunctivitis and by Hela cells culture.	Chill foods rapidly in small quantities. Cook and reheat foods thoroughly. Practice personal hygiene. Prepare foods in sanitary manner. Protect and treat water. Dispose of sewage in sanitary manner.
Yersiniosis (*Yersinia enterocolitica, Y. pseudotuberculosis* enteritis)	*Yersinia enterocolitica, Y. pseudotuberculosis*	Gram-negative, motile rod. Coccoid forms predominate in young cultures. Aerobic, facultatively anaerobic. Psychotropic. About 10^9 bacilli caused illness in volunteers.	24 to 36 hours and longer. Abdominal pain suggesting acute appendicitis, fever, headache, malaise, anorexia, diarrhea, vomiting, nausea, chills, pharyngitis, leukocytosis, erythema nodosum.	Urine and feces of infected animals, frequently rodents, dogs, pigs, chickens. Found in soil, dust, and water. Waterborne transmission.	Pork and other meat, raw milk, chocolate milk.	Feces, blood, suspect food, animal tissue. Lymph nodes. Cold enrichment, isolation, identification. Determine specific agglutinins in blood. Animal inoculations.	Cook foods thoroughly. Protect food from cross-contamination. Control rodents. Rapid chilling and refrigeration increases lag and slows growth, but may have a selective effect.

898

---

[2] Serogroups that have caused the invasive-type illness are O25, O28, O112, O124, O136, O143, O144, O147, and O512; those that have been shown to elaborate enterotoxins are O06, O15, O18, O20, O27, O44, O55, O78, O86, O111, O114, O119, O125, O126, O127, O128, O142, O146, O148, O154, O155, and O156.

Disease	Etiologic agent	Nature of organism/toxin	Incubation period/ signs and symptoms	Source, reservoir, and epidemiology	Foods involved	Specimens/ laboratory tests	Control measures
Brucellosis	Brucella melitensis, B. abortus, or B. suis	Gram-negative, encapsulated, nonmotile, coccoid to rod-shaped cells. Aerobic, but B. abortus requires CO_2.	5 to 21 days. May be several months. Insidious onset. Fever, chills, sweating, insomnia, weakness, malaise, headache, muscle and joint pain, loss of weight, anorexia.	Tissue, blood, placenta, urine, milk, vaginal discharge, and aborted fetus of infected animals (cattle, sheep, swine, goats, and horses). Main mode of transmission: contact with infected tissues.	Raw milk, cheese made from raw goat milk.	Blood, bone marrow, milk, urine, animal tissue (see Source). Isolation, identification, biochemical typing, animal inoculations, serology. Test for specific agglutinins in blood.	Eradicate brucellosis from livestock (immunize young animals, restrict movement, test, segregate or slaughter infected animals). Cook food thoroughly. Pasteurize milk and dairy products. Age cheese for at least 90 days.
Tuberculosis (extrapulmonary, of zoonotic origin)	Mycobacterium bovis	Gram-positive, nonmotile, acidfast rod. Aerobic. Grows slowly (>18-hour generation time).	Variable. Several weeks. Cervical or mesenteric lymph node involvement. Skeletal tuberculosis: pain, limp, refusal to walk, restriction of movement, night cries, fatigue, weight loss. Tuberculous endarteritis in growing bone progressing into joint space. Bone destruction leading to collapse, spinal deformity, paraplegia. Necrosis of joints, and soft tissues form paravertebral cold abscesses. Spine, hip, and knees most frequently involved.	Milk from diseased cattle. Ingestion of bacilli with milk in areas of high prevalence of bovine TB.	Raw milk.	Joint fluids, lymph nodes, bone biopsy, suspect food. Isolation, Ziehl-Neelsen staining, identification, animal inoculations, drug susceptibility testing.	Eradicate tuberculosis in animals (test and slaughter reactors). Pasteurize milk. Immunize with BCG in high-prevalence areas.

Disease	Etiologic agent	Nature of organism/toxin	Incubation period/signs and symptoms	Source, reservoir, and epidemiology	Foods involved	Specimens/laboratory tests	Control measures
Tularemia	*Francisella tularensis*	Gram-negative, nonmotile, pleomorphic rod. Aerobic. Survives quite well at low temperatures. Can penetrate unbroken skin. 10^{10} bacterial cells can cause illness by respiratory or intradermal routes.	8 to 24 hours or longer. Ulcer forms at site of pathogenic invasion. Chills, high fever, prostration, stupor, coma; swollen, tender, suppurative lymph nodes. Bronchopneumonia. Gastric form includes fever, toxemia, ulcers in the digestive tract. Course of illness may be fulminant and fatal.	Source: blood and tissue of infected mammal or infected arthropod. Reservoir: wild animals, frequently rabbits, wood ticks. Main mode of transmission: contact with infected tissue. Also transmitted by insect bites and contaminated drinking-water. Rarely transmitted by food.	Wild rabbit meat.	Blood, lymph nodes, sputum, muscle, and other tissues. Rabbit meat. Isolation, agglutination reaction, serology, animal inoculation. Demonstrate specific agglutinins in blood. Immunofluorescence test on exudate obtained from ulcers and aspirated from lymph nodes for rapid diagnosis.	Cook meat of wild rabbits thoroughly. Use rubber gloves when dressing rabbits. Wear protective clothes and use tick repellent in endemic areas.
Anthrax (intestinal)	*Bacillus anthracis*	Gram-positive, nonmotile, spore-forming, encapsulated, large rods which frequently form long chains. Aerobic, facultatively anaerobic. Morphologically and biochemically resembles *B. cereus*.	2 to 3 days. High fever, general weakness, malaise, headache, insomnia, nausea, abdominal pain, vomiting (containing bile and blood), diarrhea; progressing through general toxemia, shock, cyanosis, and death. Gastrointestinal anthrax is frequently fatal.	Tissue of opened carcasses of animals that died of anthrax. Soil contaminated by infected animals. Main mode of transmission: contact with infected animals or contaminated hides or materials. Intestinal form rare, but still occurs in developing countries.	Raw or under-cooked meat from animals dead of anthrax; sausage.	Blood, autopsy tissue (lymph nodes), animal tissue, environmental swabs, suspect food, soil. Isolation, identification, microscopic examination, animal inoculations.	Vaccinate animals in enzootic areas. Bury animal carcasses unopened. Do not consume meat from dead animals.
Haverhill fever (rat-bite fever)	*Streptobacillus moniliformis*	Gram-negative, non-spore-forming, pleomorphic rods forming chains. Requires ascitic fluid or blood for growth. Aerobic, facultatively anaerobic.	1 to 5 days. Rash. Swollen, red, and painful joints. Sore throat. Fever, muscle aches.	Nasopharynx of rats. Main mode of transmission: rat bites. One documented food-borne outbreak.	Raw milk.	Blood, joint fluid, pus, animal saliva, suspect food.	Pasteurize milk. Control rodents.

Disease	Etiologic agent	Nature of organism/toxin	Incubation period/ signs and symptoms	Source, reservoir, and epidemiology	Foods involved	Specimens/ laboratory tests	Control measures
Fecal streptococcal (enterococcal) enteritis	*Streptococcus faecalis* and *S. faecium*	Gram-positive cocci in chains. Grows in 6.5% NaCl at pH 9.6 from 10°C to 45°C. Withstands 60°C for 30 minutes. Alpha-, beta-, or non-hemolytic. Lancefield's group D streptococci. 10^{9-10} cells of a few strains of *S. faecalis* required to cause illness.	2 to 36 hours, usually 6 to 12 hours. Nausea, abdominal pain, diarrhea, sometimes vomiting. Relatively mild and similar to *C. perfringens* food-borne illness.	Feces of animals and man.	Sausage, evaporated milk, meat croquettes, meat pies, pudding.	Feces, suspect food. Selective enumeration, identification, test for Sherman's criteria, serogrouping.	Chill foods rapidly in small quantities. Cook foods thoroughly. Practice personal hygiene. Prepare food in sanitary manner.
Proteus gastroenteritis	*Proteus vulgaris, P. mirabilis, P. morganii,* and *P. rettgeri*	Gram-negative, motile rod. Aerobic, facultatively anaerobic. Produces urease.	3 to 5 hours. Diarrhea, vomiting, abdominal cramps.	Feces of animals and man.	Headcheese, ham, cheese, spaghetti.	Feces, suspect food. Isolation, identification.	Chill foods rapidly in small quantities. Cook foods thoroughly. Practice personal hygiene.
Providencia gastroenteritis	*Providencia alcalifaciens* and *P. stuartii* (*Proteus inconstans*)	Gram-negative, motile rod. Aerobic, facultatively anaerobic.	2 to 24 hours. Diarrhea, vomiting, abdominal cramps.	Feces of animals and man.	Chicken.	Feces, suspect food. Isolation, identification, serotyping.	Chill foods rapidly in small quantities. Cook foods thoroughly. Practice personal hygiene.
Klebsiella enteritis	*Klebsiella pneumoniae, K. ozaenae,* and *K. rhinoscleromatis*	Gram-negative, non-motile, encapsulated rod. Aerobic, facultatively anaerobic. Enterotoxin detected.	10 to 15 hours. Headache, dizziness, nausea, abdominal pain, watery stools.	Feces of animals and man. Respiratory tract of man.	Beef, rice.	Feces, suspect food. Isolation, identification, serotyping.	Chill food rapidly in small quantities. Cook foods thoroughly. Practice personal hygiene.

Disease	Etiologic agent	Nature of organism/toxin	Incubation period/ signs and symptoms	Source, reservoir, and epidemiology	Foods involved	Specimens/ laboratory tests	Control measures
Citrobacter gastro-enteritis	*Citrobacter freundii* (formerly *Escherichia freundii*), *C. intermedius*. Bethesda-Ballrup Group.	Gram-negative, motile rod. Aerobic. Facultatively anaerobic. Citrate positive, coli-aerogenes organism. Some antigens same as *Salmonella, Arizona, E. coli*.	1 to 48 hours, median 12 hours. Diarrhea, abdominal cramps, nausea, vomiting, fever, chills, dizziness.	Feces of animals and man.	Corn pudding, raw milk, macaroni with meat, liver sausage, smoked meat.	Feces, suspect food. Isolation, identification, serotyping.	Chill foods rapidly in small quantities. Cook foods thoroughly. Practice personal hygiene.
Enterobacter gastro-enteritis	*Enterobacter (Aerobacter) cloacae, E. aerogenes, E. hafniae,* and *E. liquefaciens*	Gram negative, (usually) non-motile rod. Aerobic, facultatively anaerobic. Enterotoxin detected.	2 to 6 hours. Diarrhea, nausea, vomiting, abdominal pain.	Feces of animals and man.	Cream-filled pastry, milk, stew.	Feces, suspect food. Isolation, identification.	Chill foods rapidly in small quantities. Cook foods thoroughly. Practice personal hygiene.
Edwardsiella enteritis	*Edwardsiella tarda*	Gram-negative rod. Aerobic, facultatively anaerobic.	Abdominal cramps, diarrhea.	Feces of animals (particularly snakes, other reptiles, seagulls, seals) and man.	Foods of animal origin including eggs and fish contaminated with animal or human feces.	Feces, suspect food. Isolation, identification.	Chill foods rapidly in small quantities. Cook foods thoroughly. Practice personal hygiene.
Listeriosis	*Listeria monocytogenes*	Gram-positive, motile rod. Aerobic, microaerophilic. Grows well in 10% NaCl media and survives in 20%. Beta-hemolytic grows well at 4°C. Survives at 80°C for 5 minutes.	Unknown. Probably 4 days to 3 weeks. Fever, headache, nausea, vomiting, monocytosis, meningitis, septicemia, abortion, localized external or internal lesions, pharyngitis.	Tissues, urine, or milk of infected animals. Environmental sources.	Milk, possibly milk products (cream, sour milk, cottage cheese), eggs, meat, poultry.	Animal tissue, milk, suspect food, blood, urine, cerebrospinal fluid, placental tissue, autopsy tissue. Isolation, identification, production of keratoconjunctivitis in rabbit's eyes, serology.	Cook foods thoroughly. Pasteurize milk.

Disease	Etiologic agent	Nature of organism/toxin	Incubation period/ signs and symptoms	Source, reservoir, and epidemiology	Foods involved	Specimens/ laboratory tests	Control measures
Erysipeloid	Erysipelothrix rhusiopathiae (E. insidiosa)	Gram-positive, non-motile rod with tendency to form long filaments. Microaerophilic, facultative. Resistant to salting, pickling, and smoking.	A few hours to 7 days. Pruritus, redness, and swelling of infected areas; lesions located on hands and fingers. Burning sensation, throbbing pain. Occasionally septicemia.	Infected animals (especially swine) and fish. Primarily an occupational disease of persons handling meat, fish, mollusks, and crustaceans. Infection via wounds and abrasions. Rodents can be important reservoir.	Foods of animal origin, including fish.	Suspect food, biopsy tissue, aspirated fluid. Isolation, identification.	Cook foods thoroughly. Avoid cross-contamination. Thorough cleaning of meat and fish processing equipment. Practice personal hygiene and treat wounds.
Pasteurellosis	Pasteurella multocida	Gram-negative, encapsulated, non-motile, bipolar, coccobacillus. Pleomorphic. Aerobic, facultatively anaerobic.	A few hours (in the case of bites). Wound infection, respiratory ailments; various organs and tissue affected. Septicemic form (rarely).	Upper respiratory tract of animals and possibly of humans. Mode of transmission: dog and cat bites; respiratory and digestive routes.	Poultry, vegetables soiled with animal feces and secretions.	Sputum, pus, cerebrospinal fluid, blood, urine, infected tissue. Isolation, identification.	Avoid dog and cat bites. Cook foods thoroughly. Protect foods from contamination by animal feces.

2. Viral and Rickettsial Diseases

Disease	Etiologic agent	Nature of organism/toxin	Incubation period/ signs and symptoms	Source, reservoir, and epidemiology	Foods involved	Specimens/ laboratory tests	Control measures
Bolivian hemorrhagic fever	Machupo virus	Arenavirdae, Tacaribe group. RNA core.	10 to 14 days. Malaise; headache; muscular pain; fever; sweats; prostration. Exanthems on throat, flanks, and soft palate. Gastrointestinal symptoms. Hemorrhages. CNS complications. Duration 1 to 2 weeks.	Urine and secretions of infected rodent (Calomys callosus). Mode of transmission to man: contact with rodent, ingestion of contaminated food or water.	Corn and other cereals. Possibly any food contaminated with rodent urine.	Blood; spleen of fatal cases. Serology, complement fixation. Intracerebral inoculation of suckling mice.	Control rodents. Protect food from contamination. Cook foods thoroughly.

Disease	Etiologic agent	Nature of organism/toxin	Incubation period/signs and symptoms	Source, reservoir, and epidemiology	Foods involved	Specimens/laboratory tests	Control measures
Russian spring-summer encephalitis (diphasic milk fever)	Virus belonging to tick-borne *Flavivirus* complex	Genus *Flavivirus*, family Togaviridae. RNA core. Two variants: oriental and occidental.	4 to 7 days (milk transmission). 8 to 20 days (tick bite). In Europe and part of Siberia (occidental variant), diphasic course. First phase is a week of fever; mild improvement, then relapse with headache, neck stiffness, vomiting. Illness by oriental variant more severe.	Transmitted to man mainly by bites of infected ticks. Also transmitted in goat or sheep milk and cheese.	Raw milk from goats or sheep; unaged cheese made from this milk.	Blood, cerebrospinal fluid, brain tissue of fatal cases. Animal inoculations, tissue culture, serology.	Pasteurize milk. Control ticks; use protective clothing and repellents. Immunize (USSR).
Q (Query) fever	*Coxiella (Rickettsia) burnetii*	Gram-negative, small, pleomorphic, nonmotile rod, frequently occurring in pairs. Obligate intracellular parasite occurring as clumps and masses within cytoplasm. Markedly resistant to desiccation. Resists 60°C for 1 hour.	2 to 4 weeks, mean 20 days. Sudden onset, chills, headache, weakness, malaise, severe sweats, high fever, pneumonia, mild cough, chest pain, nausea, vomiting, diarrhea.	Dust and aerosols from animal placental tissue, fetal membranes, amniotic fluid; milk. Bodies of patients, carcasses, wool, straw. Ticks (natural foci). Milk-borne transmission is rare.	Cow, goat, or sheep milk (rarely transmitted by this source).	Blood, sputum, urine, cerebrospinal fluid, postmortem tissues, milk. Placenta and amniotic fluid. Animal inoculation, serology, isolation (high security laboratories).	Pasteurize milk at 63°C for 30 minutes or 72°C for 15 seconds. Practice personal hygiene (animal workers). Vaccinate animals before shipping to areas having infected animals. Dispose of placentae and fetal membranes by incineration or burial.

2.1 Viral diseases which could possibly be transmitted by foods, but proof is lacking

Disease	Etiologic agent	Nature of organism/toxin	Incubation period/signs and symptoms	Source, reservoir, and epidemiology	Foods involved	Specimens/laboratory tests	Control measures
Creutzfeldt-Jakob disease	Agent similar to agent of "scrapie" and to other slow viruses	Characterized by long incubation period, resistance to heat, formalin, and other agents. Only detectable by animal inoculation.	12 months to years. Insidious onset. Dementia, severe visual and behavioral disturbances, myoclonic jerking. No remission or recovery. Always fatal.	Brains of sheep and goats with scrapie (?). Man is most probable reservoir.	Inadequately cooked sheep brains (?).	Brain tissue of fatal cases.	

Disease	Etiologic agent	Nature of organism/toxin	Incubation period/ signs and symptoms	Source, reservoir, and epidemiology	Foods involved	Specimens/ laboratory tests	Control measures
Lymphocytic chorio-meningitis	Virus of lymphocytic choriomeningitis	Arenaviridae RNA virus, genus *Arenavirus*.	8 to 21 days, 15 to 21 days to meningeal symptoms. Fever, chills, sore throat, cough, headache, vomiting, neck stiffness, photophobia, acute aseptic meningitis. Recovery in a few weeks.	Nasal secretions, urine, feces, and semen of mice (*Mus musculus*), and hamsters (*Mesocricetus auratus*) contaminate man's environment. Mode of transmission not well known. Contact, bites, contaminated foods. Virus may persist in mouse throughout life.	Unknown, could possibly be any food contaminated by mice.	Blood from febrile patients, cerebrospinal fluid, CNS tissue. Isolation, identification, serology. Animal (mouse or guinea pig) inoculations.	Control rodents. Clean home and work environments (sanitation).
Lassa fever	Lassa virus	Arenaviridae RNA virus, genus *Arenavirus*.	6 to 14 days. Malaise, asthenia, lassitude, headache, unremitting fever, sore throat, muscular aches, abdominal cramps, nausea, vomiting, diarrhea, pharyngitis, flushing, subcutaneous hemorrhages, puffed face, swollen neck, oliguria, dysuria, circulatory collapse.	Rodent (*Mastomys natalensis*) is reservoir. Contact with rodent or excreta, eating food contaminated by rodent excreta, contact with blood and excreta of patients.	Rodent flesh (?), grain or any food contaminated by rodents.	Immunofluorescence, complement fixation, neutralization, isolation in high security laboratories from blood and pharyngeal swabs.	Control rodents. Isolate patients.
Rotavirus gastroenteritis (infantile gastroenteritis)	Rotaviruses	Spherical RNA Reoviridae virus, 65 to 75 nm in diameter. Wheel-like appearance. Several serotypes. Survives months at ambient temperatures.	1 to 3 days. Vomiting, followed by diarrhea (watery green or yellow stool), malaise, fever, abdominal pain; dehydration in severe cases can cause death. Duration 2 to 16 days in infants, 24 hours or less in adults.	Person-to-person spread by fecal-oral route. Serotypes common to humans and animals indicate animals as additional source of infection.	Unknown. Could be any contaminated food, also contaminated water.	Feces. Electron microscopy. Immunoelectro-osmophoresis, ELISA, radioimmunoassay.	Practice personal hygiene. Dispose of sewage in sanitary manner. Prepare food in sanitary manner. Cook foods thoroughly.

3. Parasitic Diseases

3.1 Always or usually transmitted by foods

Disease	Etiologic agent	Nature of organism/toxin	Incubation period/ signs and symptoms	Source, reservoir, and epidemiology	Foods involved	Specimens/ laboratory tests	Control measures
Trichinosis (trichinellosis, trichinellasis)	*Trichinella spiralis* Variants: *T. spiralis* var. *domestica* (domestic and peridomestic cycle—main hosts swine); *T. spiralis* var. *nativa* (wild carnivores in Arctic); *T. spiralis* var. *nelsoni* (wild carnivores in Africa).	Delicate, thread-like roundworm (nematode). Larvae excyst in duodenum. Females invade mucosa of small intestine, larviposit. Larvae travel via blood and lymph, encyst in muscle.	1 to 43 days, usually 10 days. First stage (intestinal invasion): nausea, vomiting, diarrhea, abdominal pain. Second stage (muscle penetration): irregular and persistent fever, edema of eyes, profuse sweating, muscular pain, thirst, chills, skin lesions, weakness. Third stage (tissue repair): generalized toxemia, myocarditis. High eosinophil blood count.	Meat of infected animals. Reservoirs: swine, more than 40 species of wild animals. Pigs are primary source of trichinellae for humans.	Pork, bear meat, walrus flesh, dog meat. Frequently, homemade raw pork sausage. Meat of wild pigs in Africa.	Muscle biopsy (gastrocnemius, deltoid). Diaphragm muscle of swine. Microscopy (cysts), serology (ELISA).	Cook pork thoroughly (until it turns white) to 60°C or above. Freeze and store pork <6" thick at −15°C for 20 days or −30°C for 6 days. Cook garbage for feeding pigs at 100°C for 30 minutes. Cure meat adequately. Eliminate rodents from hog lots.
Taeniasis (beef or pork tapeworm infections)	*Taenia saginata* (beef tapeworm) *Taenia solium* (pork tapeworm). Their respective larval stages are *Cysticercus bovis* and *C. cellulosae*.	The definitive host of both cestodes is man; they inhabit the small intestine. The intermediate hosts of *T. saginata* are bovines, of *T. solium*, swine.	3 to 6 months. Often subclinical. Abdominal pain, nervousness, insomnia, nausea, weakness, diarrhea or constipation.	The source of infection for man is beef containing *Cysticercus bovis* (larva of *T. saginata*) or pork containing *C. cellulosae* (larva of *T. solium*).	Beef or pork.	Feces of patient. Beef or pork samples. Microscopy (eggs and proglottids).	Dispose of sewage in sanitary manner. Inspect meat. Cook meat thoroughly (>135°F), freeze (15°F, 10 days). Avoid pasturing cattle where human feces or sewage accumulate. Diagnose and treat cases.

Disease	Etiologic agent	Nature of organism/toxin	Incubation period/ signs and symptoms	Source, reservoir, and epidemiology	Foods involved	Specimens/ laboratory tests	Control measures
Cysticercosis	*Taenia solium* larvae, *Cysticercus cellulosae*	Larval stage. Cysticerci develop in subcutaneous tissues, muscles, and may localize in brain, eyes, heart, central nervous system.	15 days to several years. Pain at site of cysticerci development. May be subclinical. Neurocysticercosis is the most serious form; its symptomatology varies with the number of cysticerci, their location and development stage; resembles brain tumor, basal meningitis.	Human feces. Autoinfection; ingestion of food or water contaminated with *T. solium* eggs.	May be any food or water contaminated by human feces containing eggs of the parasite (especially vegetables and fruit).	Biopsy. Cerebrospinal fluid (look for high percentage of plasmocytes and eosinophils). CAT. Serologic tests.	Practice personal hygiene. Treat cases. Practice food hygiene. Raise swine under sanitary conditions.
Diphyllobothriasis (fish tapeworm infection)	*Diphyllobothrium latum, D. pacificum*	Flatworm (cestode). Adult attaches to mucosa of small intestine. Definitive host of *D. latum* is man and other mammals; that of *D. pacificum* is pinnepeds.	5 to 6 weeks. Symptoms often trivial or absent. Nausea, vomiting, weakness, dizziness, diarrhea or constipation; anemia may occur (2% of patients).	Infective eggs from human feces, dogs, and other fish-eating mammals contaminate water sources. Intermediate host: Copepods. Immediate source: Flesh of infected fish.	Raw or partially cooked or inadequately pickled freshwater fish (*D. latum*). Raw marine fish (*D. pacificum*).	Feces, fish. Microscopy (eggs).	Cook fish thoroughly. Dispose of sewage in sanitary manner. Prevent stream pollution. Freeze fish (−10°C for 24 hours). Treat cases.
Sparganosis	Second-stage larvae of *Spirometra* spp.	Tapeworm (cestode), ribbon-like larvae.	3 weeks to more than a year. Tender, puffy areas around site of parasite, irritation and migratory swelling.	Cat and dog feces. Intermediate host: water fleas (cyclops). Immediate source: water, fish, frogs, snakes. Transmission also occurs by drinking water containing water-fleas and by using animal meat as poultice.	Tadpoles, snakes, frogs, and meat of wild animals.	Infected human tissue (biopsy), fish. Microscopy (cross section of larva).	Cook foods thoroughly. Abstain from eating raw flesh of infected animals. Avoid using raw vertebrates as poultices. Protect or boil water.

Disease	Etiologic agent	Nature of organism/toxin	Incubation period/signs and symptoms	Source, reservoir, and epidemiology	Foods involved	Specimens/laboratory tests	Control measures
Angiostrongyliasis (eosinophilic meningoencephalitis)	Angiostrongylus cantonensis	Roundworm (nematode). Adult worm lives in pulmonary artery of rats and deposits eggs in blood. Larvae hatch from eggs and travel up trachea, whence they are swallowed and pass in feces, source of infection for intermediate hosts (mollusks).	14 to 16 days. Abrupt onset. Gastrointestinal upset, encephalitis (headache, stiffness of neck and back, paresthesia), low grade fever. Eosinophilia in blood and cerebrospinal fluid.	Larvae from rat feces penetrate terrestrial mollusks (snails and slugs) or marine mollusks. Man becomes infected by eating raw mollusks and paratenic hosts (crustaceans, fish).	Raw crab, prawns, garden slugs, land planarian, shrimp, snails.	Mollusks, rats, serum, autopsy tissue, cerebrospinal fluid. Microscopy (worms), serology (ELISA).	Cook foods thoroughly; freeze at −15°C. Avoid eating raw freshwater prawns, raw land mollusks, and raw crab.
Abdominal angiostrongyliasis	Angiostrongylus costaricensis	A roundworm (nematode). Definitive host is the cotton rat (Sigmodon hispidus). Intermediate host is slug Vaginulus ameghini.	Moderate fever, abdominal pain, diarrhea, vomiting. Palpable masses. Leukocytosis and eosinophilia.	Source of infection for man is probably vegetables contaminated with slug secretions containing larvae.	Salad, vegetables contaminated by slugs.	Slugs, rats, autopsy tissue and surgical specimens. Microscopy (worms), serology.	Avoid eating slugs. Wash greens carefully. Wash hands after garden work.
Anisakiasis (herring worm disease)	Larval stage of Anisakis spp., Contracaecum spp., and Phocanema spp.	Roundworm (nematode). Highly resistant to brine, easily killed by 60°C and freezing.	Gastric: 4 to 6 hours. Sudden stomach pain, nausea, vomiting, eosinophilia. Intestinal: 7 days. Severe lower abdominal pain, nausea, vomiting, fever, diarrhea, occult blood in stools, leukocytosis, ascites.	Adult worm lives in intestine of fish-eating sea mammals. Requires one or two intermediate hosts.	Marine fish or squid. Herring (raw, partially cooked, pickled, smoked).	Stools, stomach or intestinal tissue. Microscopy (worms).	Cook fish thoroughly. Freeze at −20°C within 12 hours and hold for 24 hours. Preserve with high concentrations of NaCl and hold for 10 days. Promptly clean fish to be eaten raw.

Disease	Etiologic agent	Nature of organism/toxin	Incubation period/ signs and symptoms	Source, reservoir, and epidemiology	Foods involved	Specimens/ laboratory tests	Control measures
Fasciolopsiasis	*Fasciolopsis buski*	Large intestinal fluke (trematode). Adult attaches to intestinal mucosa of humans and pigs.	3 months. Diarrhea alternating with constipation, abdominal pain, nausea, vomiting, anorexia; intestinal obstruction may occur, as well as edema of face and abdomen, weakness. Symptomatic cases are caused by large parasitic burdens.	Human, dog, or hog feces containing fluke eggs contaminate fresh water. Intermediate host: snail. Cercariae encyst on water vegetables and are ingested when skins of water vegetables are bitten into and peeled off with teeth. Occurs in Orient.	Water chestnuts, water bamboo, water hyacinths, lotus plant root.	Feces, suspect foods. Microscopy (eggs).	Avoid hulling or peeling water plants with teeth or lips— use a knife or drop in boiling water. Dry plants. Cook water-grown vegetables thoroughly. Dispose of sewage in sanitary manner. Control snails. Treat patients.
Echinostomiasis	*Echinostoma ilocanum, E. lindoense, E. malayanum, E. revolutum,* and other spp.	Small intestinal fluke (trematode). Adult attaches to small intestinal wall of mammals, birds, and reptiles.	Several months. Inflammatory reaction at site of attachment to intestinal wall, intestinal colic, diarrhea. Not very pathogenic.	Infective feces of man, dogs, fowl, rats contaminate fresh water. Immediate source: snails (intermediate hosts).	Raw snails, clams, limpets, freshwater fish, or tadpoles.	Feces, suspect foods. Microscopy (eggs).	Cook snails and other foods thoroughly. Dispose of sewage in sanitary manner.
Clonorchiasis	*Clonorchis sinensis* (Chinese liver fluke)	Slender hepatic fluke (trematode). Habitat is distal biliary passages and pancreatic duct of man and domestic and wild animals.	Probably several weeks. First stage: fever, epigastric pain. Second stage: loss of appetite, diarrhea, low grade fever, tenderness over liver, bile duct obstruction. Third stage: cirrhosis, progressive ascites and endema, jaundice. Many infections asymptomatic.	Infective feces of man, cats, dogs, hogs, or other animals which are hosts of adult flukes contaminate fresh water. First intermediate host: snails. Encyst in muscle of fish (second intermediate host). Occurs in Orient and Eastern Europe.	Raw or partially cooked fresh, dried, salted, or pickled fish (carp and 80 other species).	Feces, bile, fish. Microscopy (eggs), serology.	Cook freshwater fish thoroughly. Dispose of sewage in sanitary manner. Keep sewage out of streams. Control snails.

909

Disease	Etiologic agent	Nature of organism/toxin	Incubation period/ signs and symptoms	Source, reservoir, and epidemiology	Foods involved	Specimens/ laboratory tests	Control measures
Heterophyid infections	Many species of the family Heterophyiidae. The most common species are *Heterophyes heterophyes*, *Stellantichasmus talcatus*, and *Metagonimus yokogawai*.	Small intestinal fluke (trematode). It attaches to mucosa of upper levels of small intestine in man, other mammals, and birds.	Several weeks. Abdominal pain; diarrhea containing mucus; heart, brain, or spinal cord involvement may follow.	Infective feces of fish-eating birds and mammals contaminate fresh water. First intermediate host: snails. Encyst in fish muscle (second intermediate host). Occurs in the Orient, Egypt, and Southeast Europe.	Raw, partially cooked, salted or dried freshwater or brackish-water fish (mullet).	Feces, fish. Microscopy (eggs).	Cook fish thoroughly. Prevent stream pollution. Control snails. Dispose of sewage in sanitary manner.
Opisthorchiasis	*Opisthorchis felineus*, *O. viverrini*, and *Amphimerus pseudofelineus*	Hepatic fluke (trematode), resembles *C. sinensis*. Infects man, cats, dogs, and other mammals.	Several weeks. Cirrhosis of liver resembling clonorchiasis. Symptomatology depends on parasite burden.	Infective feces from humans and piscivorous mammals, containing eggs. Snails ingest eggs. Cercariae penetrate freshwater cyprinoid fish. Occurs in Central and Eastern Europe, Eastern Asia, and Ecuador.	Freshwater fish.	Feces, fish. Microscopy (eggs).	Cook freshwater fish thoroughly. Dispose of sewage in sanitary manner. Keep sewage out of streams. Control snails. Do not feed raw fish to animals.
Fascioliasis	*Fasciola hepatica* and *F. gigantica*	Large hepatic fluke (trematode). Fluke burrows through intestinal wall to liver. Infects domestic herbivores (definitive hosts).	Several months. Initial phase: fever, malaise, hepatomegaly, pain in right side, eosinophilia. Chronic phase: abdominal pain, dyspepsia, diarrhea, irregular fever, jaundice.	Infective feces from humans, sheep, cattle, or other herbivorous and omnivorous animals, containing eggs, contaminate fresh water. Intermediate host: snails. Cercariae encyst on aquatic vegetation.	Aquatic vegetation, watercress.	Feces. Microscopy (eggs).	Eradicate infection in sheep and other herbivorous animals. Omit watercress in salads in endemic areas. Dispose of sewage in sanitary manner. Drain pastures. Prevent stream pollution. Control snails.

Disease	Etiologic agent	Nature of organism/toxin	Incubation period/ signs and symptoms	Source, reservoir, and epidemiology	Foods involved	Specimens/ laboratory tests	Control measures
Paragonimiasis	*Paragonimus westermani, P. skrjabini,* and other species in Asia; *P. africanus* and *P. uterobilateralis* in Africa; *P. mexicanus* in Latin America	Plump, oval fluke (trematode). Penetrates intestinal wall and reaches lungs in man and other mammals.	Long and variable, many months. Cough, hemoptysis, thoracic pain, eosinophilia. Roentgenographic findings closely simulate those of pulmonary tuberculosis. Migrations and ectopic development in intestine, lymph glands, genitourinary tract, subcutaneous tissue, and brain.	Sputum and feces from man and other carnivores containing eggs contaminate fresh water. First intermediate host: snails. Cercariae encyst in freshwater crab or crayfish (second intermediate hosts). Occurs in Orient, Africa, and Latin America.	Raw or partially cooked crab or crayfish.	Feces, sputum. Microscopy (eggs), immunodiagnostic tests (intradermal, complement fixation, hemagglutination, ELISA). X-ray.	Cook crustaceans thoroughly. Heat at 55°C for 5 minutes. Dispose of sewage in sanitary manner. Prevent stream pollution. Control snails. Mass treatment in endemic areas.
Dicrocoeliasis	*Dicrocoelium dendriticum* and *D. hospes*	Small hepatic fluke (trematode) of sheep, goats, and cattle (definitive hosts).	7 weeks. Constipation, flatulence, diarrhea, abdominal pain, enlarged and tender liver.	Infective animal (cattle, sheep) feces, containing eggs, contaminate fields. Snails ingest eggs. Larvae leave snails in slime balls that infect ants. Ants are ingested by animals or accidentally by man. Occurs in tropics (rare).	Ants or foods (raw, unwashed vegetables) contaminated by ants (during picnics, camping, etc.).	Feces, bile. Microscopy (eggs).	Wash vegetables. Cook foods thoroughly. Dispose of sewage in sanitary manner. Keep sewage out of streams. Control snails and ants. Protect foods from ants.
Hymenolepiasis by *Hymenolepis diminuta*	*Hymenolepis diminuta* (rat tapeworm)	Intestinal flatworm (cestode) of rodents and, rarely, man. Length is from 20 to 60 cm.	2 to 4 weeks. Diarrhea, abdominal pain, and indefinite gastrointestinal complaints. Mainly asymptomatic.	Feces of definitive hosts, especially rats, contain eggs which are ingested by coprophilic arthropods (intermediate hosts). Source of infection for man: food containing insects.	Grains and cereals.	Feces. Microscopy (eggs).	Avoid eating insect-contaminated grains and cereals. Inspect grains and cereals. Control rodents in grain storage areas. Control insects.

911

Disease	Etiologic agent	Nature of organism/toxin	Incubation period/ signs and symptoms	Source, reservoir, and epidemiology	Foods involved	Specimens/ laboratory tests	Control measures
Hymenolepiasis by *Hymenolepis nana*	*Hymenolepis nana*	Intestinal flatworm (cestode) of man and rodents. Length is from 20–40 mm.	2 to 4 weeks. Abdominal pain, diarrhea, anorexia, dizziness, headache, pruritic rash.	Feces of mice and man contain eggs. Fleas and beetles may serve as intermediate hosts. Mainly transmitted person to person.	Grains (?).	Feces. Microscopy (eggs).	Sanitary disposal of sewage, rodent control. Protection of food from rodent and arthropod contamination.
Gastrodisciasis	*Gastrodiscoides hominis*	Trematode that lives in large intestine of man and swine.	Mucous diarrhea and colitis when parasite burden is large.	Pigs and man are reservoirs. Snails may be intermediate hosts.	Aquatic plants (?).	Feces. Microscopy (parasite or eggs).	Sanitary disposal of sewage. Avoid eating raw aquatic plants.
Dioctophymosis	*Dioctophyma renale* (giant kidney worm)	Roundworm (nematode) of domestic and wild carnivores.	3½ to 6 months. Renal disfunction or ureteral obstruction.	Urine of infected large fish-eating mammals containing eggs contaminates fish and frogs (paratenic hosts).	Raw fish and frogs.	Urine. Microscopy (eggs or worm).	Sanitary disposal of sewage, thorough cooking of fish and frog meat. Drink safe water.
Toxocariasis (visceral larva migrans)	*Toxocara canis, T. cati*	Prolonged migration of larvae in human tissue. Nematodes that inhabit the intestine of dogs and cats.	Fever, malaise, pallor, anorexia, muscle and joint pain, nausea, vomiting, convulsions, pruritic rash, hepatomegaly, pneumonitis, coughing, urticaria, chronic eosinophilia. Ocular form: loss of vision.	Infective feces of dog or cat contaminate soil.	Soil-contaminated foods.	Blood. Count eosinophils. ELISA test.	Avoid eating dirt and wash vegetables. Deworm dogs. Practice personal hygiene.

Disease	Etiologic agent	Nature of organism/toxin	Incubation period/ signs and symptoms	Source, reservoir, and epidemiology	Foods involved	Specimens/ laboratory tests	Control measures
Gnathostomiasis	*Gnathostoma spinigerum, G. hispidum*	Roundworm (nematode). Live in stomach wall of cats and dogs (*G. spinigerum*) or pigs and wild boar (*G. hispidum*). Extra-intestinal sites in humans.	1 to 2 days. Epigastric pain, nausea, vomiting, edema, fever, granulomatous lesions, stationary abscess. Infection may persist for years. Movement of larvae in abdominal and thoracic organs simulates cholecystitis, appendicitis, and other conditions.	Adult parasites in gastric tumors of definitive hosts. Eggs pass in feces to water. Intermediate hosts: Water fleas (cyclops). Immediate source: Fish muscle. Third-stage larvae migrate to muscle of species eating infected fish, frogs, birds, and snakes, and remain infective.	Raw, fermented, or partially cooked freshwater fish; snakes, birds, mammals.	Emerging worms from skin, abscesses, or natural orifices; biopsy. Microscopy (larvae).	Cook foods thoroughly.

3.2 Diseases usually transmitted by other means but sometimes food-borne

Disease	Etiologic agent	Nature of organism/toxin	Incubation period/ signs and symptoms	Source, reservoir, and epidemiology	Foods involved	Specimens/ laboratory tests	Control measures
Amebiasis (amebic dysentery)	*Entamoeba histolytica*	Intestinal protozoan. Vegetative stage (trophozoite) is very fragile; cyst stage is more resistant but does not survive drying. Invades mucosa of colon.	5 days to several months, usually 3 to 4 weeks. Variable symptoms, including abdominal discomfort, diarrhea, constipation; blood and mucus may be observed in stools; distention, headache, drowsiness, ulcers. May spread via bloodstream, causing organ infections and abscess of liver, lungs, or brain. Most infections are asymptomatic.	Human feces containing cysts. Main mode of transmission: Personal contact. Can be transmitted by food and water.	Raw vegetables and fruits.	Feces, lesion exudates, material aspirated from ulcers. Microscopy to detect vegetative and cyst stages; serology.	Practice personal hygiene (food handlers). Cook foods thoroughly. Dispose of sewage in sanitary manner. Protect and treat water. Control flies. Avoid using human excreta for fertilizer (night soil).

Disease	Etiologic agent	Nature of organism/toxin	Incubation period/ signs and symptoms	Source, reservoir, and epidemiology	Foods involved	Specimens/ laboratory tests	Control measures
Amebiasis	*Entamoeba polecki*	Intestinal protozoan of swine. Vegetative (trophozoite) and cyst stages in development.	Mainly asymptomatic. Diarrhea and abdominal pain. Does not produce extra-intestinal invasions.	Swine are the reservoir. Man is infected by ingesting cysts along with food, water, and from contaminated hands.	Any contaminated, raw food.	Feces. Microscopy to detect vegetative and cyst stages.	Practice personal and food hygiene. Protect drinking water.
Cryptosporidiosis	*Cryptosporidium* spp.	Protozoan similar to coccidia. Multiplies sexually and asexually on surface of intestine.	Possibly 10 days. Watery or mucoid diarrhea lasting 3 to more than 14 days, anorexia, vomiting, abdominal pain.	Reservoirs: cattle, sheep, goats, birds. Mode of transmission: fecal-oral.	Little is known about water- and food-borne transmission.	Feces. Identify oocysts in stained smears.	Careful management of animal feces. Personal and food hygiene. Sanitary disposal of human wastes.
Capillariasis	*Capillaria hepatica, C. philippinensis,* and *C. aerophila*	*C. hepatica* is a hepatic nematode of rodents. *C. philippinensis* is an intestinal parasite of man, and *C. aerophila* is a respiratory tract parasite of wild and domestic canids.	Hepatic form: fever, nausea, vomiting, diarrhea, edema, hepatomegaly, death. Intestinal form: diarrhea, weight loss, malabsorption, and death. Pulmonary form: asthmatic symptoms, cough, fever.	Soil contaminated with embryonated eggs. For *C. philippinensis,* freshwater fish.	Foods contaminated with soil. Raw fish.	Liver biopsy (*C. hepatica*); Coprologic exam (*C. philippinensis*); lung biopsy or sputum (*C. aerophila*).	Rodent control. Avoid eating raw fish (*C. philippinensis*).
Trichostrongyliasis	*Trichostrongylus orientalis, T. columbriformis, T. axiei,* and other spp.	Thread-like roundworm (nematode) that infects the intestine and stomach of animals and humans.	Several months. Usually asymptomatic; gastrointestinal symptoms in intense infections.	Animal and human feces contaminate soil and vegetation, especially when used as fuel or fertilizer.	Vegetables contaminated with larvae.	Feces. Microscopy (eggs). Coproculture.	Personal hygiene. Cook foods thoroughly. Food and environmental hygiene. Avoid eating raw vegetables in endemic areas.

914

Disease	Etiologic agent	Nature of organism/toxin	Incubation period/ signs and symptoms	Source, reservoir, and epidemiology	Foods involved	Specimens/ laboratory tests	Control measures
Hydatidosis (Hydatid disease)	Larval stage of *Echinococcus granulosus*	Intestinal flatworm (cestode) of dogs (definitive hosts). Eggs may survive for long periods in soil.	Several months to years. Variable, depends on site of hydatid cyst. Liver, lungs, kidney, pelvis, heart, bones, or central nervous system may be involved.	Feces (containing eggs) of carnivores (dogs and wolves) infected with adult worms. Intermediate host: larvae occur in sheep, cattle, pigs, camels, moose, deer. Dogs become infected with hydatid cysts from eating raw foods of animal origin. Main mode of transmission: contact with dogs.	Any contaminated raw food.	Serum. Surgical specimens. Serology. X-ray, CAT, ultrasound, scintigraphy.	Control slaughtering so that dogs do not have any access to scraps. Control stray dogs. Incinerate or deeply bury dead animals. Deworm domestic dogs. Practice personal hygiene.
Alveolar hydatid disease	*Echinococcus multilocularis*	Small intestinal flatworm (cestode) of foxes and other canids. Wild rodents are intermediate hosts.	Several years. Hepatomegaly, jaundice, ascites, splenomegaly. Frequently fatal.	Feces of foxes, sled dogs, wolves contaminate environment. Maintained in a fox-vole-fox cycle. The disease is transmitted to man by foods contaminated with excreta of Canidae, contaminated soil, or contact with infected animals.	Raw fruits and vegetables.	Serum, autopsy specimens. Serology, microscopy (scolices or cysts).	Control slaughtering so that dogs do not have any access to scraps. Control stray dogs. Incinerate or deeply bury dead animals. Deworm domestic dogs. Practice personal hygiene.
Balantidiasis (Balantidial dysentery)	*Balantidium coli*	Large ciliated protozoan, forms cysts. Habitat is mucosa at lower end of large intestine.	Unknown. Sometimes a few days. Diarrhea with mucus, blood, pus; constipation. Abdominal pain, nausea, vomiting.	Reservoir: swine, and possibly other animals. Feces containing cysts contaminate food and water.	Contaminated raw food.	Feces. Microscopy.	Practice personal hygiene. Cook foods thoroughly. Treat cases. Control flies. Protect water supply.

Disease	Etiologic agent	Nature of organism/toxin	Incubation period/ signs and symptoms	Source, reservoir, and epidemiology	Foods involved	Specimens/ laboratory tests	Control measures
Toxoplasmosis	*Toxoplasma gondii*	Protozoan of the order Coccidia; definitive hosts are domestic cats and wild felids. Occurs in 3 main forms: 1) tachyzoites (acute infection); 2) encysted bradyzoites (tissue); 3) oocysts, which are very resistant and form only in the intestine of felids.	5 days to more than 3 weeks. Usually subclinical. Congenital or acquired. Acquired form includes febrile or afebrile lymphadenopathy. Cures spontaneously or takes a serious course with various localizations.	Source of infection for acquired form is pork, mutton, or, more rarely, beef.	Raw or insufficiently cooked pork, mutton, or beef containing bradyzoites. Food and water contaminated with cat feces (oocysts). Goat milk (tachyzoites).	Affected tissue, blood, biopsy of lymph nodes. Serologic tests, mouse inoculation.	Cook foods thoroughly. Wash hands after handling raw meat or contact with cat feces. Freeze raw meat (3 days at −15°C) before feeding to cats.
Sarcocystosis	*Sarcocystis hominis, S. suihominis*	Coccidia, whose definitive host is man; cattle (*S. hominis*) or pigs (*S. suihominis*) are intermediate hosts.	9 to 10 days. Usually asymptomatic. Nausea, abdominal pains, diarrhea observed in volunteers.	Man contaminates the environment with feces containing sporocysts. Cattle and swine ingest contaminated pasture and develop muscular cysts (sarcocysts). Humans become infected by eating meat containing sarcocysts.	Raw or under-cooked beef or pork containing muscular cysts.	Feces. Microscopy to detect sporocysts.	Cook meat thoroughly. Freeze meat. Avoid environmental contamination with human feces.

916

APPENDIX II

Technical Meaning of Terms Used in the Text

Presented below are definitions of terms in current epidemiologic use, adapted from *Control of Communicable Diseases in Man,* 14th edition (A. S. Benenson, Editor), published by the American Public Health Association, Washington, D.C., 1985. (Reprinted with the permission of the publisher.)

DEFINITIONS

1. **Carrier**—A person or animal that harbors a specific infectious agent in the absence of discernible clinical disease and serves as a potential source of infection. The carrier state may exist in an individual with an infection that is inapparent throughout its course (commonly known as healthy or asymptomatic carrier), or during the incubation period, convalescence, and postconvalescence of an individual with a clinically recognizable disease (commonly known as incubatory carrier or convalescent carrier). Under either circumstance the carrier state may be of short or long duration (temporary or transient carrier, or chronic carrier).

2. **Case fatality rate**—Usually expressed as a percentage of the number of persons diagnosed as having a specified disease who die as a result of that illness. This term is most frequently applied to a specific outbreak of acute disease in which all patients have been followed for an adequate period of time to include all attributable deaths. The case fatality rate must be clearly differentiated from mortality rate (see Definition 30). Synonyms: fatality rate, fatality percentage.

3. **Chemoprophylaxis**—The administration of a chemical, including antibiotics, to prevent the development of an infection or the progression of an infection to active manifest disease. Chemotherapy, on the other hand, refers to use of a chemical to cure a clinically recognizable disease or to limit its further progress.

4. **Cleaning**—The removal by scrubbing and washing, as with hot water, soap, or suitable detergent or by vacuum cleaning, of infectious agents and of organic matter from surfaces on which and in which infectious agents may find favorable conditions for surviving or multiplying.

5. **Communicable disease**—An illness due to a specific infectious agent or its toxic products which arises through transmission of that agent or its products from an infected person, animal, or inanimate reservoir to a susceptible host, either directly or indirectly through an intermediate plant or animal host, vector, or the inanimate environment (see 46, Transmission of infectious agents).

6. **Communicable period**—The time or times during which an infectious agent may be transferred directly or indirectly from an infected person to another person, from an infected animal to man, or from an infected person to an animal, including arthropods.

   In diseases such as diphtheria and streptococcal infection, in which mucous membranes are involved from the initial entry of the infectious agent, the period of communicability is from the date of first exposure to a source of infection until the infecting microorganism is no longer disseminated from the involved mucous membranes, i.e., from the period before the prodromata until termination of a carrier state, if the latter develops. Some diseases are more communicable during the incubation period than during actual illness.

In diseases such as tuberculosis, leprosy, syphilis, gonorrhea, and some of the salmonelloses, the communicable state may exist over a long and sometimes intermittent period when unhealed lesions permit the discharge of infectious agents from the surface of the skin or through any of the body orifices.

In diseases transmitted by arthropods, such as malaria and yellow fever, the periods of communicability (or more properly infectivity) are those during which the infectious agent occurs in the blood or other tissues of the infected person in sufficient numbers to permit infection of the vector. A period of communicability (transmissibility) is also to be noted for the arthropod vector, namely, when the agent is present in the tissues of the arthropod in such form and locus (infective state) as to be transmissible.

7. **Contact**—A person or animal that has been in an association with an infected person or animal, or a contaminated environment which might provide an opportunity to acquire the infective agent.

8. **Contamination**—The presence of an infectious agent on a body surface; also on or in clothes, bedding, toys, surgical instruments or dressings, or other inanimate articles or substances including water and food. Pollution is distinct from contamination and implies the presence of offensive, but not necessarily infectious, matter in the environment. Contamination on a body surface does not imply a carrier state.

9. **Disinfection**—Killing of infectious agents outside the body by direct exposure to chemical or physical agents.

Concurrent disinfection is the application of disinfective measures as soon as possible after the discharge of infectious material from the body of an infected person, or after the soiling of articles with such infectious discharges; all personal contact with such discharges or articles should be minimized prior to such disinfection.

Terminal disinfection is the application of disinfective measures after the patient has been removed by death or to a hospital, or has ceased to be a source of infection, or after hospital isolation or other practices have been discontinued. Terminal disinfection is rarely practiced; terminal cleaning generally suffices (see 4, Cleaning), along with airing and sunning of rooms, furniture, and bedding. Disinfection is necessary only for diseases spread by indirect contact; steam sterilization or incineration of bedding and other items is recommended after a disease such as Lassa fever or other highly infectious diseases.

10. **Disinfestation**—Any physical or chemical process serving to destroy or remove undesired small animal forms, particularly arthropods or rodents, present upon the person, the clothing, or in the environment of an individual, or on domestic animals (see 26, Insecticide, and 41, Rodenticide). Disinfestation includes delousing for infestation with *Pediculus humanus,* the body louse. Synonyms include the terms disinsection and disinsectization when only insects are involved.

11. **Endemic**—The constant presence of a disease or infectious agent within a given geographic area; may also refer to the usual prevalence of a given disease within such area. Hyperendemic expresses a persistent intense transmission, and holoendemic a high level of infection beginning early in life and affecting most of the population, e.g., malaria in some places.

12. **Epidemic**—The occurrence in a community or region of cases of an illness (or an outbreak) clearly in excess of expectancy. The number of cases indicating presence of an epidemic will vary according to the infectious agent, size and type of population exposed, previous experience or lack of exposure to the disease, and time and place of occurrence; epidemicity is thus relative to usual frequency of the disease in the same area, among the specified population, at the same season of the year. A single case of a

communicable disease long absent from a population or the first invasion by a disease not previously recognized in that area requires immediate reporting and epidemiologic investigation; two cases of such a disease associated in time and place are sufficient evidence of transmission to be considered an epidemic. (See 38, Report of a disease, paragraph 3.)

13. **Fumigation**—Any process by which the killing of animal forms, especially arthropods and rodents, is accomplished by the use of gaseous agents (see 26, Insecticide, and 41, Rodenticide).

14. **Health education**—Health education is the process by which individuals and groups of people learn to promote, maintain or restore health. Education for health begins with people as they are, with whatever interests they may have in improving their living conditions. Its aim is to develop in them a sense of responsibility for health conditions, as individuals and as members of families and communities. In communicable disease control, health education commonly includes an appraisal of what is known by a population about a disease, an assessment of habits and attitudes of the people as they relate to spread and frequency of the disease, and the presentation of specific means to remedy observed deficiencies. Synonyms: Education; education for health; education of the public.

15. **Host**—A person or other living animal, including birds and arthropods, that affords subsistence or lodgment to an infectious agent under natural (as opposed to experimental) conditions. Some protozoa and helminths pass successive stages in alternate hosts of different species. Hosts in which the parasite attains maturity or passes its sexual stage are primary or definitive hosts; those in which the parasite is in a larval or asexual state are secondary or intermediate hosts. A transport host is a carrier in which the organism remains alive but does not undergo development.

16. **Immune individual**—A person or animal that has specific protective antibodies or cellular immunity as a result of previous infection or immunization, or is so conditioned by such previous specific experience as to respond adequately to prevent infection and/or clinical illness following exposure to a specific infectious agent. Immunity is relative; an ordinarily effective protection may be overwhelmed by an excessive dose of the infectious agent or by exposure through an unusual portal of entry; it may also be impaired by immunosuppressive drug therapy, concurrent disease, or the aging process. (See 40, Resistance.)

17. **Immunity**—That resistance usually associated with the presence of antibodies or cells having a specific action on the microorganism concerned with a particular infectious disease or on its toxin. Passive humoral immunity is attained either naturally by transplacental transfer from the mother, or artificially by inoculation of specific protective antibodies (from immunized animals, or convalescent hyperimmune serum, or immune serum globulin (human)); it is of short duration (days to months). Active humoral immunity, which usually lasts for years, is attained either naturally by infection with or without clinical manifestations, or artificially by inoculation of the agent itself in killed, modified, or variant form, or of fractions or products of the agent. Effective immunity depends on cellular immunity which is conferred by T-lymphocyte sensitization, and humoral immunity which is based on B-lymphocyte response.

18. **Inapparent infection**—The presence of infection in a host without recognizable clinical signs or symptoms. Inapparent infections are identifiable only by laboratory means or by the development of positive reactivity to specific skin tests. Synonyms: Asymptomatic, subclinical, or occult infection.

19. **Incidence rate**—A quotient (rate), with the number of new cases of a specified disease diagnosed or reported during a defined period of time as the numerator, and the number of persons in a stated population in which the cases occurred as the denominator. This is usually expressed as cases per 1,000 or 100,000 per annum. This rate may be expressed as age- or sex-specific or as specific for any other population characteristic or subdivision (see 29, Morbidity rate, and 35, Prevalence rate).

Attack rate, or case rate, is an incidence rate often used for particular groups observed for limited periods and under special circumstances, as in an epidemic, usually expressed as percent (cases per 100). The secondary attack rate in communicable disease practice expresses the number of cases among familial or institutional contacts occurring within the accepted incubation period following exposure to a primary case, in relation to the total of exposed contacts; it may be restricted to susceptible contacts when determinable. Infection rate expresses the incidence of all infections, manifest and inapparent.

20. **Incubation period**—The time interval between initial contact with an infectious agent and the appearance of the first sign or symptom of the disease in question, or, in a vector, the first time transmission is possible (extrinsic incubation period).

21. **Infected individual**—A person or animal that harbors an infectious agent and who has either manifest disease (see 33, Patient or sick person) or inapparent infection (see 1, Carrier). An infectious person or animal is one from whom the infectious agent can be naturally acquired.

22. **Infection**—The entry and development or multiplication of an infectious agent in the body of man or animals. Infection is not synonymous with infectious disease; the result may be inapparent (see 18, Inapparent infection) or manifest (see 24, Infectious disease). The presence of living infectious agents on exterior surfaces of the body, or upon articles of apparel or soiled articles, is not infection, but represents contamination of such surfaces and articles (see 8, Contamination).

23. **Infectious agent**—An organism (virus, rickettsia, bacteria, fungus, protozoa, or helminth) that is capable of producing infection or infectious disease.

24. **Infectious disease**—A clinically manifest disease of man or animal resulting from an infection (see 22, Infection).

25. **Infestation**—For persons or animals the lodgment, development, and reproduction of arthropods on the surface of the body or in the clothing. Infested articles or premises are those which harbor or give shelter to animal forms, especially arthropods and rodents.

26. **Insecticide**—Any chemical substance used for the destruction of insects, whether applied as powder, liquid, atomized liquid, aerosol, or a "paint" spray; residual action is usual. The term larvicide is generally used to designate insecticides applied specifically for destruction of immature stages of arthropods; adulticide or imagocide, to designate those applied to destroy mature or adult forms. The term insecticide is often used broadly to encompass substances for the destruction of all arthropods, but acaricide is more properly used for agents against ticks and mites. More specific terms, such as tickicide, lousicide, and miticide are sometimes used.

27. **Isolation**—As applied to patients, isolation represents separation, for the period of communicability, of infected persons or animals from others in such places and under such conditions as to prevent or limit the direct or indirect transmission of the infectious agent from those infected to those who are susceptible or who may spread the agent to others. In contrast, quarantine (see Definition 36) applies to restrictions on the healthy contacts of an infectious case.

28. **Molluscicide**—A chemical substance used for the destruction of snails and other mollusks.

29. **Morbidity rate**—An incidence rate (see Definition 19) used to include all persons in the population under consideration who become clinically ill during the period of time stated. The population may be limited to a specific sex, age group, or those with certain other characteristics.

30. **Mortality rate**—A rate calculated in the same way as an incidence rate (see Definition 17), using as a numerator the number of deaths occurring in the population during the stated period of time, usually a year. A total or crude mortality rate utilizes deaths from all causes, usually expressed as deaths per 1,000, while a disease-specific mortality rate includes only deaths due to one disease and is usually reported on the basis of 100,000 persons. The population base may be defined by sex, age, or other characteristics. The mortality rate must not be confused with case fatality rate (see Definition 2).

31. **Nosocomial infection**—An infection occurring in a patient in a hospital or other health care facility and in whom it was not present or incubating at the time of admission, or the residual of an infection acquired during a previous admission. Includes infections acquired in the hospital but appearing after discharge, and also such infections among the staff and visitors of the facility.

32. **Pathogenicity**—The capability of an infectious agent to cause disease in a susceptible host.

33. **Patient or sick person**—A person who is ill.

34. **Personal hygiene**—Those protective measures, primarily within the responsibility of the individual, which promote health and limit the spread of infectious diseases, chiefly those transmitted by direct contact. Such measures encompass a) washing hands in soap and water immediately after evacuating bowels or bladder and always before handling food or eating; b) keeping hands and unclean articles, or articles that have been used for toilet purposes by others, away from the mouth, nose, eyes, ears, genitalia, and wounds; c) avoiding the use of common or unclean eating utensils, drinking cups, towels, handkerchiefs, combs, hairbrushes, and pipes; d) avoiding exposure of other persons to spray from the nose and mouth, as in coughing, sneezing, laughing, or talking; e) washing hands thoroughly after handling a patient or his belongings; and f) keeping the body clean by sufficiently frequent soap and water baths.

35. **Prevalence rate**—A quotient (rate) obtained by using as the numerator the number of persons sick or portraying a certain condition in a stated population at a particular time (point prevalence), or during a stated period of time (period prevalence), regardless of when that illness or condition began, and as the denominator the number of persons in the population to which they belong. For example, the prevalence rate of athlete's foot in a group of boys examined on a given day may be 25 per 100; the prevalence rate of positive reactors to serologic tests performed on blood samples from a certain population group may be 10 per 1,000.

36. **Quarantine**—Restriction of the activities of well persons or animals who have been exposed to a case of communicable disease during its period of communicability (i.e., contacts) to prevent disease transmission during the incubation period if infection should occur.

　　a) Absolute or complete quarantine: The limitation of freedom of movement of those exposed to a communicable disease for a period of time not longer than the longest usual incubation period of that disease, in such manner as to prevent effective contact with those not so exposed (compare 27, Isolation).

b) Modified quarantine: A selective, partial limitation of freedom of movement of contacts, commonly on the basis of known or presumed differences in susceptibility and related to the danger of disease transmission. It may be designed to meet particular situations. Examples are exclusion of children from school, exemption of immune persons from provisions applicable to susceptible persons, or restriction of military populations to the post or to quarters. It includes personal surveillance, the practice of close medical or other supervision of contacts in order to permit prompt recognition of infection or illness but without restricting their movements; and segregation, the separation of some part of a group of persons or domestic animals from the others for special consideration, control, or observation, such as removal of susceptible children to homes of immune persons, or establishment of a sanitary boundary to protect uninfected from infected portions of a population.

37. **Repellent**—A chemical applied to the skin or clothing or other places to discourage a) arthropods from alighting on and attacking an individual, or b) other agents, such as helminth larvae, from penetrating the skin.

38. **Report of a disease**—An official report notifying an appropriate authority of the occurrence of a specified communicable or other disease in man or in animals. Diseases in man are reported to the local health authority; those in animals to the livestock, sanitary, veterinary, or agriculture authority. Some few diseases in animals, also transmissible to man, are reportable to both authorities. Each health jurisdiction declares a list of reportable diseases appropriate to its particular needs. Reports should also list suspect cases of diseases of particular public health importance, ordinarily those requiring epidemiologic investigation or initiation of special control measures.

When a person is infected in one health jurisdiction and the case is reported from another, the health authority receiving the report should notify the other jurisdiction, especially when the disease requires examination of contacts for infection, or if food or water or other common vehicles of infection may be involved.

In addition to routine report of cases of specified diseases, special notification is required of all epidemics or outbreaks of disease, including diseases not listed as reportable (see 12, Epidemic).

39. **Reservoir (of infectious agents)**—Any person, animal, arthropod, plant, soil, or substance (or combination of these) in which an infectious agent normally lives and multiplies, on which it depends primarily for survival, and where it reproduces itself in such manner that it can be transmitted to a susceptible host.

40. **Resistance**—The sum total of body mechanisms which interpose barriers to the progress of invasion or multiplication of infectious agents or to damage by their toxic products. Inherent resistance—an ability to resist disease independent of antibodies or of specifically developed tissue response; it commonly resides in anatomic or physiologic characteristics of the host and may be genetic or acquired, permanent or temporary. Synonym: Nonspecific immunity (see 17, Immunity).

41. **Rodenticide**—A chemical substance used for the destruction of rodents, generally through ingestion (compare 13, Fumigation).

42. **Source of infection**—The person, animal, object, or substance from which an infectious agent passes to a host. Source of infection should be clearly distinguished from source of contamination, such as overflow of a septic tank contaminating a water supply, or an infected cook contaminating a salad (compare 39, Reservoir).

43. **Surveillance of disease**—As distinct from surveillance of persons (see 36, Quarantine, paragraph b), surveillance of disease is the continuing scrutiny of all aspects of occurrence and spread of a disease that are pertinent to effective control. Included are the systematic collection and evaluation of a) morbidity and mortality reports; b) special reports of field investigations of epidemics and of individual cases; c) isolation and identification of infectious agents by laboratories; d) data concerning the availability, use, and untoward effect of vaccines and toxoids, immune globulins, insecticides, and other substances used in control; e) information regarding immunity levels in segments of the population; and f) other relevant epidemiologic data.

A report summarizing the above data should be prepared and distributed to all cooperating persons and others with a need to know the results of the surveillance activities. The procedure applies to all jurisdictional levels of public health from local to international. Serological surveillance identifies patterns of current and past infection using serological tests.

44. **Susceptible**—A person or animal presumably not possessing sufficient resistance against a particular pathogenic agent to prevent contracting infection or disease if or when exposed to the agent.

45. **Suspect case**—A person whose medical history and symptoms suggest that he or she may have or may be developing some communicable disease.

46. **Transmission of infectious agents**—Any mechanism by which an infectious agent is spread from a source or reservoir to a person. These mechanisms are:

a) Direct transmission: Direct and essentially immediate transfer of infectious agents to a receptive portal of entry through which human or animal infection may take place. This may be by direct contact as by touching, biting, kissing, or sexual intercourse, or by the direct projection (droplet spread) of droplet spray onto the conjunctiva or onto the mucous membranes of the eye, nose, or mouth during sneezing, coughing, spitting, singing, or talking (usually limited to a distance of about 1 meter or less). Droplet nuclei are the small residues which result from evaporation of fluid from droplets emitted by an infected host. They also may be created purposely by a variety of atomizing devices, or accidentally as in microbiology laboratories or in abattoirs, rendering plants, or autopsy rooms. They usually remain suspended in the air for long periods of time. Direct transmission can also occur by exposure of susceptible tissue to dust, the small particles of widely varying size which may arise from soil (as, for example, fungus spores separated from dry soil by wind or mechanical agitation), clothes, bedding, or contaminated floors.

b) Indirect transmission:
   1) Vehicle-borne—Contaminated inanimate materials or objects (fomites) such as toys, handkerchiefs, soiled clothes, bedding, cooking or eating utensils, surgical instruments or dressings (indirect contact); water, food, milk, biological products including blood, serum, plasma, tissues, or organs; or any substance serving as an intermediate means by which an infectious agent is transported and introduced into a susceptible host through a suitable portal of entry. The agent may or may not have multiplied or developed in or on the vehicle before being transmitted.
   2) Vector-borne—(a) Mechanical: Includes simple mechanical carriage by a crawling or flying insect through soiling of its feet or proboscis, or by passage of organisms through its gastrointestinal tract. This does not require multiplication or development of the organism. (b) Biological: Propagation (multiplication), cyclic development, or a combination of these (cyclopropagative) is required before the arthropod can transmit the infective form of the agent to man. An incubation period (extrinsic) is required following infection before the arthropod becomes infective. The infectious agent may be passed vertically to succeeding generations

(transovarial transmission); transstadial transmission indicates its passage from one stage of the life cycle to another, as nymph to adult. Transmission may be by injection of salivary gland fluid during biting, or by regurgitation or deposition on the skin of feces or other material capable of penetrating through the bite wound or through an area of trauma from scratching or rubbing. This transmission is by an infected nonvertebrate host and not simple mechanical carriage by a vector as a vehicle. However, an arthropod in either role is termed a vector.

c) Airborne—The dissemination of microbial aerosols to a suitable portal of entry, usually the respiratory tract. Microbial aerosols are suspensions of particles in the air consisting partially or wholly of microorganisms. They may remain suspended in the air for long periods of time, some retaining and others losing infectivity or virulence. Particles in the 1- to 5-μ range are easily drawn into the alveoli of the lungs and may be retained there. Not considered as airborne are droplets and other large particles which promptly settle out (see Direct transmission, above).

47. **Virulence**—The degree of pathogenicity of an infectious agent, indicated by case fatality rates and/or its ability to invade and damage tissues of the host.

48. **Zoonosis**—An infection or infectious disease transmissible under natural conditions from vertebrate animals to man. May be enzootic or epizootic (see 11, Endemic, and 12, Epidemic).

INDEX

About the authors...

Dr. Pedro N. Acha began working for the Pan American Health Organization in early 1957. In the course of his career, he served as Chief of the Department of Human and Animal Health, Chief of the Division of Disease Control, Director of Program Analysis and Operations Coordination, Country Representative in Argentina, and, most recently, Area Director of Health Systems Infrastructure until his retirement from PAHO in late 1986. He is presently in charge of inter-institutional coordination for technical programs of the Inter-American Institute for Cooperation on Agriculture. His broad and profound experience in the fields of prevention, control, and research in zoonoses and communicable diseases common to man and animals has been brought to bear in the writing of this book.

Dr. Boris Szyfres likewise began his career with PAHO in 1957, when he became one of the organizers of the Pan American Zoonoses Center in Azul, Argentina. He served as the Chief of Laboratory Services and later as Director of the Center, a position he occupied until 1971. Since then he has continued his service to the Organization as a special consultant in the areas of zoonoses and communicable diseases common to man and animals. In 1986 he was presented with PAHO's Abraham Horwitz Award for Inter-American Health for his leadership in zoonoses control activities in the Region of the Americas. His contributions in the fields of brucellosis and other bacterioses, particularly, are widely recognized.

NOTES